BIOFEEDBACK
A Practitioner's Guide

Third Edition

Edited by

Mark S. Schwartz
Frank Andrasik

THE GUILFORD PRESS
New York   London

© 2003 The Guilford Press
A Division of Guilford Publications, Inc.
72 Spring Street, New York, NY 10012
www.guilford.com

Figures 4.1–4.32, 14.A1, 14.A2, 22.1, 22.6, 22.7, 22.9, 22.10, 22.12, 22.13, 23.1–23.11,
and 27.2–27.4 are © 2003 The Mayo Foundation.

Printed in the United States of America

This book is printed on acid-free paper.

Last digit is print number: 9 8 7 6 5 4 3

Library of Congress Cataloging-in-Publication Data

Biofeedback : a practitioner's guide / edited by Mark S. Schwartz,
Frank Andrasik.—3rd ed.
    p. cm.
Includes bibliographical references and index.
    ISBN-10: 1-57230-845-1 ISBN-13: 978-1-57230-845-9 (hc : alk. paper)
    ISBN-10: 1-59385-233-9 ISBN-13: 978-1-59385-233-7 (pbk : alk. paper)
  1. Biofeedback training. I. Schwartz, Mark S. (Mark Stephen) II.
Andrasik, Frank, 1949–
RC489.B53 S39 2003
615.8'51—dc21

                      2002154975

About the Editors

Mark S. Schwartz, PhD, began his professional experience with biofeedback in 1974 at the Mayo Clinic in Rochester, Minnesota. From 1978 through 1982, he chaired the Professional Affairs Committee (PAC) of the Biofeedback Society of America (BSA). During that time, the Committee developed the original Applications Standards and Guidelines for Providers of Biofeedback Services, published in 1982. The Biofeedback Certification Institute of America (BCIA), founded in 1981, started from within the PAC. Dr. Schwartz chaired the BCIA Board for several years and then chaired the early growth of the written examination. He also served as President of the BSA from March 1987 to March 1988. He has been on the staff of Mayo Clinics since 1967, including 21 years in Rochester, Minnesota, and nearly 16 years at the Mayo Clinic in Jacksonville, Florida. He is a Senior Fellow of the Biofeedback Certification Institute of America.

Frank Andrasik, PhD, began his professional career in the Department of Psychology at the State University of New York in Albany. He later served as Associate Director for the Pain Therapy Centers in Greenville, South Carolina. His current affiliation is Senior Research Scientist at the Institute for Human and Machine Cognition and Professor of Psychology at the University of West Florida in Pensacola, Florida. He has also served the Association for Applied Psychophysiology and Biofeedback (AAPB) in numerous capacities, in particular as Chair of the Task Force on Biofeedback Treatment of Tension Headache in 1984, President from 1993 to 1994, and most recently and currently as Editor-in-Chief of the Association's journal, *Applied Psychophysiology and Biofeedback*. He is also a recipient of the AAPB's Merit Award for Long-Term Research and/or Clinical Achievements, as well as the AAPB's Distinguished Scientist Award. He is a Senior Fellow of the Biofeedback Certification Institute of America.

Contributors

Sami R. Achem, MD, Division of Gastroenterology and Hepatology, Mayo Clinic Jacksonville, Jacksonville, Florida

Frank Andrasik, PhD, Institute for Human and Machine Cognition, University of West Florida, Pensacola, Florida

John G. Arena, PhD, Department of Biofeedback/Psychophysiology, Veterans Administration Medical Center and Medical College of Georgia, Augusta, Georgia

Barbara Bailey, RN, MSN, CDE, St. Vincent Mercy Medical Center, Toledo, Ohio

Gerard A. Banez, PhD, Section of Pediatric Psychology, The Children's Hospital at The Cleveland Clinic, Cleveland, Ohio

Niels Birbaumer, PhD, Institute of Medical Psychology (retired), and Behavioral Neurobiology, University of Tuebingen, Tuebingen, Germany

Keith I. Block, MD, Block Medical Center, Evanston, Illinois

Timothy P. Culbert, MD, Integrative Medicine and Cultural Care, Children's Hospitals and Clinics, Minneapolis, Minnesota

Eugene Eisman, PhD, (retired), Department of Psychology, University of Wisconsin–Milwaukee, Milwaukee, Wisconsin

Timothy L. Fagerson, DPT, MS, Orthopaedic Physical Therapy Service, Wellesley Hills, Massachusetts

Herta Flor, PhD, Department of Neuropsychology at the University of Heidelberg; Central Institute of Mental Health, Mannheim, Germany

Eric R. Fogel, PT, BCIAC, Health West P.C. Physical Therapy, Ashland, Oregon

Richard N. Gevirtz, PhD, California School of Professional Psychology, Alliant International University, San Diego, California

Alan G. Glaros, PhD, School of Dentistry, University of Missouri–Kansas City, Kansas City, Missouri

Charlotte Gyllenhaal, PhD, Program for Collaborative Research in the Pharmaceutical Sciences, College of Pharmacy, University of Illinois at Chicago, Chicago, Illinois

David E. Krebs, DPT, PhD, MGH, Institute of Health Professions and Biomotion Lab, Massachusetts General Hospital, Boston, Massachusetts

Andrea Kübler, PhD, Institute of Medical Psychology and Behavioral Neurobiology, Eberhard-Karls-University, Tuebingen, Germany

Leonard Lausten, DDS, School of Dentistry, University of Missouri–Kansas City, Kansas City, Missouri

Paul Lehrer, PhD, Department of Psychiatry, Robert Wood Johnson Medical School, University of Medicine and Dentistry of New Jersey, Piscataway, New Jersey

Wolfgang Linden, PhD, Department of Psychology, University of British Columbia, Vancouver, British Columbia, Canada

Joel F. Lubar, PhD, Department of Psychology, University of Tennessee, and Southeastern Biofeedback and Neurobehavioral Institute, Knoxville, Tennessee

Angele McGrady, PhD, Complementary Medicine Center, Department of Psychiatry, Medical College of Ohio, Toledo, Ohio

Vincent J. Monastra, PhD, FPI Attention Disorders Clinic, Endicott, New York

Doil D. Montgomery, PhD, Center for Psychological Studies, Nova Southeastern University, Fort Lauderdale, Florida

Nicola Neumann, PhD, Institute of Medical Psychology and Behavioral Neurobiology, University of Tuebingen, Tuebingen, Germany

R. Paul Olson, PhD, Minnesota School of Professional Psychology, Minneapolis, Minnesota

Charles J. Peek, PhD, Independent Consultant in Healthcare Collaboration and Communication, Minneapolis, Minnesota

Mark S. Schwartz, PhD, Department of Psychiatry and Psychology, Mayo Clinic Jacksonville, Jacksonville, Florida

Nancy M. Schwartz, MA, Associates for Counseling and Biofeedback, Jacksonville, Florida

Keith Sedlacek, MD, Stress Regulation Institute, New York, New York

Wesley Sime, PhD, Biofeedback and Stress Management, University of Nebraska–Lincoln, Lincoln, Nebraska

Ute Strehl, PhD, Institute of Medical Psychology and Behavioral Neurobiology, University of Tuebingen, Tuebingen, Germany

Sebastian Striefel, PhD, (Emeritus), Department of Psychology, Utah State University, Logan, Utah

Jeffrey M. Thompson, MD, Department of Physical Medicine and Rehabilitation, Mayo Clinic, Rochester, Minnesota

Jeannette Tries, PhD, Aurora Women's Pavilion, Sinai Samaritan Medical Center, Milwaukee, Wisconsin; University of Illinois at Chicago Hospital and Clinics, Chicago, Illinois

Robert Whitehouse, PhD, Colorado Center for Biobehavioral Health, Boulder, Colorado

Susanne Winter, MD, Department of Neurology, Municipal Hospital, Munich Harlaching, Munich, Germany

Marcie Zinn, PhD, NCTM, Performing Arts Psychophysiology and Zinn Piano Academy, Pleasanton, California, and Illinois Institute of Technology, Chicago, Illinois

Mark Zinn, MM, PhD, NCTM, Performing Arts Psychophysiology and Zinn Piano Academy, Pleasanton, California

Preface

The responses to the first and second editions of *Biofeedback* were very rewarding in terms of acceptance and reviews. The second edition added much to the first edition, essentially doubling the size. Yet, from new research areas and interests in biofeedback that have emerged in recent years, it was clear that there were still more topics that warranted inclusion. For instance, in the past several years, there has been a substantial expansion of EEG biofeedback/neurotherapy. Pelvic floor applications have also substantially expanded in the past several years and include more than treatment of incontinence. In addition, major medical centers provide biofeedback for a variety of pelvic-floor-related disorders. Pediatric applications have always been a major research area in biofeedback and continue to be so, receiving even more interest and attention in recent years. The relatively new area of respiratory sinus arrhythmia (RSA) biofeedback has also been receiving considerable interest, with research support for several conditions. Other biofeedback applications, such as those for athletes and musicians, are also starting to garner enough interest to deserve attention in this text.

In order to address these new areas of interest, this third edition has been extensively revised and is largely a new text. There are 11 new chapters on new topics, as well as a number of new authors writing on topics covered in previous editions. The new chapters include a primer of EEG instrumentation (Chapter 5), a review chapter on EEG applications (Chapter 19), and two chapters on very specific EEG biofeedback applications developed in Germany (Chapters 20 and 21). Other new chapters include respiratory sinus arrhythmia (RSA) (Chapter 11) and applications to musicians (Chapter 24) and athletes (Chapter 25). There is a new chapter specifically on pediatric headache (Chapter 30) and one on other pediatric applications (Chapter 31). There is also a new chapter on pelvic floor applications (Chapter 28). Finally, the new chapter on professional issues (Chapter 37) reflects the condensing of several prior chapters in the second edition, along with the addition of new content.

Most of the rest of the chapters have been revised, updated, and streamlined to varying degrees. Several chapters from the second edition have been combined into new chapters and a few chapters eliminated entirely.

On the occasion of the publication of this third edition, we together thank all the readers of the previous editions for their support, ideas, dedication, and feedback and look forward to the reception of readers of this new edition.

Acknowledgments

MARK S. SCHWARTZ

In memory of Pearl Schwartz and Sol Schwartz, for their unconditional love and for providing the foundation, early confidence, encouragement, and support during my formative years. I miss both of you. In memory of my biological father, Harry S. Taylor, for providing the seeds and support for my education, and for the genetics and heritage of the Taylor family.

To my four adult children—Angie, Ian, Cindi, and David—their wonderful spouses, and my three grandchildren: my endless love, gratitude, understanding, and congratulations for all your accomplishments and the many joys you bring to me. You all continue to provide meaning and inspiration.

To Nancy M. Schwartz, for the joy she brings to her family and friends, and for her humor and infectious laughter. It is easy to love her. To her sons, for their great wit, their love and devotion to their mother, and their many talents. And to Nancy's wonderful parents, for continued life inspirations.

To the same professionals listed in the first and second editions, my thanks. And again to Donn Byrne, PhD, whose retirement Festschrift in April 2002 reminded me of how he inspired me and of my gratitude for his mentoring. To those authors from the two previous editions who did not write chapters for this new edition, I again thank you for your contributions that helped make those prior editions successful, hence allowing a third edition. And to all those professionals who reviewed the prior editions, for their thoughtful reviews. Finally, in memory, again, of Susan P. Lowery, for whom there is a Memorial Statement in the second edition. Susan was an inspiration to all who knew her.

To the Mayo Clinics and Mayo Foundation, my professional home for over 35 years, for all the reasons noted in the second edition, and to all those of the Mayo Foundation thanked in the first two editions. To Paul A. Fredrickson, MD, and T. Carey Merritt, MD, two very close friends and colleagues. A new thanks to Daniel Hubert, of Mayo Clinic Medical Photography, for help with photographs. To Kathryn Dolan of the legal department of Mayo Foundation, for her patience and skillful help.

Many thanks again to The Guilford Press, for continued acceptance, support, patience, and flexibility. Thank you, Seymour Weingarten, Editor-in-Chief, and Robert Matloff, President, for your long-term support and wonderful style. It has always been fun and comfortable working with you. To Carolyn Graham, who charmingly and tactfully managed many of the preproduction administrative matters for the book. To the wonderful copy editor, Marie Sprayberry, who also provided copy editing for the first edition, again my gratitude for your skills, tact, flexibility, and patience. To Anna Nelson, for her patience and skills at completing the final editorial and production stages for the book.

When faced with the opportunity and need for a third edition, I faced the reality that I could not do it alone again. I am incredibly thankful that Frank Andrasik agreed to coedit the text and share in the writing. His involvement clearly permitted completion of the book, and there is no doubt that he fulfilled and exceeded my hopes and needs to complete this third edition.

FRANK ANDRASIK

I begin by expressing my sincere thanks to Mark Schwartz for providing me the opportunity to assist with the revision of a text that my students and I have found invaluable for training and conducting research. I did not realize until recently that Mark and I entered the field around the same time—he in 1974, I in 1975. Over this nearly 30-year period, I have grown to admire, respect, emulate, and heed his words of wisdom. More than that, I value and appreciate his abiding friendship. I am certain that many within our fold would have readily embraced the opportunity to join Mark as coeditor. I remain flattered and honored that he extended this position to me. The many visits, e-mails, and phone calls required to pull off a task of this magnitude have enhanced my knowledge, sharpened my focus, and strengthened our friendship. For that and more, I remain forever grateful to Mark.

Let me also acknowledge those who had been instrumental to my entering the field of biofeedback (specifically headache management) and in helping me to sustain this interest over the ensuing decades. I was indeed fortunate to team up with Kenneth A. Holroyd, PhD, when I returned to graduate school from a work break. He introduced me to the then radically new nonpharmacological treatment called biofeedback, as well as the topic of headache and the equipment made by Cyborg. Little did I know that this would be the start of a lifelong career in biofeedback, many years of fruitful collaboration and continued mentoring, and a lifetime of friendship. Ken's scientific expertise, dedication, and easygoing collegial manner continue to serve me as sources of guidance and inspiration, all of which I attempt to model. John R. McNamara, PhD, another professor from my graduate school days, introduced me to clinical psychology and behavior therapy, at a time when I was struggling for direction. Working under his tutelage opened my eyes to new research possibilities and career directions. I continue to value his perspectives, career advice, and friendship. Although nearly all of my graduate professors influenced me in measurable ways, one other professor, Harry Kotses, PhD, needs to be acknowledged. He provided me with further in-depth training in psychophysiology that has enabled me to conduct the kind of research that is necessary.

In my first faculty position I was indeed fortunate to have the opportunity to work with Edward B. Blanchard, PhD, a pioneer and one of the luminaries in the field of biofeedback. Working with him exposed me to new horizons and opened doors that I did not know existed. Thanks are also due to the many undergraduate and graduate students who have worked tirelessly with me over the years, as well as to the funding agencies who made many of the clinical trials possible to complete.

It takes more than superb mentors for a successful career, however. Any successes I have had are due in great part to the many caring and supportive people behind the scenes. I begin by acknowledging Pearl, my mother, who lovingly brought me into this world, nourished my development, and supported my educational endeavors to the largest extent possible; Meghan and Kelly, my beautiful daughters, who needn't do anything but exist to remain special in my heart; Candy, my loving companion of many years, who has remained steadfastly and unfalteringly by my side through the thick and thin times since we have known one another;

and Holly and Dodge, Candy's children, whom I have come to love and admire as my own. I continue with my siblings, Cheryl, Cathy, Cindy, Candy, and John, and my many aunts, uncles, and cousins, too numerous to name, but each of whom has influenced me in unique and meaningful ways.

There are also two additional people, both now deceased but not the least bit forgotten: My father, Frank Sr., passed away nearly 15 years ago, but hardly a day goes by that I do not think of him. My drive and work ethic are his legacy to me. And Mary Andrasik, my grandmother, or "Grandma Mom" as everyone knew her, taught me the true meaning of unconditional love, long before I studied about Carl Rogers in college. My commitment to family, love of children, and appetite for Hungarian food are her legacy to me.

Finally, working on this text has introduced me to the wonderful and talented people at The Guilford Press. The polished product that you see here is a tribute to them as well.

Contents

IV. CULTIVATING LOWER AROUSAL

V. DISORDERS NEEDING LOWER TENSION AND AROUSAL

VI. ELECTROENCEPHALOGRAPHIC BIOFEEDBACK APPLICATIONS

VII. NEUROMUSCULAR APPLICATIONS

VIII. ELIMINATION DISORDERS

IX. PEDIATRIC APPLICATIONS

X. OTHER APPLICATIONS

PART I

History, Entering, and Definitions

CHAPTER 1

A Historical Perspective
on the Field of Biofeedback
and Applied Psychophysiology

MARK S. SCHWARTZ
R. PAUL OLSON[1]

This chapter conveys a rich appreciation of the converging trends that have influenced the development and journey of applied biofeedback, and the evolution of the broader field of applied psychophysiology. This historical perspective helps readers to understand not only the origins of biofeedback, but also some factors shaping its future. It also helps to illuminate the broader concept of applied psychophysiology, and to give perspective to the name changes of the primary professional membership organization and its journal.

Applied biofeedback began in the United States with the convergence of many disciplines in the late 1950s. The major antecedents and fields from which it developed include the following. (Both in this list and in subsequent text, italics on first use of a term indicate that the term is included in the glossary at the end of this chapter.)

1. Instrumental conditioning of *autonomic nervous system* (*ANS*) responses.
2. Psychophysiology.
3. Behavior therapy and behavioral medicine.
4. Stress research and stress management strategies.
5. Biomedical engineering.
6. Surface electromyography (EMG), diagnostic EMG, and control of *single* motor units.
7. Consciousness, altered states of consciousness, and electroencephalography (EEG).
8. Cybernetics.
9. Cultural factors.
10. Professional developments.[2]

The order of the items in this list reflects neither historical sequence nor importance. Other classifications and historical perspectives on biofeedback applications can be found in Gaarder and Montgomery (1977, 1981), Gatchel and Price (1979), Anchor, Beck, Sieveking, and Adkins (1982), and Basmajian (1989).

INSTRUMENTAL CONDITIONING OF AUTONOMIC
NERVOUS SYSTEM RESPONSES

Learning theory developed within experimental psychology as a means of understanding, predicting, and controlling variations in animal and human behavior. In contrast with those who emphasize heredity as the major determinant of behavior, learning theorists emphasize the importance of one's environment—specifically, of environmental contingencies, including *reinforcers*, which lead to acquisition and maintenance of learned behavior.

"Learning" means a change in behavior as the direct result of experience. Reinforcement is necessary for *operant conditioning* or *instrumental conditioning* to take place. From this perspective, both overt behaviors and covert behaviors, such as thoughts, feelings, and physiological responses, are functions of the antecedents and consequences of such behaviors. This model describes the learning of responses instrumental to obtaining or avoiding positive or negative consequences.

The prevailing scientific viewpoint for several decades was that only the voluntary musculoskeletal system, mediated by the *central nervous system* (*CNS*), was responsive to operant conditioning. This view held that the *autonomic nervous system* (*ANS*) functioned automatically beyond conscious awareness, and hence beyond voluntary control. Most scientists thought that the internal, homeostatic controls for such functions as circulation and digestion were innate and unaffected by self-regulatory learning. Most scientists assumed that ANS functioning or *visceral learning* was modifiable only via *classical conditioning*, if subject to learning at all. In this view, responses are automatic after conditioning occurs. In classical conditioning, thoughts can even become conditioned stimuli (CSs) and elicit physiological responses.

The strong biases against instrumental conditioning of the ANS and the visceral responses it controls limited the amount of experimental work in this area until about three decades ago (Miller, 1978). Later studies with humans and animals showed that instrumental training could produce increases and dereases in several body responses. These included *vasomotor* responses, blood pressure, salivation, *galvanic skin response* (*GSR*), and cardiac rates and rhythms (see reviews by Kimmel, 1979, and Harris & Brady, 1974).

Research indicated that individuals could gain volitional control over several different ANS functions without learning that could be attributed to cognitive factors. Many scientists and professionals were very skeptical of these findings. There was much disagreement concerning whether the research really demonstrated cortical control over ANS activity. As research advanced, it became clear that to show operant learning effects in the ANS, researchers needed more sophisticated designs. They had to rule out *skeletally mediated mechanical artifacts* and *visceral reflexes*.

By the 1970s, researchers began studying CNS-controlled, integrated skeletal–visceral responses and patterns. They also studied specificity and patterning of learned visceral responses and cognitively mediated strategies for producing visceral changes (Miller, 1978). The *curarized animal* studies of Miller and his associates (Miller & DiCara, 1967) countered the argument that skeletal muscle activity was mediating some visceral changes. The skeletal muscles were temporarily paralyzed.

Orne (1979), a cautious but supportive conscience of the biofeedback field, reminded us that, in terms of animal studies,

> It would be misleading, however . . . not to point out that the important studies with curarized animals . . . while initially replicated, cannot now be reproduced. Though there is no difficulty in demonstrating statistically significant changes in visceral function as a result of instrumental conditioning in curarized animals—leaving no doubt about the phenomenon—obtaining effects sufficiently large to be clinically significant eludes the present techniques. (p. 495)

The research with instrumental conditioning of visceral responses mediated by the ANS gave a major impetus to the development of clinical biofeedback. It appeared to resolve the controversy concerning whether such conditioning was a legitimate phenomenon. An assumption of clinical biofeedback is that it can help persons improve the accuracy of their perceptions of their visceral events. These perceptions allow them to gain greater self-regulation of these processes. Indeed, some professionals view some biofeedback as instrumental conditioning of visceral responses.

This operant model of biofeedback has significant heuristic value. One can apply principles of instrumental conditioning to physiological self-regulation. These principles include *schedules of reinforcement, shaping, extinction*, and *fading*.

Although it is helpful to view biofeedback primarily as instrumental conditioning of visceral responses, this model is seriously limiting. Learning theory has developed far beyond the more traditional views of operant conditioning. Other professionals believe that human learning includes major cognitive dimensions as well as environmental reinforcers. Examples include thinking, expectation, visualization and imagery, foresight and planning, and problem-solving strategies.

One can include cognitive factors within the operant conditioning model. However, professionals adhering to more stringent interpretations of the model consider cognitive factors inadmissible, because one cannot observe or objectively measure them. Nevertheless, studies of motor skill learning (Blumenthal, 1977) show that humans develop mental models ("motor programs") of what a skilled movement should be like. Furthermore, research shows that one may acquire behavior without obvious practice or even reinforcement. This evidence comes from latent learning experiments (Harlow & Harlow, 1962), studies of discovery learning (Bruner, 1966), and studies of *observational learning* involving imitation of a model (Rosenthal & Zimmerman, 1978).

Increased acceptance for the role of mental processes in learning led to cognitive-behavioral therapies and studies of cognitively mediated strategies in the changes occurring during biofeedback therapies. The emphasis on cognitive learning also supported the applications of *cybernetics* to biofeedback.

PSYCHOPHYSIOLOGY

David Shapiro offered the first academic course in *psychophysiology* at Harvard University in 1965. The *Handbook of Psychophysiology*, a major publication, appeared 7 years later (Greenfield & Sternback, 1972).

Psychophysiology involves the scientific study of the interrelationships of physiological and cognitive processes. Some consider it a special branch of physiology. Some also consider it an offspring of psychobiology, which in turn is the child of the marriage between the physical and social sciences (Hassett, 1978). Physiological psychologists often manipulate physiology and observe behavior. In contrast, psychophysiologists often facilitate, manage, guide, hinder, or obstruct human psychological variables and observe the physiological effects.

As a form of "applied psychophysiology,"[3] clinical biofeedback helps people alter their behaviors with feedback from their physiology. These include muscle activity, peripheral blood flow, cardiac activity, sweat gland activity, brain electrical activity, and blood pressure. Some providers of clinical biofeedback call themselves "clinical psychophysiologists." This name emphasizes the applied nature of their professional activities and their involvement with this scientific specialty.

BEHAVIOR THERAPY AND BEHAVIORAL MEDICINE

Related outgrowths of both learning theory and psychophysiology are the fields of behavior therapy and behavioral medicine. "Behavior therapy" developed in the 1950s as an alternative to *insight-oriented psychodynamic theories and therapies* for mental disorders. Early proponents of behavior therapies included Wolpe (1973), Paul (1966), Bandura and Walters (1963), and Ullman and Krasner (1965). The roots of behavior therapy include the notion that one learns maladaptive behaviors, and thus in most cases, one can unlearn them. The model is largely educational rather than medical as such. It applies the principles of operant and respondent conditioning, as well as of cognitive learning, to change a wide range of behaviors. Many professionals view some biofeedback applications as a form of operant learning. Others view biofeedback more cognitively within an information-processing model.

"Behavioral medicine" is another outgrowth of learning theory, psychophysiology, and behavior therapy. This specialty developed within behavior therapy and psychosomatic medicine. It appeared as a distinct entity in the late 1970s. Behavioral medicine focuses on applications of learning theories to medical disorders and other health-related topics. It does not focus on psychopathology or mental disorders. G. E. Schwartz and Weiss (1978) reported a definition of behavioral medicine proposed at the Yale Conference held in 1977:

> Behavioral medicine is the field concerned with the development of behavior science knowledge and techniques relevant to the understanding of physical health and illness and the application of this knowledge and these techniques to diagnosis, prevention, treatment, and rehabilitation. Psychosis, neurosis, and substance abuse are included only insofar as they contribute to physical disorders as an end point. (p. 379)

Behavioral medicine also developed because traditional medical approaches were insufficient for managing and treating many chronic diseases, conditions, and health-damaging or maladaptive behaviors. This new specialty goes beyond the traditional germ theory of the etiology and progression of diseases. It recognizes the important roles of stress, lifestyle, habits, and environmental variables in the development, maintenance, and treatment of medical and dental diseases and conditions.[4]

Behavioral medicine places much emphasis on the patient's role in prevention of and recovery from organic diseases and conditions. The same emphases are clear in applied or clinical biofeedback. In fact, some professionals consider clinical biofeedback to be a major specialty within the broader field of behavioral medicine.

The contributions of behavior therapy and behavioral medicine to the development and applications of applied biofeedback and applied psychophysiology are clear. The interactions among professionals from all of these fields will continue to be enriching.

STRESS RESEARCH, RELAXATION THERAPIES, AND OTHER STRESS MANAGEMENT TECHNIQUES

An important area of behavioral medicine is research on the effects of stress on causing physical symptoms and altering the immune system. However, research on stress began long before the development of behavioral medicine or biofeedback; in fact, both fields have their roots partly in stress research. Selye's (1974) report of more than 130,000 entries on stress showed the extent of stress research.

Pioneering research was conducted by the physicians Claude Bernard and Walter B. Cannon and by Hans Selye. Pi-Suner (1955) observed that Bernard developed the concept of physiological "homeostasis" as the major process by which the body maintains itself. As Langley (1965) noted, the concept became integral to the discipline of physiology. Physical and mental disease are thought to occur because some homeostatic feedback mechanism is malfunctioning. One of the major effects of such homeostatic imbalance is stress.

In his book *The Wisdom of the Body*, Cannon (1932) indicated the natural causes and results of the innate stress response. He named this response *fight or flight*. Selye's (1974, 1976, 1983) extensive research led to a triphasic conceptualization of the nature of the physiological stress response: It includes stages of alarm, resistance, and exhaustion. One first experiences stressful events as hardship; then one gets used to them; and finally one cannot stand them any longer (Selye, 1971).

The brilliant and pioneering work of Cannon and Selye contributed significantly to the development of the field of psychosomatic medicine. Their work increased awareness of the role of stress in physical and mental diseases. This awareness nurtured applied biofeedback, and many of these applications focused on stress-related disorders. Furthermore, as noted by Miller (1978), the emphasis of biofeedback on measurement and producing changes in bodily processes contributes to other behavioral techniques for relieving stress effects.

Many stress management systems evolved with the awareness of the effects of stress on health and disease. Included among these are many relaxation therapies, and some observers perceive biofeedback as a specific treatment modality within this group. In practice, the effects of relaxation have a major role in achieving the therapeutic effects with biofeedback.

A very early form of physical relaxation is "hatha yoga," a technique adopted from the Far East and popularized in Western countries in the 1960s. In the United States in the 1930s, Edmund Jacobson (1938, 1978) developed "progressive relaxation training," which is a series of muscle activities designed to teach people ways to distinguish degrees of tension and relaxation, and to reduce specific and general muscle tension. It also reduces or stops many symptoms and some causes and effects of stress.

> Muscle relaxation has long been noted as an important treatment for a variety of psychophysiological and stress-related disorders. The value of taking time to relax is becoming increasingly recognized in Western society, and we are borrowing techniques from those Eastern cultures where relaxation procedures . . . have been practiced for centuries. (Tarlar-Benlolo, 1978, pp. 727–728)

Lehrer and Woolfolk (1984) reviewed empirical and comparative studies through the early 1980s involving progressive relaxation and versions of it. Lichstein (1988) provided one of the most thorough reviews of relaxation strategies and research results. Other very useful resources are two books by Smith (1989, 1990). Modifications of progressive relaxation have been developed by Wolpe (1973), Bernstein and Borkovec (1973), and Jacobson and McGuigan (1982). A related technique developed in England by Laura Mitchell (1977, 1987) involves stretch–release procedures.

In addition to the physiological relaxation procedures, there has been a proliferation of primarily mental techniques, most of which are some form of meditation. Islamic Sufis, Hindu yogis, Christian contemplatives, and Hasidic Jews have practiced religious meditation for centuries. However, meditation was not (and still is not) a popular practice in the United States except among a very small minority.

Meditation became popularized in the United States in the 1960s as a result of the development of Transcendental Meditation (TM), practiced and promoted by a teacher from India named Maharishi Mahesh Yogi (Forem, 1974). More Westernized variations of TM were subsequently developed as "clinically standardized meditation" (Carrington, 1977) and the "relaxation response" (Benson, 1975). A modification of a meditation technique combined with physiological relaxation is Strobel's (1982) "quieting reflex."

Another meditation approach is "open focus," developed by Fehmi and Fritz (1980). This intends to promote an open, relaxed, and integrated mind–body state. It is closer to Soto Zen meditation in its goal of a content-free and quiet mind, by contrast with the focused concentration of yoga and TM. The emigration of Zen Buddhist teachers to the United States beginning in the 1940s was yet another factor contributing to the meditation movement.

There are still other approaches involving relaxation/meditation: Ira Progoff's (1980) "process meditation," José Silva's (1977) "Silva mind control," and C. Norman Shealy's (1977) "biogenics." Practitioners often use relaxation/meditation techniques with biofeedback instrumentation to enhance the learning of psychophysiological self-regulation.

Hypnosis is yet another approach developed to aid persons to control pain and stress. In the 1700s, Franz Mesmer first postulated "animal magnetism" to explain persons' responses to suggestion. Hypnosis developed slowly until the 20th century. Over the past few decades, it has become more sophisticated and empirically grounded as a set of therapeutic techniques. Liebeault, Charcot, and Freud were among the first to apply the techniques to patients (Moss, 1965). Contemporary researchers, such as Barber, Hilgard, Weitzenhoffer, and Erickson, have conducted serious investigations into the parameters of hypnosis.

In Germany early in the 20th century, J. H. Schultz developed a form of physiologically directed, self-generated therapy called "autogenic training." Wolgang Luthe (1969) reported the extensive research and therapeutic applications of this popular technique, variations of which are now also in common practice. Some, like Wickramasekara (1976, 1988), have reported integrations of hypnosis and biofeedback.

There are numerous other stress management techniques. Many of these have been summarized by Davis, Eshelman, and McKay (1980), McKay, Davis, and Fanning (1981), Charlesworth and Nathan (1985), and Lehrer and Woolfolk (1993).

BIOMEDICAL ENGINEERING

Without high-quality instrumentation for measuring physiological events accurately and reliably, there would be no biofeedback. As Tarlar-Benlolo (1978) reminds us, "prior to World War II, available equipment was not sufficiently sensitive for measuring most of the body's internally generated electric impulses" (p. 728). Progress occurred after the war, and

> technology had advanced far . . . making feasible the task of designing and constructing instruments that could accurately detect and record minute electrical discharges, integrate and amplify these responses, and produce a corresponding signal that could be interpreted by the person being monitored. (p. 728)

Biomedical engineers have developed technology that is both noninvasive and sophisticated. Surface recordings used for biofeedback measurement provide feedback for many different physiological activities. Feedback can also be provided for angles of limbs and the force of muscles and limbs. Instruments continuously monitor, amplify, and transform electronic and *electromechanical* signals into audio and visual feedback—understandable information.

Now multiple and simultaneous recordings of several channels of physiological information are available with instrumentation linked to computers. Computers allow greater storage capabilities, rapid signal and statistical analyses, simultaneous recording and integration of multiple channels, and displays impossible only a few years ago.

ELECTROMYOGRAPHY, DIAGNOSTIC ELECTROMYOGRAPHY, AND SINGLE-MOTOR-UNIT CONTROL

The workhorse of the biofeedback field is surface electromyography or simply *electromyography* (abbreviated here as *EMG*, though sEMG is also used). According to Basmajian (1983), EMG instrumentation grew out of the studies of neuromuscular and spinal cord functions. He reminds us that "it began with the classic paper in 1929 by Adrian and Bronk, who showed that the electrical responses in individual muscles provided an accurate reflection of the actual functional activity of the muscles" (p. 2).

Physicians' use of EMG in diagnosing neuromuscular disorders is many decades old. As early as 1934, reports indicated that voluntary, conscious control over the EMG potentials of *single motor units* was possible (Smith, 1934). Marinacci and Horande (1960) added case reports of the potential value of displaying EMG signals to assist patients in neuromuscular reeducation. Basmajian (1963, 1978) also reported on the control of single motor units.

Several investigators reported EMG feedback in the rehabilitation of patients after stroke (Andrews, 1964; Brudny, 1982; Basmajian, Kukulka, Narayan, & Takebe, 1975; Wolf & Binder-MacLeod, 1983; Binder-MacLeod, 1983). Such research was important in the development of applied biofeedback, especially for the field of neuromuscular rehabilitation. Thus EMG biofeedback gained solid support among researchers and clinicians.

Practitioners have also used EMG feedback for treating such symptoms and disorders as tension headaches and tension myalgias, and, more recently, incontinence.

CONSCIOUSNESS, ALTERED STATES OF CONSCIOUSNESS, AND ELECTROENCEPHALOGRAPHIC FEEDBACK

Some observers prior to the late 1960s viewed psychology as a discipline that lost its mind when it stopped studying human consciousness and lost its soul when it discarded a phenomenology of the self. Since then, however, these trends have been reversed. Humanistic psychology has reestablished the human self as a legitimate source of inquiry, and scientists in transpersonal psychology and neurophysiology have renewed the study of human consciousness. Such theorists as Tart (1969), Krippner (1972), Ornstein (1972), Pelletier and Garfield (1976), G. E. Schwartz and Beatty (1977), and Jacobson (1982) are among those who have made significant contributions to our understanding of human consciousness.

Many studies of altered states of consciousness induced by drugs, hypnosis, or meditation have added to our knowledge of the relationships between brain functioning and human behavior. Such research helped stimulate the use of *electroencephalography* (EEG) in biofeedback, which also focuses on the functional relationships between brain and behavior.

In the early 1960s, studies began appearing on the relationships between EEG *alpha wave activity* (8–12 hertz) on the one hand, and emotional states and certain states of consciousness on the other. Alpha biofeedback, commonly reported as associated with a relaxed but alert state, received its most attention in the late 1960s. Clinical applications were mostly for general relaxation.

Kamiya (1969) reported that one could voluntarily control alpha waves—a feat that was previously believed impossible. Support for these and related findings came from Brown (1977), Nowlis and Kamiya (1970), and Hart (1968). "Though these studies tended to lack systematic controls, they nonetheless caught the imagination of many serious scientists as well as the media" (Orne, 1979, p. 493). Some investigators and practitioners continued to advocate the value of alpha biofeedback through the early 1980s (e.g., Gaarder & Montgomery,

1981), despite recognizing that "there was no clear-cut and concrete rationale to explain why it should help patients" (p. 155). Interested readers can review Gaarder and Montgomery's informative discussion. In contrast, Basmajian (1983) noted that

> alpha feedback . . . has virtually dried up as a scientifically defensible clinical tool . . . it has . . . returned to the research laboratory from which it probably should not have emerged prematurely. Through the next generation of scientific investigation, it may return as a useful applied technique. (p. 3)

Other investigators studied specialized learning processes and other EEG parameters, such as theta waves, evoked cortical responses, and EEG phase synchrony of multiple areas of the cortex (Beatty, Greenberg, Deibler, & O'Hanlon, 1974; Fehmi & Selzer, 1980; Fox & Rudell, 1968). A few investigators continue this experimental work.

Specialized EEG biofeedback from selected brain areas, and selected EEG parameters (e.g., *sensorimotor rhythm* and *slow-wave activity*), became the focus of well-controlled studies. These emerged as effective therapeutic approaches for very carefully selected patients with CNS disorders such as epilepsy (Lubar, 1982, 1983; Sterman, 1982; see also Strehl, Chapter 20, this volume), as well as for some patients with attention-deficit/hyperactivity disorder (Lubar, 1991; see also Lubar, Chapter 18, this volume).

More recently, combined alpha–theta EEG feedback procedures purport to be successful in treating patients' addictive behaviors, such as alcoholism (Ochs, 1992; Rosenfeld, 1992a; Wuttke, 1992; Peniston & Kulkosky, 1989, 1990; see also Monastra, Chapter 19, this volume). Clinical applications, as well as debate and research on them, continue.

CYBERNETICS

The term "biofeedback" is a shorthand term for external psychophysiological feedback, physiological feedback, and sometimes augmented *proprioception. The* basic idea is to provide individuals with increased information about what is going on inside their bodies, including their brains.

The field that deals most directly with information processing and feedback is called *cybernetics*. A basic principle of cybernetics is that one cannot control a variable unless information about the variable is available to the controller. The information provided is called "feedback" (Ashby, 1963; Mayr, 1970).

Another principle of cybernetics is that feedback makes learning possible. Annett (1969) reviewed the evidence for this principle. In applied biofeedback, individuals receive direct and clear feedback about their physiology. This helps them learn to control such functions. For example, from an EMG instrument, persons receive information concerning their muscle activity. This helps them learn to reduce, increase, or otherwise regulate the muscle tension.

From a cybernetic perspective, operant conditioning is one form of feedback. It is feedback provided in the form of positive or negative results of a particular behavior. The point is that another significant contribution to the development of applied biofeedback is an information-processing model derived from cybernetic theory and research. Proponents of this model in the field of biofeedback include Brown (1977), Anliker (1977), Mulholland (1977), and Gaarder and Montgomery (1981).

CULTURAL FACTORS

Several cultural factors have contributed to the development of applied biofeedback. The gradual merging of the traditions and techniques of the East and West is one major factor.

The rise in popularity of schools of meditation was an expression of a cultural change providing a context in which applied biofeedback developed. Yogis and Zen masters reportedly alter their physiological states significantly through meditation. Related phenomena presumably occur in some forms of biofeedback experiences. Therefore, some have referred to biofeedback as the "yoga of the West" and "electronic Zen."

Within the United States, there are other cultural factors adding to a *Zeitgeist* encouraging biofeedback applications. These are the heightened costs of health care and the resulting need for more efficacious and cost-effective treatments. In addition, it is commonly recognized that pharmacotherapy, with all its benefits, is of limited value for many patients. Some patients cannot take medications because of untoward side effects; many patients avoid compliance; and some physicians deemphasize pharmacotherapy.

Perhaps even more significant is the current popular public health emphasis on prevention. The movement toward wellness has continued to grow since the 1960s. Practitioners of holistic health also emphasize self-regulation and self-control. The result of these emphases is that more people are involving themselves in lifestyle changes to regulate their health. These changes include enhancing physical fitness, avoiding caffeine and nicotine, reducing or stopping alcohol use, and pursuing better weight control. More people are thus assuming increased responsibility for their physical, as well as their mental and spiritual, well-being. In addition, more people are accepting responsibility for their recovery from illness. Many believe that biofeedback therapies facilitate and fit well into these efforts at greater self-regulation, wellness, and growth.

PROFESSIONAL DEVELOPMENTS

Also adding to the development of applied biofeedback are the organizations of professionals engaged in both research and clinical/educational applications. Issues considered here include the professional organizations themselves (and the various names the primary one has used); the status of the literature in this field; the professional journal of the primary organization (and the journal's name); and, finally, the scope of the field.

Professional Organizations

Homer's epic poem *The Odyssey* can serve as a metaphor for the past, present, and future of biofeedback and applied psychophysiology.[5] From the title of this epic, an "odyssey" has come to mean any long series of wanderings, especially when filled with notable experiences, hardships, and the exploration of new terrain. Just as Homer's Odysseus experienced setbacks but was ultimately successful in his journey to reach home, the journey of psychophysiological self-regulation with biofeedback has experienced and will continue to experience setbacks and successes. The Biofeedback Society of America (BSA) was entering its 20th year, thus completing one full generation of development, when similar words were first delivered (M. S. Schwartz, 1988). Twenty years constitute one generation, or the average period between the birth of parents and the birth of their offspring. Thirteen years then remained until the year 2001, the date of the famous book and movie *2001: A Space Odyssey*. However, our field does not seek the universality of something as monolithic as Arthur C. Clarke's and Stanley Kubrick's odyssey.

The Association for Applied Psychophysiology and Biofeedback, and Its Various Names

How the Journey Began. The Biofeedback Research Society (BRS) was formed in 1969, largely by a handful of research psychophysiologists. After 6 years the BRS became the BSA, with both an experimental and an applied division. Age 6 is about the age at which children go through the transition from home to school; similarly, the scope of the organization and the field broadened into applied arenas. This change in name reflected the growth and importance of the applied area.

How the Journey Continued. At age 19, as a result of the field's expanding scope, the BSA went through its second transformation—into the Association for Applied Psychophysiology and Biofeedback (AAPB). This is about the age at which many students graduate to institutions of higher learning. This organization returned to some of its roots in psychophysiology at the same interval. The consistency with the journey metaphor first struck M. S. Schwartz (1988) then, as Odysseus also took 20 years to return home.

As later reported by M. S. Schwartz (1999a, p. 3),

> the name . . . change was a hotly debated topic. Many argued for a need to expand the implied scope of the organization. One factor was that most practitioners utilized a wider array of therapy methods than biofeedback. Presentations at the annual meetings of the BSA encompassed much more than biofeedback. Researchers at universities were saying that the term biofeedback was too limiting. They maintained that the term biofeedback alone was not viewed as sufficiently credible by some individuals and that this hampered their abilities to publish their research in some quality journals and to obtain external research funding. The researchers further contended that the term "biofeedback" was insufficient for them to obtain the kind of recognition they needed in their academic departments. Thus, both applied practitioners and researchers were contending that a name change was needed.
>
> Psychophysiology was the birthplace of the field of biofeedback, and so it was time to return to these roots. The emphasis was placed on the term applied to distinguish it from [its] grandparent organization and field, the Society for Psychophysiological Research.
>
> Many members of the BSA . . . argued for dropping the term biofeedback but the supporters of the term successfully argued for the preservation of the term. . . . The term "applied psychophysiology" reflected the evolution of science and clinical practice.

The AAPB continues to be a productive, intellectually stimulating, clinically useful, scientifically sound, and vibrant organization.

Disagreement has continued, however, about the most appropriate name for both the membership organization and its journal (see below). Some argue for only "Association for Applied Psychophysiology." Others argue for maintaining the terms "Biofeedback" and "Self-Regulation." There is good reasoning on both sides. Those supporting "Association for Applied Psychophysiology" as sufficient emphasize a broader scope. This is more acceptable conceptually and politically to many psychophysiologically oriented researchers with close ties to biofeedback. Those who advocate keeping the term "Biofeedback" in the names of the organization and journal focus on the established place of this term in the minds of professionals and the lay public, as well as on its history, brevity, and ease of communication. Why change horses in midstream, they argue, especially from a familiar one that is doing so well?

Other Membership Organnizations

Another national membership organization, the American Association of Biofeedback Clinicians, started in 1975 but went out of existence in the late 1980s. This left the BSA, now the AAPB, as the only organization with a major emphasis on biofeedback. However, many other professional and scientific societies also devote space in their publications and time at their meetings to biofeedback and applied psychophysiological research.

The Biofeedback Certification Institute of America

A professional organization that influenced the continued development of the field is the Bio-feedback Certification Institute of America (BCIA). As its name indicates, the BCIA maintains a credible credentialing program. Before 1979, credentialing was in the hands of a few state biofeedback societies. These societies, well-meaning as they were, suffered from the understand-able problems of small groups of professionals who typically had little or no training and expe-rience with the complexities of credentialing. Thus there was considerable variability in the credentialing across states. In most states, there was no credentialing at all or the hope of any.

Ed Taub, then president-elect of the BSA, had the foresight and wisdom to inspire the development of an independent, credible, nationwide credentialing program. The BSA spon-sored and supported the official establishment of the BCIA (named by Bernard Engel, later the first chair of the BCIA board) in January 1981. Three months later, when Engel became President of the BSA, he graciously relinquished the chair of BCIA to Schwartz. The BCIA evolved with more stringent criteria for education, training, experience, and recertification. Professionals continue to seek and earn the BCIA's credential as the only one of its kind.

Although the BCIA holds primacy in credentialing, educational opportunities exist in many undergraduate and graduate courses in biofeedback. Private training programs and work-shops are offered by national, state, and regional professional organizations. There are also many companies manufacturing biofeedback instrumentation, and several companies selling and servicing a variety of instruments from different manufacturers.

The Journey of a Family or Separate Journeys?

All professionals in this field share some joint responsibility and custody for the young adult we call "biofeedback and applied psychophysiology." Some individual professionals proceed on their own journeys; they seek their own destinations, their own Ithacas, instead of com-mon ones. However, the AAPB continues as the leading administrative, facilitative, educa-tional, and coordinating organization dedicated to integrating professional disciplines and conceptual frameworks that involve varied scientific and applied areas of psychophysiology and biofeedback. It is the nuclear family for biofeedback.

Status of the Literature in the Field

The number of publications is one barometer of the history, growth, and possibly the future of a field. The first bibliography of the biofeedback literature (Butler & Stoyva, 1973) contained about 850 references. The next edition, 5 years later, listed about 2300 references (Butler, 1978). Thousands more have appeared since 1978 (Hatch & Riley, 1985; Hatch & Saito, 1990). There was a downward trend in journal publications in English from 1985 through 1991 (Hatch, 1993). However, about 150 per year continue appearing with no decline between the years 1987 through 1991. (See M. S. Schwartz & Andrasik, Chapter 39, this volume, for more discussion.)

Note there are dozens of papers published each year in non-English-speaking countries. For example, the important Japanese literature was still in its early stages in 1979, but rap-idly increased in the 1980s (Hatch & Saito, 1990). There is also a rich history of research publications and clinical applications in Russia and other countries that were formerly part of the USSR (Sokhadze & Shtark, 1991; Shtark & Kall, 1998; Shtark & Schwartz, 2002). This foreign literature is not well known in the United States.

A perspective on the issues of history, publications, and past and current interest, and a full appreciation for roots, research, and applications, all require awareness of and access to foreign publication databases.

The Primary Journal, and Its Name

A measure of the maturity of a field is the existence of and quality of its primary professional journal. The journal *Biofeedback and Self-Regulation*, published by Plenum Press, was started in 1976. The journal's name was changed to *Applied Psychophysiology and Biofeedback* as of Volume 22, 1997. The editors, board, and publisher noted that "the journal has long had a broader focus than the title implied, and this new name more accurately reflects its expanded scope" (Andrasik, 1997, p. 1).

Defining "Applied Psychophysiology"

Defining the term "applied psychophysiology" still remained a need, goal, and challenge as of 1998, several years after the AAPB's and the journal's name changes. As noted by M. S. Schwartz (1999a, p. 4), "One can only surmise that everyone apparently *knew* what applied psychophysiology meant. . . . What everyone apparently knew, no one had written. What everyone apparently knew, was unclear."

J. Peter Rosenfeld, in his AAPB presidential address (Rosenfeld, 1992b), was the first to address a definition of "applied psychophysiology." He identified some of its elements, "and touched on elements of a definition" (M. S. Schwartz, 1999a, p. 4). Sebastian Striefel, a later president of AAPB, again raised the question of a definition of applied psychophysiology in his 1998 presidential address (Striefel, 1998). At the same meeting, "Paul Lehrer, chairperson of the AAPB Publication Committee, convened an ad hoc committee to deal with a wide array of topics. . . . One of these topics was . . . the lack of a formal . . . definition of 'applied psychophysiology'" (M. S. Schwartz, 1999a, p. 4). The committee assigned the task of establishing an operational definition for the term. The initial paper by M. S. Schwartz (1999a), responses and critiques by an array of notable professionals, and the response by Schwartz (1999b) are all contained in the journal (1999, Vol. 24, pp. 1–54). (See N. M. Schwartz & Schwartz, Chapter 3, this volume, for the definition and selected comments.)

The development of a definition that is acceptable to everyone is unlikely. Just as there were broader and narrower definitions for "biofeedback," there probably will remain broader and narrower definitions for "applied psychophysiology." This is not a problem, as long as one considers definitions as operational entities developed for specific purposes. Perhaps the AAPB will adopt an official definition eventually.

SUMMARY

The field of biofeedback has a very rich history with multiple roots. Awareness of this background can be helpful in understanding the beginnings of biofeedback, its status, and salient factors shaping its future. From feedback research and applications of the past, one may find inspiration and momentum for a creative future in this exciting field. The scope and contributions of biofeedback encompass many professional fields. For some professionals, biofeedback remains a field in itself. For many other professionals, biofeedback is part of the broader field of "applied psychophysiology"—now the term that is part of the primary national organization's name and the title of the primary journal. However, it is still too early to forecast how the applied psychophysiology concept and term will affect the metamorphosis of the broader field and the biofeedback component. "Biofeedback" remains a viable and enduring term with a rich and complex history, present status, and future. This is true whether, by implication or design, it is independent of, linked to, or subsumed by broader terms and conceptual models.

GLOSSARY[6]

ALPHA WAVE ACTIVITY. Electroencephalographic (EEG) activity (8–12 hertz) commonly, but not always, thought to be associated with an alert but relaxed state.

AUTONOMIC NERVOUS SYSTEM (ANS). The part of the nervous system that is connected to all organs and blood vessels, and transmits signals that control their functioning. It consists of two branches, the sympathetic and parasympathetic, which usually produce opposite responses. Once thought to be totally involuntary, it is now known to be under some significant voluntary control, although less so than the CNS.

CENTRAL NERVOUS SYSTEM (CNS). The part of the nervous system including human thought, sense organs, and control of skeletal muscles. Once believed to be totally separate from the ANS, it is now known to interact with the ANS.

CLASSICAL CONDITIONING. Originating with Pavlov, the type of conditioning or learning that assumes that certain stimuli (unconditioned stimuli, or UCSs) evoke unconditioned or unlearned responses (UCRs) (e.g., acute pain evokes crying, withdrawal, and fear), and that other, previously neutral stimuli (conditioned stimuli, or CSs) associated with the pairing of these events develop the capacity to elicit the same or similar responses or conditioned responses (CRs).

CURARIZED ANIMALS. Animals intentionally paralyzed by the drug curare to control for body movements during visceral conditioning, such as biofeedback of heart rate.

CYBERNETICS. The science of internal body control systems in humans, and of electrical and mechanical systems designed to replace the human systems.

ELECTROENCEPHALOGRAPHY (EEG). The measurement of electrical activity of the brain.

ELECTROMECHANICAL. A term describing devices that measure mechanical aspects of the body (e.g., position of a joint or degree of pressure or weight placed on it), rather than a property of the body (e.g., its direct electrical activity or temperature). Examples of these mechanical aspects include degrees that a knee bends in a person after knee surgery, steadiness of the head of a child with cerebral palsy, and the weight pressure placed on a leg and foot by someone after a stroke. Instruments transform these mechanical forces into electrical signals.

ELECTROMYOGRAPHY (EMG). The use of special instruments to measure the electrical activity of skeletal muscles. In recent years, also called "surface electromyography" and sometimes abbreviated as sEMG.

EXTINCTION. The behavioral principle predicting that abruptly and totally stopping all positive reinforcements after specified behaviors will lead to the behavior's no longer occurring.

FADING. Gradually changing a stimulus that controls a person's or animal's performance to another stimulus. As a behavioral procedure, it does not always mean disappearance of a stimulus.

FIGHT OR FLIGHT. Walter Cannon's well-known concept of the body's psychophysiological arousal and preparation for fighting or fleeing actual or perceived threatening stimuli.

GALVANIC SKIN RESPONSE (GSR). A form of electrodermal activity—increased resistance of the skin to conducting tiny electrical currents because of reduced sweat and dryness. Older term less ofen used now, but still accepted. Opposite of "skin conductance" (SC).

INSIGHT-ORIENTED PSYCHODYNAMIC THEORIES AND THERAPIES. A wide range of psychological theories and therapies, starting from the time of Sigmund Freud. A basic assumption is that patients need to gain insight into the psychological origins and forces motivating their current psychological problems and behaviors before they can achieve adequate relief of symptoms.

INSTRUMENTAL CONDITIONING. Same as operant conditioning (see below). The behavioral theories and therapies originated by B. F. Skinner. For example, reinforcers are said to be instrumentally linked to the recurrence of behaviors.

OBSERVATIONAL LEARNING. Learning that takes place by means of the organism's observing another organism doing the task to be learned.

OPERANT CONDITIONING. The same as instrumental conditioning (see above), originating with B. F. Skinner. "Operant" means that a response is identified and understood in terms of its consequences rather than by a stimulus that evokes it. Stimuli and circumstances emit responses rather than evoke them, as in classical conditioning.

PROPRIOCEPTION. Perception mediated by sensory nerve terminals within tissues, mostly muscles, tendons, and the labyrinthal system for balance. They give us information concerning our movements and position. Examples include (1) the sense of knowing when we are slightly off balance; and (2) the ability to perceive (even with eyes closed) the difference between, and approximate weights of, objects weighing 5 ounces and 7 ounces held in each hand.

PSYCHOPHYSIOLOGY. The science of studying the causal and interactive processes of physiology, behavior, and subjective experience.

REINFORCERS. Events or stimuli that increase the probability of recurrence of behaviors they follow.

SCHEDULES OF REINFORCEMENT. Usually, forms of intermittent reinforcement of an operant behavior. A common schedule in life, and most resistant to extinction, is a variable-ratio schedule—one in which the number of times a reinforcement follows a specific behavior varies randomly, so the person or animal never knows when the reinforcer will occur. This contrasts with variable-interval, fixed-interval, and fixed-ratio schedules.

SENSORIMOTOR RHYTHM. An EEG rhythm (12–14 hertz) recorded from the central scalp and involving both the sensory and motor parts of the brain, the sensorimotor cortex. Used in the EEG biofeedback of some persons with seizure disorders.

SHAPING. A behavioral principle from operant conditioning, referring to procedures designed to help learning of complex new behaviors by very small steps. Also known as "shaping by successive approximations."

SINGLE MOTOR UNITS. Individual spinal nerves or neurons involved in movement. Biofeedback training of single spinal motor neurons was a major advance in the late 1950s and early 1960s. This training requires fine-wire EMG electrodes.

SKELETALLY MEDIATED MECHANICAL ARTIFACTS. Artifacts in instrumentation-recorded signals that are caused by intentional body movements. Examples include moving a body part such as the head or neck during recordings of resting muscle activity, or clenching the teeth during EEG recordings.

SLOW-WAVE ACTIVITY. EEG activity (3–8 hertz) included in the frequency range often called theta activity, also reported as 4–7 hertz.

VASOMOTOR. Affecting the caliber (diameter) of a blood vessel.

VISCERAL LEARNING. Learning that takes place by body organs, especially those in the abdominal cavity, such as the stomach and bowels.

VISCERAL REFLEXES. Reflexes in which the stimulus is a state of an internal organ.

ZEITGEIST. The spirit or general trend of thought of a time in history. Often used to refer to a time in history when new ways of thinking and technologies are more likely to be accepted by the culture in question.

NOTES

1. R. Paul Olson's name is retained as coauthor of this chapter because most of it remains from the original first and second editions. The current version has added content but essentially has not altered existing content. Dr. Olson graciously withdrew from the third edition because of other commitments and a different focus of his professional life. However, his name is retained out of respect and recognition for his earlier contributions, and because of his old friendship with Mark S. Schwartz, who takes responsibility for the new content.

2. The 25th-anniversary meeting of the primary professional membership organization, the Association for Applied Psychophysiology and Biofeedback (AAPB), was held in 1994. The commemorative *AAPB Silver Anniversary Yearbook* published for that meeting contains articles about the history and development of the biofeedback field and the organization. Reading it is enriching and informative. It is available from the AAPB, 10200 West 44th Ave., Suite 304, Wheat Ridge, CO 80033; (303) 422-2615; fax (303) 422-8894. The Web site is http://www.aapb.org.

3. Note that this sentence appeared in the first edition of this book in early 1987. It does not seem to be a coincidence that the Biofeedback Society of America (BSA) went through the process of changing its name to include "applied psychophysiology" during that year while one of us (Mark S. Schwartz) was president of the BSA. However, it is a coincidence! Long after the name change and during a review of this chapter in preparation for the second edition, Schwartz noted the term here. Its presence in this chapter was never raised or discussed

during any of the board meetings or other public or private meetings concerning the name change. The term was written into an early draft of this chapter several years before 1987.

4. "Health psychology" is a more recent field with similar roots and ties to behavioral medicine. The focus is more on prevention and health enhancement.

5. Although the term "applied psychophysiology" is now usually given first in this pairing, the order is reversed here to reflect the emphasis on biofeedback in this book.

6. The intent of the glossaries in this and several other chapters is to provide enough information to give the reader a reasonable idea of the meaning of selected terms.

REFERENCES

Anchor, K. N., Beck, S. E., Sieveking, N., & Adkins, J. (1982). A history of clinical biofeedback. *American Journal of Clinical Biofeedback*, 5(1), 3–16.

Andrasik, F. (1997). Editorial. *Applied Psychophysiology and Biofeedback*, 22, 1.

Andrews, J. M. (1964). Neuromuscular re-education of the hemiplegic with aid of electromyograph. *Archives of Physical Medicine and Rehabilitation*, 45, 530–532.

Anliker, J. (1977). Biofeedback from the perspective of cybernetics and systems science. In J. Beatty & H. Legewie (Eds.), *Biofeedback and behavior*. New York: Plenum Press.

Annett, J. (1969). *Feedback and human behavior*. Baltimore: Penguin Books.

Ashby, W. R. (1963). *An introduction to cybernetics*. New York: Wiley.

Bandura, A., & Walters, R. (1963). *Social learning and personality development*. New York: Holt.

Basmajian, J. V. (1963). Conscious control of individual motor units. *Science*, 141, 440–441.

Basmajian, J. V. (1978). *Muscles alive: Their functions revealed by electromyography* (4th ed.). Baltimore: Williams & Wilkins.

Basmajian, J. V. (Ed.). (1983). *Biofeedback: Principles and practice for clinicians* (2nd ed.). Baltimore: Williams & Wilkins.

Basmajian, J. V. (Ed.). (1989). *Biofeedback: Principles and practice for clinicians* (3rd ed.). Baltimore: Williams & Wilkins.

Basmajian, J. V., Kukulka, C. G., Narayan, M. G., & Takebe, K. (1975). Biofeedback treatment of foot drop after stroke compared with standard rehabilitation technique: Effects on voluntary control and strength. *Archives of Physical Medicine and Rehabilitation*, 56, 231–236.

Beatty, J., Greenberg, A., Deibler, W. P., & O'Hanlon, J. F. (1974). Operant control of occipital theta rhythm affects performance in radar monitoring task. *Science*, 183, 871–873.

Benson, H. (1975). *The relaxation response*. New York: Morrow.

Bernstein, D. A., & Borkovec, T. D. (1973). *Progressive relaxation training: A manual for the helping professional*. Champaign, IL: Research Press.

Binder-MacLeod, S. A. (1983). Biofeedback in stroke rehabilitation. In J. V. Basmajian (Ed.), *Biofeedback: Principles and practice for clinicians* (2nd ed.). Baltimore: Williams & Wilkins.

Blumenthal, A. L. (1977). *The process of cognition*. Englewood Cliffs, NJ: Prentice-Hall.

Brown, B. (1977). *Stress and the art of biofeedback*. New York: Harper & Row.

Brudny, J. (1982). Biofeedback in chronic neurological cases: Therapeutic electromyography. In L. White & B. Tursky (Eds.), *Clinical biofeedback: Efficacy and mechanisms*. New York: Guilford Press.

Bruner, J. S. (1966). *Toward a theory of instruction*. Cambridge, MA: Belknap Press of Harvard University.

Butler, F. (1978). *Biofeedback: A survey of the literature*. New York: Plenum Press.

Butler, F., & Stoyva, J. (1973). *Biofeedback and self-control: A bibliography*. Wheat Ridge, CO: Biofeedback Society of America.

Cannon, W. B. (1932). *The wisdom of the body*. New York: Norton.

Carrington, P. (1977). *Freedom in meditation*. Garden City, NY: Doubleday/Anchor.

Charlesworth, E. A., & Nathan, R. G. (1985). *Stress management: A comprehensive guide to wellness*. New York: Atheneum.

Davis, M., Eshelman, E., & McKay, M. (1980). *The relaxation and stress reduction workbook*. Richmond, CA: New Harbinger.

Fehmi, L. G., & Fritz, G. (1980, Spring). Open focus: The attentional foundation of health and well being. *Somatics*, pp. 24–30.

Fehmi, L. G., & Selzer, F. (1980). Attention and biofeedback training in psychotherapy and transpersonal growth. In S. Boorstein & K. Speeth (Eds.), *Explorations in transpersonal psychotherapy*. New York: Aronson.

Forem, J. (1974). *Transcendental meditation*. New York: Dutton.

Fox, S. S., & Rudell, A. P. (1968). Operant controlled neural event: Formal and systematic approach to electrical coding of behavior in brain. *Science*, 162, 1299–1302.

Gaarder, K. R., & Montgomery, P. S. (1977). *Clinical biofeedback: A procedural manual for behavioral medicine*. Baltimore: Williams & Wilkins.

Gaarder, K. R, & Montgomery, P. S. (1981). *Clinical biofeedback: A procedural manual for behavioral medicine* (2nd ed.). Baltimore: Williams & Wilkins.

Gatchel, R. J., & Price, K. P. (1979). *Clinical applications of biofeedback: Appraisal and status*. New York: Pergamon Press.

Greenfield, N. S., & Sternback, R. A. (1972). *Handbook of psychophysiology*. New York: Holt, Rinehart & Winston.

Harlow, H. F., & Harlow, M. K. (1962). Social deprivation in monkeys. *Scientific American, 207*, 136–146.

Harris, A. H., & Brady, J. V. (1974). Animal learning: Visceral and autonomic conditioning. *Annual Review of Psychology, 25*, 107–133.

Hart, J. T. (1968). Autocontrol of EEG alpha [Abstract]. *Psychophysiology, 4*, 506.

Hassett, J. (1978). *A primer of psychophysiology*. San Francisco: Freeman.

Hatch, J. P. (1993, March). Declining rates of publication within the field of biofeedback continue: 1988–1991. In *Proceedings of the 24th Annual Meeting of the Association for Applied Psychophysiology and Biofeedback, Los Angeles*. Wheat Ridge, CO: Association for Applied Psychophysiology and Biofeedback.

Hatch, J. P., & Riley, P. (1985). Growth and development of biofeedback: A bibliographic analysis. *Biofeedback and Self-Regulation, 10*(4), 289–299.

Hatch, J. P., & Saito, I. (1990). Growth and development of biofeedback: A bibliographic update. *Biofeedback and Self-Regulation, 15*(1), 37–46.

Jacobson, E. (1938). *Progressive relaxation*. Chicago: University of Chicago Press.

Jacobson, E. (1978). *You must relax*. New York: McGraw-Hill.

Jacobson, E. (1982). *The human mind: A physiological clarification*. Springfield, IL: Thomas.

Jacobson, E., & McGuigan, F. J. (1982). *Principles and practice of progressive relaxation: A teaching primer* [Cassette]. New York: BMA Audio Cassettes.

Kamiya, J. (1969). Operant control of the EEG alpha rhythm and some of its reported effects on consciousness. In C. T. Tart (Ed.), *Altered states of consciousness*. New York: Wiley.

Kimmel, H. O. (1979). Instrumental conditioning of automanically mediated responses in human beings. *American Psychologist, 29*, 325–335.

Krippner, S. (1972). Altered states of consciousness. In J. White (Ed.), *The highest state of consciousness*. Garden City, NY: Doubleday.

Langley, L. L. (1965). *Homeostasis*. New York: Van Nostrand Reinhold.

Lehrer, P. M., & Woolfolk, R. L. (1984). Are all stress reduction techniques equivalent, or do they have differential effects?: A review of the comparative empirical literature. In R. L. Woolfolk & P. M. Lehrer (Eds.), *Principles and practice of stress management*. New York: Guilford Press.

Lehrer, P. M., & Woolfolk, R. L. (Eds.). (1993). *Principles and practice of stress management* (2nd ed.). New York: Guilford Press.

Lichstein, K. L. (1988). *Clinical relaxation strategies*. New York: Wiley.

Lubar, J. F. (1982). EEG operant conditioning in severe epileptics: Controlled multidimensional studies. In L. White & B. Tursky (Eds.), *Clinical biofeedback: Efficacy and mechanisms*. New York: Guilford Press.

Lubar, J. F. (1983). Electroencephalographic biofeedback and neurological applications. In J. V. Basmajian (Ed.), *Biofeedback: Principles and practice for clinicians* (2nd ed.). Baltimore: Williams & Wilkins.

Lubar, J. F. (1991). Discourse on the development of EEG diagnostics and biofeedback treatment for attention-deficit/hyperactivity disorders. *Biofeedback and Self-Regulation, 16*, 201–225.

Luthe, W. (Ed.). (1969). *Autogenic therapy* (Vols. 1–6). New York: Grune & Stratton.

Marinacci, A. A., & Horande, M. (1960). Electromyogram in neuromuscular re-education. *Bulletin of the Los Angeles Neurological Society, 25*, 57–71.

Mayr, O. (1970). *The origins of feedback control*. Cambridge, MA: MIT Press.

McKay, M., Davis, M., & Fanning, P. (1981). *Thoughts and feelings: The art of cognitive stress intervention*. Richmond, CA: New Harbinger.

Miller, N. E. (1978). Biofeedback and visceral learning. *Annual Review of Psychology, 29*, 373–404.

Miller, N. E., & DiCara, L. (1967). Instrumental learning of heart rate changes in curarized rats: Shaping and specificity to discriminative stimulus. *Journal of Comparative and Physiological Psychology, 63*, 12–19.

Mitchell, L. (1977). *Simple relaxation: The physiological method for easing tension*. New York: Atheneum.

Mitchell, L. (1987). *Simple relaxation: The Mitchell method for easing tension* (rev. ed.). London: Murray.

Moss, C. S. (1965). *Hypnosis in perspective*. New York: Macmillan.

Mulholland, T. (1977). Biofeedback as scientific method. In G. E. Schwartz & J. Beatty (Eds.), *Biofeedback: Theory and research*. New York: Academic Press.

Nowlis, D. P., & Kamiya, J. (1970). The control of electroencephalographic alpha rhythms through auditory feedback and the associated mental activity. *Psychophysiology, 6,* 476–484.

Ochs, L. (1992). EEG treatment of addictions. *Biofeedback,* 20(1), 8–16.

Orne, M. T. (1979). The efficacy of biofeedback therapy. *Annual Review of Medicine, 30,* 489–503.

Ornstein, R. E. (1972). *The psychology of consciousness.* San Francisco: Freeman.

Paul, G. L. (1966). *Insight versus desensitization in psychology.* Stanford, CA: Stanford University Press.

Pelletier, K. R., & Garfield, C. (1976). *Consciousness: East and west.* New York: Harper & Row (Harper Colophon Books).

Peniston, E. G., & Kulkosky, P. J. (1989). Alpha–theta brainwave training and endorphin levels of alcoholics. *Alcoholism: Clinical and Experimental Research,* 13(2), 271–279.

Peniston, E. G., & Kulkosky, P. J. (1990). Alcoholic personality and alpha–theta brainwave training. *Medical Psychotherapy, 3,* 37–55.

Pi-Suner, A. (1955). *The whole and its parts in biology.* New York: Philosophical Library.

Progoff, I. (1980). *The practice of process meditation.* New York: Dialogue House Library.

Rosenfeld, J. P. (1992a). "EEG" treatment of addictions: Commentary on Ochs, Peniston, and Kulkosky. *Biofeedback,* 20(2), 12–17.

Rosenfeld, J. P. (1992b). New directions in applied psychophysiology. *Biofeedback and Self-Regulation, 17,* 77–87.

Rosenthal, T. L., & Zimmerman, B. J. (1978). *Social learning and cognition.* New York: Academic Press.

Schwartz, G. E., & Beatty, J. (Eds.). (1977). *Biofeedback: Theory and research.* New York: Academic Press.

Schwartz, G. E., & Weiss, S. M. (1978). What is behavioral medicine? *Psychosomatic Medicine,* 39(6), 377–381.

Schwartz, M. S. (1988). The biofeedback odyssey: Nearing one score and counting (Presidential address). *Biofeedback and Self-Regulation,* 13(1), 1–7.

Schwartz, M. S. (1999a). What is applied psychophysiology?: Toward a definition. *Applied Psychophysiology and Biofeedback, 24,* 3–10.

Schwartz, M. S. (1999b). Responses to comments and closer to a definition of applied psychophysiology? *Applied Psychophysiology and Biofeedback, 24,* 43–54.

Selye, H. (1971). The evolution of the stress concept: Stress and cardiovascular disease. In L. Levi (Ed.), *Society, stress, and disease* (Vol. 1). New York: Oxford University Press.

Selye, H. (1974). *Stress without distress.* Philadelphia: Lippincott.

Selye, H. (1976). *The stress of life* (rev. ed.). New York: McGraw-Hill.

Selye, H. (Ed.). (1983). *Selye's guide to stress research* (Vol. II). New York: Scientific and Academic Editions.

Shealy, C. N. (1977). *Ninety days to self-health.* New York: Dial Press.

Shtark, M. B., & Kall, R. (1998). *Biofeedback-3: Theory and practice.* Novosibirsk, Russia: CERIS.

Shtark, M. B., & Schwartz, M. S. (2002). *Biofeedback-4: Theory and practice.* Novosibirsk, Russia: CERIS.

Silva, J. (1977). *Silva mind control method.* New York: Simon & Schuster.

Smith, J. C. (1989). *Relaxation dynamics.* Champaign, IL: Research Press.

Smith, J. C. (1990). *Cognitive behavioral relaxation training.* New York: Springer.

Smith, O. C. (1934). Action potentials from single motor units in voluntary contraction. *American Journal of Physiology, 108,* 629–638.

Sokhadze, E. M., & Shtark, M. B. (1991). Scientific and clinical biofeedback in the USSR. *Biofeedback and Self-Regulation,* 16(3), 253–260.

Sterman, M. B. (1982). EEG biofeedback in the treatment of epilepsy: An overview circa 1980. In L. W. White & B. Tursky (Eds.), *Clinical biofeedback: Efficacy and mechanisms.* New York: Guilford Press.

Striefel, S. (1998). Creating the future for applied psychophysiology and biofeedback: From fantasy to reality. *Applied Psychophysiology and Biofeedback, 23,* 93–106.

Stroebel, C. (1982). *The quieting reflex.* New York: Putnam.

Tarlar-Benlolo, L. (1978). The role of relaxation in biofeedback training: A critical review of the literature. *Psychological Bulletin, 85,* 727–755.

Tart, C. T. (Ed.). (1969). *Altered states of consciousness: A book of readings.* New York: Wiley.

Ullmann, L., & Krasner, L. (Eds.). (1965). *Case studies in behavior modification.* New York: Holt, Rinehart, & Winston.

Wickramasekera, I. E. (Ed.). (1976). *Biofeedback, behavior therapy and hypnosis: Potentiating the verbal control of behavior for clinicians.* Chicago: Nelson Hall.

Wickramasekera, I. E. (1988). *Clinical behavioral medicine: Some concepts and procedures.* New York: Plenum Press.

Wolf, S. L., & Binder-MacLeod, S. A. (1983). Electromyographic biofeedback in the physical therapy clinic. In J. V. Basmajian (Ed.), *Biofeedback: Principles and practice for clinicians* (2nd ed.). Baltimore: Williams & Wilkins.

Wolpe, J. (1973). *The practice of behavior therapy* (2nd ed.). New York: Pergamon Press.

Wuttke, M. (1992). Addiction, awakening, and EEG biofeedback. *Biofeedback,* 20(2), 18–22.

CHAPTER 2

Entering the Field and Assuring Competence

MARK S. SCHWARTZ
DOIL D. MONTGOMERY

Biofeedback and applied psychophysiology constitute a multidisciplinary and heterogeneous field of many professional disciplines and types of applications. Educational and training opportunities in the field range from courses at universities and individual workshops to comprehensive biofeedback training programs. The Biofeedback Certification Institute of America (BCIA) provides accreditation for the biofeedback programs that are independent of universities. For many, the sources of education are the annual meetings and workshops of the Association for Applied Psychophysiology and Biofeedback (AAPB) and the Society for Neuronal Regulation; workshops sponsored by state and regional societies; and private training programs that offer multiday programs.

GENERAL SUGGESTIONS FOR ENTERING AND MAINTAINING COMPETENCE

The development and maintenance of clinical competence require active participation in a variety of educational and training experiences. Responsible professionals seek continuing education and training. Supervisors and others involved with the education and training of professionals in their setting have the responsibility to support attendance at educational and training programs. Professionals providing clinical services also have a responsibility to request time and financial support to attend these programs. The following general suggestions are made, without any order or preference, as ways to obtain and maintain competence. We urge you, our readers, to consider them seriously and to try as many as are feasible.

　　1. Enroll in carefully selected workshops, private programs, and academic courses. Ask sponsors and presenters for the names of those who have attended in the past, and talk to them.
　　2. Read recommended books, journal articles, manuals, AAPB publications, and patient education booklets. Consider the BCIA references as a resource. Furthermore, listen to audiotapes, such as those from national meetings.

3. When feasible, visit with credible professionals to discuss and observe their clinical approaches. These opportunities are very limited.

4. Study the BCIA Blueprint Knowledge Statements, and prepare for and attain BCIA certification.

5. Regularly read the principal journal in this field, *Applied Psychophysiology and Biofeedback*, and other journals that publish pertinent articles. Subscribe to abstracting services.

6. Attend the annual meetings of the AAPB. These meetings are the best chance to attend a wide variety of symposia, panels, and workshops. They also present an excellent chance to talk with professionals in this field. These meetings are high in caliber and attended by many clinicians and researchers who are interesting, competent, academically sound, and especially sociable. The address for the AAPB office is 10020 West 44th Ave., Suite 304, Wheat Ridge, CO 80033; (303) 422-2615; fax (303) 422-8894. The Web site is http://www.aapb.org.

7. Become involved in a state or regional biofeedback society.

8. Contact credible professionals who have experience. Ask their advice about treatment of selected patients.

9. Invite highly credible and experienced professionals who are good therapists, educators, and/or researchers to your professional setting. Institutions or other groups of professionals can cooperate to absorb the costs.

10. Beginners should usually limit the number of biofeedback modalities used. Consider starting with surface electromyographic (EMG) and skin temperature feedback. Trying to learn and use several modalities often unduly complicates assessment and therapy sessions.

11. Be familiar with a few instrumentation manufacturers before purchasing instruments and discuss instrumentation with professionals experienced with different manufacturers and models. The AAPB annual meetings and some state and regional meetings usually provide such exposure to new equipment. A number of independent distributors sell instruments from several manufacturers. Shop around and get good advice about what will ideally meet your setting's particular needs and be most cost-effective. Avoid getting more instruments than needed for your setting; on the other hand, avoid getting less than is needed.

12. EMG instrumentation that allows multiple simultaneous recording sites often enhances evaluation and therapy.

13. Locate a competent biomedical engineer and familiarize him or her with existing instruments. A competent local engineer can reduce time lost in sending instruments away for needless checking.

14. Consider initially limiting the number of disorders for which to offer services. It is logical to choose among disorders that are more prevalent and those for which the research on biofeedback's effectiveness is more supportive. Consider those disorders that are of the most interest to you and that are likely to generate referrals.

15. Be prepared and willing to accept patients with difficult problems, to invest more time with these patients, and to adjust therapeutic goals accordingly. Even some improvement can be very satisfying to such patients and to the referral source. Referral sources will probably appreciate a practitioner's willingness to accept such patients.

16. Review sample assessment and therapy protocols from highly credible and experienced professionals. Standardized assessment and therapy protocols have a place in some practices. However, it is equally true that successful and cost-efficient services benefit from tailoring assessment and treatment to individual patients. Practitioners can always alter the protocols of other therapists to fit their own needs, preferences, and situations. Again, isolation breeds limited competence.

17. Review the patient education documents and presentations of others.

18. Make every effort to see that supervised therapists attain certification by the BCIA or are seriously working toward certification.

19. Those who are supervising others and those who are being supervised should maintain close and frequent communications about patients and services. Supervision varies with circumstances, such as competence, type, and complexity of patients, and specific responsibilities or job functions. Some therapists who practice biofeedback are supervised by professionals with little or no biofeedback expertise. Some well-meaning professionals do not know what they do not know.

Competent use of biofeedback obviously requires an understanding of the symptoms and disorders treated. Interpretation of psychophysiological and clinical data must be proper and responsible. Clear, accurate, and responsible interprofessional communications must be provided. Proper interpretation of publications is yet another part of competent practice. All this is a lot to expect from many biofeedback therapists, so proper supervision by qualified professionals is often necessary to guarantee all of it. Furthermore, none of us should avoid self-scrutiny and reappraisal. All of us must be willing to update and change our practices.

20. Supervisory professionals with expertise in biofeedback should usually provide at least some sessions with biofeedback and other applied psychophysiological therapies. There is no substitute for this type of direct experience, at least periodically. Prudent supervising professionals avoid allowing too much distance from patients. One exception occurs when the person providing therapy with limited supervision is clearly highly qualified, competent, and highly experienced.

EDUCATION AND TRAINING PROGRAMS

Selecting courses, workshops, and training programs is often difficult. One source of information about training programs is the BCIA Didactic Education Accreditation Program, which was established in January 1990. Contact the BCIA for accreditation criteria, and the names and addresses of accredited educational and training programs. The phone number for the BCIA is 303-420-2902. The Web site is http:www.bcia.org. If you are considering educational and training programs without BCIA accreditation, the following steps are essential:

1. Consider the presenter's reputation as a clinical practitioner.

2. Consider the presenter's experience. This includes number of years using biofeedback and other applied psychophysiological therapies, number of patients treated, and percentage of time devoted to using biofeedback and other applied psychophysiological therapies.

3. Select a program sponsored or accredited by a credible organization, such as the American Psychological Association or your state professional agency.

4. Consider the presenter's qualifications and experience to teach about the specific topic, as well as the number of workshops, courses, and other presentations provided by the presenter.

5. Consider comments by previous recipients of the specific education and training program.

6. Check the time available for the topics listed in the program. A minimum of 1 hour is often necessary to cover even very specific topics. Half-day and full-day workshops are often necessary for covering topics thoroughly. It is desirable for presenters to know the needs and preferences of enrollees a few weeks ahead of time.

7. Ask about the meaning of the term "hands-on experience." Will the presenter observe enrollees preparing a subject, attaching electrodes and thermistors, adjusting the instruments, and providing a few minutes of physiological monitoring and biofeedback? If you only need or want to observe and briefly become familiar with an instrument, then you do not need much hands-on experience. However, if you need or want to learn more about using the

instruments in assessment and therapy, then more time with the instruments is preferable and necessary.

8. Be sure that the presenter clearly specifies specific goals.

9. Verify which instrumentation will be available for demonstration or use.

10. Ask about time for audience questions and discussion.

11. Consider the cost–benefit ratio of attending. Very experienced and talented professionals deserve and have the right to expect reasonable compensation for their educational services. Promotional materials, space, administrative factors, transportation for the presenter, and daily expenses are all expensive items. It is also necessary to consider preparation time, even if the presenter has presented the same or similar content before. Most workshop presenters are usually underpaid and rarely overly compensated.

12. Check whether the instructor has BCIA certification. This is not necessary; however, it is one piece of useful information about the presenter's broader knowledge and skills, and involvement in the field.

13. Some manufactures offer training on their equipment. Check with the manufacture of your equipment, and then ascertain the qualifications of the presenters in your area of interest for applications.

University-based educational opportunities are available at various regionally accredited universities and colleges, at both the undergraduate and graduate levels. Examples of such institutions and their opportunities are as follows:

• Truman State University in Kirksville, Missouri, offers an undergraduate course titled Applied Psychophysiology that can be a part of the bachelor's degree in psychology.

• The University of Texas in Austin, Texas, offers master's-level and doctoral-level training (a few bachelor's-level students are also allowed to enroll each year) in general biofeedback and electroencephalographic (EEG) biofeedback. It also offers supervised clinical supervision in both areas.

• The California School of Professional Psychology in San Diego, California, also offers a master's degree in clinical psychophysiology and biofeedback.

• Nova Southeastern University in Fort Lauderdale, Florida, offers a graduate-level semester course in clinical biofeedback and a year-long clinical practicum.

Since the AAPB has recently approved a model curriculum master's degree program in applied psychophysiology and biofeedback, it is anticipated that training at this level will be offered at other academic institutions in the future.

CERTIFICATION OF BIOFEEDBACK PROFESSIONALS

Rationale

The primary reason for certification is to provide the public with some assurance that a provider has met the fundamental training and experience to provide biofeedback services. The BCIA was established to set minimal standards for service providers, because providers have varied training histories in different professions, and no one profession has identified specific training and experience for providers.

Attaining BCIA certification has several advantages for providers of biofeedback services (these include researchers, practitioners, and presenters of biofeedback educational and training programs). Certification is valuable for both supervised and supervisory professionals. There are competent practitioners without certification; certification is not a guarantee of competence, and it was never intended to guarantee a full range of competencies. However, certification provides a useful index of fundamental knowledge and basic instrumentation proficiency.

Reasons vary for avoiding certification. Sometimes professionals with excellent credentials and extensive experience do have a philosophical or economic basis for the avoidance. For example, some such professionals oppose any certification for themselves and others, and some say they cannot financially afford it. In other cases, the avoidance serves to evade examination anxiety. Some practitioners harbor doubts about their competence to practice in this field. However, for many responsible professionals, these are not sufficient justifications to avoid the process. There are several compelling reasons why most practitioners using biofeedback should seriously consider attaining and maintaining BCIA certification:

1. Certification reflects involvement in this field and increases professional credibility.
2. It attests that the certified individual meets specified criteria to use biofeedback.
3. It increases "market value" and mobility for many.
4. It gives employers a credible index of competence.
5. Some reimbursement systems view the BCIA credential as an important criterion for reimbursement.
6. A credible certification program is a cornerstone and important sign of the maturation of the field. It improves the image of biofeedback to health care professionals, referral sources, and others outside the field. We should not undervalue the importance of this.
7. Preparing for and maintaining certification involve considerable studying and learning—a benefit for applicants, certificants, and patients.

The History of the Certification Program

There is only one established national certification program, the BCIA, which was established in 1981. A brief history of the beginning of the BCIA and the establishment of its credential process is presented for those interested in aspects of this professional credential process.

The National Commission for Health Certifying Agencies (NCHCA) was started in 1977, with strong recommendations from and initial financial support from the federal government. Its mission was to provide "certification of certifying agencies." The NCHCA required such agencies to fulfill extensive, demanding, and challenging criteria. To the credit of the early BCIA board, it achieved full membership in 1983. The BCIA later dropped its membership in the NCHCA because of the weakened state of the NCHCA. As a small certifying agency, BCIA had concerns about investing thousands of dollars in a weak and uncertain NCHCA.

The weakening of the NCHCA occurred for at least two major reasons. First, the criteria for membership were stringent and extensive. It allowed up to 5 years for fulfillment of all the criteria, but many organizations striving for certification could not or would not do what was necessary. Second, the NCHCA had a dynamic and highly competent executive director who was very successful in obtaining financial support for projects and keeping the organization together; however, a tragic car accident changed all that. Nevertheless, the NCHCA deserves our thanks for establishing both a vision and admirable criteria. It was very helpful to the early credibility and success of the BCIA.

There are lessons to be learned from the NCHCA experience. First, a certifying agency should avoid credential criteria so extensive and strict that many potential applicants cannot fulfill them in the time frame required. Second, such an agency should apply the basic learning principles of successive approximation or shaping, and use small steps over a long enough time to allow participants to learn, change, and maintain their gains. Third, no organization should rely on a single leader; accidents happen. Finally, leaders should make every possible effort to acquire and wisely invest enough money to sustain an organization over at least 2 years of hard times. However, they must be realistic about the fees for members and certificants. Is anyone listening?

Aspects of Certification

The BCIA now offers both general biofeedback certification and certification in the specialty area of EEG biofeedback.

In the general area, the requirements include an earned degree in a health-care-related field, a course in anatomy and physiology, didactic training in a core curriculum, supervised self-regulation training, supervised clinical biofeedback experience (which includes experience with EMG and thermal modalities), and biofeedback case conferences. The applicant must also successfully complete an examination on the materials covered in the Blueprint Knowledge Statements.

The BCIA's Blueprint Knowledge Statements provide a detailed outline of knowledge needed to enter the biofeedback field and prepare for the examinations. The BCIA completed a revision of the original 1981 Blueprint Knowledge Statements in 1990, and again in 1999.

Certification for EEG biofeedback became an official part of the BCIA's offerings in 1997. There are corresponding training and experience requirements, and a detailed set of Blueprint Knowledge Statements for this certification. Contact the BCIA for the requirements and the detailed Blueprint Knowledge Statements.

Briefly, the Blueprint Knowledge Statement areas for general certification include the following:

    I. Introduction (including definitions, history, learning principles)
   II. Preparation for Clinical Interventions (e.g., intake tasks, psychophysiological profiling, ongoing assessment)
  III. Neuromuscular Interventions—General
  IV. Neuromuscular Interventions—Specific
   V. Central Nervous System Interventions—General
  VI. Autonomic Nervous System Interventions—General
 VII. Autonomic Nervous System Interventions—Specific
VIII. Biofeedback and Distress
  IX. Instrumentation
   X. Adjunctive Therapeutic Interventions
  XI. Professional Conduct

Briefly, the Blueprint Knowledge Statement areas for the EEG certification are as follows:

    I. Introduction to EEG Biofeedback
   II. Research
  III. Basic Neurophysiology and Neuroanatomy
  IV. EEG and Electrophysiology
   V. Instrumentation
  VI. Psychopharmacology Considerations
 VII. Treatment Planning
VIII. Other Therapeutic Techniques
  IX. Professional Conduct

The certification process acts to deter the least competent practitioners and is an incentive for increasing competence. It is an objective and acceptable criterion for would-be practitioners to assess their entry-level competence.

SUMMARY

This chapter provides ideas and suggestions for persons entering the biofeedback field. For those already in the field, these ideas and suggestions may help them maintain and enhance their competence. Biofeedback is a broad, heterogeneous, and complex field. Practitioners need infusions of new knowledge, ideas, and skills. Deciding when and where these infusions are to take place, and determining who is to provide them, are not always easy. In this chapter, we have offered some guidance.

The AAPB and the BCIA continue to be the national resources and centers for continued maturation of the field. Those who are not presently members of the AAPB should join or rejoin. Those who are not certified by the BCIA should consider this credential for themselves. Those currently certified should continue to stay certified. Those who were certified in the past but are not currently certified should return.

Definitions[1] of Biofeedback and Applied Psychophysiology

NANCY M. SCHWARTZ
MARK S. SCHWARTZ

HISTORICAL REVIEW OF DEFINITIONS

The history of biofeedback has witnessed many definitions. Olson (1987, 1995) noted 10 definitions starting from 1971 (Basmajian, 1979; Birk, 1973; Brown, 1977; Gaarder & Montgomery, 1977; Green & Green, 1977; Hassett, 1978; Kamiya, 1971; Ray, Raczynski, Rogers, & Kimball, 1979; G. E. Schwartz & Beatty, 1977; M. S. Schwartz & Fehmi, 1982). Olson (1995) divided those definitions into "operational" definitions (emphasizing the processes or procedures involved), "teleological" definitions (stressing the aims or objectives of biofeedback), and "combined" definitions (synthesizing elements of both). Olson (1995) noted that the theoretical models influencing past definitions differed in emphasis.

Different opinions exist about whether or not the specific feedback signals as such result in changes. However, even the critics of biofeedback agree that many of the feedback procedures are part of something that works. The disagreement focuses on the ingredients and process that result in changed outcomes.

The debate between Furedy (1987) and Shellenberger and Green (1987) was an invigorating exchange. Attempts to moderate and create perspective were valuable and appreciated by many (Rosenfeld, 1987). Practitioners, students, and critics of biofeedback should be familiar with these issues and the references.

In writing this chapter, we have also derived guidance from Middaugh (1990), who focused on patient selection, treatment protocol selection, instrumentation, and patient–therapist interactions, in combination with other techniques. This fits well with the aptitude × treatment interaction (ATI) model (Holloway & Rogers, 1988; Dance & Neufeld, 1988) of therapy effectiveness. This interaction of the person and treatment often accounts for the outcome. It is similar to the still vibrant idea from Paul (1966): Briefly, treatments work for selected patients in selected conditions.

ASSUMPTIONS

Many assumptions form a background for the discussion that follows. We divide the assumptions into three groups headed "Biofeedback," "Patient Education," and "Integration."

Biofeedback

• Many patients improve significantly during and after exposure to biofeedback and the therapy context in which it is a part. This is true for many disorders.
• Many patients do not improve with biofeedback treatment packages.
• Similar studies and procedures in different settings lead to different results.
• Similar procedures, delivered by the same therapist in the same study or office, lead to different results among different patients or subjects.
• The same treatment delivered by different professionals to the same type of patient, and in a similar manner, often yields different results.

Patient Education

• Patients, especially those with medical disorders, are often skeptical about therapies perceived as psychological.
• Patients forget most of what they hear.
• Patients often do not understand patient education information.
• The quality and clarity of communications vary across patients and professionals.
• Expectations affect satisfaction, compliance, mood, motivation, arousal, attention and concentration, and therefore outcome.
• Patient education and knowledge affect expectations, satisfaction, and compliance.

Integration

• Practitioners differ widely in education, training, interpersonal skills, instruments used, knowledge of and skills with the instruments, and choices of theoretical models.
• Most professionals agree that biofeedback, like other treatments, contains many different elements. They also assume that for many applications of biofeedback, one needs multiple elements. The relationship between the elements is probably synergistic. In gestalt terms, "the whole is greater than the sum of its parts."
• Most professionals further assume that some elements or factors are more important than others in some applications and with some patients. For example, in some cases the feedback signal is more important for the physiological information it conveys to the patient. In other situations, its value is the information it provides for the therapist. In still others, the signal helps shape or reinforces cognitive changes that result in symptom changes.

A PATIENT EDUCATION MODEL: SEVEN LEVELS OR FACETS OF INFORMATION ABOUT BIOFEEDBACK

Our model proposes that patient education is an active ingredient of biofeedback, regardless of the discipline within which one uses it. In physical therapy, a patient can find it helpful to see a small change in muscle activity before the patient can feel it. In turn, this information can help the patient generate the physiological change required to show a larger change in the feedback signal. Thus the therapist can vary the range displayed. This is comparable to using a microscope with different powers of magnification: One sees smaller changes with higher magnification. Computer-based instruments expand the choices for presenting feedback signals. Feedback choices are extensive.

Signal Presentation

The first challenge for the therapist is to choose signal displays that convey necessary and sufficient information to help the patient meet his or her session and therapy goals, without presenting distracting or anxiety-producing signal information.

By definition, the signal should have some reinforcing properties. Therapists should be familiar with the instruments and with patients' needs and limitations. This facilitates selection of the signals and displays that help ease patients' information processing. For example, if the range is too large in biofeedback, initial tiny changes in the desired direction go undetected. If a patient is primarily a visual learner, then audio feedback with eyes closed is not the ideal choice. Therapists will enhance patient education by selecting feedback signals and displays that tailor these to each patient's needs and therapy goals. The signal as the basic and lowest level of information is complex. It varies across studies, clinical practitioners, patients, and sessions. By itself, the signal provides limited systematic and reliably useful information.

Explanation of the Signal

The second level of information is the explanation of the signal and display. At this level, the information might be as simple as "the red line is temperature, the blue one is muscle activity, and the green one is perspiration." It is possible for the patient to learn through trial and error how to make changes in the signal and therefore in their physiology. The signal can provide enhanced proprioception at this point and more information than a person is aware of from internal cues.

There has been much discussion about what biofeedback is and whether or not it works. Furedy's (1987) focus was on only our first two levels of information. Shellenberger and Green (1987) suggest that these two levels are not biofeedback. Neither is correct. The first two levels are biofeedback, but they usually do not provide enough information to accomplish desired goals in clinical practice.

Explanation of the Signal in Relation to Physiology

The third information level relates the signal to physiology. Examples of some therapist statements[2] are as follows: "When your hand temperature is above 92°F, you are more relaxed," "If you have the blue line below this dotted blue line, then you are below 2.0 microvolts and you are showing that you can relax that muscle group," and "If you can keep the blue line above 30 microvolts for 10 seconds, you will show that you have increased your strength."

Again, computer-based instruments expand the potential ability to convey information. The ability to freeze the screen allows therapists to review events and discuss the signal in more detail.

All of this is also biofeedback. It is therapist feedback using stop action and/or summarized and visually displayed psychophysiological data. Starting at this level, from a patient education viewpoint, some verbal instruction or education about physiology can enhance a patient's understanding of the signal. This should increase the usefulness of the information provided by the signal.

Explanation of the Signal in Relation to Symptoms

The fourth level requires the therapist to inform the patient about how the signal display relates to the patient's symptoms. A therapist might say,

> "Keeping the blue line down means your muscles are more relaxed. Notice that it only takes you a few moments to reach this level. It took much longer when you started. When you relax your muscles like this often enough, you can have fewer headaches. Relaxing often and quickly throughout the day prevents the excess tension that leads to headaches."

Therapist Suggestions

At the fifth information level, the therapist gives suggestions and coaches the patient to help achieve the desired feedback. Examples are instructions in posture, releasing muscle tension, slow and deep abdominal breathing, visualization, or ways to increase muscle strength. A therapist might say,

> "Allow your arms to feel heavy and relaxed. Visualize relaxing at the beach on a warm, bright day. You are in a comfortable recliner chair. No one is close by. All you hear are the waves lapping at the shore and sea gulls in the distance. You may feel your hands warming."

Suppose that Fred keeps his head shifted forward when he works at his computer and often when he is standing. He also often clenches his teeth while working. All of this increases the tension in the muscles in the back of his neck. A therapist might say to Fred,

> "Change your posture slightly. Keep your head level and shift your head back slightly. Drop your chin slightly. Let your jaw drop slightly. This can reduce the muscle tension in the back of your neck."

Instructions may be to relax very briefly many times a day. Patients should be encouraged to use this information and their internal cues, rather than be dependent on external feedback. A therapist might advise, "Notice how you feel right now. You can reproduce that feeling in your daily life."

Information to the Therapist

The sixth level is the information available to the therapist. Biofeedback instruments allow therapists to improve their ability to assess psychophysiological baselines, reactivity to stress challenges, and recoveries. Therapists can adjust treatment as needed to meet physiological goals. If a patient is attaining these goals, a therapist informs the patient to attend to the body cues and sensations associated with the desired physiological activity.

The therapist may see that one relaxation procedure is not as helpful as another. For example, releasing muscle tension without first tensing the muscle group may be better than tensing the muscles first. One type or style of autogenic-like or self-generating phrases may lower arousal more effectively than other phrases.

Accurately measuring changes in physiology helps these therapies be more scientific. The therapist can see from the feedback what helps and what does not. A therapist might say, "I see that this relaxation procedure is not very helpful for you. There are several others we can try. Let's start with this one."

Informing Patients That They Are Successful

The issue of feedback versus feedforward is also a subject of discussion and disagreement. The seventh information level underscores the feedforward aspect of treatment.

Suppose that Mary has panic disorder and feels that her physiology is out of control. She is learning relaxation skills. With the feedback signals, she sees that she can control her physiology. She feels more confident about her relaxation skills and less threatened when she notices physiological arousal cues. She learns to use the cues to prompt herself to employ self-regulation procedures. The confidence she gains helps her interrupt the negative self-talk that previously made her symptoms worse.

Suppose also that Fred (described above) sees how the changes in posture affect the tension in his neck. He now knows how this affects his neck pain and headaches. He sees that simple adjustments of his posture lower the surface electromyographic (EMG) activity. He could make the adjustments without the feedback. However, the feedback serves to show him the result immediately and reinforces his confidence.

There is also disagreement about whether symptom changes result from changes in physiology or changes in thoughts. Both are probably valid views. Both probably occur to varying degrees in different patients at different times in the therapy process. For example, seeing self-generated changes in physiology helps alter thoughts; it increases thoughts of self-efficacy and decreases cognitions of helplessness. This can help encourage compliance. Knowledge of results is therefore helpful for achieving treatment goals (Salmoni, Schmidt, & Walter, 1984).

EXPLANATIONS, MODELS, AND MODEL BUILDING

The discussion above of information levels in biofeedback is a step in the direction of model building. We now turn to other models. Detailed discussion of the various explanations or models for how biofeedback works is beyond the intent of this chapter and the space allotted. However, mention of these is germane to give perspective. We also borrow ideas and models from other fields. The models are not listed below in any order of preference.

Prior models used in the biofeedback literature include the following:

Model 1. Physiological changes result in symptom changes.
Model 2. Cognitive changes (beliefs and expectations) lead to symptom changes.
Model 3. Placebo/nonspecific effects account for symptom changes.
Model 4. Feedforward processes account for symptom changes.

Other models with relevance for biofeedback are as follows:

Model 5. Bandura's self-efficacy model
Model 6. The patient education model
Model 7. The R. Rosenthal interpersonal expectancy model
Model 8. The Omer and London model
Model 9. The ATI model

Prior Models Used in the Biofeedback Literature

Model 1

Physiological changes result in symptom changes. This is the traditional model. It suggests that making information from the target physiological system available to the patient will allow the patient to gain control. A common example is reducing muscle tension to reduce tension-type headaches. Another example is increasing muscle awareness and tension in pelvic floor muscles to reduce urinary or fecal incontinence. Reducing peripheral vasoconstriction to reduce vasospastic episodes is a third example. Some professionals allow for an important revision of this model, which proposes that the feedback encourages the person to attend more to the specific body area and its functioning. This heightened awareness of sensations and circumstances that precede the symptoms results in developing other voluntary behaviors to manage and reduce the symptoms. Examples include relaxing more often or remembering to tighten sphincters.

Model 2

Cognitive changes (beliefs and expectations) result in symptom changes (Holroyd et al., 1984; Meichenbaum, 1976). This model suggests that the process of biofeedback with its performance feedback and verbal encouragement from a therapist result in cognitive changes. These include positive expectations, perceived success, and reduced anxiety and symptoms associated with a reduced sense of helplessness. These cognitive factors are the mediators and necessary elements in change. The therapeutic value of self-efficacy fits well into this model.

Model 3

Placebo or nonspecific effects account for symptom changes (Furedy, 1987; Roberts, 1985, 1986). Such concepts as expectations, therapist credibility, and the therapist–patient relationship are among the concepts interwoven with, and inseparable from, placebo and nonspecific factors. This overlaps with the cognitive model; however, it attributes the changes to unspecified or miscellaneous factors that are not directly related to the active ingredients in the biofeedback. This explanation is no different from that proposed to explain some other therapies. Although they have received extensive attention for decades, views of placebo and nonspecific factors are now undergoing a major metamorphosis (Critelli & Neumann, 1984; White, Tursky, & Schwartz, 1985; Omer & London, 1989).

Model 4

Feedforward processes account for symptom changes. In this view (Dunn, Gillig, Ponsor, Weil, & Utz, 1986; LaCroix, 1984), the person already can execute a response and uses the feedback signals as confirmation and reinforcement.

Other Models with Relevance for Biofeedback

Model 5

Bandura's self-efficacy model (Bandura, 1997) states that performance and mastery experiences are among the most potent in their effects on efficacy expectations and behavior. In other words, what I do and clearly see that I can do has a more significant impact on my beliefs and behavior than what other people tell me they think I can do.

Model 6

A patient education model encompasses and implies more and different concepts, elements, and processes than other models do, including those involving cognitive and information processing. The elements and emphases include many components within the rubrics of knowledge, communication, patient, professional, memory, patient satisfaction, competing factors, and social support.

Model 7

The R. Rosenthal interpersonal expectancy model focuses on interpersonal expectancy effects and outcome. This research shows that a teacher's expectations about a student change the teacher's affect concerning the student. This results in a partially independent change in the teacher's degree of effort while teaching the student. The belief that a student can learn reinforces the belief that the teacher's efforts are worthwhile. Rosenthal and colleagues (Harris & Rosenthal, 1985; Rosenthal, 1990; Learman, Avorn, Everitt, & Rosenthal, 1990) have extended this model to clinical situations.

Model 8

The Omer and London model represents a metamorphosis of the concepts of placebo and nonspecific effects. "Now . . . nonspecific factors are not noise to be filtered out of 'real' treatment, but are important signal events in it" (Omer & London, 1989, p. 239). These authors conceptualize these factors into four groups: "relationship," "expectancy," "reorganizing," and "impact."

1. Under "relationship," Omer and London include trust, warmth, understanding, and a secure atmosphere for exploration, learning, and change.

2. They emphasize cognitive factors, such as "expectancy" and self-efficacy. Patients' beliefs about their abilities to develop and apply recommended physiological skills and changes affect their success. Health care professionals who believe in a treatment and in the patients' abilities to be successful will probably convey this confidence to the patients.

3. The "reorganizing" element involves health care professionals' trying to help patients dismantle or "unfreeze" dysfunctional patterns. Treatments, such as biofeedback, give patients new views and new logical versions of their problems—new "conceptual schemes of the change process" (Omer & London, 1989, p. 243). This resembles Wickramasekara's (1988) proposal that practitioners using biofeedback shape the cognitions of patients into accepting a new role and a revised perspective with new vocabulary.

4. "Impact" refers to successful treatments' and professionals' ability to "overcome . . . [patients'] . . . tendencies to ignore . . . [a problem or] . . . neglect it, habituate to it, or forget it" (Omer & London, 1989, p. 244).

Model 9

An ATI model adds much to our model building (Holloway, Spivey, Zismer, & Withington, 1988). It permits inclusion of all aptitudes and personal characteristics of patients that might interact with treatments or informational strategies.

This model has the capability to describe better treatments for selected clients (Dance & Neufeld, 1988). One can use this as a framework to subdivide patients on a pertinent attribute. One then assigns patients to different forms of intervention or focuses on certain educational components. Although the ATI model is a single-interaction model, one expects more than one level of interaction. Others include professional variables, competing variables, social support variables, and reinforcers.

Increased information and patient education are common elements in all models. We suggest a conceptualization that includes different levels and types of information received by patients during biofeedback sessions. This discussion acknowledges the contributions of Gary E. Schwartz (1982, 1983), who emphasized the contextual, organistic, multicategory, and multicausal approach to understanding biofeedback. We also borrow from Middaugh's (1990) synthesis. For her, the question is not simply "How does biofeedback work?" Rather, the question is "How does it work for different people and under what circumstances?"

TOWARD A MORE INCLUSIVE DEFINITION OF "BIOFEEDBACK"

Furedy (1987, p. 180) asks whether the information provided by biofeedback is really helpful. If one employs only the first two information levels, it is probable that the limited information provided is not sufficiently helpful. A better question might be "Is all the information provided by the therapist sufficiently helpful?" By Olson's (1995) definition, a competent therapist is an important part of biofeedback therapies. Moreover, computerized biofeedback is like having a high-tech electronic chalkboard for teaching and a built-in ability to measure progress. It is up to the therapist to use this technology to be the best possible teacher and communicator.

In much research, it is difficult to assess whether biofeedback as such was helpful. It often is not clear how many and which information levels or facets the therapists employed. It would be helpful to tease apart these levels or facets. The aim is not to see whether the biofeedback has been useful but which levels or facets of information are most helpful and how we can expand and optimize each. In other words, the question is not "Is the signal helpful?" but "How can we improve upon the information from the signal?"

In essence, biofeedback, used in the broad sense of signals, explanations, and patient education, *provides missing or deficient information in the therapy context. This information is helpful for the patient, the therapist, or the interaction.* One does not evaluate a school book when it is presented to students by itself. Some students have the following:

- Sufficient motivation
- Sufficient capabilities
- No significant interference
- Sufficient times and places to study
- Other resources to use as references
- An experiential background conducive to independent learning
- Confidence in their ability
- A teacher for help if they reach an impasse

Some students thus do well with self-study and never need to go to class. Others need classroom instructions and review of the text. Some of these others need text review paragraph by paragraph, page by page, and chapter by chapter. Some learn it for an average grade. Others seek or need a grade of A. Some never learn it. None of this is news. However, the point is that we do not attribute the problem to the book unless it is written poorly and/or not tailored well to the student.

A comprehensive definition includes statements of both the process and purpose of biofeedback. As a synthesis, the following list includes seven procedural elements (1–7) and three goals (8–10). Thus we propose slight but important additions to Olson's (1995) definition (these additions are given in italics in the list here). As a process, "applied biofeedback" is

1. a group of therapeutic procedures that
2. uses electronic or electromechanical instruments
3. to accurately measure, process, and feed back, to persons *and their therapists,*
4. information with *educational and* reinforcing properties
5. about their neuromuscular and autonomic activity, both normal and abnormal,
6. in the form of analog or binary, auditory, and/or visual feedback signals.
7. Best achieved with a competent biofeedback professional,
8. the objectives are to help persons develop greater awareness *of, confidence in, and an increase in* voluntary control over their physiological processes that are otherwise outside awareness and/or under less voluntary control,
9. by first controlling the external signal,
10. and then by using *cognitions, sensations, or other cues to prevent, stop, or reduce symptoms.*

Here is a discussion of each element of the definition.

1. "a group of therapeutic procedures that": Biofeedback is not one generic therapeutic modality. It can involve different sites, modalities, and procedures. Even when feedback is provided through only one modality, such as EMG, there are many dimensions and steps. These include verbal instructions, focused attention, relaxation procedures, feedback, stress challenges, and motor skill learning.

2. "uses electronic or electromechanical instruments": Most internal physiological systems involve natural feedback mechanisms to maintain homeostatic balance. The body's internal biofeedback or "living feedback" systems have limits and malfunctions that result in impaired functioning and symptoms. Some areas of the body have fewer or less efficient feedback systems. For example, the sensory and motor nerves connecting most head muscles to the brain are fewer in number than the nerves connecting the hands and lips to the brain. Biofeedback therapy does not usually refer to the body's internal biological feedback systems, but, rather, to external electronic or electromechanical feedback systems.

"Biofeedback" does not refer to physiological self-regulation that omits external instrumentation and feedback.

"Applied biofeedback" typically refers to electronic modalities, such as EMG, skin temperature, electrodermal activity or perspiration, heart rate, blood volume, blood pressure, respiration, and electroencephalography. In addition, it can involve the use of electromechanical instruments, such as pressure transducers and goniometers.

3. "to accurately measure, process, and feed back, to persons *and their therapists,*": One unique feature of applied biofeedback is to provide accurate and meaningful physiological information directly to the patient. The signals are fed back to the patient, to enable him or her to assume a greater and different role in treatment than a patient does in other therapies. "The patient is no longer an object of treatment, he is the treatment" (Brown, 1977, p. 13). There is also a shift in the role of the therapist, who sometimes becomes a coach or instructor as well as a therapist.

4. "information with *educational and* reinforcing properties": This phrase integrates the perspectives of both cybernetics and learning theory. The biofeedback signals fed back to a person convey information, and this information often contains reinforcing properties. In a learning theory model, biofeedback is instrumental or operant conditioning of physiological activity, and feedback signals are viewed as positive reinforcers of physiological changes. In a cybernetics model, the information in biofeedback signals completes an external feedback loop. Admittedly, the therapist often needs to explain to the patient the meaning of the information, and thus the information becomes educational as well. From a behavioral perspec-

tive, the person learns to self-regulate his or her physiological processes with the help of feedback information. Feedback information reinforces, facilitates, augments, and encourages physiological and cognitive learning.

The term "feedback" comes from the mathematician Norbert Weiner, who defined it as "a method of controlling the system by reinserting the results of its past performance" (quoted in Birk, 1973, p. 3). The physiological information fed back can be with or without awareness. In either case, it is information that is fed back.

5. "about their neuromuscular and autonomic activity, both normal and abnormal,": The somatic processes recorded are both neuromuscular and visceral activities, innervated by either the central or the autonomic nervous system or both.

6. "in the form of analog or binary, auditory, and/or visual feedback signals,": Feedback may be visual and/or auditory, and sometimes kinesthetic. Visual feedback may be continuous (analog), as in a numerical meter or on a computer display. It may be discrete (discontinuous), as in a sound that can be turned on or off by changing the level of one's physiological activity. One can present both continuous and discrete signals graphically on computer-generated displays.

7. "Best achieved with a competent biofeedback professional,": For example, a person does not usually learn to reduce respiration rate and make it smooth, effortless, and diaphragmatic by simply listening to or watching feedback signals. Attachment to biofeedback instruments without proper cognitive preparation, instructions, and guidance is not appropriate biofeedback therapy.

Some professionals consider biofeedback as a form of education (see item 4 above). For many applications, it is psychophysiological education. As with all education, the results are partly the result of the teacher's skills, personality, and attention to the student. Other professionals consider biofeedback as therapy. As with all forms of therapy, the therapist's skills, personality, and attention to the patient affect the outcome. The important point is that the professional conducting biofeedback therapy sessions is an integral part of the intervention.

8. "the objectives are to help persons develop greater awareness *of, confidence in, and an increase in* voluntary control over their physiological processes that are otherwise outside awareness and/or under less voluntary control,": A basic premise of the biofeedback field is that a person can develop or enhance significant self-regulation for any accurately measured physiological process or activity. One reason for skepticism about biofeedback is the belief that many of the body's systems function without awareness and involuntarily. This is only a partial truth. Humans are much more capable of developing physiological self-regulation than has been previously believed.

It is no longer tenable to assert that humans have little or no capacity for some self-regulation of organs and functions mediated by the autonomic nervous system. Neither can one assume this for muscles and nerves malfunctioning because of injury or disease. However, neither is it tenable to argue that there are no limits to the degree of physiological self-regulation. There clearly are such limits, but those limits are less than once believed. Biofeedback is neither a placebo nor a panacea.

9. "by first controlling the external signal,": The finite sensory feedback and control systems of humans limit the development of physiological self-regulation. For example, most persons are unaware of changes in muscle activity corresponding to a few or several microvolts. Most are unaware of blood pressure changes of a few to several millimeters of mercury, or of changes in the electrical activity of the brain. Minute changes in skin temperature or sweat gland activity are too small for awareness. Biofeedback instruments detect minute changes in bioelectrical activity that human sensory systems cannot detect or are not detecting. Theoretically, the person first learns to control the external signal, and then develops more control over his or her physiological processes.

10. "and then by using *cognitions, sensations, or other cues to prevent, stop, or reduce symptoms.*" The final goal is for persons to maintain physiological self-regulation without feedback from external instruments. People learn to apply self-regulation in their daily lives by learning to identify undesirable internal cues, cognitions, or sensations and reproducing those desired and associated with physiological changes learned and reinforced with external feedback. An effective biofeedback program includes methods to help people transfer and generalize the acquired self-regulation responses.

A PROPOSED DEFINITION OF "APPLIED PSYCHOPHYSIOLOGY"

Our discussion now turns to the definition of "applied psychophysiology," as this term is more recent than, much broader than, and subsumes "biofeedback." A series of papers in 1999 (Vol. 24, pp. 1–54) in the journal *Applied Psychophysiology and Biofeedback* involved the initial steps in the direction of developing such a definition, including critiques, responses, and modifications. In the first paper, M. S. Schwartz (1999a) discussed the background of the debate (see M. S. Schwartz & Olson, Chapter 1, this volume, for a summary of this discussion). Briefly, the Publication Committee of the Association for Applied Psychophysiology and Biofeedback (AAPB) asked Schwartz (1999b, p. 43) to initiate a process for developing a definition "for use by the AAPB and the journal of the organization." This chapter presents the revised proposed definition. Amendments and modifications were expected. The published discussions of the key elements, examples of topics included and excluded, rationale for these choices, critiques, and responses are best read in their originals. At present, there is still no formal and agreed-upon definition of "applied psychophysiology"—only the proposed operational definition (Schwartz, 1999b). Here is the proposed definition as given by Schwartz (1999b, p. 54):

> Applied psychophysiology reflects an evolving scientific discipline and specialty involving understanding and modifying the relationship between behavior and physiological functions by a variety of methods including noninvasive physiological measures. The term "applied psychophysiology" is a rubric encompassing evaluation, diagnosis, education, treatment, and performance enhancement.
>
> Applied psychophysiology includes a group of interventions and evaluation methods with the exclusive or primary intentions of understanding and effecting changes that help humans move toward and maintain healthier psychophysiological functioning. [Applied psychophysiology] involves helping people change physiological functioning and psychological functioning (measured, theoretical, and potential) and/or to achieve sensorimotor integration and motor learning within physical rehabilitation.
>
> The group of interventions use all forms of biofeedback, relaxation methods, breathing methods, cognitive behavioral therapies, patient/client education, behavioral changes, hypnosis, meditative techniques, and imagery techniques [some commentators would add: *when directed at changing physiological functioning*]. In some situations, dietary and other biochemical (nonmedication) changes and some truth detection research and applications may be considered under the rubric of applied psychophysiology.
>
> Evaluation methods use all forms of physiological measurements. The physiological functioning includes but is not limited to accurately measured changes in skeletal muscles, all autonomic physiology, breathing measures, biochemistry, electroencephalographic activity, both normal and abnormal and imaging techniques. Autonomic measures include electrodermal, skin temperature, blood pressure, heart rate, gastrointestinal motility, and vasomotor.
>
> The interventions need to be part of or have implications for applications to humans. These could, but do not need to, involve the raw procedures and/or symptoms of medical and psychophysiological disorders.

NOTES

1. The original chapter on definitions that appeared in the first edition, and one of the two chapters on this topic in the second edition, were by R. Paul Olson. Those chapters are still wonderful and excellent historical pieces for readers interested in historical origins of the term "biofeedback." We will always be indebted to and appreciative of Dr. Olson's many contributions to prior editions, and to him personally.

2. The therapist statements in this and the following sections are provided only for illustrative purposes.

REFERENCES

Bandura, A. (1997). *Self-efficacy: The exercise of control*. New York: Freeman.

Basmajian, J. V. (Ed.). (1979). *Biofeedback: Principles and practice for clinicians*. Baltimore: Williams & Wilkins.

Birk, L. (Ed.). (1973). *Biofeedback: Behavioral medicine*. New York: Grune & Stratton.

Brown, B. (1977). *Stress and the art of biofeedback*. New York: Harper & Row.

Critelli, J. W., & Neumann, K. F. (1984). The placebo: Conceptual analysis of a construct in transition. *American Psychologist*, 39(1), 32–39.

Dance, K. A., & Neufeld, R. W. (1988). Aptitude–treatment interaction research in the clinical setting: A review of attempts to dispel the "patient uniformity" myth. *Psychological Bulletin*, 104(2), 192–213.

Dunn, T. G., Gillig, S. E, Ponser, S. E., Weil, N., & Utz, S. W. (1986). The learning process in biofeedback: Is it feed-forward or feedback? *Biofeedback and Self-Regulation*, 11(2), 143–156.

Furedy, J. J. (1987). Specific versus placebo effects in biofeedback training: A critical lay perspective. *Biofeedback and Self-Regulation*, 12, 169–184.

Gaarder, K. R., & Montgomery, P. S. (1977). *Clinical biofeedback: A procedural manual for behavioral medicine*. Baltimore: Williams & Wilkins.

Green, E., & Green, A. (1977). *Beyond biofeedback*. New York: Delta.

Harris, M. J., & Rosenthal, R. (1985). Mediation of interpersonal expectancy effects: Thirty-one meta-analyses. *Psychological Bulletin*, 97, 363–386.

Hassett, J. (1978). *A primer of psychophysiology*. San Francisco: Freeman.

Holloway, R. L., & Rogers, J. C. (1988). Aptitude × treatment interactions in family medicine research. *Family Medicine*, 21(5), 374–378.

Holloway, R. L., Spivey, R. N., Zismer, D. K., & Withington, A. M. (1988). Aptitude × treatment interactions: Implications for patient education research. *Health Education Quarterly*, 15(3), 241–257.

Holroyd, K. A., Penzien, D. B., Hursey, K. G., Tobin, D. L., Rogers, L., Holm, J. E., Marcille, P. J., Hall, J. R., & Chila, A. G. (1984). Change mechanisms in EMG biofeedback training: Cognitive changes underlying improvements in tension headache. *Journal of Consulting and Clinical Psychology*, 52(6), 1039–1053.

Kamiya, J. (1971). Preface. In T. Barber, L. DiCara, J. Kamiya, N. Miller, D. Shapiro, & J. Stoyva (Eds.), *Biofeedback and self-control*. Chicago: Aldine-Atherton.

LaCroix, J. M. (1984). *Mechanisms of biofeedback control: On the importance of verbal (conscious) processing*. *Psychophysiology*, 18, 573–587.

Learman, L. A., Avorn, J., Everitt, D. E., & Rosenthal, R. (1990). Pygmalion in the nursing home: The effects of caregiver expectations on patient outcomes. *Journal of the American Geriatric Society*, 38(7), 797–803.

Meichenbaum, D. (1976). Cognitive factors in biofeedback therapy. *Biofeedback and Self-Regulation*, 1, 201–216.

Middaugh, S. J. (1990). On clinical efficacy: Why biofeedback does—and does not—work (Presidential address). *Biofeedback and Self-Regulation*, 15(3), 191–208.

Olson, R. P. (1987). Definitions of biofeedback. In M. S. Schwartz (Ed.), *Biofeedback: A practitioner's guide*. New York: Guilford Press.

Olson, R. P. (1995). Definitions of biofeedback and applied psychophysiology. In M. S. Schwartz & Associates, *Biofeedback: A practitioner's guide* (2nd ed.). New York: Guilford Press.

Omer, H., & London, P. (1989). Signal and noise in psychotherapy: The role and control of non-specific factors. *British Journal of Psychiatry*, 155, 239–245.

Paul, G. L. (1966). *Insight versus desensitization in psychotherapy*. Stanford, CA: Stanford University Press.

Ray, W. J., Raczynski, J. M., Rogers, T., & Kimball, W. H. (1979). *Evaluation of clinical biofeedback*. New York: Plenum Press.

Roberts, A. H. (1985). Biofeedback. *American Psychologist*, 40, 938–941.

Roberts, A. H. (1986). Biofeedback, science, and training. *American Psychologist*, 41, 1010.

Rosenfeld, J. P. (1987). Can clinical biofeedback be scientifically validated?: A follow-up on the Green–Shellenberger–Furedy–Roberts debates. *Biofeedback and Self-Regulation*, 12(3), 217–222.

Rosenthal, R. (1990). *Experimenter expectancy, covert communication, and meta-analytic methods* (Donald T. Campbell Award presentation, American Psychological Association Meeting, August 14, 1989). (ERIC Document Reproduction Service No. TMO 14556, 317551)

Salmoni, A. W., Schmidt, R. A., & Walter, C. B. (1984). Knowledge of results and motor learning: Area view and critical reappraisal. *Psychological Bulletin, 95*(3), 355–386.

Schwartz, G. E. (1982). Testing the biopsychosocial model: The ultimate challenge hcing behavioral medicine? *Journal of Consulting and Clinical Psychology, 50*(6), 1040–1053.

Schwartz, G. E. (1983). Social psychophysiology and behavioral medicine: A systems perspective. In J. T. Cacioppo & R. E. Petty (Eds.), *Social psychophysiology: A sourcebook*. New York: Guilford Press.

Schwartz, G. E., & Beatty, J. (1977). *Biofeedback: Theory and research* New York: Academic Press.

Schwartz, M. S. (1999a). What is applied psychophysiology?: Toward a definition. *Applied Psychophysiology and Biofeedback, 24*, 3–10.

Schwartz, M. S. (1999b). Responses to comments and closer to a definition of applied psychophysiology. *Applied Psychophysiology and Biofeedback, 24*, 43–54.

Schwartz, M. S., & Fehmi, L. (1982). *Applications standards and guidelines for providers of biofeedback services*. Wheat Ridge, CO: Biofeedback Society of America.

Shellenberger, R., & Green, J. (1987). Specific effects and biofeedback versus biofeedback-assisted self-regulation training. *Biofeedback and Self-Regulation, 12*(3), 185–209.

White, L., Tursky, B., & Schwartz, G. E. (1985). Proposed synthesis of placebo models. In L. White, B. Tursky, & G. E. Schwartz (Eds.), *Placebo: Theory, research, and mechanisms*. New York: Guilford Press.

Wickramasekara, I. E. (1988). *Clinical behavioral medicine: Some concepts and procedures*. New York: Plenum Press.

PART II

Instrumentation

CHAPTER 4

A Primer of Biofeedback Instrumentation

CHARLES J. PEEK

MONITORING PSYCHOPHYSIOLOGICAL AROUSAL: THE CENTRAL FOCUS OF BIOFEEDBACK

A major application for biofeedback is to provide tools for detecting and managing psychophysiological arousal. As health care fields matured, it became clear by the early 1970s that frequent, excessive, and sustained psychophysiological tension and overarousal cause or exacerbate many health problems. Interest in detecting and managing these states intensified. By the same time, improved biomedical electronics had made it practical to monitor previously invisible physiological processes associated with overarousal.

The natural combination of these developments in health and technology found expression in the new field of biofeedback, in which the languages and concepts of psychology, physiology, and electronics freely intermingle. The terms "stress," "anticipation," "autonomic arousal," and "muscle fibers" are found in the same sentences as "electromyography" (EMG), "microvolts," "bandwidths," and "filters." Such hybrid sentences usually contain at least some mystery to those (i.e., most of us) who are not fluent in all these languages. Probably the greatest mystery among biofeedback devotees and beginners is in the language of electronics. Of the three languages spoken in biofeedback, this is the least similar to ordinary language.

This chapter aims to put into ordinary language basic technical matters of practical importance in biofeedback. Technical concepts are introduced through analogy or heuristic description, such that they can become a usable part of the reader's biofeedback language. This chapter contains many judgments on the practical importance of things encountered in biofeedback, and to that extent represents my own views on the subject, especially in matters where no definitive conceptual, empirical, or practical view holds sway in the field.

This chapter is focused on basic electronic and measurement concepts for EMG, temperature, and electrodermal biofeedback. (Electroencephalographic biofeedback is covered by Neumann, Strehl, & Birbaumer in Chapter 5 of this volume.) It is focused on the "front end," where electrodes, basic electronics, and feedback modes interact with clinicians and clients. Other chapters address the "back end," where computers and myriad forms of feedback and data recording are devised for clinical biofeedback or research. Although computerized biofeedback is very common and can be very sophisticated, a great many biofeedback users still work with free-standing biofeedback instruments or simple devices, such as those used in this chapter as vehicles for illustrating basic electronic and measurement principles. Moreover, users with sophisticated computer systems still need to understand the fundamental principles and methods for detecting and measuring physiological processes, even at times when much may be automated and invisible behind the computer screen.

This chapter is therefore created as a primer. It is practically focused, rather than comprehensive. It is simplified, rather than highly technical. It stays with basic principles and methods that are foundational to highly technological approaches, rather than delving into today's advanced technology. It is heuristically presented, with emphasis on principle as well as fact, and contains practical judgments rather than being strictly objective.

CORRELATES OF AROUSAL: THREE PHYSIOLOGICAL PROCESSES OF INTEREST IN BIOFEEDBACK

Three physiological processes commonly associated with overarousal are skeletal muscle tension, peripheral vasoconstriction, and electrodermal activity. These three, especially the first two, are the most common biofeedback modalities. This is no surprise, as these processes have been recognized all along as intimately involved in anger, fear, excitement, and arousal.

This association can be seen by recalling common expressions or idioms that have found their way into everyday language. For example, when a person is said to be "braced" for an onslaught, one gets a picture of muscles "at the ready." The person is tense and may have fists "clenched" and jaw "set"; in a word, the person is "uptight." If this tension were unrealistic or simply habitual, commonplace advice would be to loosen up," "relax," or "let go."

The expression "my blood ran cold" evokes the connection between fear and cold extremities, as does the image "cold hands, warm heart." In both is the recognition that having cold hands is a sign of emotional responsivity—in other words, the common knowledge that peripheral vasoconstriction is a sign of arousal. In referring to electrodermal activity, a person might illustrate fear with the image of "a cold sweat" or of "sweating bullets." A picture of calm and ease is drawn by the term "no sweat."

As these idioms illustrate, people already know that muscle tension, peripheral vasoconstriction, and electrodermal activity are related to arousal. The systematic study and modification of these processes are in the domain of biofeedback. Biofeedback devices exist to aid in the study and especially in the modification of these processes.

BIOFEEDBACK EQUIPMENT

Terminology

A piece of biofeedback hardware may be referred to as "instrument," "machine," "device," "equipment," "apparatus," "unit," and even "gadget" or "gizmo." Most of these terms are used interchangeably and with little or no uniformity or consistency; often the choice is based simply on preference or whim. This is not offered as a criticism, for people often have many terms for things that are interesting to them. It may simply be a case of the ancient Chinese proverb, "A child who is loved has many names."

In any case, it is worthwhile to outline the connotations for the more popular terms for biofeedback hardware. "Instrument" is the most formal of the terms, denoting a measuring device for determining the present value of a quantity under observation. Many items of bio-feedback hardware do not qualify as "instruments" under this definition, since actual measurements are not being made; only changes or relative magnitudes are being monitored. For example, "mood rings" and other simple biofeedback "gadgets" or "gizmos" are not considered instruments. The terms "apparatus," "equipment," and "device" leave unspecified whether or not measurement is made, and hence are safe general terms, although "device" implies the performance of a highly specific function. The term "unit" is even more neutral, claiming nothing more than an entity is being referred to. The term "machine" denotes a mechanism that transmits forces, action, or energy in a predetermined manner. Those familiar with electronics see electronic equipment abstractly transmitting forces, motion, and energy within their circuits, and hence often use the term "machine" in describing biofeedback equipment.

In this chapter, most of these terms are used, and (as in common practice) they are used more or less interchangeably. Nothing beyond the ordinary meanings and connotations is intended.

What Biofeedback Instruments Are Supposed to Do

A biofeedback instrument has three tasks:

1. To monitor (in some way) a physiological process of interest.
2. To measure (objectify) what is monitored.
3. To present what is monitored or measured as meaningful information.

The following sections outline how access is gained to three important psychophysiological processes in biofeedback.

EMG: An Electrical Correlate of Muscle Contraction

A biofeedback device cannot measure muscle contraction in a simple, direct way. When a muscle contracts, it tries to pull its two anchor points together; this is what is meant by "muscle contraction." It is a kinetic phenomenon involving force and sometimes movement. Practically speaking, this is not easily monitored. One cannot insert a strain gauge between one end of a muscle and its anchor point to measure grams of pull. (Force and movement gauges, called "goniometers," are used as muscle contraction monitors in physical medicine applications, but these are not sensitive to the levels or locations of muscle contraction involved in relaxation and low-arousal applications of biofeedback.)

Because muscle contraction itself is inaccessible, some aspect or correlate of it will have to do. Biofeedback exploits the electrical aspect of muscle contraction. Muscle contraction results from the more or less synchronous contraction of the many muscle fibers that constitute a muscle. Muscle fibers are actuated by electrical signals carried by cells called "motor units," and muscle contraction corresponds to the aggregate electrical activity in these muscle fibers (see Fogel, Chapter 23, this volume). This electrical activity can be sensed with fine wire or needle electrodes that actually penetrate the skin above the muscle. More commonly, it is sensed with surface electrodes that contact the skin above the muscle, where there exist weakened electrical signals from muscle fibers beneath the skin. This is the preferred biofeedback method for monitoring muscle contraction, because it is practical and corresponds well to actual muscle contraction. Note that this electrical method, surface EMG, does not directly monitor muscle contraction, but monitors an electrical aspect of muscle contraction that bears a more or less regular relationship to muscle contraction.

The important point is this: Surface EMG (hereafter referred to simply as EMG) is the preferred method for monitoring muscle contraction, but does not directly measure muscle contraction. An EMG device does not read out in units of force or movement, such as grams or millimeters. Instead, it measures an electrical correlate of muscle contraction and reads out in electrical units (microvolts—millionths of a volt). This is because it is making an electrical, not a kinetic, measurement. This explains the initial puzzlement that often comes over the biofeedback novice upon learning that muscle contraction is measured in volts—electrical units that, at face value, seem to have little to do with muscle contraction.

Peripheral Temperature: A Correlate of Peripheral Vasoconstriction

A biofeedback device cannot directly measure the changing diameter of peripheral blood vessels or the smooth muscle activity that brings about these changes. Therefore, some correlate of vascular diameter will have to do. Dilated vessels pass more warm blood than constricted vessels do. Therefore, surrounding tissue tends to warm and cool as vascular diameter increases and decreases, providing a good correlate of vascular diameter. This effect is most pronounced in the extremities (especially the fingers and toes), where changes in vascular diameter are pronounced, and where the relatively small amount of surrounding tissue warms and cools rapidly in response to changes in the blood supply.

Here again the physiological process of interest (peripheral vasoconstriction) is inaccessible, but an accessible correlate (peripheral temperature) is a practical indicator. Biofeedback devices typically read out in degrees Fahrenheit as the indirect indicator of peripheral vasoconstriction. This shows that only indirect access to peripheral vasoconstriction is possible in biofeedback.

Finger Phototransmission: Another Correlate of Peripheral Vasoconstriction

A second indirect way to gain access to peripheral vasoconstriction takes advantage of the fact that a finger or toe having less blood in its vessels allows more light to pass through than an extremity with more blood. That is, pale skin passes more light than infused skin. A small light is shone through the flesh of a finger and is reflected off the bone back to a light sensor. The variation in light intensity at the sensor, and the resulting electrical signal, indicate variation in blood volume.

This device is commonly called a "photoplethysmograph" and is sometimes used in biofeedback. It monitors pulse, and (with appropriate circuitry to average out the pulses) can give an indication of relative blood volume, another correlate of vasoconstriction. Such devices read out only in relative units. That is, they read changes but are not anchored to some outside standard reference point. Photoplethysmography is not employed nearly as often as peripheral temperature to indicate peripheral vasoconstriction. Further description of photoplethysmography is beyond the scope of this chapter. For more information, see Jennings, Tahmoush, and Redmond (1980). For more on the psychophysiology of peripheral blood flow, see Cacioppo, Tassinary, and Berntson (2000).

Skin Conductance Activity: A Correlate of Sweat Gland Activity

Sweat gland activity is another physiological process that is not directly accessible. One cannot tell whether a sweat gland is "on," how much sweat is being secreted, or how many such glands are active. However, sweat contains electrically conductive salts that make sweaty skin more conductive to electricity than dry skin. Hence skin conductance activity (SCA) corresponds well to sweat gland activity. SCA, along with other electrical phenomena of the skin, is known as electrodermal activity (EDA); historically, it has also been known as "galvanic skin response" (GSR). A skin conductance device applies a very small electrical pressure (voltage) to the skin, typically on the volar surface of the fingers or the palmar surface of the hand (where there are many sweat glands), and measures the amount of electrical current that the skin will allow to pass. The magnitude of this current is an indication of skin sweatiness and is read out in units of electrical conductance called "micromhos."

Here again, an electrical unit (conductance) serves as the indirect measure of a physiological phenomenon (sweat gland activity). This explains what might initially seem odd: that EDA is measured in electrical units that at face value have nothing to do with sweat gland activity.

Objectification and Measurement

As described above, direct monitoring of muscle contraction, peripheral vasoconstriction, and sweat gland activity is not feasible. Therefore, biofeedback devices gain access indirectly through monitoring more accessible correlates of these physiological processes. This means that a biofeedback reading should be taken as a convenient indication of a physiological process, but should be understood as separate from the physiological process itself. Practitioners must distinguish the physiological process beneath the skin from the instrumentation schemes outside the skin used to gain access to it. This distinction is important for understanding measurement, objectification, artifact, and the interpretation of biofeedback data.

To compare a person's biofeedback readings from one occasion to another, or to compare readings between different individuals, an objective scale permitting such measurement is advantageous. "Measurement" takes place when the device is calibrated to and reads out in standardized quantitative units that show how the monitored process is varying. An example is a thermometer calibrated to the Fahrenheit temperature scale.

On the other hand, what I'll call "indication of relative magnitude" takes place when an observable signal such as a meter reading is made to correspond to a particular process such as skin temperature or muscle contraction, but the correspondence is not displayed in standardized quantitative units. An example is a homemade thermometer that reads out on an arbitrary "warm–cool" scale of 1–10.

The advantage of measurement is that different observers can make direct quantitative comparisons. Without measurement, observers can only compare relative magnitude or change. Measurement tends to increase replicability of procedures and comparability of results. Measurement in this sense is often not possible in biofeedback, due to the lack of clearly defined and/or widely accepted standardized scales for measurement.

For example, EMG devices typically have meters or scaled outputs that give readings in microvolts. Because numbers appear on the meters, this appears to give objectivity to the readings and to permit actual measurement. In fact, however, there is no widely accepted and standardized scale for EMG microvolts. In effect, each model or brand of EMG device becomes its own reference standard. Consequently, different equipment gives different readings for the very same degree of muscle contraction. Therefore, EMG readings can be compared only when the same (or very similarly designed) equipment is used for all the readings. Explanations for this will become clear later, when the design of the EMG device is described. The important point to remember now is that EMG readings are better thought of as indications of relative magnitude than as measurements. The same is true for skin conductance readings. Skin temperature readings, however, are measurements, as long as the temperature device is properly calibrated to a temperature scale such as degrees Fahrenheit.

OPERATION OF THE EMG INSTRUMENT

The EMG instrument picks up weak electrical signals generated during muscle action. Each muscle consists of many muscle fibers, with "motor neurons" electrically connected to higher levels of the nervous system. Muscle contraction occurs when these motor neurons carry electrical activating signals to the muscle fibers. A small part of this electrical energy leaves the muscle and migrates through surrounding tissue. Some of this energy becomes available for monitoring at the surface of the skin. The tasks of an EMG machine are as follows:

1. To receive the very small amount of electrical energy from the skin.
2. To separate EMG energy from other extraneous energy on the skin, and to greatly magnify the EMG energy.
3. To convert this amplified EMG energy into information or feedback that is meaningful to the user.

Receiving EMG Energy from the Skin: Electrodes

"Surface electrodes" (usually small metallic discs mounted on plastic or rubber) contact the skin through an electrically conductive cream or gel. Wires complete the electrical pathways from the skin to the EMG machine. Some electrodes are quite small and designed for precise locations. Some are individually attached with tape or double-stick adhesive washers. Others come on strips or on a headband for simultaneous application of the three electrodes generally required for EMG biofeedback. Some electrodes are permanently attached to electrode cables, whereas others are made to snap onto the cable, permitting changes of electrodes without changing the cable.

Many electrodes are made of simple materials, such as nickel-plated brass or stainless steel; others are made of rare materials, such as gold or silver chloride over silver (silver/silver chloride). The precious-metal electrodes have historically been the materials of choice for physiological monitoring, because the materials do not interact significantly with skin or other substances with which they are in contact. However, the simpler and cheaper electrodes have been found to be quite satisfactory for biofeedback EMG applications and are now in widespread use. Modern equipment can well tolerate imperfect electrodes and skin preparation, and thus has reduced the need for precious-metal electrodes for EMG biofeedback.

Electrode Cream or Gel

Common to nearly all EMG electrodes is the use of an electrode gel or cream. Because this conductive substance flows into the irregularities of the skin and the electrode, it establishes a stable and highly conductive connection between them (see Figure 4.1).

Skin Preparation

A standard part of electrode application is to remove dirt, oil, dead skin cells, and makeup. These impede the travel of bioelectric signals from the skin to the electrode. Some manufacturers have suggested using an abrasive skin cleaner for this purpose, while others suggest wiping the skin with an alcohol swab. The risk in underpreparing the skin is that EMG readings will be erroneously high, but usually the skin must be oily or covered with makeup for this to result. The risk of overpreparing the skin, particularly with the abrasive compounds, is that the skin (and client) will become irritated. There is nothing to be gained by actually scrubbing skin unless there is significant dirt, oil, or makeup present. In fact, some special-

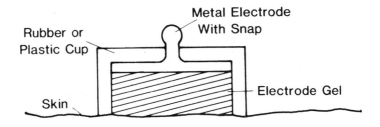

FIGURE 4.1. EMG electrode and gel.

ized EMG biofeedback equipment (used in neuromuscular rehabilitation) operates not only with simple metal electrodes, but with no electrode gel or skin preparation. This is not to say, however, that one can just forget about skin preparation.

Separating EMG Energy from Extraneous ("Noise") Energy

"Noise" is the general term for unwanted or extraneous signals. In EMG machines, there are two kinds of noise: electrical interference and internally generated noise.

Electrical Interference and the Differential Amplifier

The environment is continuously saturated with electrical energy transmitted through space from power lines, motors, lights, and electrical equipment. Human bodies and EMG electrodes pick up this energy. The EMG apparatus therefore receives unwanted electrical noise signals, in addition to the desired bioelectric signals from the muscles. The EMG unit must therefore find a way to reject the noise so that only EMG signals remain.

Interference is rejected in an ingenious way, using an electrical subtraction process in a "differential amplifier." The electrodes establish three independent pathways from an area of the skin to the EMG instrument. One pathway, called the "reference," is used by the instrument as a point of reference from which the minute electrical pressure (voltage) exerted from the other two "active" electrodes is gauged. (Remember that any electrical pressure or voltage measurement is defined as a pressure difference between one point and another point. There is no such thing as a voltage measurement without respect to some second point of reference.) This results in two "sources" feeding the instrument, each using the reference electrode as the point of reference (see Figure 4.2). Note that the reference electrode can be placed

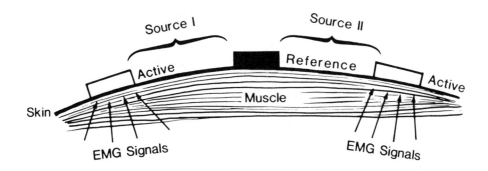

FIGURE 4.2. Active and reference EMG electrodes.

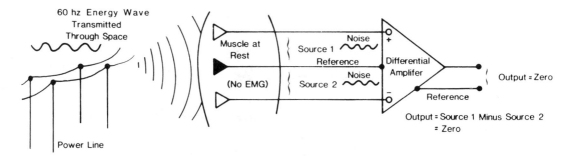

FIGURE 4.3. Differential amplifier eliminating the electrical interference picked up by the body acting as an antenna.

nearly anywhere on the body, but it is shown in Figure 4.2 between the two active electrodes for the sake of illustration, and because it is a common arrangement.

The differential amplifier requires these two sources in order to separate the EMG energy from the extraneous energy. To see why, we must remember that this extraneous energy is the hum or noise transmitted through space from power lines, motors, and appliances that is picked up by the body acting as an antenna. Most of this extraneous electrical noise energy rises and falls rhythmically at 60 cycles per second. At any given moment, this energy is in exactly the same place in its rhythm ("in phase") at any point on the body and at any point that an electrode can be placed. Hence it is possible for the differential amplifier to continuously subtract the voltage at source 1 from that at source 2. This cancels the noise voltage. Only slightly simplified, this is illustrated graphically in Figure 4.3; it is assumed that the muscle is at rest and giving off no EMG signals. The following steps explain Figure 4.3:

1. Electrical interference is received by the body acting as an antenna.
2. The interference is in the same place in its rhythm for both active electrodes.
3. Therefore, the active inputs (from source 1 and source 2) of the differential amplifier "see" exactly the same interference signal at any given moment (interference is in the "common mode").
4. Because the output of the differential amplifier is proportional to the difference between the signals at its two active inputs (from sources 1 and 2),
5. and the interference signals are always identical (restatement of point 3),
6. then the output of the differential amplifier is zero for electrical interference.

But What about EMG Signals? Suppose that motor neurons now signal the resting muscle to contract. Each electrode receives signals most strongly from the area of muscle directly beneath it. Since electrodes are spaced along the muscle, they each receive a different pattern of EMG signals. Here is an analogy: If two microphones were placed in a room full of speaking people, each one would pick up a different pattern of sounds, even if the overall loudness of sound in each microphone were the same. Therefore, at any given moment, the electrodes feed "differential" EMG signals superimposed on the previously discussed identical "common-mode" signals.

Now, as the differential amplifier continuously subtracts the signal at source 2 from that at source 1 (thus amplifying only differences between them), the common-mode noise signals will be canceled, while the differential EMG signals will always leave a remainder to be amplified and ultimately displayed on a meter. The operation of the differential EMG amplifier with the desired EMG signals is shown graphically in Figure 4.4 and is summarized below.

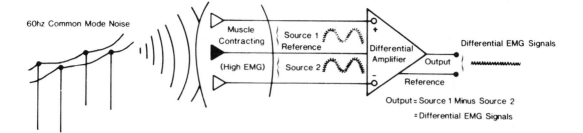

FIGURE 4.4. Differential amplifier amplifying the common-mode interference while amplifying differential EMG signals.

1. Different EMG signals arrive at the two electrodes as the muscle beneath them contracts.
2. Therefore, sources 1 and 2 feed "differential" EMG signals to the inputs of the differential amplifier.
3. At the same time, identical ("common-mode") interference signals are superimposed on the differential EMG signals.
4. Thus the inputs (from sources 1 and 2) "see" composite signals that have an identical component (common-mode noise) and a differing component (differential EMG signals).
5. Since the output of the differential amplifier is proportional to the difference between the signals at its two inputs (from sources 1 and 2),
6. and a portion of the signals are identical (common-mode) and a portion are different (differential-mode) (restatement of point 4),
7. then the output of the differential amplifier is zero for common-mode interference and high for differential-mode EMG signals.

The Chemist's Balance Analogy. The operation of the differential amplifier can be illustrated by another analogy. Imagine a sensitive chemist's balance scale, with its two pans, center fulcrum, and a set of weights. With no weights in the pans, the scale balances. With equal weights in the pans, it also balances. Even if we stretch our imaginations to envision the weights constantly changing (but always remaining equal in both pans), the scale will remain balanced. However, a fly landing on one pan during this process will upset the balance, and the pointer will move off center. Moreover, if two flies of equal weight hop up and down, one on each pan, each with its own idiosyncratic rhythm, the pointer will move from side to side. The deflection indicates, at any given moment, the difference in weight on the two pans. Only differences in total weights can lead to a pointer deflection.

By now, the reader will recognize the differential amplifier as an electronic version of the chemist's balance. Figure 4.5 and Table 4.1 spell out the correspondence between the two.

The preceding discussion of the differential amplifier makes it easier to see why deteriorated electrodes or high-resistance contact with the skin can lead to erroneously high EMG readings. For example, if one of the active electrodes makes poor contact with the skin, it will feed a reduced signal to the differential amplifier. Since the other electrode is feeding a full-sized signal to the differential amplifier, the common-mode noise signals applied to the two inputs are of different size. Therefore, when the subtraction process takes place, there is a noise remainder that artificially elevates the reading. Figure 4.6 illustrates this.

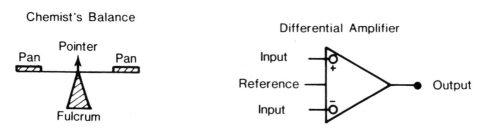

FIGURE 4.5. Graphic representation of data in Table 4.1.

TABLE 4.1. Correspondence between Chemist's Balance and Differential Amplifier

Chemist's balance	Differential amplifier
1. Pans	1. Inputs
2. Pointer	2. Output
3. Fulcrum	3. Reference
4. Equal weights in the pans → balance (pointer remains straight)	4. Common-mode signals → zero output
5. Different weights in the pans → imbalance (pointer deflects)	5. Differential signals → nonzero output
6. Two equal weights in the pans *and* Two unequal weights in the pans → imbalance (pointer reflects the difference between the unequal weights only, as equal weights cancel out)	6. Common-mode signals *and* Differential signals → nonzero output (output reflects the difference between the differential signals only, as equal signals cancel out)

The ratio of differential signal amplification to common-mode signal amplification for a particular differential amplifier is the "common-mode rejection ratio." "Input impedance" is the differential amplifier specification that indicates its level of protection from inaccuracy due to unequal electrode contact. Both are quite high for reputable instruments. Further discussion of these specifications is beyond the scope of this chapter.

Internal Noise: Filters and Bandwidth

The task of removing extraneous signals is still not complete. Electrical "filters" further reduce interference from power lines, and also limit the noise inevitably generated within the circuits of the EMG amplifier itself. These filters are comparable to tone controls on a stereo amplifier, except that they are usually set in one position at the factory. Their purpose is to make the EMG amplifier sensitive to some frequencies (or pitches) of incoming signals and insensitive to others.

Speech or music consists of a wide range of frequencies or pitches, all combined to give us the familiar sounds. Tone controls alter these by increasing or decreasing bass and treble, depending on the listener's preference. For example, turning down the treble may improve the sound of a particularly hissy tape or scratchy old phonograph record by reducing some of the high-frequency scratch and hiss sounds. Turning down the bass may improve the sound

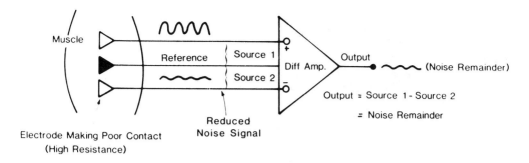

FIGURE 4.6. Unequal common-mode noise inputs leading to a noise remainder.

of an amplifier that has a boomy bass or hums. In both cases, a modification of the amplifier's "frequency sensitivity" or "bandwidth" or "bandshape" is being made.

There are reasons to do something similar with an EMG device. For example, much of the electrical interference or noise from power lines is concentrated at a narrow pitch of 60 cycles or vibrations per second (hertz). Anyone with a stereo or electric guitar with a bad patch cord knows this humming or buzzing sound. To further reduce this noise signal, a special filter can make the EMG amplifier much less sensitive to this pitch. More typically, the entire bass response of the amplifier is "rolled off" to further reduce electrical interference remaining after the differential amplifier. A typical "bass" or low-frequency bandwidth limit is about 100 hertz.

There is also good reason to limit the EMG amplifier's "treble" frequency sensitivity. All amplifiers unavoidably generate high-pitched noise within their own circuits that sounds like hiss (a sound also familiar to users of stereo equipment). The EMG amplifier's treble response is typically "rolled off" (e.g., above 1000 hertz) to diminish internal noise contributions to EMG readings.

The EMG instrument's range of sensitivity between the bass frequency limit and the treble limit is called the "bandwidth." Like speech and music sounds, EMG signals are comprised of a range of frequencies or pitch. They tend to vary from about 10 to 1000 hertz. The graph in Figure 4.7 shows two idealized bandwidths superimposed on a hypothetical EMG frequency distribution. This shows that even with treble and bass limits, an EMG amplifier is sensitive to significant amounts of EMG energy.

In both cases, the amplifier's bandwidth (range of sensitivity) includes a significant area of EMG energy. However, the wide bandwidth shown in Figure 4.7 includes more EMG energy (and noise) than the narrower bandwidth. This means that (other things being equal) the instrument set with a wider bandwidth will give higher readings than the one with the narrower bandwidth. A stereo can also illustrate this. Turning the bass and treble controls all the way down narrows the bandwidth and produces not only a different tone, but less volume of both sound and noise.

Other things being equal, the wider the bandwidth, the higher the readings for both EMG and noise. The proportion of the reading that is noise (the "signal-to-noise ratio") may be the same in both cases, but the levels of both EMG and noise will be higher with a wide-bandwidth EMG amplifier.

EMG biofeedback devices are made with different bandwidths, due to differing design philosophies. The most important message here is that *different bandwidths lead to different readings.* This has to be taken into account when one is comparing readings and noise specifications between different models of EMG equipment. For example, an instrument with a

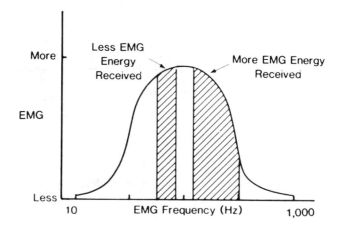

FIGURE 4.7. Two hypothetical bandwidths.

lower noise or sensitivity specification may not really be any more sensitive or noise resistant than another; it may just have a narrower bandwidth. Readers who wish to know more about EMG frequency distribution, filters, and bandwidth are referred to Mathieu and Sullivan (1990).

Converting EMG Energy to Information

At this point in our story, EMG energy has been picked up from the skin and separated from extraneous noise energy. The resulting signal is proportional to the electrical activity of the motor neurons in the muscle being monitored, and is often referred to as "raw EMG."

Raw EMG

Raw EMG resembles auditory static; it is a rushing sound that rises and falls in loudness in proportion to muscle contraction. This "raw" or "raw filtered" EMG is one form of audio feedback. Commercial EMG units usually do not provide raw EMG audio output. Instead, they generate an audio tone or series of beeps. The pitch or repetition rate is made proportional to the amplitude or "loudness" of the raw EMG, and therefore to the muscle contraction. Raw EMG amplitude can also be displayed on a meter.

Smoothing and Integration

"Smoothing" and "integration" refer to two ways of quantifying EMG energy over time. Smoothing refers to continuously averaging out the peaks and valleys of a changing electrical signal. Integration refers to measuring the area under a curve over a time period. Both require processing the raw EMG signal, as described in the next section.

Alternating Current and Pulsating Direct Current. Raw EMG is an alternating current (AC) signal. Alternating current pushes alternately back and forth or "vibrates" like a reed in the wind or a swinging clock pendulum, as represented in Figure 4.8. The curve represents the change in electrical pressure over time, first in one direction and then in the opposite direction. The "+" represents pressure in one direction, and the "−" represents pressure in the other direction. The center line represents the point of zero voltage, analogous to the position

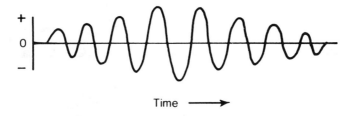

FIGURE 4.8. Gradually increasing, then decreasing alternating voltage.

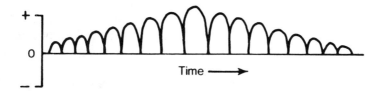

FIGURE 4.9. Rectified alternating voltage.

of the reed at rest or the clock pendulum in its straight-down position. The height of a wave represents its peak amplitude or peak voltage. Figure 4.8 shows an electrical signal "vibrating" at a specific frequency (number of oscillations per second, or hertz).

Not only is the electrical signal oscillating, but the amplitude or magnitude of the oscillations first builds to a high point and then diminishes. It is the measurement of this overall increase and then decrease that is significant for EMG biofeedback. The first step in accomplishing this is to "flip" the negative peaks up above the zero line with the positive peaks, a process called "rectification." Without rectification, the sum of the negative peaks and positive peaks would always equal zero (they would cancel each other). Without rectification, it would be hard to recognize overall trends in magnitude unless one was viewing the oscillations on an oscilloscope screen or listening to the raw EMG over a speaker. Figure 4.9 shows the rectified EMG wave. The negative peaks have been electronically "flipped" up with the positive peaks, so that all the peaks are positive. This means that the electrical signal now pushes in just one direction; hence the term "direct current" (DC). In this case, the signal is pulsating DC.

Smoothing the EMG Signal for Moment-to-Moment Quantification. If the voltage in Figure 4.9 is applied to a needle-type DC voltmeter, the meter mechanism and attached needle will move, while mechanical inertia will prevent the mechanism from following each rapid voltage pulse. It will, in effect, smooth out the pulses by displaying a voltage value somewhat less than the peak voltages of the successive, positive-going EMG pulses. This changing voltage level is called "rectified smoothed" or "filtered" EMG, as illustrated in Figure 4.10. Its voltage value is the mathematical average of the rectified EMG voltage for a constant-amplitude EMG signal.

Most mechanical meters respond too fast for optimal smoothing of EMG amplitude. Fortunately, electronic smoothing or filtering can be performed on the rectified EMG signal. The outputs of smoothing circuits are then used to drive analog or digital meters, as well as audio feedback circuitry (see Figure 4.11 and discussion below). Electronic smoothing is essential for digital meters, because they have no mechanical inertia to smooth out the pulses. A great advantage to electronic smoothing or filtering circuits is the wide choice of time con-

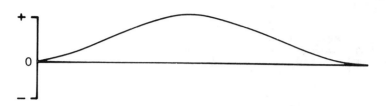

FIGURE 4.10. Rectified filtered or smoothed EMG.

stant or response time. The designer has wide choice of how fast the digital or analog meter will respond to momentary changes in EMG level (tracking time).

The most common form of smoothing or filtering found in commercial EMG equipment employs a fixed time constant (or tracking time) suitable for general-purpose use. Some EMG instruments and computer-based systems have selectable tracking times, which require the user to decide how much smoothing of the curve is desired. Long tracking time leads to a smoother output that is less responsive to momentary ups and downs in the EMG level. Unsmoothed output may seem too jumpy for relaxation training, and overly smoothed output may cover or delay information. There is no generally agreed-upon optimum tracking time. The choice is based on application, technique, and subjective preference. It does not appear that any one tracking time is particularly advantageous for relaxation training. This view is apparently shared by the manufacturers, who build their instruments with various fixed or adjustable tracking times.

Integration for Cumulative EMG or Average EMG over a Fixed Time Period. A second quantification scheme involves letting the area under the EMG curve (in microvolt minutes) accumulate over a period of time, such that the reading starts at zero and continually builds until the time period ends, as shown in Figure 4.12. The accumulated area under the curve at the end of the trial indicates the accumulated number of microvolt minutes of EMG received over that time. Dividing the accumulated microvolt minutes of integrated EMG by the accumulated time in minutes yields the average level of EMG (in microvolts) during that time. Then the timer and integrator are reset to zero, and a new time period or trial begins. Integration establishes relaxation trials of many seconds (e.g., 30, 60, 120, or more seconds). Comparisons can then be made over multiple trials—something that is more difficult to do when only moment-to-moment EMG levels are used.

Audio Feedback

Audio feedback encodes the EMG level in auditory form and is very important in biofeedback, because it transmits information without the need for visual attention. A common way to do this is to use the smoothed EMG signal to vary the pitch of an electronic tone generator. The higher the EMG level, the higher the pitch. A continuous audio tone feedback derived from the smoothed EMG signal has been shown in Figure 4.11.

Audio Tone
(Continuous
Tone)

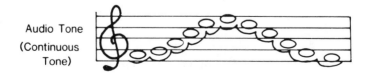

FIGURE 4.11. Audio tone derived from smoothed EMG.

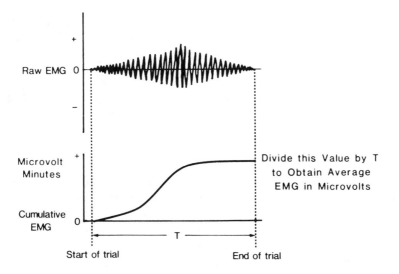

FIGURE 4.12. Integration for cumulative EMG or average EMG over a fixed time period.

Another form of audio feedback consists of a "pulsed tone," in which the tone is interrupted so it comes in beeps separated by silence. The higher the EMG level, the higher the tone's pitch, and the more frequent the beeps. Small changes in level are very apparent with this form of feedback.

The range of possibilities for audio feedback is virtually limitless, and many forms have appeared on commercial units. There is no one optimum form of audio feedback. Preferences develop on the basis of purely subjective criteria as well as application requirements.

Visual Feedback: Meters and Computer Displays

A meter that displays the smoothed EMG signal provides visual indication of the strength of muscle contraction at that moment. This is used for making moment-to-moment quantified readings. Most EMG meters are calibrated with scales that show quantified units such as microvolts. Others give only a relative scale without quantification.

Biofeedback devices use both analog and digital meters. A digital meter displays information in changing numbers, which are read directly like an automobile odometer. An analog meter has a continuous scale and a moving needle like an auto speedometer. The user reads an analog meter by estimating the quantity to which the needle points. Although digital meters are associated with high technology, analog meters should not be summarily dismissed as obsolete. Each type has its advantages.

For example, digital meters excel at precise quantification of readings over a very wide range. But the user must actually read the meter's numbers to get the information. The changing digits of a digital meter are not as comfortable or instinctively meaningful to some users.

On the other hand, the relative position and movement of an analog meter needle communicates a great deal without actually requiring the user to read any figures. Feedback requires minimum effort from the user; even peripheral vision is sufficient for recognizing levels and changes. The swing of a needle on a large meter scale can be a very simple and inherently meaningful way to present information. Moreover, the analog meter scale implicitly brackets the range of obtainable readings and therefore provides a quantitative context for any given reading. The expression "off the scale" refers to this feature of an analog meter scale. With a digital meter, one may not know whether the reading is in the high or low part of the range unless one remembers the actual numerical range that is obtainable.

In summary, digital meters are better for some purposes, and analog meters are better for others. Computer-generated visual displays also differ in how much attention is required to grasp and use the information. Some display numbers or other information that requires more focused attention than simpler displays, such as bar or line graphs.

Objective Units of Measurement

Several factors besides degree of muscle contraction affect the number of microvolts an EMG device displays. A brief review of the earlier section on objectification and measurement may be helpful. The microvolt is the unit of EMG measurement; this is an electrical term used as a measure of muscle contraction. The microvolt is not literally a measure of muscle contraction, but a measure of an electrical correlate of muscle contraction. Therefore, microvolt readings involve the characteristics of the electrical apparatus (the EMG unit) that monitors and processes the EMG signals. Because of differences in design philosophy, EMG devices differ from one another, and so do the readings obtained for any given degree of muscle tension at a given site on a given person. Consequently, microvolt readings are only objectively comparable from one model to another if the instruments are known to have the same bandwidth and quantification method.

For the technically inclined, EMG instruments are AC voltmeters that make objective AC voltage measurements. However, the internal characteristics of bandwidth or bandshape and quantification method affect these measurements. Accuracy, if specified, is only at a given frequency within the bandwidth. Because EMG voltages sensed by surface electrodes are composed of an ever-changing blend of frequencies (see Figure 4.7), the bandwidth or bandshape of any particular unit will affect the readings. (This has been discussed in the section on internal noise, filters, and bandwidth.)

Quantification method also affects EMG instrument readings. First of all, there is no standardized EMG signal for calibrating EMG instruments. Instead, calibration is done using conveniently available constant-amplitude AC signals called "sine waves." (Figure 4.8 shows a changing-amplitude sine wave.) Accordingly, the use of sine waves rather than actual EMG signals is the basis for the following discussion.

The term "peak-to-peak microvolts" refers to the voltage difference between the positive peaks and the negative peaks of the unrectified AC sine wave. Quantification by the "averaging" method usually involves rectification, smoothing, and then moment-to-moment display on a meter or integration and division by time, both described earlier. The "average" voltage of a sine wave after rectification as displayed on a meter is equal to just less than one-third of the "peak-to-peak" value. Conversely, the peak-to-peak value is just over three times the average value. Some early commercial EMG instruments responded to average EMG amplitude but had meters scaled in peak-to-peak microvolts. For consistency, many EMG instruments may still use this method. To convert from peak-to-peak values to average values, divide by 3.14.

Quantification by the "root mean square" (RMS) method involves electronically making a mathematical computation on either the alternating or rectified version of the filtered EMG signal to arrive at an RMS voltage. RMS quantification is necessary to determine the electrical *power* as contrasted with *voltage,* carried by the signal. This is usually not important in biofeedback. RMS values for EMG are usually within 20% of average values.

There is little practical difference between these quantification methods or in the action of the meter needle—just different scales on the meter's face. In any case, the user of EMG equipment should become familiar with the range of readings obtained under various conditions, and should be cautious about comparing microvolt readings between units that are not known to have similar characteristics. The lesson here is that even though EMG instruments are AC voltmeters, EMG readings are not made on standardized scales and are not standardized measurements of muscle contraction. Variability exists between EMG instruments, and there is no standardized scaled correspondence between EMG microvolts and muscle contraction.

Thresholds

A threshold control allows the user to set a particular EMG level as a criterion for some form of feedback (e.g., to turn on audio feedback only when EMG exceeds the threshold). Visual feedback, such as lights or a computer display, may indicate when EMG exceeds or drops below the chosen threshold level. Thresholds are adjusted over time as training goals change.

Other Feedback Modes

The smoothed EMG level can be used to operate virtually any feedback method, including lights, sound, appliances, computers, or tactile feedback devices. All forms of feedback are ways of encoding EMG level as meaningful information or consequences. Choice of feedback mode depends on the requirements of the application and the people using the feedback. Although complex or novel feedback may be interesting, the best feedback modes for a given application are the ones that get the information across with a minimum of distraction and ambiguity. Simple, well-designed feedback usually fits this criterion. Practitioners often settle on a limited number of practical feedback modes.

Safety

EMG equipment makes direct electrical connection to a person via surface electrodes, thereby establishing a path for bioelectric signals between the person and the instrument. Although this path is intended for bioelectric signals, electricity from other sources can also take this path under some conditions. The presence of other currents in the signal path is a risk. Consequently, great care is taken in the design and manufacture of top-grade biomedical instruments to minimize the possibility of exposing patients to extraneous electrical currents. Despite this, no equipment, no matter how well made and installed, is 100% immune from electrical hazards for all time.

The chance of risky electrical faults' developing is small, especially in battery-operated equipment, but the manner in which an equipment user sets up and maintains the equipment is at least as important to patient safety as the soundness of the equipment design. It is therefore your responsibility as a professional using these instruments to be aware of potential electrical hazards and to take standard safety precautions in installing, using, and maintaining the equipment. If there is any question about the safety of a particular installation, you, the professional, must consult the manufacturer of the equipment or a qualified biomedical engineer or technician. *This is particularly important when there are multiple instruments or any connections to power-line-operated equipment or accessories.*

A good rule of thumb is to be skeptical of the safety of all setups involving power-line-operated auxiliary equipment, such as audio amplifiers, computers, and oscilloscopes, until you positively establish the safety of the installation. This is because the potential consequences of leakage current from the AC power line can be extreme. For example, it takes only 0.009

amperes (9 milliamperes) or less to cause a person to be unable to release his or her grasp on an object through which the leakage current flows. Respiration may be affected at approximately 18 milliamperes, and heart fibrillation (and death) may occur at about 50 milliamperes. This is hundreds of times less than the current required to blow a standard household fuse or circuit breaker, so they provide no protection. There are several precautions you should take, some of which require the consultation of a biomedical engineer or technician:

1. Each power-line-operated piece of auxiliary equipment should be periodically evaluated technically and certified by a biomedical technician for electrical safety. Power-line-operated EMG equipment should also be periodically tested for leakage currents. Consult the manufacturer or your biomedical technician.

2. Keep all patients or subjects out of arm's reach of all metal building parts, such as radiators and plumbing.

3. Ground all equipment properly. Use a "ground fault interrupter," a device that senses a diversion of electricity from the normal pathway established by the two legs of the standard power circuit. This device shuts down power to the equipment if more than about 5 milliamperes of current is "lost" through non-normal pathways, such as leakage current to ground through a person.

Troubleshooting with a "Dummy Subject"

High-grade EMG circuitry is quite reliable, but electrodes, cables, and batteries may need frequent service in heavily used installations. Diagnosing failure of these parts is usually simple and requires few tools.

Faulty electrodes or electrode contact usually leads to spuriously high readings. Follow the electrode maintenance and application instructions supplied with the instrument. If unexpected or suspiciously high readings are observed, determine whether the problem is in the electrodes, the electrode contact, the cable, or the EMG unit. Use a "dummy subject," which is nothing more than two resistors that can be snapped to the electrode cable in place of the normal electrodes. This simulates a subject with zero EMG (see Figure 4.13).

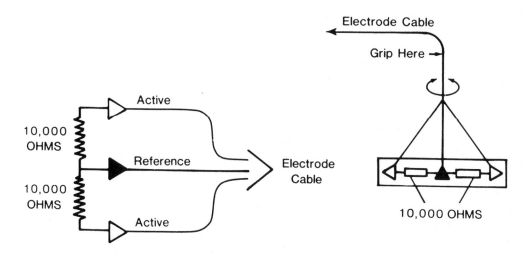

FIGURE 4.13. Dummy subject.

The dummy subject supplies about the same "input resistance" as actual electrodes on skin, but generates no EMG signals. With the dummy subject in place, the readings should therefore be close to the residual noise level of the instrument as given in its specifications. For a fair test, hold the electrode cable between the fingers at least a foot away from the dummy subject as it dangles toward the floor. This distance prevents excessive noise from being coupled from your body to the dummy subject. EMG readings with the dummy subject typically vary as you twist the cable between the fingers, much as television reception on "rabbit ears" varies as one rotates the antenna.

If a dummy subject test done in the patient area results in a reading near the instrument's residual noise specification, then it is safe to conclude that electrical noise in the area is not overpowering. This means that suspiciously high readings with the real subject are not the result of failure of the EMG unit or electrode cable. In this case, the fault is most likely with the electrodes or electrode contact.

If the reading goes off scale and stays there while the dummy subject is rotated, there is likely to be a break in the electrode cable. Verify this by substituting another cable. If the repeat test still leads to off-scale or very high readings, then it is likely that the fault is with the EMG unit itself, or that the work area is saturated with electrical noise. High dummy subject readings that don't go off scale may be attributable to excessive noise from nearby electrical equipment. Check this by moving the machine to other locations and repeating the dummy subject test.

If the dummy subject test indicates that the instrument and cable are working properly, but abnormally high readings with the real person being tested remain, consider removing the electrodes, cleaning the person's skin again, and reapplying the electrodes.

Construct a dummy subject if you don't have one already. Experiment with the dummy subjects when you know that your instrument and cables are working properly. You will then be in a better position to judge test results with dummy subjects when actual failures occur.

Battery Failure

Abnormally high or low readings may result from battery failure. Most instruments have a built-in battery check. Use it whenever there is doubt about the accuracy of the readings. Units without a battery check usually include battery-checking instructions in the user's manual. Aging batteries may pass the check and work fine early in a session, deteriorate during the session, and then "self-rejuvenate" after a few idle hours. The usable time after these "self-rejuvenations" gets shorter and shorter, until the batteries are unable to power the equipment at all.

Summary

A summary block diagram of a hypothetical EMG instrument with several outputs is presented in Figure 4.14.

OPERATION OF THE TEMPERATURE BIOFEEDBACK INSTRUMENT

Temperature biofeedback instruments measure changing skin temperature, which is significant because it is linked, through vasoconstriction, to sympathetic arousal. Vasoconstriction affects perfusion of blood and therefore skin temperature, particularly in the extremities (especially the fingers and toes). Typically, sympathetic arousal leads to increased vasoconstriction, which leads to a reduction in blood volume and hence to a cooling effect at the skin.

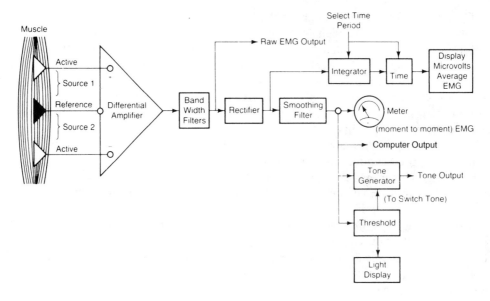

FIGURE 4.14. Block diagram of hypothetical EMG instrument with several outputs.

Although this neurovascular phenomenon involves the constriction and dilation of vessels, the single term "vasoconstriction" is used here to denote all changes in vascular diameter. For example, "reduced vasoconstriction" is used to express the idea of vasodilation. The tasks of a temperature biofeedback instrument are as follows:

1. To let the skin heat a temperature-sensitive probe.
2. To make the probe serve as a temperature-sensitive electrical "valve" that modulates an electric sensing current applied to the probe.
3. To display temperature-dependent variations in probe current as temperature in degrees, and to provide other temperature feedback or information meaningful to the user.

Letting the Skin Heat a Probe

A typical temperature probe is made of one or more small pieces of heat-sensitive electrical material (called "thermistors"), encased in electrically insulating material with wires protruding for connection to the temperature unit. A temperature probe is not an electrode. It is specifically designed to make only *thermal* contact, not *electrical* contact with the skin, where it is usually taped or strapped. The probe accepts heat from the skin and remains at nearly the same temperature as the skin immediately beneath it. As the skin warms and cools, the probe warms and cools accordingly—but with a slight delay, as probe temperature takes a little time to "catch up" with the skin temperature.

The probe is attached to either side of a finger. No single site is standard, nor has any particular site been shown to be superior. However, consistency from session to session is important, because temperature or speed of response may vary from site to site. The dorsal surface (back side) of the fingers is a common site. This permits the person to rest the hand on the chair or lap without artificially warming the probe between the finger and the chair or body. Furthermore, the dorsal surface has fewer sweat glands, so the chance of evaporative cooling is less. It is no doubt possible to make a case for the use of other sites as well, but consistency will probably remain more important than the specific choice of finger site.

Making the Probe Serve as a Temperature-Sensitive Electrical Valve

The heat-sensitive probe acts like a "valve" for electricity applied to it from the instrument, analogous to a water valve that gradually opens and closes to regulate water flow. But in this case, probe temperature operates the "valve" and regulates the flow of electricity. As the probe heats, its electrical resistance decreases, and more electric current flows. As the probe cools, its resistance increases (the "valve" closes a little), and less electric current flows. In this way, probe (and skin) temperature is encoded in the electrical flow through the probe.

Displaying Temperature and Other Feedback

The temperature instrument measures the current flow through the probe and displays this quantity (properly scaled) as degrees or as other feedback.

Internal Workings of Temperature Feedback Devices

Temperature feedback instruments can perform the required operations in more than one related way. Intelligent use of temperature biofeedback equipment does not require detailed knowledge of internal workings. However, it is important to understand the basic scheme shared by all temperature feedback devices.

Ohm's Law. Temperature feedback devices operate on one or another form of Ohm's law. Georg Ohm was the Bavarian scientist who, in 1827, specified the quantitative relationships among three basic elements of an electrical circuit: voltage, resistance, and current. In 1891, the Electrical Congress in Paris agreed that electrical pressure would be measured in volts, after Volta, an Italian; electrical flow volume in amperes, after Ampère, a Frenchman; and resistance in ohms, after Ohm, a German. Since there is a convenient hydraulic analogy to Ohm's law, the law and the analogy are presented together in Table 4.2.

Ohm's Law and a Temperature Feedback Device. Ohm's law says that the amount of current flowing in a circuit powered by a constant voltage depends entirely upon the resistance in the circuit. The resistance of the probe varies with its temperature. Therefore, when the probe is the only resistance element in a constant-voltage circuit, the current flow in the circuit is proportional to the temperature of the probe. The quantitative relationship between temperature and probe resistance is a property of the probe and varies greatly from one model to another. For this reason, probe models are usually not interchangeable. A suitable current-sensing circuit with meter displays a reading in degrees. Figure 4.15 shows a hypothetical temperature feedback device.

Parameters of Temperature Feedback Devices: Ways They Differ from One Another

Temperature feedback devices come in a wide range of performance and cost. The following three parameters—response time, absolute accuracy, and resolution—provide a basis for judging or comparing the performance of temperature feedback devices.

Response Time. "Response time" indicates how rapidly the unit responds to a change in skin temperature. It is mostly a property of the probe; if a probe responds quickly, feed-

TABLE 4.2. Ohm's Law: Voltage, Resistance, and Current

Electrical law	Hydraulic analogy
Units	
Volt: Unit of electrical pressure	Pounds per square inch: Unit of water pressure
Ampere: Unit of electric current flow	Gallons per minute: Unit of water flow
Ohm: Unit of resistance to electric current flow	Unspecified unit of resistance to water flow
Circuit description	
Pressure (in volts) pushes the current (in amperes) through the resistance (in ohms) of the circuit	Pressure (in pounds per square inch) pushes the water flow (in gallons per minute) through the resistance of the pipes
Quantification	
Current = pressure/resistance; that is, Amperes = volts/ohms (Ohm's Law)	
Algebraic formulas	
Volts = amperes × ohms Ohms = volts/amperes	
Conventional abbreviations	
Voltage: V or E Current: I Resistance: R	

back delay is minimal, and small temperature changes are readily apparent. However, quick response time is usually gained at the expense of increased cost and fragility. A very fast-responding probe (e.g., 0.3 seconds) is very small and light, encased in a material that gains or loses heat very rapidly in step with skin temperature. Larger, bulkier probes are cheaper and more durable, but they take more time to heat and cool as skin temperature changes.

A very fast-responding probe is not thought necessary in most applications. To understand why, recall that skin temperature is important because it provides indirect access to

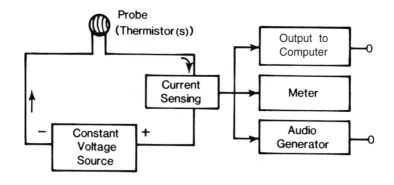

FIGURE 4.15. A hypothetical temperature feedback device.

peripheral vasoconstriction. There is already a considerable time delay between a change in vascular diameter and the resultant change in skin temperature. Probe response time adds a second delay to the overall delay between the vascular event and the resulting temperature event. One could argue that because of these delays, it is important to minimize probe response time so that further delay is kept to a minimum. A counterargument is that skin temperature is a relatively slow-changing phenomenon to which rapid response time does not add value for relaxation applications. Neither view holds obvious sway. Successful thermal biofeedback appears to have been conducted with temperature devices of widely differing response times. Calculations of "tracking error" based on conditions expected in biofeedback suggests that probe response times on the order of 1 second are probably adequate.

Absolute Accuracy. "Absolute accuracy" refers to how closely the displayed temperature corresponds to the actual probe temperature. Virtually any temperature machine will follow temperature changes (delayed by its particular response time), but there is variation between instruments in the accuracy of the temperature readings. Although a given unit may respond very sensitively to *changes* in temperature, it is unlikely that readings will exactly equal the *true* temperature of the probe; it may read up to a few degrees higher or lower than the true temperature.

Furthermore, two identical units monitoring the same site will probably not give exactly the same readings. This variability in absolute accuracy is to be expected, and the error range for a given unit is usually included in its specifications. Absolute accuracy of ±1°F is considered sufficient. Absolute accuracy is a tradeoff against cost, because a high degree of absolute accuracy tends to be very expensive to assure. And practical advantages of highly accurate temperature equipment for clinical biofeedback are not evident. Successful biofeedback takes place with widely differing degrees of absolute accuracy—including devices that are not calibrated to the Fahrenheit or Celsius standard at all, giving only relative indications of warming and cooling.

The question of accuracy arises for temperature feedback equipment, because there exist standardized temperature scales (Fahrenheit and Celsius). In contrast, the question of accuracy is less pertinent for EMG equipment, because there is no standardized EMG scale for reference, comparable to the standardized temperature scales. Remember that although *temperature* is measured on a standardized scale, *vasoconstriction* is not. An absolutely accurate temperature reading does not imply an absolutely accurate gauge of vasoconstriction, much less sympathetic arousal.

Resolution. "Resolution" refers to the smallest temperature change that the instrument can discern and display. Resolution affects length of feedback delay. For example, a digital unit that resolves to 1°F will feed back that a temperature change has taken place when a 1° change has occurred. Since temperature change occurs over time, the feedback will be delayed by however long it takes for the temperature to change 1°F. A resolution of 0.1°F will provide much more rapid feedback, since it takes far less time for the temperature to move 0.1° than 1°. Instruments can be built to resolve 0.01°F, and this reduces feedback delay even further. However, extremely high resolution also increases the risk of mistaking artifact for vasoconstriction-caused temperature change. For example, the effects of movement, a light breeze, and room cooling are much more likely to affect the readings from an instrument with exceedingly fine resolution than from one with coarser resolution. Furthermore, a high-resolution temperature instrument must be manufactured with much more exacting tolerances and increased expense. Otherwise, it may create discernible change in the readings through "drift" in its own circuits. An instrument with exceedingly high resolution is more likely to display distracting information or artifacts superimposed on true vasoconstrictive effects. A resolution of 0.1°F is a typical resolution value for temperature instruments and appears to be a suitable general-purpose value.

Digital and analog feedback have different resolving power. For example, a digital meter with three digits (tens, ones, and tenths) can resolve to 0.1°F. However, an audio tone (such as the sensitive pulsed-tone feedback described in the EMG section) indicates even finer differences that occur during the interval between changes of the tenths digit on the meter.

Artifacts

Because peripheral temperature is an indirect index of peripheral vasoconstriction, there are several sources of misleading readings. In looking for sources of artifact, the question to ask is this: "What conditions lead to temperature changes that are not linked to vasoconstrictive changes?"

Cool Room Temperature. Air temperature in the room where measurements are being made may affect the readings. For a given degree of vasoconstriction, skin temperature may be cooler in a cool room than in a warm room, simply because the cool air absorbs more heat from the skin. Cool air may also directly cool the probe.

Breeze. Moving air exaggerates the cooling effect mentioned above in two ways. First, breeze removes heat from the skin more rapidly than still air. Second, breeze evaporates sweat more rapidly than still air.

Warm Room Temperature. Room temperature sets an approximate lower limit for hand temperature. That is, a hand cannot cool very much below the temperature of the air around it. This is because cooling takes place through the dissipation of heat from the hand to the air. As soon as the hand cools down to the temperature of the air, there is no longer any place for heat to go. The hand remains at about that temperature regardless of further vasoconstriction, unless the skin cools a little further as sweat evaporates.

Warm-air effect is usually not a problem, because room temperature is usually below 72°F (close to the low end of the skin temperature range for most persons). However, in the event of a high room temperature, higher skin temperature will be observed than in a cooler room, even with an identical degree of vasoconstriction. For example, using thermal biofeedback in a 90°F room will lead to warmer hands for everyone, regardless of the degree of vasoconstriction. In this case, even the hand temperature of a cadaver, which has no warm blood at all, would be 90°F!

Room Temperature and the Temperature Feedback Instrument. Even if the temperature of the probe is held constant, temperature readings may change as the temperature unit *itself* is heated and cooled. The performance of electronic circuitry is vulnerable to change or "drift" as surrounding air temperature changes. This is a well-known phenomenon that designers take into account. Such "temperature compensation" is very important for temperature instruments, because they are required to resolve exceedingly small changes in electric current from the probe. If temperature compensation is inadequate, then readings vary with room temperature as well as skin temperature. This source of artifact is not practically significant unless room temperature is known to vary over a wide range.

Probe Contact and "Blanketing." Changes in probe contact caused by movement also affect temperature readings. If the probe begins to lift from the skin when pulled by its leads, lower readings are likely. The opposite occurs when the probe is covered by a hand, clothing, or materials used to secure the probe to the skin, all of which have the effect of "blanketing" the probe.

Chill. If the person to be monitored comes in chilled from the outside, cold hands are likely. Cold hands should be allowed to restabilize indoors before training begins. Otherwise, the natural warming of the hands after being exposed to cold may be mistaken for a training effect.

Testing for Absolute Accuracy. Test the accuracy of temperature instruments by immersing the probe in a glass of water along with a lab thermometer of known accuracy and then stirring the water. Compare the readings after they have stabilized. This test is useful when the accuracy of the instrument or probe is questioned, or when the actual interchangeability of "identical" probes is assessed.

If done carefully, this method can be used to test for temperature drift in the temperature instrument itself. With probe temperature stabilized in a thermos of water, heat and cool the instrument while noting any change in its reading.

Other Feedback

Different models of stand-alone or computerized temperature biofeedback instruments employ different variations on the basic audio and visual feedback described in this chapter, as well as different levels of response time, absolute accuracy, and resolution. A question remains about which combinations of these parameters and feedback modes are most effective for training various skills. There is some evidence that signficant differences may exist (Otis, Rasey, Vrochopoulos, Wincze, & Andrasik, 1995), although a systematic research base on these many variations does not exist.

Audio Feedback. Digital meters are often used for visual feedback, because they resolve small differences over a very wide range. Audio tones cannot provide the same resolution over such a wide range. If a usable range of audio pitches is simply distributed over the working range of skin temperature, then persons with very low or high skin temperature will have to listen to feedback in the extremes of the audio range. This will be uncomfortable to listen to for long. Moreover, small changes in temperature will lead to only slight changes in the pitch of the tone. A good solution to this problem is to let the user move the entire pitch range of audio tones up and down the temperature range, so that high-resolution audio feedback in a comfortable pitch range can be obtained, regardless of the actual skin temperature. Moving the audio range is accomplished by turning a control that affects the pitch of the audio feedback but not the meter readings. In this way, the user adjusts the audio feedback for a comfortable pitch range around any temperature.

Some temperature machines have an audio "slope" control that allows the user to select whether the pitch rises or falls with temperature. This encourages the user to fit the audio feedback to his or her warming images. For example, some users feel that the image of increasing blood flow through the fingertips calls for an increasing audio pitch. Others find decreasing pitch more natural as relaxation occurs.

Derivative Feedback. "Derivative" or "rate" feedback is sometimes found on temperature instruments. "Derivative" is a mathematical term referring to rate of change. In a temperature machine, this usually takes the form of a light or tone that turns on when skin temperature is changing at a certain rate. For example, a red light turns on when the person's hand temperature is climbing at 1°F or more per minute. Another light or tone might come on if the person's hand temperature were falling at that rate. This establishes a target hand-warming rate and permits a summary quantification such as the percentage of time above the target warming rate.

Safety

Because no electrodes are used, temperature biofeedback equipment may not pose the same electrical safety challenges as EMG equipment. The probe is deliberately electrically insulated from the subject, so the chances of a risky electrical fault's developing may be lower than with EMG equipment. Nevertheless, temperature equipment should not be considered exempt from the safety precautions discussed earlier for EMG equipment. If, for example, a probe fails (internally or through a break in its insulation) so that it is no longer insulated from the skin, it becomes in effect an electrode. This increases the potential for electric shock or leakage currents, particularly since the temperature device is probably not specifically designed to operate safely with a direct electrical connection to a person. Therefore, to be as safe as possible, follow the safety guidelines for EMG equipment. Moreover, *safety guidelines are best thought of as applying to entire biofeedback installations, not just the individual units in isolation.*

ELECTRODERMAL BIOFEEDBACK

Early History of Electrodermal Research

The early history of electrodermal research is an interesting story recounted by Neumann and Blanton (1970). They begin the story with Galvani's discovery of the electrical processes in nerve and muscle action, which quickly stimulated research into the medical applications of electricity. By 1840, it was widely believed that electrical processes provided a basis for explaining disease and generating diagnoses and therapies. The authors note that this was strongly consistent with the physicalistic thinking of the day, in reaction to the vitalistic thinking of earlier times. By 1870, then-sophisticated instrumentation and procedures had been developed as part of electrophysiological research methodology. (A fascinating collection of such literature and instrumentation exists at the Bakken Museum of Electricity in Life, Minneapolis, MN.)

As the field developed, investigators noted that skin resistance varied over the body. Since investigation focused on the physical effects of electrical currents and static fields, the early workers noted that variations in skin resistance introduced variations in current flow through the body; hence they viewed variations in skin resistance as a source of artifact, and they built instruments that controlled for this artifact. Most researchers continued to regard variations in skin resistance as artifact encountered while applying electric current or static fields for diagnostic or therapeutic purposes.

But in 1879, Romain Vigouroux measured skin resistance as an experimental variable in cases of hysterical anesthesias. This, according to Neumann and Blanton (1970), is generally regarded as the first observation of psychological factors in electrodermal phenomena. In 1888, Vigouroux's colleague, Charles Fere, studied the effect of physical stimulation on skin resistance, noting increases in current flow following stimulation. This, the reviewers say, was the first study of what by 1915 was called galvanic skin response (GSR), and was probably the first statement of an arousal theory.

It is noteworthy that by Fere's time, the French physicist D'Arsonval had developed silver chloride nonpolarizable electrodes for physiological research, as well as a sophisticated "galvanometer" (needle-type meter), a forerunner of modern meter movements that still bear D'Arsonval's name. The German investigator Hermann linked GSR with sweat gland activity in 1881, thus establishing a physiological basis for the phenomenon. In 1889, the Russian investigator Ivan Tarchanoff, while investigating skin potentials, showed that not only physical stimuli but also mental activity (such as mental arithmetic and the recollection of upsetting events) led to skin potential changes. Moreover, he linked this phenomenon to the distribution of sweat glands and proposed that it was related to the action of "secretory nerves." Neumann and Blanton (1970) report that Tarchanoff's and Fere's papers were followed by "several years of oblivion." GSR was rediscovered in 1904.

At that time, a Swiss engineer, E. K. Mueller, noticed that skin resistance changed with psychological events. He showed this to the Swiss neurologist Veraguth, and both believed this to be a newly discovered phenomenon. Mueller went on to assume the role of a psychological expert and to address the technical problems of measurement, reliability of electrode design, and experimentation with the use of AC. By 1905, Veraguth had finished some preliminary experiments when he embarrassedly discovered the earlier work of Tarchanoff and others.

Veraguth and Carl Jung were friends, and somehow (each claimed to have suggested it to the other), GSR was used in Jung's word association experiments. Jung then provided most of the impetus for further studies in this area. By 1907 he considered GSR, known to Veraguth and Jung as "psychogalvanic reflex," a means of objectifying heretofore invisible "emotional tones." Jung embarked on extensive studies and exported this idea to friends in the United States. Neumann and Blanton (1970) report that a "flood" of papers in America appeared over the next two decades and established this field as a major research area. Since then, GSR has been recognized as a way to gain objective access to psychophysiological arousal.

This physiological variable has appeared in countless psychological experiments, in clinical practice, in "lie detector" equipment, and even in toys and parlor games. Biofeedback has used it for access to autonomic arousal. GSR is recognized as distinctively sensitive to transitory emotional states and mental events, while often remaining more or less independent of other biofeedback measures such as muscle tension and skin temperature. It is a complex variable, responsive to a wide range of overt and covert activities and external and internal stimulation. Its responsivity to psychological content in actual or laboratory human situations apparently prompted Barbara Brown (1974) to dub GSR "skin talk." This is an apt metaphor that does justice to its psychological responsivity, while legitimizing its often complex and seemingly unpredictable variations and individual differences. Like any actual language, "skin talk" must be studied and experienced to be understood. EMG and temperature biofeedback are, in comparison, more easily understood by virtue of their less articulated response to mental events. That is, EMG and temperature biofeedback tend not to reflect mental events as quickly or with as much resolution as GSR.

Electrodermal phenomena are often less well conceptualized and more disparagingly discussed than other biofeedback measures because of complexity, individual variability, methodological challenges in measurement, and the multiplicity of technical approaches. The purposes of this section are to conceptualize the skin conductance phenomenon, and to describe and critique some of the approaches to skin conductance measurement and instrumentation.

As revealed in the history given above, two forms of EDA have been studied. The most common is the *exosomatically* recorded activity of Fere, Veraguth, and Jung, in which an external electric current is passed through the skin. Activity is indicated by the skin's electrical resistance (or its reciprocal, conductance). The second method, that of Tarchanoff, is *endosomatically* recorded activity (skin potentials), which involves monitoring voltage differences between electrodes at two points on the surface of the skin. The endosomatic method is not covered in this chapter, because it is much less common in biofeedback than exosomatically recorded skin conductance. For more on the endosomatic method, see Venables and Christie (1980). For more on EDA, see Dawson, Schell, and Filion (2000) and Boucsein (1992). Dawson et al.'s work is a chapter in Cacioppo et al.'s (2000) *Handbook of Psychophysiology*, 2nd edition. This handbook is also recommended for basic information relevant to biofeedback.

TABLE 4.3. Organization of Electrodermal Terms

| | Endosomatic or exosomatic | Exosomatic | | |
		Conductance	Resistance	Endosomatic
Activity	EDA	SCA	SRA	SPA
Response	EDR	SCR	SRR	SPR
Level	EDL	SCL	SRL	SPL

Terms

GSR is no doubt the most universally recognized term for EDA. Perhaps this is because the term has been used for a long time to refer to a variety of exosomatic and endosomatic phenomena, and to both levels and responses. Although the term GSR will probably continue in widespread use, other terminology has been suggested that is more descriptive of specific electrodermal phenomena. Adopted from Venables and Christie (1980), the following nomenclature is used in this chapter.

Electrodermal activity (EDA), electrodermal response (EDR), and electrodermal level (EDL) are used as general terms for either exosomatic or endosomatic phenomena. EDL refers to baseline levels; EDR refers to responses away from baselines; and EDA is the most general term, referring to levels and/or responses.

Skin conductance activity (SCA), skin conductance response (SCR), and skin conductance level (SCL) specify the exosomatic method and the conductance (in contrast to resistance) scale. Again, SCL refers to baseline levels; SCR refers to changes from baselines; and SCA refers to either or both.

Parallel terms for skin resistance and skin potentials are sometimes used: skin resistance activity (SRA), skin resistance response (SRR), and skin resistance level (SRL); skin potential activity (SPA), skin potential response (SPR), and skin potential level (SPL).

Table 4.3 clarifies the meaning of all these terms and their interrelationships. Although the table contains a dozen terms, this chapter is concerned only with SCA—that is, SCL and SCR. These are clearly the prevalent forms of electrodermal biofeedback.

Electrical Model of the Skin

The skin is electrically complex, and no one claims to have perfect knowledge of the physiology of EDA. But the following electrical model of the skin brings out the essential features of practical importance in biofeedback.

The skin on the palm or volar surface of the hand contains up to 2000 sweat glands per square centimeter. Each sweat gland when activated can be considered a separate electrical pathway from the surface of the skin, which normally has high resistance, to deeper and more conductive layers of the skin. This is shown in Figure 4.16, based on Venables and Christie (1980).

Each resistor represents the conductive pathway of a sweat gland. For illustrative purposes, a sweat gland is considered "on" or "off." When it is "on," it forms a low-resistance path from the skin surface to deeper layers. When it is "off," it makes a very high-resistance pathway. In Figure 4.16, some glands are shown "on" and others are shown "off." The inner layers of skin are highly conductive, but the outer layer is highly resistive. This means that the resistors are electrically tied together at the deeper layers within the skin, but are electrically isolated from each other at the surface. This presents an opportunity to monitor sweat gland activity electrically. If two electrodes are placed over skin laden with sweat glands, and

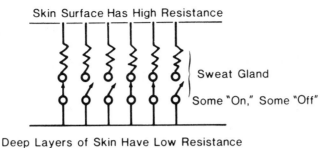

FIGURE 4.16. Electrical model of the skin. (Based on Venables & Christie, 1980.)

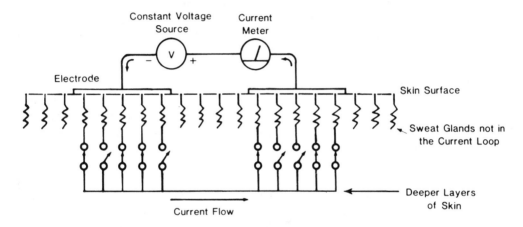

FIGURE 4.17. Basic skin conductance current loop.

a voltage is applied to the electrodes, a circuit is formed, and an electric current will flow. The size of the current will depend (according to Ohm's law) on the resistance of the skin, which in turn depends on the number of sweat glands turned "on." See Figure 4.17 for an illustration.

As more and more sweat glands turn "on," more and more conductive pathways switch into the circuit, and (since some current flows through each pathway) more and more total current flows. In this case, Ohm's law determines current flow, just as it does in temperature instruments. The difference is that the skin (instead of a temperature probe) acts as a variable resistor that regulates current flow through the circuit. The meter measures current flow in the circuit, and the reading is proportional to sweat gland activity. (Review this circuit in the section on temperature biofeedback instruments by substituting "skin resistance" for "probe resistance" in the explanation of Ohm's law.)

Scales and Measurement: Resistance and Conductance

At this point, I distinguish resistance from conductance and explain why conductance is the preferred measurement unit. "Resistance" and "conductance" are defined as reciprocals of each other, and they represent the same basic electrical property of materials. As discussed earlier, the ohm is the unit of resistance. The unit of conductance is the "mho" ("ohm" spelled backward); it is defined as the reciprocal of resistance (i.e., 1 divided by resistance). Therefore, resistance is also the reciprocal of conductance (1 divided by conductance). These are two scales for measuring the same phenomenon (see Table 4.4).

A newer term for micromhos (one millionth of a mho) is "microsiemens." This term appears in recent textbooks and is synonymous with "micromhos." This chapter continues to use "micromhos" because the older term is more familiar to most readers.

Although resistance and conductance scales measure the same property, there is a good reason to use the conductance measurement scale. Recall that as sweat glands turn "on," they add conductance pathways within the skin. This means that conductance increases in a linear relationship to the number of activated sweat glands. Resistance, on the other hand, decreases in a nonlinear fashion as more and more sweat glands are activated. This is shown graphically in Figure 4.18.

The linear relationship between sweat gland activity and skin conductance is statistically preferable for scaling and quantification. This is why skin conductance is now the standard unit. There are times (e.g., when one is using Ohm's law or testing electrodes) when it is more convenient to think in terms of resistance rather than conductance. Once the relationship between these two scales is understood, shifting from one scale to the other presents no problem.

Speaking of scales and measurement, note that skin conductance is not a direct measure of sweat gland activity (i.e., how many are turned on). Rather, it is an *indirect* measure that, except for artifact, correlates highly with sweat gland activity. That is, conductance is an electrical concept, not a physiological concept; it is not a direct measure of how many sweat glands are in operation.

Because skin conductance results only when an electrical voltage is imposed from outside, the measurement apparatus is inextricably tied into the skin conductance phenomena and contributes heavily to the observations. For the technically inclined, skin resistance or skin conductance biofeedback instruments are designed to be ohm-measuring or mho-measuring meters.

TABLE 4.4. Correspondence between Conductance and Resistance

Conductance	Resistance
Units	
Mho	Ohm
Micromho (millionth)	Megohm (million)
Conversion formulas	
Conductance = 1/resistance	Resistance = 1/conductance
Mho = 1/ohm	Ohm = 1/mho
Micromho = 1/megohm	Megohm = 1/micromho

Sample correspondences

1 micromho ~ 1 megohm
10 micromhos ~ .1 megohm
100 micromhos ~ .01 megohm

Range of skin conductance values

Approx. 0.5 micromho to 50 micromhos	Approx. 0.02 megohm to 2 megohms

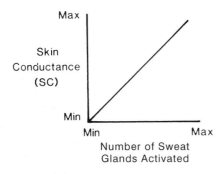
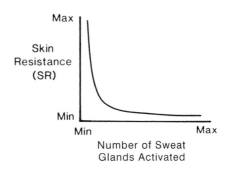

FIGURE 4.18. Comparison of skin conductance (left) and resistance (right) scales.

As such, they objectively measure whatever electrical equivalent network is presented to their inputs. They are characterized in part by the means of applying electrical excitation to the skin—either a steady-state voltage (DC) or an alternating voltage (AC)—and by their readout in either ohms or mhos. If a calibrated readout is provided, calibration is usually done by presenting a known value or values of simple electrical resistors and by verifying that the unit displays those values to within the specified accuracy of the instrument.

The problem is that skin presents a far more complex electrical network than simple calibration resistors. Sweat glands are not uniformly distributed in skin tissue, so sensing sites and electrode surface areas affect readings. If DC current loops are used, electrode material may be very important, because voltage may accumulate at the skin–electrode interfaces, which then act like tiny batteries and influence the readings. This is called "electrode polarization" and is discussed later. The use of silver/silver chloride electrodes will minimize but not eliminate this artifact. If AC current loops are used, polarization effects are minimized, but "reactive" components of the electrical equivalent network of the skin will cause an apparent increase in skin conductance. (These and other artifacts are discussed in a later section.) Finally, the electrical resistance of skin tissue may vary with the magnitude of the current in the current loop.

In summary, biofeedback users should not assume that each other's or published quantified SCA readings are actually comparable. Specifications of the conditions outlined above (plus the technical knowledge required to interpret the effects of these conditions) are necessary in order to compare SCA readings from different contexts.

Parameters of SCA

The hypothetical 20-second SCA record in Figure 4.19 yields three primary and two secondary parameters. Similar descriptions of measurement and typical waveforms appear in Stern, Ray, and Quigley (2001).

Primary Parameters

SCL or Tonic Level. SCL expressed in micromhos represents a baseline or resting level. Although this level may change, in a resting, quiescent person it is likely to hover around a value identified as the tonic level. SCL or tonic level is thought to be an index of baseline level of sweat gland activity, an inferred indication of a relative level of sympathetic arousal. For example, conductance values above 5–10 micromhos are thought to be relatively high, whereas those below 1 micromho are thought to be low. Remember that these estimates depend on a number of other variables and should be taken only as a rule of thumb based on the use of $3/8$-inch dry electrodes on the volar surface of fingertips.

SCR or Phasic Changes. Phasic changes are noticeable episodes of increased conductance caused by sympathetic arousal generated by a stimulus. For example, in the case of the stimulus introduced after 5 seconds, there is a 1- or 2-second delay and then an increase in conductance that peaks, levels out, and falls back to the baseline or tonic level. This is a phasic change, and its magnitude (height) is expressed as the number of micromhos reached above baseline. The size of phasic changes is thought to be an indication of the degree of arousal caused by stimuli (e.g., a startle or orientation to novel internal or external stimulus).

SCR Half-Recovery Time. "SCR half-recovery time" is defined as the time elapsed from the peak of the phasic change to *one-half* of the way back down to baseline. SCR half-recovery time is thought to be an index of a person's ability to calm down after a transitory excitation. It has been hypothesized that persons with chronic overarousal may have difficulty returning to relaxed baselines after even minor stimulation.

Secondary Parameters

"SCR latency" is defined as the time from stimulus onset until the beginning of an SCR. "SCR rise time" is defined as the time elapsed from the beginning of an SCR to its peak. These parameters have carried little significance in biofeedback, and therefore they are not discussed in detail here.

Normative Values for the Parameters

The hypothetical SCA record in Figure 4.19 shows specific values for the parameters. These values are actual mean values taken from normative samples of SCA records for tropical nonpatients, summarized in Venables and Christie (1980). However, these are not necessarily representative of values obtainable in ordinary biofeedback practice. Since large individual differences in SCL and SCR are common, readings far different from those cited in Figure 4.19 should come as no surprise. Furthermore, potential sources of normative variation include differences between patient and nonpatient groups, the effects of medications on SCL and SCR, differing procedures for establishing baselines and especially SCRs, and the great differences in instruments and electrodes likely to be used. For a discussion of the effects of such variables as temperature, humidity, time of day, or season, see Venables and Christie (1973, 1980).

My advice to you, the reader, is this: To increase your confidence in norms, find or build normative samples specific to the instruments you are using and to the populations you are working with. At this time, there is no solid substitute for systematically accumulated experience with your own patient group, purposes, and equipment. This is not meant to be discouraging to the clinician or disparaging to the field; it is only a reflection of the present state of the art.

Scales and Measurement: The "Percentage Increase" Scale for SCR Amplitude

Displaying SCR amplitude as an increase in the number of micromhos is not the only alternative. SCR amplitude can also be expressed as a percentage change from the tonic level. For

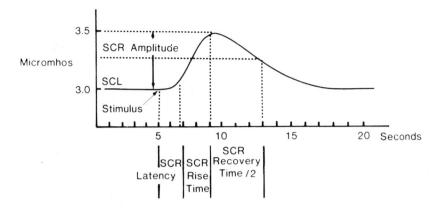

FIGURE 4.19. Parameters of skin conductance. (SCA values shown are taken from Venables & Christie, 1980.)

example, an SCR consisting of a 1-micromho change from 3 to 4 micromhos is expressed as a 33% change. This has the effect of "relativizing" the SCR to the baseline from which it occurs. With this method, a change from 6 to 8 micromhos is also a 33% change, and so is a change from 1.5 to 2 micromhos.

The rationale for this scale is the assumption that a given increase in autonomic arousal leads to a given percentage increase in conductance over the baseline level, and that this holds for all baseline levels. The following hypothetical examples and the electrical model of the skin illustrate this. Imagine that 200 sweat glands are turned on, giving an SCL of 2 micromhos. Now a stimulus comes along that turns on an additional 100 sweat glands, thus leading to a 1-micromho or a 50% increase. Now imagine another case in which there are 600 sweat glands turned on for an SCL of 6 micromhos. According to the percentage model, a stimulus with the same arousing properties as in the first case will lead again to a 50% increase in conductance by turning on an additional 300 sweat glands, for a 3–micromho increase in conductance.

The assumption here is that changes in arousal are better gauged as percentage increases in conductance over existing baselines than as absolute increases in conductance with no regard to initial baselines. This is analogous in the economic domain to expressing a year's growth in the gross domestic product as a percentage increase over the previous year's level, rather than as an increase in the number of dollars.

Loudness perception also provides an analogy: Achieving a given increase in perceived loudness takes a larger absolute increase in loudness above a noisy background level than above a quiet background level. If an SCR is some sort of "orienting response," it is plausible that to be psychophysiologically "noticeable," a stimulus must lead to a significant increase in conductance relative to existing baseline arousal—parallel to what occurs in loudness perception.

Pitch perception supplies a third analogy. The difference in pitch between the note C and the note A above it sounds the same in any octave. (It is the musical interval of a sixth.) The difference between middle C (256 hertz) and the A above it (440 hertz) is 184 hertz, a 72% increase in frequency. The difference between the next C (512 hertz) and the next A (880 hertz) is 368 hertz, but it is also a 72% increase in frequency. In this case, the percentage increase in frequency, rather than the number of vibrations per second, leads to the perception of equal increases in pitch.

The absolute-micromho increase scale for SCR amplitude rests on an assumption opposite to that of the percentage increase scale: Namely, a micromho increase in conductance indicates a given increment in arousal, no matter where it is observed on the continuum of

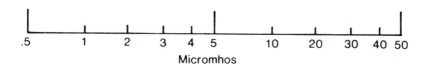

FIGURE 4.20. Logarithmic scale for SCA values.

possible initial baselines—a fixed increment of arousal, regardless of initial baseline. This assumption is also plausible.

There are, to my knowledge, no published data or definitive conceptual arguments to support or disconfirm either of the assumptions presented above. Each of these scales has plausibility and appeal, and it is apparently yet to be discovered whether either has distinct practical advantages or greater psychophysiological appropriateness. However, I prefer the assumptions supporting the use of the percentage increase scale for SCR amplitude. This is because the method of relating the magnitude of changes to initial baselines is appropriate and useful in perceptual contexts that to me are analogous to SCR. In addition, my informal observations suggest that persons with low SCL baselines often show fewer micromhos of SCR than persons with average SCL baselines. For me, intrinsic plausibility and these informal observations tip the balance toward the percentage increase scale for SCR amplitude. However, at very high SCLs, the percentage increase scale probably loses appropriateness, because most of the available sweat glands are already turned on to make the high SCLs.

Convenient scaling follows from the percentage increase scale assumption. If the skin conductance continuum is plotted along a line, a logarithmic scale conveniently contains all possible SCL values while retaining a useful degree of resolution for SCRs all along the line. This scale is illustrated in Figure 4.20. It has the advantage of providing adequate resolution at the low end while avoiding excessive resolution at the high end. Recall that the percentage increase scale supposes that the difference between 1 and 2 micromhos is more significant than the difference between 10 and 11 micromhos, and is equivalent to the difference between 10 and 20 micromhos. On the logarithmic scale, equal distances along the line represent equal percentage changes. That is, the distance from 1 to 2 is the same as that from 10 to 20; both are 100% changes. This means that an SCR amplitude of any given percentage is represented by the same distance along the line, regardless of initial baseline.

Skin Conductance Record Interpretation

The three primary parameters discussed earlier help professionals describe actual skin conductance records and extract data from them. But because records usually contain compounded changes in both responses and levels, interpretation is often required to specify values for the parameters. Below are paradigmatic descriptions of complex skin conductance records and interpretive hypotheses.

Upward Tonic Level Shift

The sample record in Figure 4.21 reveals a phasic change away from the beginning tonic level and incomplete return to that level. Think of this as an SCR that did not recover and led to a

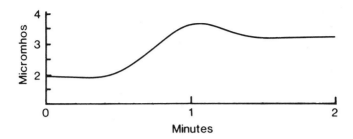

FIGURE 4.21. Upward tonic level shift.

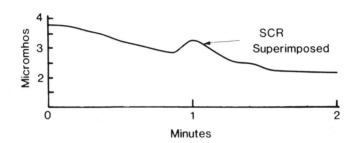

FIGURE 4.22. Downward tonic level shift.

new and higher tonic level from which subsequent phasic changes depart. A hypothesis is that whatever arousal led to the phasic change did not completely "wear off," thereby leaving the person with a new and elevated tonic level. Increase in conductance may be slow like "drift," rather than rapid like a typical SCR.

Downward Tonic Level Shift

The arousal leading to the new or elevated tonic level discussed above may in time "wear off" or be "relaxed away," leading to a downward trend in skin conductance. As shown in Figure 4.22, this record has downward slope to it, although SCRs may be superimposed. In this way, a new lower tonic level may eventually be reached.

Stairstepping

With multiple excitatory stimuli, especially for persons who show high-magnitude phasic changes and slow recovery time, a phenomenon called "stairstepping" may occur. As shown in Figure 4.23, this results when an excitatory stimulus occurs before the phasic changes from previous stimuli have had time to return to the prior tonic level. The SCA may then "stairstep" higher and higher. This stairstepping process could theoretically be implicated in development of overarousal. Figure 4.24 illustrates how individuals who show lower magnitude phasic changes and more rapid return to baseline are less susceptible to stairstepping from repeated stimulation.

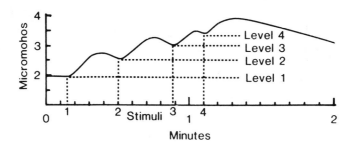

FIGURE 4.23. Stairstepping.

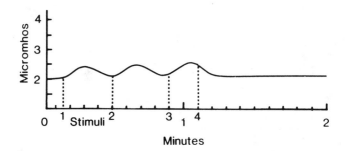

FIGURE 4.24. Rapid return to baseline, reducing stairstepping.

Nonresponsive Pattern

A "nonresponsive pattern" is an unusually flat conductance level (see Figure 4.25), which does not respond to typically arousing stimuli even when there is a reason to believe that arousal or emotion is or should be present. A hypothesis for this pattern, when extreme, is inappropriate detachment, overcontrol, or helplessness rather than relaxation (Toomin & Toomin, 1975).

Optimal Skin Conductance Patterns

Skin conductance is linked to arousal, but optimal SCA patterns are not necessarily the lowest or flattest patterns. This is because persistent minimal arousal, overcontrol, inattention, or flattened affect is not usually considered healthy or adaptive. There is a time for minimizing arousal during deep relaxation, in which a steady, low level of skin conductance may be desired, but uniformly invariant or flat levels are not necessarily desirable.

For example, encountering a novel stimulus calls for recognizing and treating it appropriately. Habitual blunting of the arousal associated with orientation or action is not thought to be healthy or adaptive. However, after a person orients to the novel stimulus and takes appropriate action, arousal should drop to baseline levels, avoiding unnecessary arousal or wasted energy. It is possible for a person to react too vigorously to novel stimuli, so that the reaction is out of proportion. In this case, the person is treating stimuli as more alarming, dangerous, or exciting than warranted, and is paying a price in energy and physical tension.

SCA is not something to be minimized but something to be optimized, and this requires judgment about what is appropriate for a given person in a given circumstance. At this time, no one claims to know optimum tonic levels and SCRs, or to be able to show that there is any

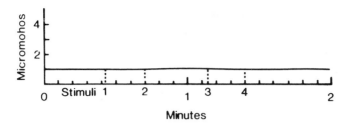

FIGURE 4.25. Nonresponsive pattern.

such thing as specifiable optimums. What is clear is that it is possible to have overreaction and underreaction, and that this holds for both the tonic levels and phasic changes. Quick return to baseline after an SCR may be consistently desirable except when it is part of an underresponsive pattern.

Because of large individual differences in SCA patterns and the lack of normative data under various standard paradigms of stimulation and measurement, it is difficult to specify clear and widely accepted procedures for relaxation training with SCA. Useful SCA biofeedback requires experience and judgment on the part of the clinician. The best way to acquire the "feel" of how SCA works under various conditions is to observe it within and between individuals, especially oneself. Those who work regularly with SCA are often quick to point out its ambiguities and uncertainties, but, undiscouraged, are also eager to discuss its unique responsiveness to transitory emotional states and thoughts. Its apparent complexity and ambiguity may conceal a wealth of valuable psychological as well as physiological information to those who have the patience to learn and further describe its patterns.

Operation of the Skin Conductance Instrument

Most Basic Constant DC Voltage Scheme

Figure 4.26 shows the *most* basic SCA monitoring scheme. A constant voltage is impressed across the two electrodes. The variable resistance of the skin leads to a variable current through the circuit. A current amplifier monitors this current, and, through proper scaling, drives a

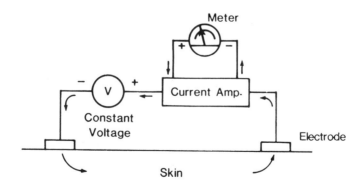

FIGURE 4.26. Most basic SCA monitoring scheme.

meter that reads out in micromhos. In this most basic form, it is similar to temperature instruments as shown in Figure 4.15. However, to be practical, it must be refined.

Adjustable Viewing "Window"

SCL baselines are spread over a wide range, yet it is important to distinguish small SCRs (e.g., a 5% change from any SCL) from all possible baselines. If the entire range of possible SCA values were made to fit on a meter face, SCL values would show, but an SCR would barely deflect the needle. Figure 4.27 illustrates how a 5% SCR from a 1-micromho SCL would be barely discernible. It would take a much larger SCR to move the needle enough to accurately gauge SCR amplitude and recovery time. This is the familiar issue of "resolution," discussed earlier in connection with temperature biofeedback instruments. A digital meter overcomes resolution problems simply by having enough digits (e.g., tenths or even hundredths). However, a digital meter is not suitable for observing SCRs, because changing digits during an SCR are hard to read. In contrast, the swing of a meter needle or light bar up and then back down is much more meaningful for SCRs.

A common solution to this problem is to use an analog meter for SCR display, but to restrict its range to form a "viewing window" that looks on only a portion of the SCA continuum. Of course, this "window" must be movable to any part of the SCA continuum, so an SCR can be monitored regardless of initial baseline SCL. This is shown graphically in Figure 4.28. The "window," which looks upon a small portion of the SCA range, is expanded on the entire meter scale. This way, small SCRs result in significant meter deflections. The center zero point on the meter in the figure represents the center of the window. The meter scale is calibrated so that the extent of the needle swing indicates the percentage change from a starting baseline.

In the illustration, the meter is calibrated for a +50% or −50% change. The user operates a calibrated control that moves the window up and down the SCA continuum until the SCL of the person being monitored "comes into view." If this level is approached from the left, the needle will remain off scale to the right until the window moves over the SCL. Once the SCL is in view, the needle falls back to the left as the window moves toward the center zero point. With the needle at zero, the window is centered over the person's SCL. The SCL value is read off a digitally calibrated control that moves the window up and down the SCA continuum. When an SCR occurs, the meter needle moves upward. At maximum deflection, the needle points to the percentage change. The digital control remains in place during SCRs, so it "remembers" the starting SCL baseline. If a person's SCL changes a lot or "drifts," the

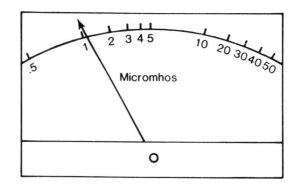

FIGURE 4.27. Lack of resolution when entire SCA range is squeezed onto a meter face.

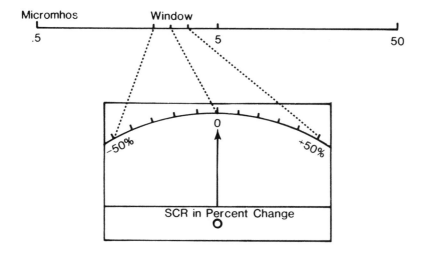

FIGURE 4.28. Movable viewing window.

user moves the window along the SCA continuum with the digital control. The SCL is kept "in view," and the digital control indicates the new baseline. If a computer is used, equivalent functions can be programmed to occur automatically.

To reduce how often the window must be moved to keep the SCL reading on scale, some instruments have adjustable window "widths" or choice of resolution. A very wide window width (e.g., 100% change) will cover more of the SCA continuum and hence will require readjustment less often during periods of SCL drift or for very large SCRs. Wider windows also reduce resolution. That is, small SCRs will be less pronounced on the meter scale. When a very stable SCL with very small SCRs is being observed, switching to a narrow window width (e.g., ±10%) expands small changes on the meter face, thus increasing visual resolution of the response.

Electrical Operation of the Movable Viewing Window

Figure 4.29 shows a skin conductance instrument with a movable viewing window. The constant-voltage source feeds two current loops. First is the familiar loop through the electrodes and skin, described earlier. The second loop is identical, except that a calibrated variable resistance (or variable conductance) takes the place of the electrodes and skin. In each loop, a current-to-voltage amplifier produces an output voltage proportional to the current through its loop.

Whenever current flow through the loops is equal, the outputs of the amplifiers are equal. Whenever the current flow through the loops is unequal, the outputs of the loop amplifiers are unequal in proportion to the difference in loop current flow. A meter measures the difference between the two loop amplifier outputs. This meter has a needle that is normally at rest in the center of the scale, pointing to zero. When current through the loops is equal, the outputs of the amplifiers are equal, and the needle remains at rest in the center, pointing to zero. When current through the loops is unequal, the meter needle will swing left or right, depending on which loop has the greater current. The extent of the deflection indicates the magnitude of the difference in current through the loops and reads out in percentage. The meter measures only *differences* in current flow in the two loops. The reader may notice the similarity between this circuit and the differential amplifier discussed in the EMG section.

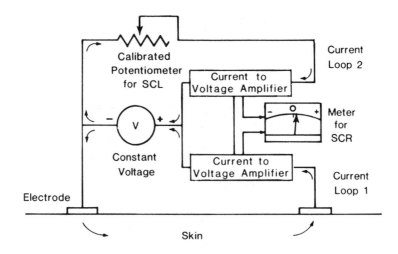

FIGURE 4.29. Skin conductance device with movable viewing window.

The user adjusts the control (the variable conductance) so that the meter balances at its zero point. This means that current through the loops is equal. This, in turn, means that the micromho value set on the control equals the person's SCL. Now suppose an SCR comes along. Skin conductance increases, but the calibrated control remains at the same position (i.e., at a value that equals the previous SCL). Because skin conductance has just increased over the previous level, current flow through the loops is unequal, and the meter deflects to the right in proportion to SCR magnitude. The needle points to the percent increase above the SCL shown on the calibrated control. As recovery from the SCR takes place, the needle moves back toward its center balance point, where loop currents are equal.

This is how the viewing window is electrically moved along the SCA continuum to accommodate any person's baseline SCL. Changing window width is accomplished electrically by changing the "gain" or sensitivity of the current-to-voltage amplifiers, so that a given difference in loop current leads to greater or lesser meter deflections. This is why the window width switch is usually called a "sensitivity control," though "resolution control" would be a better term for it. Audio feedback follows SCR, shifting along with the viewing window.

The previous section illustrates the basic design. Filtering or smoothing can be used to minimize the need to manually readjust the position of the viewing window as SCA drifts to a much different baseline SCL. (Smoothing and filtering have been discussed in the section on EMG.)

Simple SCR Devices

Simple SCR devices use a manual, noncalibrated baseline adjustment and feed back SCR with an audio tone or noncalibrated meter scale. These devices quantify neither SCL nor SCR and are more susceptible to artifact than full-sized instruments. Even so, they are very convenient and provide very interesting and useful information to a person about patterns of SCR.

For example, the rise and fall of an audio tone communicates a great deal about the person's responsivity in actual situations, even when quantified SCL or SCR is absent. These devices have distinct advantages when it comes to ambulatory use in real life. Pocket-sized miniaturization, dry finger electrodes, and an earplug for private feedback permit a person to wear the unit conveniently while walking, talking, driving, phoning, writing, thinking, reading, or carrying out other real activities. This provides insight into patterns of responsivity in active situations that are not obtainable in the clinic setting. It is a very good way for a person (including the therapist!) to discover his or her own patterns of responsivity. In any application, the therapist involved must provide adequate instruction in the use and limitations of the device and in the interpretation of results.

Artifact

There are many ways to process and display SCA, and there is no firm consensus on the most appropriate way to do it. Historically, the most common method is probably the one shown in Figure 4.29, with a manual calibrated baseline control and an analog zero center meter for SCR. Simple SCR devices certainly have a useful place in clinical biofeedback, even though quantitative measurements are usally not possible. The following points about artifact are important for all SCA devices.

Electrode Size. Different-sized electrodes lead to different readings. A larger electrode covers more skin and therefore places more sweat glands in the current loop. This leads to a higher SCL than does a smaller electrode that places fewer sweat glands in the loop. Therefore, electrode size must be standardized in order to assure comparability of quantified SCL readings.

Movement. Because electrode size affects SCA, anything that alters the effective contact area of an electrode also alters SCA. Finger or hand movement causes variations in contact pressure. The electrode may lift slightly and diminish the contact area, or press harder against the skin and increase the contact area. These effects are more pronounced for dry electrodes than for precious-metal electrodes with electrode gel. The practitioner should encourage the monitored person to minimize hand movements and arrange the electrodes and cables for a reasonably stable position. When hand movement cannot be avoided (e.g., monitoring while the person is doing something with both hands), corresponding sites on the toes could be used. This would require exploring new norms for SCL and SCR on those sites. Fortunately, movement artifact is usually easy to spot, because the resultant patterns are often abrupt and uncharacteristic of true SCA patterns, and because movement can often be observed.

Skin Condition. Skin condition can affect conductance readings. For example, if a person has a skin abrasion or a fresh cut through the high-resistance skin surface, a high-conductance path may be established from the electrode to deeper layers of the skin and lead to an increased SCL. If a person has developed a callus, the high-resistance surface layer increases in thickness and dryness, leading to a much lower SCL and diminished SCR amplitude. Venables and Christie (1980) note that SCL falls markedly after a washing with soap and water, as residual salt is removed. Because salt builds up over time since the last wash, they recommend that persons begin sessions with freshly washed hands. It is not clear how important this is to clinical biofeedback, but it is clear that this standardizing procedure is not universally followed.

Room Temperature. There is some evidence (Venables & Christie, 1980) that SCA is affected when individuals feel cold, and that warmer-than-usual office conditions appear to produce what they call more "normal" responsivity. It is also plausible that the temperature-regulating function of sweating in an overly warm room leads to increases in SCL that are not psychophysiologically significant.

Electrode Polarization Potentials and Electrode Design. The exosomatic method involves the passage of current through the skin via surface electrodes. Polarization potentials develop at the skin–electrode interface as DC passes, and the polarization effect builds up over time. The size of polarization potential is variable and unknown. EDA units have historically varied widely in their susceptibility to the effects of electrode polarization. But in general, this is probably not a major problem, especially with DC instruments that apply very small electrical currents to the skin. Nevertheless, biofeedback clinicians who are interested in EDA and the devices that have been employed to assess it over the years should probably be aware of the issues concerning electrode polarization and methods that have been used to minimize it. A somewhat technical discussion of this follows.

Dry electrodes are often used for EDA. They are made from various materials, including lead, zinc, chrome, stainless steel, gold, or silver-coated fuzz, and are often secured by Velcro straps that conveniently adjust to different finger sizes. They are simpler, cheaper, and more convenient than silver/silver chloride electrodes, especially in clinical practice. However, when used with DC EDA equipment, the simple dry electrodes suffer from polarization potentials to various degrees.

When polarized, the skin–electrode interface is like a tiny battery charged by the passing current. Polarization voltage is thereby added to (or subtracted from) the constant voltage applied by the instrument. Because the polarization potential (voltage) is variable, the voltage in the current loop is no longer constant. Therefore, what appear to be changes in SCL may be due in part to variable electrode polarization potentials. Drift in skin conductance level due to the buildup of polarization potential causes artifact, but this effect may not be all that significant, for practical purposes. Nevertheless, silver/silver chloride electrodes have sometimes been used, because they develop minimal polarization potentials and therefore add minimal polarization artifact. But they are more expensive and less convenient than dry electrodes, and the gel used with silver/silver chloride electrodes may prolong the recovery phase of SCRs. A similar prolongation may occur in very humid climates even when dry electrodes are used. Artifactual prolongation of SCR recovery could lead to results mistakenly interpreted as "stairstepping."

Use of AC to control electrode polarization artifact. Instrument designs have been evolved to circumvent the effects of polarization potentials. The most obvious way to minimize electrode polarization artifact in EDA equipment is to use an AC voltage source rather than the DC voltage source described earlier. Using AC in the current loop helps in two ways. First, the constantly reversing polarity of AC first charges and then discharges the electrode–skin interface "battery," thus reducing the buildup of polarization voltage. Second, any remaining polarization voltage is blocked by capacitors in the current loop. Capacitors permit only the AC to pass. This is illustrated in Figure 4.30.

A "capacitor" is an electronic component with conductive plates separated by an insulating membrane. Alternating attraction and repulsion of charges across the insulating membrane

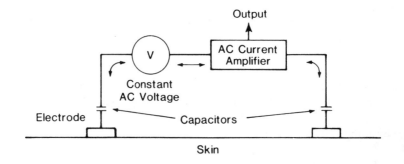

FIGURE 4.30. AC current loop with DC-blocking capacitors.

permits AC to pass through a capacitor. No current actually flows through the membrane. This can be illustrated by analogy. Imagine a fluid-filled cylinder fitted with an elastic diaphragm in the middle and an opening at each end (Figure 4.31). If the fluid pressure at opening A is greater than at B, then fluid flows into the cylinder at A and bulges the membrane, forcing fluid out through opening B. If the pressure diminishes, the membrane begins to move back to its original position as fluid returns to the cylinder through opening B and the same amount of fluid leaves through opening A. If pressure at A continues to drop, then more fluid leaves through opening A; the membrane bulges to the left, drawing fluid into the cylinder through opening B. So long as there is a cycle of pressure changes at A, then there will be a corresponding cycle of changes at B. This is analogous to how a capacitor passes AC.

However, suppose that a modest unchanging pressure is introduced at A. The membrane bulges a little and then stops. Fluid flows from A only while the pressure is building and the membrane is in motion. After it stops in a bulged position, no more fluid moves at B. This is analogous to how a capacitor blocks DC.

This analogy shows how a capacitor blocks small residual DC polarization potentials in an AC loop while passing the AC unrestricted. This does remove polarization potential artifact. However, it generates another kind of artifact, which is probably more of a problem. It turns out that the skin itself forms a capacitor. Although this fact is of no consequence when a constant DC voltage is used, as in the designs described earlier, it does become a significant factor when AC is used. Figure 4.32 shows the location of this natural capacitor.

Skin capacitance forms a second "reactive" pathway for AC in the current loop. If AC is applied to the skin, a portion of the current flows as usual through the diminished resistance of the activated sweat glands, but some additional current flows through the skin capacitance. This means that total current flow is greater (and the readings show greater SCL). This effect can be quite pronounced and cannot be neglected. A note for the technically inclined is that an AC measurement in which skin capacitance contributes to the reading should be called "skin impedance" (analogous to resistance) or "skin admittance" (analogous to conductance).

To make matters worse, impedance or admittance varies with the frequency of the AC, because higher frequencies pass through a capacitor more easily than lower frequencies. The reader need not worry, because there are still other ways to minimize polarization artifact without generating capacitance artifacts. Explanation of these systems is beyond the scope of this chapter. Such systems have been commercially available and minimize these artifacts even when simple dry electrodes are used. A wise buyer who is very concerned about repeatable quantified SCL data inquires about how these artifacts are handled or avoided. As for the miniature SCR devices described earlier, their lack of quantification makes polarization artifact much less relevant than for instruments capable of quantification. Skin capacitance artifact is generally not an issue with the miniature devices, because they almost always use simple DC loops.

Safety

Electrical safety precautions for SCA devices are the same as for EMG devices. Both are electrically connected to the person via electrodes; therefore, the same stringent standards for

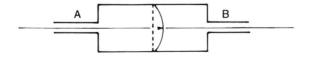

FIGURE 4.31. Fluid analogy to the capacitor.

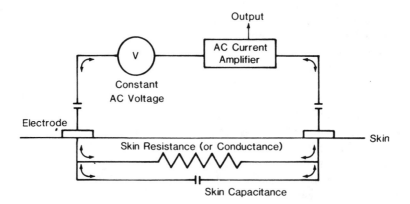

FIGURE 4.32. AC current loop and skin capacitance.

design, manufacture, installation, and maintenance should be followed for SCA and EMG devices, and for the entire installation of which any of these instruments are a part. The passage of DC from an electrode to the skin over a prolonged time may lead to the formation of chemical by-products on the skin if the voltage drop across the skin exceeds about 3 DC volts, such as might be encountered in "toy" or very early EDA gizmos (Leeming, Ray, & Howland, 1970). This effect is normally negligible, but if the current passed is high enough and is passed long enough, then skin irritation could develop. This effect is unlikely to occur in modern skin conductance instruments, but very old units, those that were made as novelties or toys, or those that have developed leakage currents may be more likely to create this effect. As a rule of thumb, a device that passes current of 10 microamperes or less per square centimeter of electrode area in its current loop, and applies under 3 DC volts to the skin, will not lead to the accumulation of irritating chemicals on the skin.

ACKNOWLEDGMENTS

My thanks go to the late Wallace A. Peek, the late Roland E. Mohr, and John B. Picchiottino, who have acted so generously as my engineering mentors. I give special thanks to John B. Picchiottino, whose suggestions for this chapter in its first edition marked a long and much-appreciated history of helpfulness with biofeedback projects. A special thanks must also go to Mark S. Schwartz, without whose enthusiasm the first edition's chapter and subsequent revisions would doubtless have remained on my list of things to do someday.

REFERENCES

Boucsein, W. (1992). *Electrodermal activity*. New York: Plenum Press.

Brown, B. (1974). *New mind, new body: New directions for the mind*. New York: Harper & Row.

Cacioppo, J. T., Tassinary, L. G., & Berntson, G. G. (Eds.). (2000). *Handbook of psychophysiology* (2nd ed.). New York: Cambridge University Press.

Dawson, M. E., Schell, A. M., & Filion, L. (2000). The electrodermal system. In J. T. Cacioppo, L. G. Tassinary, & G. G. Berntson (Eds.), *Handbook of psychophysiology* (2nd ed.). New York: Cambridge University Press.

Jennings, J. R., Tahmoush, A. J., & Redmond, D. D. (1980). Non-invasive measurement of peripheral vascular activity. In I. Martin & P. H. Venables (Eds.), *Techniques in psychophysiology* (pp. 70–131). New York: Wiley.

Leeming, M. N., Ray, C., & Howland, W. S. (1970). Low-voltage, direct-current burns. *Journal of the American Medical Association, 214*(9), 1681–1684.

Mathieu, P. A., & Sullivan, S. J. (1990). Frequency characteristics of signals and instrumentation: Implication for EMG biofeedback studies. *Biofeedback and Self-regulation*, *15*(4), 335–352.

Neumann, E., & Blanton, R. (1970). The early history of electrodermal research. *Psychophysiology*, *8*(4), 463–474.

Otis, J., Rasey, H., Vrochopoulos, S., Wincze, J., & Andrasik, F. (1995). Temperature acquisition as a function of the computer-based biofeedback system utilized: An exploratory analysis. *Biofeedback and Self-Regulation*, *20*(2), 185–190.

Stern, R. M., Ray, W. J., & Quigley, K. S. (2001). *Psychophysiological recording* (2nd ed.). New York: Oxford University Press.

Toomin, M., & Toomin, H. (1975, February). *Psychological dynamic correlates of the paradoxically invariant GSR*. Paper presented at the Fifth Annual Convention of the Biofeedback Research Society, Monterey, CA.

Venables, P. H., & Christie, M. J. (1973). Mechanisms, instrumentation, recording techniques, and quantification of responses. In W. F. Prokasy & D. C. Raskin (Eds.), *Electrodermal activity in psychological research*. New York: Academic Press.

Venables, P. H., & Christie, M. J. (1980). Electrodermal activity. In I. Martin & P. H. Venables (Eds.), *Techniques in psychophysiology* (pp. 3–67). New York: Wiley.

A Primer of Electroencephalographic Instrumentation

NICOLA NEUMANN

UTE STREHL

NIELS BIRBAUMER

Understanding *electroencephalography* (EEG) and EEG instrumentation requires a basic knowledge of the recorded parameters. This chapter begins with a description of *event-related potentials*, the main EEG frequency bands, and their behavioral significance. EEG instrumentation proper is then elucidated, with a particular emphasis on biofeedback practitioners' interests and questions. (Italics on first use of a term in text indicate that the term is included in the glossary at the end of this chapter.)

NEUROPHYSIOLOGICAL BASIS OF THE EEG AND BEHAVIORAL CORRELATES

The EEG results from the summation of excitatory and inhibitory *postsynaptic potentials* (PSPs) in the *pyramidal cells* of the upper layers of the cerebral cortex, with some contribution of granular and *glia cell* activity (for reviews, see Creutzfeldt, 1974; Lopes da Silva, 1991; Speckmann & Elger, 1999). Extracellular current flow associated with such postsynaptic activity leads to large field potentials that can be recorded on the surface of the scalp (see Figure 5.1).

The EEG rhythms are defined as regularly recurring waveforms of similar shape and duration. They are of cortical origin, but subcortical structures (particularly the *thalamus*) contribute to their special characteristics. The dominant EEG frequency bands are called *alpha* (8–13 hertz [Hz]), *beta* (13–30 Hz), *gamma* (30–100 Hz), *theta* (4–7 Hz), and *delta* (0.5–4 Hz). In addition, direct current (DC) shifts of less than 1 Hz are referred to as *slow cortical potentials*.

EEG Synchronization and Desynchronization

Generally, the normal adult waking EEG can be classified into two main patterns. The synchronized EEG pattern measured in a relaxed, eyes-closed state is characterized by rhythmic,

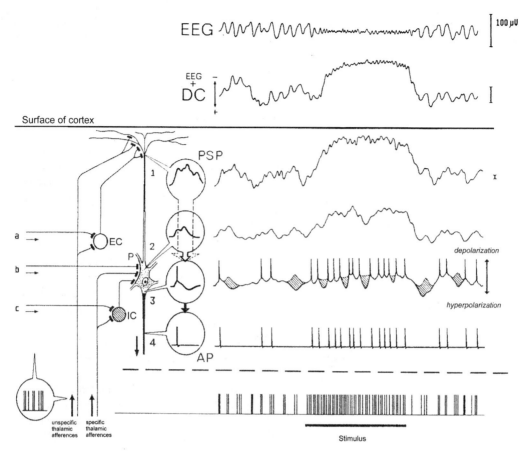

FIGURE 5.1. Summation of postsynaptic potentials (PSPs) as the potential source of the EEG. Afferent fibers (a, b, c,) are shown with connections to an excitatory nerve cell (EC), to a large pyramidal cell (P), and to an inhibitory nerve cell (IC). The course of the potential is depicted in the area of the apical dendrites (1), the basal dendrites (2), the axon hillock (3), and the axon (4). Action potentials (APs) become more frequent with the presentation of a stimulus. At the apical dendrites, the summation of excitatory PSPs leads to a negative direct current (DC) shift, which often does not pass filtering in the routine EEG. From Zschocke (1995). Copyright 1995 by Springer Verlag. Reprinted by permission.

high-amplitude, low-frequency activity, whereas the desynchronized pattern recorded during visual attention with eyes open is composed of irregular, lower-voltage, higher-frequency waves. The synchronization of the EEG, as recorded in the alpha band, results from oscillations in thalamic relay nuclei whose cells discharge rhythmically in bursts of high-frequency spikes. The mechanisms generating these oscillations are still a matter of controversy. Andersen and Andersson (1968) claimed that intrinsic properties of a thalamic network can lead to spindling with a main role for inhibitory interneurons; Steriade and Buzsáki (1990) postulated that neurons in the thalamic reticular nucleus possess pacemaker properties. The desynchronization (or acceleration) of the EEG corresponds to an enhancement of cortical activity (e.g., by sensory input) and to dissolution of the synchronized pacemakers. Thalamic and cortical neurons fire in a tonic mode, implying sustained and high spontaneous activity (Glenn & Steriade, 1982). This variable discharge pattern with a low synchronization between cells is the reason why EEG electrodes, which summate the electrical activity of many cells, only record small but irregular and fluctuating waves. Desynchronization is caused by activation of the reticular formation, which in turn leads to the disinhibition of specific thalamic relay nuclei accompanied by increased diffuse excitatory projections onto the cortex.

Event-Related EEG Changes

Changes in the activity of neuronal populations time-locked to a specific event, such as a sensory stimulus, are traditionally studied via event-related potentials (ERPs). These are deflections in the EEG that have a fixed time delay to the stimulus, while the ongoing EEG activity behaves as additive noise. To detect ERPs, averaging techniques are used. An averaged ERP is composed of a series of large, biphasic waves, lasting a total of 500 to 1000 milliseconds (ms). Generally, the ERP is subdivided into early and late components, with the boundary drawn at about 100 ms. The early components are mainly determined by the physical qualities of the stimulus (such as intensity and duration), while the late components are strongly influenced by endogenous factors (i.e., information-processing activities). Thus ERPs are employed to study human information processing under the assumption that a selective change in a specific ERP component might reveal a change in a specific cognitive process. An example is the P300, the positive deflection appearing about 300 ms after a rare, task-relevant stimulus is presented. It is associated with such cognitive operations as context updating (Donchin & Coles, 1988) or perceptual closure (Verleger, 1988).

However, the model assuming that an ERP can be represented by a signal added to uncorrelated noise is just an approximation of the real situation. Following a stimulus, there are additional ("induced" rather than evoked) changes in the EEG that are time-locked but not phase-locked, and that consequently cannot be detected by averaging, but must be determined by frequency analysis. These changes can be regarded as either decreases or increases of power in given frequency bands. Pfurtscheller and Aranibar (1977) called the decrease in synchrony of the underlying neuronal populations *event-related desynchronization* (ERD), and the increase in synchrony *event-related synchronization* (ERS) (for a review, see Pfurtscheller & Lopes da Silva, 1999). ERD/ERS phenomena following an external event can be observed in nearly every frequency band (Basar, Basar-Eroglu, Karakas, & Schürmann, 1999). In the remainder of this chapter, these oscillation changes and their behavioral correlates are not discussed further, because they require extensive filtering and computerized data analysis usually not available to the biofeedback practitioner.

Functional Correlates of Frequency Components

In this section, the main EEG frequency bands are described. Typical waveforms are depicted in Figure 5.2.

Alpha activity (8–13 Hz) is recorded over the posterior regions of the head, with higher voltage over the occipital areas. It is usually characterized by sinusoidal waveforms. Amplitudes of alpha waves vary considerably between individuals and wax and wane over time, but are mostly about or below 50 microvolts (μV) in adults. Alpha activity is associated with a state of physical calmness and the lack of visual/oculomotor activity. Stimulation (particularly visual) or mental effort can lead to its attenuation or suppression—a phenomenon referred to as "alpha blocking." "Alpha dropout" can be observed in the earliest stage of drowsiness, when alpha waves become more and more discontinuous, giving way to a low-voltage pattern in sleep stage 1. It can be concluded that alpha is highly dependent on vigilance and particularly related to the visual system. Enhanced alpha activity has also been observed during meditation and hypnosis (Anand, China, & Singh, 1961). As mentioned above, synchronized EEG activity such as the alpha rhythm was originally attributed to thalamocortical circuits

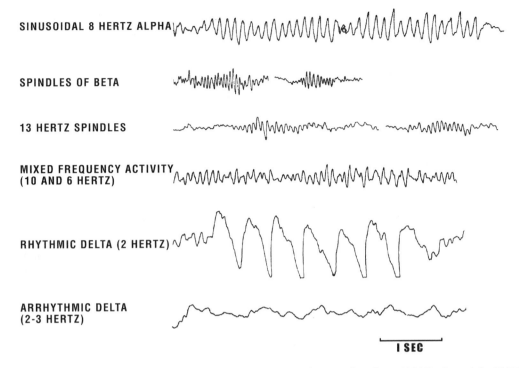

SINUSOIDAL 8 HERTZ ALPHA

SPINDLES OF BETA

13 HERTZ SPINDLES

MIXED FREQUENCY ACTIVITY
(10 AND 6 HERTZ)

RHYTHMIC DELTA (2 HERTZ)

ARRHYTHMIC DELTA
(2-3 HERTZ)

I SEC

FIGURE 5.2. Various waveforms in the human EEG. From Blume and Kaibara (1995). Copyright 1995 by Lippincott Williams & Wilkins. Reprinted by permission.

(Andersen & Andersson, 1968). However, more recent findings seem to indicate that the alpha rhythm is primarily cortical in origin. The results indicate that the alpha rhythm can be recorded both from the visual cortex and from visual thalamic (lateral geniculate and pulvinar) nuclei (Lopes da Silva, Van Lierop, Schrijer, & Storm van Leeuwen, 1973), and that the coherence between alpha rhythms recorded in adjacent foci of the visual cortex is larger than any thalamocortical coherences measured in the same animal (Lopes da Silva, Vos, Mooibroeck, & Van Rotterdam, 1980). Steriade (1999, p. 69) states in his review that "these data led to the conclusion that a system of surface-parallel intra-cortical connections is mainly involved in the spread of alpha activity, while the influence of visual thalamic nuclei over the cerebral cortex is only moderate."

Another rhythm in the alpha frequency band is the *rolandic mu rhythm*. It is located in the central (rolandic) region, and is best recorded with C_3 and C_4 electrodes (according to the *International 10-20 System*; see below). The mu rhythm is not present in every subject, but only visible in between 3% and 14% of subjects (see Niedermeyer, 1999b, p. 156), reaching values close to 100% when a frequency analysis is conducted (Schoppenhorst, Brauer, Freund, & Kubicki, 1980). The mu rhythm predominantly shows a sharp negative and a rounded positive compound, with a dominant frequency of 10 Hz. In contrast to the alpha rhythm, the mu rhythm does not block with eye opening, but with movement or intended movement of the contralateral extremity (ERD; see above). The desynchronization of the mu rhythm starts about 1–2 seconds (s) prior to movement onset, like the desynchronization of central beta rhythms (12–22 Hz; see below) (Pfurtscheller & Berghold, 1989). Sterman (1977) described a low-amplitude rhythm recorded from central locations between 12 and 15 Hz as "sensorimotor rhythm," which may be identical to mu. Pfurtscheller (1989) concludes that a variety of rhythms within the alpha and beta bands are attenuated when cortical structures become activated during either internal or external events, especially movements. After termination of the movements, these rhythms show a recovery within 1–3 s. Thus synchronization of these motor-related rhythms seems to indicate the immobilization or "idling" (Kuhlmann, 1978) of the pyramidal motor system.

Beta activity (13–30 Hz) represents the desynchronized state of the EEG recorded in a state of alertness or during active dreaming. It consists of a mixture of different low-amplitude frequencies. Beta activity is recorded mainly over frontal and central regions, with amplitudes seldom exceeding 30 μV. It can be differentiated according to its frequency and spatial characteristics (Niedermeyer, 1999b). Frontal beta is common and may be very fast (~30 Hz). Central beta is mixed with the rolandic mu rhythm (see above) and can be blocked by motor activity or tactile stimulation.

Gamma activity consists of synchronized, higher-frequency oscillations ranging from about 30 to 100 Hz. It can be recorded in widely distributed brain structures and appears to have specific cognitive and behavioral correlates (see reviews by Basar-Eroglu, Strüber, Schürmann, Stadler, & Basar, 1996; Tallon-Baudry & Bertrand, 1999). Different categories of gamma responses can be distinguished (Galambos, 1992). The 40-Hz transient evoked response is time-locked to external stimuli, such as auditory clicks or flashing lights (Basar, Rosen, Basar-Eroglu, & Greitschus, 1987; Pantev & Elbert, 1994). Another category of gamma oscillations is the induced gamma response (30–80 Hz), which consists of oscillatory bursts whose latency fluctuates from trial to trial. It has been observed in response to sensory stimuli and during motor tasks in a variety of experiments (e.g., Kaiser, Lutzenberger, Preissl, Ackermann, & Birbaumer, 2000; Lutzenberger, Pulvermüller, Elbert, & Birbaumer, 1995; Pulvermüller, Birbaumer, Lutzenberger, & Mohr, 1997; Pulvermüller, Keil, & Elbert, 1999); it is enhanced with increasing attention and during complex tasks (Basar-Eroglu, Strüber, Kruse, Basar, & Stadler, 1996). Gamma activity has been related to "binding" (i.e., the brain's ability to integrate different stimuli into a coherent whole). It is exclusively of cortical origin and indicates functional associative connections between cell assemblies, as suggested by Hebb (1949).

The frequency range from 4 to 8 Hz is referred to as theta activity. In early childhood (between 12 and 36 months of age), it is the basic rhythm of wakefulness over the posterior cortex. After the third year, it moves into the alpha range. Intermingled mild to moderate theta activity at posterior scalp locations is still seen in young adults until the age of 30. From that age on, posterior slow activity is only observed occasionally, except in sleep and pathological conditions. Schacter (1977) suggested that two different types of theta activity exist: one associated with drowsiness, and another frontally located theta rhythm associated with attention and alertness. The anterior theta in the range of 6–7 Hz over the frontal midline region has been recorded during mental tasks, such as problem solving (Mizuki, 1982; Mizuki, Tanaka, Isozaki, Nishijima, & Inanaga, 1980). Takahashi, Shinomiya, Mori, and Tachibana (1997) found the same theta rhythm during drowsiness in individuals who revealed this pattern during the performance of mental tasks. For this reason, Niedermeyer (1999b) suggested the possibility that the theta activity noted during drowsiness and mental tasks may be of the same origin, if it is assumed that the tasks are boring enough to induce light drowsiness instead of attention. Theta activity dominates the activity in the hippocampus in mammals, but it is controversial whether this hippocampal activity is related to frontal theta in humans (Steriade, Gloor, Llinás, Lopes da Silva, & Mesulam, 1990). Some experimental results have suggested that the master structure controlling at least one type of theta activity is the septohippocampal cholinergic system, driven from the brainstem reticular core (see Steriade, 1999).

The delta band comprises frequencies from 0.5 to 4 Hz. Thalamocortical relay neurons are involved in the generation of these high-voltage, low-frequency waves. Delta activity is associated with deep sleep in healthy humans, as well as with pathological conditions such as brain lesions. It is also commonly observed in human infants during the first 2 years of life (see Niedermeyer, 1999a).

Slow cortical potentials (*SCPs*) are changes in cortical polarization of the EEG lasting from 300 ms to several seconds. On the scalp, the amplitude of SCPs may vary from several microvolts (e.g., during cognitive tasks) to more than 100 μV during seizures. Functionally, SCPs reflect a threshold regulation mechanism for local excitatory mobilization. Negative SCP shifts, such as the "Bereitschaftspotential" (Kornhuber & Deecke, 1965) or contingent negative variation (Walter, Cooper, Aldridge, McCallum, & Winter, 1964), indicate local excitatory mobilization, whereas positive potential shifts indicate disfacilitation. A consistent relationship between cortical negativity on the one hand and reaction time, signal detection, and short-term memory performance on the other has been found in many studies of both humans and monkeys (Birbaumer, Elbert, Lutzenberger, Rockstroh, & Schwarz, 1981; Lutzenberger, Elbert, Rockstroh, & Birbaumer, 1979; Lutzenberger, Elbert, Rockstroh, & Birbaumer, 1982; Lutzenberger, Roberts, & Birbaumer, 1993; Rockstroh, Elbert, Lutzenberger, & Birbaumer, 1982). Tasks requiring attention are performed significantly better when presented during spontaneous or self-induced cortical negativity. Neurophysiologically, negative surface SCPs result from a sink caused by synchronous slow excitatory PSPs in the apical dendrites of layer I in the cortex with a source being located in layers IV and V. Surface positivities are less easy to explain, but may result from sinks in deeper layers or inhibitory sources in layer I.

EEG INSTRUMENTATION

Although procedures for recording EEG activity have been improved greatly over the past 20 years with the incorporation of computer-controlled and digital amplifiers, there is still a need to consider carefully how the EEG is recorded. Artifacts can occur at every step of the recording procedure, from the electrodes to the recording system, and interfering electrical potentials can be easily mistaken for the proper EEG signal. Specific problems are described in the "Artifacts" section, below.

Electrode Placement

The system of locating electrodes is referred to as the International 10-20 system (Jasper, 1958) and originally comprised 19 electrodes (see Figure 5.3). The name "10-20 System" derives from the fact that electrodes are placed at sites separated by 10% or 20% of the distance from one of four anatomical landmarks on the head to another. There are two landmarks at the front (the nasion, or bridge of the nose) and back (the inion, or bump at the back of the head), and two landmarks on the right and left sides (the preauricular points, or depressions in front of the ears above the cheekbones). Between each pair of these landmarks, electrode positions are determined by measuring distances that are 10% or 20% of the total distance between the landmarks. The standard numbering in the 10-20 System places odd-numbered electrodes on the left and even-numbered electrodes on the right, with a letter designating the anatomial area. Such electrode placement can be replicated consistently over time, as well as between laboratories. The American Electroencephalographic Society (1991) added electrode placement nomenclature guidelines that designate specific locations and identifications of 75 electrode positions. Which and how many electrodes are used depends very much on the research question or clinical considerations. For further information, see Reilly (1999).

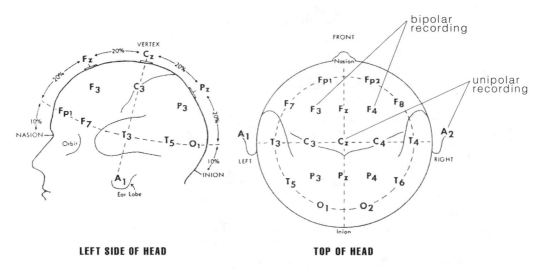

LEFT SIDE OF HEAD   TOP OF HEAD

FIGURE 5.3. International 10-20 System of electrode placement. In monopolar recording, one electrode site is (preferably) electrically silent, whereas in bipolar recording both sites are electrically active. From Blume and Kaibara (1995). Copyright 1995 by Lippincott Williams & Wilkins. Reprinted by permission.

The Issue of Electrode Reference

Since EEG potentials are always recorded as the voltage difference between two electrodes, one can distinguish between two types of recording, referred to as *monopolar* and *bipolar recording* (see Figure 5.3). In monopolar recording, the site of the reference is chosen in such a way that the corresponding electrode is preferably electrically silent. Common sites are the ear lobe, the mastoid (the prominence behind the ear), or the nose. The disadvantage of the ear reference is that it is contaminated by the temporobasal activity of the brain. Noncephalic reference sites have the disadvantage that they pick up more electrocardiographic and electromyographic (EMG) activity than do electrodes placed on the head. To avoid these disadvantages, the mathematical average of one electrode on each side of the head, or the electrically combined activity from two or more electrodes, is taken as a reference. Artifacts that might occur at the site of one single reference electrode are better controlled in this case. In the common average reference method, the average value of the entire electrode montage is taken as the reference. If the entire head is covered by equally spaced electrodes and the potential on the head is generated by point sources, the common average reference should result in a spatial voltage distribution with a mean of zero.

In bipolar recording, each electrode is located at an active site on the scalp. Therefore, bipolar recording is useful to compare the activity in corresponding electrodes of the two hemispheres or different locations within one hemisphere.

In EEG feedback, spatial and temporal filtering methods can increase the *signal-to-noise ratio*. Feeding back the 8- to 12-Hz mu rhythm, McFarland, McCane, David, and Wolpaw (1997) compared a conventional ear reference, a common average reference, and two different Laplacian derivations. With the *Laplacian method*, the value at each electrode location is calculated by subtracting the value at that location from the values of a set of surrounding electrodes. The common average reference and the large Laplacian derivation (a 6-centimeter circle of surrounding electrodes) showed maximum signal-to-noise ratio.

Signal Acquisition

Electrodes

Inside the tissue, electric charges are transported by ions (i.e., electrically charged atoms). These charges have to be transmitted to the recording system. For this transmission, a conductive electrolyte paste is required. The electrodes, which may be made out of different metals, are directly in contact with the electrolyte paste, and ions move across the boundary. Initially after the electrodes are fixed, electric charges move and generate an unstable signal. When a balance is reached, a charged double layer is formed between the electrolyte and the metal surface of the electrode. This corresponds to a DC voltage source, with the electric potential difference referred to as "electrode potential."

It is important that the electrode potential is stable after a few minutes; this should be the case if clean, nonpolarizable electrodes are used. The electrode potential should also be the same for all electrodes, and this presupposes that all electrodes are made of the same material. Disturbances of the potential gradient may be caused by alterations in temperature, by sweating, or by mechanical displacement of the electrodes (see below).

Electrode Application

Electrodes have to be attached very firmly. When one is recording SCPs, it is especially important to exclude slow potential shifts that derive from artifacts or polarization. A good *impedance* of less than 5 kiloohms can be obtained by removing oil, hair, and dead skin with alcohol, acetone, or an abrasive cream. An electrode paste (usually containing sodium chloride as the electrolyte) is applied to the skin under each electrode. A similar procedure is used with electrode helmets, in which a blunted needle is used to move the hair away from the electrode and a syringe-like device is used to inject electrode paste between the electrode and the scalp. The electrodes and instruments should be disinfected after each usage, to avoid the spread of pathogens between users.

Amplification and Filters

In modern amplifiers, only signal differences between the two inputs of the amplifier are processed. The main advantage is that technical noise, primarily caused by 60-Hz (in Europe, 50-Hz) household power and arriving at both amplifier inputs, is canceled. The common-mode rejection accomplishes the same purpose, excluding signals swinging in phase. Thus the *common-mode rejection ratio* constitutes a quality characteristic of amplifiers, being defined as the ratio between amplification of out-of-phase signals and (residual) amplification of in-phase signals.

It is important that the amplifier records all desired EEG frequencies from 0.01 up to 100 Hz. Most commercially available systems, however, cannot record slow potential shifts and high-frequency rhythms. The limited frequency range amplified adequately by a certain type of amplifier is called its "bandwidth." Often, unwanted frequency ranges are additionally suppressed by filters. Determining the lower frequency limit, the high-pass filter lets higher frequencies pass and attenuates lower ones. This filter is also called the "time constant" and describes the time an alternating current (AC) signal needs to decay two-thirds of its initial amplitude (see Figure 5.4). The low-pass filter determines the upper frequency limit; it lets lower frequencies pass and attenuates higher ones. All filters, including the 60-Hz (in Europe, 50-Hz) notch filter, should be carefully considered and set, as they are not precise and may remove frequencies of activity below and/or above the unwanted frequency.

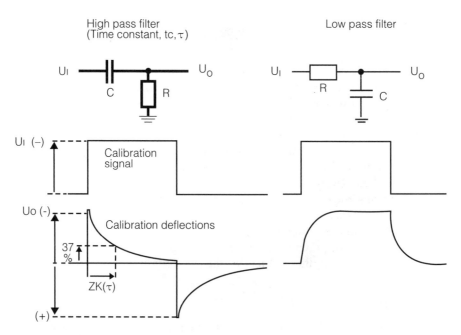

FIGURE 5.4. High-pass and low-pass filtering and its influence on a rectangular calibration signal. The high-pass filter is also referred to as the "time constant" (tc) and determines the time an alternating current (AC) signal needs to decay two-thirds of its initial amplitude. From Zschocke (1995). Copyright 1995 by Springer Verlag. Reprinted by permission.

Artifacts

In EEG recording, artifacts consist of potential shifts that do not originate in the brain. The exact knowledge of artifacts is as important as the knowledge of EEG activity itself, as some artifacts can easily be mistaken for EEG activity. Artifacts can be of biological or of technical origin, with the former deriving from extracerebral sources in the organism, and the latter arising from electrical noise or disturbances inside the recording system.

Vertical eye movements (see Figure 5.5) are the most frequent artifacts occurring in EEG recording. The neurons in the human retina generate electrical potentials that constitute an electric dipole, with the inner (caudal) side of the bulbus being negative. Eye movements lead to a change of the dipole, thereby influencing potential changes recorded in the EEG, particularly at frontal sites. Blink potentials usually occur in the absence of ocular rotation. The eyelid, like a sliding electrode, picks up a positive potential when moving over the positively charged cornea. Eye movement and blinks can be measured by *electrooculography* (*EOG*), the recording of potential differences from electrodes placed around the eyes. Before an EEG pattern can be interpreted, ocular influences have to be removed from it. A common method to account for ocular potentials picked up by the EEG electrodes is to subtract a fraction of the EOG. (For EOG correction algorithms, see, e.g., Gratton, Coles, & Donchin, 1983; Kotchoubey et al., 1996.)

Muscle activity and movements can also lead to artifacts in the EEG (see Figure 5.6). When patients are instructed to relax and not move, artifacts may still originate in muscles that are close to the recording electrodes (e.g., the frontalis, orbicularis oculi, and temporalis muscles). Neck tensions can lead to artifacts at occipital sites. Swallowing, tongue movements, and breathing can also cause low-frequency artifacts. Since EMG activity may have frequen-

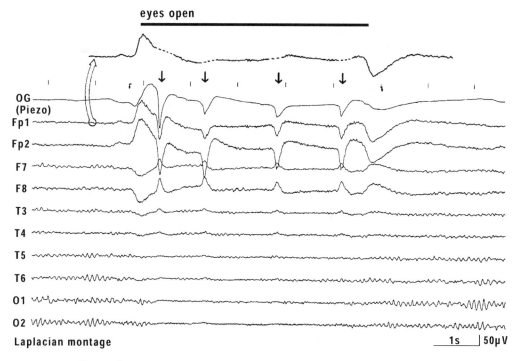

FIGURE 5.5. Effects of eye movement on the EEG. Arrows indicate blinks. From Zschocke (1995). Copyright 1995 by Springer Verlag. Reprinted by permission.

cies up to 1000 Hz, it is often interpreted as beta or gamma waves. EMG activity is particularly difficult to recognize and to remove: One possibility is to compare the activity at nearby electrodes. If frequency differences in the 30–100 Hz range exist between these electrodes, widespread EMG activity is unlikely. In biofeedback, movement-contaminated trials can be excluded by introducing an amplitude offset around 100 μV. Thereby, trials with amplitudes surpassing a certain value are invalid.

Other sources of biological artifacts are changes of skin resistance caused by sweating. These changes are not necessarily visible, and can also be caused by psychological factors. In the EEG, changes of skin resistance are reflected by slow potential shifts referred to as "drifts." Especially when slow brain activity is recorded, drifts can be misinterpreted and have to be avoided. This can be done by very careful electrode attachment and a thorough cleaning of the skin.

The most frequent technical artifact is the 60-Hz (in Europe, 50-Hz) noise caused by AC household power, mentioned earlier. Inductive 60-Hz noise can be reduced by switching off electrical devices. If there are electrical systems being connected to the patient, 60-Hz noise can result from ground loops when different pieces of apparatus used are connected to different grounds. Therefore, all devices used should be connected to one single ground. For this reason, a common socket should be used. Electrostatic interference may be caused by power supplies in the walls. It is recommended to seat the patient as far away from affected walls as possible. The metal parts of the chair must be connected to the ground. Many amplifiers have a 60-Hz notch filter to suppress 60-Hz noise selectively. Since notch filters produce a dampened oscillatory response to a transient input, their use is only recommended for specific applications.

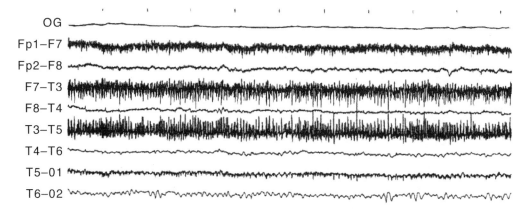

FIGURE 5.6. Muscle artifacts in the EEG. From Zschocke (1995). Copyright 1995 by Springer Verlag. Reprinted by permission.

Digitizing

After proper recording and amplification of the bioelectric measures, the signals can be fed into the *analog-to-digital (A/D) converter* of a digital computer. The A/D converter measures the voltage at regular intervals (e.g., every 10 ms). The frequency of measurements per second is referred to as "sampling rate." The original analog signal can be reconstructed from the digital information (i.e., numerical values) only if the original signal does not contain any frequency above half of the sampling frequency. Otherwise, the occurrence of fast frequencies would simulate oscillations on the lower frequency range. This effect is called *aliasing* (see Figure 5.7). Therefore, an adequate high-frequency filter is mandatory for the input of the signal into a digital computer (i.e., prior to A/D conversion).

EEG BIOFEEDBACK: HOW TO CHOOSE THE RIGHT PROGRAM

The effectiveness of the chosen device has to be evaluated on several dimensions.

Validity of the Feedback Parameter

The field of application (see the chapters in Part VI of this book) should be specific. For example, the decision to change the amount of certain spectral power frequencies has to be substantiated theoretically and empirically, and the empirical evidence should rely on controlled studies. Baseline data should be representative, and the feedback signal should be easily understood.

Reliability of the Instrumentation

To reduce artifacts (see above), the filtering capacities have to be considered carefully. The susceptibility to behaviorally or physiologically induced artifacts should be checked in test sessions by the therapist.

Electrical interference from the instrumentation as well as from the environment may distort the signal. The feedback signal should be as accurate and stable as possible, because the patient's learning depends on this information. This holds especially for EEG feedback as compared with feedback of peripheral parameters, since humans normally cannot perceive

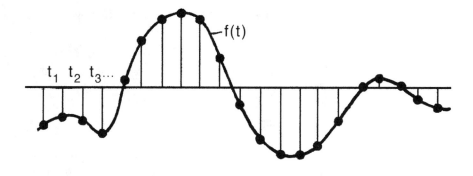

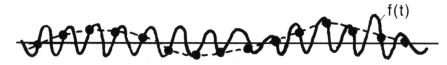

· Sampling points

FIGURE 5.7. Analog-to-digital (A/D) conversion. The signal f(t) is sampled regularly (at t_1, t_2, t_3, etc.) and stored digitally. Frequencies of above half of the sampling frequency simulate oscillations of lower EEG frequency range (depicted as dashed line). From Birbaumer and Schmidt (1999). Copyright 1999 by Springer Verlag. Reprinted by permission.

their brain waves. To ensure accuracy, the calibration of the instrument has to be checked; for stability reasons, the power source (in case of batteries or accumulators) has to be controlled.

Flexibility of the Software

The software should allow adaptations to individual characteristics. If the aim of therapy is to obtain changes in frequency bands, it should be possible to define the target (e.g., the "alpha spectrum" of a specific patient).

When progress is lacking, the therapist must be able to lower thresholds for positive feedback to initiate shaping (or even prompting) procedures. A selection of different screen surfaces improves the motivation in some cases; in other cases, it may be important that the screen surface does not interfere with the task.

Access to sophisticated data processing and data storage can be an important feature if more parameters are of interest. For instance, it might be useful to analyze the consequences of feedback of SCPs for the power spectra.

GLOSSARY

ALIASING. A potential error in the conversion of analogue to digital signals; variation in fast EEG activity may mimic slow potential changes if the original signal contains frequencies above half of the sampling frequency.

ALPHA. EEG frequency band from 8 to 13 hertz (Hz).

ANALOG-TO-DIGITAL A/D CONVERTER. Device within a digital conversion of analogue to digital signals.

BETA. EEG frequency band from 13 to 30 Hz.

BIPOLAR RECORDING. EEG derivation with an electrically active reference.

COMMON-MODE REJECTION RATIO. The ratio between amplification of out-of-phase signals and (residual) amplification of in-phase signals.

DELTA. EEG frequency band from 0.5 to 4 Hz.

ELECTROENCEPHALOGRAPHY (EEG). Recording, amplification, and analysis of the electrical activity of the brain.

ELECTROOCULOGRAPHY (EOG). Recording of electrical signals evoked by eye-movement.

EVENT-RELATED DESYNCHRONIZATION (ERD). Amplitude attenuation or blocking of rhythmic components within the alpha and beta bands time-locked (not necessarily phase-locked) to an internal or external event.

EVENT-RELATED POTENTIAL (ERP). A series of deflections in the EEG time- and phase-locked to an internally or externally paced event.

EVENT-RELATED SYNCHRONIZATION (ERS). The opposite of ERD; rhythmic, high-amplitude, low-frequency brain activity time-locked to an internal or external event.

GAMMA. EEG frequency band from 30 to 100 Hz.

GLIA CELL. Nonconducting cell that serves as support cell in the nervous system and helps to protect neurons.

IMPEDANCE. The total opposition to alternating current by an electric circuit.

INTERNATIONAL 10-20 RECORDING SYSTEM. System of locating electrodes at sites separated by 10% or 20% distance from four anatomical landmarks on the head to another.

LAPLACIAN METHOD. An EEG derivation method; the value at each electrode location is calculated by subtracting the value at that location from the values of a set of surrounding electrodes.

MONOPOLAR RECORDING. EEG derivation with an electrically silent reference.

POSTSYNAPTIC POTENTIAL (PSP). Potential that arises behind the junction site between two nerve cells, or between a nerve cell and an effector cell.

PYRAMIDAL CELL. Vertically oriented cell in the cerebral cortex with a pyramid-shaped soma.

ROLANDIC MU RHYTHM. EEG rhythm of the sensorimotor areas around 10 Hz.

SIGNAL-TO-NOISE RATIO. Ratio of the intensity of the signal of interest to that of the background noise.

SLOW CORTICAL POTENTIAL (SCP). Direct current shift of less than 1 Hz.

THALAMUS. Diencephalic brain structure; a major relay center for both sensory and motor signals.

THETA. EEG frequency band from 4 to 7 Hz.

REFERENCES

American Electroencephalographic Society. (1991). Guidelines for standard electrode position nomenclature. *Journal of Clinical Neurophysiology, 8*, 200–222.

Anand, B. K., China, G. S., & Singh, B. (1961). Some aspects of electroencephalographic studies in yogis. *Electroencephalography and Clinical Neurophysiology, 13*, 452–456.

Andersen, P., & Andersson, S. A. (1968). *Physiological basis of the alpha rhythm*. New York: Meredith.

Basar, E., Basar-Eroglu, C., Karakas, S., & Schürmann, M. (1999). Are cognitive processes manifested in event-related gamma, alpha, theta and delta oscillations in the EEG? *Neuroscience Letters, 259*, 165–168.

Basar, E., Rosen, B., Basar-Eroglu, C., & Greitschus, F. (1987). The associations between 40 Hz-EEG and the middle latency response of the auditory evoked potential. *International Journal of Neuroscience, 33*, 103–117.

Basar-Eroglu, C., Strüber, D., Kruse, P., Basar, E., & Stadler, M. (1996). Frontal gamma-band enhancement during multistable visual perception. *International Journal of Psychophysiology, 24*, 113–125.

Basar-Eroglu, C., Strüber, D., Schürmann, M., Stadler, M., & Basar, E. (1996). Gamma-band responses in the brain: A short review of psychophysiological correlates and functional significance. *International Journal of Psychophysiology, 24*, 101–112.

Birbaumer, N., Elbert, T., Lutzenberger, W., Rockstroh, B., & Schwarz, J. (1981). EEG and slow cortical potentials in anticipation of mental tasks with different hemispheric involvement. *Biological Psychology, 13*, 251–260.

Birbaumer, N., & Schmidt, R. F. (1999). *Biologische Psychologie*. Berlin: Springer-Verlag.

Blume, W. T., & Kaibara, M. (1995). *Atlas of adult encephalography*. New York: Raven Press.

Creutzfeldt, O. D. (1974). The neuronal generation of the EEG. In A. Remond (Ed.), *Handbook of electroencephalography and clinical neurophysiology: Vol. 2B. Electrical activity from the neuron to the EMG*. Amsterdam: Elsevier.

Donchin, E., & Coles, M. G. H. (1988). Is the P300 component a manifestation of context updating? *Behavioral and Brain Sciences, 11*, 357–374.

Galambos, R. (1992). A comparison of certain gamma band (40-Hz) brain rhythms in cat and man. In E. Basar & T. H. Bullock (Eds.), *Induced rhythms in the brain*. Boston: Birkhäuser.

Glenn, L. L., & Steriade, M. (1982). Discharge rate and excitability of cortically projecting intralaminar thalamic neurons during waking and sleep states. *Journal of Neuroscience, 2*, 1387–1404.

Gratton, G., Coles, M. G. H., & Donchin, E. (1983). A new method for off-line removal of ocular artifacts. *Electroencephalography and Clinical Neurophysiology, 55*, 468–484.

Hebb, D. O. (1949). *The organization of behavior: A neuropsychological theory*. New York: Wiley.

Jasper, H. H. (1958). The ten-twenty electrode system of the International Federation. *Electroencephalography and Clinical Neurophysiology, 20*, 371–375.

Kaiser, J., Lutzenberger, W., Preissl, H., Ackermann, H., & Birbaumer, N. (2000). Right-hemisphere dominance for the processing of sound-source lateralization. *Journal of Neuroscience, 20*(17), 6631–6639.

Kornhuber, H., & Deecke, L. (1965). Hirnpotentialänderungen bei Willkürbewegungen und passiven Bewegungen des Menschen: Bereitschaftspotential und reafferente Potentiale. *Pflügers Archiv, 284*, 1–17.

Kotchoubey, B., Schneider, D., Schleichert, H., Strehl, U., Uhlmann, C., Blankenhorn, V., Fröscher, W., & Birbaumer, N. (1996). Self-regulation of slow cortical potentials in epilepsy: A retrial with analysis of influencing factors. *Epilepsy Research, 25*, 269–276.

Kuhlmann, W. (1978). Functional topography of the human mu rhythm. *Electroencephalography and Clinical Neurophysiology, 44*, 83–93.

Lopes da Silva, F. (1991). Neural mechanisms underlying brain waves: From neural membranes to networks. *Electroencephalography and Clinical Neurophysiology, 79*, 81–93.

Lopes da Silva, F., Van Lierop, T. H. M. T., Schrijer, C. F. M., & Storm van Leeuwen, W. (1973). Organization of thalamic and cortical alpha rhythm: Spectra and coherences. *Electroencephalography and Clinical Neurophysiology, 35*, 627–639.

Lopes da Silva, F., Vos, J. E., Mooibroeck, J., & Van Rotterdam, A. (1980). Relative contribution of intracortical and thalamo-cortical processes in the generation of alpha rhythms, revealed by partial coherence analysis. *Electroencephalography and Clinical Neurophysiology, 50*, 449–456.

Lutzenberger, W., Elbert, T., Rockstroh, B., & Birbaumer, N. (1979). The effects of self-regulation of slow cortical potentials on performance in a signal detection task. *International Journal of Neuroscience, 9*, 175–183.

Lutzenberger, W., Elbert, T., Rockstroh, B., & Birbaumer, N. (1982). Biofeedback produced slow brain potentials and task performance. *Biological Psychology, 14*, 99–111.

Lutzenberger, W., Pulvermüller, F., Elbert, T., & Birbaumer, N. (1995). Visual stimulation alters local 40-Hz responses in humans: An EEG-study. *Neuroscience Letters, 183*, 39–42.

Lutzenberger, W., Roberts, L. E., & Birbaumer, N. (1993). Memory performance and area-specific self-regulation of slow cortical potentials: Dual-task interference. *International Journal of Psychophysiology, 15*, 217–226.

McFarland, D. J., McCane, L. M., David, S. V., & Wolpaw, J. R. (1997). Spatial filter selection for EEG-based communication. *Electroencephalography and Clinical Neurophysiology, 103*, 386–394.

Mizuki, Y. (1982). Frontal midline theta activity during performance of mental tasks [Abstract]. *Electroencephalography and Clinical Neurophysiology, 54*, 25P.

Mizuki, Y., Tanaka, O., Isozaki, H., Nishijima, H., & Inanaga, K. (1980). Periodic appearance of theta rhythm in the frontal midline during performance of a mental task. *Electroencephalography and Clinical Neurophysiology, 49*, 345–351.

Niedermeyer, E. (1999a). Maturation of the EEG: Development of waking and sleep patterns. In E. Niedermeyer & F. Lopes da Silva (Eds.), *Electroencephalography: Basic principles, clinical applications, and related fields* (4th ed.). Baltimore: Williams & Wilkins.

Niedermeyer, E. (1999b). The normal EEG of the waking adult. In E. Niedermeyer & F. Lopes da Silva (Eds.), *Electroencephalography: Basic principles, clinical applications, and related fields* (4th ed.). Baltimore: Williams & Wilkins.

Pantev, C., & Elbert, T. (1994). The transient auditory evoked gamma-band field. In C. Pantev, T. Elbert, & B. Lütkenhöner (Eds.), *Oscillatory event-related brain dynamics*. New York: Plenum Press.

Pfurtscheller, G. (1989). Functional topography during sensorimotor activation studied with event-related desynchronization mapping. *Journal of Clinical Neurophysiology, 6,* 75–84.

Pfurtscheller, G., & Aranibar, A. (1977). Event-related cortical desynchronization detected by power measurements of scalp EEG. *Electroencephalography and Clinical Neurophysiology, 42,* 817–826.

Pfurtscheller, G., & Berghold, A. (1989). Patterns of cortical activation during planning of voluntary movement. *Electroencephalography and Clinical Neurophysiology, 72,* 250–258.

Pfurtscheller, G., & Lopes da Silva, F. (1999). Event-related EEG/MEG synchronization and desynchronization: Basic principles. *Clinical Neurophysiology, 110,* 1842–1857.

Pulvermüller, F., Birbaumer, N., Lutzenberger, W., & Mohr, B. (1997). High-frequency brain activity: Its possible role in attention, perception and language processing. *Progress in Neurobiology, 52,* 427–445.

Pulvermüller, F., Keil, A., & Elbert, T. (1999). High-frequency brain activity: Perception or active memory. *Trends in Cognitive Sciences, 3,* 250–252.

Reilly, E. L. (1999). EEG recording and operation of the apparatus. In E. Niedermeyer & F. Lopes da Silva (Eds.), *Electroencephalography: Basic principles, clinical applications, and related fields* (4th ed.). Baltimore: Williams & Wilkins.

Rockstroh, B., Elbert, T., Lutzenberger, W., & Birbaumer, N. (1982). The effects of slow cortical potentials on response speed. *Psychophysiology, 19*(2), 211–217.

Schacter, D. L. (1977). EEG theta waves and psychological phenomena: A review and analysis. *Biological Psychology, 5,* 47–82.

Schoppenhorst, M., Brauer, F., Freund, G., & Kubicki, S. (1980). The significance of coherence estimates in determining cerebral alpha and mu activities. *Electroencephalography and Clinical Neurophysiology, 48,* 25–33.

Speckmann, E.-J., & Elger, C. E. (1999). Introduction to the neurophysiological basis of the EEG and DC potentials. In E. Niedermeyer & F. Lopes da Silva (Eds.), *Electroencephalography: Basic principles, clinical applications, and related fields* (4th ed.). Baltimore: Williams & Wilkins.

Steriade, M. (1999). Cellular substrates of brain rhythms. In E. Niedermeyer & F. Lopes da Silva (Eds.), *Electroencephalography: Basic principles, clinical applications, and related fields* (4th ed.). Baltimore: Williams & Wilkins.

Steriade, M., & Buzsáki, G. (1990). Parallel activation of thalamic and cortical neurons by brainstem and basal forebrain cholinergic systems. In M. Steriade & D. Biesold (Eds.), *Brain cholinergic systems.* Oxford: Oxford University Press.

Steriade, M., Gloor, P., Llinás, R. R., Lopes da Silva, F. H., & Mesulam, M.-M. (1990). Basic mechanisms of cerebral rhythmic activities. *Electroencephalography and Clinical Neurophysiology, 76,* 481–508.

Sterman, M. B. (1977). Effects of sensomotor EEG feedback training on sleep and clinical manifestations of epilepsy. In J. Beatty & H. Legewie (Eds.), *Biofeedback and behavior* (pp. 167–200). New York: Plenum Press.

Takahashi, N., Shinomiya, S., Mori, D., & Tachibana, S. (1997). Frontal midline theta rhythm in young healthy adults. *Clinical Electroencephalography, 28,* 49–54.

Tallon-Baudry, C., & Bertrand, O. (1999). Oscillatory gamma activity in humans and its role in object representation. *Trends in Cognitive Sciences, 3,* 151–162.

Verleger, R. (1988). Event-related potentials and cognition: A critique of the context updating hypothesis and an alternative interpretation of P3. *Behavioral and Brain Sciences, 11,* 343–356.

Walter, W. G., Cooper, R., Aldridge, V. J., McCallum, W. C., & Winter, A. L. (1964). Contingent negative variation: An electric sign of sensorimotor association and expectancy in the human brain. *Nature, 203,* 380–384.

Zschocke, S. (1995). *Klinische Elektroencephalographie.* Berlin: Springer-Verlag.

PART III

Office Assessment and Compliance

Intake Decisions and Preparation of Patients for Therapy

MARK S. SCHWARTZ

This chapter discusses intake decisions and the preparation of patients for therapy. It begins with considerations and guidelines for making decisions about the selection of patients and the planning of appropriate interventions. It continues with discussions of both the importance of tailoring therapy goals and the cognitive preparation of patients, or patient education. Additional sections focus on interviewing, history taking, and selected self-report measures.

One basic intake decision in the therapeutic setting is whether or not to use biofeedback with a specific patient. This chapter discusses many factors in this decision-making process.

Practitioners can benefit from being aware of the information and guidelines set forth in this chapter before and during assessment interviewing. Although the selection of topics is not exhaustive, it is sufficient for many of the situations a practitioner is likely to encounter. For more intake information and considerations about specific disorders discussed in this book, the reader is referred to specific chapters (especially to Arena & Schwartz, Chapter 7, and M. S. Schwartz & Andrasik, Chapter 14).

DISORDERS FOR WHICH BIOFEEDBACK AND RELATED TREATMENTS ARE APPROPRIATE

Arriving at a list of disorders for which biofeedback and other applied psychophysiological treatments are appropriate is not an easy task. One must consider both the individual to be treated and the specific features and stage of the disorder. There are many practical considerations, including the accuracy of the diagnosis. Prudent practitioners first consider the published literature and current clinical practice.

Published Literature and Current Clinical Practice

Good research is one cornerstone of clinical practice and a basis for deciding which disorders, symptoms, and patients to treat. One must therefore read many journals and books and attend professional meetings. However, research often does not capture the essence of clinical applications, and good research is lacking for many disorders. Therefore, practitioners need not wait for well-controlled research to support all procedures and applications before using biofeedback and associated therapies. However, they do need to base decisions on logical and responsible criteria. Other considerations become more important when adequate research is lacking.

Prudent professionals know their limitations. They can also recognize the limits of others' experience and the limitations of published research. As practitioners, we must guard against the problem of "not knowing what we do not know." Each of us should place ourselves in the role of the patient and even a third-party payer: "Suppose I were the patient, or Suppose someone asked me to pay for the treatment of this patient. What questions would I ask? What compromises and accommodations would I ask for and regard as proper?" Prudent practitioners consider several sources of data.

Disorder Lists

Agreement on a list of disorders for which biofeedback is appropriate is a formidable task, especially considering the diversity of health care professionals and issues. Complete agreement is unlikely even among practitioners who endorse and use biofeedback. Whether or not a disorder is on an indication list depends on the diagnostic criteria, the individual patient, and the degree of caution exercised. Practitioners consider many sources when selecting disorders for which, and patients for whom, to recommend treatment.

I was very tempted to avoid presenting any lists of disorders. Doing so is subjective, somewhat arbitrary, and subject to criticism, and the lists themselves can soon become obsolete. However, I offer the lists in the three columns of Table 6.1 as examples and guidelines. The three lists convey degrees of confidence in the current literature and clinical practice. These lists are merely guidelines and are not etched in granite. Mindful practitioners never automatically accept or reject for treatment all or most patients with a disorder on any list.

Disorders on the A list in Table 6.1 are those about which there is the most confidence. Research on biofeedback for these disorders is usually the best and most abundant, and agreement among practitioners and researchers is probably easiest to get. It is the "best" list by these criteria. Inclusion in this list does not imply that biofeedback alone is always the treatment of choice or the sole or primary treatment. One exception is nocturnal enuresis, for which forms of biofeedback can be the primary or sole treatment.

The disorders on the B list enjoy research support, although the number of studies is smaller and/or the methodologies are less well studied than for those on the A list. Forms of biofeedback are often a legitimate part of a treatment plan for these disorders. However, other treatments usually play a larger role than for the disorders in the A list.

The disorders on the C list are promising, and case studies of biofeedback treatment for them have been conducted. There are other disorders that could appear on this list.

Although I have not done this in Table 6.1, one also can include disorders for which relaxation and other applied psychophysiological techniques are effective and one uses biofeedback instruments to get a more complete assessment. Biofeedback can help some of these patients change their beliefs about themselves, including their self-confidence about making changes. For some patients, biofeedback helps improve their self-regulation. Instrumentation also allows practitioners to assess and document progress.

One could also properly include several other symptoms and conditions on the three lists in Table 6.1 from the field of physical medicine and rehabilitation; omission reflects my limited knowledge and experience. Such lists would be better treated separately by other professionals.

TABLE 6.1. Selected Disorders for Which Biofeedback Can Be Considered

A. Best	B. Good	C. Maybe
Tension-type headache	Insomnia, psychophysiological	Writer's cramp; occupational cramps of musicians
Migraine headache	Anxiety disorders: Generalized anxiety disorder, phobias, posttraumatic stress disorder	Other dystonias (torticollis)
Nocturnal enuresis		Blepharospasm
Fecal incontinence	Attention-deficit/hyperactivity disorder	Dermatological disorders
Urinary incontinence		Diabetes
Other pelvic floor disorders	Epilepsy	Posture training
Essential hyptertension	Nausea/vomiting	Menopausal hot flashes
Phantom limb pain	Irritable bowel syndrome	Hyperfunctional dysphonia
	Asthma	Vasovagal or stress-induced syncope
	Temporomandibular disorders and bruxism	Essential tremor
	Tinnitus	Reflex sympathetic dystrophy/ complex regional pain syndrome II
	Raynaud's disease and Raynaud's phenomenon	Psychoactive substance abuse/ dependence
	Chronic pain	
	Fibromyalgia	
	Hyperventilation	

Note. For all symptoms and diagnoses, careful patient selection and tailoring of treatment combinations to the individual are needed. Inclusion of a disorder in this table is not intended to imply that biofeedback is suitable for all or most patients with this diagnosis.

Cautions and Contraindications

Practitioners must consider various cautions and contraindications before using biofeedback and other physiological self-regulatory therapies. Experts generally agree about many of these; however, there is no single, agreed-upon document listing or discussing all cautions and contraindications. Adler and Adler (1984, 1989a, 1989b) have offered sage opinions regarding limitations of biofeedback. I encourage all practitioners to read their chapters.

Most practitioners consider the following disorders and conditions as outright contraindications to biofeedback, or at least as indicating the need for much caution. These include severe depression; acute agitation; acute or fragile schizophrenia (or a strong potential for psychotic decompensation); mania; paranoid disorders with delusions of influence; severe obsessive–compulsive disorder (OCD); delirium; acute medical decompensation; or a strong potential for a dissociative reaction, fugue state, or depersonalization. There is very little or no literature on biofeedback or other applied psychophysiological interventions for patients with these disorders, as logic has precluded such interventions with these patients.

In the rare cases when a practitioner can justify using relaxation and biofeedback with a patient who has one of these diagnoses or conditions, then prudent standards of practice dictate using special assessment and treatment procedures. For example, one might treat tension or migraine headaches in a patient with OCD.

Caution must also be employed in using some forms of biofeedback and relaxation therapies for patients with certain other conditions. These are not contraindications; however, providers must be very knowledgeable and experienced with these conditions, and must be well versed in using special approaches. They include moderate to severely impaired attention or memory (as in dementia and mental retardation), as well as some seizure disorders. One also needs to be cautious with patients with significant "secondary gain" from symptoms.

Practitioners should inform patients taking medications for certain medical disorders (e.g., diabetes mellitis, hypothyroidism, seizure disorders, hypertension, glaucoma, and asthma) that relaxation therapies may result in a need for reduced dosage, and should discuss this possibility with the patients' physicians. However, it should be noted that reports documenting adverse effects or altered medication requirements associated with relaxation therapies and biofeedback are very rare.

Medical Conditions Masquerading as Psychological Symptoms

Most practitioners know and understand that many symptoms "masquerade" as psychological or functional ones, but actually are caused by an organic medical disorder requiring different treatments (Rosse, Deutsch, & Deutsch, 2000; Othmer & Othmer, 2002; Hall, 1980). All health care professionals must be aware of this possibility. They must be familiar with the symptoms and other manifestations of diagnosed conditions and other possible diagnoses. Nonmedical practitioners are particularly in need of extra caution and consultations from medical specialists. Prudent practice standards dictate working closely with competent and proper physicians who have already ruled out other causes and diagnoses, and who will reevaluate patients as indicated.

The scope of this chapter does not permit a detailed discussion of this subject, which has been well treated by others. I trust that the present discussion is helpful and sufficient for the scope of this volume. The reader is referred to the reference list for sources of excellent and more detailed information.

Neurological, endocrine, cardiovascular, connective tissue, and other disorders often produce psychological or psychiatric symptoms. It is in the early stages of many of these disorders that practitioners are more likely to be misled.

For older patients, we must consider that irritability and depressive symptoms are often part of the early stages of a progressive dementia such as Alzheimer's disease. These patients most often do not recognize or admit to their neurocognitive impairments, including their memory problems. For some patients, expressive language or spatial problems rather than memory problems are the earliest neurocognitive impairments. We must also recognize that anxiety, depression, occasionally hyperactivity, and/or grandiose behavior occur among persons with hyperthyroidism (Graves's disease, thyrotoxicosis) long before a confirmed diagnosis. Connective tissue disorders such as systemic lupus erythematosus develop over a long time, often many years. This disease produces anxiety, depression, and multiple symptoms in many body systems.

Anxiety and/or depression are often manifestations of a wide variety of neurological disorders, such as Wilson's disease, multiple sclerosis, and cerebral ischemia. Panic and other anxiety symptoms are common symptoms of oat-cell lung cancer, Menière's disease, hyperparathyroidism, hypoparathyroidism, and hyperadrenalism (Cushing's disease). Panic, anxiety, and headaches are among the symptoms of pheochromocytoma. Very rapid heart rate and pounding, with all or several of the classic symptoms of panic disorder, can occur with supraventricular tachycardia. This includes rapid onset of a heart rate often above 140 and up to about 200 beats per minute.

Medications not used for psychiatric disorders also produce a wide variety of symptoms. These include irritability, restlessness, insomnia, anxiety, lethargy, and/or depression. For example, note the associations of one or more of these symptoms reported by Othmer and Othmer (2002) and Hall (1980). They list some or many of these symptoms for some anti-infection agents, autonomic nervous system drugs, stimulants, hormones, diuretics, and others (including antihistamines, vitamin B complex, and nicotinic acid).

Recommendations

The following recommendations are intended to help you, as a practitioner, avoid important mistakes:

- Become familiar with the special features of the medical disorders seen in your practice, and the unusual symptoms for disorders specific to the practice.
- Become familiar with the features of psychiatric disorders, for those patients with one or more of these disorders.
- Make sure that your patients will soon have or recently have had a competent medical examination; maintain a close relationship with your patients' physicians and/or other physicians who can help.
- Recommend to patients that they maintain regular or periodic contact with their physicians.
- Encourage patients to report any new symptoms, new and unusual behaviors, and changes in existing symptoms.
- Know the drugs your patients take, to understand possible symptoms and side effects.

OTHER CONSIDERATIONS IN CHOOSING TREATMENTS

Stepped Care

The stepped-care approach usually involves first using less complicated, less expensive, and sometimes less time-consuming treatments. There is a strong precedent for this approach in medicine and other health care fields. For example, practitioners consider less potent medications or lower doses before more potent or higher doses, and changes in diet and exercise before medication.

There are situations when an even more conservative approach than biofeedback is appropriate and preferable to try first. Patients and referral sources will usually be grateful and respectful when practitioners are conservative and successful with "less" rather than "more" treatment. For example, one can consider audiotaped relaxation before live instructions.

One can also consider dietary changes, especially cessation of caffeine use, before relaxation and biofeedback. All patients need not stop caffeine use before starting biofeedback and related therapies (see Block, Schwartz, & Gyllenhaal, Chapter 9, this volume, for a detailed discussion of this topic). However, patients with headaches, anxiety, Raynaud's disease, irritable bowel syndrome (IBS), psychophysiological insomnia, and hypertension should seriously consider this issue. At a minimum, one should discuss with such patients the rationale for eliminating caffeine to reduce interference with relaxation and biofeedback. If stopping caffeine before other treatments leads to improvement, there will be a credible demonstration of the effects of caffeine. However, even when eliminating caffeine does not result in symptom relief, it still allows for a more meaningful symptom baseline. Patients also may be more motivated to comply with later recommendations, and better able to do so, if they have first made indicated dietary changes.

Stepped care also includes other factors that are often simple to change. For example, stopping gum chewing is sometimes proper before relaxation and biofeedback. Consider the patient who chews gum a few hours per day and has tension-type headaches in the temporalis muscles or facial pain from probable daytime bruxism. This simple change is a necessary first step and may be sufficient.

Practical considerations often compel me to use the stepped-care model. It is very consistent with advocating and using biofeedback, and very consistent with the cost containment

Zeitgeist. Many patients get significant and often sufficient benefit with less rather than more treatment. Many disorders lend themselves to the stepped-care approach. Among these are headaches, essential hypertension, anxiety, IBS, psychophysiological insomnia, temporomandibular disorders, tinnitus, and Raynaud's disease.

Alternative Treatments Tried and/or Available

Among the important initial factors to consider are the prior therapies tried and their outcomes. If relaxation or biofeedback therapies were previously unsuccessful, the practitioner should ask about the following:

- Exactly which therapies were used, to avoid providing the same or similar therapies.
- The patient's understanding of the rationale and treatment procedures, and his or her compliance with these.
- The patient's comfort with the prior therapist.
- The presence or absence of the prior therapist during sessions.
- The instrumentation and modalities used, and the placement sites of electrodes.
- The types of relaxation instructions and body positions during relaxation and biofeedback.
- The patient's understanding and demonstration of desired breathing techniques.
- The patient's past generalization and transfer of training procedures.

A therapist can usually get the answers to these and related questions within a few minutes. A prior unsuccessful trial need not prevent another trial. However, there need to be indications that another trial could improve upon important therapy procedures.

An adequate trial of proper medication can often offer a less expensive, yet effective option that is acceptable to the patient. This suggestion may sound like heresy from an advocate of behavior therapies and biofeedback. However, the cost of some medications that result in significant improvement can be less than a series of office visits.

Our patients, referral sources, and third-party payers appreciate concern for treatment costs. They respect biofeedback practitioners who are alert to and facilitate alternative effective and less expensive treatments first. In some cases, an adequate trial of an appropriate medication is a correct option. For example, some patients do not yet use preferred medications. Some use inadequate doses of an appropriate medication. Others use the medication incorrectly, such as at the wrong times. Some use the wrong medications. Some use too much medication and need to reduce or stop it. Others use incorrect combinations of medications. Some use only over-the-counter medications. It often may be better to try medication if the patient is willing to do so and there are no medical cautions or contraindications.

If an adequate trial of medication is ineffective or achieves insufficient improvement, the patient's motivation for such options as relaxation and biofeedback can increase. Biofeedback and associated therapies are often more easily justified after an unsuccessful trial of other proper and cost-efficient therapies. This assumes an adequate rationale for biofeedback, a competent provider, and the presence of other necessary criteria for such therapies.

Severity and/or Seriousness of Symptoms or Disorders

The practitioner also needs to consider the seriousness or severity of the patient's symptoms and disorder when deciding whether to offer biofeedback. Physiological self-regulatory therapies, including biofeedback, should be considered for a patient with serious or severe symptoms even when there is scant, insufficient, or equivocal research and/or clinical experience to support its use. This is especially true when options are nonexistent, more risky, or far more expensive. Again, this assumes an adequate rationale for biofeedback, a competent provider, and the presence of other necessary criteria for such therapies.

For example, a patient presented with hyperemesis gravidarum, a serious disorder involving unrelenting nausea and vomiting during pregnancy. Antiemetic medications were either contraindicated because of her pregnancy or were no longer available in the United States. Research studies on the use of biofeedback and relaxation therapies for this disorder did not exist. However, the clinical rationale was sound. Practitioners and research supported the successful use of such therapies for patients with functional emesis not associated with pregnancy (e.g., patients with anticipatory emesis associated with chemotherapy for cancer). Alternative therapies for this patient were far less practical. The only other option consisted of hospitalization and intravenous nutritional therapy for the remaining 6 months of her pregnancy or until the hyperemesis stopped. A brief and intensive therapy program proved successful in substantially reducing the emesis.

A practitioner might reasonably consider avoiding or deferring treatment if a patient's symptoms are mild or infrequent enough that he or she can live comfortably with minimal or no treatment. This category for example, might include patients with vascular headaches once every 2–3 months that last a few hours and respond well to a safe medication; patients with very mild tension-type headaches two or three times a month for a few hours each; or patients with bruxism without pain or damage to the teeth or other oral structures or tissues. Some practitioners encourage such people to live with their symptoms unless a brief and inexpensive therapy program has a good chance of success.

Geographical (or Other) Distance between Patients and Treatment Facilities

Some patients live beyond a reasonable driving distance from treatment facilities. Often a suitable referral in the patients' home area is not available. Other patients prefer treatment away from their home area, because they have had bad experiences there. Still others prefer or need to maintain strict confidentiality away from their home area. Some prefer the type of therapy, professional care, and credibility of a specific facility. In some large medical centers, a patient can only stay for a very short time.

When there are good indications for biofeedback and related therapies, and more regularly spaced treatment options are impractical, inappropriate, or nonexistent, a practitioner might consider a "massed-practice" therapy program. Such a program involves one or two daily office sessions for a few or several days. There are advantages to this schedule, and sometimes it is the only or the best option available. It can also serve to encourage the patient to continue when he or she returns home.

A limitation of massed-practice therapy away from a patient's home environment and usual routine is that the patient is usually experiencing much less stress. There also may be self-imposed or implied pressure to accomplish more than is reasonable in a short period of time.

Professional's Confidence and Competence with Biofeedback

The practitioner's confidence and competence with using necessary instrumentation during evaluation and therapy are important. It may be moot whether other professionals believe they can attain the same results without instrumentation. If a professional is competent to use instrumentation and prefers to do so, then it is acceptable to do so, regardless of whether non-instrumentation-based procedures might result in similar results.

There is considerable precedent for this philosophy of practice in medicine and psychology. For example, some psychologists and psychiatrists prefer to rely usually or solely on detailed interviews and direct observations to make diagnoses and recommendations. This is a common and acceptable approach. In contrast, many professionals prefer to add and often rely on psychological assessments and testing, which can add significant costs to evaluations. However, the additional assessments are common practice, and many believe that they add to the quality of the diagnostic and therapy plan.

Similarly, many neurologists and other physicians get neuropsychological assessments to help confirm a diagnosis or add information about a patient's functioning. Sometimes these merely confirm the practitioners' clinical impressions. This is acceptable and common clinical practice. Other neurologists and other physicians believe such assessments are unnecessary. This, too, is acceptable clinical practice.

Alternative therapies and procedures may be equally effective. Some studies show one treatment to be better, whereas other studies show a second treatment to be better than the first; still other studies may show them to be equal. Practitioners have the right to choose among evaluative and therapeutic approaches that are consistent with their interest and confidence, since a practitioner's interest and confidence are crucial to the therapeutic outcome. Of course, practitioners must also keep in mind risks, costs, and efficacy.

Initial Physiological Evaluation and Baseline Session(s)

The results of the psychophysiological baseline assessment constitute an important source of information for making therapy decisions. For example, suppose that a practitioner observes consistently low levels of muscle activity from multiple muscle areas during rest and stressor segments. In this situation, the practitioner should consider deferring biofeedback or omitting it from the treatment plan.

In such a case, the instrumentation-based monitoring serves a very useful purpose. It reveals that the patient can relax to a therapeutic range. The practitioner then clearly explains the meaning of that finding and gives instructions, encouragement, and supervision for using relaxation. This includes using relaxation frequently enough, long enough, and at the right times for it to be of therapeutic value.

It may be that selected muscular tension is occurring in the patient's daily life but not in the practitioner's office. Without demonstration of tension in the office, it is still proper to use non-instrumentation-based physiological self-regulatory procedures in the patient's daily activities.

Another question that arises in the present context concerns the criteria for being sufficiently relaxed. There are no hard and fast rules, and few on which professionals can agree except at the extremes. The level and duration of physiological activity needed for a positive therapeutic effect differ among patients. Practitioners often do not agree on necessary physiological criteria for relaxation to result in positive results for the symptoms and disorders treated. Reaching clear or ideal criteria during biofeedback-assisted relaxation office sessions is probably often unnecessary. Patients often improve despite somewhat tense levels in early and later baselines.

The practitioner should consider recommending to the patient that he or she needs to avoid excess tension, especially for sustained periods. A patient might benefit from reproducing the reduced tension observed in the baselines, even if he or she has not reached the ideally relaxed range. Indeed, the therapist should suggest this and help the patient learn to do it frequently, rapidly, for various durations, and at the right times.

Baselines need to be long enough to observe increasing or decreasing physiological activity over several minutes. Baselines that are too short or those integrated over long periods can obscure such trends. (See Arena & Schwartz, Chapter 7, for more discussion of baselines.) Also, one should consider varying the conditions under which one conducts baselines. Baselines with only the patient's eyes closed can be very misleading and inadequate, because many patients show much higher tension with their eyes open. In addition, monitoring only during resting conditions without stressors provides unrealistic results. Such recordings often show little or no tension or arousal, whereas with anticipation of or during stressful stimuli, tension and arousal are often greater.

It should also be noted that psychophysiological measurements are often unreliable across sessions. Thus the activity in one session does not reliably occur in other sessions. In the first session, the patient may be more tense because of the novelty of the situation. This is one reason for additional baseline segments to base decisions about the need for biofeedback.

Furthermore, some patients relax adequately at home and in their real-life situations; however, they have difficulty relaxing in professionals' offices. No matter how a practitioner may present it, there is an implied evaluation atmosphere in an office that some patients find difficult to overcome. If the practitioner suspects this, he or she should evaluate how the patient views the session and what the patient feels like during office sessions. Then he or she should check the patient's physiological activity during practice periods outside the office.

Other useful data include the patient's physiological responses to feedback and after feedback segments. The questions to be asked include the following:

- Does the patient lower tension and arousal significantly with the feedback?
- Are the lowered arousal and tension maintained after the feedback?
- Does the feedback increase the arousal and tension?
- Do the stressors increase the arousal or precipitate arousal?

There are several questions and types of information on which one may base the decision to provide more biofeedback. Here are a few examples:

- Are there much excess tension and arousal during resting baseline and self-regulation segments without feedback?
- Are much tension and arousal precipitated or worsened with office stressors?
- Does feedback result in significantly lowered tension and arousal?
- Does the person return to baseline tension and arousal after feedback?

It is instructive to remember that such logical questions and criteria have not yet been clearly shown to predict the necessity of biofeedback-assisted therapies for achieving positive therapeutic outcomes. Until research supports such evidence, practitioners need to remain cautious and conservative in making such decisions and recommendations.

Symptom Changes in the First Weeks

Symptom changes during the first weeks of therapy are important for deciding whether to continue sessions and determining which therapy procedures to pursue. Such improvements often occur early before patients reach ideal physiological mastery. If the initial intervention results in a clinically significant reduction of symptoms, practitioners need to justify more office-based therapy.

The primary goal is to decrease or stop symptoms, and not to reduce microvolts or increase hand temperatures. When there are clinically significant changes in the first few weeks, practitioners should consider deferring more biofeedback sessions, even if they assume that some patients need specific physiological mastery for reliable therapeutic changes. In addition to cost considerations, another reason for this determination is credibility to the patient, the referral source, and the third-party payer. If biofeedback has a "placebo component" for some patients, premature extended use may "use up" that component. (Note that the use of the term "placebo component" here is not a statement that biofeedback itself is a placebo.)

Patients need preparation for the possibility that more office therapy may be needed later. As an example, here is a statement that might be made to a patient who has shown clinically significant improvement of symptoms in the early weeks of therapy.

> "I am happy for your improvement in such a short time. I am sure that you too are very pleased. You significantly reduced the hours of severe headache, increased the hours without headaches, and reduced your use of medications. You also are showing improved ability to reduce muscle tension in your face and head muscles. It sounds like you are applying the therapy very well.
>
> "The muscle tension in your head is still tense when we measure it in the office. In the long run, it might be better to relax these muscles deeper and faster, and maintain the lower levels longer.
>
> "I do not want to overdo the biofeedback sessions. More sessions now could speed more improvement, but I cannot predict that with certainty. Consider this conservative option: Continue applying the therapy and keep records of your symptoms for another few weeks. We can review your situation at that time. If your improvement does not continue, we can resume the biofeedback."

Patient Characteristics

There are several studies of the association between patient characteristics and benefit from biofeedback and related therapies. Even when some characteristics are found to have significant correlation with outcome, there is usually much overlap between groups.

The results of these studies are interesting and have academic and heuristic value. The studies identify patient characteristics that differentiate more successful from less successful results. One inference sometimes drawn is that the patient variables provide criteria for who should not receive biofeedback or related therapies. However, there are many variables that influence the relationships between patients and therapy results. These studies need replications in a variety of clinical settings and with potential "moderator variables" before one can conclude that some patients should not receive therapy.

Practitioners should ask themselves what to do with patients with different characteristics. For example, do the practitioners need to add more patient education? Will more frequent or more closely spaced sessions work better for some patients? Will procedural variations help?

Patient's Motivation and Compliance: Enhancement with Biofeedback

Patients need to maintain motivation for practice and application of physiological self-regulatory therapies. Relaxation therapies alone can be successful without biofeedback for many patients.

For other patients, feedback is confirming and encouraging. It helps them gain or maintain confidence in the treatment and their abilities. Some question and dispute the idea that they are physically tense or autonomically aroused; others doubt that their thoughts affect their physiological tension and arousal; still others doubt that they can control their physiology. All these patients need concrete and credible evidence. Using instrumentation with physiological self-regulation procedures is not a rejection of the value of relaxation alone. It is not an either–or choice, as some portray it.

Patient's Choice and Cost of Therapy

Practitioners always need to respect each patient's needs and treatment choices. They must discuss the patient's options, time needed, desired results, prognosis, and costs realistically.

As practitioners, we obviously want to see as much improvement as practical for patients. We often measure success against research criteria such as 50+%, 70+%, or 90+% reduction of symptoms, along with reduced medications when indicated. Indeed, we strive for these ideal goals and encourage our patients accordingly. However, such goals are often unrealistic and even inappropriate. They may not match the patients' own goals. Some patients welcome an improvement of 20–50%, especially after years of very little change.

Financial costs and time invested are important considerations for patients. Some patients may decide that additional improvement is not worth the additional investment. Such patients show concern with the number of office visits, time away from work, and financial costs. There are also the costs and inconvenience of transportation and child care to consider. Practitioners need not always measure success against the criteria of what is possible. Realism allows patients to participate in choosing how much benefit they desire or will accept for how much investment.

AN INTRODUCTION TO PATIENT EDUCATION

Rationale

Some patients have difficulty accepting the potential benefits of relaxation, biofeedback, and other applied psychophysiological treatments. They are sometimes skeptical, critical, and resistant. That should not surprise us practitioners or lead us to become defensive. Nor should we dismiss patients as unsuitable candidates because they question treatment or appear resistant. Many patients have already seen other health care professionals who were optimistic about their therapy, yet the results were unsuccessful. We are now asking them to accept a different approach, often perceived as the last one of a series.

However, patients are often unfamiliar with behavioral and self-regulatory strategies. These represent approaches that are often very different from those with which patients are more familiar. Patients often do not have adequate and understandable information about the rationale for these therapies. They need information they can understand and accept. Furthermore, some patients are skeptical or defensive about nonmedical health care professionals.

If we think about it from the patients' standpoint, relaxation and biofeedback therapies can appear as rather simplistic solutions. Explanations can appear very complex. Some patients probably think to themselves something like the following:

> "You mean I have these pains in my head [or other symptoms] for years, went to several good doctors, took thousands of pills, and continued to suffer? Now you tell me that relaxing each day, and watching and listening to a machine measuring my muscle tension, are all that I needed all this time? I would like to believe that, but I have been down this road before. Convince me!"

We should not assume that patients understand and accept the rationale for therapy or that brief explanations are usually sufficient. Nor should we assume that patients spontaneously ask questions or directly tell us their concerns. They usually do not!

Furthermore, we should not assume that patients accept and remember explanations and recommendations. Thus we must seriously consider well-planned and well-executed patient education to increase patients' attention, understanding, recall, confidence, satisfaction, and compliance. We must devote adequate time early in the therapeutic relationship and thereafter to prepare and teach patients adequately. The values of good patient education and its varied methodologies are often underestimated or neglected.

Patient education can also reduce anxiety, increase the credibility of the professional and the therapy procedures, and facilitate positive expectations. As Shaw and Blanchard (1983) concluded,

> Giving participants a high initial expectation of therapeutic benefit from stress management training has significant benefit in terms of self report of change and reduced physiological reactivity[,] and . . . these improvements are mediated at least in part by increased compliance with home practice instructions. . . . the procedures, per se, are not especially powerful without the appropriate set. (p. 564)

They noted as well that "a certain degree of salesmanship and trainer enthusiasm certainly can make a difference in outcome" (p. 564).

Some practitioners rush into the therapy phase with limited patient education. This is often understandable, considering the high costs of health care and demands on professionals' schedules. However, there are cost-efficient methods for providing good patient education.

Good patient education can improve patients' knowledge and attitudes about the causes of their symptoms and about therapy. It can enhance a patient's perceptions of a practitioner as an expert, and as being credible and trustworthy. Compliance and therapy effectiveness partly depend on patient knowledge, beliefs, perceptions, and a positive therapeutic alliance.

Metaphors

Tailoring patient education to a specific patient depends on that patient's intelligence, education, reading ability, sophistication, and psychological-mindedness. Health care professionals commonly use metaphors to communicate with and educate patients. One of the major reasons for using metaphors is to help simplify information, concepts, and procedures. Metaphors are excellent for presenting the rationale, concepts, and ideas that patients need to understand at an experiential and indirect level. This presentation can make the ideas easier to accept and use (Combs & Freedman, 1990, pp. 59–60).

The struggle for an agreed-upon definition of "metaphor" is ancient. The lack of agreement continues to the present (Ortony, Reynolds, & Arter, 1978; Muran & DiGiuseppe, 1990). One view is that "a *metaphor* is a way of writing or speaking figuratively and of describing something in terms of something else" (Morris & Morris, 1985, p. 387). Synonyms include "figure of speech," "image," and "symbol."

In contrast, the interactive view (Richards, 1936; Black, 1962) posits that metaphors are much more than simply analogies. Metaphors are valuable for learning and understanding new knowledge blueprints. Muran and DiGiuseppe (1990) summarize this view and describe it as a radical constructivist view, in which

> metaphors are seen as "cognitive instruments" by which similarities are created that previously were not known to exist . . . (Boyd, 1979). . . . [They are] one way of breaching the epistemological chasm between old and new knowledge by affording different ways of perceiving and organizing the world (Petrie, 1979). (p. 71)

> [Metaphor] has been used for centuries as a method of teaching and communicating in many fields. (p. 70)

> Metaphorical communication conceptualized as both a heuristic and epistemic device makes it a highly persuasive means of conveying and altering thought . . . not only a vehicle for communication but also a vehicle for change. (p. 73)

Furthermore, Siegelman (1990) starts her book on the subject by stating, "Most of us, and our patients . . . find ourselves cleaving to metaphor to communicate experience that is hard to convey in any other way" (p. 1).

Practitioners of cognitive-behavioral therapies also advocate analogies and metaphors. McMullin (1986) describes in detail many examples of perceptual shift techniques for cognitive restructuring therapy. These techniques "make a creative use of analogies to help clients who are preoccupied with damaging beliefs to understand the nature of the perceptual transition that they must undergo" (p. 73). For example, reversible drawings or embedded figures provide stimuli to help patients perceive how they can perceive situations differently or in a perceptually shifted way with practice. Many other examples for the use of analogies in cognitive therapy can be found in McMullin (1986).

Although professionals use many metaphors, further discussion or examples of them are beyond the scope of this book.

Cautions in the Use of Metaphor

Many linguists and psychologists warn about the potential misuse and misleading potential of metaphors. For example, the use of metaphor can foster careless thought "by acting as a substitute for the hard, analytic work of determining precisely what to say, a point previously raised by Aristotle . . . when he warned of the ambiguity and obscurity inherent in metaphor" (Muran & DiGiuseppe, 1990, p. 72).

Muran and DiGiuseppe (1990) review the cautions of other writers (Petrie, 1979; Beardsley, 1972; Fraser, 1979). People interpret metaphors in many different ways, and metaphors are very context-sensitive, thereby increasing the chances of mistakes. Thus practitioners need to be careful about *why* they are using a metaphor, *with whom,* and *in what context.*

One premise of this section is that metaphors can improve cognitive preparation and education of patients. Improved cognitive preparation improves compliance for maintaining many behaviors necessary for effective therapy results (Levy, 1987).

EVALUATION/ASSESSMENT: INTERVIEWING, HISTORY TAKING, AND SELF-REPORT MEASURES

Psychological Evaluation

Deciding where to begin history taking, and whether or not (and, if so, how soon) to include psychological inquiries, depends on the patient, the circumstances, and clinical judgment. With many medical patients, mental health practitioners are often wise to begin with a history of physical symptoms. However, exceptions abound. Often all or most of the symptom history information is available in the recorded history.

With medical patients, practitioners often do not need much time for psychological evaluation. Practical constraints are often created by the patient's schedule or by the distance from home of the therapeutic center. Many have limited psychological-mindedness and resist such an evaluation. However, even a brief psychological evaluation is often better than none. One should at least ask something like this: "What are the pressures and frustrations in your life?"

Asking a few psychological questions can help with rapport. It can help assess the patient's receptiveness or resistance to this type of question and treatment. Furthermore, it can determine whether or not more evaluation is needed.

I have culled and revised the following list of psychological factors from one by Adler and Adler (1987), who provide an erudite, insightful, refined, and skilled commentary on history taking. One must read their original text to appreciate their style and clinical wisdom. Although it was written as a guide for interviewing people with headaches, their list and discussion are useful for other disorders. The Adlers (1987) suggest considering evaluation of many factors:

- Patient's expectations of themselves.
- Perceived expectations by others.
- Existence of past or present family conflicts.
- Sensitivity to criticism and to emotional expressions.
- Comfort with and skills at being assertive.
- Illnesses and hospitalizations.
- Past or present grief, or anticipated grief.
- Medication misuse.
- Perceptions of health care professionals.
- Perceived emotional triggers or factors increasing the risk of a symptom.

Do patients' personality features and psychopathology worsen or maintain current symptoms, or are they the effects of chronic symptoms? How necessary is it for practitioners to assess and treat psychopathology to significantly reduce current physical symptoms? Also, do life stressors in the past cause or contribute to current symptoms? For example, what is the role of past sexual abuse or grief in current symptoms? How necessary is it for practitioners to assess and treat these factors to reduce current physical symptoms significantly? (See the section below on sexual abuse. Also, see M. S. Schwartz & Andrasik, Chapter 14, and M. S. Schwartz & Achem, Chapter 29, for discussion of such assessment and treatment for headaches and IBS, respectively.)

History Taking and Interviewing

There are many resources for history taking and interviewing. Good examples include Hersen and Turner (1985) and Othmer and Othmer (2002).

Practitioners often use interview outlines as guides. For example, the reader should review Lacks (1987) for insomnia. The topics and specific items covered and the time invested for each depend on many factors:

- Professional setting.
- Professional specialty.
- Referral source.
- Referral information available.
- Whether there will be continuing care by another professional, such as the referral source.
- Results from screening measures.
- Stepped-care considerations.
- Cost consideration for the patient.
- Time available by the patient and the practitioner.
- Purpose of the consultation or evaluation.[1]

Medical and other practitioners responsible for assessment and treatment are wise to get at least some of their own history information, rather than to rely exclusively on information from others. This is true even when the other sources are competent professionals, including physicians. It is tempting and sometimes necessary and acceptable to forgo this process because of time and cost constraints. However, a practitioner needing specific information often needs to get it directly from the patient. The practitioner can review the prior reports aloud with the patient for his or her confirmation and elaboration. Even seemingly clear information, such as onset, location, frequency, and duration, can differ when one carefully asks the questions and listens carefully to the answers.

Even competent and experienced professionals can overlook potentially important items. This does not mean that they are careless or incompetent. Patients tell different professionals different information and give different answers to the same types of questions. Practitioners can also misunderstand patients' statements. Furthermore, practitioners, including physicians, sometimes get only the information needed for the purpose of their consultation—which may be to make a diagnosis; rule out serious organic pathology; prescribe medication; and/or make referrals for psychological evaluations, biofeedback, physical therapy, or other treatments.

Physicians and other practitioners with special interests and expertise in specific symptoms and disorders often get more detailed information than do other professionals. For example, for headaches, these areas of information include dietary factors, gum-chewing habits, use of bed pillows, sleep habits, stress, work postures and other ergonomic factors, driving habits, beliefs, and sexual and physical abuse. A practitioner sometimes observes discrepancies between the recorded history information and the information he or she now gets from the patient. The practitioner must be alert to such inconsistencies and address them tactfully.

Sexual and Physical Abuse[2]

Research reports that sexual and/or physical abuse is often part of the history of patients with functional[3] gastrointestinal disorders, primarily IBS (Delvaux, Denis, & Allemand, 1997; Drossman et al., 1990; Drossman, Talley, Leserman, Olden, & Barreiro, 1995; Talley, Fett, Zinsmeister, & Melton, 1994; Talley, Fett, & Zinsmeister, 1995); gynecological disorders, most notably chronic pelvic pain (Walker et al., 1992; Lampe et al., 2000) and possibly severe premenstrual syndrome (Golding, Taylor, Menard, & King, 2000); somatization (Morrison, 1989); possibly nonepileptic attack disorder (so-called "pseudoseizure") (Moore & Baker, 1997; Harden, 1997); and chronic pain (Haber & Roos, 1985; Domino & Haber, 1987; Toomey, Hernandez, Gittleman, & Hulka, 1993). Percentages vary with at least the definition of abuse, the ages selected, assessment methods and questions asked, and the type of abuse (sexual, physical, or both). See Berkowitz (1998) for a review of the medical consequences of childhood sexual abuse (CSA).

The question is whether a history of abuse, especially CSA, is more common among adults with these disorders than in more heterogeneous and general population samples. First, consider that CSA and other sexual abuse are very common. See Salter (1988, pp. 16–24, especially Table 1.1, p. 18) for a review of several prevalence studies of sexual abuse. Also, see Berkowitz (1998) for comments about incidence and prevalence. There are reports that 20–25% of women and 10–15% of men have been sexually abused (Berkowitz, 1998). The National Committee for Prevention of Child Abuse reported 3 million suspected cases of CSA in the United States in 1992 (Ireland, Freeman, & Shore, 1996). This committee also reported the estimate that one in three girls and one in seven boys are sexually abused before age 18 in the United States (Ireland et al., 1996).

Russell (1984) reported that 28% of females under age 16 experienced sexual abuse; Badgley (1984) noted that 15% of females experienced such abuse before age 16. These figures are very representative of studies in the 1980s. The Badgley study also reported sexual abuse for 6% of males under the age of 15. Older studies, mostly done in the 1950s and earlier, reported higher percentages. This discrepancy may result from differences in definitions, assessment methods, and questions. Furthermore, among female medical patients, the estimated history of sexual or physical trauma is between 25% and 75% of women (Domino & Haber, 1987; Drossman et al., 1990; Springs & Friedrich, 1992).

There are concerns that incidence and prevalence estimates are often low, because some believe that the vast majority of cases are unreported (Arnold, Rogers, & Cook, 1990; Russell, 1984). These reports estimate that up to 98% of sexual abuse is not reported. Medical patients typically do not spontaneously report a history of CSA. At least one report noted that about one-third of the women surveyed had never told anyone of the abuse, and only 17% had discussed it with their physicians (Drossman et al., 1990). Another report (Lechner, Vogel, Garcia-Shelton, Leichter, & Steibel, 1993) noted that only 5% of the women studied had disclosed this information to a physician.

In the original study of chronic pain and abuse by Bradley and colleagues (reviewed by Bradley, McDonald-Haile, & Jaworski, 1992), abused patients, relative to those who had not been abused, were "twice as likely to have suffered pain without a specific precipitating injury or identified cause and to have a significantly greater number of previous medical problems for which they had sought treatment" (p. 198). In the next study by this group, abused patients, relative to those who were not abused, were "significantly more likely to report constant daily headaches . . . [and a] significantly greater number of medical problems for which they had been hospitalized as well as previous surgical procedures" (p. 198).

Therefore, the Bradley et al. (1992) review recommends "that assessments of all chronic pain patients should include a careful evaluation of possible sexual and physical abuse" (p. 199). The interview questions from Drossman et al. (1990) included in that review are one set of possible questions. Practitioners should review other sources and guidelines for self-report and interview questions, and consult with specialists in this field, before deciding how to assess this complex and delicate topic.

Evaluating this topic and considering proper intervention are of potential value to biofeedback practitioners. One potential advantage of knowing about abuse is the opportunity to consider its possible influence on the development and/or maintenance of medical and psychophysiological problems.

However, no data show that abuse is an etiological or contributory factory for disorders commonly referred for applied psychophysiological therapies. I have found no studies of these disorders in which the treatment focused on abuse, and no studies that examined abuse as a factor in relaxation and biofeedback treatment failures. There is also the question of whether there are specific behaviors (such as promiscuity, substance abuse/dependence, or other health risk behaviors) that might be consequences of or affected by CSA, and thus contribute to the medical conditions associated with/correlated with a history of CSA (Springs & Friedrich, 1992). Long-term prospective studies are still lacking, and are very challenging to conduct.

Nevertheless, giving a patient a chance to discuss this openly with an appropriate professional is often helpful (Cahill, Llewelyn, & Pearson, 1991). Referral to a specialist in abuse may be necessary to "resolve issues such as poor self-image, self-blame for the abuse, sexual dysfunction, and suppressed anger and rage" (Bradley et al., 1992, p. 199).

Furthermore, there are now substantial legal concerns for health care professionals when questioning patients about a history of sexual abuse, and when providing psychotherapy for such a history (Scheflin & Spiegel, 1998; Cannell, Hudson, & Pope, 2001). This concern is particularly important if a professional is inquiring about and/or suspecting a history of CSA that the patient is not reporting as having occurred. Prudent health care professionals guard against overzealousness, are well informed about the topic of CSA and so-called "repressed memories," the needs for careful informed consent, and the other legal issues and recommendations.

> Clinicians are well-advised to practice defensively in cases involving memory or dissociative disorders, especially by keeping extracautious notes and the more frequent use of informed consent forms. Books on legal risk management are important preventive guides that could help avoid costly and unnecessary law suits. (Scheflin & Spiegel, 1998, p. 860)

However, the history of abuse in some patients may be significant, and sometimes very significant. "Failing to inquire about a history of trauma, and therefore assuming that it did not occur or if it did is unimportant, can be as damaging as insisting that a trauma history must lurk behind any symptom" (Scheflin & Spiegel, 1998, p. 861). Perhaps it influences tolerance for symptoms? Perhaps it contributes to those factors that motivate people with these symptoms to seek medical help? Perhaps it contributes to the factors that motivate people to avoid treatment? Self-blame, poor self-image, control issues, shame, trust, vulnerability, dependency conflicts, sexual dysfunction, and suppressed anger could affect all of these.

Interview Outline

The following outline or checklist offers a guideline to consider and one from which to glean ideas for interviewing and other intake procedures. Most of these questions and items are useful in the general clinical practice of applied psychophysiology, and especially in the treatment of headache and anxiety disorders. Some items and questions do not apply to other disorders, such as incontinence. (See M. S. Schwartz & Andrasik, Chapter 14, for a more detailed discussion of taking a headache history.)

1. Symptom(s). [Note: A patient's highest-priority symptoms are not always the reason for referral.]
   a. Description. "What are the symptoms like?" [Offer choices.]
   b. Location(s). "Where does it begin? Show me. Does it move around?"
   c. Frequency. "How often does it occur? When does it increase/decrease?"
   d. Timing. "When do the symptoms occur? What time of day do they occur? Do they always or usually occur then?"
   e. Duration. "How long do the symptoms last? Do they last for . . . ? What are the shortest, longest, and usual durations?"
   f. Intensity. [Consider rating scales.] "Are the symptoms slight, mild, moderate, severe, or very severe?"
   g. Origin. "When did the symptom originally begin?"
   h. Development. "Has it changed over weeks, months, or years?"
   i. Course/progression. "Does it change over minutes/hours after it starts?"
   j. Precipitants/antecedents. [Look for dietary, environmental, postural, hormonal, emotional, work/family stress, and time factors.] "What do you think causes or starts the symptoms? Do you suspect that anything might be triggering it? Is there anything that often seems to precede it?"
   k. Aggravating/worsening factors. "Does anything increase the severity? What makes it worse?"
   l. Alleviating/helping factors. "Does anything decrease the severity? What makes it better? What do you do that reduces the symptoms?"
   m. Medications. [Note when and why medications are taken. Are medications taken when the patient is anticipating situations? Does the patient take medications

with minimal symptoms?] "When do you take medications? How soon do you get relief after taking . . . ?"

    n. Nonrelief. "What has not worked for you? When was it taken?"

    o. Periods of remission. "Are you ever totally free of symptoms for days, weeks, longer?"

    p. Associated symptoms. "What other symptoms do you get with the main one? Do you get . . . ?" [Ask specific questions about specific symptoms.]

    q. Reactions of others. "What does your family do when you have symptoms?"

    r. Behaviors before, during, and after onset, including behaviors and attitudes on days without the symptoms. "On days when you are feeling much better or have no symptoms, do you try and catch up with house/yard work, and other activities? Do you typically have worsening or resumption of symptoms soon after or the next day? Do you feel you need to live up your responsibilities on good days?"

    s. Limitations in life due to symptoms.

    t. Family members with similar or the same symptoms (optional).

2. Prior treatments.

    a. Prior psychological treatments. [Ask when, where, with whom; number of sessions, duration, results; patient's reactions and views.]

    b. Prior experience with relaxation therapies. [Ask about prior relaxation therapies, what was done, for how long this was used, what is still done, when it is done, what seems to work, what does not work. Ask for demonstration, especially breathing.]

    c. Prior experience with biofeedback. [Ask who provided it, where on body sensors were placed, whether eyes were open or closed, what body positions were used, what was done during sessions, and whether patient was alone or with therapist. Ask about perceptions and attitudes about this treatment.]

    d. Other treatments. [Ask about other therapies, including other applied psychophysiological therapies; when, number, and what helped; and patient's attitudes about these treatments, including either desperation or open-mindedness.]

3. Current treatments. [Psychological and medical. Get names and addresses of professionals seen, and ask about attitudes, comfort, expectancies, content, preferences, questions, and plans.]

4. Attitudes about health care professionals, treatments, and symptoms.

    a. Symptoms. "What do you think is causing your symptoms? Do you think anything has been overlooked?" [This is when one learns of a patient's beliefs and fears about a cause not yet found.] "What are your thoughts when symptoms start and worsen?" [Cognitive factors.] "How would your life be different without these symptoms or with greatly reduced symptoms?"

    b. Treatments. "What do you expect from _____ treatments ? What have you heard or read about this treatment? What did your physician tell you?"

    c. Professionals. "What do you think/feel about coming to a _____ [e.g., psychologist]?"

5. Reasons for seeking treatment now. "Why have you come for treatment now? Are your symptoms worse? Have new features? Is your depression worse, or is your job or marriage at risk?" [Is the patient planning life changes, such as pregnancy, that entail a need to stop medications? Is the patient returning to school, changing jobs, getting married, or making other major changes calling for better treatment for the symptoms? Is there another agenda, such as secondary gain, or seeking help as a socially acceptable means of access to the practitioner?]

6. Stressors. [Check past and current stressors in interview and/or questionnaires. Stressor areas include interpersonal, work, schedule overload, perfectionism, procrastination, disorganization, inefficient time use, lack of goals and priorities, family, financial, health, sexual, living conditions, legal, existential.]

7. Emotions. [Observe, ask, and consider measures for depression, anxiety, anger.]

8. Neurocognitive factors. [Observe, review records, ask, and consider assessing for long-term limitations or acquired impairments in memory, attention/concentration, intellectual, language, academic achievement. Check for head/brain injuries and surgeries with residual effects.]

9. Physical factors. [Observe, check records. Ask about hearing, vision, and physical limitations.]

10. Dietary and chemical intake. [Check records and ask for past and current use of caffeine, tobacco, alcohol, other vasoactive substances (e.g., tyramine and monosodium glutamate, other stimulants and depressants, gum chewing, other foods and dietary substances, and so-called "street" or "recreational" substances/drugs.]

11. Medications. [Check records. Ask about all prescription and over-the-counter medications, results, and side effects.]

12. Health-promoting behaviors. [Check records. Ask about exercise, time use management, dietary, vacation.]

13. Social support systems. [Check on family and friends, church/synagogue activities, volunteer and other organizational activities. Ask where children and other family members live, their relationships with the patient, frequency of visits with them.]

14. Education and work history. [Recent and current.]

15. Sleep. [Check for at least basics, such as bedtime and awake time, sleep onset latency, sleep interruptions and durations, sleeping partner's observations (e.g., snoring, breath stopping, teeth grinding). Check for feelings after morning awakening and daytime sleepiness. Consider Epworth Daytime Sleepiness questions (Johns, 1991; www.daytimesleep.org).]

16. Abuse. [Check for physical and sexual abuse in childhood, adulthood. If recorded history or other sources provide insufficient information, consider asking. The intake interview is usually not the time for detailed discussion of this topic or probing unless the patient wants to talk about it then. Gaining this information is a very delicate matter fraught with complex subtleties. Factors guiding whether to obtain this information and how much include presenting symptoms; purposes of the interview; time available;, likelihood of seeing the patient again; and your own experience, skills, and comfort. Consider asking at least: "Did you experience any abuse, sexual or physical, as a child or adolescent?" or "Is it possible that you experienced anything as a child or adolescent that one might consider sexual or physical abuse?"

   A patient's equivocal response, such as "Not that I remember," is a cue to a history of possible abuse. Consider inquiring further, or wait for or create chances for further inquiry in later sessions—for example, "When I asked you about abuse, you said you didn't think so as far as you could remember. Some patients with questions about possible abuse recall more as therapy progresses. Is there anything you want to ask me about definitions of abuse, and the meaning and implications of possible memories?" [If this leads to the possibility, probability, or confirmation of abuse, consider a consultation with or referral to specially trained and experienced professionals.]

17. Recommendations: Considerations and discussions. [Further evaluation with interview, inventories, self-report measures, or neurocognitive assessment. Referral, psychophysiological assessment, multiple types of relaxation therapies and demonstra-

tion, symptom log, biofeedback-assisted therapies. Consider "prudent limited office treatment" (PLOT), stepped-care options, and so forth. Discussion/patient education on varied topics tailored to patient.]

Self-Report Measures as Part of Intake

Rationale, Uses, and Issues

The usefulness of self-report measures in clinical practice is not news, nor is it debated among most practitioners. Their use has many advantages, summarized in a list below. These measures can provide information about topics not obtained during interviews and observations. They can shed light on unclear behaviors and provide hypotheses to explain these. They provide quantification and documentation of many variables of interest and are often necessary for reports to other professionals and third-party payers. The usual issues are selection of measures, when and how to use them, interpretation, and costs.

Some professionals argue persuasively that there are situations in which it is prudent to administer sets of such measures routinely. Bradley et al. (1992) state that in their inpatient program they educate, prepare, and reassure patients before the evaluation that

> the psychological evaluation [is] part of the medical diagnostic process. In order to reduce patients' concerns that their symptoms are not viewed as legitimate . . . they are informed that the psychological assessment is mandatory for all patients . . . performed . . . prior to completion of the medical diagnostic procedures. . . . required to identify interactions between pathophysiological and psychologic[al] processes that affect patients' physical symptoms, disabilities, and social and familial activities . . . [and] also may suggest interventions that might help to reduce the patients' suffering. (p. 194)

However, there are clinical situations in which such measures are unnecessary and not cost-efficient. They sometimes do not add enough to clinical decision making and treatment plans to justify the required time and expense. They also sometimes can interfere with desired rapport and the therapeutic alliance between practitioner and patient. Many practitioners are skilled interviewers and highly experienced clinicians; self-report paper-and-pencil measures often do not provide much more information than such practitioners can gain in a good interview.

Let us consider, for example, a consultation to decide the appropriateness of biofeedback for tension-type headaches for a probable work-posture-related tension myalgia. Let us further assume that this is a consultation with a patient who is resistant to seeing a psychologist. Now consider the potential perceptions and reaction of this patient to a series of self-report mood and personality measures.

The decision to proceed or not to proceed with biofeedback and related therapies will be the same, regardless of information gained from paper-and-pencil self-report measures. Skilled practitioners can often base such decisions on prior recorded information and an interview. This sounds like an argument against the use of the measures. That is not my point at all; however, I maintain that one must use them prudently and not routinely in all clinical situations. The merits of self-report measures include their ability to do the following:

- Document symptoms, personality, beliefs, and behaviors.
- Document changes or lack of changes.
- Direct practitioners to areas needing more time and effort.
- Increase patients' awareness of their beliefs, behaviors, and personality factors.
- Provide a basis for feedback to patients about attending to their beliefs, behaviors, and personality factors.

- Correct some patients' self-misperceptions.
- Provide cautions for practitioners.
- Confirm or disconfirm impressions from interviews.
- Correct practitioners' misperceptions of some patients.
- Generate hypotheses about possible problems and treatments.
- Assist less experienced practitioners.
- Potentially save interviewing and treatment time.
- Raise topics, beliefs, and behaviors for discussion.
- Select patients needing special attention.

The selection of measures is the prerogative of individual practitioners and depends on many factors. A detailed discussion of these factors is beyond the scope of this chapter; a brief listing will suffice:

- Availability of the measures.
- A patient's motivation and availability for the time needed.
- A practitioner's experience with the measures.
- Brevity of the measures and ease of administration and scoring.
- Reading level of the measures, and reading ability of the patient.
- Useful and/or important clinical and treatment plan questions needing information obtainable from the measures.

Selecting Measures and Selected Measures

The categories and selected measures listed in Table 6.2 of the second edition of this book (Schwartz, 1995, pp. 133–137) were provisional selections. The list and references are not reproduced here because of space considerations.

CONCLUSION

This chapter discusses topics and guidelines for selecting whom to treat with biofeedback or other applied psychophysiological interventions (including other physiological self-regulation therapies). It includes topics and guidelines for intake interviewing and patient education.

NOTES

1. Practitioners' evaluations of patients for therapy with other professionals will differ from their evaluations of patients they intend to see for therapy themselves.
2. I extend loving appreciation for help and insights for this section to Nancy M. Schwartz, MA, LMHC, whose significant experience and expertise includes evaluating and treating both survivors and perpetrators of sexual abuse.
3. "Functional" here signifies the absence of a structural, infectious, or metabolic cause (Berkowitz, 1998).

REFERENCES

Adler, C. S., & Adler, S. M. (1984). Biofeedback. In T. B. Karasu (Ed.), *The psychiatric therapies: The American Psychiatric Association Commission on Psychiatric Therapies*. Washington, DC: American Psychiatric Association.

Adler, C. S., & Adler, S. M. (1987). Evaluating the psychological factors in headache. In C. S. Adler, S. M. Adler, & R. C. Packard (Eds.), *Psychiatric aspects of headache*. Baltimore: Williams & Wilkins.

Adler, C. S., & Adler, S. M. (1989a). Biofeedback and psychosomatic disorders. In J. V. Basmajian (Ed.), *Biofeedback: Principles and practice for clinicians* (3rd ed.). Baltimore: Williams & Wilkins.

Adler, C. S., & Adler, S. M. (1989b). Strategies in general psychiatry. In J. V. Basmajian (Ed.), *Biofeedback: Principles and practice for clinicians* (3rd ed.). Baltimore: Williams & Wilkins.

Arnold, R. P., Rogers, D., & Cook, A. G. (1990). Medical problems of adults who were sexually abused in childhood. *British Medical Journal, 300,* 705–708.

Badgley, R. (1984). *Sexual offenses against children: Report of the Committee on Sexual Offenses Against Children and Youths.* Ottawa: Government of Canada.

Beardsley, M. C. (1972). Metaphor. In P. Edwards (Ed.), *The encyclopedia of philosophy* (Vol. 5). New York: Macmillan.

Berkowitz, C. D. (1998). Medical consequences of child sexual abuse. *Child Abuse and Neglect, 22*(6), 541–550.

Black, M. (1962). *Models and metaphor.* Ithaca, NY: Cornell University Press.

Boyd, R. (1979). Metaphor and theory change: What is metaphor for? In A. Ortony (Ed.), *Metaphor and thought.* New York: Cambridge University Press.

Bradley, L. A., McDonald-Haile, J., & Jaworski, T. M. (1992). Assessment of psychological status using interviews and self-report instruments. In D. C. Turk & R. Melzack (Eds), *Handbook of pain assessment.* New York: Guilford Press.

Cahill, C., Llewelyn, S. P., & Pearson, C. (1991). Treatment of sexual abuse which occurred in childhood: A review. *British Journal of Clinical Psychology, 30,* 1–12.

Cannell, J., Hudson, J. I., & Pope, H. G., Jr. (2001). Standards for informed consent in recovered memory therapy. *Journal of the American Academy of Psychiatry and the Law, 29,* 138–147.

Combs, G., & Freedman, J. (1990). *Symbol, story, and ceremony: Using metaphors in individual and family therapy.* New York: Norton.

Delaux, M., Denis, P., & Allemand, H. (1997). Sexual abuse is more frequently reported by IBS patients than by patients with organic digestive diseases or controls: Results of a multicentre inquiry. *French Club of Digestive Mobility, 9*(4), 345–352.

Domino, J., & Haber, J. (1987). Prior physical and sexual abuse in women with chronic headache: Clinical correlates. *Headache, 27,* 310–314.

Drossman, D., Lagerman, J., Nachman, G., Li, Z., Gluck, H., Toomey, T., & Mitchell, C. (1990). Sexual and physical abuse among women with functional and organic gastrointestinal disorders. *Annals of Behavioral Medicine, 113,* 828–833.

Drossman, D. A., Talley, N. J., Leserman, J., Olden, K. W., & Barreiro, M. A. (1995). Sexual and physical abuse and gastrointestinal illness: Review and recommendations. *Annals of Internal Medicine, 123,* 782–794.

Fraser, B. (1979). The interpretation of novel metaphors. In A. Ortony (Ed.), *Metaphor and thought.* New York: Cambridge University Press.

Golding, J. M., Taylor, D. L., Menard, L., & King, M. J. (2000). Prevalence of sexual abuse history in a sample of women seeking treatment for premenstrual syndrome. *Journal of Psychosomatic Obstetrics and Gynecology, 21,* 69–80.

Haber, J. D., & Roos, C. (1985). Effects of spouse abuse and/or sexual abuse in the development and maintenance of chronic pain in women. *Advances in Pain Research and Therapy, 9,* 889–895.

Hall, R. C. W. (Ed.). (1980). *Psychiatric presentation of medical illness.* New York: Spectrum.

Harden, C. L. (1997). Pseudoseizures and dissociative disorders: A common mechanism involving traumatic experiences. *Seizure, 6*(2), 151–155.

Herson, M., & Turner, S. M. (1985). *Diagnostic interviewing.* New York: Plenum Press.

Ireland, N., Freeman, T., & Shore, H. (Eds.). (1996). *The directory of critical information for helping children.* King of Prussia, PA: The Center for Applied Psychology.

Johns, M. W. (1991). A new method for measuring daytime sleepiness: The Epworth Sleepiness Scale. *Sleep, 14*(6), 540–545.

Lacks, P. (1987). *Behavioral treatment for persistent insomnia.* New York: Pergamon Press.

Lampe, A., Solder, E., Ennemoser, A., Schubert, C., Rumpold, G., & Sollner, W. (2000). Chronic pelvic pain and previous sexual abuse. *Obstetrics and Gynecology, 96*(6) 929–933.

Lechner, M. E., Vogel, M. E., Garcia-Shelton, L. M., Leichter, J. L., & Steibel, K. R. (1993). Self-reported medical problems of adult female survivors of childhood sexual abuse. *Journal of Family Practice, 36,* 633–638.

Levy, R. L. (1987). Compliance and clinical practice. In J. A. Blumenthal & D. C. McKee (Eds.), *Application in behavioral medicine and health psychology: A clinician's source book.* Sarasota, FL: Professional Resource Exchange.

McMullin, R. E. (1986). *Handbook of cognitive therapy techniques.* New York: Norton.

Moore, P. M. & Baker, G. A. (1997). Non-epileptic attack disorder: A psychological perspective. *Seizure, 6,* 429–434.

Morris, W., & Morris, M. (1985). *Harper dictionary of contemporary usage* (2nd ed.). New York: Harper & Row.

Morrison, J. (1989). Childhood sexual histories of women with somatization disorder. *American Journal of Psychiatry, 146,* 236–241.

Muran, J. C., & DiGiuseppe, R. A. (1990). Towards a cognitive formulation of metaphor use in psychotherapy. *Clinical Psychology Reviews, 10,* 69–85.

Ortony, A., Reynolds, R., & Arter, J. A. (1978). Metaphor: Theoretical and empirical research. *Psychological Bulletin, 85*(5), 919–943.

Othmer, E., & Othmer, S. C. (2002). *The clinical interview using DSM-IV-TR* (Vol. 1). Washington, DC: American Psychiatric Press.

Petrie, H. G. (1979). Metaphor and learning. In A. Ortony (Ed.), *Metaphor and thought.* New York: Cambridge University Press.

Richards, I. A. (1936). *The philosophy of rhetoric.* London: Oxford University Press.

Rosse, R. B., Deutsch, L. H., & Deutsch, S. I. (2000). Medical assessment and laboratory testing in psychiatry. In B. J. Sadock & V. A. Sadock (Eds.), *Kaplan and Sadock's comprehensive textbook of psychiatry* (7th ed.). Philadelphia: Lippincott Williams & Wilkins.

Russell, D. (1984). *Sexual exploitations: Rape, child sexual abuse, and workplace harassment.* Beverly Hills, CA: Sage.

Salter, A. C. (1988). *Treating child sex offenders and victims: A practical guide.* London: Sage.

Scheflin, A. W., & Spiegel, D. (1998). From courtroom to couch: Working with repressed memory and avoiding lawsuits. *Psychiatric Clinics of North America, 21*(4), 847–867.

Schwartz, M. S. (1995). Intake decisions and preparations of patients for therapy. In M. S. Schwartz & Associates, *Biofeedback: A practitioner's guide* (2nd ed.). New York: Guilford Press.

Shaw, E. R., & Blanchard, E. B. (1983). The effects of instructional set on the outcome of a stress management program. *Biofeedback and Self-Regulation, 8*(4), 555–565.

Siegelman, E. Y. (1990). *Metaphor and meaning in psychotherapy.* New York: Guilford Press.

Springs, F. E., & Friedrich, W. N. (1982). Health risk behaviors and medical sequelae of childhood sexual abuse. *Mayo Clinic Proceedings, 67,* 527–532.

Talley, N. J., Fett, S. L., & Zinsmeister, A. R. (1995). Self-reported abuse and gastrointestinal disease in outpatients with irritable bowel-type symptoms. *American Journal of Gastroenterology, 90,* 366–371.

Talley, N. J., Fett, S. L., Zinsmeister, A. R., & Melton, L. J. (1994). Gastrointestinal tract symptoms and self-reported abuse: A population-based study. *Gastroenterology, 107,* 1040–1049.

Toomey, T. C., Hernandez, J. T., Gittleman, D. F., & Hulka, J. F. (1993). Relationship of sexual and physical abuse to pain and psychological assessment variables in chronic pelvic pain patients. *Pain, 53,* 105–109.

Walker, E. A., Eaton, W. J., Hanson, J., Harrop-Griffiths, J., Holm, L., Jes, M. L., Hickok, L., & Jamelka, R. P. (1992). Medical and psychiatric symptoms in women with childhood sexual abuse. *Psychosomatic Medicine, 54,* 658–664.

CHAPTER 7

Psychophysiological Assessment and Biofeedback Baselines

A Primer

JOHN G. ARENA

MARK S. SCHWARTZ

We hope that this chapter will successfully demystify psychophysiological assessment and enhance applied psychophysiologists' ability to formulate clinical questions and employ psychophysiological assessments to answer them.

The process of learning how to use psychophysiological assessments to answer relevant clinical questions first involves the review of some basic concepts in applied psychophysiology: (1) the measures that are generally used by applied psychophysiologists; (2) basic concepts in psychophysiology that are most relevant to applied psychophysiologists; and (3) general conditions that biofeedback therapists are likely to employ in such assessments. We stress what is perhaps the most important methodological issue in any type of assessment—that is, the temporal stability (i.e., reliability) of psychophysiological measures. We emphasize two conditions that are of essential importance to any psychophysiological assessment: baselines and adaptation periods.

MEASURES USED IN PSYCHOPHYSIOLOGICAL ASSESSMENTS

The measures generally employed in psychophysiological assessments are surface electromyography (EMG); skin surface temperature (e.g., fingers, hands); electrodermal response; cardiovascular activity (heart rate, blood pressure, and vasomotor activity); and respiration (generally respiration rate and depth). Electroencephalography (EEG) requires specialized training and is outside the expertise of the average biofeedback clinician (as well as ourselves!), and therefore is not discussed in this chapter (but see Neumann, Strehl, & Birbaumer, Chapter 5, this volume, for such a discussion). For references about how surface EMG (hereafter referred to simply as EMG), skin temperature, and electrodermal responses are recorded and interpreted, see Peek, Chapter 4, this volume. For more on EMG, see Basmajian and DeLuca (1985). For measures of cardiovascular activity, see Larsen, Schneiderman, and DeCarlo Pasin (1986). For respiration, see Fried (1993), Kaufman and Schneiderman (1986), and Timmons and Ley (1994).

BASIC CONCEPTS IN PSYCHOPHYSIOLOGY

Basic concepts in applied psychophysiology and the scientific method in general with which biofeedback clinicians need to be familiar are autonomic balance, individual response stereotypy, stimulus–response specificity, the law of initial values, homeostasis, orienting and defensive responses, carryover effects, and (especially) temporal stability of the measures. Again, because of the importance of temporal stability, it is discussed at some length here.

"Autonomic balance" refers to response patterning of the autonomic nervous system (ANS) (Sturgis & Arena, 1984). It has long been believed that individuals who are exposed to a stimulus of some sort will respond with either a sympathetic or a parasympathetic response activation. In 1917, Eppinger and Hess were the first to classify individuals as "vagotonic" (parasympathetic) and "sympatonic" (sympathetic) responders. In 1966, Wenger created a score of autonomic balance based on how an individual's electrodermal response, heart rate, diastolic blood pressure, and salivation output responded to various stimuli. Autonomic balance scores have been used for a variety of disorders, including anxiety disorders, schizophrenia, hypertension, headache, antisocial personality disorder, and attention-deficit/hyperactivity disorder; low scores tend to be related to increased susceptibility to both physical and psychological disease, whereas high scores are associated with greater mental and physical health.

"Individual response stereotypy" and "stimulus–response specificity" are somewhat complex categorization schemes that also involve the use of various psychophysiological measures and a search for patterns in the responses. Stimulus–response specificity is seen when different stimuli, such as a cognitive versus a physical stressor, produce idiosyncratic patterns of responding. Individual response stereotypy, on the other hand, is seen when an individual evidences a single, distinctive response pattern to all stimuli (Sternbach, 1966). For example, one individual may characteristically respond to stressful events with increased heart rate, whereas another evidences lowered hand surface temperature (stereotypy); alternatively, one individual may reliably respond to a mental arithmetic task with increased respiration rate and lowered respiration depth, while responding to an ischemic pain stressor with increased frontal EMG.

The "law of initial values" refers to the effect that prestimulus values of a particular psychophysiological measure have on that response's magnitude of psychophysiological reactivity to a specific stimulus (Wilder, 1950). The higher the level of the measure prior to presentation of a stressful stimulus, the smaller the increase in response to the stressor (often referred to as a "ceiling effect"). Conversely, the higher the level of the measure prior to presentation of a relaxing stimulus, the larger the decrease in response to the relaxing stimulus (when prestimulus response values are low prior to the presentation of a relaxing stimulus, this will lower the magnitude of the response and is often referred to as a "floor effect"). Although the law has been shown to hold generally for measures of respiration and cardiovascular activity (such as heart rate and the vasomotor response), other measures, such as salivation and electrodermal response, have nor been found to be influenced by prestimulus values.

"Homeostasis" refers to the tendency of any organism to strive to maintain a state of equilibrium or rest. Homeostasis is believed to be maintained by a negative feedback loop, which is a hypothesized bodily mechanism that provides information directing the physiological system to decrease activity if levels of functioning are higher than normal, or to increase activity if levels are below normal. Thus all organisms strive to return to prestimulus levels of physiological arousal when presented with any stimulus. Applied psychophysiology research has demonstrated that there are limits beyond which increases and decreases in the physiological response cannot be trained.

The "orienting response" and the "defensive response" refer to the ways organisms react to unique and novel stimuli; these responses are both behavioral and physiological. The orienting response can be viewed as the "What is it?" response. It typically involves "an increased sensitivity of the sensory organs, body orientation towards the stimulus, increased muscle tone with a reduction of irrelevant motor activity, EEG activation, vasoconstriction of the peripheral vascular system, vasodilatation of the cranial vascular system, increased skin conductance, respiration amplitude increase accompanied by decreased respiration rate, and a slowing of the heart rhythm" (Sturgis & Arena, 1984, p. 16). It is impossible to ascertain which portions of the initial response to a stimulus are an orienting responses and which are the actual response to the stimulus; applied psychophysiologists generally disregard the initial responses to stimuli when analyzing response patterns. The orienting response generally habituates quickly, but it has been shown that responses to both psychologically and physiologically relevant stimuli habituate at much slower rates. As contrasted to the increased attention toward a stimulus that is the orienting response, the defensive response is defined as a turning away of attention, usually from a painful stimulus or a stimulus that is too intense. Physiologically it is similar to the orienting response, but with increased heart rate and constriction of the cranial vascular system. It is generally believed that the orienting response habituates more quickly than the defensive response.

The term "carryover effect" is a basic research methodology notion referring to the effect that prior research conditions can have on subsequent conditions. It is important to note that in addition to carryover effects from the actual experience of the condition, a temporal factor may also be causing participants to tire over time (see below) and show a change in response pattern unrelated to the condition being evaluated (Sturgis & Arena, 1984). For example, a biofeedback therapist may present a variety of stressful conditions in a psychophysiological assessment; the presentation of stressor 1 may affect stressor 2, and the presentation of stressors 1 and 2 may affect stressor 3. In addition to the specific carryover effects of stressors 1 and 2, stressor 3 may have been affected by the patient becoming fatigued over time.

There are two generally acceptable solutions to the problem of carryover effects in research methodology. First, and most conservative, is to avoid the use of a repeated-measures design and use only an independent-groups design. The primary limitations of this design for clinical biofeedback therapists are that large sample sizes are needed, and, of course, the average clinician does not have the resources, the time, or the patience to conduct such studies. A second solution to the problem of carryover effects is to use a counterbalanced design— that is, to vary the order of the conditions in a random manner. This is something that the average clinician can do, since it does not involve large numbers of patients. One major concern about this design is the inherent assumption that carryover effects are equivalent between the differing conditions. That is, the carryover effect of stressor 1 is exactly the same as the carryover effects of stressor 2 and of stressor 3. The possibility of interactions among the conditions and differential practice effects are not controlled. Unfortunately, there has been little research examining the possibility of carryover effects in applied psychophysiology, and the limited available data are inconclusive.

"Temporal stability," or "reliability," of the measures used in psychophysiological assessment and treatment has been a topic of increasing importance in the past 20 years. If an assessment measure is not stable over time, it is a poor indicator of what is purportedly tested. Given the wide range of factors that can affect the magnitude of the various psychophysiological responses, it is not surprising that there can be difficulties in obtaining stable recordings across time. Moreover, when limits are set on the reliability of a measure, there is generally an inability to obtain a high estimate of "validity" (whether the measure actually records a true representation of the concept supposedly assessed).

To illustrate the difficulties involved in temporal stability of psychophysiological assessment, consider the following scenario: Ms. X, a single mother who suffers from chronic headaches, comes to her therapist's office for a pretreatment psychophysiological assessment. The appointment is at 5:30 P.M. on a cold January day. Ms. X has gotten little sleep the night before because she has been up all night taking care of her 6-year-old son, who has a stomach virus. Work that day is extremely difficult (she is a secretary in a lawyer's office); she must guzzle coffee all day just to stay alert; and she has an argument with a coworker about who is responsible for a botched copying job just before leaving at 5:00 P.M. Traffic is horrible, and she gets stuck behind a slow driver in the left lane. Ms. X arrives at the office just in time, after finding a parking place two blocks away and running there. She is promptly ushered into the biofeedback and psychophysiological assessment lab, and given a brief explanation by a therapist she has only met once. Sensors are attached to her forehead, neck, shoulders, and two of her fingertips, and placed around her chest. She is asked to perform several tasks—including immersing her hand in a bucket of ice water and counting backward from 999 by 7's—by the therapist, who is speaking to her over an intercom from an adjacent room. She wonders the entire time how long the session will last, as the sitter must leave by 7:00. At the end of the assessment, she is asked whether she has any questions, and responds, "No." An appointment is scheduled for treatment.

Halfway through treatment, on a rather warm day in mid-March, the therapist retests Ms. X to "determine if treatment has had any effects yet on your body's responses to stressful situations." This time, however, in contrast to the testing in January, Ms. X has had a great night's sleep. Her 6-year-old has come home the day before with all A's on his report card. The appointment is at 9:30 A.M., and she receives permission from her boss to take the morning off. She finds a parking spot directly in front of the office and, while waiting for 10 minutes, plans a shopping trip for later that morning (as she has lost 10 pounds since beginning therapy, and her clothes are now loose). She is ushered into the biofeedback and psychophysiological assessment lab by her therapist, and they are both joking, as they are now well acquainted with each other. The procedures are repeated. Her reactions to the stressors are greatly reduced, and the therapist states, "We now have hard evidence that the treatment has already had an effect on your body's responses to stress." Is this actually the case? Can we truly arrive at that conclusion? Could the reduction in magnitude of the responses to the stressors merely be a result of repeating the test? Could it be a result of more sleep? Weight loss? Differences in time of day? Comfort with the therapist? Seasonal temperatures? Such questions underscore the vital importance of temporal stability research and relevance of such factors as age, gender, race, weight loss, situational and trait anxiety, and many others.

Review of the Temporal Stability Literature

Because of the topic's importance, we comprehensively review the essential literature concerning temporal stability of psychophysiological responses. We focus on measures of EMG and surface skin temperature, as those are the two non-EEG responses most often used in biofeedback training.

Sturgis (1980) was one of the first researchers to investigate temporal stability. She examined the frontal EMG response, bilateral cephalic vasomotor response, and digital vasomotor responses in 10 patients with migraine and 10 with tension headache. Overall test–retest reliability of the measures was .31, which, albeit statistically significant, accounted for a small proportion of the variance.

Arena, Blanchard, Andrasik, Cotch, and Myers (1983) began studying reliability with a normal population. Fifteen undergraduate subjects were assessed on multiple response measures (frontal and forearm flexor EMG, heart rate, skin resistance level, hand surface temperature, and cephalic vasomotor response) under multiple stimulus conditions (baseline, relaxing whole body deeply, warming hands, relaxing forehead, mental arithmetic, positive imagery, stressful imagery, cold pressor) on multiple occasions (days 1, 2, 8, and 28). Subjects were screened for medical conditions, and all assessments occurred at approximately the same time of day. Three forms of reliability coefficients were computed for each response measure: coefficients on absolute scores, and two coefficients on relative measures (percent change from baseline, and change scores from baseline to stressful conditions). ("Relative measures" are any measures other than the actual raw value of the response; in other words, the actual raw score of the psychophysiological response has been changed or transformed in some manner. This is typically done to decrease the wide variability that is often found in psychophysiological responses, as well as to control, in EMG studies particularly, in differences between various equipment brands, etc.)

Results indicated that for absolute values of the measures, only frontal EMG seemed consistently reliable, while hand surface temperature was reliable if sessions were repeated within 1 week. Heart rate and forearm flexor EMG were somewhat less consistently reliable. Lower reliability coefficients were generally obtained when responses were treated as relative measures. Further analysis indicated that, with the exception of forearm flexor EMG and hand surface temperature, the experimental conditions led to the desired responses. Forearm flexor EMG did not respond to any of the experimental manipulations (i.e., verbal instructions), but even baseline comparisons were unreliable. It did seem, however, that hand surface temperature habituated after the third session or after 1 week, because the experimental manipulations produced the desired results for the first three sessions, with associated high reliability.

It was concluded that investigators must first ascertain the reliability of these measures on their respective subject population, and subsequently must employ in their research only those measures that are found to be reliable with that population. Another conclusion was that since frontal EMG and hand surface temperature were the primary biofeedback modalities, and they were fairly reliable, clinicians merely need to be wary of falsely attributing baseline hand temperature increases solely to biofeedback training, which may be partly resultant from habituation to the clinical situation. Arena et al. (1983) also argued for the necessity of examining reliability as a function of, for example, demographic variables, clinical populations, laboratory versus nonlaboratory settings, and such characteristics as depression, anger, and anxiety.

Other investigators suggested examining a more complex patterning of the responses. Waters, Williamson, Bernard, Blouin, and Faulstich (1987) built upon the work of Manuck and Schaifer (1978). These experimenters differentiated groups of "reactors" and "non-reactors" based on cardiovascular responses to difficult cognitive tasks, and found stability in these designations when subjects were retested a week later.

Waters et al. (1987) compared 30 college students, using 5 stimuli and 10 psychophysiological measures over 2 weeks. The magnitude and range of correlations were similar to those found in the Arena et al. (1983; Arena, Goldberg, Saul, & Hobbs, 1989a) studies. They also analyzed individual response specificity with the Profile Similarity Index (PSI; Buco & Blouin, 1983), providing a single index of overall similarity or reliability of the two response profiles. For reactivity, at least 87% of the subjects showed similarity as indicated by the PSI.

Probably their most revealing analysis resulted from comparing the subjects' ranks (on a 10-to-1 scale) with a ranked hierarchy of standardized physiological scores for each subject and for the 10 psychophysiological measures. Waters et al. averaged the ranks across the stimulus procedures. Fifteen of 30 subjects ranking 10th in one session, and 14 ranking 9th, were ranked 10th or 9th in the second session. Similarly, 29 of the subjects ranked 2nd or 1st in the first session were ranked 2nd or 1st in the second session. Those ranked between these extremes in the first session varied considerably in the second, and some went to the other extreme. Waters et al. (1987) concluded that "it is thus clear that the most extreme responses in an individual's psychophysiological response hierarchy are the most stable (reliable) across experimental sessions" (p. 219).

Building on the work of Waters et al. (1987), Arena et al. (1989a) argued that analysis of both individual response stereotypy and stimulus–response specificity might provide a perspective on reliability not available from the traditional Pearson correlational procedures commonly employed, or from an analysis of only individual response stereotypy. A multivariate response pattern approach might have some predictive validity. For example, some (Engel, 1960) might argue that clinical populations would have more stability than normal individuals in the particular response system presumed to be abnormal (e.g., patients with low back pain in the paraspinal muscles, patients with headache in the forehead or upper trapezius muscles), whereas others (Sternbach, 1966) would argue the opposite.

Arena et al. (1989a) therefore examined the temporal stability of three response measures (forehead EMG, hand surface temperature, heart rate) on 64 college and community volunteers during four sessions over a month's interval. Each session consisted of an adaptation period, a baseline condition, a cognitive stressor (serial 7's), and a physical stressor (a cold pressor task). Reliability coefficients on the absolute scores across conditions were, for the most part, modest and statistically significant. Treating the responses as relative measures produced smaller and less frequently significant correlational coefficients. The data were also examined in a multidimensional manner, using z-scores to determine whether each subject showed any consistencies across sessions with respect to which response system was maximally aroused. This analysis led to identifying three groups of subjects: those who responded primarily within a single system across sessions regardless of stressor (individual response stereotypy, 42%); those who responded differentially across sessions to the two stressors (stimulus–response specificity, 20%); and those whose profiles were not readily classifiable (38%).

Results supported the notion that psychophysiological measures achieve some degree of meaningful reliability over time. Arena et al. (1989a) also argued that identification of clinical patients who fit the stimulus–response specificity pattern may have great clinical relevance. For example, a patient with headache who responds to physical stressors with hand surface temperature, but to mental stressors with EMG, may require psychophysiological intervention targeting both response systems. Moreover, a clinician may need to investigate these response patterns in terms of the stimuli most readily eliciting them. This may explain why some patients with headache fail to respond to a single modality biofeedback intervention. Presumably, a less complex therapeutic approach would suffice for the more common stereotypical responder.

Following a challenge that researchers should examine reliability in clinical populations, and to determine whether such populations have greater or lesser reliability than normals, Arena, Sherman, Bruno, and Young (1990) recorded bilateral surface paraspinal EMG in 29 patients with lower back pain and 20 normal subjects in six different positions (standing, bending from the waist, rising, sitting with back supported, sitting unsupported, prone) on two occasions. Measures were highly reliable when examined via analysis-of-variance procedures. Statistically significant reliability coefficients were obtained when the absolute values of the measures were examined. When the data were examined as relative (percent change from prone condition) values, differences between the two groups were observed: The normal subjects were statistically more reliable than the patients with lower back pain during every condition. It was suggested that investigators use primarily absolute values of the paraspinal EMG responses for patients with lower back pain.

Shaeffer, Sponsel, Kice, and Hollensbe (1991) studied the 1-week reliability of resting baseline psychophysiological activity for several ANS variables assessed for 5 minutes after a

15-minute stabilization period. The 21 male and female undergraduates, aged 18 to 21, reclined with their legs supported and their eyes open. The stability was high for skin conductance level ($r = .89$); moderate and statistically significant for heart rate ($r = .63$), abdominal amplitude ($r = .63$), finger temperature ($r = .54$), and respiration rate ($r = .49$); and low and nonsignificant for blood volume pulse ($r = .23$).

Speckenback and Gerber (1999) replicated the results of Arena's group (Arena et al., 1983; Arena, 1984) and those of others (Sturgis, 1980; Shaeffer et al., 1991) concerning the reliability of blood volume pulse. Twenty healthy individuals with a mean age of 28.3 years were seen on two separate occasions for a 30-minute baseline period with the probe positioned over the terminal branch of the external carotid artery, the superficial temporal artery. The probe was then removed and repositioned as closely as possible to the original position. One week later, the process was repeated. Results indicated that blood volume pulse within a single session was highly reliable, but unreliable from session to session. Repositioning the probe within the session resulted in lower, but still significant and sizable, correlation coefficients. The authors concluded, "How best to compare PVA [pulse volume amplitude] data from different sessions needs further exploration" (p. 264).

As did most investigators in studies examining the temporal stability of psychophysiological measures, in studies before 1990 Arena and colleagues had employed the Pearson product–moment correlation coefficient as the primary correlational measure of psychophysiological intersession reliability. Statisticians would argue that the intraclass correlational coefficient (Kirk, 1982) is a more appropriate reliability statistic to use when one is employing more than two test–retest intervals. Intraclass correlations take into account changes in values, not just the relative proportion, of scores. This is especially useful in psychophysiological measures on which initial intensities commonly vary. More importantly, intraclass correlations allow simultaneous incorporation of more than one set of values on the same subjects. Therefore, Arena and Hobbs (1995a) reanalyzed their 1989 study data using the intraclass correlation, and found that with the exception of EMG during the physical stressor (cold pressor task), the absolute values of the responses (forehead EMG, hand surface temperature, heart rate) had quite significant reliability (.70 or greater). They concluded that statistical estimates of psychophysiological response reliability are functions of the study design and particular reliability analysis employed. But, even though intraclass correlational estimates of reliability are significantly higher than the traditional Pearson product–moment correlational estimates, Arena and Hobbs argued then (and continue to advance) the proposal that this does not vitiate the call for more research into factors that affect the reliability of psychophysiological responding, because much of the test–retest variance in psychophysiological responses is still unexplained.

Therefore, Arena and Hobbs (1995b) divided the subjects from their 1989 study into two groups: 17 subjects with high Spielberger Trait Anxiety Inventory scores and 17 with low scores. Results indicated that reliability coefficients for the two anxiety groups did not differ on frontal EMG or heart rate responses; however, hand surface temperature responding was considerably less reliable for highly anxious individuals than for individuals low in anxiety. Magnitudes of the three physiological responses did not significantly differ as a function of trait anxiety. We strongly recommend to both clinicians and researchers that they employ additional measures of arousal and relaxation, instead of relying solely on hand surface temperature response.

One major limitation of this study was the lack of controls for nicotine and caffeine. Arena and Hobbs (1995b) mentioned this at the time, but suggested that this "would not typically occur in practice settings" (p. 35). However, as Schwartz (1995) noted, "both caffeine and nicotine are more commonly used by high-anxious people and both affect hand temperatures through peripheral vasoconstriction. Therefore, one needs to control for these"

(p. 162). The two of us (Arena and Schwartz) are now in agreement that this is a major oversight, and we would call for further reliability research on clinically anxious individuals that controls for caffeine and nicotine use.

Gerin et al. (1998), in what may prove to be a seminal article, looked at the reliability of cardiovascular responses (blood pressure and heart rate) and the generalizability of these responses across various settings. Twenty-four female students in college (age range 17–26) were given a mental arithmetic task (serial 13's) following a 12-minute baseline twice in the laboratory (to examine test–retest reliability), once in a classroom, and once at home. Adequate test–retest reliability was found for the baseline condition (.81 for systolic blood pressure, .63 for diastolic blood pressure, and .68 for heart rate). However, poor reliability was found in change scores from baseline to the mental arithmetic task (absolute values were not given in the report) for heart rate response (.09), while systolic blood pressure (.68) and diastolic blood pressure (.62) had adequate reliability. When the investigators examined for generalizability, smaller correlation coefficients were obtained on all three measures for the nonlaboratory settings than for the laboratory setting. The authors concluded, "This suggests that even a minor variation in procedure, such as a change in setting, can affect generalizability" (p. 209). They further stated:

> If we are to find predictive power from the laboratory to the natural environment, there is no dimension of variability so trivial that it can be dismissed without investigation. If simply changing the location of the test site can reduce the lab-to-life associations, then altering more significant aspects of the test situation, such as the task or the subject's motivation, is likely to do even more damage to the stability of reactivity as an individual difference. (p. 217)

(For those interested in the topic of heart rate variability, we recommend the Committee Report on Heart Rate Variability [Berntson et al., 1997], an exhaustive review of the topic.)

Veit, Brody, and Rau (1997) in a very interesting study, examined the stability of cardiovascular measures (heart rate, systolic and diastolic blood pressure) to a laboratory psychological stressor (mental arithmetic) in 75 adults over a 4-year test–retest interval. They found adequate reliability for both absolute and change scores from baseline for heart rate (.81 absolute, .76 change score) and systolic blood pressure (.52 absolute and .66 change score) measures. However, the absolute value correlation for diastolic blood pressure was .27, and the change score coefficient was only .16.

Finally, Arena et al. (1994) also looked at the temporal stability of an ambulatory monitoring device for surface EMG levels. Twenty-six healthy controls wore a lightweight (24-ounce) device that measured bilateral upper trapezius EMG, as well as peak and integral motion, for 5 consecutive days for up to 18 hours each day. Intraclass correlational coefficients for the two EMG variables across the 5 days were both significant, with alpha levels set at .01. The two EMG measures were highly correlated ($r = .77$); the two motion measures were also highly correlated ($r = .60$). Reliability coefficients for the EMG measures were similar to those found in laboratory studies. It was concluded that the test–retest reliability of the ambulatory monitoring device was within acceptable limits.

Temporal Stability Conclusions

Some tentative conclusions can be drawn from the results of the studies reviewed above.

1. For forehead EMG, heart rate, blood pressure, and hand surface temperature, the majority of the studies indicate at least statistically significant reliability coefficients of modest magnitude.

2. The amount of variance explained, even by those measures with the correlations of greatest magnitude, suggests that other factors are accounting for more variance than the experimental manipulation (i.e., retesting).

3. Reliability is affected significantly by the statistical approach employed (i.e., analysis of variance, absolute-value Pearson product–moment correlations, relative-value [percent change from baseline, raw change scores from baseline] Pearson correlations, intraclass correlations, or analysis of response patterns such as individual response stereotypy or stimulus–response specificity), with most studies suggesting that relative-value procedures produce lower correlations than absolute-value procedures.

4. It is probably prudent to use multiple measures of arousal rather than to rely on any one measure.

5. Hand surface temperature appears to be a very complex response that may be affected by repeated measurement and patients' trait levels of anxiety.

6. More research is vitally needed, especially on the temporal stability of such measures as electrodermal response, digital blood volume pulse, respiration, and EMG other than forehead.

7. More research is needed on reliability as a function of demographic factors (such as age, gender, and race), clinical populations, laboratory versus nonlaboratory settings, caffeine and nicotine consumption, and psychological characteristics (such as anger, anxiety, depression, etc.).

8. Finally, we would urge you, our readers, to gather some rudimentary baseline data on the reliability of the measures routinely employed in clinical practice. This provides some general indication of equipment reliability, as well as the effect of a particular clinical setting (type of room where measures are routinely obtained, pictures, the therapist variables, quietness, etc.). Although this may seem arduous, the reverse is true. First, obtaining this information from a clinical population is easy. At intake, ask your first 10 or so patients with headache, low back pain, anxiety, or the like whether they would mind sitting 15 minutes for some baseline readings of a few measures now and at the beginning of the next treatment session (which is usually within 7–10 days). We have never been refused, and patients are very interested in this information. We also have done this with friends and colleagues for a normal (relatively normal, if you are aware of our friends and colleagues!) population. Obtaining this normative data is usually a little bit trickier, but often can be done in a few months if you are in a hospital, clinic, or academic setting, and a year or so if you are in a private practice setting. This method will provide a wealth of information, enhance your confidence in the equipment's data, and indicate which measures produce more reliable recordings.

CONDITIONS GENERALLY EMPLOYED IN PSYCHOPHYSIOLOGICAL ASSESSMENTS

Adaptation Period

The importance of an adaptation period in psychophysiological research has long been a topic of discussion; unfortunately, there has been little empirical research to date indicating the optimum duration of an adequate adaptation period. An "adaptation period" is defined as the duration of time the subject spends in the experimental situation prior to the onset of baseline measures or the experimental conditions. The function of an adaptation period in psychophysiological research and clinical work is threefold:

1. It allows the subject to become familiar with the novel experimental situation, as most people are unaccustomed to having sensors attached to various parts of their anatomy while they sit with their eyes closed in a sound- and light-attenuated room.

2. It allows presession effects to dissipate. Such effects may include stress, rushing to the appointment, walking up flights of stairs, and significant temperature discrepancies between the outdoors and the office.

3. It allows habituation of the orienting response and permits the stabilization of psychophysiological responses. If these responses fluctuate prior to the experimental manipulation or the recording of tonic levels of physiological functioning, there is uncertainty whether the independent variable (e.g., diagnosis, experimental instructions, biofeedback training) led to the findings, as opposed to random variations secondary to an insufficient period of stabilization. Thus an adaptation period is especially salient in early sessions of biofeedback training.

Likewise, an adaptation period is especially important if advocacy of the law of initial values yields a need to examine a patient's physiological responses by using relative rather than absolute scores (Wilder, 1950). If baseline or prestimulus levels are unstable, the relative measures—generally raw change scores (pre minus post) or percent change scores from baseline—may be drastically influenced and results potentially vitiated.

There have been only a few studies investigating what constitutes an adequate adaptation period. Meyers and Craighead (1978), in a rather confusing study, found that respiration rate, finger pulse volume, heart rate, and basal skin resistance could reach stability in an average of about 5–6 minutes; however, there was a great deal of variability between subjects, with some needing almost no adaptation period and others requiring a lengthy one. Taub and School (1978), in an anecdotal study, found that some individuals required as long as 30 minutes to stabilize on hand surface temperature response. Frontal EMG stabilization occurred in an average of 11 minutes across a very small group of 17 undergraduate, nonclinical students (Sallis & Lichstein, 1979). However, among these subjects, there was "considerable idiosyncrasy of the EMG adaptation response" (p. 339). This suggests that there would probably be much variability among clinical patients, especially for those with high levels of forehead muscle tension. Lichstein, Sallis, Hill, and Young (1981) reported a gender effect for heart rate response, in which males were adapted from onset and females required 13 minutes for an adequate adaptation period. They also found that adaptation periods of 7 and 13 minutes were necessary for, respectively, skin resistance level and frontal EMG.

Many factors merit consideration during planning and implementation of adaptation and baseline (see below) recordings, as well as for psychophysiological feedback. Even after these global changes are made, individual differences in responses and patterns will still exist, and clinical judgment must enter into the picture. One size (or adaptation) does not fit all.

In practice, the clinician usually tailors the cognitive preparation and adaptation time to the patient and situation, although there is no standard. Practitioners need to be aware of the potential impact of instructional set on their patients, and should consider standardizing it as much as possible and always documenting the instructions they used. Other practitioners will appreciate a clinical or research report that includes this information. It can ease replication and application to clinical practice.

The total duration of the stabilization phase varies and depends on several factors, including time in the waiting room. Other practical factors include the physical condition of the patient arriving at the office, the physiological activity monitored, the therapist's purpose, and the number of prior sessions. Rashed, Leventhal, Madu, Reddy, and Cardoso (1997) suggested that cardiovascular responses (heart rate, blood pressure, and hand surface temperature) to cold pressor stress are significantly attenuated by exercise. Thus an adaptation period is especially important when a cold pressor task is part of a psychophysiological assessment.

Practitioners should monitor and record moment-by-moment physiological functioning to check the potential effects of brief orienting responses and should, for example, watch for such events as abrupt noises. Brief orienting responses are of potential clinical use as well. For example, the person who is more physiologically responsive to low-level environmental stimuli may require different procedures. Habituation is rapid after orienting responses, but can affect summary scores of adaptation and other periods.

Psychophysiological arousal can occur if either perceived or bona fide threatening stimuli are present. Habituation of this type of response is usually slow and variable (Sturgis & Gramling, 1988). Several potentially threatening factors associated with office visits can increase muscle tension and autonomic arousal. An example occurs in a person who feels threatened by physicians or mental health professionals. Sitting quietly for several minutes, reclining, and connection to the instruments are other examples of stimuli that can be threatening for some persons. Practitioners should check these factors when planning and interpreting adaptation and other baseline periods. Repeated exposure to potentially threatening stimuli within a longer initial session or repeated sessions may be necessary to obtain adequate adaptation. Additional research is needed to develop more standard guidelines for adaptation.

We suggest that a person commonly needs at least 5 minutes for adaptation. However, sitting quietly for up to 20 minutes may be necessary for some patients. For example, Taub and School's (1978) anecdotal report suggests that for some persons, even 30 minutes is not enough for stabilization of hand temperature. Shorter times are probably enough for most people seen in clinical practice. Adaptation time is often between 3 and 5 minutes with instruments attached, especially for patients who have waited several minutes in a waiting room.

Neutral conversation is acceptable if the goals are adjustment of body position and adjustment to the instruments. Therapists should consider omitting conversation if the goal is allowing the physiological systems of interest to settle down. During this phase, therapists typically give no specific instructions to the patients except to sit quietly and get comfortable. Arena et al. (e.g., 1983, 1989a) usually tell their patients to "sit quietly with your eyes closed for the next couple of minutes." Other therapists may wish to have patients sit with their eyes open (see discussion in the section on baselines, below). The basic goal is to get a patient to sit quietly and get used to the clinical or experimental situation.

Another perfectly acceptable criterion is a floating adaptation period, which has no prescribed length. Rather, the clinician or investigator has a preset criterion for stabilization of each response (e.g., heart rate must remain plus or minus 3 beats per minute for a full minute, or EMG response cannot fluctuate by more than 5% for a full minute), advancing to another condition once that criterion is met. This saves time with those individuals who are already stable, is tailored to the patient's physiological responding, and assures that all patients achieve stabilization. However, disadvantages also exist: The therapist must focus deeply on a patient's responding (instead of getting a cup of coffee during the adaptation period!), and must risk the patient's needing, as Taub and School (1978) noted, 30 minutes to stabilize. Fortunately, the latter problem is solved with a modified floating adaptation period—that is, patients meet the floating criterion or the 10-minute time limit, whichever comes first. Regardless of the adaptation period used, we urge clinicians to employ a specific strategy consistently. That is, they should avoid using a 2-minute adaptation period one day, a 10-minute the next, a floating criterion the next, and a 5-minute adaptation period another day. In psychophysiological assessment and treatment, consistency is half the battle!

Psychophysiological Baselines

Although the actual instructions given during a baseline period are usually identical to those provided for adaptation, the two conditions serve different functions. A "baseline period" is defined as the period following adaptation, where psychophysiological response measures have stabilized (prior to the onset of any experimental or clinical manipulation, such as a stressor condition or biofeedback). The purpose of this condition is to observe and measure resting basal physiological activity. This condition is essential, because nearly always a practitioner compares the baseline or resting condition values to the experimental or treatment conditions. As noted above, relative values (most generally raw change scores from baseline or percent change from baseline) are dependent on a baseline condition. A baseline is essential in cardiovascular research, where nearly all measures of cardiovascular reactivity use relative scores.

Whether a patient's eyes are open or closed during baseline is an area of disagreement among clinicians and researchers. There are no available data on this subject, so personal preference determines choice. Here, the two of us mildly disagree. Arena conducts baselines with eyes closed during nearly all psychophysiological assessments and most biofeedback training sessions. He reserves an eyes-open baseline period for biofeedback when patients express a preference for visual feedback or generalization training (usually, after a patient is sufficiently skilled in producing the biofeedback response, instruction advances to reproduce more challenging "real-world" factors). Schwartz (1995) believes that eyes-closed baselines are suitable for conditions such as insomnia, and are less realistic for assessing baseline physiology for headaches and other symptoms that occur with eyes open. For example, he argues that using only an eyes-closed baseline can lead a therapist to conclude incorrectly there is no excess muscle activity. Commonly, more muscle activity in the head and facial muscles exists when eyes are open.

Schwartz (1995) has stated:

> Therapists should get baseline data with eyes open when patients' symptoms start with their eyes open and when biofeedback with eyes open is planned. Observing lower arousal with eyes open than with eyes closed is potentially useful. It provides cues about what it means for patients to close their eyes. It raises questions to answer about what patients are thinking about and doing when they close their eyes. When eyes are kept open, therapists should consider instructing patients to include time calmly gazing at an object such as a picture or plant. They should remind patients to avoid staring or examining the object they are looking at as well. (p. 152)

Regardless of which baseline recording strategy professionals choose, both of us urge careful consideration and consistent application during both clinical and research practice. This ensures a large database, and the larger a database is—and we would argue that clinical experience creates a very strong database, indeed—the surer professionals can be of their observations and conclusions.

As noted above, there are few data about what constitutes an adequate baseline, and much of the research confuses baseline with adaptation periods. For example, Hastrup (1986) reviewed the methodology and duration of baseline conditions in an exhaustive review of cardiovascular reactivity studies, and found almost no agreement among the studies in terms of methodology and duration of the baseline periods. She recommended that the baseline period be at least 15 minutes in duration for cardiovascular reactivity experiments, to ensure the lowest possible baseline recordings. Jennings, Kamarck, Stewart, Eddy, and Johnson (1992) found similar results, with 5 of 24 studies reviewed having baseline periods of 10 minutes or more, 5 between 6 and 10 minutes, and the remaining 24 being less than 5 minutes in duration.

For those interested in conducting methodologically complex psychophysiological research, Jamieson (1999) has written an excellent article concerning baseline differences in psychophysiological recording, indicating that (1) relative values such as change scores are confounded with baseline values whenever data are skewed; and (2) when baseline differences are real, analysis of covariance has a directional bias that magnifies differences in one direction and minimizes those in the other direction. Jamieson provides suggestions for identifying and correcting these problems. Finally, Piferi, Kline, Younger, and Lawler (2000), arguing that simply resting quietly does not assure equivalency between individuals, present data suggesting that showing a relaxing video of the sea achieves a greater degree of relaxation and a more accurate recording of baseline measures than does the traditional baseline condition, at least for measures of cardiovascular reactivity. We would argue, however, that the baseline condition should not "obtain the lowest possible resting rates along the same point on the continuum of excitement" (Piferi et al. 2000, p. 215), and Piferi and her colleagues are actually creating a relaxation condition (see below).

Clinical Considerations in Psychophysiological Baselines

For resting baselines and for office-based stressors, clinical practitioners need to be very cautious when interpreting physiological data. Comparisons of resting baselines across sessions are complex for many patients. Knowledge of this fact is important when clinicians generalize to other situations or compare data across sessions. Many practitioners view each session's resting baselines as largely new situations, at least for most ANS-mediated variables.

Marked shifts in muscle and autonomic activity often occur after a patient is sitting quietly for several minutes. Muscle activity can steadily or suddenly drop. Finger temperature can gradually or suddenly increase. Heart rate can plummet. Therefore, baseline periods up to 15 minutes should be considered in a very early biofeedback session and in some therapy sessions that can capture these changes. This will also help a therapist check for physiological changes that occur in the extended relaxation periods outside the therapist's office. There is no fixed or proper time for all people and all circumstances.

Realizing that these changes can occur before therapy can help to increase a patient's confidence. It is also important to document the lack of change, especially when changes begin to occur later during feedback and nonfeedback phases. This information is useful for the therapist, because such changes in an initial session do not mean that a patient needs therapy less. Among the important therapeutic goals are shortening the time before the therapeutic changes occur and increasing the degree and replicability of such changes.

Shorter baseline phases, such as 1–3 minutes, are also feasible and proper under some conditions. For example, if we consider the patient sitting quietly with eyes closed, his or her muscle activity may remain low and steady with very little variability for about 1–2 minutes among multiple muscles in the head and neck. The muscle activity will probably not change significantly over the next few minutes. Cost containment and other pragmatic factors argue for the shortest baseline phases that can typically answer evaluative and therapy questions

There are circumstances in which a clinician wants or needs additional baseline data. Obtaining such data can entail more than one baseline session and extending some baseline phases even beyond 15 minutes. For example, when there is much variability within or between sessions, one can justify longer resting baselines. Another example occurs for disorders such as sleep-onset insomnia, when the relaxation sessions at home are long.

Some patients show increasing roused activity, cooling hands, increasing pulse, and/or restlessness during the first few minutes of a baseline. More than several minutes of a baseline may be unnecessary and counterproductive. Even about 5 minutes may be enough. In such a case, the therapist should consider that relaxation-induced anxiety (RIA) may be present (see M. S. Schwartz, Schwartz, & Monastra, Chapter 12, this volume, or Arena & Blanchard, 1996, for a detailed discussion of RIA). When this occurs, the clinician should consider the therapeutic goal of gradually increasing periods of sitting quietly without increases in physiological arousal.

Pretreatment and periodic physiological baselines are less practical under some circumstances. For example, there are limitations in the schedules of some patients; consider the case of a patient who lives a few hundred miles from the therapist, in a location where there is no qualified professional to whom to refer the patient. The therapist is consulting only for one session, and that session focuses on the intake interview and patient education for treatments thought to help reduce physical symptoms. There is time for a brief biofeedback session—but not enough time for a desired baseline. The therapist decides instead to get only a brief baseline of about 5 minutes and to invest the remaining instrumentation time in providing feedback. The therapist instructs the patient in relaxation techniques and provides education booklets and audiotapes. The patient then goes home and practices as instructed.

The lack of physiological baseline data does not always compromise therapy. One can properly adjust priorities, maintain the patient's best interests, and initiate therapy. If this patient returns for further therapy, the therapist can still get a physiological baseline. Practitioners can discuss the ideal with their patients and note in their reports the reasons for proceeding differently.

Conversely, there are conditions for which one can justify multiple physiological baseline segments or sessions. One such situation occurs when a therapist suspects that a patient's symptoms fluctuate in intensity at different times. Examples of such times are soon after specific eliciting or emitting events (e.g., eating, upsetting discussions, physical activity) and certain times of day. Therapists should consider scheduling office sessions to coincide with or immediately follow such events.

The absence of excess tension or arousal during a resting baseline does not mean that a person has adequate control. This is also true for patients who show a lack of significant reactivity to a stressor. Therapists should always consider such factors as the possible effects of medications, the office environment, baseline conditions, and the limitations of simulated stressors. For example, some people do not react to office stressors. There are individual differences in how therapists present stressors. Presentation style can influence a stressor's effect.

Physiological tension and arousal, reactivity, and slow recoveries in one office session often do suggest similar functioning in daily life. That is, one can generalize from the psychophysiological assessment setting to real-life settings. However, office sessions do have limits. Tension, physiological reactivity, and slow recovery in one session does not mean that the person reacts the same way in other situations. At best, these are snapshots or glimpses of a person's psychophysiological activity in daily life. Office procedures are sources of hypotheses and information for productive discussions. However, they are not always reliable evidence for a patient's daily functioning.

Conditions Involving Assessment of Self-Control Abilities

1. *"Relax deeply" condition.* As many psychophysiological interventions are believed to work through the final common pathway of relaxation, obtaining some measure of the patient's ability to relax on his or her own prior to any treatment and periodically during treatment is often useful. The instructions that Arena and colleagues have used for this condition (Andrasik, Blanchard, Arena, Saunders, & Barron, 1982; Arena et al., 1983) are simply "Please try to relax as deeply as you possibly can." Schwartz (1995) uses the following instructions:

"Now, rest quietly a little longer. Use whatever methods you think best to relax. Focus on the muscles of your face, head, and shoulders. Let yourself go and release the tension in different parts of your body. If you feel that you have to move, scratch, sneeze, or something else, go ahead and do it. This phase lasts a few minutes. Don't think of problems or upsetting events and do not worry about how well you are doing. Whatever degree of relaxation achieved is all right." (p. 154)

2. *"Warm hands" condition.* This condition is directly relevant to thermal biofeedback therapy, which involves teaching hand warming through mental means. Obtaining some measure of a patient's ability to increase hand temperature prior to treatment is useful, particularly when one is assessing whether the skills have developed or been learned. There are many ways to test or prepare the patient for psychophysiological learning. The most common by far is a "self-control" condition that is interspersed between a baseline and a feedback segment. During the self-control period, the patient is asked to control the desired psychophysiological response (in this instance, hand temperature—"Please try to warm your hands through purely mental means") without any feedback. If the patient can control the response, the clinician may infer that between-session learning has occurred. Such a phase can be routinely added after the second or third biofeedback session. Sometimes this condition is presented following the biofeedback portion. If a patient can control the response, then the practitioner may infer that within-session learning has occurred.

Generalization involves preparing the patient to, or determining whether or not the patient can, apply the learning that may have occurred during the biofeedback session to the "real world." One can partially or tentatively infer this from the procedures described above, and can also obtain temperature measurements in other situations.

3. *"Relax muscles" condition.* This condition is directly relevant to EMG biofeedback, which involves teaching reduction of muscle activity. Obtaining some measure of a patient's ability to decrease muscle activity prior to treatment is useful. The instructions are adapted to the muscle group recorded.

4. *Personally meaningful positive imagery condition.* This condition is often included as a control condition to compare to the negative imagery condition. This is frequently useful, because individuals' abilities to imagine vary greatly; and without this phase, a practitioner may mistakenly believe that a patient has no reactivity to a negative imagery condition, when in reality he or she is merely poor at imagining. Consider asking the patient for a vividness score of the scene after the condition is over. Prior to the assessment, consider asking him or her to describe a very pleasant scene experienced previously, with descriptors of images targeting a majority of the five senses. Also, consider requesting that the scene rates a 9 or 10 on a 1–10 scale of pleasantness. Information is recorded and modified to refine the scene until consensus is reached. During the assessment, the instructions used are as follows: "I'd like you to try to imagine, to picture in your mind's eye . . ." (the pleasant scene is then read). In addition to variable imaging skills, another problem is the absence of control for the experimenter effect. That is, some therapists or experimenters are rather low-key and likely to read the image in a monotone, while others (like the two of us!) are outgoing hams who usually read the image with dramatic flair. Thus some researchers and practitioners provide more standardized negative imagery tasks that use tape recorded instructions/imagery. However, standardization or a one-size-fits-all approach is imperfect, as the reader shall see below.

Stressor Reactivity or the Stimulation Phase

It is often useful to introduce cognitive and physical stressors to check for psychophysiological reactivity and rate of recovery. Both reactivity effects and recovery can help identify causes and correlates of biobehavioral disorders, and can potentially help predict those persons at risk for these disorders (Haynes, Gannon, Orimoto, O'Brien, &Brandt, 1991). Haynes et al. also note that assessing reactivity can help develop effective interventions. This section discusses reactivity, while the next section focuses on recovery.

Although many providers use stress stimuli routinely before starting therapy, some do not. However, using stress stimuli may help therapists answer some patients' questions about the ways that their physiology reacts to stimuli, and some patients benefit from seeing their reactivity and recovery.

For some patients there is very little, if any, excess tension or arousal while they are sitting quietly or relaxing. The therapist may suspect that this is not typical for specific patients. Stimulation allows one to examine such patients during and following a stressor presentation, and to compare and contrast them to normal individuals and individuals with the same biobehavioral problems.

There are two interdependent pathways in which physiological stress occurs (Haynes et al., 1991). One is the ANS pathway, especially the sympathetic nervous system division. The other is the hypothalamic–pituitary–adrenal cortex system pathway. The hypothalamus organizes the ANS pathway with input from cortical and subcortical brain structures. This tends to have a rapid onset and a short equilibrium time that is the duration of maximum effect. The effects are mostly the results of nerve endings releasing epinephrine and norepinephrine and from the adrenal medulla. In the second pathway, the hypothalamus also regulates the release of adrenocorticotropic hormone (ACTH) from the pituitary gland. This promotes the release of cortisol from the adrenal cortex. These effects are slower and have a longer equilibrium latency or time until maximum effects. The time is longer than that resulting from epinephrine and norepinephrine.

Thus the duration of a stressor strongly influences its impact. Many studies show that short-duration stressors elevate neurotransmitters, but longer-duration stressors suppress them. Longer-duration stressors deplete norepinephrine, lift the inhibition of ACTH, release cortisol, and suppress the immune system. Transient stressors often used in laboratory studies and clinical practice may not be sufficient for health-inhibiting effects.

The nature of the stress—physiological or psychological—is important. For measuring primarily psychological stressors, therapists should be aware that serum cortisol responds more to subjectively distressing, uncontrollable, and psychologically prominent stress (Dienstbier, 1989). In contrast, the ANS-mediated catecholamine responses, such as epinephrine and norepinephrine, respond to nearly all stimuli—including startle, cognitive stimuli, exercise, and mild electric shock (Haynes et al., 1991). See Asterita (1985) and Haynes, Falkon, and Sexton-Radik (1989) for more detailed discussions of this topic.

Stress and stimulation constitute part of evaluations and treatments for conditions other than those treated with relaxation. For example, when evaluating patients with fecal incontinence, therapists should use simulated stimulation to the lower bowel. This checks for reactivity of the internal and external anal sphincters. It also checks for ineffective tensing of the gluteal and abdominal muscles.

With patients with urinary incontinence, therapists sometimes introduce fluid into the bladder to check for sphincter control. During this procedure, practitioners also check for ineffective tensing of abdominal muscles. Other examples involve patients undergoing muscle reeducation. Therapists often ask them to hold, carry, walk, push, or bend to evaluate their muscle activity (see Arena, Sherman, Bruno, & Young, 1989b, 1991).

Response magnitude, such as peak reactivity during a stressor, is a commonly used psychophysiological response parameter for assessing the effects of stress (Haynes et al., 1991). Researchers and practitioners use cognitive and physical stressors to examine reactivity mediated by the ANS or the central nervous system. A variety of stimuli are in use in clinical practice, and practitioners assume that the stimuli are stressful; however, for some individuals this may not be the case. In some cases, it is merely orienting or mild stimulation. The following are a few stimuli in clinical and research use, as well as abbreviated sample instructions. For each, if instructions are not included with the description of the stressor, the therapist should assume that an introductory phrase (such as "In a few moments I will ask you to . . ." or "When I ask you to, please . . .") should be used.

1. *Mental arithmetic.* "When I tell you to, please start at (an arbitrarily chosen large number such as 986) and count backward by 7's [or 8's, 9's, or 13's], keeping your eyes closed." Alternatively, "Please read silently (or aloud) each math problem and write down [or call out] the answer" (e.g., 121 + 767 = ?; 326 − 74 = ?; 18 × 12 = ?) (Linden, 1991).

This is probably the most commonly used office stressor in research and clinical practice. Advantages (Linden, 1991) of a mental math stressor are ease of administration and lack of equipment requirements (unlike video games, reaction times, or cold pressor tasks). At most, only a method of visually presenting equations is necessary. No ethical concerns should be raised by an institutional review board, human subjects research review committee, ethics committee, or clinical practices committee. In addition, the technique of mental arithmetic offers a wide range of variations for adaptations to specific patients and for repeated presentations. However, a potential problem for comparing studies and procedures stems from the lack of universally accepted standardized procedures.

Linden (1991) provides a useful review and a series of studies of the effects of vocal versus written versions, noise distraction, and different types of math tasks. The most arousing, at least for cardiovascular reactivity, are those involving vocal responding, noise distraction, and solving visually presented equations (Linden, 1991). One may expect some attenuation of the reactivity with repeated presentations of the same math task (Sharpley, 1993). Thus the therapist should consider different math tasks if he or she uses repeated stressor presentations involving math.

2. *Tensing muscles.* "Make a fist." "Clench your teeth." "Try to open this tightly closed jar." "Shrug your shoulders." "Bend slightly at the waist." "Hold this package with both hands."

3. *Personally meaningful negative imagery.* This is similar to personally meaningful positive imagery (see above), except that the patient is asked to imagine something very unpleasant for him or her.

4. *Memory tasks.* "Remember this story exactly as I say it."

5. *Hyperventilation.* "Inhale and exhale very quickly and deeply for 2 minutes." Or "Inhale and exhale through both your mouth and nose. Each time you inhale try to fill your lungs completely. Each time you exhale try to empty your lungs completely." Or "Inhale every time I say 'In.' Exhale every time I say 'Out.'" One can use an audiotape to signal inhalations and exhalations. (See Gevirtz & Schwartz, Chapter 10, this volume, for discussion of hyperventilation, hyperventilation provocation test, and cautions.)

6. *Prerecorded loud noises or other unpleasant sounds.* Examples are a baby crying, car horns repeatedly blowing, or listening to people screaming at each other. For combat-related posttraumatic stress disorder, often sounds of war (such as helicopters and machine guns) are used.

7. *Cold exposure and cold pressure.* "Hold this glass of ice water for 2 minutes. When I say 'Start,' I'd like you to place your right hand up to your wrist in the bucket of ice water. Then close your eyes. Please keep your hand in the ice water until it hurts so badly [or becomes too uncomfortable] that you want to remove it, or until I tell you to remove it. Any questions? OK. Start." For an excellent review of the methodology of the cold pressor test (certainly the most widely used physical stressor in psychophysiology today), as well as the physiology involved, see Velasco, Gomez, Blanco, and Rodriguez (1997).

8. *Action and challenging video games.*

9. *Slides of stressful scenes or videotaped trauma.* "Look at these slides [or this video]."

10. *Difficult quizzes.* "Complete this quiz. Most people get a score of at least ____."

11. *Your Everyday Life Pressures task and Holmes–Rahe visualizations*. Rosenthal et al. (1989) have developed two brief and practical stressor tasks for research that are of potential clinical use. The first involves a number of stressful vignettes based on the Holmes and Rahe (1967) Social Readjustment Scale, which ranks a number of stressful life events in terms of severity. Instructions are as follows: "Please close your eyes. Visualize yourself in the following situation[s]. Try to see yourself in the situation. Feel just how this situation hits you. Really get into it! Try to make it as real and vivid as you can, including the sights, sounds, smells, and emotions. Imagine how you would react, as clearly as possible."

The second stressor task, which involves generally stressors of lesser intensity, is termed the Your Everyday Life Pressures (YELP) task. The YELP task involves eight selected vignettes depicting "frustrating, disappointing, or otherwise noxious" (Rosenthal et al., 1989, p. 551) situations. Many doctoral-level clinicians selected the eight YELP vignettes from among 48 potential items (Schwartz, 1995). Interested readers should refer to Rosenthal et al. (1989) or Schwartz (1995) for additional information regarding the YELP task items, including sample vignettes.

12. *Ischemic (blood pressure tourniquet) pain* (e.g., Pinerua-Shuhaibar et al., 1999).

13. *Exercise step-up test* (e.g., Feinstein et al., 1999; Lim, Shields, Anderson, & McDonald, 1999).

Obviously, one does not use all or most of these techniques with each patient. Research and clinical practice usually include from one to three stressors. Most require at least 1 minute and usually up to 4 minutes for each presentation. There are individual differences in reactivity; hence the rationale for using multiple stimuli of different types.

Instructions probably have an arousal effect for at least some physiological responses, such as heart rate (Furedy, 1987; Sharpley, 1993). This probably results from several factors, such as attending to the instructions and anxiety associated with the uncertainty and challenge of the task. This additional arousal effect can confound the assessment of reactivity of the stressor. Therefore, the therapist should consider measuring the reactivity during the instructions and separating this from the stressor task data. With computer-based psychophysiological systems, one can create periods or trials designated as instructions.

Some practitioners insert another period of about 1 minute after giving the instructions and before instructing the patient to start the task. They assume that this allows the patient to relax and allows for measuring the effects of instructions and anticipation. However, some patients may prematurely start some cognitive task during this period. Therapists can circumvent this easily by instructions such as these: "In a few moments I will ask you to . . . keep relaxing until I say to begin." For counting backward, therapists should wait until after the interspersed postinstruction period to give the numbers.

One vitally important area of research that has been nearly overlooked is that of which stressor is best for which type of patient under what condition. Yoshida et al. (1999) compared the cold pressor, hyperventilation, mental arithmetic, and exercise step-up stressors in their ability to induce an angina attack in 29 patients with vasospastic angina pectoris. They found that the hyperventilation task was least effective (13%), with cold pressor and mental arithmetic equally effective (27 and 28%, respectively) and the step-up test most effective (55%). Similar research needs to be conducted for other types of disorders (such as headache, panic, Raynaud's disease, etc.).

Poststress Adaptation Periods

Psychophysiological and other biobehavioral disorders often have important physiological components. Implicated as causal factors are environmental and other stressors. However, the interactions among behavioral, cognitive, and physiological factors are complex.

The strength of the relationship between the magnitude of reactivity and other indices of psychological functioning is often modest (Haynes et al., 1991). Haynes et al. also observed a modest ability for reactivity to distinguish persons with a disorder from those without it. Hence there is interest in both the rate and degree of recovery to help explain etiology and plan clinical interventions.

The goal of many clinical interventions is changing the psychophysiological response to stress (Cacioppo, Berntson, & Anderson, 1991; Haynes et al., 1989). Therefore, psychophysiological poststress recovery is of crucial importance.

Implications include etiology and treatment of psychophysiological disorders. Specifically, recovery indices may help identify causal mechanisms of many biobehavioral disorders. They may help identify persons at risk for these disorders, and may help professionals develop effective interventions and evaluations of treatment. For example, if a patient reacts in a normal fashion during a variety of stressors, but takes much longer than normal to return to baseline levels following these stressors, two reasonable inferences can be made. One is that this individual has an impairment in his or her physiology that causes the return to baseline to be slower than in normal individuals. Two, this person needs to develop psychological and psychophysiological coping strategies immediately following a stressor, to reduce physiological arousal as quickly as possible and help him or her return to a basal quiescent state.

Within-study differences between stressor and poststress recovery results constitute a very important index of the importance and potential use of poststress recovery. This implies that these two indices stem from different mechanisms. Of 180 statistical analyses reported by Haynes et al. (1991), 81 showed nonsignificant effects of stressors. Of these 81, 74% showed significant recovery phase effects. Conversely, when stressor effects were significant in 74 analyses, recovery phases showed nonsignificant effects for 42% of the same variables. Stress effects and recovery are very often different and of differential sensitivity and potential utility.

Impaired recovery or slowness of recovery after psychophysiological reactivity to one or more stressors is the focus of using poststress recovery stages. Nearly all theories of psychophysiological disorders have as one of their central tenets or include in their definition of psychophysiological abnormality an impaired recovery process. Specific definitions of "poststress recovery" vary in the literature. Arena, Blanchard, Andrasik, Applebaum, and Myers (1985) defined recovery as a return to the quiescent baseline state after stress-induced reactivity. The EMG recovery was a return to 5% of the mean of the initial resting baseline. Hand temperature recovery was a return to within 5% of the baseline mean. Heart rate recovery was recovery to within 2 beats per minute of the baseline.

Other definitions of recovery are "changes in stressor-induced responses following stressor termination" and "the rate and degree to which a psychophysiological response approaches pre-stress levels following a stressful experience" (Haynes et al., 1991, p. 356). These definitions allow for nonlinear and bidirectional changes. It is different from a return to a prestressor quiescent baseline state. The time course of recovery is the magnitude of the response over time after a stressor is stopped. It is sometimes nonlinear and may diverge from prestressor levels. For example, arousal sometimes increases or becomes unstable.

Very few studies specifically address the optimal time period for assessing poststress recovery (Arena, 1984; Arena, Bruno, Brucks, & Hobbs, 1992). The physiological variables in these two studies included cephalic vasomotor response, frontal and forearm flexor EMG, hand temperature (left hand), heart rate, and skin resistance.

Arena (1984) studied 15 college undergraduates (about age 20) and reported that a 3-minute poststress period was adequate to return to a basal quiescent state for most of several psychophysiological measures. Frontal EMG, however, needed more than 3 minutes to recover. This study "indicated good intrasession reliability on all measures except frontal EMG, whereas there was inadequate intersession reliability" (Arena, 1984, p. 247).

A more recent study (Arena et al., 1992) did not completely replicate or support the major findings of the earlier study. This study examined heart rate, hand surface temperature and frontal EMG following a cognitive (serial 7's) and a physical (cold pressor task) stressor, and had 6-minute poststress adaptation periods. Most subjects (about 78%) returned to baseline within 6 minutes for heart rate. Average times were 3.7 and 2.9 minutes for the two poststress periods. However, for forehead EMG, only 48% returned to baseline in the 6 minutes. The average times were 4.6 minutes and 5.1 minutes for the two poststress periods.

For hand surface temperature, a 6-minute period was clearly inadequate (Arena et al., 1992) for most subjects. Only about 38% returned to baseline in this period. The average times were about 4.5 minutes and 5.6 minutes during the two poststress periods. The percentages returning to baseline appeared higher in the first poststress period. For example, hand temperatures returned to baseline in nearly 48% of subjects after the first, cognitive stressor (mental arithmetic), compared to only about 26% after the second, physical stressor (cold pressor task).

Although the earlier study suggested that about 3 minutes are required for cardiovascular and heart rate modalities to recover to a prestress basal level, the latter study indicates that much longer times are necessary. The authors speculation about the differences focuses on the larger sample size and the wider age range of the second study. The age range was 17–75, and the mean age was nearly 33. (The Arena et al. [1992] abstract included analyses of only 20 subjects. Interested readers can write to Arena for a copy of the paper, based on the analyses of all 62 subjects.)

These two studies used serial 7's from a large random three-digit number as the cognitive stressor, and cold pressor (to the right hand) as the physical stressor. Exposure was 4 minutes for the cognitive task, and up to that for the physical task. This cognitive stressor was probably milder than many others use, and the cold pressor was a more intense physical stress than most clinicians use (and more likely to evoke cardiovascular effects prolonging recovery than most other office-based physical stressors). The subjects were college students and community volunteers of various ages; hence caution should be used in generalizing to patients. However, a reasonable assumption is that implications from the more recent study are more applicable to patients.

Except for the limitations described above concerning these studies, we believe that this type of research is important and useful. The findings support the need for recovery periods. They show the differences in the durations of these periods among modalities, and document the duration of the recovery periods under specified conditions. Poststress periods should be at least 6 minutes if patients must return to a baseline. This is feasible in clinical practice, if two or three stress periods are used during an evaluation session. However, it is typically impractical during routine therapy sessions if multiple stressors or intense stressors are used. The cognitive stress in the Arena et al. studies was only serial 7's for 4 minutes. This is not universally stressful for everyone. As Arena (2000) has recently noted concerning laboratory and office-based stressors,

> There are many other inferences that applied psychophysiology researchers make. One is that laboratory stressful conditions are comparable to stressors found in the everyday world. Having both a) placed my hand in a bucket of ice water up to my wrist and kept it there until I couldn't stand it any longer, and b) been in an airplane for three hours with screaming children in the seats directly in front and in back of me, I can tell you that equivalence of laboratory and "real world" stressors is a very dubious proposition, indeed. (p. 22)

SELECTED EXAMPLES OF PSYCHOPHYSIOLOGICAL ASSESSMENTS TO ANSWER CLINICAL QUESTIONS

We now present a number of examples in which a biofeedback therapist or clinical researcher might use psychophysiological assessments to answer clinical questions. An example from the published literature is described; the remainder of the scenarios are selected case illustrations. We highlight pain problems (headache and lower back pain) because of our own expertise. First, though, some caveats are in order.

In his recent article, Arena (2000) has asserted that "much of the research and clinical pain work that utilize psychophysiological assessments or 'stress profiling'—including those that employ surface EMG measures—are based on inferences which have not been empirically tested and nearly all psychophysiological assessments have not been empirically demonstrated to have any clinical utility" (p. 21). He has further stated:

> The biggest inference that clinicians routinely proceed upon is that conducting a psychophysiological assessment or a "stress profile" will give them important information in helping to determine how to proceed in treatment. . . . This assumption has never been empirically tested. That is, no study has shown that if you have a pain patient who demonstrates one particular EMG abnormality, compared to a different EMG abnormality or no abnormality, that that person does better in one type of treatment compared to a different type of treatment. Such research is vitally important and must be conducted if our field is to continue to grow and flourish. (pp. 22–23)

Such research is especially important when standard treatments are expected to produce very high rates of success, as is the case with psychophysiological treatments for headache (Arena & Blanchard, 2000; Blanchard & Arena, 1999). When we achieve such high rates of success by providing everyone the same standard treatment, the psychophysiological assessment must add significant predictive value, or the justification for its use is lacking.

The fact that such research has not yet been conducted, though, does not mean that clinicians should stop conducting psychophysiological assessments. Clinicians are often making inferences and going where "no literature has gone before." The inferences that we and other clinicians make are our and their best judgments, based on clinical experiences, assessment literature, and the indication that the presence of certain abnormalities or findings warrants a specific treatment direction. We should be humble and understand the limits of our interpretations. A little tentativeness goes a long way. With that very important caveat discussed, we proceed with some examples.

Research Example: Stress Profiling of Patients with Chronic Back Pain

Flor, Turk, and Birbaumer (1985) provide an excellent study of the value of stress profiling (from Flor's doctoral dissertation at the University of Tuebingen). The data do not address stability of responses, but do provide valuable information on logical and predicted muscle reactivity differences between groups, the importance of office stressors, and the value of recovery data. Another important asset is the inclusion of the diathesis–stress model of chronic back pain (CBP) for conceptualizing the procedures and explaining the results.

There were 17 subjects each in the three groups: patients with CBP, patients with chronic general pain (GP) unrelated to the back, and hospital patients with non-pain-related medical problems such as diabetes. Of the 51 patients, 40 were male, with an age range of 23 to 73 (average age = 47). The CBP group included seven patients with degenerative disc disease/ spondylosis, four with low back pain of unknown origin, and three with disc herniation. Nine of the patients with CBP showed X-ray evidence of moderate to severe degenerative changes, and the other patients showed minimal or no changes.

The EMG recordings were made with Cyborg Biolab instrumentation. Electrodes were placed on the lumbrosacral erector spinae muscles for the 14 patients with CBP in the lower back and on the trapezius muscle of the three with CBP in the upper back. The fixed bandpass filter was 100–250 hertz.

Recording of frontal EMG, a theoretically irrelevant muscle site, was made to assess the response specificity of the stressors for patients with back pain. Heart rate recordings from the second digit of the right hand, and skin resistance level recorded from the left hand, helped check the stressor manipulations (i.e., assured that the stressors were achieving increased arousal).

The Pain Experience Scale (PES; Turk, 1981) assessed emotional and cognitive reactions to pain. The PES and the Beck Depression Inventory were found to be the most useful measures for predicting EMG reactivity, accounting for almost 76% of the variance of EMG reactivity. Readers should refer to the original article for information about the other measures employed in the study.

The authors did not specify an adaptation period. However, they did record 10 minutes of a resting baseline with the subjects sitting still with their eyes open. The average resting EMG activity was higher for the CBP group. However, this came from only four of the patients with CBP, who showed extreme baseline muscle activity that was very different from that of the other patients in this group.

A number of experimental tasks were given. Stressors consisted of recalling and describing for 1 minute a recent personally stressful event or a recent pain episode, as well as counting backward by 7's from 758. A neutral task was reciting the alphabet. The order of the tasks varied among the subjects. The ANS measures of heart rate and skin resistance level, and the self-report ratings of the stressors, served as validity checks of the stressor conditions (i.e., did they actually bring about increases in subjective levels of stress and physiological arousal levels?).

EMG data were averaged across the full minute of each stressor task. The EMG reactivity of patients with CBP was significantly greater only to the personal stressors. For example, for the stress task, the CBP group showed 4.5 microvolts ($SD = 5.1$), compared to the prestress 2.6 microvolts. In contrast, the other groups showed 1.8 and 1.4 microvolts of reactivity, compared to their prestress EMG activity of 1.5 and 1.1 microvolts. The pain recall stressor showed about the same result (an average increase of 2.2 microvolts, compared with essentially no increase for the other groups). The other tasks showed significantly lower increases of about 0.6 for the patients with other medical problems and 0.3 microvolts for the CBP group.

Flor et al. (1985) defined recovery from a stressor as the average number of seconds for a patient's muscle tension to return to the level of the 1-minute pretrial baseline (up to the maximum of the 5-minute recovery period). The patients with CBP showed slower recoveries of bilateral back muscles after the personal stressors than the other two groups.

The authors note the possible limitation of using a fixed 100- to 250-hertz bandpass filter. This does not discredit the reactivity results, but implies that a wider bandpass would capture more muscle activity. The inability to control for the potential effects of analgesic medications may be a limitation of the study. However, the CBP and GP groups did not differ in type and amount of these medications. The published account also does not specify the exact trapezius muscle electrode placement.

There are some other limitations to this study. The investigators combined patients with widely variable causes for their CBP. Depression and reactions to pain might be related to the type of CBP diagnosis, and other factors may be associated with both pain and diagnosis. The study also did not report which aspects of depression were more predictive of reactivity. The details of the sitting position were vague in the published report; for example, we do not know whether there was back support.

However, the strengths of the study outweigh the limitations. The use of clinical populations is unique and applauded. The comparison among a group with back pain, a clinical control group with general pain, and a control group of medical patients without pain deserves more accolades. Providing stressors with clinical practicality and relevance eases clinical application. Controlling for order and body movement effects adds to the strength of the conclusions (excessive movement resulted in excluding only two subjects!). Further adding to the clinical utility is the inclusion of measures of mood and self-reported emotional effects of symptoms to predict physiological changes. Finding no differences between the groups for a theoretically irrelevant muscle site (forehead EMG) helps support a response specificity model.

The study controlled for the possible effects of surgery, as well as the possible effects of denervation potentials. Comparing personal stressors with a general stressor and a neutral task is yet another strength.

This study demonstrates that the impact of stress on physiological reactivity among clinical patients can be effectively investigated to provide practically applicable data for clinician/investigators and front-line clinicians. Future research should assess the aspects of depression and self-reported attitudes on paraspinal EMG levels and on pain intensity. This could help better predict psychophysiological reactivity and recovery. We also need assessment of more intense and longer-duration stressors. This would help ascertain whether such stressors result in more reactivity and more significant delays in recovery, and could help bridge the gap from office procedures to daily life. Assessing a wider bandpass that captures more of the electrical activity of the muscles is another research need.

These procedures should be studied with more homogeneous causes for CBP. The authors also noted the need for further investigation of the potential effects of surgery, medication effects, and denervation of muscles.

There are several clinical implications of this study. Measuring muscle reactivity to personal stressors and measuring recovery after these stressors can be useful and may be necessary (at least with some patients with CBP). Therapists should consider using and comparing the effects of multiple stressors, including personally meaningful stress, general stress (such as serial 7's and 9's), and a neutral task.

Measuring logically related muscles in the target areas of the pain is appropriate. The use of frontal EMG is of limited value for assessing patients with CBP with these procedures. Although the levels of muscle reactivity were low, they were enough to justify patient education about their reactivity and recovery in daily life situations.

Aspects of depression (and quite possibly other emotions, such as anger and anxiety) probably interact with psychophysiological reactivity. Thus psychological factors among patients with CBP should be incorporated into clinical decision making. There may be subgroups of patients with CBP for whom these psychophysiological measures are more useful. Patient reactions and perceptions of the effects of pain probably interact with reactivity. Depression and reactions to pain may be the results of the type of CBP diagnosis or other variables associated with the pain and diagnosis. Practitioners should consider this when they assess depression and pain reactivity, rather than relying solely or primarily on self-ratings alone. For example, depression and pain reactivity ratings may change with various interventions. We do not yet know whether this would alter their relationships with psychophysiological reactivity and recovery.

Clinical Vignettes

Straightforward EMG Assessment of a Patient with Tension Headache

A therapist wants to ascertain in the intake whether Mrs. Smith, a patient with tension headache, is likely to benefit from biofeedback, and, if so, whether feedback from one muscle site is more likely to achieve treatment success than feedback from another muscle site. Her reported tension and pain are primarily in the forehead and in the upper back and/or posterior neck. In a psychophysiological assessment, he measures forehead EMG and bilateral upper trapezius EMG levels during two baseline conditions—a 5-minute eyes-open and a 5-minute eyes-closed condition—which are preceded by a 10- to 15-minute adaptation period to the room and sensors with eyes open. He decides to stop at this point and not continue with other aspects of an assessment, as he observes that Mrs. Smith has approximately four times the normal EMG levels in both forehead and upper trapezius muscle groups, based on his office normative data; he does not notice any left–right upper trapezius muscle differences. He tentatively concludes that (1) EMG biofeedback is likely to help Mrs. Smith, due to her elevated muscle tension; and (2) at least the forehead and bilateral upper trapezius should be used. Being a careful clinician, he conducts the same assessment prior to the first biofeedback session. He obtains the same results; he thus has a greater level of certainty concerning his findings, and feels more confident in following his treatment plan. There is probably no need for additional assessment at this point.

Throwing a Monkey Wrench into This Straightforward EMG Assessment

Let us suppose the same scenario as above, except that the therapist on the second assessment comes up with different results than on the first assessment. Now forehead EMG levels remain at the same magnitude, but trapezius readings are different: The right-side trapezius levels are about 4 times higher than those of his normative group, but the left-side trapezius levels are 10 times the normative levels. What can the therapist do in this situation (other than curse himself for repeating the assessment!)?

There are multiple possible strategies in this situation, and there are no clearly right or wrong answers. First, the therapist could decide that he needs more information and conduct a more detailed psychophysiological assessment, including stressor conditions and assessment of various postures and positions, either immediately or at the next session. Athough this would give more information, it would add significant cost to the treatment regimen, and although it could simplify the treatment picture, it could also cloud it even more. Second, he could follow his original treatment plan, as forehead EMG abnormalities have been found, and forehead EMG biofeedback is a standard treatment for tension headache (Blanchard & Arena, 1999). He is still left, however, with the nagging question of what to do about the trapezius findings. He could still give trapezius feedback, should Mrs. Smith's headache prove refractory or should she obtain insufficient relief from forehead feedback. Third, he could continue with his plan of forehead feedback, and monitor (but not have the patient attempt to control) bilateral trapezius levels. If on repeated biofeedback sessions this asymmetry continues, he may wish to change the focus of the feedback to correcting the left–right trapezius asymmetry if it does not dissipate (as, following a general relaxation theory of frontal biofeedback, it is likely to do). Fourth, he could decide to use the second assessment results and change the focus of Mrs. Smith's feedback to correcting the left–right trapezius asymmetry. He could then give forehead feedback, should Mrs. Smith's headache prove refractory or should she obtain insufficient relief from trapezius feedback. Fifth, he could decide to give Mrs. Smith feedback from all three EMG sites. This has the advantage of giving her a clearer picture of her psychophysiological abnormalities, but might provide too much information, interfering with the psychophysiological learning process. Sixth, he might devote part of each session to each muscle area or focus on the different areas in different sessions.

If our readers are getting confused by the wide variety of treatment options posed by the psychophysiological assessment results, then we have been successful in our endeavors to point out that even simple assessments often do not have simple answers. However, it is important to note that all of the options described above are perfectly defensible. Arena would probably choose the third option, and Schwartz the fifth or sixth. We urge readers to document in each report the rationale for selecting a particular treatment direction, so others can understand their thought processes.

A More Involved EMG Psychophysiological Assessment of the Patient with Tension Headache

The psychophysiological assessment of Mrs. Smith assumes no abnormalities during the adaptation and baseline conditions. The therapist plans another assessment next week, consisting of the same adaptation and baseline conditions, three stressors (personally meaningful stressful imagery, mental arithmetic [serial 9's], and a cold pressor task) of 4 minutes each, interspersed with 3-minute poststress adaptation periods, followed by assessments in six different positions (standing, bending from the waist, rising, sitting with back unsupported, sitting with back supported, and prone). Mrs. Smith again is within normal limits during both baselines, but during the personally meaningful stressful imagery she has about 6 times the normal forehead EMG levels. During both cognitive stressors she takes longer to return to baseline on forehead EMG, and during the standing and sitting unsupported positions she has approximately 10 times the upper trapezius EMG levels of normal subjects. There are no left–right upper trapezius muscle differences during any condition.

Based on this data, the therapist can tentatively conclude the following:

- EMG biofeedback is likely to help Mrs. Smith, due to the abnormal patterns of EMG responding during the psychophysiological assessment.
- Since her forehead EMG levels have been more elevated during the stressor and poststress recovery conditions, the therapist decides to use forehead EMG biofeedback initially.
- Following Mrs. Smith's learning the forehead EMG biofeedback response, he will switch to the upper trapezius muscle group.
- When he teaches generalization of the biofeedback response, the therapist will make sure that Mrs. Smith learns to reduce her muscle tension levels when she is standing and sitting with her back both supported and unsupported, as abnormalities in trapezius EMG have been noted during the standing and sitting unsupported positions. Given the fact that an impaired recovery process was found during both cognitive stressors for forehead EMG, the therapist will have Mrs. Smith repeatedly practice rapidly decreasing her forehead EMG levels, and he will emphasize the extreme importance of her reducing forehead muscle tension levels immediately after a stressful situation in her daily living.

Repeated assessment of the stressor and position conditions would be helpful, but cost-effectiveness and the practicalities of clinical work probably preclude another assessment. Also, given that the portion of the assessment he has repeated has remained unchanged, there is more confidence in the stability of the psychophysiological responding. One could reasonably question why the therapist has not included measures of other responses, such as heart rate, respiration, and hand surface temperature. Inclusion of these measures might enhance the clinical picture and allow examination of stimulus–response specificity and individual response stereotypy. His line of reasoning is probably that he has found in his clinical practice that these measures do not add anything to the tension headache patient assessment, and that they would be prohibitive in terms of time.

Psychophysiological Assessment of a Patient with Refractory Migraine

A therapist conducts 12 sessions of thermal biofeedback with Mr. Jones, a 49-year-old accountant with migraines since age 16. Mr. Jones has mastered the hand warming with thermal biofeedback in the office and outside the office, but he has not experienced any headache relief. Therefore, she conducts a psychophysiological assessment with Mr. Jones, consisting of a variety of psychophysiological measures (forehead, upper trapezius, posterior neck, and frontal posterior neck EMG; heart rate; hand temperature from multiple sites; respiration; cephalic blood volume pulse; electrodermal response) in a variety of conditions: adaptation, baseline, a relaxed body condition, and stressors (such as an exercise step-up test, fists, mental arithmetic, and personally meaningful negative imagery), with poststress adaptation periods following each stressor. Mr. Jones responds generally within normal limits during all conditions; however, when examined for individual response stereotypy and stimulus–response specificity during each stressor, he responds with maximal arousal in some of the EMG measures, and he is able to relax these responses the least during the relaxed body condition. On the basis of the psychophysiological assessment, the therapist begins EMG biofeedback from the EMG sites listed above (including frontal), focused daily relaxation instructions for those sites, and reinforced frequent daily practice of varying durations.

This is a logical and defensible treatment plan, based on the psychophysiological data. One could postulate that the assessment is contaminated by the thermal biofeedback, and perhaps this is the reason why Mr. Jones does not respond abnormally during the assessment. One could also advance the hypothesis that this explains his not responding stereotypically with hand surface temperature. The reader may also wonder why the therapist has taken so long to question the effectiveness of the earlier treatment (although some therapists have had patients who do not receive any headache relief until more than 12 sessions). Also, although repeated assessments might shed further light on Mr. Jones's psychophysiology, cost-effectiveness and clinical practicalities probably preclude another assessment.

Another Scenario for the Patient with Refractory Migraine

In an alternative scenario, the therapist finds Mr. Jones responding within normal limits in the psychophysiological assessment. There are no patterns in the examination of individual response stereotypy and stimulus–response specificity. Defensible possible responses are as follows:

- Refer him elsewhere, because all likely possible approaches are exhausted, and he is not improving.
- Repeat the psychophysiological assessment with different stressors, in hope of identifying abnormalities.
- Begin searching for other causes of the head pain, such as secondary gains (e.g., days off from work, children keeping quiet when headache is present, etc.), dietary factors, or psychological characteristics (such as depression, anger, or anxiety).
- Assume that the stressors used are insufficient, and consider other relevant stressors for another assessment (e.g., playing a tape of Mr. Jones arguing with his wife, etc.).
- Attempt a psychophysiological assessment in the natural environment (through ambulatory recordings, accompanying him to work and conducting an assessment in his office, etc.).
- Check on and focus instructions on daily relaxation practice in terms of frequency, durations, and timing.
- Consider including other muscle sites and other skin temperature sites.

Routine EMG Assessment of a Patient with Low Back Pain

Some research shows significant paraspinal EMG differences between patients with low back pain and controls without pain, as well as between patients with low back pain of differing etiologies (Arena et al., 1989b, 1991). Arena often conducts psychophysiological assessments of his patients with back pain, using right- and left-sided L4–L5 paraspinal activity and bilateral biceps femoris (a muscle located in the back of the thigh; see Arena & Blanchard, 1996, for a detailed figure depicting the sensor placement) activity in six different positions. He looks for three possible muscle tension abnormalities:

- Unusually low muscle tension levels (perhaps from nerve damage with resultant muscle atrophy).
- Unusually high muscle tension levels (the most frequent abnormality).
- Asymmetry, in which one side of the back or thigh muscles has normal muscle tension levels, while the other side has unusually low or high readings.

He may use biofeedback to decrease muscle tension in the respective muscle group(s). If an asymmetry is found, he will use biofeedback to help patients increase and/or decrease the abnormal sides. One goal is balanced bilateral values within normal ranges.

Mr. Doe is a 26-year-old bank clerk and an amateur weightlifter. His paraspinal EMG are 5–6 times normal levels on all positions except lying prone, which does not show any abnormalities. There are also no abnormalities with biceps femoris EMG. While he is sitting with his back unsupported, his left paraspinal muscles are over 30 times normal, and his right side are about 5 times normal. This is the only time any left–right asymmetry is found during the assessment. Based on the psychophysiological assessment, the therapist conducts paraspinal EMG biofeedback to correct for the asymmetry.

An Evaluation of a Patient with Low Back Pain in the Work Setting

We cannot overemphasize the importance of tailoring psychophysiological assessments and treatments to each patient. Clinicians must be creative and flexible. Take the example of Mr. Doe; let us assume that he goes through the regimen as described and achieves 40% reduction in his back pain, but not as much as he and his therapist want and think possible. The therapist then explores Mr. Doe's lifestyle in greater detail. The therapist focuses on the weightlifting as an obvious and probable area of inappropriate muscle usage, but the therapist knows that Mr. Doe has been lifting weights for only 2 years, whereas his back problems began 4 years ago. He knows that Mr. Doe began working at a bank 5 years ago. Further inquiry now about his job reveals that one of his major job functions is to assist customers in accessing their safe deposit boxes.

The therapist accompanies Mr. Doe to work and notes that many of the safe deposit boxes are quite high, and although there is a ladder in the vault, Mr. Doe uses the ladder only for those boxes he cannot reach. Moreover, there are other safe deposit boxes that are nearly at floor level, and to access them, Mr. Doe must either bend, squat, kneel, or sit on the floor (the last of which he never does). A workplace psychophysiological assessment (with a portable EMG device) of the paraspinal muscles when Mr. Doe is either reaching up for a safe deposit box, or bending or squatting for a safe deposit box near the floor reveals massive paraspinal EMG activity.

The therapist then does the following:

- He instructs Mr. Doe to use the ladder when accessing any safe deposit box that is higher than head level.

- He uses the portable EMG biofeedback device to instruct Mr. Doe on proper ways to access boxes on the lower wall levels.
- He provides Mr. Doe with office-based paraspinal feedback of simulated access to safe deposit boxes, reinforcing what has been learned during the evaluation in the vault.
- He instructs Mr. Doe to become much more aware of his muscle tension levels whenever he performs his safe deposit box duties, and to conduct relaxation exercises following his accessing the boxes, in addition to maintaining the correct form and posture.

As a result, Mr. Doe's back pain is significantly reduced. Although the therapist's standard psychophysiological assessment includes bending from the waist and rising, it is not comprehensive enough to identify Mr. Doe's problems. This is because bending from the waist in the office assessment goes from straight to about 30 degrees; generally, this is all that the typical patient with lower back pain can do without experiencing significant increases in pain levels. Mr. Doe's youth and overall physical fitness have allowed him to bend much lower than the typical patient with back pain, demonstrating the importance of tailoring psychophysiological assessment and treatment to the needs of each patient. (Please note that Mr. Doe is not a real patient, but a mixture of three patients combined together for illustration purposes.)

CONCLUSION

Our intent in this chapter has been to present readers with a reasonably detailed "how-to" discussion of conducting psychophysiological assessments, as well as to provide an understanding of the major pitfalls and questions that arise during such procedures, especially with some patients with headaches or other chronic pain.

We have hoped to demystify the concept of psychophysiological assessment. Good clinical/common sense, and a basic understanding of the general concepts of psychophysiology, are required. We urge clinicians to utilize psychophysiological assessments when they have questions about their patients' treatment plans, or when they are confused about what may be causing or maintaining their patients' symptoms. Such evaluations can often shed light on complex clinical questions.

At the same time that we advocate practitioners employ such techniques, we caution readers to recognize the limitations of psychophysiological assessments, and to avoid using them to obtain simple answers to complex questions. We are especially concerned that applied psychophysiologists will give the same assessment to all patients, not tailoring it to the individual patient and disorder. We are even more concerned with practitioners who give every patient a psychophysiological assessment. Such a practice is neither necessary nor fruitful. We cannot rely solely upon equipment for decision making and practical application. As anyone familiar with computers knows, the technology is only as good as our related abilities and knowledge. Still, after the best equipment is purchased, clinicians must formulate appropriate questions and develop valid methods to answer them.

ACKNOWLEDGMENTS

This chapter was supported by a Department of Veterans Affairs MERIT-Review awarded to John G. Arena, who gratefully acknowledges the assistance of Steven J. Goldberg, MS, and Susan L. Hannah, MS, in the preparation of this chapter.

REFERENCES

Andrasik, F., Blanchard, E. B., Arena, J. G., Saunders, N. L., & Barron, K. D. (1982). Psychophysiology of recurrent head pain: Methodological issues and new empirical findings. *Behavior Therapy, 13*, 407–429.

Arena, J. G. (1984). Inter- and intra-reliability of psychophysiological poststress adaptation periods. *Journal of Behavioral Assessment, 6*, 247–260.

Arena, J. G. (2000). Surface electromyographic psychophysiological assessment for chronic pain disorders: The necessity for clinical and research inferences to be empirically verified. *Biofeedback, 28*, 21–24.

Arena, J. G., & Blanchard, E. B. (1996). Biofeedback and relaxation therapy for chronic pain disorders. In R. J. Gatchel & D. C. Turk (Eds.), *Psychological approaches to pain management.* New York: Guilford Press.

Arena, J. G., & Blanchard, E. B. (2000). Biofeedback therapy for chronic pain disorders. In J. D. Loeser, D. Turk, R. C. Chapman, & S. Butler (Eds.), *Bonica's management of pain* (3rd ed.). Baltimore: Williams & Wilkins.

Arena, J. G., Blanchard, E. B., Andrasik, F., Applebaum, K., & Myers, P. E. (1985). Psychophysiological comparisons of three kinds of headache sufferers during and between headache states: Analysis of post-stress adaptation periods. *Journal of Psychosomatic Research, 29*, 427–441.

Arena, J. G., Blanchard, E. B., Andrasik, F., Cotch, P. A., & Myers, P. E. (1983). Reliability of psychophysiological assessment. *Behaviour Research and Therapy, 21*, 447–460.

Arena, J. G., Bruno, G. M., Brucks, A. G., & Hobbs, S. H. (1992, March). What is an adequate psychophysiologic post-stress adaptation period? In *Proceedings of the 23rd Annual Meeting of the Association for Applied Psychophysiology and Biofeedback, Colorado Springs.* Wheat Ridge, CO: Association for Applied Psychophysiology and Biofeedback.

Arena, J. G., Bruno, G. M., Brucks, A. G., Searle, J. D., Sherman, R. A., & Meador, K. J. (1994). Reliability of an ambulatory electromyographic activity device for musculoskeletal pain disorders. *International Journal of Psychophysiology, 17*, 153–157.

Arena, J. G., Goldberg, S. J., Saul, D. L., & Hobbs, S. N. (1989a). Temporal consistency of psychophysiological stress profiles: Analysis of individual response stereotypy and stimulus response specificity. *Behavior Therapy, 20*, 609–618.

Arena, J. G., & Hobbs, S. N. (1995a). Temporal stability of psychophysiological stress profiles: A re-analysis using intraclass correlation coefficients. *Psychological Reports, 76*, 171–175.

Arena, J. G., & Hobbs, S. N. (1995b). Reliability of psychophysiological assessment as a function of trait anxiety. *Biofeedback and Self-Regulation, 20*, 19–37.

Arena, J. G., Sherman, R. A., Bruno, G. M., & Young, T. R. (1989b). Electromyographic recordings of five types of low back pain subjects and non-pain controls in different positions. *Pain, 37*, 57–65.

Arena, J. G., Sherman, R. A., Bruno, G. M., & Young, T. R. (1991). Electromyographic recordings of five types of low back pain subjects and non-pain controls in different positions: Effect of pain state. *Pain, 45*, 23–28.

Arena, J. G., Sherman, R. A., Bruno, G. M., & Young, T. R. (1990). Temporal stability of paraspinal electromyographic recordings in low back and non-pain subjects. *International Journal of Psychophysiology, 9*, 31–37.

Asterita, M. F. (1985). *The physiology of stress.* New York: Human Sciences Press.

Basmajian, J. V., & DeLuca, C. J. (1985). *Muscles alive: Their functions revealed by electromyography* (5th ed). Baltimore: Williams & Wilkins.

Berntson, G. G., Bigger, J. T., Jr., Eckberg, D. L., Grossman, P., Kaufmann, P. G., Malik, M., Nagaraja, H. N., Porges, S. W., Saul, J. P., Stone, P. H., & Van Der Molen, M. W. (1997). Heart rate variability: Origins, methods, and interpretive caveats. *Psychophysiology, 34*, 623–648.

Blanchard, E. B., & Arena, J. G. (1999). Biofeedback, relaxation training and other psychological treatments for chronic benign headache. In M. L. Diamond & G. D. Solomon (Eds.), *Diamond's and Dalessio's The practicing physician's approach to headache* (6th ed.). Philadelphia: Saunders.

Buco, S. M., & Blouin, D. C. (1983). *Use of similarity coefficients when populations parameters are unknown.* Paper presented at the Meeting of the Southeastern Psychological Association, New Orleans, LA.

Cacioppo, J. T., Berntson, G. G., & Anderson, B. L. (1991). Psychophysiological approaches to the evaluation of psychotherapeutic process and outcome: Contributions from social psychophysiology. *Psychological Assessment, 3*(3), 321–336.

Dienstbier, R. A. (1989). Arousal and physiological toughness: Implications for mental and physical health. *Psychological Review, 96*, 84–100.

Engel, B. T. (1960). Stimulus–response and individual response specificity. *Archives of General Psychiatry, 2*, 305–313.

Eppinger, H., & Hess, L. (1917). *Vagotonia.* New York: Nervous and Mental Disease Publications.

Feinstein, R. A., Hains, C. S., Hemstreet, M. P., Turner-Henson, A., Redden, D. T., Martin, B., Erwin, S., & Bailey, W. C. (1999). A simple "step-test" protocol for identifying suspected unrecognized exercise-induced asthma (EIA) in children. *Allergy and Asthma Proceedings, 20*(3), 181–188.

Flor, H., Turk, D. C., & Birbaumer, N. (1985). Assessment of stress-related psychophysiological reactions in chronic back pain patients. *Journal of Consulting and Clinical Psychology, 53*(3), 354–364.

Fried, R. (1993). The role of respiration in stress and stress control: Toward a theory of stress as a hypoxic phenomenon. In P. M. Lehrer & R. L. Woolfolk (Eds.), *Principles and practice of stress management* (2nd ed). New York: Guilford Press.

Furedy, J. J. (1987). Beyond heart rate in the cardiac psychophysiological assessment of mental effort: The T-wave amplitude component in the electrocardiogram. *Human Factors, 29,* 183–194.

Gerin, W., Christenfeld, N., Pieper, C., DeRafael, D. A., Su, O., Stroessner, S. J., Deich, J., & Pickering, T. G. (1998). The generalizability of cardiovascular responses across settings. *Journal of Psychosomatic Research, 44*(2), 209–218.

Hastrup, J. L. (1986). Duration of initial heart rate assessment in psychophysiology: Current practices and implications. *Psychophysiology, 23,* 5–17.

Haynes, S. N., Falkin, S., & Sexton-Radek, K. (1989). Psychophysiological measurement in behavior therapy. In G. Turpin (Ed.), *Handbook of clinical psychophysiology.* Chichester, England: Wiley.

Haynes, S. N., Gannon, L. R., Orimoto, L., O'Brien, W. H., & Brandt, M. (1991). Psychophysiological assessment of poststress recovery. *Psychological Assessment, 3*(3), 356–365.

Holmes, T. H., & Rahe, R. H. (1967). The Social Readjustment Scale. *Journal of Psychosomatic Research, 11,* 213–218.

Jamieson, J. (1999). Dealing with baseline differences: two principles and two dilemmas. *International Journal of Psychophysiology, 31,* 155–161.

Jennings, J. R., Kamarck, R., Stewart, C., Eddy, M., & Johnson, P. (1992). Alternate cardiovascular baseline assessment techniques: Vanilla or resting baseline. *Psychophysiology, 29,* 730–742.

Kaufman, M. P., & Schneiderman, N. (1986). Physiological bases of respiratory psychophysiology. In M. G. H. Coles, E. Donchin, & S. W. Porges (Eds.), *Psychophysiology: Systems, processes, and applications.* New York: Guilford Press.

Kirk, R. E. (1982). *Experimental design: Procedures for the behavioral sciences* (2nd ed.). Belmont, CA: Brooks/Cole.

Larsen, P.B., Schneiderman, N., & DeCarlo Pasin, R. (1986). Physiological bases of cardiovascular psychophysiology. In M. G. H. Coles, E. Donchin, & S. W. Porges (Eds.), *Psychophysiology: Systems, processes, and applications.* New York: Guilford Press.

Lichstein, K. L., Sallis, J. F., Hill, D., & Young, M. C. (1981). Psychophysiological adaptation: An investigation of multiple parameters. *Journal of Behavioral Assessment, 3,* 111–121.

Lim, P., Shields, P., Anderson, J., & MacDonald, T. (1999). Dundee step test: A simple method of measuring the blood pressure response to exercise. *Journal of Human Hypertension, 13*(8), 521–526.

Linden, W. (1991). What do arithmetic stress tests measure?: Protocol variations and cardiovascular responses. *Psychophysiology, 28*(1), 91–102.

Manuck, S. B., & Schaifer, B. C. (1978). Stability of individual differences in cardiovascular reactivity. *Physiology and Behavior, 21,* 675–678.

Meyers, A. W., & Craighead, W. E. (1978). Adaptation periods in clinical psychophysiological research: A recommendation. *Behavior Therapy, 9,* 355–362.

Piferi, R. L., Kline, K. A., Younger, J., & Lawler, K. A. (2000). An alternative approach for achieving cardiovascular baseline: Viewing an aquatic video. *International Journal of Psychophysiology, 37,* 207–217.

Pinerua-Shuhaibar, L., Prieto-Rincon, D., Ferrer, A., Bonilla, E., Maixner, W., & Suarez-Roca, H. (1999). Reduced tolerance and cardiovascular response to ischemic pain in minor depression. *Journal of Affective Disorders, 56*(2–3), 119–126.

Rashed, H. M., Leventhal, G., Madu, E. C., Reddy, R., & Cardoso, S. (1997). Reproducibility of exercise-induced modulation of cardiovascular responses to cold stress. *Clinical Autonomic Research, 7*(2), 93–96.

Rosenthal, T. L., Montgomery, L. M., Shadish, W. R., Edwards, N. B., Hutcherson, H. W., Follette, W. C., & Lichstein, K. L. (1989). Two new, brief, practical stressor tasks for research purposes. *Behavior Therapy, 20,* 545–562.

Sallis, J. F., & Lichstein, K. L. (1979). The frontal electromyographic adaptation response: A potential source of confounding. *Biofeedback and Self-Regulation, 4,* 337–339.

Schwartz, M. S. (1995). Baselines. In M. S. Schwartz & Associates, *Biofeedback: A practitioner's guide* (2nd ed.). New York: Guilford Press.

Shaeffer, F., Sponsel, M., Kice, J., & Hollensbe, J. (1991, March). Test–retest reliability of resting baseline measurements. In *Proceedings of the 22nd Annual Meeting of the Association for Applied Psychophysiology and Biofeedback, New Orleans.* Wheat Ridge, CO: Association for Applied Psychophysiology and Biofeedback.

Sharpley, C. F. (1993). Effects of brief rest periods upon heart rate in multiple baseline studies of hear rate reactivity. *Biofeedback and Self-Regulation, 18*(4), 225–235.

Speckenback, U., & Gerber, W. D. (1999). Reliability of infrared plethysmography in BVP biofeedback therapy and the relevance for clinical application. *Applied Psychophysiology and Biofeedback*, 24(4), 261–265.

Sternbach, R. S. (1966). *Principles of psychophysiology*. New York: Academic Press.

Sturgis, E. T. (1980, November). *Physiological lability and reactivity in headache activity*. Paper presented at the 14th Annual Convention of the Association for Advancement of Behavior Therapy, New York.

Sturgis, E. T., & Arena, J. G. (1984). Psychophysiological assessment. In M. Hersen, R. Eisler, & P. M. Miller (Eds.), *Progress in behavior modification* (Vol. 17). New York: Academic Press.

Sturgis, E. T., & Gramling, S. (1988). Psychophysiological assessment. In A. S. Bellack & M. Hersen (Eds.), *Behavioral assessment: A practical handbook* (3rd ed.). New York: Pergamon Press.

Taub, E., & School, P. J. (1978). Some methodological considerations in thermal biofeedback training. *Behavioral Research Methods and Instrumentation*, 10, 617–622.

Timmons, B. H., & Ley, R. (1994). *Behavioral and psychological approaches to breathing disorders*. New York: Plenum Press.

Turk, D. C. (1981). *The Pain Experience Scale*. Unpublished questionnaire, Yale University.

Veit, R., Brody, S., & Rau, H. (1997). Four-year stability of cardiovascular reactivity to psychological stress. *Journal of Behavioral Medicine*, 20(5), 447–460.

Velasco, M., Gomez, J., Blanco, M., & Rodriguez, I. (1997). The cold pressor test: Pharmacological and therapeutic aspects. *American Journal of Therapeutics*, 4(1), 34–38.

Waters, W. F., Williamson, D. A., Bernard, B. A., Blouin, D. C., & Faulstich, M. E. (1987). Test–retest reliability of psychophysiological assessment. *Behaviour Research and Therapy*, 25(3), 213–221.

Wenger, M. A. (1966). Studies of autonomic balance: A summary. *Psychophysiology*, 2, 173–186.

Wilder, J. (1950). The law of initial values. *Psychosomatic Medicine*, 12, 392–400.

Yoshida, K., Utsunomiya, T., Morooka, T., Yazawa, M., Kido, K., Ogawa, T., Ryu, T., Ogata, T., Tsuji, S., Tokushima, T., & Matsuo, S. (1999). Mental stress test is an effective inducer of vasospastic angina pectoris: Comparison with cold pressor, hyperventilation and master two-step exercise test. *International Journal of Cardiology*, 70(2), 155–163.

CHAPTER 8

Compliance

MARK S. SCHWARTZ

Patients must cooperate with recommendations if the recommendations are to be effective. Being able to educate, persuade, and motivate patients enhances the effectiveness of health care professionals. This is true regardless of the treatments' efficacy, the professionals' knowledge, or the professionals' good intentions.

This chapter discusses factors that affect compliance, and summarizes ideas and conclusions from the extensive literature on compliance with medical and psychological treatments (DiMatteo & DiNicola, 1982). It also presents considerations about conducting a professional practice. This chapter's guidelines and considerations apply to most settings in which practitioners provide biofeedback. Prudent professionals aware of these factors adjust their behaviors toward patients accordingly. We can all strive to change our behaviors and office environments so as to improve our effectiveness.

The term "compliance" is complex and suggests an approach to patient care that implies a duty by patients to follow practitioners' orders blindly (DiMatteo & DiNicola, 1982). Other terms include "adherence," "cooperation," "collaboration," and "therapeutic alliance." The term "compliance" is still a commonly employed term and is the one used by DiMatteo and DiNicola (1982). However, they correctly point out that compliance should not "imply varying power relationships between the practitioner and patient" (p. 8).

"Adherence" involves holding fast to a plan, and is thus the behavior of supporting or following ideas and recommendations (Buchmann, 1997). "Compliance" is sometimes thought of more as a willingness to follow or consent. However, both compliance and adherence are processes and goals, and they are very often treated interchangeably (although sometimes distinguished). For example, sometimes compliance is thought of as less voluntary and adherence as more voluntary; thus some prefer the term "adherence," as it does not connote coercion (Erlen, 1997). As Erlen (1997) concludes, changing the terminology is like changing window dressing: The end result and the process toward achieving that goal may not change. Erlen (1997) discusses various ethical questions involved in compliance, including whether the patient or the health care provider knows best, and whether and how providers listen, assess, ask, and plan for patients. Recommended therapy plans often require significant lifestyle changes that providers need to consider. However, overzealousness or coercive efforts by health care professionals when patients are less than ideally compliant can result in demeaning, counterproductive communications.

Do our patients understand and accept our recommendations? Do they feel comfortable to admit their lack of understanding and acceptance? Do they always tell us the truth? Suggesting that patients sometimes do not tell us the truth may appear callous. I do not intend this as criticism. Many of us professionals realize that some patients distort and slant the truth to please us and to avoid embarrassment. They also do this to avoid perceived and expected criticism and for other reasons. They also often simply forget. Some patients do not understand or accept much of what we have asked them to remember and do.

For the purposes of this chapter, the topic of compliance is divided into three major categories and 11 subcategories, outlined as follows:

1. The professional
   A. Professional setting, and nontherapy and therapy personnel
   B. Referral source's attitudes and behaviors
   C. Practitioner's characteristics and behaviors
   D. Interaction and relationship between the practitioner and patient
   E. Cognitive preparation of the patient
2. The patient
   A. Patient's perceptions
   B. Patient's expectations
   C. Patient's affect
   D. Other patient factors
3. Evaluation and intervention
   A. Selected methods of assessing compliance
   B. Selected methods of increasing compliance

THE PROFESSIONAL

Professional Setting, and Nontherapy and Therapy Personnel

Personnel who are friendly, efficient, and professional in their appearance and behaviors affect patients' impressions, comfort, confidence, satisfaction, and compliance. Comfortable, neat, and uncluttered office rooms, with comfortable temperatures, also probably help. Short waiting times and consistency of therapists are additional factors that promote compliance. Prudent practitioners consider all of these recommendations, and strive to establish and maintain an office environment consistent with them.

Referral Source's Attitudes and Behaviors

Practitioners should consider asking patients about their perceptions of what the referral source conveyed to them about referring them. Did the referral source convey that the referral for biofeedback and related therapies is a logical next step, or did the decision to refer seem based on desperation? Practitioners should also consider discussing with referral sources their viewpoints about biofeedback and related therapies. This helps a practitioner know how much attention to direct toward building a patient's confidence in the therapy rationale, recommendations, and procedures.

Therapists should consider sending educational reading materials and including useful, informative, and sensible content in letters to referral sources. Well-written letters to referral sources, and well-written notes in patients' records, influence referral sources' attitudes and behaviors. A well-informed referral source can be an ally.

One can avoid both writing a long report or letter, and repeating what the reader already knows about the patient. The following is a sample letter to a referral source; one could include data and graphs with this letter. Another option is to send a copy of the intake evaluation and therapy session notes.

> Dear Dr. _____,
> Thank you for referring Ms. _____ for treatment of her tension headaches. I will not repeat her history, of which you are aware. I saw her first on ____/____/03. My evaluation of her head and neck muscle activity used four sites: bifrontal, bilateral posterior neck, and right and left frontal posterior neck. Baseline measures were taken with her eyes open and closed while she was sitting with her back and head supported, and while she was standing. The assessment involved rest and mild office stressors. The procedures then included feedback to measure her response and begin to develop her physiological self-regulation.
>
> Muscle activity from the neck while she was sitting with her eyes open showed excess muscle activity, mostly 4 to 6 microvolts (100- to 200-hertz bandpass). While standing and trying to relax, she showed higher excessive muscle activity, mostly 9 to 12 microvolts. Muscle activity from the other sites was only slightly tense for resting muscles while she was sitting, and only slightly higher while she was standing. Visual feedback helped her reduce muscle activity, especially while standing. Without the feedback, muscle activity increased and remained elevated.
>
> I discussed the rationale for therapy and the procedures. Evaluation of psychosocial factors did not suggest enough to warrant other forms of stress management, and she was not receptive to other forms of stress management. I provided audiotapes and patient education booklets to her.
>
> She was seen for five more sessions. She is working on weaving physiological self-regulation into her daily activities. She continues to increase her ability to lower muscle activity during resting conditions, and to maintain lower muscle activity after feedback stops. In the last two sessions, her muscle activity during some phases was in a therapeutic range below 2 microvolts.
>
> Her symptom log for the last 4 weeks shows a 75% reduction in severe headaches, a 50% reduction in total hours of headaches, and an 80% decrease in medication use compared to her initial reports.
>
> Thank you for referring this pleasant lady. I am happy to be of help to her. Contact me with any questions.
>
> Sincerely yours,
>
> _____

Practitioner's Characteristics and Behaviors

Our credibility as practitioners is a major element in patients' attitudes, and thus it affects compliance. We enhance or detract from our credibility by our presentation, as well as the amount and quality of time we spend with patients. Our appearance, behaviors, and personality all affect credibility. The recommendations and patient education we provide also influence our credibility. We cannot rely solely on our reputations or the reputation of the treatment.

Trustworthiness is another major factor in achieving attitude changes and compliance. Practitioners increase and maintain patients' trust in them by being on time, maintaining confidentiality, and being consistent in their approach. They realistically discuss therapy goals and expectations. They also discuss expected and possible changes in therapy well in advance.

The appearance of a relaxed therapist, or one who effectively shows relaxation when needed, conveys an important teaching model. It also influences credibility. The therapist might consider some self-disclosure about how he or she has used physiological self-regulation to prevent and manage symptoms.

Effective communication is also important for compliance. A therapist's presentations need to be logical and coherent in order to be understood, accepted, and remembered. Effective communication must also be within the patient's "latitude of acceptance." A provider with a rigid conceptual framework and a rigid approach to therapy may not evoke compliance from patients whose attitudes are outside the limits of the information and therapy plan. Patients' attitudes must be taken into account when therapists are framing explanations about the causes of their symptoms, as well as descriptions of the therapy rationale, procedures, and recommendations. Both the wording and the content of these explanations and descriptions must be considered. For example, therapists must consider how such phrases as "letting go" and a "nonstriving attitude" sound to many patients. Similarly, some recommendations (e.g., changing work schedules) are outside the acceptance range for some patients.

It is often not advisable to insist on total early compliance for nearly everything. Instead, the professional should clearly explain the role of each factor and develop a flexible stepped-care approach. Consider the following sample explanation to a patient:

> "Mrs. _____, we talked about the potential advantages of stopping caffeine, managing your time use more effectively, and using relaxation therapies. Caffeine interferes with effective relaxation. More effective use of time will help you make time for enough relaxation to help you reduce anxiety and tension in your life. I know you might not feel ready for some of these changes. I am not saying that all of them are completely necessary for you to reduce or stop your symptoms. However, some are necessary. Seriously consider these recommendations. The decision about what to do, both now and later, is up to you. You can start with _____ for a trial, and then see how far you get."

Flexibility, laced with clear communication and empathy, is often more likely than rigid insistence to lead to acceptance.

Interaction between the Practitioner and Patient

A professional's interaction with a patient is a major cornerstone and necessary part of therapy. Here is a checklist of selected considerations for the professional:

1. Attend to your personal characteristics and behaviors.
2. Spend enough time with the patient.
3. Provide an active interaction.
4. Acknowledge the legitimacy of the patient's complaints.
5. Present an organized, systematic, and flexible approach.
6. Include appropriate, but limited, social conversation.
7. Provide reassurance, support, and encouragement
8. Provide and reinforce realistic positive expectations.
9. Provide choices for the patient.
10. Allow the patient to question recommendations.
11. Tailor therapy whenever indicated and practical.
12. Demonstrate and model selected procedures.
13. Provide appropriate self-disclosure.
14. Show attention and interest in the patient through tone of voice, facial expression, and physical posture.
15. Convey appropriate affect.
16. Maintain frequent eye contact.
17. Touch the patient appropriately.
18. Observe for signs of anxiety, resistance, and confusion.

Some of the items in this list are discussed elsewhere in this chapter. Others are so obvious that they need no elaboration. The following discussion elaborates on items 9, 11, 13, 14, and 17.

Providing Choices for the Patient; Tailoring Therapy

Discussed together are items 9 and 11—the closely related topics of providing the patient with choices and tailoring therapy whenever possible. Although there may be a place for predesigned therapy programs, they may detract from compliance. For example, for patients with headaches, there are several ways to begin: with a baseline symptom log, a medication trial, dietary changes alone, relaxation therapy alone, or a few biofeedback sessions followed by a few weeks of practice. Or treatment could start with several office sessions combining biofeedback and relaxation therapies. Or it could start with cognitive stress management, time use management, or other psychotherapy.

"Tailoring therapy" means basing a plan on interview information, the patient's individual situation and preferences, and psychophysiological assessment. Tailoring also includes consideration of the patient's attitudes, schedule, and finances. In addition, the therapist considers the symptoms during the first days and weeks of therapy and the first few biofeedback sessions.

Having choices and knowing the potential advantages and disadvantages of each give a patient the sense of actively participating in the design of his or her program. Such an approach also conveys that the practitioner is considering the patient's situation, preferences, and needs. I assume that such tailoring helps compliance. Consider these factors:

1. Improvement of symptoms sometimes occurs after a physician gives convincing reassurance to a patient about the nonserious nature of his or her symptoms.

2. Starting a new medication or changing dosage can improve symptoms.

3. Making changes in lifestyle, work, exercises, and/or dietary intake can result in a significant decrease in symptoms.

(Note: In these first three examples, compliance with a time-consuming treatment will often be less than ideal, especially if the patient believes that the symptom changes result from these factors. In such circumstances, tailoring the therapy plan can involve deferring more biofeedback.)

4. Another factor that alerts practitioners to the need for tailoring is a lack of physiological tension and arousal, and/or a rapid return to a "therapeutic range"[1] after intentional arousal during office sessions. This suggests that the patient can relax adequately but needs to apply his or her ability to do so.

5. Some patients show significant improvement of symptoms in the first weeks of therapy, regardless of the physiological self-regulation shown in the office. It is sometimes difficult to explain rapid improvement of symptoms. The scientist in each of us wants to know why and how this is occurring; the skeptical and cautious part of us is suspicious. However, the clinician in us, especially the cost-conscious and pragmatic part, accepts the progress and may defer more office therapy. If the symptoms increase later, patients may better accept the role of the therapy and the need for compliance.

6. Therapists should consider deferring or stopping office-based biofeedback sessions with patients who continue noncompliance with necessary parts of therapy. For example, some patients do not practice relaxation at all, or do so for much less time than suggested. Many continue lifestyle behaviors (such as caffeine usage, stressful work habits, and overburdened schedules) that are inconsistent with making progress.

7. Assessment and feedback sites may need tailoring. For example, a patient may perceive repeated sessions semireclined, with eyes closed, and with feedback from only one area as meaningless. Tailoring the sites, body positions, and conditions can make the sessions more sensible to the patient and can increase the patient's confidence and compliance.

8. Physiological arousal to cognitive stressors and activities offers data with which to tailor therapy. For example, let us suppose that a patient shows good relaxation in multiple muscle areas, warm hands, and low skin conductance during resting baselines. Furthermore, suppose that the patient can do this during a standard cognitive stressor and in different positions. Now let us suppose that this patient has significantly decreased finger temperatures while imagining or talking about work or family stress. The therapist may consider repeating the arousal scenes several times with and without feedback and exploring the content. Or the therapist may encourage relaxation before, during, and immediately after work situations.

9. Long geographic distance between the patient and the treatment office will require tailoring of the therapy. Office sessions twice a day for 2 or more consecutive days, with a few weeks between such phases, may be preferable for some patients who live too far away for weekly sessions. Such a "massed-practice" schedule conveys that the therapist is willing to extend him- or herself, and may help increase patient compliance.

Providing Appropriate Self-Disclosure

Limited, appropriate self-disclosure by practitioners (item 13 in the list above) includes brief and proper descriptions of how they effectively use applied psychophysiology in their own lives. In this manner, therapists can communicate that they know firsthand that this works.

Showing Attention and Interest in the Patient through Tone of Voice, Facial Expression, and Physical Posture; Touching the Patient Appropriately

Items 14 and 17 in the list above are discussed together because they have overlapping features. The practitioner's voice, facial expressions, body posture, and other nonverbal behaviors all convey interest, trust, sincerity, experience, and confidence.

Touch is also important. Touching patients is part of the practice of physicians, nurses, physical therapists, occupational therapists, dentists, and some other health care professionals. Psychologists and some other persons providing biofeedback do not typically use physical contact in their other contacts with patients. Even those with experience may not know how to use touch to help convey sincerity, support, and encouragement.

There are several obvious chances to use touch properly, aside from the initial handshake. They include times when the therapist is attaching electrodes and other transducers to a patient, and when he or she is directly helping in relaxation or muscle reeducation. For example, the therapist might consider how he or she moves a patient's hair and grasps the patient's arm. It can be enlightening for the practitioner to ask, "How would this contact feel if I were the patient?"

Another opportunity for the careful use of touch that supports and enhances rapport between a practitioner and a patient who needs much reassurance and hope is near the end of a supportive statement. The practitioner can gently but firmly place a hand on the patient's forearm, and may give a mild squeeze or brief pat on the arm, but for no longer than about 2 seconds. A therapist must always be sensitive about contact; some patients may not like such contact or may distrust it. However, if not overdone in intensity or frequency, the technique can have positive effects.

Other chances for reassuring with touch include occasions when patients express frustration, fear, life stress, and difficulty with physiological self-regulation. Proper use of touch can help a practitioner convey caring about such a patient's welfare.

It bears repeating that touch should not be overdone, because touch can have a negative effect. For example, consider the possible impressions of female patients touched by male practitioners. I am not suggesting that one should avoid such contacts altogether. However, the duration and frequency of the contacts can convey the wrong message. Consider the difference between a possible undesirable message from a touch of about 5 seconds, and a desirable one of about 2 seconds. I do not need to elaborate on this point. If the practitioner's hands are cold, moist, or both, he or she should consider touching clothed parts of the arm and not bare skin. This also probably needs no elaboration.

Cognitive Preparation of the Patient

Cognitive preparation includes correcting misperceptions and misinformation. Topics include (1) the rationale for physiological self-regulation, (2) therapy process, (3) therapy goals, (4) use of medications, (5) generalization, (6) therapy options, (7) stepped care, and (8) a symptom log.

A therapist should try to avoid overloading a patient during one session. Some information may need presentation during the first few sessions and then need to be repeated later for emphasis and to help patients recall. Carefully developed patient education scripts, booklets, and audiotapes help. A checklist can help a therapist organize presentations and help avoid overlooking some information. This is useful for the neophyte and practitioner with limited experience.

Because most patients forget much of what they hear, therapists should consider repeating some information. Most patients will have at least some compliance problems. Shaping acceptance of self-responsibility is one of the challenging aspects of clinical practice.

Cognitive preparation also includes expecting slow progress, plateaus, and setbacks. Practitioners want to communicate realistic positive expectations. It can be useful to show patients graphs of developing physiological self-regulation and symptom changes from prior patients. In addition, it can be helpful to tell a patient something like the following:

> "You have a good chance of making progress in reducing or stopping your symptoms. I do not know how long this will take. Some patients show much improvement within days or weeks. Others progress gradually over several weeks or a few months. Plateaus and even temporary reversals happen. If they occur, remember that they are normal and a natural part of learning. You need not feel discouraged. You know athletes and musicians expect unevenness in developing and keeping their skills. Also, keep in mind that even accomplished athletes have off days. Not even a great baseball player, golfer, or tennis player always hits the ball well."

Patients often display resistance, skepticism, and pessimism. Often they have gone to several doctors and have tried various treatments. They have had positive expectations, but have felt disappointment with the results. For some patients, our treatment approach appears too simplistic, despite careful explanations and even our reputations. If their healthy skepticism leads to our being defensive or rejecting of them, then we unnecessarily risk losing them and not starting therapy.

Prudent therapists will consider investing extra time checking and discussing the perceptions of selected patients. They offer creative explanations of the rationale for a therapeutic trial and discuss options. They gently, compassionately, and empathetically overcome patient resistance. It is too easy to give up and label such patients unsuitable for therapy. For such patients, the challenge to their therapists is greater. The challenge is to establish a therapeutic alliance and mobilize these patients realistically. In addition, the challenge is to shape their attitudes and perceptions of the therapy. Thus the therapists shape their self-confidence, their optimism, and their willingness to engage in a realistic therapy trial. A therapist should consider saying something like the following to show that he or she understands a patient:

"If I put myself in your place, I would be skeptical too. I know you went to several doctors and tried several treatments without success. I understand that you were hopeful and then disappointed. Part of you is asking yourself, 'Why is this going to be any different?' You do not want to get your hopes up, because you do not want that disappointment again. I understand that, and I think it is perfectly normal.

"You know I cannot promise that you will improve or tell you how much improvement you will have. However, I can tell you that many patients treated did well, despite being unsuccessful with past therapies. Thousands of professionals all over the country report the same experiences with their patients.

"There are several approaches we can take. If the first is less than ideal, then there are variations and other approaches. Biofeedback and related therapies involve many therapies. Ask me any questions you wish, or express any concerns and doubts you may have.

"Some parts of the therapy may appear to you as too simple to work. I do not want them to appear complicated. They are not as simple as they appear, but neither are they very complicated. Even long-term symptoms often do not require complex solutions.

"For example, I treated many patients with [this patient's symptoms] for years. [Practitioners can also insert their personal experiences.] These treatments helped most of them. Many of those patients thought these treatments were probably not enough for them, and yet they got better. Relaxation and biofeedback treatments are often enough alone. However, sometimes we also need other therapies."

Therapists should consider using patient education booklets and audiotapes that contain much of the necessary and useful information. One can get booklets and tapes prepared by others or develop one's own. Therapists who develop their own patient education materials should consider consultations with professional writers and editors about readability, style, and grammar. Compliance counseling begins during or after the initial session.

THE PATIENT

A patient's perceptions, expectations, and mood are among the important aspects of therapy and compliance. This assumes that the patient's cognitions affect compliance—an assumption with which few professionals would disagree. The list below provides a catalogue of many specific patient perceptions, expectations, affective and symptom-related factors, and other factors. All of these can affect compliance and therapy results. Their order, and the space devoted to discussing each topic, do not indicate relative importance. This list should be considered during evaluation, cognitive preparation, and treatment.

I. Perceptions
    A. Biofeedback/relaxation. Patients may perceive this treatment as:
        1. Psychological treatment.
        2. Insufficient or useless therapy.
        3. A waste of time.
        4. The last chance for help, thus increasing stress.
    B. Therapy. Patients may perceive:
        1. Therapy as preprogrammed, and may resist such a program.

2. The need for alternative therapies, based on prior medical consultations.
3. Aspects of biofeedback/relaxation as silly or embarrassing.
4. The therapy as too costly and impractical.
5. The therapy program as taking too long.
6. The explanations of the rationale and therapy procedures as too complex.
7. Self-report symptom logs as impractical.
8. The time needed daily as interfering with other priorities.
   C. The therapist. Patients may:
1. Distrust doctors and health care professionals in general.
2. Not perceive their professionals/therapists as allies.
   D. Symptoms. Patients may perceive their symptoms as:
1. Organic, and hence requiring alternative therapy.
2. Out of their control.
   E. Self and others. Patients may:
1. Fear using passive therapies.
2. Expect loss of control with relaxation therapy.
3. Perceive a lack of cooperation from significant others.
II. Expectations. Patients may have:
   A. Unrealistic negative expectations.
   B. Unrealistic positive expectations.
   C. Experienced inadequate biofeedback/relaxation and may expect to do so again.
III. Affective and symptom-related discomfort. The following may interfere with patients' attention and compliance:
   A. Anxiety.
   B. Physical symptoms.
   C. Depression.
IV. Other factors.
   A. Patients may be reluctant to speak candidly about psychological, interpersonal, and other stressful matters.
   B. Symptoms may be reinforcing, and symptom relief may be perceived as threatening.
   C. Patients may resist stopping the use of caffeine, nicotine, alcohol, or other vasoactive dietary chemicals; chewing gum; and/or unnecessary, ill-advised, and risky medications.
   D. Patients' neurocognitive functioning may be impaired enough to interfere with their attention.

Perceptions

Perceptions of Biofeedback / Relaxation

Patients May Perceive Biofeedback/Relaxation as Psychological Treatment. Because mental health professionals commonly provide biofeedback-assisted relaxation, it is understandable that many patients perceive biofeedback as a psychological approach. Many health care professionals also consider biofeedback a psychological technique. However, these therapies are multidisciplinary and not uniquely or exclusively within the province of psychology.

The important points here are patients' perceptions and feelings about psychological therapies, especially many patients' resistance to psychological therapies. A therapist should consider explaining that many professionals do not view biofeedback and relaxation as psychological treatments.

Such a discussion is pertinent when one is treating patients with medical disorders. One may not need to discuss the multidisciplinary nature of biofeedback with patients who voluntarily seek mental health help. Furthermore, nurses, physical therapists, occupational therapists, and other non-mental-health professionals providing or supervising these therapies need not have this type of discussion with patients. A mental health professional might consider portraying physiological self-regulation and biofeedback as having many unique features in addition to any psychological aspects.

Patients May Perceive Biofeedback/Relaxation as Insufficient, Useless, or a Waste of Time. Relaxation and biofeedback-assisted relaxation may appear to some patients as insufficient or useless, especially when they think of the intensity, frequency, and chronicity of their symptoms. Prior unsuccessful therapies can diminish the credibility of self-regulation therapies. Patients may harbor these perceptions and yet not openly express them. One result can be an extreme form of noncompliance—dropping out of treatment early.

A corollary of the insufficiency/uselessness perception is that relaxation is simply a waste of time. Such a perception is especially common among medical patients who have chronic physical symptoms. A therapist should consider showing awareness of these perceptions—for example, by saying:

> "You may be thinking, 'How is this therapy going to help me? I have had these symptoms so long and tried so many treatments. I got my hopes up before and the treatments did not help. How is this going to be different? I have a busy schedule. I am having trouble believing this is not a waste of time.' If you are having thoughts like this, let's discuss them."

The therapist can then explain the rationale for therapy and discuss how it can help the patient, despite the chronicity of his or her symptoms and any prior unsuccessful treatments. Time spent in the present treatment can be described as an investment.

Compliance with homework assignments is often crucial within many types of therapies, including applied psychophysiology. See Kazantzis (2000) for a recent review and references. Some studies support the role of homework compliance and improvement in therapy, whereas other studies have not found such support. Kazantzis (2000) studied the statistical power of homework research in 27 studies from 1980 through 1998 in which homework was specifically examined and sufficient statistical information was provided. He concluded that power levels were weaker than desired, and that this could account for the inconsistent findings. The mean sample size was about 48, and all but 3 studies involved much fewer than 100 subjects (the other 3 had 150–175). Kazantzis (2000) reported that 780 subjects would be needed to detect a small effect with 80% power between two groups; thus the contribution of homework is likely to be clinically trivial.

Homework compliance had a large causal effect on depression in two samples of 122 and 399 patients (Burns & Spangler, 2000). Homework compliance will continue to be a focus of attention and is probably helpful for many patients.

Patients May Perceive Biofeedback/Relaxation as the Last Chance for Help. Some patients who have tried several therapies without adequate success may perceive relaxation and biofeedback as therapies of "last resort." This perception is especially common among patients seen in tertiary medical centers. As with other misperceptions, patients are usually hesitant to report this perception spontaneously.

Such a perception is an added source of anxiety. It can interfere with patients' attending to what professionals present and complying with recommendations. The increased tension and symptoms that sometimes result can lead to more frustration and discouragement. Some patients then consider giving up entirely and dropping out of therapy.

One can change and even stop this perception by conveying to the patient that several different therapies and approaches are available. There are lifestyle changes, dietary changes, cognitive stress management therapies, other stress management approaches, and various combinations of these. This information can significantly alter the perception of biofeedback as the therapy of last resort.

Patients may resist or be less than ideally cooperative with therapy recommendations if they are perceived as the last resort. Implicitly, such patients may be saying that they would rather not try very hard than try and fail. Rather than saying, "It is better to have tried and lost," these patients act according to a different belief: "It is better not to try and still have some hope that a good therapy might still exist."

Perceptions of Therapy

Patients May Perceive Therapy as Preprogrammed, and May Resist Such a Program. Practitioners sometimes provide biofeedback and related therapies in preprogrammed packages. This sometimes includes a specified number of sessions, standard placements of transducers, standard body positions, and therapy session conditions. There are often specific physiological criteria for proceeding to the next stage or changing to a different strategy. Some patients (and practitioners) resist preprogrammed packages and prefer tailored therapy. Therapists need to be aware of these potential perceptions and adjust their treatments accordingly.

Patients May Perceive That Other Therapies Are Needed, Based on Prior Medical Consultations. Physicians with whom a patient has consulted have probably discussed and recommended therapy options. These include new or different medications, dosage changes, surgery, or psychotherapy. Before pursuing those other therapies, the patient has come to a provider who uses biofeedback and related therapies. However, the other options often remain in the patient's perceptions as viable and possibly effective. The biofeedback therapist should uncover these perceptions and deal with them as soon as practical.

Patients May Perceive Aspects of Biofeedback/Relaxation as Silly or Embarrassing. Some patients perceive certain aspects of relaxation as silly or embarrassing. These include tensing and releasing facial muscles, diaphragmatic breathing, listening to audiotaped relaxation, and relaxing in public places. Patients will usually not spontaneously voice such perceptions and feelings. The next question is how to revise them.

Some practitioners and therapists model some aspects of biofeedback and relaxation. A therapist's self-disclosure that he or she uses these procedures in daily life can be reassuring. Some patients also may feel more comfortable once they know that many professionals, executives, athletes, entertainers, and others also often use these procedures. Providing a credible rationale for, and explaining the application of, each procedure can help to put it in better perspective as well.

Patients May Perceive the Therapy as Too Costly and Impractical, or the Therapy Program as Taking Too Long. Some patients perceive the costs and duration of treatment as beyond their capabilities and patience. This discourages them, and hence decreases compliance. Solving this problem is not easy, because therapy can extend over several months. The steppedcare approach offers a model within which to adjust the number of office sessions.

The relationship between a practitioner and a patient can help the patient accept the costs and duration of therapy. A practitioner can support reduced fees when standard fees are a hardship for a patient, when there is a clear need for therapy, and when fee reduction is allowable. Such humane and generous adjustments result in appreciation and can increase compliance. However, fee adjustments have become more difficult in recent years because of reimbursement problems throughout the health care system.

Patients May Perceive the Explanations of the Rationale and Therapy Procedures as Too Complex. Patients need to relate the procedures logically to symptom reduction. Otherwise, they may perceive treatment as being too complex or irrelevant for them. This can affect compliance.

Patients May Perceive Self-Report Symptom Logs as Impractical. Self-report symptom logs should be practical and easy for patients to use. If not, then patients will perceive keeping such logs as too much of a chore. This perception can lead to a lack of records, contrived data, or withdrawal from therapy.

Patients May Perceive the Time Needed Daily as Interfering with Other Priorities. Biofeedback/relaxation therapy often involves considerable time commitments by patients. These can take time away from other important activities. Taking an hour or more daily for applying recommendations—which therapists often suggest—is more than some patients can do. Of course, when patients' schedules are very full, there is often a greater need for balance and therapy. However, patients may not perceive their situations that way.

Examples of people whose schedules do not permit time for ideally applying treatments are farmers, tax accountants, and other seasonal workers whose schedules change significantly. In such cases, therapists need to be flexible and wait, rather than "beating their [professional] heads against a stone wall." Shorter daily relaxation sessions, and/or instructions for blending therapy activities into daily activities, should be considered.

Another strategy would be to defer some treatment and focus therapy on altering the patient's schedule and priorities—in other words, to practice "time use therapy." For example, some people need to delegate, to drop items from their daily and weekly lists, to learn to do some tasks with less perfection, and/or to get better organized.

Perceptions of the Therapist

Patients May Distrust Doctors and Other Health Care Professionals. Some patients have learned to mistrust health care professionals. Such distrust often stems from their experiences or others' opinions. Many such patients have experienced mistreatment, have been misled, or have received treatment from insensitive providers.

Professionals who have added to the negative perceptions of patients may include some who have provided inadequate relaxation, biofeedback, and associated therapies. For example, many patients react negatively to being alone for most or all sessions. These patients report feeling abandoned, anxious, confused by what to do, and frustrated. These feelings have added to their negative perception of biofeedback and of professionals offering such services. Professionals can modulate such experiences by the quality of interactions with their patients. They should inquire about prior experiences if the patients do not volunteer the information.

Some patients will candidly describe their negative experiences. Other patients either sit quietly with distrustful looks on their faces, or provide no obvious clues of their distrust. Some people simply do not want to be in therapists' offices or follow therapists' advice—no matter who the therapists are, what they say, and how pleasant they are.

Patients May Not Perceive Their Practitioners as Allies. Even patients without negative experiences may not perceive us practitioners as their allies in the battle against their symptoms. We may be credible and even highly competent. However, they may see us as too formal, too distant, not devoted enough, or too busy to provide the time they perceive as needed.

We need to get out from behind our desks and our formality, and convey that we do care about patients as people, not only as patients or cases. It is difficult for some of us professionals to adopt Will Rogers's dictum, "I never met a man [or woman] I didn't like." However, it helps to keep striving to show our liking for all patients . . . perhaps with a few exceptions!

Perceptions of Symptoms

Patients May Perceive Their Symptoms as Organic, and Hence Requiring Alternative Therapy. A patient's perception may be that "if only my doctors believed me and did more tests, they would find the cause of my problems." Such patients continue to believe that an organic cause is the major factor explaining their symptoms. They may hold this perception despite the fact that highly expert medical examinations and laboratory tests have ruled out an organic explanation for the symptoms.

Patients often limit their compliance in such cases. To comply properly, patients need to believe that stress, tension, or arousal could cause or worsen their symptoms. They need to believe that organic factors are minor or nonexistent, or can be overcome. Superficial compliance with the mechanics of therapy may still occur; however, these patients only "go through the motions." They often wait for another chance to get more medical tests. They may even view such compliance as a chance for them to show that the symptoms indeed are organic. They do this by failing to improve. Such a situation is typically very difficult to manage.

Such patients often go to highly credible tertiary medical centers. Resulting examinations and tests sometimes do find organic disease explanations for some patients' symptoms. Ruling out organic causes by the best and credible medical examinations can help patients accept physiological self-regulation and related therapies.

It is often wiser to defer applied psychophysiological therapies if a patient does not yet sufficiently accept these therapies. Otherwise, one risks souring the patient's experience with failure from a treatment that might later be successful when the patient is more accepting. However, the presence of some patient skepticism does not prevent starting applied psychophysiological therapies.

Patients May Perceive Their Symptoms as Out of Their Control. Patients can believe that their symptoms are beyond their control, even if they accept a functional or psychophysiological explanation and believe that psychophysiological therapies can ameliorate symptoms in many people. This sometimes involves the perception of themselves as inadequate to relieve their symptoms. They lack sufficient self-efficacy. They also may perceive the intensity or chronicity of the symptoms as so severe that these therapies could not possibly work for them. A skilled clinician can convince patients of the potential for help, despite the chronicity and severity of their symptoms, and can mobilize these patients for enough compliance to achieve successful results.

Perceptions of Self and Others

Patients May Fear Using Passive Therapies. Some patients perceive relaxation therapies as tantamount to becoming passive; this is a threatening perception for those patients who avoid anything passive. Therapists should look for this fear if patients are avoiding relaxation practice. Such patients need to be reassured that relaxation is not equal to, nor does it increase, passivity. Therapists can try briefer periods of relaxation, or consider suggesting that patients periodically raise themselves out of the relaxed state. The latter can reassure patients that they can do this any time they need to.

Patients May Expect Loss of Control with Relaxation Therapy. Some patients fear losing control even without a history of such a loss. Such patients require extra reassurance and gradual exposure to treatment procedures. Therapists should communicate early that physiological self-regulation therapies increase self-control rather than lessen it.

Patients May Perceive a Lack of Cooperation from Significant Others. Patients often need support and cooperation from their family members and others. Some patients believe that these people will not be understanding, accepting, and cooperative. Such perceptions are often accurate. These other people may misunderstand, and this can decrease patients' compliance.

Therapists should consider four options. The first of these is giving patient education booklets and/or tapes to patients, and encouraging patients to share these with their significant others to help convey the rationale and procedures. Some patients can explain the rationale and procedures directly to the others. Increasing the patients' assertiveness to gain the understanding, acceptance, and cooperation of others is ideal.

Second, a therapist may consider directly contacting the other people, with the patient's permission. This option can be pursued when cooperation from the other people is necessary, but the patient is not getting it. A third approach is to suggest that the patient use relaxation procedures only when other people are not around. This is the least desirable option.

Finally, for some patients, therapists may consider enlisting others to give direct cooperation and help. For example, others can take care of some household or work responsibilities, reduce noise, and answer phone calls for a few minutes. Others can remind the patient about body postures and relaxation. However, cooperation and help may threaten some patients' perceptions of self-sufficiency. Many patients want to conduct their therapy without help from other people. Some such patients get along poorly with other people in their lives and may have a history of poor cooperation from those people. Other patients have a strong preference and capability for independence and a good history of self-discipline. Still others have ample chances to apply the treatment procedures without the cooperation and help from others.

Expectations

Patients May Have Unrealistic Positive or Negative Expectations

Unrealistic negative expectations often interfere with compliance, as noted in several contexts above. However, unrealistic positive expectations are also common and involve expecting greater or faster benefit than usual. Unrealistic positive expectations can result in disappointment and later noncompliance when the expectations do not match reality. Cognitive preparation includes promoting realistic positive expectations.

Patients May Have Experienced Inadequate Biofeedback/Relaxation and May Expect to Do So Again

Patients may perceive biofeedback/relaxation therapy as inadequate when they did not get successful results with it in the past. However, the prior therapy may have been less than ideal. Reversing negative expectations requires extra care, especially if one is to avoid disparaging the prior practitioner. A therapist should consider saying something like the following:

"The treatment you received in the past sounds like what many professionals provide. Some professionals devote more time to developing specialized knowledge, skills, and procedures. Others are less specialized. Some professionals are not in places that allow them to get preferred instruments. Most practitioners mean well, but often they do not know what they do not know. There is much we can add to the therapy you had in the past. This can be important and helpful for you."

Affective and Symptom-Related Discomfort

Practitioners usually know that patients' affect and physical symptoms have an impact on what they remember from spoken patient education. Affective and symptom-related discomfort can interfere with patients' attention and experience during feedback. This point probably does not need more discussion.

Other Factors

Patients May Be Reluctant to Speak Candidly about Psychological, Interpersonal, and Other Stressful Matters

Some patients view a referral for relaxation and biofeedback therapies as "face-saving" by comparison with a psychological evaluation. These patients sometimes expect that psychological topics will not be a focus of the evaluation and treatment. They are often reluctant to speak candidly about psychological matters that are of potential importance in the formulation of an effective treatment program.

For some of these patients, practitioners can skirt such topics, at least in the early sessions. It is often sufficient to focus on physiological self-regulation therapies, reducing or stopping the use of chemical stressors, and making related changes.

Symptoms May Be Reinforcing, and Symptom Relief May Be Perceived as Threatening

Most practitioners know that symptoms can serve reinforcing value, despite the discomfort and impairment they cause. Some patients expect that significant symptom relief will result in threatening effects. Practitioners often struggle with ways to discuss this delicate topic with patients. Without ample caution and tact, the result can be loss of a patient's confidence and trust.

Discreet practitioners consider using examples when discussing this topic and checking for the possible role of this factor in maintaining patients' symptoms and in compliance problems. For instance, persons with chronic obesity (often from their adolescence onward) often face very different heterosexual situations when they lose considerable weight and their figures approach normal size. They may not believe that they have the interpersonal skills and stress management strategies to adjust to such conditions. They may or may not be aware of the approach–avoidance conflict; in either case, they will probably be reluctant to discuss their feelings spontaneously. A common result is lack of continued compliance with a weight loss program.

Some practitioners have experienced severe physical symptoms themselves, and have thereby gained an awareness for and increased empathy with patients' expectations and behavior. Some practitioners have even experienced the temptation for others to take care of them, so that they could gain temporary relief from onerous responsibilities and escape distasteful situations. They know firsthand the temptation to maintain this state. If such practitioners are comfortable with limited self-disclosure, then sharing these experiences may be helpful. It may encourage the patients to admit such thoughts.

Patients May Resist Stopping the Use of Vasoactive Dietary Chemicals, Chewing Gum, and/or Unnecessary Medications

Typically, many (though by no means all) patients accept stopping caffeine, chewing gum, and some foods with vasoactive chemicals. However, patients do commonly resist stopping nicotine, alcohol, and many unnecessary medications. What do therapists do when patients plan to continue ingesting chemicals that are known to detract from the effectiveness of physiological self-regulation therapies?

Practitioners advise patients of these substances' potential negative effects on treatment. They explain the physiological effects of caffeine, nicotine, and other chemicals. They try to persuade patients to avoid such chemicals during at least the hour or so before relaxation and biofeedback sessions. The effects of gum chewing on temporalis muscles are not clear to most patients, and hence there is a need for patient education and demonstration. A general statement to patients about these substances may be something like the following:

> "I know your symptoms are very distressing to you, and you want to reduce or stop them. I've explained how _____ interferes with therapies and self-regulation of your body. I know you want to make progress as fast as practical. You probably want to limit the number of office sessions you need. Continuing to consume these chemicals can detract from your progress and prolong therapy. The decision about whether you stop them or not is yours. However, I do not want you to waste your time and money. I will do everything I can to help you withdraw from and stop these chemicals. Please give this some thought, and we can discuss this further."

Patients' Neurocognitive Functioning May Be Impaired Enough to Interfere with Their Attention

Impaired neurocognitive functioning often results in patients' inability to remember instructions and therapy recommendations, and to attend to therapy tasks. Practitioners can sometimes successfully treat such patients, with help from cooperative persons living with the patients.

EVALUATION AND INTERVENTION

There are several methods for assessing compliance:

1. Patient self-monitoring of frequency and durations of relaxation, and the times when relaxation is used.
2. Self-report log of symptoms.
3. Self-monitoring of subjective physiological sensations associated with relaxation.
4. Self-monitoring of cognitions associated with relaxation.
5. Self-monitoring of caffeine, nicotine, and other chemical use.
6. Self-monitoring of physiological parameters, such as skin temperatures, pulse rates, and blood pressure. Patients can do this before, during, and after relaxation sessions.
7. Practitioner interviews.
8. Periodic psychophysiological assessments.
9. Practitioner observation of a patient's breathing and body postures.
10. Reports from other people in a patient's daily life.

11. Patients' motor functioning.
12. Patients' daily activities.

Each patient should be encouraged to maintain a self-report log. This conveys the importance of the information requested, as well as the intent of the therapist to review this information. However, requesting too much or too complicated record keeping can be counterproductive. In addition, patients' records do not need to be 100% accurate for practitioners to obtain useful information and assess compliance. A log is often enough to allow practitioners to check on compliance and to stimulate discussion.

Some portion of each office session should be devoted to reviewing the log. If necessary, therapists can use interviews to get information about patients' compliance. Clinicians who are competent interviewers know that simple questions are often not enough to elicit needed and useful information, since patients often provide incorrect and misleading responses in interviews. For example, consider the value of the response "yes" to the following questions:

- "Are you practicing your relaxation?"
- "Are you practicing your relaxation as instructed?"
- "Are you feeling relaxed when you use the relaxation?"
- "Are you practicing your relaxation daily?"
- "Are you practicing your relaxation at various times each day?"

These and similar questions are inadequate alone to elicit useful information. Patients can answer such questions with a "yes" or "no," but they may be interpreting the questions in ways they prefer, which are not always the ways the practitioner intends. For instance, when patients say "yes" to "practicing daily," does this really mean "daily," or does it mean "most days" or just "some days"?

Limited time to question patients in detail, or limited interviewing skills, can result in not enough information for assessing compliance and progress. If there is no self-report log or it is incomplete, the therapist might consider the following examples of interview questions. One might start in this manner:

"Let's review your relaxation practice. As accurately as you can recall, please tell me how often and when are you using relaxation procedures [or other procedures]."

Depending on the completeness of the patient's response to such a question, the therapist might consider more specific questions:

- "How many times each day, during the past week, did you relax for 15–20 minutes each? How many brief relaxations of 2–10 minutes each?"
- "Are there days on which you were not been able to relax? How many days?"
- "Let's talk about those days. What are the problems?"
- "How do you feel during your relaxation sessions? What sensations are you experiencing during relaxation? What do you experience after your relaxation sessions? How long do those sensations and feelings last?"
- "In what situations did you use relaxation during the past week?"
- "When could you benefit from relaxation but are not using it?"

Therapists should avoid misusing and misinterpreting physiological measures during office sessions to assess compliance. It is reasonable to assume that warmer baseline skin temperatures, faster increases in skin temperature, lower baseline muscle activity, and/or faster drops of muscle activity reflect good relaxation experiences between office sessions. However, a therapist cannot assume that these are clear signs of compliance. Improved psychophysiological functioning during baselines in office sessions can reflect increasing comfort or habituation to the office, instrumentation, and the therapist. Psychophysiological data are often consistent with verbal reports of compliance with relaxation, reduction of undesired chemicals, and/ or other lifestyle changes. In such cases, the therapist can use the data as a valuable basis for positive verbal reinforcement of the patient. Conversely, a lack of compliance cannot be assumed from the lack of psychophysiological progress during baselines.

Observations of patients by persons living or working with the patients may help therapists assess compliance. These can include observation of patients' restlessness, posture, breathing, facial muscles, and other visible cues of tension and relaxation.

INCREASING COMPLIANCE AND SUMMARY

This chapter helps answer a common question asked by practitioners: "What can I do to help assure, or increase the likelihood, that my patients will do what I recommend?" Some of the answers appear throughout the chapter. Three arbitrary divisions of the methods and considerations for increasing compliance have been discussed. The most pertinent points are summarized below.

Persons and factors that prevent or decrease noncompliance are as follows:

- Professional setting and office personnel.
- Professional's characteristics and behaviors.
- Interaction between the professional and patient.
- Cognitive preparation of the patient.
- Patient's perceptions, expectations, and affect.
- Patient's family members and other significant individuals.

Specific interventions include the following:

- Use readily accessible, easy-to-use self-report record systems.
- Ask patients to record readily observable and meaningful behaviors.
- Instruct patients why and how to self-monitor.
- Reinforce patients' accuracy and completeness.
- Convey that the patient's records will be reviewed.
- Encourage patients to record behaviors, experiences, and symptoms when they occur.
- Establish subgoals, and review and revise them as needed.

Important general considerations include these:

- Be willing to accept less than ideal compliance and therapeutic progress.
- Successively approximate and shape compliance.
- Allow patients to set their own goals and subgoals, and discuss cost–benefit considerations.

I conclude the chapter by elaborating on a few of these various points.

A therapist should give positive verbal reinforcement to those parts of self-report logs that appear accurate. One can also encourage or shape more accuracy and completeness. For example, one might say:

"These records are a good beginning. You have the idea. Allow me, please, to suggest [or ask] that you add and develop your records a little more by . . ."

Patients ideally record their symptoms and behaviors when they occur, and not hours later. Exceptions are when the symptoms are very severe for hours or when there are no symptoms for hours. Preaddressed and prestamped envelopes can ease communications for those patients who are not seen often in the office.

In reviewing the data with patients, therapists can share tabulations and graphs derived from the data. This reinforces the usefulness and importance of the records, as well as the professionals' interest in the patients. Therapists need to be patient with patients, and to avoid conveying negative criticism, displeasure, or disappointment. Implied scolding or expressions of disappointment may signal reappraisal of the question "Who is treating whom?"

It is useful for us practitioners to remind ourselves that we are here to serve our patients— and not the reverse. We fulfill many of our responsibilities when we provide a good rationale for our recommendations and present practical and achievable methods to reach therapy goals. We fulfill other responsibilities by maintaining our credibility in the views of our patients and preserving positive rapport with them.

Patients often know the degree of symptom improvement that is enough for them. They know the limits of the time, money, and inconvenience they are willing and able to invest for the desired benefits. Determining and reviewing subgoals can enhance compliance. For example, the goal of eliminating symptoms is too distant and too unrealistic for many patients. In such cases, subgoals—such as a specific number of minutes of relaxation and separate relaxation periods per day, reduced caffeine and nicotine use, symptom-free hours, and/or time use changes—may be helpful.

It is abundantly clear that compliance is a complex and many-sided concept. Patient compliance requires great care, preparation, ingenuity, persistence, and patience by practitioners. It requires professionals to review their own professional behaviors, setting, and procedures. It requires tailoring interventions and giving patients adequate time to apply recommendations. Practitioners also need to tolerate and function with ambiguity and within the less than ideal world of clinical practice. All of us need to continue to strive toward further cultivation and growth of our skills to help our patients cultivate compliance, healthy attitudes, and health-promoting behaviors.

NOTE

1. I prefer the term "therapeutic range." This term may or may not be the same as a "relaxed range." The criteria for a relaxed range differ among practitioners; they also differ at different stages of therapy and for different therapeutic goals.

REFERENCES

Buchmann, W. F. (1997). Adherence: A matter of self-efficacy and power. *Journal of Advanced Nursing*, 26, 132–137.

Burns, D. D., & Spangler, D. L. (2000). Does psychotherapy homework lead to improvements in depression in cognitive-behavior therapy or does improvement lead to increased homework compliance? *Journal of Consulting and Clinical Psychology*, 68(1), 46–56.

DiMatteo, M. R., & DiNicola, D. D. (1982). *Achieving patient compliance*. New York: Pergamon Press.

Erlen, J. A. (1997). Ethical questions inherent in compliance. *Orthopaedic Nursing*, 16(2), 77–80.

Kazantzis, N. (2000). Power to detect homework effects in psychotherapy outcome research. *Journal of Consulting and Clinical Psychology*, 68(1), 166–170.

PART IV

Cultivating Lower Arousal

CHAPTER 9

Dietary Considerations
Rationale, Issues, Substances, Evaluation, and Patient Education

KEITH I. BLOCK
MARK S. SCHWARTZ
CHARLOTTE GYLLENHAAL

Many health care professionals believe, and many patients report, that certain dietary elements and patterns aggravate or trigger some physical or psychological symptoms. Professionals advise their patients to alter those dietary elements that they believe cause or aggravate those symptoms, many of which are symptoms treated with applied psychophysiological interventions (e.g., migraine headaches, anxiety, irritable bowel syndrome [IBS], insomnia). This chapter helps readers assess dietary factors in clinical practice. It emphasizes the relationship between diet and migraine because of the work in this area, although it does not exclude the other conditions just listed.

MECHANISMS OF MIGRAINE

There are disagreements about the proposed links between diet and migraine headache, but there is research support for including dietary recommendations in clinical practice with some patients with migraine headaches. One reason for the disagreements is that the association between dietary factors and migraine headaches is variable. Even for a specific individual, a particular food may not trigger headaches every time he or she ingests it, possibly because of differences in stress levels and recent consumption of other aggravating foods.

Nevertheless, most people susceptible to migraines appear to be unusually reactive to events and substances that trigger vasoconstriction or vasodilation. Serotonin plays a major role. Serotonin (also known as 5-hydroxytryptamine or 5-HT) is an important neurotransmitter with vasoconstrictor activity. It seems to be released in large quantities from blood platelets in migraine; its metabolites appear in the urine following migraine, and platelet serotonin level has been shown to decrease by 40% during migraines (Humphrey, 1991). It has also been suggested that immunoglobulins (especially immunoglobulin E [IgE], which is frequently involved in allergic reactions), or other components of the immune system, may be involved in the pathogenesis of migraines. To date, however, evidence for an IgE mechanism in food-induced migraine is doubtful, and too little work has been done with other immune mechanisms to implicate them in migraine causation (Pradalier & Launay, 1996).

Many migraine triggers and inhibitors have activities related to serotonin. Red wine, a common migraine trigger, has been shown to cause release of serotonin from platelets *in vitro* (Jarman, Glover, & Sandler, 1991). Many antimigraine drugs react with serotonin receptors, including sumatriptan, ergot derivatives, and methysergide. However, these drugs also show other relevant activities, such as vasoconstriction (Saxena & DenBoer, 1991). Giving serotonin intravenously abolishes migraine symptoms. Feverfew (*Chrysanthemum parthenium* Bernh., Family Asteraceae), an herb in the daisy family that is potentially useful in migraine prophylaxis (Ernst & Pittler, 2000; Pittler, Vogler, & Ernst, 2000), blocks release of serotonin from platelets in the laboratory. It also reduces platelet aggregation induced by serotonin in migraine patients who use it regularly. Feverfew also, however, blocks prostaglandin synthesis, another possible migraine-inhibiting mechanism (der Marderosian & Liberti, 1988). Ginger (*Zingiber officinale* Roscoe) is another botanical product reported useful in aborting migraine headaches in a case study; it also inhibits prostaglandin synthesis as well as thromboxane generation (Mustafa & Srivastava, 1990).

Exactly what serotonin does in the brain neurovascular system to cause migraines is not clear. Some theorize that migraine is a manifestation of serotonin deficiency in the brain, possibly caused by factors that trigger serotonin release from storage sites in platelets and other tissues, and consequent depletion. The depletion may cause vasodilation and the pain of migraine. The situation may, however, be more complex. Serotonin receptors also help to modulate release of plasma from brain blood vessels, which could cause inflammation in surrounding brain tissue (Moskowitz & Buzzi, 1991). Other substances, including prostaglandins, histamine, and hormones, also play a role in migraine symptoms, although their activities are even less well worked out than that of serotonin. How migraine trigger foods fit into the picture is not well understood, except that most of them have some vasoactive components.

METHODOLOGICAL ISSUES

Several important factors must be considered in any discussion of the relationships between what people consume and their symptoms. For example, Kohlenberg (1980) presented interesting and valuable arguments supporting the theory that an interaction or combination of substances causes migraine, rather than one substance alone. His idea was that multiple dietary substances and other risk factors such as stress can result in migraine symptoms in some persons. "Stress" includes a wide variety of environmental, psychological, and somatic factors. Olesen (1991), for instance, lists emotional upset, hormonal changes, fatigue, smoke, strong light, weather, and high altitudes as some of the nondietary physical stresses that may trigger migraines. Missed meals or erratic blood sugar may also trigger migraines (Egger, 1991). Martin and Seneviratne (1997), in an experimental context, studied food deprivation in combination with emotional stress. They noted that both food deprivation and stress caused headaches, but that there was no evidence for an interaction between the two. The combinations and interactions of these factors, as well as those of diet, vary significantly both within and between individuals. This makes it more difficult to determine what relationships are active in each case.

Furthermore, for some persons the circumstances surrounding the consumption of suspected substances may be as important as, or even more important than, the substances themselves. For example, people commonly consume many of the suspected foods and beverages in the evenings, on weekends, at parties, or at sports events. Examples of such foods are red wine, aged cheeses, sausages, chocolate, and hot dogs. Social activities and sporting events often involve additional sources of tension, arousal, and fatigue. These may lead to symptom onset via sympathetic arousal, general muscle tension, or both.

In addition, people are more likely to recall times when symptoms began soon after ingestion of specific foods and beverages. They are less likely to recall the times when symptoms did not occur or when they occurred several hours later. Once a person experiences symptoms soon after ingestion of specific foods or beverages, he or she may expect the symptoms the next time—regardless of whether the food or beverage actually has anything to do with symptom onset. This expectancy itself can increase the chance that symptoms will occur. Alternatively, an inconsistent or variable association can lead patients to believe mistakenly that there is no relationship between the dietary element and their symptoms.

The complex interactions among potential migraine triggers can manifest themselves in puzzling research results. Salfield et al. (1987), for instance, randomized a group of children with migraines to either a diet low in vasoactive amines or a high-fiber diet that served as a placebo. Both groups had significant reductions in headache, and headaches were reduced in the placebo and low-amine groups by the same amount. This could have been a result of placebo or nonspecific effects. It could also have resulted from a reduction in hypoglycemia by the high fiber content of the placebo diet, since fiber frequently stabilizes blood sugar levels. The higher fiber content may have assisted in natural detoxification mechanisms. The children on the high-fiber diet may also have previously eaten "junk food" high in other potential vasoactive substances, such as monosodium glutamate (MSG) and sodium nitrate, which were displaced by the high-fiber foods (Radnitz, 1990).

A further complication in determining the causes of migraine headaches is the time lag that often follows intake of migraine trigger foods. Gettis (1987a) described an excellent example of this in his case report of a male in his late 30s, a vegetarian who suffered from common migraines. Eventually the subject isolated three foods that triggered his headaches: bananas, citrus, and cheese (all of which are vasoactive via serotonin, dopamine, and tyramine; e.g., Riggin, McCarthy, & Kissinger, 1976). His detailed records and careful plan of food introduction also revealed that he had a delayed reaction to his trigger foods: His headaches occurred 48–72 hours following ingestion of the offending foods. Patients with migraine may fail to observe the relationship between specific foods and migraines because of such time lags, and may therefore assume that there is no connection between foods and their headaches.

Gettis (1987b) has discussed the importance of this meticulously documented time lag in research on food-related migraines. In the light of this phenomenon, many studies did not leave adequate time for the development of migraines after intake of the foods or compounds under study. Many appear to have assumed that migraines triggered by food or chemicals would appear within 24–48 hours. This assumption led investigators to administer test substances and placebos within 48 hours of each other. If some subjects are reacting to test substances after 48 hours, this would lead to headaches following placebo administration that were actually due to the test substance—explaining in part the high rate of reaction to placebo seen in many migraine studies (Radnitz, 1990). Gettis (1987b) also points out that some studies do not control the intake of other potentially migraine-causing foods by their subjects, and suggests that control of diet during the testing period could lead to more consistent results. Finally, subjects must eliminate all migraine-causing foods from their diets to give accurate results (Gettis, 1987a). If the subject described above had eliminated bananas, citrus, and cheese one at a time and reintroduced them before eliminating the other foods, he never would have been able to determine the causes of his headaches, since his diet would never have been free from his migraine trigger foods.

Finally, the possibility that the gelatin capsules used to administer experimental and placebo foods in tests of migraine triggers in a single- or double-blind research situation may themselves cause headaches has been raised. An investigator who suffers from food-induced migraines took gelatin capsules and other migraine triggers (e.g., tyramine) mixed with foods, or took the foods themselves without the experimental substances. He found that gelatin (a hydroyzed animal protein) was able to cause headaches in amounts as small as a single capsule (Strong, 2000). Use of gelatin capsules in experimental situations may thus erase significant differences between placebo and control groups, and impart to the food trigger concept less validity than it deserves.

THE ISSUE OF ALLERGY AND MIGRAINE

Speer (1977), a pediatric allergist, argued for an allergic etiology for many migraines. He discussed in detail many dietary and nondietary factors. The literature he referred to is mostly from the 19th and early 20th centuries and anecdotal in nature. Nevertheless, Speer's book contains some potentially useful information about dietary and nondietary factors that are worth keeping in mind.

There were no well-controlled studies showing that vascular headaches represented an allergic reaction until the ambitious study by Egger, Wilson, Carter, Turner, and Soothill (1983a). This study supported an allergic pathogenesis for migraines among many children aged 3–16. Children were put on a diet low in foods known to be commonly allergenic for 2 weeks. Of the 88 children who completed the diet, 78% reported full recovery from migraines. Forty of the children then underwent double-blind challenges at weekly intervals with allergenic foods. Of these 40, 39% reported migraines from cow's milk, 31% from wheat, 36% from eggs, and 17% from corn—all foods commonly found to be highly allergenic. Adverse reactions, however, were idiosyncratic for each child. Other commonly allergenic foods found to trigger migraines were orange, tomato, rye, fish, and soy. Some foods suspected to contain vasoactive substances also caused migraines, including chocolate, cheese, coffee, and malt (Egger, 1991). Podell (1984) provided an excellent summary of the study.

Identifying food sensitivities is not easy in clinical situations. Comprehensive dietary elimination-and-challenge procedures are often not practical, especially as one of the first evaluative and treatment approaches. Many professionals described the Egger et al. (1983a) study as a landmark. We need, however, to be careful not to overgeneralize or overinterpret the findings from even such a well-done study. We need replications and extensions of these findings with other samples of children and adults.

Letters to *Lancet* in response to this study noted questions and caveats (Cook & Joseph, 1983; Stephenson, 1983; Gerrard, 1983; Hearn & Finn, 1983; Peatfield, 1983; Feldman, 1983). Egger, Wilson, Carter, Turner, and Soothill (1983b) responded to some of the questions. There are several reasons for not easily extrapolating these findings to adults. The percentage of adults who are prone to atopic diseases is lower than that of children. There is no compelling theoretical basis explaining how the immune system mediates migraines. The children in this study (Egger et al., 1983a) had many other behavioral and somatic symptoms, creating some doubt about the representativeness of the sample. Egger (1991) argues that the effect of allergenic foods may be to increase gut permeability, allowing increased vasoactive substances in other foods to enter the circulation in greater quantities. Radnitz (1990) points out that the response to the diet could have been a placebo effect, especially since the trial period was only 2 weeks. Food allergies were not confirmed with more sophisticated tests, such as IgE or skin tests. Finally, childhood migraine responds well to a number of manipulations (including biofeedback), so that the response rate could represent a nonspecific effect.

Immune cell counts obtained from duodenal biopsies of patients with migraine who did or did not have food allergies were used in one study as a means of investigating migraine–allergy relationships. Proportions of cells containing IgA, IgM, IgE, and IgG were similar between the two groups, raising doubt about the IgE-mediated allergic mechanism for food migraines (Pradalier, de Saint Maur, Lamy, & Launay, 1994).

Other researchers, however, have argued for the validity of the food allergy hypothesis. Mansfield, Vaughn, Waller, Haverly, and Ting (1985) eliminated wheat, milk, corn, eggs, and other foods to which individuals had positive skin tests from the diets of selected adults. Of 16 subjects with positive skin tests, 11 experienced relief of migraines; of 27 who had negative skin tests, only 2 experienced relief. In a later paper, Mansfield (1990) argued for histamine-mediated causes of allergic migraines. Specialized immune cells in the gut, termed "mast cells," release histamine in the presence of allergenic foods. Histamine inhibits uptake of serotonin by brain cells, possibly leading to depletion of serotonin and consequent migraine. Intravenous infusions of histamine lead to throbbing headaches in normal individuals and patients with migraine; the latter usually develop pain first on the side that is clinically affected in migraine, and respond to lower doses of histamine than normal individuals.

Guariso et al. (1993)and colleagues tested children with migraine headaches using a low-antigen diet of eight simple foods. Of 12 children who completed the diet trial, 6 had complete remission of headache, and 5 had a significant improvement in migraine incidence. Children who were only followed with a food diary did not manifest such improvement (Guariso et al., 1993). Among the foods that were recognized as responsible for attacks were chocolate, banana, egg, and hazelnuts.

Giacovazzo and Martelletti (1989) tested 24 patients with food-triggered migraine who had a positive skin test or radioallergosorbent test (RAST—a sophisticated method of detecting allergies) to relevant foods. The foods identified as migraine triggers were eliminated from the diet, and dosing with sodium cromolyn begun (sodium cromolyn is a drug given prophylactically to block allergic responses). At the start of the trial, before drug dosing or diet, the trigger foods were tested to develop baseline headache index values for each food. After 1 and 2 months on the diet–drug trial, and 1 month after the trial was ended, foods were tested again. Headache index values fell during the first and second months, and rose again after the trial, although not to the baseline values.

Immune complexes are commonly formed in the blood after sensitive persons ingest allergenic foods. Sodium cromolyn inhibits histamine release from gut mast cells, which is triggered by the presence of immune complexes. Giacovazzo and Martelletti (1989) suggested that such inhibition blocks a sequence of events leading to release of serotonin from circulating platelets.

Weber and Vaughan (1991) reviewed several studies that correlated the release of allergic mediators (such as histamine) with migraine headaches, and then attempted to relate these reactions to skin test data. Migraines, they noted, have been reported to be associated with increases in histamine following exposure to known allergenic foods. For instance, in a patient with beef-induced migraine, beef ingestion tripled histamine levels preceding a migraine headache. Skin tests and RAST for beef were both negative. A study of five patients with food-induced migraines showed major increases in histamine levels following challenges with allergenic foods. The increased histamine levels were followed by migraine headaches. Skin tests for the allergenic foods, however, were negative.

Other investigators reporting evidence of headache relief after elimination of foods shown to be allergenic include Monro, Carini, Brostoff, and Zilkha (1980), Grant (1979), Radnitz and Blanchard (1991), Lucarelli et al. (1990), and Hughes, Gott, Weinstein, and Binggeli (1985). Egger, Carter, Soothill, and Wilson (1989) found that elimination of allergenic foods brought relief in epilepsy–migraine syndrome. Pradalier, Weinman, Launay, Baron, and Dry (1983) and Wilson, Kirker, Warnes, and O'Malley (1980), however, found no relation between food allergy and migraine. Some of the variability in results may arise because allergy-triggered migraines probably affect only a small (and unknown) percentage of migraine sufferers. There do, however, appear to be enough data to regard the food allergy–migraine hypothesis as one worth clinical consideration. Skin tests and RAST, however, may be of less value than food elimination and challenge in detecting allergy-related migraine trigger foods, as the studies reviewed by Weber and Vaughan (1991) suggest.

VASOACTIVE CONTENTS (NOT INCLUDING CAFFEINE) OF FOODS AND BEVERAGES

Aside from caffeine (discussed separately later), other vasoactive chemicals may trigger or increase the likelihood of migraine headaches. Commonly mentioned substances are tyramine, sodium nitrate, phenylethylamine, MSG, levodopa, alcohol, and the noncaloric sweetener aspartame. These substances are found in many foods and beverages, and may lead to migraine headaches in a variety of ways. The effectiveness of foods containing vasoactive substances in triggering migraine was shown by Lai, Dean, Zigler, and Hassanein (1988). Subjects who reported migraines associated with red wine, chocolate, and sharp cheddar cheese ate these foods for the study. Of the 38 subjects, 42% reported migraines after eating the offending foods in this situation.

Tyramine

Tyramine is the most commonly discussed vasoactive substance. Chemically, it is an amine (i.e., a breakdown product of an amino acid). Amines result when proteins are chemically altered by decarboxylation by enzymes during metabolism, or by bacterial contamination after death. The pressor amines are a group of amines that can stimulate the sympathetic nervous system. This group includes serotonin, tryptophan, histidine, and tyramine, the amine derivative of the amino acid tyrosine (interestingly, the Greek word *tyros*, from which "tyrosine" and "tyramine" are derived, means "cheese").

Health care professionals became aware of tyramine's vasoactive properties when investigators discovered its interaction with monoamine oxidase inhibitors (MAOIs), drugs used in the treatment of depression and hypertension. Serious adverse biochemical interactions (even death) have occurred when patients consume tyramine while taking these medications. Tyramine and other pressor amines are usually harmless, as they are detoxified in the liver and intestines. Monoamine oxidase mediates this oxidative mechanism. The MAOI drugs significantly interfere with detoxification, allowing large amounts of amines to reach the bloodstream, triggering hypertensive crises and migraine-like headaches.

The mechanism by which tyramine may trigger migraine headaches may be analogous to the activity of MAOI drugs. Some workers hypothesized that 5–10% of migraine sufferers have a genetic deficiency of monoamine oxidase activity, allowing excessive amounts of tyramine to reach the bloodstream. The vasoactive effect of this pressor amine may then cause a migraine headache (Gettis, 1987b).

Hanington (1980; Hanington, Horn, & Willkinson, 1969) and colleagues were the first to investigate the relationship of tyramine to migraine headaches. They gave patients with migraine capsules containing tyramine or placebo. Over the series of trials they conducted, headaches resulted after tyramine 80% of the time, and after placebo only 8% of the time (Radnitz, 1990). Several other research groups were unable to replicate these studies, possibly because tyramine sensitivity may affect only 5% of patients with migraine (or perhaps because of the use of gelatin capsules that themselves caused headaches). Relationships between tyramine-containing foods and headache can, however, be documented (as shown, e.g., in the case report by Gettis, 1987a). Tyramine sensitivity must therefore be considered clinically when one is treating migraines that appear to be food-related. Tyramine, however, is not the only vasoactive amine that may cause migraine headaches, although it receives the most attention because of its interaction with MAOI drugs. Other agents, such as the octopamine in citrus fruits, must also be considered.

Tyramine content varies significantly not only among foods, but even between samples of the same food. For example, in yogurt and sour cream, the manufacturing process and contamination may or may not result in vasopressor amines (see *Nutrition Reviews*, 1965, cited in McCabe & Tsuang, 1982). For instance, Horowitz, Lovenberg, Engelman, and Sjoerdsma (1964) found no detectable tyramine in the yogurt they analyzed. One should instruct persons with tyramine-related migraines that if they eat dairy foods, they should consume only fresh products manufactured by a reputable source and stored appropriately. Some such individuals may then tolerate moderate servings of yogurt and sour cream, even though they commonly contain small amounts of tyramine.

Tyramine usually increases with the aging process in cheeses. However, cheese with an aged and mature appearance does not always contain more tyramine than pale, mild-flavored cheese (McCabe & Tsuang, 1982). Although increased maturation times usually increase tyramine level, other factors also affect it. Such factors include types of microorganisms or decarboxylating enzyme levels. Thus a short-maturation cheese, such as Camembert, can contain high levels of tyramine. Likewise, a long-maturation cheese can contain low amounts of tyramine if there is lower decarboxylation or if other enzymes transform the tyramine. Moreover, the bacteriological quality of the milk is a major factor affecting the final concentration of tyramine (Antila, Antila, Mattila, & Hakkarainen, 1984).

Furthermore, cheese closer to the rind of a block can contain much more tyramine than samples from the center of the block (Price & Smith, 1971). They reported a difference in tyramine concentration from 11 to 1184 micrograms per gram with distances of 7 to 0 centimeters from the rind of several pieces of Gruyère cheese. Most tyramine was close to the rind—about 3 centimeters or less. Concentrations near the rind varied widely nearer the rind (e.g., 250 to 1184) among the samples, but the gradients of distance were similar.

Sen (1969) suggested that tyramine content of fish may be the result of bacterial contamination. Meat can also undergo such contamination. There are reports, for example, of hypertensive crises among persons taking MAOIs who consumed ground beef 3 days after cooking it. Problems have resulted from eating tuna fish 2 days after opening the can or eating beef liver stored for 1 week before preparation (Boulton, Cookson, & Paulton, 1970; Lovenberg, 1973). Any food with much protein has the potential of undergoing degradation from tyrosine to tyramine if contaminated and consumed after storage of a few to several days. The implication is that one should instruct patients to avoid leftover foods and potentially spoiled foods.

Bananas are often in lists of food for patients with migraines to avoid or reduce. Although there are several amines in banana peels that could produce pressor activity, the banana pulp contains smaller concentrations of the amines. Dopamine levels of 22–48 micrograms per gram for fruit pulp and 210–720 micrograms per gram for fruit peel, for instance, have been reported (Riggin et al., 1976). Banana peels also contain much more tyramine than banana pulp (see Table 9.1). One published report of a hypertensive crisis associated with bananas was that of a patient who consumed whole green bananas stewed in their skins (Blackwell & Taylor, 1969). The case report by Gettis (1987a) shows that some patients with migraine do react to bananas. Perhaps the cumulative effect of the several amines in combination with other amine-containing foods was the problem in this subject, who ate two to three servings of bananas, citrus, and cheese daily. Some lists discourage eating significant quantities of other fruits such as oranges, which have small tyramine concentrations but may contain other potentially problematic amines.

Yeast extracts are also commonly on the lists in question. Published reports from the British literature have referred to brands that do contain very large concentrations of

TABLE 9.1. Tyramine-Containing Foods, Beverages, and Condiments, and Tyramine Concentrations (in Micrograms per Gram or Micrograms per Milliliter, Unless Otherwise Noted)[a]

Cheeses

Cheddar (Highest: old, center-cut Canadian and New York State, approx. 1500; Canadian aged in ale, approx. 1000) (Others: English, up to 953; New Zealand, 471–580; Australian, 226; other Canadian, most 120–192)

Gruyère (American, 516; British, 11–1184; Finland, 102)

Stilton (American, 466; English, 2170)

Emmenthal (225); Emmentaler (225–1000)

Brie (American, 180; Danish, nil)

Camembert (American, 86; Danish, 23–1340; Mycella [Camembert type], 1304; Cuban, 34–425)

Roquefort (French, 27–520)

Blue (Danish, 31–256; French, 203; Bourmandise [blue type], 216)

Boursault (French, 1116)

Parmesan (Italian, 65; American, 4–290)

Processed (American, 50; Canadian, 26)

Romano (Italian, 238)

Provolone (Italian, 38)

Cracker Barrel (Kraft brand, American, 214)

Brick (natural Canadian, 524)

Mozzarella (Canadian, 410)

Gouda (Canadian, 20; Cuban, 40–280)

Cream cheese and cottage cheese (nil except South African cottage, 6.6)

Cuban (Fontina, 54–167; Broodkaase, 0–163; Dambom, 26–100; Carré, 52–200)

Spanish (Mahon old, 369; Cáceres cured, 225; Cáceres, 102; Malaga fresh, 22)

Dry/fermented sausage

Salami (hard, average 210, up to 392; farmer, average 314; Genoa, average 534, up to 1237)

Sausage (summer, up to 184; dry, up to 244; semidry, up to 85.5)

Others (pepperoni, average, up to 195; smoked landjaeger, up to 396; dry fermented, 102–1506)

Others

Herring (Marinated [pickled], 3030; Canadian, 470)

Caviar (estimated high, but no published analysis found)

Sour cream, yogurt (variable but often nil, especially from reputable brands)

Chicken liver (cooked, not kept refrigerated, 94–113; fresh cooked, nil)

Beef liver (fresh or frozen, approx. 5)

Raspberries, fresh (13–92)

Yeast products (English: unspecified brand, 2100; Marmite, 1087–1639; Yex, 506; Befit, 419; Barmene, 152; Yeastrel, 101) (Canadian: unspecified brand, 66–84; plain, nil)

Bananas (peel, 63–65; pulp, 7)

Soya beans (fermented, Singapore, 713 [50 q]; Taiwan, 878 [10 ml]; Swiss soya sauce, Dr. Dunners, 293 [10 ml], Formosa soya bean condiment, 939 [20 g]; Korea soya bean paste fermented, 206 [50 g][b]

Red wine (highly variable, some nil)

Note. See Block and Schwartz, 1995, Table 10.1, for many other foods and beverages, most of which have very small amounts of tyramine. All tyramine < 1 mg/portion unless specified. Portions of most meat/vegetables, 50–75 g (1.8–2.6 oz.).

[a]Normal portions of cheese are variable. As a guide, Vidaud, Chaviano, Gonzales, and Garcia Roche (1987) note that a normal portion of Camembert cheese is about 23 g (0.8 oz., avoirdupois) and of Gouda is about 30 g (1.06 oz.).

The data on concentrations are from the following sources: Maxwell (1980), reporting the concentrations as reported by Horowitz, Lovenberg, Engelman, and Sjoerdsma (1964), McCabe (1986), Sen (1969), Boulton, Cookson, and Paulten (1970), Coffin (1970), Hedberg, Gordon, and Glueck (1966), Marley and Blackwell (1970), Orlosky (1982), Udenfriend, Lovenberg, and Sjoerdsma (1959); Cuban and Spanish data from Vidaud, Chaviano, Gonzales, and Garcia Roche (1987); Rice, Eitenmiller, and Kohler (1975, 1976); Rice and Kohler (1976), Rivas-Gonzalo, Santos-Hernandez and Marine-Font (1983); cited by McCabe, 1986).

Vidaud et al. (1987) reviewed eight studies with ranges of 13–2000 milligrams per kilogram. All but one study (Asatoor, Levi, & Milne, 1963) reported average tyramine content of less than 211.

[b]The amounts given here are those consumed in a normal serving.

tyramine. Brewer's yeast in pill or liquid form does contain significant concentrations of tyramine; this is found in health food and drug stores as a vitamin supplement. Although reports about plain yeast-leavened bakery products show negligible tyramine concentrations, some headache clinics recommend that patients with food-related migraine avoid hot, fresh homemade bread.

Levodopa or dopamine, another pressor amine, is found in fava beans in significant amounts (Hodge, Nye, & Emerson, 1964). Fava beans or broad beans, often marketed as "Italian" green beans, are much wider (more than ½ inch) than common green beans.

Many foods and beverages contain tyramine and other vasoactive amines, and these frequently appear on lists of foods for patients with dietary migraine to avoid. One finds differences among lists by different sources, although most such lists are quite similar. The concentrations of vasoactive substances vary significantly among listed foods and beverages. However, most lists treat items as about equal and do not refer to the wide variations in concentrations. A major reason for the absence of such information in most lists is that it is difficult to obtain. There are many factors that result in differences, even for the same food or beverage. The information available about concentrations is important; this is especially true if we assume the importance of the interaction or additive effects among factors. Selected tyramine concentrations for many foods are given in Table 9.1. We have added information about the published tyramine concentrations of many items. This provides readers with a sense of the wide variations among items even within the same food group. The implication is that the items are not necessarily of equivalent potential in causing or increasing the likelihood of migraines or contributing to other problems (e.g., negative interactions such as hypertensive crisis with MAOI antidepressants).

Phenylethylamine

Phenylethylamine is a compound found in chocolate and in red and white wines (Ibe et al., 1991) that may be a cause of diet-related migraines. It is similar in chemical structure to epinephrine, norepinephrine, dopamine, ephedrine, amphetamine, tyramine, and numerous other sympathomimetic drugs with vasoconstrictor and pressor activities. All these compounds, in fact, share a basic chemical structure (Gilman, Rall, Nies, & Taylor, 1990).

Chocolate has been reported clinically to trigger migraines. Sandler, Youdim, and Hanington (1974) gave phenylethylamine capsules to 36 patients who reported migraines after eating chocolate, and found that phenylethylamine triggered three times as many headaches as placebo capsules. Other workers attempted to trigger migraines using chocolate in placebo-controlled studies but did not duplicate these results, perhaps because of insufficiently high dosages of phenylethylamine (Dalessio, 1980; Moffet, Swash, & Scott, 1974). Gibb et al. (1991), however, challenged 12 patients with chocolate and a closely matched placebo in a double-blind, parallel-group study. Chocolate was followed by migraine in 5 of the 12 patients who received chocolate and none of the 8 patients who received placebo. On the other hand, Marcus, Scharff, Turk, and Gourley (1997) reported that chocolate was not more likely to trigger headaches than carob in a group of patients with migraine, tension, and combined headaches. The relationship between chocolate and migraine was not apparent in subjects who reported sensitivity to chocolate (Marcus et al., 1997). The variability in results might, of course, have been due to differences in processing of chocolate used by different experimenters, although Marcus and colleagues used a chocolate preparation that had previously caused migraines in another study. It should be noted that octopamine, another potentially bioactive amine, has been isolated from chocolate beans (Kenyhercz & Kissinger, 1978).

Monosodium Glutamate

The reality of the "Chinese restaurant syndrome" is still under challenge (Radnitz, 1990; Geha et al., 2000). Some of the difficulty certain researchers have found in documenting the syndrome may be due to different dosages of MSG employed. Variability may also arise from the amounts of background dietary intake of MSG, which is almost ubiquitous in processed foods. It is possible that other substances than MSG, such as histamine, may cause headaches in persons complaining of this syndrome (Chin, Garriga, & Metcalfe, 1989).

This syndrome is characterized by facial tightness, sweating, and a throbbing headache. Most of the work validating the syndrome was done in healthy subjects, but more recent double-blind tests have used subjects claiming sensitivity to MSG (Geha et al., 2000). It is not certain that MSG is a specific trigger for migraine headaches. Neverthless, Scopp (1991) presents a case study of a patient who came close to eliminating her migraine headaches, plus a constant muscle contraction headache, by removing MSG from her diet. Merritt and Williams (1990) have investigated the effect of MSG on rabbit aorta, and indicated a possible mechanism by which MSG may trigger migraines in sensitive subjects. Solutions of MSG were applied to strips of rabbit aorta. MSG or glutamine was observed to cause contraction of the blood vessels when applied at high concentrations. It also relaxed contractions induced by serotonin, norepinephrine, prostaglandin, and histamine, and subsequently contracted the vessels. Tyramine potentiated the effects of glutamine by over 200%. Although the concentrations used were high, Merritt and Williams (1990) stated that they can occur in humans. These experiments show a clear vasoactive potential for this substance.

Eliminating MSG from the diet is not an easy task within the context of contemporary American eating habits. The substance appears in nearly all processed foods (under a variety of names; see below). The fact that from 3 to 5 grams of MSG may now be present in a typical American meal takes MSG effects out of the Chinese restaurant and into the culture at large; this figure is similar to amounts that have been used experimentally.

MSG—the sodium salt of glutamine, a naturally occurring amino acid—is typically made from hydrolyzed plant proteins. It is used to impart a fresh or savory flavor to processed foods, and is widely used as a flavor enhancer in Asian cooking. MSG typically constitutes 10–30% of such hydrolyzed plant proteins. After 1986, the U.S. Food and Drug Administration permitted the food industry to drop the name "MSG" from flavor enhancers containing glutamine. MSG is thus now known under a variety of names, including "hydrolyzed vegetable protein," "natural flavor," "flavoring," and "kombu extract." Table 9.2 shows a variety of foods and food components containing MSG. Amounts of MSG are not listed specifically in most cases, as this information is industrially sensitive and varies widely with the processor.

Other Substances

"Hot dog headache" may be a reaction to sodium nitrate and ingestion of nitrite, by persons sensitive to it, also can result in headaches. Henderson and Raskin (1972) gave 10 milligrams of sodium nitrate or placebo to one patient with migraine. Headache occurred in 8 of 13 trials of sodium nitrate, and no headaches occurred after placebo. Ten healthy volunteers had no headaches after nitrate or placebo. Amyl nitrite, formerly used in treatment of angina, often caused vascular headaches, possibly because of vasodilator action. Nitrites used in the munitions industry cause headaches in some individuals (Diamond, Prager, & Freitag, 1986).

Headaches followed ice cream ingestion in 31% of 49 subjects without migraine, and 93% of 59 patients with migraine, in one experiment. This phenomenon may result from the sudden cooling of the oral pharynx. It represents an excessive vasomotor reaction to cold,

TABLE 9.2. Possible Migraine-Inducing Dietary Factors: Monosodium Glutamate (MSG)

Food ingredients containing MSG

Autolyzed yeast
Calcium caseinate
Hydrolyzed oat flour
Hydrolyzed protein
Hydrolyzed vegetable protein (HVP)
Hydrolyzed plant protein
Kombu extract
Sodium caseinate
Textured protein
Yeast extract
Yeast food

Food ingredients usually containing MSG

Barley malt
Bouillon
Malt extract
Malt flavoring
Natural flavoring
Natural beef flavoring
Natural chicken flavoring

Food products usually containing MSG or HVP

Beef bouillon cubes	40–46% HVP
Poultry bouillon cubes	30–50% HVP
Canned cream soups	0.25–0.6% HVP
Canned beef broths	0.5–2.0% HVP
Canned gravies	0.5–2.0% HVP
Dehydrated soups	
Meat type (oxtail, kidney)	15–25% HVP in dry product
Poultry type	5–10% HVP in dry product
Vegetable (mixed vegetable, pea)	3–10% HVP in dry product
English sausage	0.15–0.35% HVP
Frozen dinner entrees	
Gravy powders	20–40% HVP in dry product
International foods	
Liver sausage	0.25–0.5% HVP
Luncheon meats	0.25–0.5%HVP
Most diet foods and weight loss powders	
Most sauces in jars and cans (e.g., tomato and barbecue)	
Most salad dressings and mayonnaises	
Potato chips and prepared snacks	
Prepared beef products (e.g., beef stews, beefburgers,	
hot pot, hashes etc.)	0.5–1.0% HVP

Note. The data are from Scopp (1991) and the National Organization Mobilized to Stop Glutamate (NoMSG; 1992).

and could be a manifestation of the erratic vasomotor regulation common in patients with migraine (Diamond et al., 1986).

Alcohol is a known vasodilator, and may trigger headaches or worsen existing ones. Certain types of alcoholic drinks contain other vasoactive substances as well; for instance, red wine is a well-known migraine trigger with serotonin-releasing properties (Jarman et al., 1991). Littlewood et al. (1988), for instance, compared red wine and vodka, and found that red wine triggered headaches in 11 patients with dietary migraine, while vodka did not. The migraine-triggering activity of red wine has sometimes been attributed to phenolic flavonoids, which may result in increased catecholamine concentrations by inhibiting catechol-O-methyltransferase. This hypothesis has not been thoroughly examined (Radnitz, 1990).

The artificial sweetener aspartame may cause headaches in some people. Lipton, Newman, Cohen, and Solomon (1989) queried 171 patients with headache about whether aspartame, alcohol (a positive control), and carbohydrates (a negative control) caused headaches. Nearly 50% reported headaches caused by alcohol, 8% by aspartame, and 2% by carbohydrates. Patients with migraine were significantly more likely to report alcohol, and three times more likely to report aspartame, as headache triggers than were patients without migraine. Koehler and Glaros (1988) studied 25 subjects with migraine in a double-blind, placebo-controlled trial, in which 300 milligrams per day of aspartame or placebo were given for 4 weeks, separated by a week-long washout period. Significantly more headaches occurred during the aspartame period than during the baseline or placebo periods.

Harrison (1986) suggests that copper may be a unifying factor in several migraine-related foods. These foods either contain large amounts of copper or increase its absorption into the body. Chocolate, glutamate, nuts, shellfish, whiskey, wheat germ, and citrate are examples of copper-containing or copper-transporting foods. Histamine, produced in allergic reactions, may also transport copper ions into the bloodstream. The mechanism by which copper might trigger migraines could be through a defect in a copper-containing enzyme, ceruloplasmin. The enzyme defect may reduce inactivation of vasoactive amines such as serotonin and tyramine. Table 9.3 summarizes the other possible migraine-inducing foods discussed here.

CAFFEINE

Status of Effects on Health and Disease

Caffeine is the focus of considerable attention by health care professionals and the public. One major concern here is that caffeine, as a psychotropic stimulant, elicits or aggravates physiological symptoms associated with several disorders—including migraine headaches, anxiety, Raynaud's disease, IBS, hypertension, premenstrual syndrome, and sleep-onset insomnia. Caffeine use is inconsistent with the overall goals of reducing sympathetic arousal (Hibino, Moritani, Kawada, & Fushiki, 1997) and general muscle tension. Furthermore, in-

TABLE 9.3. Possible Migraine-Inducing Dietary Factors: Other Items

Item	Substance contained or action in the body
Alcohol	Nonspecific vasodilator
Chocolate	Phenylethylamine
Hot dogs	Nitrate
Ice Cream	Cooling of oral pharynx

take of caffeine-containing beverages may be associated with the development of hot flashes in perimenopausal women (Lucero & McCloskey, 1997). Reduction of caffeine is one part of therapy for urinary incontinence (Arya, Myers, & Jackson, 2000; Iqbal & Castleden, 1997). The effects of withdrawal, however, constitute another cause for concern.

Action, Metabolism, and Toxicity

Caffeine is a bitter-tasting crystalline substance and the world's most popular drug (James, 1997). In North America, an average person's consumption is estimated at about 200 milligrams a day (Griffiths et al., 1990; Barone & Roberts, 1996), with an estimated 85% of Americans consuming caffeine. In usual doses, caffeine stimulates the central nervous system. The effects vary from pleasant stimulation and alertness to unpleasant stimulation and tension. Caffeine can reduce fatigue by increasing skeletal muscle contractions. Higher doses can stimulate breathing and increase heart rate.

Caffeine causes vasoconstriction in cerebral circulation. This effect helps explain its presumed efficacy in relieving some headaches (i.e., reducing cerebral vasodilation from other sources). Presumably, the timing of the ingestion of caffeine can be important for the latter. At other times, one would not seek to constrict cerebral blood vessels.

Caffeine spreads rapidly through the body, where body tissues and fluids quickly absorb it. About 90% metabolizes in the liver, and people excrete the rest unchanged in the urine. Individuals differ in sensitivity and tolerance to caffeine. It reaches all tissues of the body within about 5 minutes. Peak plasma levels vary widely and range from 15 minutes to as long as 2 hours, with one report of 20–30 minutes (Kalow, 1985).

Half-life estimates also vary, with some estimates from about 1.5 hours to as long as 7.5 hours; they are reported as 3–6 hours by Kalow (1985). The average is about 3–4 hours (Curatolo & Robertson, 1983; Gilbert, 1981). Some variation results from individual differences, tolerance, smoking, and a person's usual consumption of caffeine. For example, people who smoke metabolize caffeine more rapidly than those who do not smoke (Gilbert, 1981). There is no day-to-day accumulation of caffeine in the body.

Caffeine metabolism appears to be related to dosage (Denaro, Brown, Wilson, Jacob, & Benowitz, 1990). Denaro et al. observed disproportionate increases in blood levels with increasing daily doses, which may be a factor adding to the observed adverse effects seen among persons consuming higher levels. The dosage-dependent relationship occurred even in low-dose conditions, with doses only moderately higher than the average consumption of adults.

Toxicity occurs at about 1 gram. A lethal dose in adults requires 5–10 grams orally. For drip coffee, such a dose would require 34 to 68 five-ounce cups. Toxicity, however, could occur with 7–14 cups drunk in a very short period. For highly caffeinated carbonated beverages, a lethal dose requires 77–150 twelve-ounce cans. It is unlikely and uncommon for a toxic or lethal dose to occur. Caffeine is nevertheless a potent chemical that can have harmful effects.

Caffeine Effects

Headaches

The role of caffeine in migraine headaches is not precisely defined (Radnitz, 1990). Caffeine may cause migraines because of its actions on cerebral veins. Consuming caffeine causes vasoconstriction: It can thus be useful in stopping headaches. This vasoconstriction, however, is later followed by a rebound vasodilation, which may cause headache. Matthew and Wilson (1985) studied cerebral blood flow changes induced by caffeine. Increased cerebral blood flow is correlated with migraine headaches. They found that caffeine intake in a group of caffeine users with high daily intake was immediately followed by a decrease in cerebral blood flow.

For episodic tension-type headache, "caffeine-containing analgesics were significantly superior both to placebo and to 1000 mg acetaminophen, and . . . acetaminophen was significantly superior to placebo. The significant analgesic adjuvant effect of caffeine was independent of patients' usual caffeine use or their caffeine consumption in the 4 hours before medication" (Migliardi, Armellino, Friedman, Gillings, & Beaver, 1994, p. 576). Thus there is "good evidence that the adjuvant effect of caffeine cannot be attributed to relieving caffeine withdrawal headache" (Migliardi et al., 1994, p. 585). These conclusions were based on six randomized, double-blind, two-period crossover studies involving over 2500 patients. However, the data also indicate that the improvement from placebo appears to account for most of the improvement, and the side effects (such as nervousness and dizziness) were greater with caffeine included than without it. In a study of chronic daily headaches (Spierings, Schroevers, Honkoop, & Sorbi, 1998), caffeine was not supported as a significant factor.

Anxiety, High Blood Pressure, Insomnia, and Other Conditions

Several reports support the effect of caffeine on anxiety (Bruce & Lader, 1989; Bruce, 1990; Bruce, Scott, Shine, & Lader, 1992). In an uncontrolled series, 24 patients diagnosed with generalized anxiety disorder or panic disorder withdrew from caffeine. Six of these patients showed significant reductions of anxiety symptoms with only caffeine abstention, and remained improved for at least 6 months. Not all reports support the relationship between caffeine and anxiety among anxiety patients (Matthew & Wilson, 1990), although those reports were based on dosages of 250 milligrams. There is another report of anxiety induced by similarly low doses of caffeine (Griffiths et al., 1990).

Caffeine's impact on other conditions commonly treated with applied psychophysiology may be substantial. A syndrome termed "caffeinism," which is difficult to differentiate from anxiety attacks, is brought on by excess caffeine consumption. Some evidence has been adduced that people with panic disorder have unusual sensitivity to caffeine. Because of increased heart rate and force of contraction, caffeine may potentiate cardiovascular responses to stress. Caffeine stimulates gastric secretion and may cause chronic stomach pain. It may also aggravate IBS and ulcers (Sargent & Solbach, 1988).

Caffeine doses of 250 to 500 milligrams can raise systolic and diastolic blood pressure significantly by a few to several millimeters of mercury (Lane, Adcock, Williams, & Kuhn, 1990; Lane, 1997; Lane, Phillips-Bute, & Pieper, 1998) independent of posture, activity, or perceived stress. Implications include interpreting blood pressure collected during caffeine-deprived conditions.

Caffeine has long been thought to improve alertness, improve mood, and enhance psychomotor and cognitive performance on such tasks as tapping speed, simple reaction time (SRT), sustained attention, memory and logical reasoning, and simulated driving (Rogers & Dernoncourt, 1998, cited in Robelin & Rogers, 1998). Placebo-controlled studies have provided support for this hypothesis, but have added a note of caution. A review by Pritchard, Robinson, deBethizy, Davis, and Stiles (1995) concluded that "caffeine enhances overall performance . . . [of] . . . relatively simple tasks requiring speeded responding or moderately complex tasks that have been practiced," but that "for very complex tasks and moderately complex but unpracticed tasks, caffeine appears to either have no effect or may actually impair performance" (p. 20). This review also found "no interactive effects . . . between caffeine and smoking for any measure" (p. 25) (rapid visual information-processing task). There was increased muscle tension and a trend toward increased anxiety due to the caffeine.

However, testing was after caffeine deprivation, usually overnight. Thus it was not known confidently whether the beneficial effects were from caffeine or in contrast to the deleterious effects after deprivation. In a dose–response study by Robelin and Rogers (1998), mood and SRT performance improved by the same degree for three different spaced doses of 86, 172, and 258 milligrams, the second administered 75 minutes after the first and then the third given 150 minutes after the second with placebo-controlled groups; thus a flat dose–response relationship was observed. This suggests that there is "little net benefit to be gained from frequent caffeine use" (Robelin & Rogers, 1998, p. 611). The smallest dose is less than one small cup of coffee and less than two cans of most sodas.

In a retrospective chart review, there were no significant effects of three levels of caffeine intake on global experience and disability from chronic low back pain. The three levels were less than 100, 100–400, and more than 400 milligrams per day (Currie, Wilson, & Gauthier, 1995).

Stimulation of colonic motor activity by caffeine has received support from Rao, Welcher, Zimmerman, and Stumbo (1998). The degree of stimulation is similar to that caused by a meal, and stronger than that caused by warm water or decaffeinated coffee.

For sleep-onset insomnia, persons age 65 and older should avoid caffeine (Brown et al., 1995). This is based on a large in-person survey comparing 155 (5.4% of 2885) persons surveyed about their use of caffeine-containing medications, typically over-the-counter (OTC) analgesics. There were methodological limitations—primarily unspecified period of time for the sleep problems, unknown diseases or other drugs that might interfere with sleep, and unknown amount of caffeine-containing medications and timing of use. However, after adjustment for factors that add to trouble starting sleep, caffeine in the medications increased the risk by about 60%. Brown et al. (1995) conclude that persons in this age range should avoid caffeine if possible.

Some reports (Rossignol, 1985; Rossignol & Bonnlander, 1990) support the relationship between premenstrual symptoms and caffeine consumption, with a dose–response relationship not explained by total fluid intake. This relationship was clearer for those women with more severe symptoms. Methodological factors limit definitive conclusions. However, the clinical implication is for women with these symptoms to stop consuming caffeine for at least several months before and with other treatments.

Reduction of caffeine is reported in a follow-up questionnaire as helpful in diminishing symptoms of urinary incontinence in older women with stress incontinence, those with detrusor muscle overactivity, and those with mixed incontinence (Weinberger, Goodman, & Carnes, 1999). Arya et al. (2000), in a case–control study, found that women consuming a mean of about 500 milligrams per day of caffeine were more likely than women consuming a mean of about 200 milligrams per day, or an amount about midway between these amounts, to have detrusor muscle instability.

Caffeine Contents of Beverages and Foods

Estimates of the caffeine content in coffees vary significantly. This depends upon the strain of coffee bean and the condition of the beans (whether they are green or roasted). It also depends on the type of coffee (e.g., drip, instant). Brewing time also affects caffeine content. There are several studies of the caffeine content of coffees and other beverages. Table 9.4 provides estimates of caffeine content for selected beverages. See Barone and Roberts (1996) for an extensive review, list of references, and summaries of contents. See also the Internet web sites of the Mayo Clinic and the Center for Science in the Public Interest for additional information.

Longer percolation of coffee (e.g., 10 minutes vs. 5 minutes) usually increases caffeine by about 4–15 milligrams per 150 milliliters. In general, the ratio of ground coffee to water is about 71–78 grams to 48 ounces of water.

TABLE 9.4. Caffeine Contents[a]

Beverage	Estimated[b] milligrams per 1 ounce
Coffee	
Drip	8–25 mg, use estimate = 20
Instant	4–15, use estimate = 10
Flavored from mixes	3–13, mostly 6–11
Espresso	50–67 mg, use estimate = 50
Tea (black more than green, instant, and premixed)	3–17 mg
Carbonated beverages:	
Most colas	2–6 mg, mostly 3–4
Jolt, Mountain Dew, Mellow Yellow, Mr. Pibb	4.4–4.75 mg
AfriCola	8
Barols-Guarana (Brazil)	6.7
Frozen desserts (with coffee)	1–11 (mostly 5–8)
Chocolate (e.g., semisweet, sweet dark, special dark)	3–8
Chocolate bars	7–21 per 1.2–1.5 oz
Coffee nips	3 per piece
Guarana[c] "Magic Power"	25 per capsule

[a]Selected and summarized. See original references (journals, books, and Internet sites) for extensive lists (Pennington & Church, 1985, 1998; Barone & Roberts, 1996).
[b]Rough and rounded generously for ease of calculation.
[c]Common in Germany; 15 ml alcohol with 5 g guarana seeds; capsules with 500 mg guarana seeds.

A small chocolate bar contains about 25 milligrams of caffeine. Soft drinks contain between 33 and 65 milligrams of caffeine. Consider the example of a child weighing about 27 kilograms (59–60 pounds) who ingests three caffeinated soft drinks and three small chocolate bars. This is about 7.2 milligrams per kilogram and is the equivalent of about eight cups of instant coffee for a 174-pound (79-kilogram) adult.

A practitioner need not know the exact amount of caffeine in a specific patient's coffee. It does not pay to invest expensive professional time exploring the strain of coffee beans and brewing time used by the patient. One can estimate the caffeine intake from coffee from the general type (e.g., instant, drip) and the number of ounces drunk. One should also inquire about the size of the cup used, as most people use the term "cup" when they are actually drinking from larger-sized mugs. A mug can vary from about 5 to 12 ounces or even more.

The value of using questionnaires to estimate patterns of caffeine consumption received qualified support from James, Bruce, Lader, and Scott (1989). Self-report and saliva assays were significantly but modestly correlated. However, a practitioner must be cautious about relying entirely on questionnaire sources. Careful clinical interviewing and attempts at precise daily record keeping may be necessary if one needs accuracy.

Caffeine Withdrawal

Regular use of as little as 100 milligrams of caffeine per day can induce a form of physical dependence, interruption of which elicits characteristic withdrawal symptoms in some people

(Griffiths et al., 1990). Until recently, the most conspicuous feature of caffeine withdrawal was noted to be a severe headache, relieved by consuming more caffeine (Greden, Victor, Fontaine, & Lubetsky, 1980). Fennelly, Galletly, and Purdie (1991) reported that "headache after general anesthesia is related to preoperative caffeine withdrawal consequent upon moderate daily levels of caffeine intake" (p. 453). Among 287 patients, they found "a highly significant difference in caffeine consumption" between patients with and without headache (p. 449). The more caffeine, the greater the probability of headaches developing both preoperatively and postoperatively. Increases of 100 milligrams resulted in 12% and 16% increases in headaches, respectively. Other articles support this relationship between caffeine withdrawal and postoperative headache (Weber, Ereth, Danielson, & Ilstrup, 1993; Harper, 1993).

The importance and implications of the studies by Griffiths and his colleagues (Griffiths et al., 1990; Silverman & Griffiths, 1992; Mumford et al., 1994) provide strong support for the presence of more types of withdrawal symptoms and a higher incidence of symptoms. People can discriminate low doses of caffeine (below 20 milligrams). These researchers' data support "an orderly, time-limited caffeine withdrawal syndrome after abstinence from low dietary doses of caffeine" (Griffiths et al., 1990, p. 1129). They also report their findings as "the first evidence that caffeine withdrawal produces craving for caffeine-containing foods" (p. 1130).

Readers should examine this group's reports, especially that of Griffiths et al. (1990), which is the most convincing study in the series. Although it was based only on seven subjects, the methodology and results are impressive. One phase was a simple ABA (baseline–treatment–baseline), double-blind design with "exposure to 100 mg/day of caffeine for 9 to 14 days, substitution of placebo for 12 days and . . . re-exposure to 100 mg/day of caffeine for 7 to 12 days" (p. 1125). The subjects knew there would be one or more times when caffeine would start and restart, but did not know the number or durations. They ingested 10 capsules of 10 milligrams each at hourly intervals from about 8:00 A.M. to 5:00 P.M., and rated 33 dimensions of mood and behavior four times each day. Four of the seven subjects showed strong evidence of withdrawal, peaking on either the first or second day and decreasing progressively over about 1 week.

Before the next phase, the investigators reviewed the data from all the subjects. Then they repeatedly substituted placebo for a series of five "1-day periods separated by an average of 9 days" and 15–19 days with caffeine. The subjects again did not know when they ingested placebo. All subjects showed withdrawal effects.

In the first phase, the subjects reported the following:

> a significant decrease in ratings of alert/attentive/observant, well being, social disposition, motivation for work, able to concentrate, energy/active, self-confidence, urge to do task/work-related activities and content/satisfied, and a significant increase in ratings of headache, irritable/cross/grumpy, depressed, muscle pain or stiffness, lethargy/fatigue/tired/sluggish, cerebral fullness, craving for caffeine-containing foods . . . and flu-like feelings. (Griffiths et al., 1990, p. 1127)

The strong withdrawal effects might be the result of the relatively long abstinence (39 hours in Phase II), the repeated withdrawal testing of each subject, multiple symptoms, and "subjects who were conscientious about avoiding all dietary sources of caffeine and in whom caffeine abstinence was verified biologically" (p. 1131). Note that some withdrawal effects did not peak until 27 hours after caffeine was stopped. The important points are that it requires very little daily use of caffeine to create physical dependence and withdrawal symptoms, and that there are probably many more withdrawal symptoms than headaches. (Table 9.5 lists selected symptoms.)

Another study (Van Dusseldorp & Katan, 1990) supported the high frequency of caffeine withdrawal headaches in 19 of their 45 recruited subjects in their double-blind study of

TABLE 9.5. Selected Caffeine Withdrawal Symptoms

Increased:

Headache[a,b]

Heart rate

Sleep onset problems

Nausea

Analgesic use

Dysphoria

Flu-like feelings

Cerebral blood flow volume

EEG theta (primarily in back of head)

Tiredness and fatigue (lessening over 7+ days)

Vigilance in visual monitoring (slowed response speed)[c]

Decreased:

Motor activity

Wakefulness

Alertness

Upset stomach

Well-being

Pulse

Note. Caffeine withdrawal symptoms often begin 12–24 hours after caffeine cessation and reach maximum intensity after 20–48 hours. Gradual withdrawal results in minimial, if any, withdrawal symptoms.

The data are from the following sources: Hofer and Battig (1994); Richardson, Rogers, Elliman, and O'Dell (1995); Schuh and Griffiths (1996); Jones, Herning, Cadet, and Griffiths (2000); Dews, Curtis, Hanford, and O'Brien (1999); Lane (1997); Lane and Phillips-Bute (1998); Phillips-Bute and Lane (1998); and Couturier, Laman, van Duijn, and van Duijn (1997).

[a]Doses of 250 and 70 mg prevented or alleviated headaches, often within 1 hour.

[b]High caffeine consumers (e.g., average 12 cups of coffee per day) report withdrawal headaches up to 17 days after cessation.

[c]This has implications for jobs demanding constant vigilance.

other effects of caffeine withdrawal. Six weeks of drinking coffee with an average of 435 milligrams of caffeine per day were counterbalanced with 6 weeks of drinking decaffeinated coffee with a total of 30 milligrams of caffeine per day. It is instructive to note also that five of these patients recorded fewer headache complaints during withdrawal. The withdrawal was accomplished by having an independent source switch the caffeinated and decaffeinated coffee. Only seven of the subjects reported awareness of the switch. Unfortunately, the analyses reported did not eliminate these subjects.

A patient's medication alone can contain enough caffeine to create or add to the problem. Even some migraine medications, notably certain ergotamine tartrate preparations, contain caffeine (Sargent & Solbach, 1988). Table 9.6 presents the caffeine content in several prescription and OTC preparations. The American Drug Index (ADI), (Billups & Billups, 2002), a comprehensive source, indicated fewer such preparations compared to the more than 200 such preparations located for this chapter in the second edition. The second author (M.S.S.) visually reviewed over 140 pages of the 891 pages that listed drugs, and saw no preparations with caffeine.

TABLE 9.6. Caffeine Content of Selected Prescription and Nonprescription Preparations (by Trade Names)

Trade name	Manufacturer	Caffeine content (milligrams)
	Prescription	
Cafergot	Novartis	100
Ergocaf	Rugby Labs	100
Esgic	Forest; Gilbert	40
Ezol	Stewart Jackson	40
Fioricet	Novartis	40
Fiorinal	Novartis	40
Medigesic	U.S. Pharm	100
Norgesic	3M	30
Norgesic Forte	3M	60
Orphengesic	Various	60
Orphengesic Forte	Various	40
Repan tablets	Everett	32
Synalgos-DC	Wyeth	30
Tencet	Roberts	40
Triad	Forest	40
	Nonprescription	
Anacin	Whitehall	32
Aqua Ban	Thompson Medical	100
Aqua Ban Plus	Thompson Medical	200
Caffedrine	Thompson Medical	200
Cope	Mentholatum	32
Energets	Chilton	75
Excedrin		
Extra strength	Bristol-Myers	65
ASA free	Bristol-Myers	65
Migraine	Bristol-Myers	65
Lerton	Vita Elixer	250
Midol Original		
(for cramps)	Bayer	32.4
No Doz	Squibb	100 and 200
Quick-Pep	Thompson Medical	150
Stay-Alert	Apothecary	200
Stay Awake	Whiteworth	250
Summit Extra strength	Pfeiffer	65
Vanquish	Bayer	200
Vivarin	Smith, Kline, Beecham	200
Wakespan	Weeks & Lea	250

Note. In appreciation for the current revision, we thank Petra Schultz, Pharm. D., Department of Pharmacy, Mayo Clinic/St. Luke's Hospital, Jacksonville, for providing the American Drug Index to help us update this table.

Caffeine is also found in several of the increasingly popular herbal medicines and other dietary supplements for weight control, muscular development, and increasing feelings of energy. The use of supplements for weight loss stemmed from the finding that a combination of ephedrine, caffeine, and aspirin assisted in weight loss (Daly, Krieger, Dulloo, Young, & Landsberg, 1990). This combination, called ECA and sometimes referred to as an "ECA stack," has become popular in the body-building community as a means to increase muscle definition. Many supplements containing the ECA stack are available at body-building sites on the Internet. Reports of excess stimulation from ephedrine and caffeine, and of gastrointestinal bleeding due to overuse of ECA stack products, have appeared. The ECA stack has also been put into an herbal version, which may contain ephedra (the herb source of the drug ephedrine), willow bark (willow contains salicin and related compounds, analogues of aspirin), and any of a variety of caffeine-containing herbs. These herbs include green tea, guarana, kola, and yerba maté. The caffeine content of the herbal preparations is variable. Caffeine-containing herbs (as well as other herbal stimulants, such as ephedra and ginseng) may also appear in herbal energy-promoting products. The herbal stimulants, as well as several herbal sedatives that may be of interest to patients with anxiety, have been reviewed elsewhere (Gyllenhaal, Merritt, Block, Petersen, & Gochenour, 2000; Merritt, Gyllenhaal, Petersen, Block, & Gochenour, 2000). Caffeine contents of herbal products are not listed in Table 9.6, as they are seldom shown on the products themselves.

Practitioners should thus discuss with patients all OTC and prescription drugs, as well as dietary supplements and herbal preparations, in determining total caffeine intake. Patients should also be informed of the potential for caffeine withdrawal headaches and other withdrawal symptoms. Some patients may have to be advised to reduce their consumption of caffeine-containing foods, beverages, and other products gradually, in order to diminish severe withdrawal symptoms.

DIETARY FAT

Several studies report that serotonin release from platelets during migraine headaches is correlated with elevated levels of platelet aggregability and high blood lipid levels (Anthony, 1978; Bic, Blix, Hopp, & Leslie, 1998; Mezei et al., 2000). Inhibiting platelet aggregation is considered one strategy for prevention of migraines (this may be a reason for the possible effectiveness of ginger, an anticoagulant herb). High levels of high-density lipoprotein cholesterol also appear to be related to migraine attacks. Moreover, diets high in particular types of fat that contain large amounts of linoleic acid (a fatty acid) result in the production of high levels of prostaglandins, including prostaglandin E_2, a powerful vasodilator that may be involved in the pathogenesis of migraines.

One study examined the potential contribution of a high-fat diet to the etiology of migraine headaches (Bic, Blix, Hopp, Leslie, & Schnell, 1999). In the study, 54 subjects who had migraines at least once per month were instructed in how to lower their dietary fat, and then maintained their low-fat dietary pattern for 12 weeks after an initial baseline period of 28 days. They were urged to eat more fruit, vegetables, and legumes, and were advised to limit their caffeine intake. The subjects were not counseled about reducing tyramine-containing foods. Body fat was measured using skinfold thickness measurements, and a headache scale with a 6-point rating for pain was used to measure migraine frequency and discomfort. Blood lipids were analyzed for most of the subjects. A questionnaire was used to determine adherence to the diet. Body fat, weight, serum cholesterol, daily fat and cholesterol intake, and linoleic acid intake all dropped after the 12-week intervention, indicating success in implementing the diet. Daily fat intake dropped from a median of 69 grams per day to a median of 27. Headache frequency, headache intensity, and frequency of medication all dropped significantly by the end of the study, indicating that the intervention was successful in reducing headaches.

It is not clear whether other aspects of the intervention (e.g., reductions in cheese, other tyramine-containing foods, chocolate, sausages, hot dogs, and MSG-laden foods) may have accounted for the reduction in headaches. Caffeine intake was also reduced, and this too might have affected headaches. However, note that during the baseline period, those subjects consuming less than 69 grams per day of fat had a mean of 5.4 headaches, while those consuming over 69 grams per day had a mean of 10.0 headaches per month. This study was not randomized and is thus subject to a placebo effect from the diet changes. Its findings are provocative, nevertheless, and indicate a need for further research.

THERAPEUTIC STRATEGIES

The proportion of patients with migraine whose headaches are triggered by diet or by caffeine-containing products is not known. Some estimate that 5% of migraine sufferers are sensitive to tyramine (Radnitz, 1990). Owen, Turkewitz, Dawson, Casaly, and Wirth (1992) reported that 60% of patients with head pain seen at their clinic had food-related headaches, but they did not distinguish migraines from other headache types. Thus a health care professional cannot simply assume that migraine symptoms are related to diet. It may also be unwise, however, to assume that diet plays no role. Some patients, if they have been informed of the diet–migraine connection, may be able to correlate their symptoms with particular foods on their own. Treatment principles applicable to migraine can also, of course, be applied to other potentially diet-related conditions commonly treated with applied psychophysiological interventions.

Different practitioners offer suggestions for treating headaches that are possibly diet-related. Owen et al. (1992) have described a comprehensive nutritional assessment to assess intake of possible trigger foods. These foods are systematically eliminated from the diet for 4 weeks and reintroduced one by one. Food intakes and headache are monitored to determine which foods trigger headaches. When the trigger foods have been identified, instruction is given in recognizing them on product ingredient labels and in restaurants. Low blood sugar and eating under stress are discussed, as well as overuse of vitamin supplements, as headaches are symptoms of vitamin A and vitamin D toxicity (Gilman et al., 1990).

Many professionals provide a comprehensive list of foods to avoid and foods to eat as a migraine treatment diet. Patients are told to eat and sleep at regular times; they are also instructed to keep headache diaries to help discover links between diet (or other factors) and headache. In reintroducing prohibited foods, patients should be cautioned that the absence of headache in one trial should not be considered evidence that a food is definitely harmless. Medication that patients are taking may have protected them from headache, and even foods known to provoke migraines do not do so on all occasions for some patients.

Radnitz and Blanchard (1991) used a two-step program to treat 10 patients with vascular headache who had previously had unsuccessful biofeedback training. In the first phase, patients were given a list of foods to avoid that included both allergenic foods (e.g., wheat, corn, dairy products, etc.) and foods with caffeine or other vasoactive compounds (e.g., citrus, cheese, MSG, coffee, etc.). If patients did not report a 50% decrease in headaches following this diet, they were enlisted in a comprehensive elimination diet followed by challenges with suspected trigger foods. By means of food diaries, adherence to the diets was assessed. Six of the subjects noted substantial reductions in headaches on this program, while four did not. Those who did not achieve reductions were found to be younger than those who did, to have previously reported more suspected food sensitivities, and to have adhered to the dietary restrictions less faithfully. Thus, even though they claimed more food sensitivity, they were less methodical in avoiding the foods to which they might have been sensitive.

There are, as this study shows, many problems in introducing dietary advice into the comprehensive treatment of migraine. The fact that for a possibly large percentage of patients food will have no relation to migraines is only the first of these. Diet changes are difficult to accomplish, even for what should be highly motivated patients. Other problems revolve around conflicts that patients may feel between dietary advice and other treatment modes, such as physiological self-regulation or stress management.

Much of the dietary counseling in migraine treatment is based on lists of prohibited foods. Some health care professionals advise patients to stop consuming all foods and beverages on a list at the start of a treatment program, without efforts either to use the list as a preliminary elimination diet or to take into account the relative concentrations of offending chemicals in foods on the list. For many patients this tactic is inconvenient, may be unnecessary, and may result in adherence problems. Professionals making such blanket recommendations may compromise their credibility and their therapist–patient relationships unless they make clear to patients the strong effect that diet appears to have on migraines in many people. They must give a thorough explanation of the place of an elimination diet in therapy, and must be prepared to deal with adherence issues.

For instance, making such recommendations at the beginning of a treatment that also involves other interventions may cloud or at least delay understanding the relationships of dietary factors and symptoms. Such combinations of treatments, when started simultaneously, can lead a patient to perceive the treatment program as a shotgun approach. This can diminish the patient's view of the relative importance and usefulness of the other applied psychophysiological treatments, including biofeedback.

Insisting that patients stop consuming everything that conceivably might result in symptoms on a permanent basis early in treatment also creates a demand that patients may not be ready to accept. Diet is, after all, fraught with psychological, familial, and sociocultural complications and implications. Patients may not accurately report problems in following the diet (i.e., may show lack of adherence) to a health care professional who is not sensitive to the emotional dynamics of dietary change.

However, these concerns must be weighed against the increased possibility of success if diet is indeed an important factor in the symptoms of any particular patient. Success and rapid relief of symptoms are, after all, paramount in a patient's point of view and should be equally prominent in that of a therapist. If a patient's migraines are related to diet, symptoms will disappear much more quickly with proper dietary change—possibly within days (Gettis, 1987a) or a few weeks. If the symptoms are not related to diet, a few weeks of avoiding certain foods will not hinder relief of migraines. Indeed, since many of the foods that seem to trigger migraines are not healthful (chocolate, MSG-laden processed foods, sausages, cheese, alcohol, hot dogs), such patients may note improvements in general health or learn valuable lessons about the possibility of productive diet changes.

From this point of view, integrating self-regulation training with diet gives patients both short-term benefits and long-term prophylactic effects, whether their symptoms are diet-related or not. This can be considered a highly positive and appropriate therapeutic strategy for migraines, IBS, and the other multifactorial conditions treatable with self-regulation.

Integrating the dietary and self-regulation components of a comprehensive migraine treatment program can be done in several different ways. One option in evaluating dietary connections to migraine symptoms is to query patients about their own observations on diet, medications, and symptoms. If they have not considered the question, they can perhaps be allowed a few weeks to make such observations (at the risk of delaying symptom relief), bearing in mind suggestions about foods that patients with migraine commonly find troublesome. More typically, however, the therapist should consider the following strategies of implementing the comprehensive approach. The order in which they are presented does not imply preference.

1. *Self-regulation only.* The patient does not stop using suspected substances before or while carrying out applied psychophysiological treatments. This approach assumes that the professional does not accept the potential validity of dietary or allergy factors.

2. *Diet first.* The patient stops using all or most of the suspected substances. At a minimum, the patient alters the diet and medication use of the items with higher concentrations of suspected elements and those with more suspected potential of adding to symptoms. True evaluation of the potential of the dietary approach requires, of course, a thorough (if temporary) elimination diet. The practitioner and patient can then proceed with challenges as possible. No other treatment occurs until the results of this approach alone have been adequately checked. This requires several weeks, or possibly longer.

3. *Stepped care.* The patient starts a physiological self-regulation treatment program for at least several weeks. Depending on the results, dietary treatment is begun later if it is still of potential additional benefit. This is proper, for example, if there is not enough improvement in symptoms.

4. *Self-regulation plus trigger avoidance.* The professional may start the patient on an applied psychophysiological treatment program and a few patient-acceptable dietary restrictions. Although this approach leaves unclear the relative contribution of each approach, it nevertheless is not likely to interfere with adherence. The focus of the intervention is still nondietary.

5. *Self-regulation plus elimination diet.* The patient stops using all or most of the suspected substances and proceeds with other applied psychophysiological treatments at the same time. The therapist should clearly explain to the patient the rationale and need for such an approach, along with the strategy for gradual reintroduction of initially prohibited foods. This approach is common, but confounds the relative contributions of the two treatments. The possibility of such confusion could be discussed with the patient in light of the potentially more rapid symptom relief (which may be a particular consideration in severe and frequent headaches). Later, when there are clinically significant symptom reductions, the patient may change the dietary regimen and test him- or herself by reintroducing suspected trigger foods at weekly intervals (e.g., Gettis, 1987a).

The professional may, of course, combine cognitive and other stress management treatments with other applied psychophysiological treatments. These may also be deferred in the stepped-care model of intervention, for a more adequate assessment of their relative contribution.

There are advantages and disadvantages for each of the alternative strategies we have presented for integrating list-based dietary counseling with physiological self-regulation treatment. All are justifiable and reasonable under specific circumstances. We do not favor omitting dietary considerations entirely from presentations to patients. By understanding the advantages and disadvantages of each strategy, professionals and patients can make adequately informed decisions. Table 9.7 describes selected advantages and disadvantages of each strategy.

Certain migraine cases have proven refractory to list-based dietary counseling. Some of these have been helped by comprehensive diet revision based on a positive program emphasizing whole, natural foods (preferably locally grown) and vegetarian protein sources, and radically excluding processed foods, dairy products, and refined sugar. It is also low in fat and may thus benefit from the lowered platelet aggregability and decreased prostoglandin synthesis discussed above. One of us (Block) has implemented this program as a comprehensive health regimen in his practice. It certainly does not exclude the appropriate use of medications, but does

TABLE 9.7. Advangages and Disadvantages of Five Strategies for Including Dietary Changes in Therapy Programs of Selected Patients

Strategy	Advantages	Disadvantages
Self-regulation only	No need to do without selected foods and beverages; no inconvenience from checking the ingredients of foods and beverages.	May decrease chances of ameliorating symptoms sooner; may eventually cost more for other therapies, such as medications.
Diet first	May be sufficient for clinically significant symptom reduction in some patients; may save the expenses of other therapies.	May take longer to reduce or eliminate symptoms; may be inconvenient to check dietary factors; requires patient's compliance with dietary regimen; may defer symptom reduction if dietary factors are unimportant or only part of the problem.
Stepped care	No initial need to do without desired foods and beverages; no initial inconvenience from checking ingredients; opportunity to evaluate the relative effects of physiological self-regulation and dietary therapy at separate times; may increase later compliance with either or both types of therapy when their relative contributions are better identified.	May cost more because of longer physiological self-regulation therapy; may defer symptom reduction if dietary factors are important.
Self-regulation plus trigger avoidance	No initial need to do without all or most of the foods and beverages; may result in faster reduction of symptoms if both therapies are relevant and needed; may be more acceptable to some patients, hence increasing compliance with dietary changes.	May be impossible to determine the relative contributions of each type of therapy; may decrease compliance with one approach if patient relies on the other; may cost more if more dietary changes are needed; may defer symptom reduction if more dietary changes are needed.
Self-regulation plus elimination diet	May decrease or eliminate symptoms faster.	May be impossible to determine the relative contributions of each type of therapy; may decrease compliance with either or both if the patient relies on one or does not take either seriously.

emphasize the need for self-care and self-reliance, and does discourage the overreliance on medications seen in some patients with migraine. The diet is high in fiber. It avoids many sources of vasoactive compounds, such as tropical fruits (bananas, citrus), cheese, chocolate, caffeine sources, and processed foods that contain MSG or artificial sweeteners. It is also low in many allergenic foods, including cow's milk and eggs. Wheat and corn (common grain allergens), are present in the diet but are deemphasized in favor of whole-grain rice, a staple of the program. The high fiber content of the diet, the emphasis on vegetable proteins, and the absence of refined sugars may assist those whose headaches are related to low blood sugar. In addition, the diet is fully compatible with emerging recommendations for general health and prevention of cancer and heart disease. The high intake of fiber may also assist those with IBS, since increases in fiber intake are recommended for patients with constipation (Camilleri, 2001).

The positive diet program revolves around five food groups: grains, vegetables, fruits, proteins, and fats. Carbohyrates are the main source of calories, so grains are the centerpiece of the diet. Recommended grains for daily use are brown rice, barley, oats, millet, and kasha. Grains are to be eaten as whole cooked grains, with less emphasis on flours and other processed forms.

Vegetables recommended for daily use are leafy vegetables (kale, collards, mustard greens, but not spinach), squashes, carrots, onions, turnips, and cruciferous vegetables (broccoli, cauliflower, cabbage, Brussels sprouts). Tomatoes (often allergenic and high in sugar) are deemphasized.

Fruits recommended for daily use are apples, apricots, melons, pears, cherries, peaches, and other temperate-zone fruits. Citrus fruits, bananas, figs, papaya, mango, avocado, and other tropical fruits are to be reduced and if necessary eliminated (many of these are on lists of migraine trigger foods).

Proteins include aduki beans, garbanzos, soy foods (e.g., tofu and soy milk, both good calcium sources), lentils, and other small beans; larger beans may be eaten less frequently. Fish may be eaten two or three times weekly if desired (chicken may be used when patients are making the transition to the full program). If patients feel they must eat dairy products, and are found not to be sensitive to them after elimination and reintroduction, skim milk products and low-fat yogurt are preferable to other forms. Modifications in this part of the regimen may be necessary in the case of allergies to fish, to soy, or to other beans.

Fats include nuts, seeds, and oils; canola and olive oils are emphasized. Sweetners used include brown rice syrup, maple syrup, and natural fruits. Recommended drinks include water (preferably spring water), teas such as bancha or herbal tea, or grain coffee substitutes. Caffeine-containing beverages and wines are to be avoided. Practical suggestions for meal plans are found in a few cookbooks (e.g., Colbin, 1979). Formalized nutritional need assessment and exchange lists are available for the diet.

People using the diet must be certain to obtain enough calcium from such sources as leafy green vegetables, calcium-fortified soy milk, garbanzo beans, tofu, broccoli, and other natural calcium sources. Calcium supplements are allowable if patients are not able to structure their diets adequately; vitamin B_{12} supplements are needed for those who may choose strict vegetarian diets; good-quality multivitamin supplements are also allowable.

This diet has also proven successful with many patients presenting with IBS and other bowel diseases. As noted earlier, some patients with IBS have been found to respond well to increases in dietary fiber, which is greatly increased in this diet. Some authors have noted that high-fiber diets tend to normalize bowel function, diminishing both constipation and diarrhea, both of which are features of IBS (Harvey, Pomare, & Heaton, 1973; Payler, Pomare, Heaton, & Harvey, 1975). It should be noted that some patients who present with symptoms resembling IBS are actually lactase-deficient or lactose-intolerant; this makes either a hydrogen breath test for lactase deficiency or a trial elimination of dairy products a good strategy. Not all patients with IBS respond to diet, however, and there remains some controversy concerning the impact of fiber on bowel disease (Ritchie, Wadsworth, Lennard-Jones, & Rogers, 1987; Heaton, Thornton, & Emmett, 1979; Hillman, Stace, Fisher, & Pomare, 1982). Nevertheless, a trial of increasing dietary fiber—preferably through overall diet changes that include elimination of dairy products, rather than simply fiber supplements (Soltoft, Krag, Gudmand-Hoyer, Kristensen, & Wulff, 1986)—is justified in patients with IBS who have not previously attempted it.

Some patients may be interested in the botanical migraine remedies mentioned earlier in the chapter. Feverfew can be taken as a migraine preventive. It has been studied in dosages of 50 milligrams per day, or two fresh leaves chewed daily (der Marderosian & Liberti, 1988). Some patients experience mouth ulcerations while taking fresh leaves and may need a capsule form. Dried ginger, available in supermarkets, was taken by one patient to abort migraine headaches (Mustafa & Srivastava, 1990). At the onset of aura, 500–600 milligrams of powdered ginger were mixed with water and consumed. An abortive effect was noticeable in

30 minutes. Following this, the same dose was taken twice every 4 hours until the attack was over, and for 3–4 days after. The subject experienced no ill effects, and eventually began including fresh ginger in her daily diet, which proved to be an effective migraine preventive.

Regardless of which alternative a professional and patient select, there are additional considerations to incorporate into treatment plans. First, most patients can easily avoid heavy caffeine consumption, even if they were previously heavy consumers. Second, patients should avoid dietary items they strongly suspect cause symptoms. This will be acceptable to most patients. Third, patients should avoid dietary substances known from the literature or strongly suspected to cause headaches (e.g., alcohol, MSG). Finally, if list-based dietary counseling is used, professionals should be very specific about the foods to avoid. Therapists should periodically assess how well patients are adhering to their dietary restrictions, and be prepared to offer practical suggestions for making dietary changes. As in any therapeutic situation, therapists must equip themselves to handle adherence problems.

CONCLUSION

In the last decade, studies of diet and migraine have progressed considerably. We still need, however, much more information about the concentrations of tyramine, MSG, caffeine, and other substances in the products listed in various tables of this chapter. The relative lack of such information is probably due to the complexity of such analyses. The variations within a given item depend on such factors as how one prepares it and where it comes from. We also suspect that there may be other reasons for the limited research about the concentrations of these substances. One such reason is the presumed equivocal nature of the research about the relationships between these substances and migraines. There are professional disagreements about the importance of this area. We hope to eventually better identify and adjust concentrations of vasoactive substances for persons who are or may be susceptible to the effects of such substances. Further research on the nature and physiology of diet-related migraine is also warranted; such research might take advantage of certain new technical methods, such as Enzyme-linked immunosorbent assay/Activated cell test (ELISA/ACT) testing for food allergies.

Discussion of migraine headache prevention may seem beside the point at this date, since sumatriptan and related drugs have entered the U.S. pharmaceutical market. These drugs are highly effective migraine abortives (even for debilitating headaches), with minimal side effects, in approximately 80% of patients. Obviously, the remaining 20% of patients still need to concern themselves with prevention of migraines; moreover, for many patients, sumatriptan and related medications eventually cease to be effective.

Is the elimination of migraine-triggering foods or the control of migraines through physiological self-regulation still a reasonable goal for the 80% who do benefit from the newer drugs? We feel that it is. For patients who suffer from frequent migraines, the yearly cost of some medications (e.g., sumatriptan), becomes high. We feel it is of more importance than ever that patients learn to control the incidence of migraines. Practitioners involved in dietary or physiological self-regulation treatment of migraine headaches should feel no embarrassment in continuing to advocate their treatment strategies.

In conclusion, there are many factors to consider when one is checking the possible contribution of dietary factors in patients' symptoms and when advising dietary changes. However, the data available to date suggest that unifocal care of migraines and other diet-related conditions is never complete care. This evidence warrants serious consideration of dietary changes for at least some patients. How one conveys this information and carries out the changes should involve careful thought and planning. It is not as simple as telling patients to abstain from certain foods. Dietary change is emotionally and socially difficult. Changing ingrained eating patterns requires both practical help and technical knowledge. Clinicians and researchers can be most effective if they are thoroughly familiar with dietary considerations when providing biofeedback and other applied psychophysiological treatments.

ACKNOWLEDGMENT

Marissa Oppel, Program for Collaborative Research in the Pharmaceutical Sciences, College of Pharmacy, University of Illinois at Chicago, contributed to the revision of the tables.

REFERENCES

Anthony, M. (1978). Individual free fatty acids and migraine. *Clinical and Experimental Neurology, 15,* 190–196.

Antila, P., Antila, V., Mattila, J., & Hakkarainen, H. (1984) Biogenic amines in cheese: 1. Determination of biogenic amines in Finnish cheese using high performance liquid chromatography. *Milchwissenschaft, 39,* 81–85.

Arya, L. A., Myers, D. L., & Jackson, N. D. (2000). Dietary caffeine intake and the risk for detrusor instability: A case–control study. *Obstetrics and Gynecology, 96,* 85–89.

Asatoor, A. M., Levi, A. J., & Milne, M. P. (1963). Trancylpromine and cheese. *Lancet, ii,* 733–734.

Barone, J. J., & Roberts, H. R. (1996). Caffeine consumption. *Food and Chemical Toxicology, 34*(1), 119–129.

Bic, Z., Blix, G. G., Hopp, H. P., & Leslie, F. M. (1998). In search of the ideal treatment for migraine headaches. *Medical Hypotheses, 50,* 1–7.

Bic, Z., Blix, G. G., Hopp, H. P., Leslie, F. M., & Schell, M. J. (1999). The influence of a low-fat diet in incidence and severity of migraine headaches. *Journal of Women's Health and Gender-Based Medicine, 8,* 623–630.

Billups, N. F., & Billups, S. M. (2002). *American drug index 2002* (46th ed.). St. Louis: Facts & Comparisons/ Walters Kluwer.

Blackwell, B., & Taylor, D. C. (1969). "Cold cures" and monoamine-oxidase inhibitors. *British Medical Journal, ii,* 381–382.

Block, K. I., & Schwartz, M. S. (1995). Dietary considerations: Rationale, issues, substances, evaluation, and patient education. In M. S. Schwartz & Associates, *Biofeedback: A practitioner's guide* (2nd ed.). New York: Guilford Press.

Boulton, A. A., Cookson, B., & Paulten, R. (1970). Hypertensive crisis in a patient on MAOI antidepressants following a meal of beef liver. *Canadian Medical Association Journal, 102,* 1394–1395.

Brown, S. L., Salive, M. E., Pahor, M., Foley, D. J., Corti, M. C., Langlois, J. A., Wallace, R. B., & Harris, T. B. (1995). Occult caffeine as a source of sleep problems in an older population. *Journal of the American Geriatrics Society, 43,* 860–864.

Bruce, M. S. (1990). The anxiogenic effect of caffeine. *Postgraduate Medical Journal, 66*(Suppl. 2), 18–24.

Bruce, M. S., & Lader, M. (1989). Caffeine abstention in the management of anxiety disorders. *Psychological Medicine, 19,* 211–214.

Bruce, M. S., Scott, N., Shine, P., & Lader, M. (1992). Anxiogenic effects of caffeine in patients with anxiety disorders. *Archives of General Psychiatry, 49,* 867–869.

Camilleri, M. (2001). Management of irritable bowel syndrome. *Gastroenterology, 120*(3), 652–68.

Chin, K. W., Garriga, M. M., & Metcalfe, D. D. (1989). The histamine content of Oriental foods. *Food Chemistry and Toxicololgy, 27,* 283–287.

Coffin, D. C. (1970). Tyramine content of raspberries and other fruit. *Journal of the Association of Official Analytic Chemists, 53,* 1071–1073.

Colbin, A. (1979). *The book of whole meals.* Brookline, MA: Autumn Press.

Cook, G. E., & Joseph, R. (1983). Letter. *Lancet, ii,* 1256–1257.

Couturier, E. G. M., Laman, D. M., van Duijn, M. A. J., & van Duijn, H. (1997). Influence of caffeine and caffeine withdrawal on headache and cerebral blood flow velocities. *Cephalalgia, 17,* 188–190.

Curatolo, P. W., & Robertson, D. (1983). The health consequences of caffeine. *Annals of Internal Medicine, 98,* 641–653.

Currie, S. R., Wilson, K. G., & Gauthier, S. T. (1995). Caffeine and chronic low back pain. *Clinical Journal of Pain, 11,* 214–219.

Dalessio, D. J. (1980). Migraine therapy. In D. J. Dalessio (Ed.), *Wolff's headache and other head pain.* New York: Oxford University Press.

Daly, P. A., Krieger, D. R., Dulloo, A. G., Young, J. B., & Landsberg, L. (1993). Ephedrine, caffeine and aspirin: safety and efficacy for treatment of human obesity. *International Journal of Obesity, 17*(Suppl. 1), S73–S78.

Denaro, C. P., Brown, C. R., Wilson, M., Jacob, P., III, & Benowitz, N. L. (1990). Dose-dependency of caffeine metabolism with repeated dosing. *Clinical Pharmacology and Therapeutics, 48,* 277–285.

der Marderosian, A., & Liberti, L. (1988). *Natural product medicine.* Philadelphia: George F. Stickley.

Dews, P. B., Curtis, G. L., Hanford, K. J., & O'Brien, C. P. (1999). The frequency of caffeine withdrawal in a population-based survey and in a controlled, blinded pilot experiment. *Journal of Clinical Pharmacology, 39,* 1221–1232.

Diamond, S., Prager, J., & Freitag, F. G. (1986). Diet and headache: Is there a link? *Postgraduate Medicine, 79*(4), 279–287.

Egger, J. (1991). Psychoneurological aspects of food allergy. *European Journal of Clinical Nutrition, 45*(Suppl. 1), 35–45.

Egger, J., Carter, C. M., Soothill, J. F., & Wilson, J. (1989). Oligoantigenic diet treatment in children with epilepsy and migraine. *Journal of Pediatrics, 114,* 51–58.

Egger, J., Wilson, J., Carter, C. M., Turner, M. W., & Soothill, J. F. (1983a). Is migraine food allergy?: A double-blind controlled trial of oligoantigenic diet treatment. *Lancet, ii,* 865–869.

Egger, J., Wilson, J., Carter, C. M., Turner, M. W., & Soothill, J. F. (1983b). Letter. *Lancet, ii,* 1424.

Ernst, E. & Pittler, M. (2000). The efficacy and safety of feverfew (*Tanacetum parthenium* L.): An update of a systematic review. *Public Health Nutrition, 3,* 509–514.

Feldman, W. (1983). Letter. *Lancet, ii,* 1424.

Fennelly, M., Galletly, D. C., & Purdie, G. I. (1991). Is caffeine withdrawal the mechanism of postoperative headache? *Anesthesia and Analgesia, 72,* 449–453.

Geha, R. S., Beiser, A., Ren, C., Patterson, R., Greenberger, P. A., Grammer, L. C., Ditto, A. M., Harris, K. E., Shaughnessy, M. A., Yarnold, P. R., Corren, J., & Saxon, A. (2000). Review of alleged reaction to monosodium glutamate and outcome of a multicenter double-blind placebo-controlled study. *Journal of Nutrition, 130*(Suppl. 4), 1058S–1062S.

Gerrard, J. W. (1983). Letter. *Lancet, ii,* 1257.

Gettis, A. (1987a). Serendipity and food sensitivity: A case study. *Headache, 27,* 73–75.

Gettis, A. (1987b). Viewpoint: Food induced "delayed reaction" headaches in relation to tyramine studies. *Headache, 27,* 444–445.

Giacovazzo, M., & Martelletti, P. (1989). Letter. *Annals of Allergy, 63,* 255.

Gibb, C. M., Davies, P. T., Glover, V., Steiner, T. J., Clifford Rose, F., & Sandler, M. (1991). Chocolate is a migraine-provoking agent. *Cephalalgia, 11,* 93–95.

Gilbert, R. M. (1981). Caffeine: Overview and anthology. In S. A. Miller (Ed.), *Nutrition and behavior: The proceedings of the Franklin Research Center's 1980 Working Conference on Nutrition and Behavior. New research directions.* Philadelphia: Franklin Institute Press.

Gilman, A. G., Rall, T. W., Nies, A. S., & Taylor, P. (Eds.). (1990). *Goodman and Gilman's The pharmaceutical basis of therapeutics* (8th ed.). New York: Pergamon Press.

Grant, E. C. G. (1979). Food allergies and migraine. *Lancet, i,* 966–968.

Greden, J. F., Victor, B. S., Fontaine, P., & Lubetsky, M. (1980). Caffeine-withdrawal headache: A clinical profile. *Psychosomatics, 21*(5), 411–413, 417–418.

Griffiths, R. R., Evans, S. M., Heishman, S. J., Preston, K. L., Wannerud, C. A., Wolf, B., & Woodson, P. P. (1990). Low-dose caffeine physical dependence in humans. *Journal of Pharmacology and Experimental Therapeutics, 255*(3), 1123–1132.

Guariso, G., Bertoli, S., Bernetti, R., Battistella, P. A., Setari, M., & Zacchello, F. (1993). Emicrania e intolleranza alimentare: Studio controllato in eta evolutiva. *Pediatrica Medica Chirugia, 15,* 57–61.

Gyllenhaal, C., Merritt, S. L., Block, K., Petersen, S. D., & Gochenour, T. (2000). Safety and efficacy of herbal stimulants and sedatives in sleep disorders. *Sleep Medicine Reviews, 4*(3), 229–251.

Hanington, E. (1980). Diet and migraine. *Journal of Human Nutrition, 34,* 175–180.

Hanington, E., Horn, M., & Wilkinson, M. (1969). Further observations on the effects of tyramine. In A. L. Cochrane (Ed.), *Background to migraine: Third symposium.* New York: Springer.

Harper, J. V. (1993). For want of a cup of coffee [Editorial]. *Mayo Clinic Proceedings, 68,* 928–929.

Harrison, D. P. (1986). Copper as a factor in the dietary precipitation of migraine. *Headache, 26,* 248–250.

Harvey, R. F., Pomare, E. W., & Heaton, K. W. (1973). Effects of increased dietary fibre on intestinal transit. *Lancet, i,* 1278–1280.

Hearn, G., & Finn, R. (1983). Letter. *Lancet, ii,* 1081–1082.

Heaton, K. W., Thornton, J. R., & Emmett, P. M. (1979). Treatment of Crohn's disease with an unrefined-carbohydrate, fibre-rich diet. *British Medical Journal, ii,* 764–766.

Hedberg, D. L., Gordon, M. W., & Glueck, B. C. (1966). Six cases of hypertensive crisis in patients on tranylcypromine after eating chicken livers. *American Journal of Psychiatry, 122,* 933–937.

Henderson, W. R., & Raskin, N. (1972). Hot dog headache: Individual susceptibility to nitrite. *Lancet, ii,* 1162–1163.

Hibino, G., Moritani, T., Kawada, T., & Fushiki, T. (1997). Caffeine enhances modulation of parasympathetic nerve activity in humans: Quantification using power spectral analysis. *Journal of Nutrition, 127*, 1422–1427.

Hillman, L. C., Stace, N. H., Fisher, A., & Pomare, E. W. (1982). Dietary intakes and stool characteristics of patients with the irritable bowel syndrome. *American Journal of Clinical Nutrition, 36*, 626–629.

Hodge, J. V., Nye, E. R., & Emerson, G. W. (1964). Monoamine-oxidase inhibitors, broad beans, and hypertension. *Lancet, i*, 1108.

Hofer, I., & Battig, K. (1994). Cardiovascular, behavioral, and subjective effects of caffeine under field conditions. *Pharmacology Biochemistry and Behavior, 48*(4), 899–908.

Horowitz, D., Lovenberg, W., Engelman, K., & Sjoerdsma, A. (1964). Monoamine-oxidase inhibitors, tyramine and cheese. *Journal of the American Medical Association, 188*(13), 1108–1110.

Hughes, E. C., Gott, P. S., Weinstein, R. C., & Binggeli, R. (1985). Migraine: A diagnostic test for etiology of food sensitivity by a nutritionally supported fast and confirmed by long-term report. *Annals of Allergy, 55*, 28–32.

Humphrey, P. P. A. (1991). 5-Hydroxytryptamine and the pathophysiology of migraine. *Journal of Neurology, 238*, S38–S44.

Ibe, A., Saito, K., Nakazato, M., Kikuchi, Y., Fujinuma, K., & Nishima, T. (1991). Quantitative determination of amines in wine by liquid chromatography. *Journal of the Association of Official Analytic Chemists, 74*, 695–698.

Iqbal, P., & Castleden, C. M. (1997). Management of urinary incontinence in the elderly. *Gerontology, 47*, 151–157.

James, J. E. (1997). *Understanding caffeine: A biobehavioral analysis.* Thousand Oaks, CA: Sage.

James, J. E., Bruce, M. S., Lader, M. H., & Scott, N. R. (1989). Self-report reliability and symptomatology of habitual caffeine consumption. *British Journal of Clinical Pharmacology, 27*, 507–514.

Jarman, J., Glover, V., & Sandler, M. (1991). Release of (^{14}C) 5-hydroxytryptamine from human platelets by red wine. *Life Sciences, 49*, 2297–2300.

Jones, H. E., Herning, R. I., Cadet, J. L., & Griffiths, R. R. (2000). Caffeine withdrawal increases cerebral blood flow velocity and alters quantitative electroencephalography (EEG) activity. *Psychopharmacology, 147*, 371–377.

Kalow, W. (1985). Variability of caffeine metabolism in humans. *Arzneimittelforsch, 35*, 319–324.

Kenyhercz, T. M., & Kissinger, P. T. (1978). Determination of selected acidic, neutral and basic natural products in cacao beans and processed cocoa: Liquid chromatography with electrochemical detection. *Lloydia, 412*, 130–139.

Koehler, S. M., & Glaros, A. (1988). The effect of aspartame on migraine headache. *Headache, 28*, 10–14.

Kohlenberg, R. J. (1980). *Migraine relief: A personal treatment program.* Seattle, WA: Biofeedback and Stress Management Clinic.

Lai, C. W., Dean, P., Ziegler, D. K., & Hassanein, R. S. (1989). Clinical and electrophysiological responses to dietary challenge in migraineurs. *Headache, 29*, 180–186.

Lane, J. D. (1997). Effects of brief caffeinated-beverage deprivation on mood, symptoms, and psychomotor performance. *Pharmacology, Biochemistry and Behavior, 58*(1), 203–208.

Lane, J. D., Adcock, R. A., Williams, R. B., & Kuhn, C. M. (1990). Caffeine effects on cardiovascular and neuroendocrine responses to acute psychosocial stress and their relationship to level of habitual caffeine consumption. *Psychosomatic Medicine, 52*, 320–336.

Lane, J. D., & Phillips-Bute, B. G. (1998). Caffeine deprivation affects vigilance performance and mood. *Physiology and Behavior, 65*(1), 171–175.

Lane, J. D., Phillips-Bute, B. G., & Pieper, C. F. (1998). Caffeine raises blood pressure at work. *Psychsomatic Medicine, 60*, 327–330.

Lipton, R. B., Newman, L. C., Cohen, J. S., & Solomon, S. (1989). Aspartame as a dietary trigger of headache. *Headache, 29*, 90–92.

Littlewood, J., Gibb, D., Glover, V., Sandler, M., Davies, P. T., & Rose, F. C. (1988). Red wine as a cause of migraine. *Lancet, i*, 558–559.

Lovenberg, W. (1973). Some vaso- and psychoactive substances in food: Amines, stimulants, depressants and hallucinogens. In National Research Council Food Protection Committee (Ed.), *Toxicants occurring naturally in foods* (2nd ed., rev.). Washington, DC: National Academy of Sciences.

Lucarelli, S., Lendvai, D., Frediani, T., Finamore, G., Grossi, R., Barbato, M., Zingdoni, A. M., & Cardi, E. (1990). Hemicrania and food allergy in children. *Minerva Pediatrica, 42*, 215–218.

Lucero, M. A., & McCloskey, W. W. (1997). Alternatives to estrogen for the treatment of hot flashes. *Annals of Pharmacotherapy, 31*, 915–917.

Mansfield, L. E. (1990). The role of antihistamine therapy in vascular headaches. *Journal of Allergy and Clinical Immunology, 86*, 673–676.

Mansfield, L. E., Vaughn, T. R., Waller, S. F., Haverly, R. W., & Ting, S. (1985). Food allergy and adult migraine: Double blind and mediator confirmation of an allergic etiology. *Annals of Allergy, 55*, 126–129.

Marcus, D. A., Scharff, L., Turk, D., & Gourley, L. M. (1997). A double-blind provocative study of chocolate as a trigger of headache. *Cephalalgia, 17*, 855–862.

Marley, E., Blackwell, B. (1970). Interactions of monoamine oxidase inhibitors, amines, and foodstuffs. *Advances in Pharmacology and Chemotherapy, 8*, 185–349.

Martin, P. R., & Seneviratene, H. M. (1997). Effects of food deprivation and a stressor on head pain. *Health Psychology, 16*, 310–318.

Matthew, J., & Wilson, W. H. (1985). Caffeine consumption, withdrawal and cerebral blood flow. *Headache, 25*, 305–309.

Maxwell, M. B. (1980). Reexamining the dietary restrictions with procarbazine (an MAOI). *Cancer Nursing, 3*, 451–457.

McCabe, B. J. (1986). Dietary tyramine and other pressor amines in MAOI regimens: A review. *Journal of the American Dietetic Association, 86*(8), 1059–1064.

McCabe, B. J., & Tsuang, M. T. (1982). Dietary considerations in MAO inhibitor regimens. *Journal of Clinical Psychiatry, 43*, 575–580.

Merritt, J. E., & Williams, P. B. (1990). Vasospasm contributes to monosodium glutamate-induced headache. *Headache, 30*, 575–580.

Merritt, S. L., Gyllenhaal, C., Petersen, S. D., Block, K. I., & Gochenour, T. (2000). Herbal remedies: Efficacy in controlling sleepiness and promoting sleep. *Nurse Practitioner Forum, 11*, 87–100.

Mezei, Z., Kis, B., Gecse, A., Tajti, J., Boda, B., Telegdy, G., & Vecsei, L. (2000). Platelet arachidonate cascade of migraineurs in the interictal phase. *Platelets, 11*, 222–225.

Migliardi, J. R., Armellino, J. J., Friedman, M., Gillings, D. B., & Beaver, W. T. (1994). Caffeine as an analgesic adjuvant in tension headache. *Clinical Pharmacology and Therapeutics, 56*, 576–586.

Moffet, A. M., Swash, M., & Scott, D. F. (1974). Effect of chocolate in migraine: A double-blind study. *Journal of Neurology, Neurosurgery and Psychiatry, 37*, 131–162.

Monro, J. A., Carini, C., Brostoff, J., & Zilkha, K. (1980). Food allergy in migraine. *Lancet, ii*, 1–4.

Moskowitz, M. A., & Buzzi, M. G. (1991). Neuroeffector functions of sensory fibres: Implications for headache mechanisms and drug actions. *Journal of Neurology, 238*, S18–S22.

Mumford, G. K., Eans, S. M., Kaminski, B. J., Preston, K. L., Sannerud, C. A., Silverman, K., & Griffiths, R. R. (1994). Discriminative stimulus and subjective effects of theobromine and caffeine in humans. *Psychopharmacology, 115*(1–2), 1–8.

Mustafa, T., & Srivastava, K. C. (1990). Ginger (*Zingiber officinale*) in migraine headache. *Journal of Ethnopharmacology, 29*, 267–273.

National Organization Mobilized to Stop Glutamate (NoMSG). (1992). *Hidden sources of MSG*. Santa Fe, NM: Author.

Olesen, J. (1991). A review of current drugs for migraine. *Journal of Neurology, 238*, S23–S27.

Orlosky, M. (1982). MAO inhibitors in sickness and in health. *Massachusetts General Hospital Newsletter: Biological Therapies in Psychiatry, 5*, 25–28.

Owen, M. L., Turkewitz, J., Dawson, G. A., Casaly, J. S., & Wirth, O. (1992). Nutritional education as a part of a multidisciplinary behavior modification approach to the treatment of head pain [Abstract]. *Headache, 32*, 265–266.

Payler, D. K., Pomare, E. W., Heaton, K. W., & Harvey, R. F. (1975). The effect of wheat bran on intestinal transit. *Gut, 32*, 209–213.

Peatfield, R. C. (1983). Letter. *Lancet, ii*, 1082.

Pennington, J. A. T., & Church, H. N. (1985). *Bowes and Church's food values of portions commonly used*. (14th ed.). New York: Perennial Library.

Pennington, J. A. T., & Church, H. N. (1998). *Bowes and Church's food values of portions commonly used*. (17th ed.). New York: Lippincott Williams & Wilkins.

Phillips-Bute, B. G., & Lane, J. D. (1998). Caffeine withdrawal symptoms following brief caffeine deprivation. *Physiology and Behavior, 63*(1), 35–39.

Pittler, M. H., Vogler, B. K., & Ernst, E. (2000). Feverfew for preventing migraine (Cochrane Review). *Cochrane Database Systematic Reviews, 3*, CD002286.

Podell, R. N. (1984). Is migraine a manifestation of food allergy? *Postgraduate Medicine, 75*(4), 221–225.

Pradalier, A., de Saint Maur, P., Lamy, F., & Launay, J. M. (1994). Immunocyte enumeration in duodenal biopsies of migraine without aura patients with or without food-induced migraine. *Cephalalgia, 14*, 365–367.

Pradalier, A., & Launay, J. M. (1996). Immunological aspects of migraine. *Biomedicine and Pharmacotherapy, 50*, 64–70.

Pradalier, A., Weinman, S., Launay, J. M., Baron, J. F., & Dry, J. (1983). Total IgE, specific IgE and prick tests against foods in common migraine: A prospective study. *Cephalalgia, 3*, 231–234.

Price, K., & Smith, S. E. (1971). Cheese reaction and tyramine. *Lancet, i*, 130–131.

Pritchard, W. S., Robinson, J. H., deBethizy, J. D., Davis, R. A., & Stiles, M. F. (1995). Caffeine and smoking: Subjective, performance, and psychophysiological effects. *Psychophysiology, 32*, 19–27.

Radnitz, C. L. (1990). Food-triggered migraine: A critical review. *Annals of Behavioral Medicine, 12*(2), 51–71.

Radnitz, C. L., & Blanchard, E. B. (1991). Assessment and treatment of dietary factors in refractory vascular headache. *Headache Quarterly: Current Treatment and Research, 2*(3), 214–220.

Rao, S. S. C., Welcher, K., Zimmerman, B., & Stumbo, P. (1998). Is coffee a colonic stimulant? *European Journal of Gastroenterology and Hepatology, 10*, 113–118.

Rice, S. L., Eitenmiller, B. R., & Kohler, P. E. (1975). Histamine and tyramine content of meat products. *Journal of Milk Food Technology, 38,* 256–258.

Rice, S. L., Eitenmiller, B. R., & Kohler, P. E. (1976). Biologically active amines in food: A review. *Journal of Milk Food Technology, 39,* 353–358.

Rice, S. L., & Kohler, P. E. (1976). Tyrosine and histidine decarboxylase activities of *Pediococcus cerevisiae* and *Lactobacillus* species and the production of tyramine in fermented sausages. *Journal of Milk Food Technology, 39,* 166–169.

Richardson, N. J., Rogers, P. J., Elliman, N. A., & O'Dell, R. J. (1995). Mood and performance effects of caffeine in relation to acute and chronic caffeine deprivation. *Pharmacology Biochemistry and Behavior, 52*(2), 313-320.

Riggin, R. M., McCarthy, M. J., & Kissinger, P. O. (1976). Identification of salsolinol as a major dopamine metabolite in the banana. *Journal of Agricultural and Food Chemistry, 24,* 189–191.

Ritchie, J. K., Wadsworth, J., Lennard-Jones, J. E., & Rogers, E. (1987). Controlled multicentre trial of a unrefined carbohydrate, fibre-rich diet in Crohn's disease. *British Medical Journal, 295,* 517–520.

Rivas-Gonzalo, J. C., Santos-Hernandez, J. G., & Marine-Font, A. (1983). Study of the evolution of tyramine content during the vinification process. *Journal of Food Science, 48,* 417–418.

Robelin, M., & Rogers, P. J. (1998). Mood and psychomotor performance effects of the first, but not of subsequent, cup-of-coffee equivalent doses of caffeine consumed after overnight caffeine abstinence. *Behavioral Phamacology, 9,* 611–618.

Rossignol, A. M. (1985). Caffeine-containing beverages and premenstrual syndrome in young women. *American Journal of Public Health, 75,* 1335–1337.

Rossignol, A. M., & Bonnlander, H. (1990). Caffeine-containig beverages, total fluid consumption, and premenstrual syndrome. *American Journal of Public Health, 80*(9), 1106–1110.

Salfield, S. A. W., Wardley, B. L., Houlsby, W. T., Turner, S. L., Spalton, A. P., Bekles-Wilson, N.R., & Herber, S. M. (1987). Controlled study of exclusion of dietary vasoactive amines in migraine. *Archives of Disease in Childhood, 62,* 458–460.

Sandler, M., Youdim, M. B. H., & Hanington, E. (1974). A phenylethylamine oxidising defect in migraine. *Nature, 250,* 335–337.

Sargent, J., & Solbach, P. (1988). Stress and headache in the workplace: the role of caffeine. *Medical Psychotherapy, 1,* 83–86.

Saxena, P. R., & DenBoer, M. O. (1991). Pharmacology of antimigraine drugs. *Journal of Neurology, 238,* S28–S35.

Schuh, K. J., & Griffiths, R. R. (1997). Caffeine reinforcement: The role of withdrawal. *Psychopharmacology, 130,* 320–326.

Scopp, A. L. (1991). MSG and hydrolyzed vegetable protein induced headache: Review and case studies. *Headache, 31,* 107–110.

Sen, N. P. (1969). Analysis and significance of tyramine content in foods. *Journal of Food Science, 34,* 22–26.

Silverman, K., & Griffiths, R. R. (1992). Low-dose caffeine discrimination and self-reported mood effects in normal volunteers. *Journal of the Experimental Analysis of Behavior, 57,* 91–107.

Soltoft, J., Krag, B., Gudmand-Hoyer, E., Kristensen, E., & Wulff, H. R. (1976). A double-blind trial of the effect of wheat bran on symptoms of irritable bowel syndrome. *Lancet, i,* 270–272.

Speer, F. (1977). *Migraine.* Chicago: Nelson-Hall.

Spierings, E. L., Schroevers, M., Honkoop, P. C., & Sorbi, M. (1998). Presentation of chronic daily headache: A clinical study. *Headache, 38,* 191–196.

Stephenson, J. B. P. (1983). Letter. *Lancet, ii,* 1257.

Strong, F. C., III. (2000). Why do some dietary migraine patients claim they get headaches from placebos? *Clinical and Experimental Allergy, 30,* 739–743.

Udenfriend, S., Lovenberg, W., & Sjoerdsma, A. (1959). Physiologically active amines in common fruits and vegetables. *Archives of Biochemistry and Biophysics, 85,* 487–490.

Van Dusseldorp, M., & Katan, M. B. (1990). Headache caused by caffeine withdrawal among moderate coffee drinkers switched from ordinary to decaffeinated coffee: A 12 week double blind trial. *British Medical Journal, 200,* 1558–1559.

Vidaud, Z. E., Chaviano, J., Gonzales, E., & Garcia Roche, M. O. (1987). Tyramine content of some Cuban cheeses. *Die Nahrung, 31*(3), 221–224.

Weber, J. G., Ereth, M. H., Danielson, D. R., & Ilstrup, D. K. (1993). Prophylactic oral caffeine and postoperative headache. *Mayo Clinic Proceedings, 68,* 842–845.

Weber, R. W., & Vaughan, T. R. (1991). Food and migraine headache. *Immunology and Allergy Clinics of North America, 11*(4), 831–841.

Weinberger, M. W., Goodman, B. M., & Carnes, M. (1999). Long-term efficacy of nonsurgical urinary incontinence treatment in elderly women. *Journal of Gerontology A: Biological Sciences and Medical Sciences, 54,* M117–M121.

Wilson, C. W., Kirker, J. G., Warnes, H., & O'Malley, M. (1980). The clinical features of migraine as a manifestation of allergic disease. *Postgraduate Medical Journal, 56,* 617–621.

The Respiratory System
in Applied Psychophysiology

RICHARD N. GEVIRTZ

MARK S. SCHWARTZ

The respiratory system is unique among physiological systems in that it is both voluntary and involuntary. This fact probably explains the predominance of breathing in meditation and healing traditions. Practitioners very commonly use relaxed breathing therapies[1] for reducing physiological tension and arousal, and for treating a wide variety of specific symptoms and disorders. Some researchers and practitioners consider many symptoms as breathing-related (Janis, Defares, & Grossman, 1983; Lichstein, 1988; Fried, 1987a, 1993a, 1993b; Ley, 1988a, 1988b, 1992, 1993; Timmons & Ley, 1994). This view asserts that breathing in anomalous ways frequently increases the risk for developing or triggering many symptoms. Therefore, breathing therapies are essential in the treatment of patients with many different symptoms and disorders.

Those symptoms directly implicated for breathing therapies include panic, functional chest pain, and asthma. Breathing therapy is also part of the treatment of many other symptoms and disorders, including migraine headaches, hypertension, and anxiety. Practitioners use breathing therapies alone or use them in combination with other relaxation therapies, behavioral therapies, and other forms of stress management. Some authors (e.g., Janis et al., 1983) speculate that altered breathing patterns may mediate some of the positive effects of relaxation therapies and biofeedback-assisted relaxation through autonomic nervous system (ANS) changes.

In this chapter, we attempt to provide an overview of respiratory physiology in both the normal case and in cases where some form of *hyperventilation* (HV) or anomalous breathing may occur. We then review the controversy concerning *hyperventilation syndrome* (HVS) and its role in many functional disorders. This is followed by a description of breathing therapies as they are often used in applied psychophysiological treatment. (Throughout the chapter, italics on first use of a term in text indicate that the term is included in the glossary at the chapter's end.)

ANATOMY AND PHYSIOLOGY

The respiratory system is among the most complex organ systems in the body. Descriptions of the anatomy and especially the physiology of this system are provided in medical textbooks (e.g., Guyton & Hall, 1996) and in abbreviated forms in Fried (1993b) and Naifeh (1994). A practitioner of applied psychophysiology must often be able to provide a simple but comprehensive explanation for a client, and thus we offer a rationale for respiratory function that may be useful for such purposes. The reader is urged to consult more comprehensive sources for a more thorough understanding.

The job of the respiratory system is to facilitate the exchange of vital gases in the body. Oxygen is taken in through the trachea or windpipe and pumped through a vast system of increasingly smaller tubes, which have the characteristic of letting some gases through to the blood and in turn taking waste gases (mostly carbon dioxide, or CO_2) back to be exhaled. This process is called "gas exchange." This takes place in the lungs. The lungs themselves have no intrinsic muscles for breathing; instead, the diaphragm is the major muscle for breathing. It is a sheet-like muscle stretching from the backbone to the front of the rib cage that separates the chest cavity from the abdominal cavity. It forms a flexible, moving floor for the lungs. When the diaphragm is at rest, its shape is a double dome, and it extends upward into the chest under the lungs.

To start inhalation, the diaphragm contracts, flattens downward, and descends. This allows the lungs to fill. It displaces the abdominal contents, expanding the belly. The natural return of the diaphragm to its resting state occurs with exhalation. Other muscles involved in breathing include the intercostal muscles (which act on the rib cage) and the scalene muscles (which raise the chest by lifting the first and second ribs). In some cases, the muscles of the abdominal area contract to push the abdominal contents upward and push upward on the diaphragm.

In the heart–lung system, special large molecules of a substance called "hemoglobin" carry the fresh oxygen to every part of the body. We are all aware of the problems that ensue when not enough oxygen gets across the respiratory tubules called *pulmonary alveoli*. Life-threatening conditions such as emphysema can cripple the body's ability to get enough oxygen and thus diminish function markedly. The role of CO_2 is often overlooked, however. CO_2 plays an important role in how the hemoglobin releases the oxygen. As blood *pH* changes, based on breathing changes, the hemoglobin molecule releases its oxygen cargo. If too little CO_2 is present, the oxygen is overbound to the hemoglobin and not available to fuel body organ tissue.

To understand this process more clearly, consider the analogy of a milk truck trying to deliver individual bottles of milk to local stores. The oxygen is represented by the milk; the hemoglobin is the milk truck, and the store is the body tissue needing fuel to function properly. The dairy (the heart–lung system) loads the truck up with an excess of milk bottles, and the truck sets off on its appointed rounds. Once the truck arrives at the store, the cargo door must be opened wide enough to make an adequate delivery. Since CO_2 controls the release of the oxygen from the hemoglobin, it would be seen as regulating the width of the door, so that in the scheduled time enough milk can be dropped off at the store. Not enough CO_2 means an inadequate delivery and shortages. In physiology, this oxygen dissociation function is known as Bohr's Law. It says that the oxygen can be "overbound" to the hemoglobin, creating *hypoxia* or lack of oxygen, which can produce symptoms such as lightheadedness, heart pounding, cold hands, nervous emotional states, or even mental "fog." Figure 10.1 illustrates how normal cortical blood flow is interrupted by only a few minutes of HV.

HV means that the lungs are releasing too much CO_2, because breath rate and/or *tidal volume* (the amount of air that is breathed out) exceed the level needed for the present conditions. This is often referred to as "overbreathing," *hyperpnea*, or *hypocapnia*. As can be seen in Figure 10.1, the shift in blood flow to the outer shell of the brain, where most complex thought is processed, can be dramatic. In fact, HV is used as an emergency room procedure to reduce bleeding in the brain.

HV can be obvious or subtle. The image of a person who is nervous breathing rapidly in his or her upper chest and needing a paper bag is well known. But few people realize that sighing or breath holding and gasping can produce some of the same effects.

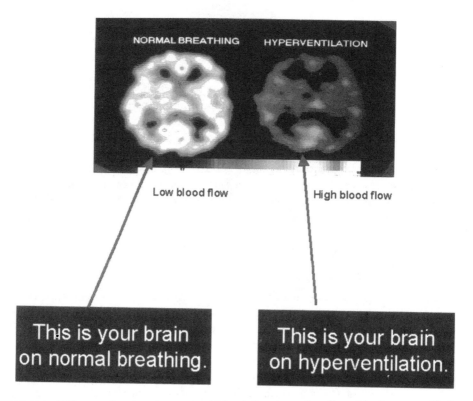

FIGURE 10.1. PET scan showing that coritcal blood flow is easily affected by hyperventiliation.

When someone overbreathes frequently, as might happen in a very stressful period, the person can create a condition in which his or her body gets used to the low level of CO_2 and maintains it with continuing sighs, yawns, and the like. When this individual slows down his or her breathing, the respiratory center in the brain may try to reestablish the previous CO_2 levels by using the sighs, yawns, or shallow breaths to blow off excess CO_2. Although this is usually not extremely dangerous, it does create a chronic condition with many potential symptoms (see Table 10.1). This chronic overbreathing is sometimes called HVS. A medical device called a "capnometer" is sometimes used to measure the amount of CO_2 in the expired (exhaled) breath. Normal levels are 40 millimeters of mercury (mm Hg) or 40 *torr*. A level under 30 mm Hg or 30 torr can be considered low.

It should now be clear that breathing patterns are a powerful force within the body, and that learning to alter these patterns can be a powerful force for change.

HYPERVENTILATION AND HYPERVENTILATION SYNDROME

Some definitions of HV focus on rapid cycles of inhaling and exhaling (*tachypnea*) and/or breathing voluminous amounts of air in each breath (*hyperpnea*). Ley (1993) asserts that one also must consider the amount of air breathed per unit of time (*minute volume*) and compare this to the person's metabolic demand for oxygen at the time. Thus, for some experts, HV is breathing beyond what the body needs to meet the immediate needs for oxygen and removal of CO_2. For others, HV is low CO_2 for any reason. Thus the physiological definition of HV is low CO_2—specifically, partial pressure of CO_2 in alveolar (lung) air (pCO_2) less than an

TABLE 10.1. Symptoms of Hyperventilation

Central neurological

Unreality
Dizziness
Faintness
Unsteady feelings
Lightheadedness
Disturbance of consciouisness
Feeling far away
Confused or dream-like feeling
Concentration impairment/trouble thinking clearly
Disturbance of vision (blurred, double vision)

Peripheral neurological

Numbness (tongue, face, hands, feet)
Coldness (general, hands or feet)
Shivering/cold shudders
Heat/warmth, feeling of (e.g., head, general)
Paresthesia (tingling) (fingers, arms, face, circumoral [around mouth], body legs, feet), pins and
   needles
Tetany (hyperexcitability of nerves and muscles, with spasms, twitching, and cramps—rare)

Musculor skeletal

Tremor (e.g., hands)
Shakiness
Tight muscles
Muscle pain (and cramps, e.g., toes, legs)
Stiffness (finger, arms, legs)
Hands tight and hard to open

Cardiovascular

Heart racing—tachycardia
Heart pounding—palpitations
Irregular heartbeat
Precordial pain (chest, over heart, lower thorax)
Raynaud's phenomenon

Gastrointestinal

Nausea
Vomiting
Diarrhea
Globus/pressure, lump, or knot in throat
Epigastric pain
Stomach feels blown up
Stomach cramps
Aerophagia

Other somatic

Dry mouth and throat
Headache
Sweating
Weakness (general)
Fatigue (general, low stamina, tires easily)

Respiratory/thoracic

Shortness of breath (while awake or from sleep)
Suffocating feeling/need for air
Unable to breathe deeply enough
Chest pain, atypical (around heart region)

(continued)

TABLE 10.1. (*continued*)

Chest tightness
Yawning
Faster or deeper breathing than normal
Sighing

Affective

Apprehension
Fear of inability to breathe
Anxiousness/nervousness
Unrest or panic feelings
Tension
Nightmares
Giddiness/feeling excited without reason
Crying fits without obvious reason

Response bias

Catarrh[a]
Drowsiness
Stinging
Choking
Earache
Ringing in ears/tinnitus

Others

Talking difficulty

Note. The data are primarily from Missri and Alexander (1978), Clark and Hemsley (1982), Lewis and Howell (1986), and Fried (1987b, 1993b).
[a]Inflamed mucous membranes and discharges in air passages of head and throat.

average of 38 torr at sea level. There is a range of values dependent on individual fitness (R. Ley, personal communication, 1996).

The implications of this for HVS, panic, relaxation-induced anxiety (RIA), and other symptoms will become clearer later in the chapter. For now, the implication is that one need not necessarily be breathing rapidly or deeply to create a state of HV. If HV lasts long enough, it can lead to "constriction of arteries of the brain and hand, increased neural excitability, increased production of lactic acid, and lowering of [the] phosphate level in arterial blood" (Garssen, deRuiter, & van Dyck, 1992, p. 142).

HVS is a variety of somatic symptoms associated with hypocapnia and induced by HV (*Dorland's Illustrated Medical Dictionary*, 1988; Lewis & Howell, 1986; see Table 10.1). Many people with HVS are unaware of their HV. They often attribute their symptoms to other causes and worry unnecessarily. Voluntary HV usually reproduces some or all of the symptoms.

A useful distinction is that between "chronic" and "acute" or "periodic" HV (Ley, 1988a, 1988b). Periodic HV is often normal as a part of reactivity to stress and physical demands. However, chronic HV is abnormal and troublesome. In addition to the variety of symptoms, it produces physiological conditions that can explain the paradoxical reactions of RIA and panic during sleep (Ley, 1988a, 1988b). Briefly, people who chronically hyperventilate are frequently in a continuous state of reduced plasma *bicarbonate* with a low level of pCO_2. Reduced plasma bicarbonate is a necessary compensatory homeostatic mechanism. This results in being near the threshold of severe hypocapnia or low alveolar CO_2. Low blood CO_2 is "hypocarbia." These are definitions and not disease states, although they may contribute to diseases. According to one view (Ley, 1988a, 1988b), when people in a chronic state of HV and low pCO_2 reduce their metabolism further during relaxation or sleep, they increase their risk of symptoms. (See the section on mechanisms for more details.)

In recent years, the concept of HVS has come under attack by many researchers. The title of one article, "Hyperventilation Syndrome: An Elegant but Scientifically Untenable Concept" (Hornsveld & Garssen, 1997), is descriptive. The criticism stems from many studies using respiratory measures with groups of patients diagnosed as having HVS. Many studies fail to see meaningful differences in respiratory rate or partial pressure of CO_2 in end-tidal breath ($ETCO_2$) in this diagnostic group, compared to normal subjects or other diagnostic groups. A debate held at the International Society for the Advancement of Respiratory Psychophysiology highlighted this controversy (Third International Society on Respiratory Psychophysiology, [ISARP] 1997). More recent work has focused on the mediational nature of respiration, without the insistence on a syndrome per se (Wilhelm, Gevirtz, & Roth, 2001).

Assessing HV

Methods for assessing HV include observations, interviews, self-report questionnaires, HV provocation, blood assays, a transcutaneous instrument that roughly estimates CO_2, and a noninvasive instrument that measures the percentage of exhaled CO_2. The last instrument is an infrared gas analyzer called a "capnometer" that can produce a "capnograph." Physiological monitoring can be done during rest and during office stress challenges. It can be performed while the patient is supine, seated, or standing.

During HV provocation, one compares the similarity of the symptoms during the provocation with the presenting complaints. Voluntary HV during provocation results in considerable individual variability of symptoms and patterns (Clark & Hemsley, 1982; see Fried, 1993b, for adverse effects, dangers, and contraindications for HV provocation).

Relying on patients to report all the symptoms is insufficient. They often do not recall or report many of the symptoms unless these are provoked in the office. Observing unprovoked breathing patterns in the office is also insufficient.

Criteria for Diagnosing HV

Criteria for diagnosing HV vary, but typically involve measures of CO_2. Physiology textbooks do not disagree, according to Fried (personal communication, March 14, 1994). It is low CO_2, less than an average of 38 torr (less than 5% $PetCO_2$, or the percentage of end-tidal CO_2) at sea level. This criteria is independent of symptoms. However, symptoms can emerge with higher and lower levels of $PetCO_2$ (Fried, 1993b). Practitioners typically focus on symptoms rather than CO_2 level. One view (Fensterheim, 1994) is that clinicians want and need to avoid failing to diagnose HV when it is present. Fensterheim also agrees with the belief of Bass and Gardner (1985) and Gardner (1994) that no symptom or clinical definition of HVS is widely accepted. Thus clinicians can be less precise than researchers, who wish to avoid including a person without HV in a group with HV, and hence must use a strict physiological criterion.

Some practitioners and researchers use a criterion of a respiration rate at rest equal to or more than a specified number of breaths per minute (b/min), such as 16. There is no universally accepted normal breathing rate. A resting breathing rate of 8–14 b/min, reported by Holloway (1994), is a commonly accepted criterion. However, there are reports of 16–17 b/min (nearly 3 b/min greater) (Tobin, Mador, Guenther, Lodato, & Sackner, 1988) for younger and older persons monitored without their awareness. Other reports suggest that men and people in their early 20s show slightly lower rates than women or older people (Qammes, Auran, Gouvernet, Delpierre, & Gimaud, 1979, as reported in Fried, 1993b). Fried (1993b) suggests a goal of "no more than 9 to 12 b/min" (p. 246) for a person at rest. He assumes normal tidal volume and pCO_2. People with organic diseases that affect respiration typically show faster respiration rates, from about 18–28 b/min (Fried, 1993b).

Therefore, using a breathing rate above 16 is a crude and insufficient criterion for HV, and one cannot rely on this. Ley (1993), Fried (1993b), and Timmons and Ley (1994) provide good discussions of this topic. For example, Ley (1993) states that even sound operational definitions are often insufficient unless they include information about the person's conditions at the time.

HV Provocation Test

The "HV provocation test" (HVPT) involves directed, intentional, and very rapid and usually deep breathing. Instructions often include something like filling the lungs with each inhalation and exhaling as completely as possible. The purpose is to reproduce the patient's symptoms and complaints as a diagnostic aid. There are cautions and criticisms, but this technique remains in common clinical practice.

Methods reported usually involve a specified breathing rate of at least 20 b/min, and sometimes as many as 60 b/min. Patients do this for a specified time of at least 60 seconds and usually 2–3 minutes. There are guidelines, but no standard protocol exists (Timmons & Ley, 1994). Howell (1990) suggests the 20 Deep Breaths Test. Folgering and Colla (1978) use "one minute of deep breathing" (Timmons & Ley, 1994, p. 218). Bonn, Readhead, and Timmons (1984) have added breathing with the upper chest and 60 b/min.

Some researchers and many practitioners rely only on the rate-and-time method. This can be very unpleasant for some patients. Therefore, practitioners sometimes stop when many of the symptoms appear. Some use a pacing device such as a fast metronome or audiotape (Salkovskis & Clark, 1990). Others also specify a percentage (e.g., 50%) drop in pCO_2 as an alternative criterion (Craske & Barlow, 1990).

One can specify a specific level of alveolar pCO_2. Criteria vary—for example, less than 19 mm Hg (19 torr) (Nixon & Freeman, 1988) to below 38 torr (Fried, 1993b). Gardner (1994) uses the criterion of "below about . . . 30 mm Hg at rest or during or after exercise, or remains low 5 minutes after voluntary over-breathing" (p. 1093). Opinions of normal pCO_2 include 38 and 40 mm Hg. There are individual differences in the level below which symptoms appear. This also always depends on other factors, such as whether the office is at sea level or at much higher altitudes. Measures of $PetCO_2$ are usually sea-level measures. The measurement drops as altitude increases because of decreased air pressure at higher altitudes; $PetCO_2$ is a percentage of CO_2 relative to air pressure in the surrounding environment. $PetCO_2$ is less at higher altitudes and in cities such as Denver.

Some consider a patient's awareness of the similarity of naturally occurring symptoms to HVPT-induced symptoms as "the most important element in the diagnosis of HVS" (Garssen et al., 1992, pp. 149–150; see also Lewis & Howell, 1986). However, studies of this criterion are rare. In the few studies available, "the response to the HVPT does not predict the occurrence of HV during panic attacks" (Garssen et al., 1992, p. 150). This review summarized studies that concluded there was no difference between the recognized symptoms typical for HV during the HVPT and to those occurring during a stressful time-pressured task without decreased $PetCO_2$. One should read Ley's (1993) comments about these studies and the Garssen et al. (1992) review. Ley is more favorable about the HVPT. However, he points out that the absence of an HVPT effect does not mean that a patient does not have a HV-related problem.

Garssen et al. (1992) note that although some patients recognize symptoms during an HVPT, CO_2 does not always drop during ambulatory monitoring of panic. He is referring to the study by Hibbert and Pilsbury (1989), who used a transcutaneous estimate of the partial pressure of CO_2 ($p_{tc}CO_2$). Furthermore, this study concluded that some patients do not recognize the provoked symptoms. These include patients who show large drops in $p_{tc}CO_2$ during panic. One interpretation is that panic can cause HV, rather than HV always causing panic. The transcutaneous method is slow in showing changes that usually occur for each breath. Thus some practitioners and researchers who have tried it have not found it useful, especially for office assessments.

In a study with nonclinical subjects, Huey and West (1983) avoided raising expectations of anxiety and avoided using the term "hyperventilation" in the instructions to overbreathe. Nevertheless, HV led to more symptoms than during a modified overbreathing technique that avoided hypocapnia. They called the technique the *isocapnic overventilation technique (IOT)*. It artificially prevents lowered PetCO$_2$ during HV by using a mixture of air enriched with CO$_2$. Under these conditions, the patients did not differ from subjects who were not over-breathing. This supports the HVS explanation.

One view is that HV is a necessary factor for most of the somatic symptoms associated with HVS, but is not sufficient for panic symptoms. For example, cognitive factors are also necessary, according to Garssen et al. (1992). Thus cognitive therapy is necessary for treatment. Ley (1992) agrees with this for a subset of patients.

A problem is that HVPT does not always evoke the symptoms in question for a specific person. For example, chest pain is not easy to reproduce. Other views are critical about the role of HV for panic and the value of HVPT as the only or best criterion. For example, stressful mental tasks with only small decreases in alveolar CO$_2$ can also evoke HVS symptoms (Garssen et al., 1992). However, the decreases in PetCO$_2$ were 1.2 mm Hg. Furthermore, a mental task of thinking about various stressful topics led to HV and decreased pCO$_2$[2] among more subjects (33/54, or 61%) than did the HVPT (7/54, or 13%) (Nixon & Freeman, 1988).

Some practitioners (Fried, 1993b) are far more cautious about HVPT. Fried considers it hazardous and recommends against this procedure. However, he provides no exceptions and guidelines about when it may be acceptable. He is cautious partly because he is a nonphysician. He is very concerned about inducing changes in blood acid–*base* balance, coronary and cerebral vasoconstriction, and ischemic hypoxia. This is worrisome to him, as it should be to everyone, because a patient could have an undiscovered and undiagnosed organic disease that places the patient at risk. For example, the patient with diagnosed "functional chest symptoms" might turn out to have an organic cardiac disease for which induced biochemical and cardiovascular changes increase the risks. However, he adds that "in fairness to my colleagues . . . a number of them use the procedure and have reported no consequent ill effects in their clients" (p. 42).

Compernolle, Hoogduin, and Joele (1979) caution against using voluntary HV with patients with chronic anemia or vascular diseases. They refer to loss of consciousness and fatal accidents when HV is followed by breath holding during underwater swimming and diving competition (Hill, 1973; Craig, 1976). Neurological impairment and fatal accidents have also occurred following HV in children with sickle cell anemia (Allen, Imbus, Powars, & Haywood, 1976). However, aside from the examples cited, Compernolle et al. (1979) noted "nothing in the literature to substantiate the fear that provoking hyperventilation may be dangerous. There are no reports of accidents resulting from two to five minutes of hyperventilation followed by breathing into a bag" (p. 616).

Prudent practitioners are extra cautious with people at risk for syncope. Causes for syncope include certain cardiovascular, metabolic, or neurological disorders, such as seizures. Remember that hypocapnia-induced vasoconstriction from HV reduces cerebral blood flow (Berkow & Fletcher, 1992). Thus caution is necessary for many elderly patients and those with compromised cerebral blood flow. The clinician should also be aware that many organic medical conditions can cause HV (Gardner, 1994). Thus practitioners must be very careful lest they provoke unintended and potentially risky symptoms. For example, even psychologically distressed patients who hyperventilate as a result of habit and anxiety can also have diabetes. Induced HV may affect or at least interact with blood glucose (Guthrie, Moeller, &

Guthrie, 1983; Lum, 1994; Lum, 1995). If blood glucose is very low because of poorly controlled diabetes, induced HV can add to the acidosis and intensify symptoms.

Nonmedical practitioners and researchers who believe they need to use the HVPT or intend to do so for other clinical or research reasons must get medical clearance. This is crucial particularly in patients with a history of respiratory, cardiovascular, or some neurological diseases. For example, a history of or evidence for coronary artery disease or unexplained chest pain raises clear caution.

A related caution stems from the potential for some patients to self-initiate breath holding or the "Valsalva maneuver"[3] to abort symptoms, including those from HVS and panic. Quiet breath holding combined with irregular breathing is a pattern associated with just as many problems as the obvious HV pattern (Holloway, 1994). There is one report (Sartory & Olajide, 1988) of the use of the Valsalva maneuver as a potential treatment for panic symptoms. Physicians suggest using the Valsalva to abort paroxysmal atrial tachycardia for selected patients. Such information may encourage patients to try these without proper consultation. For example, the case reported by Rapee (1985) began aborting her panic symptoms by holding her breath without instructions to do so. In most people, these attempts are not dangerous, but one must be cautious and complete in patient education instructions.

In some weight lifters, "hyperventilation before lifting causes hypocapnia, cerebral vasoconstriction, and peripheral vasodilation" (Berkow & Fletcher, 1992, p. 432). The lifting involves the Valsalva maneuver, which affects blood return to the heart, reducing cardiac output and altering CO_2 levels. Potentially, systemic vasodilation and decreased blood pressure may occur, increasing the risk of syncope for some people engaged in similar activities.

Although for most people the risks do not exist, there are enough reasons to be very cautious and obtain approval from a qualified physician. Prudent practitioners, especially nonmedical ones, may decide to avoid the procedure unless it is absolutely necessary to make a diagnosis or to convince a patient of the diagnosis.

Exclusion Diagnoses and Organic Causes of HV

Prudent practitioners consider the many medical disorders (Gardner, 1994) for which altered breathing and symptoms can be expected. This underscores the importance of an appropriate medical examination and tests before one concludes that a patient's symptoms are the result of HV. This does not eliminate the role of breathing therapies totally, but it does raise cautions about diagnosis and therapy procedures. Readers may find a partial list of such conditions useful. Examples of drugs that can cause HV are salicylate compounds (e.g., aspirin) and stimulants such as caffeine, nicotine, and amphetamines. Examples of diseases are hepatic (liver) and renal failure, even mild asthma, interstitial lung diseases, and various pulmonary and vascular diseases. Focal lesions of the respiratory centers of the brainstem constitute another example. See medical texts for further discussion of this topic.

SYMPTOMS OF HV

Consulting different references results in differences in the lists of HV symptoms. The list in Table 10.1 contains symptoms reported by at least some patients diagnosed with HVS, and thought to be associated with HVS. Obviously, patients do not present most of these symptoms, and many of them do not differentiate between people with HVS and those without HVS.

Nevertheless, this list alerts or reminds practitioners about the scope of symptoms associated with HV. It reflects the complexity of making the HVS diagnosis. It may also serve as a source for patient education. It is useful to divide the list into areas, although there is over-lap. Several of the specific symptoms could be placed under different headings.

Such lists presumably imply that the symptoms stem from HV. However, many symptoms often accompany HV and could result from other physiological and cognitive events that often coexist with HV (Clark, Salkovskis, & Chalkley, 1985; Garssen et al., 1992).

According to this view, cognitive factors can increase the risk of developing HV and HV-related symptoms. This can occur after other causes for physiological arousal and the onset of other symptoms. For example, anticipation of symptoms, perceptions of lack of control over symptoms or feelings of helplessness, and a lack of understanding of symptom origin can increase the risk of developing various symptoms and HV.

All practitioners should remember that many of these symptoms also accompany medical and neurological disorders as well as other stress disorders. Diagnosis is by exclusion as well as inclusion.

SYMPTOMS, DISORDERS, MECHANISMS, AND BREATHING THERAPY

Symptoms and disorders for which relaxed breathing therapy is part of the treatment plan include HVS, functional chest pain, panic, and the combination of panic and functional chest pain. We also include a discussion of RIA in this section. See other chapters of this volume for the use of breathing therapies for menopausal hot flushes, hypertension, and other symptoms.

Hyperventilation Syndrome

There is a surprising paucity of studies using breathing therapies alone for HVS. Reports and studies of breathing therapy alone for HVS do show clinically significant reductions of HVS symptoms (Grossman, De Swart, & Defares, 1985; Fried, 1993b; Timmons & Ley, 1994). However, methodological problems and equivocal results of studies detract from firm conclusions. Studies of cognitive restructuring, relaxation, breathing, feedback for respiration rate, and patient education indicate that these approaches also lead to significant improvements (Bass, 1994; Ley, 1994). Although, using breathing therapies alone for HVS remains a logical and sound approach, practitioners probably will continue to combine breathing therapy with good patient education, other relaxation procedures, and cognitive approaches. The specific need for biofeedback-assisted breathing therapy (e.g., respiration rate, diaphragmatic breathing, CO_2 feedback, and volumetric feedback) also remains logical, although unsubstantiated. Psychophysiological measurements and feedback are valuable at least for therapist information, documentation, and information for patient motivation and confirmation.

Functional Chest Pain and Functional "Cardiac" Symptoms

There are many patients with noncardiac chest pain. Often there is no objective or probable organic cardiac pathology explaining these symptoms. One correctly assumes that psychophysiological factors play a role in these symptoms for many patients (Clouse, 1992; Hegel, Abel, Etscheidt, Cohen-Cole, & Wilmer, 1989). However, chest pain associated with symptomatic HV is not "psychogenic" in the sense of being purely cognitive in origin. There are physical reasons, albeit often psychophysiological ones. Muscle tension, spasm, and fatigue in the intercostal muscles constitute one such mechanism (Bass, Gardner, & Jackson, 1994). Many physicians refer to this musculoskeletal explanation as "chest wall pain."

Some physicians suggest that a distended stomach caused by aerophagia places excess pressure on the diaphragm and can cause chest pain (Bass et al., 1994). Diaphragmatic spasms may create chest symptoms. For some, esophageal involvement contributes to these symptoms (Clouse, 1992). Here too psychophysiological factors often play a role, as noted by Drossman et al. (1990). This international panel of clinical investigators provided a preliminary consensus report of functional gastrointestinal disorders. Included among these disorders was "functional chest pain of presumed oesophageal origin" (Drossman et al., 1990, p. 163)—that is, "midline chest pain with or without dysphagia for at least three months; and no evidence for oesophagitis, cardiac or other disease to explain symptoms" (p. 163). Although esophageal disorders are common in these "chest" symptoms, the authors recognized the etiological potential for psychological factors.

One also must consider reduced blood flow to the heart (Fried, 1993b); HV can trigger paroxysmal vasospasms in the heart (and the brain). The effects of HV on cardiac functioning are not in question. They are real and accepted by all experts. In fact, HV and high arousal contribute to many occurrences of cardiac symptoms of organic origin, such as angina pectoris and infarction (Nixon, 1989; Fried, 1993b).

However, a question of clinical significance for practitioners is whether the cardiac changes with HV indicate an organic cardiac diagnosis. They often do not. Saying that breathing changes and thoughts affect various parts of the brain does not mean that a patient has an organic brain disorder.

Another question of clinical significance is whether there are noncardiac reasons to explain functional chest pain that may appear to patients (and practitioners) as having a cardiac origin. The answer is yes. There are musculoskeletal, diaphragm-related, and esophagus-related causes often stimulated and provoked by psychophysiological factors. Many people are hypervigilant and focus on their bodily sensations more keenly than is needed or desired. These people attribute dire causes to sensations and symptoms that are within the range of normal physiological sensations and events, or at least not at all dangerous. Such attributions can result in cognitive anxiety and worry, as well as in physical musculoskeletal tension and ANS arousal. These in turn can lead to or accompany the physical changes that produce the chest symptoms.

Treatments of potential value include psychopharmacological therapy, such as low-dose antidepressants (Clouse, 1992); cognitive therapy (Salkovskis, 1992); behavioral therapies, similar to those for chronic pain (Bradley, Richter, Scarinci, Haile, & Schan, 1992); and breathing therapies (DeGuire, Gevirtz, Kawahara, & Maguire, 1992; DeGuire, Gevirtz, Hawkinson, & Dixon, 1996; see also the review by Garssen et al., 1992). There are no studies of the combination of these therapies, and no comparisons among the therapies.

This chapter focuses on the study by DeGuire et al. (1992), in which breathing therapies and patient education led to significantly reduced symptoms among patients with functional cardiac symptoms who showed signs of HV. Patients received one of three breathing therapies: (1) without physiological feedback, (2) with visual biofeedback from thoracic and abdominal strain gauges, or (3) with ETCO$_2$ feedback. A control group receiving no therapy was also studied. Therapy common to all patients in the three treated groups consisted of the following:

1. Verbal patient education about respiratory physiology and the hypothesized effect of HV on functional cardiac symptoms.
2. Instructions for diaphragmatic breathing, and the therapist's demonstration of diaphragmatic breathing.
3. Office practice and correction of errors.
4. Encouragement to endure, and reassurance about the expected decline of the discomfort of slow diaphragmatic breathing often reported by patients.

5. Encouragement to avoid increasing tidal volume or amount of air inhaled to compensate for changes in rate of respiration.
6. Encouragement of a slow-paced rate of respiration (less than 14 b/min).[4]
7. Encouragement to practice this during conversations and while visualizing situations in which patients were having problems maintaining the new breathing.

In the two conditions that included feedback, physiological monitoring and feedback typically occurred in later sessions.

Several criteria for improvement included the number of days with symptoms and the frequency of cardiac symptoms. Patients completed self-reported ratings of symptom frequency and severity. There were six treatment sessions over 3 weeks. The study partly based improvement on symptom changes between a 2-week baseline and the 2 weeks after treatment. The three breathing therapy groups reduced the days on which symptoms occurred from 8–10 of 14 days down to 4–5 of 14 days. The control group showed no drop from 10 of 14 days with symptoms.

The treated groups reduced their frequency of cardiac symptoms from an average of 21 symptoms (range 15–25) down to about 9 (range 4–15). All three groups showed reduced symptoms compared to the control group, which did not change. The three treatment groups dropped from 23 to 4, from 15 to 9, and from 25 to 15 symptoms after treatment, respectively (compared to the control group, which only went from 27 to 26 symptoms). The authors note that they did not measure duration of symptoms, and that this resulted in underestimating the effect. For example, some patients recorded one episode of chest pain all day and others episodic mild pain. They thus appeared to show increased symptoms rather than improvement, which would be a more accurate interpretation. Reduced respiratory rate and increased $ETCO_2$ also occurred. Respiratory rate dropped from 15–18 to 8–9 b/min. compared to the control group, which showed no change from 15 b/min.

The breathing therapies led to $ETCO_2$ increases. They started with 34–38 torr and increased to 39 to 41 torr, showing a more normal level of CO_2. Reduction of cardiac symptoms and increased $ETCO_2$ occurred to a greater extent among those with reduced breathing rate. The reduced respiration rate correlated with reduced frequency of symptoms ($r = .53$, $p < .001$), number of days with symptoms ($r = .59$, $p < .001$), and increased $ETCO_2$ ($r = .38$, $p = .018$). DeGuire et al. (1992) note that, "the use of end-tidal CO_2, abdominal and thoracic strain gauge monitors did not add significantly to either reducing the frequency of cardiac symptoms or facilitating changes in physiology" (p. 676).

However, there was a trend for patients using strain gauge monitors with computer-based visual biofeedback to produce the largest effect. The authors caution that the extent to which physiological feedback information added to the new attributions about symptoms is unclear. The presence of mitral valve prolapse did not detract at all from the success of these subjects.

In a follow-up study, 40% of the patients (representative of the entire sample) were contacted again 3 years later. Symptom reductions were maintained or improved. Similarly, $ETCO_2$ and respiration rate measures stayed in the normal range (DeGuire et al., 1996).

Practitioners should consider including breathing therapies for patients diagnosed with functional chest pain and functional cardiac symptoms. However, functional chest symptoms and HVS are not synonymous (Bass, 1994). These authors also remind us that HV only provokes chest pain in less than half the patients assessed. Using breathing therapy for these patients is logical, considering the successful use of this therapy for many patients with panic symptoms and the frequency of panic symptoms among these patients (see below).

We can also note the potential benefit of relaxation therapies with breathing therapy during cardiac rehabilitation for patients after myocardial infarctions (van Dixhoorn, Duivenvoorden, Staal, Pool, & Verhage, 1987; van Dixhoorn & Duivenvoorden, 1989; Duivenvoorden & van Dixhoorn, 1991). They report fewer second-coronary events, rehospitalizations, unstable angina episodes, and other serious cardiac events. van Dixhoorn (1992, 1993, 1994) presents variations of breathing therapy that emphasize attentional states and total body involvement.

In a 1999 study, van Dixhoorn and Duivenvoorden randomly assigned 156 patients with myocardial infarction to a standard physical training or to the same training with a breathing awareness and retraining therapy (six sessions). The breathing group failed physical testing less often, returned to work more often, lowered respiration rates, increased cardiac variability, and had fewer cardiac events at a 2-year follow-up. Seventeen of 76 patients had a significant reinfarction (5 died) in the breathing group, while 29 of 80 experienced a similar poor outcome in the exercise-only group (7 died). The breathing group had fewer hospitalizations and lower medical costs as well. These data are consistent with other trials around the world (Blumenthal et al., 1997; Patel et al., 1985).

Relaxation-Induced Anxiety

RIA is the paradoxical arousal response that a small percentage of people experience during various relaxation procedures. HV as a cause of RIA seems contradictory, but there are logic and support for this. The assumption and hypothesis of excess hypocapnia occurring during relaxation together constitute one possible explanation for RIA. This phenomenon appears to occur mostly in people who often hyperventilate. However, this explanation cannot and does not account for all RIA, as one realizes from the detailed discussions of RIA by M. S. Schwartz, Schwartz, and Monastra in Chapter 12 of this volume, and by Ley (1988b). However, HV may be a factor for some or many such people. Thus practitioners should consider this during evaluation and treatment with relaxation therapies.

Panic

Breathing therapy constitutes a basic part of current treatments for many patients with panic symptoms and panic disorder. The debate continues as to whether HV causes panic or merely accompanies it in some patients with panic symptoms. Ley (1993) is a prolific, tenacious, and persuasive advocate of the role of HV in panic and the necessity of breathing therapy for these patients (see Ley, 1987, 1988a, 1988b, 1991, 1992). Contrary views by Garssen et al. (1992), Clark and his colleagues (Salkovskis & Clark, 1990), and Barlow and his colleagues (Barlow, 2002) provide balance and perspective. Ley's (1992, 1993) proposal helps resolve some differences in opinion.

Some studies report more benefit from respiratory control with exposure to situations in which symptoms occur, compared to only exposure without breathing therapy. However, breathing therapy often leads to mixed results, whether or not one includes cognitive components. This contrary view is that "recent studies do not support the idea that HV is an important causal mechanism in producing panic attacks" (Garssen et al., 1992, p. 149). Rather, HV accompanies panic in some patients with panic, according to this view. Garssen et al. (1992) conclude that methodology problems make for impossible interpretations and conclusions for the specific role of breathing therapy. Examples of problems include combining therapies, very small samples, and lack of controls. The specificity and mechanism of breathing therapy are unclear and elusive.

> The majority of the studies point to a therapeutic effect of breathing retraining and cognitive reattribution of physical symptoms to hyperventilation for patients suffering HVS and the closely related panic disorder with or without agoraphobia. . . . The conclusion seems warranted that both . . . [treatments] help alleviate anxiety in patients with HVS or related disorders. (Garssen et al., 1992, pp. 148–149)

However, Ley (1992, 1993) provides a studious resolution to the disagreement about the relationship of HV and panic. He has proposed three types of panic attacks (Ley, 1992). He calls the classic panic attack "Type I" or "Classic PA." He distinguishes this from "Anticipatory PA (Type II)" and "Cognitive PA (Type III)." Type I has distinctive and objective physiological features, especially compared to Type III. These features are (1) sharp drops in pCO_2 (>10 mm Hg), (2) sharp increases in respiration rate and/or tidal volume, (3) sharp increases in heart rate (>10 beats per minute), (4) sharp increases in electrodermal activity, and (5) low finger temperature (<80°F. Two more recent studies support this position. Biber and Alkin (1999) divided 51 patients diagnosed with panic disorder into two groups: those with predominantly respiratory symptoms, and others. The respiratory group had more sensitivity to inhaled CO_2, scored higher on panic and anxiety scales, and had longer duration of illness. Moynihan and Gevirtz (2001) divided patients with panic disorder by symptoms as described above and compared the respiratory group with the cognitive group on a number of respiratory parameters, during various conditions. As expected, the respiratory group had lower $ETCO_2$ (especially during a stressor) and more rapid respiratory rates.

Ley (1992, 1993) suggests that practitioners should expect the most benefit from breathing therapy for patients with Type I symptoms and expect the most benefit from cognitive therapies for Type III. One should read at least these two references to appreciate his position. A discussion of the proposed relationship between HV and panic is considered in a later section of this chapter.

Panic and Functional Chest Pain

Panic symptoms occur in many patients with unexplained or functional chest pain (Beitman, 1992) and among patients with unexplained cardiac symptoms in some cardiac care units (Carter et al., 1992). Another study found that patients with panic disorder reported more panic symptoms than patients with chest pain but no coronary artery disease (Beck, Berisford, Taegtmeyer, & Bennitt, 1990). However, both groups reported similar severity of "chest pain, dyspnea, paresthesias, and fear of having a heart attack" (p. 249).

Respiratory Mechanisms in Panic

Recently, a group of researchers at Stanford University has used more advanced technologies (including ambulatory measures) to elucidate the respiratory mechanisms in panic disorder (Wilhelm, Gevirtz, et al., 2001). Since the evidence for HV as a cause of panic is equivocal, they have examined a broader range of systems and have looked at recovery more closely. They have found that $ETCO_2$ recovers more slowly in patients with panic disorders than in patients with social phobia or normal subjects; that sighing is more frequent in patients with panic disorder (Wilhelm, Trabert & Roth, 2001a, 2001b; Roth, Wilhelm, & Trabert, 1998a, 1998b); and that patients with panic disorder exhibited more instability of ambulatory measured tidal volume. Together, these studies point to some instability in the cardiorespiratory system in panic.

Based on these findings, the emphasis here is on Ley's and related views. Whether entirely valid or not, this view has both good logic and support. HV is probably an important factor and therefore is a cornerstone in the rationale for this chapter.

First, let us follow Ley's line of thinking. If we assume constant metabolism, significantly increased volumes[5] of air inhaled (and exhaled) can lead to an excessive loss of CO_2. This results in the sensations that typify many panic attacks. Ley states that even a person's metabolism attempting to compensate, by increasing the CO_2 level, does not keep up with the effects from the increased volumes of air (Ley, 1987, 1988a, 1988b). Thus hypocapnia can occur despite the body's attempt to regain balance and a desired level of CO_2.

People with chronic and severe HV maintain low levels of CO_2 in their blood and normal blood pH. The low level of CO_2 is only slightly above the threshold of nonspecific sensations produced by hypocapnia. The lowered CO_2 from HV increases the pH. It moves the pH toward alkalinity and away from a normal pH of 7.4.[6] The kidneys compensate for this by excreting bicarbonate to lower the pH, and thus produce normal pH despite the low CO_2.

However, there is a problem for people who chronically hyperventilate. That is, there is a physiological lag between metabolic regulation of CO_2 and the breathing regulation of it. As Ley (1988a) reminds us, "breathing is a slave to metabolism" (p. 255). Thus decreases in metabolism lag behind the decreases in respiration. The reverse is true as well.

Relaxation reduces metabolic demands. However, the temporal lag in the respiratory adjustment produces a temporary drop in CO_2 and a rise in pH (respiratory *alkalosis*). This depends on the degree and rate of decreased metabolism. These people cannot easily adjust to the sudden difference. They do not adjust well to the lag between respiratory changes and the metabolic production of CO_2. Thus it takes less overbreathing to reach a low level of CO_2 in these people than in asymptomatic people who maintain a normal CO_2 level at rest. When symptomatic people overbreathe, CO_2 drops further, and depleted *bicarbonate buffers* cannot compensate fast enough. The kidneys control a small part of the acid–base balance, but most is mediated by the lungs. When a person sits or reclines to relax, the metabolic production of CO_2 can suddenly drop. If the volumes of air remain steady, there is an increase in the intensity of sensations of hypocapnia and in symptoms of panic or HV.

Exercise

Ley (1988a) also states that there are other situations when metabolism drops and when volumes of air inhaled per minute are steady or increase. He cites the common example of abruptly stopping somewhat vigorous exercise. This assumes that the person does not also voluntarily and rapidly reduce the volume of air per minute.

Exercise leads to a rise of CO_2 and decreased pH, into the acid range (respiratory *acidosis*). Thus CO_2 is higher and pH is lower during exercise. The degree of these shifts depends on the degree and rate of the metabolism increases. When the person who chronically hyperventilates stops the exercise, the problem develops. The metabolic production of CO_2 drops. The lag in respiratory adjustment also adds to the fall in CO_2 and creates a temporary state of elevated pH (respiratory alkalosis). The degree of this depends on the degree and rate of metabolic decrease. Part of the problem occurs because people who chronically hyperventilate typically overbreathe longer than others after stopping the required overbreathing during exercise. Combining the overbreathing from exercise and that from their chronic breathing habit causes larger drops in CO_2. This leads to hypocapnia and potentially to panic. The problems develop after the stimulation rather than during it. This reasoning could account for the finding that patients with panic symptoms often avoid exercise and excitement (Ley, 1988a).

Habituation and/or Homeostatic Changes in Electrolytes and Blood Gases

Some investigators observe that panic symptoms often become less pronounced during persisting and clinically significant hypocapnia; at least, this was true of the nonpatients studied by van den Hout, De Jong, Zandbergen, and Merckelbach (1990). Van den Hout et al. speculate that this may be the result of a "special case of habituation" (p. 447), as the symptoms lose their novelty over time. However, this explanation may have less application to clinical patients who continue to worry about their symptoms.

Another view involves a physiological explanation for the gradual reduction and cessation of some sensations that often accompany HV and panic. These sensations include *paresthesia*, dizziness, and depersonalization. This view has more relevance for clinical practice.

Briefly, van den Hout et al. (1990) suggest that internal and natural biological changes occur and cause changes in internal feedback. These changes alter the sensations that often lead to anxiety and more HV. This explanation focuses on natural and homeostatic changes in calcium and potassium that affect changes in paresthesia, and changes in bicarbonate and pH that result in dizziness and a sense of depersonalization. This view states that despite continued very low CO_2, there are compensatory mechanisms that change the body's electrolytes (calcium and potassium). These changes can result in decreased symptoms or cessation of some symptoms in less than an hour in some people.

This view does not negate the hypocapnic explanation for the onset of symptoms. However, it suggests that physiological stabilization and homeostasis often occur in about 30–90 minutes, and this reduces symptoms. Interventions may need to work in less time to show their specific therapeutic value.

Chronic versus Acute or Periodic HV

It is crucial to distinguish between "chronic" HV and "acute" or "periodic" HV, to understand the mechanisms underlying many of the symptoms discussed in this chapter. Chronic HV is hypothesized to produce a "steady state of diminished plasma bicarbonate" (Ley, 1988a, p. 257). One expects all patients who chronically exhibit HV to show many classic symptoms. These include "breathlessness, other respiratory complaints, low pCO_2 but normal pH, dizziness, low finger temperature, nausea, fatigue, malaise, dry mourh, and frequent micturation" (Ley, 1988a, p. 258). Relaxation during periods of HV results in reduced metabolism. However, without reduced ventilation, the increased intensity in hypocapnia produces the unpleasant, anxiogenic effects of respiratory alkalosis. The implication is that one does not expect the effects during relaxation and related conditions for people who periodically hyperventilate.

Breathing Therapy as a Treatment for Panic

Whatever the mechanism, breathing therapy has been shown to be an effective treatment mode for panic. Earlier studies indicated its effectiveness, but lacked adequate controls to isolate the breathing component (Rapee, 1985; Hibbert & Chan, 1989). Berger and Gevirtz (2001) recently compared a standard cognitive protocol to eight sessions of breathing therapy and found the two treatments equivalent on all measures except depression (where the cognitive therapy seemed to have an advantage). On the other hand, a recent study by Schmidt et al. (2000) tried to "dismantle" the breathing component within a cognitive therapy protocol, and found groups with and without breathing therapy to be equivalent. They concluded that "specific components of these protocols, such as respiratory-control techniques, are extraneous" (p. 423). Future research is needed to resolve this question.

PROPOSED MECHANISMS OF ACTION FOR BREATHING THERAPY

Historical-Interest Views

Calming Effect of Air from Nasal Inhalations

An old idea of historical interest is that warming and humidifying inhaled air through the nose exerts a soothing function (Ballentine, 1976, cited in Lichstein, 1988, p. 35). This view suggests that the airflow through the nasal passages stimulate nerve endings, and that this has a calming effect.

Yoga masters instruct trainees to alternate nostrils. One belief is that this results in shifts in cerebral lateral dominance (Chandra, 1994; Backon, 1989). Another interpretation of the calming effect is that breathing through the nose (or pursed lips, as discussed below) slows ventilation. The airways are smaller and offer more resistance (R. Ley, personal communication, March 23, 1994; Baretti, 1994). Fried (1993b) agrees and points out that "one cannot easily hyperventilate when breathing through the nose" (p. 238).

Calming Effect of Vagal Stimulation and Parasympathic Dominance via Nasal Breathing and Diaphragm Movements

The second view of historical interest suggests that in breathing therapy the regularity of the diaphragm's motion and/or of the lungs' actions causes the abdominal contents to stimulate the vagus nerve gently. This promotes increased parasympathetic functioning (Hirai, 1975, Ajaya, 1976; and Rama, 1979—all cited in Lichstein, 1988). See the review by Lichstein (1988), who notes that this view is "plausible but unvalidated" (Lichstein, 1988, p. 353).

Contemporary Views

Contemporary views involve CO_2 changes or cognitive changes. The CO_2 view is the dominant one.

Carbon Dioxide

Briefly, part of CO_2 passes out in each exhalation. The blood must maintain a certain level of CO_2 for regulating bodily processes such as blood pH, and for stimulating automatic or involuntary respiration.

When the level of CO_2 is too high, the resulting condition is *hypercapnia*. This has important implications for relaxation. Insufficient breathing increases the CO_2 level. *Hypoventilation* leads to elevated arterial CO_2—that is, hypercapnia. Breath holding for several seconds (e.g., 5–10) and shallow, slow breathing producing hypoventilation are two common examples of how people create mild hypercapnia. The first increases the CO_2 much faster.

Mild hypercapnia occurs from an increase of only about 10%. It starts a complex central and peripheral body process with several effects. These include slowing heart rate, dilation of peripheral vasculature, stimulation of gastric secretions, depressed cortical activity, and global sensation of mild somnolence (Lichstein, 1988, pp. 36–37; Ley, 1988a). This normally occurs in the transitions from wakefulness to drowsiness to sound sleep (Lichstein, 1988; Naifeh, Kamiya, & Sweet, 1982).

Too much breathing is too much of a good thing. As noted earlier, hypocapnia means not enough CO_2 in the blood. This brings us to HV, or too much breathing. Ley (1988a, 1988b, 1993) asserts that hypocapnia occurs when the total amount of air breathed exceeds the metabolic needs of the body. Breathing with more than the number of breaths needed at a particular time (respiration rate) and/or taking in larger volumes of air than needed (tidal volume) per minute (minute volume) reduces the CO_2 in the blood.

Hypocapnia also involves increased pH or the alkalinity level of the blood. The kidneys automatically compensate by excreting bicarbonate (base), which in turn helps maintains the pH balance. In essence, this model suggests that when a person breathes too much air and does so too often, it creates a chronically altered level of pCO_2. This gives rise to increased risk for HV symptoms when CO_2 drops further during rapid, deep breathing or during relaxation and sleep.

Cognitive Views

There are two models of how cognitive activity could be the active process explaining how breathing therapy reduces symptoms. We refer to these as "cognitive diversion" and "cognitive restructuring."

Cognitive Diversion. The first view proposes that shifting attention away from worrisome, annoying, irritating, and similar thoughts results in a temporary, although incomplete, reduction of anxiety. This process is inherent in all relaxation therapies (Lichstein, 1988; Rosenthal, 1980). One explanation of how relaxation procedures are successful for helping people with sleep-onset insomnia is that they divert attention from cognitive activity that contributes to the patient's staying awake. That does not mean that relaxation procedures have no physiological relaxation properties that are necessary for some patients. The cognitive explanation for how relaxation procedures help facilitate sleep onset means that for some patients, cognitive activity is probably more important than physiological tension and arousal for maintaining wakefulness. Furthermore, cognitive activity often has arousal properties. For these people, relaxation procedures that successfully divert attention away from this cognitive activity help reduce the latency to sleep onset.

As Lichstein (1988) states, "breath manipulations fill our mind with unprovocative content . . . like any other emotionally neutral act capable of consuming attention" (p. 38). If this is true, then "more difficult or complex breathing patterns that naturally command more careful attention should prove to be more powerful relaxation techniques" (Hirai, 1975, cited in Lichstein, 1988, p. 38). There is some indirect support, albeit incomplete, for this hypothesis (Worthington & Martin, 1980, cited in Lichstein, 1988, p. 38). Many Eastern and Western relaxation procedures (e.g., breath meditation, breath mindfulness, yoga, Zen, Benson's relaxation response, autogenic training, and Jacobson's progressive muscle relaxation) focus on or include breathing. The reader is referred to Lichstein (1988) for an extensive discussion of this topic.

Cognitive Restructuring. Another cognitive model focuses on the anticipation of symptoms and cognitive beliefs or attributions about the symptoms. These cognitions can increase the risk of developing HV after physiological activation (see Garssen et al., 1992). For example, many people feel helpless and believe that they have no control over their symptoms. They often lack understanding of the origin of the symptoms and attribute them to a serious disease. They often anticipate symptoms and engage in the type of cognitive activity that results in physiological arousal and some symptoms. Therefore, according to this model, these cognitions can increase the risk of developing HV after physiological activation.

Cognitive therapies include cognitive reattribution of the symptoms to HV rather than to a serious disease. Therapy also involves developing beliefs of self-efficacy and control over the symptoms. The implication is that patient education and cognitive-behavioral therapies can be useful and sometimes essential parts of therapy. Breathing therapies often provide immediate relief, and relief can lead to cognitive restructuring that helps prevent future arousal and symptoms.

For a practitioner, it may not matter whether a patient's improvement is the result of practicing corrected breathing regularly, the diversion properties of relaxed breathing, altered cognitions, or a combination of these. For that matter, it may not matter to many patients. Prudent practitioners include both the physiological and cognitive components.

BREATHING THERAPY TECHNIQUES: NON-INSTRUMENTATION-BASED/NONFEEDBACK AND PROPOSED MECHANISMS

There are several types of breathing therapy techniques that are used without psychophysiological monitoring and biofeedback. These include slow diaphragmatic breathing, paced respiration, breath meditation/breath mindfulness, rebreathing, and pursed-lip breathing (PLB) (Berkow & Fletcher, 1992, p. G32).

Slow Diaphragmatic Breathing

Slow diaphragmatic breathing is a very common technique used by practitioners. In fact, it probably is the most common. Using it, one teaches the patient to breathe with the diaphragm and to minimize or stop the use of mid- to high-chest and accessory breathing muscles (e.g., shoulder raising). One standard goal is slowing respiration to about 6–8 b/min. This is much less than the 12–15 b/min typical for most people. Some practitioners strongly recommend 3–5 b/min. This often includes widening of the lower ribs. There is often a short pause after each exhalation.

Proposed mechanisms include increases in pCO_2. Cognitive elements of distraction and restructuring may also be important. Practitioners often use various types of biofeedback instruments with this technique. These include stretch gauges for chest and abdominal movements, electromyography (EMG) from accessory breathing muscles, volume devices, and capnographic measures of pCO_2 and oxygen.

Paced Respiration

Inhaling and exhaling at a predetermined rate is called "paced respiration" (Clark & Hirschman, 1990; Lichstein, 1988). Therapists who use this technique suggest that patients coordinate the rate with a device (such as a metronome) that allows a preset rhythm. A summary of the rationale of, value of, and research with paced respiration (Clark & Hirschman, 1990) justifies its use. For example, reduced electrodermal responsiveness and lowered ratings of subjective discomfort in response to threat both occur with paced respiration below the baseline rate of nonclinical and clinical subjects (Clark & Hirschman, 1990).

Clark and Hirschman (1990) point to the potential advantage of using respiratory cues over other somatic and ANS cues. They note the evidence supporting the generalized ANS effects accompanying respiratory changes because of the coupling of the somatic and ANS systems. They also note the association of anxiety and tension with respiratory changes, and the fact that various stress reduction techniques include variations of paced respiration. They understandably focus on the reduction of symptoms such as panic attacks and HV that can accompany use of paced respiration.

This rationale for paced respiration is the same for most or all relaxed breathing therapies, which involve (1) slowing the respiratory rate to below the usual or baseline rate and (2) using a regular breathing rhythm. The advantage of so-called "paced respiration" is the use of an external pacing device. This may be especially useful when people are in the early stages of breathing therapy, or when the clinician is providing abbreviated office therapy in a stepped-care protocol.

In a sample of alcohol-dependent male inpatients with high trait anxiety, Clark and Hirschman (1990) used a 10-minute pacing procedure. This resulted in significantly more reduction of self-reported tension and state anxiety than an attention control procedure. The use of an external cue with tones helped the patients pace themselves better than without it. The external cue was an audiotaped alternation of two tones (800 and 900 hertz) changing every 3 seconds, providing a rate of 10 respiration cycles per minute. The investigators have suggested longer training periods, especially to consolidate the learned pacing rate, which drifted back to baseline without the external pacing signal.

One may wonder about the 10-cycles-per-minute pacing procedure. It was slower than the typical baseline of about 16+ b/min in the subjects of Clark and Hirschman (1990)—a rate often associated with anxiety. However, it was not as slow as the more common goal of 6–8 b/min used in other breathing therapies. Clark and Hirschman (1990) report the average rate for these subjects as 11, but their table shows a rate of 13–14. Both figures are slower than the control group average of 18, but not the 10 b/min specified. One wonders how relaxing it is to breathe at a rate of 11 or 13 b/min while listening to alternating tones at a rate of 10 per minute. Last, this study examined only intrasession relaxation.

Caution

Some authorities (R. Fried, personal communication, March 13, 1994; E. Peper, personal communication, March 20, 1994) express concern about the potential for harm from fixed-pace breathing. Part of their concern is that this technique alone ignores the vital role of increased tidal volume with normal pCO_2. When tidal volume rises, breathing rate drops proportionately, assuming constant metabolism. Slowing breathing without raising tidal volume can result in hypoventilation. In a patient with emphysema, oxygen drops abruptly.

Breath Meditation and Breath Mindfulness

Methods of meditation noted by Lichstein (1988) include passive breath mindfulness and breath meditation. The origins of these methods include yoga and Zen Buddhism. Western-derived relaxation procedures such as progressive muscle relaxation also include being mindful of breathing. Lichstein (1988) provides a review of the theories, methods, and research for breath meditation and mindfulness, as well as other meditative methods. Practitioners should have access to that book.

In breath mindfulness and breath meditation, as their names indicate, patients focus their attention on breathing. This allows the emergence of natural breathing and thus facilitates altered breathing. In meditative techniques, one often combines the breathing focus with "a mantra, counting, fixed gaze on an external object, or a relaxation cue word" (Lichstein, 1988, p. 163). Other schools of meditation also include breathing, but with less focus upon it.

The methods of slow diaphragmatic breathing and paced respiration are more contemporary and secularized versions. Unlike the meditation methods, these allow open eyes and do not require imagery. These changes probably make the methods more practical and acceptable to more people.

Various theories attribute the positive therapeutic effects of these breathing techniques to improvement in right-hemisphere functioning, nasal airflow, and diaphragm movement, as well as to gentle stimulation of the vagus nerve, CO_2 changes, and cognitive distraction. Most research supports the CO_2 hypothesis. The research for the other theories and methods is less supportive and equivocal at best. However, this should not detract from consideration of the use of breath meditation and breath mindfulness procedures with selected patients. One matches procedures with patients and symptoms.

Rebreathing

Rebreathing is obviously not a relaxation technique. However, it is a non-instrumentation-based technique for stopping HV and physiological panic symptoms. It is an old and very common technique recommended by many physicians (Compernolle et al., 1979) and some respiratory therapists and physiotherapists (Holloway, 1994). Interestingly, there were no controlled studies of rebreathing found before an analogue study by van den Hout, Boek, van der Molen, Jansen, and Griez (1988). This study of medical students supported the value for rapidly raising pCO_2.

However, restoring pCO_2 faster in a closed system did not reduce physical symptoms faster than when subjects were rebreathing in an open system that they thought was closed. In other words, rebreathing expired air into a bag that was in a semiclosed system yielded symptom changes similar to those of the closed system. Thus this study did not reliably support the physiological rationale for the effectiveness of the technique among healthy young medical students. The interpretation was that distraction and/or instructions, and patients' expectations, may be important factors in its success. The authors acknowledged the limits of generalizing this to clinical patients. This study should not discourage practitioners from using the paper bag technique for some patients. It does support the role of expectation and other cognitive factors for at least some patients. It casts some doubt on the necessary relationship of restoring CO_2 and the subsiding of symptoms.

Holloway (1994, pp. 170–171) suggests using the paper bag rebreathing method in emergencies when other methods are not successful. She recommends 6–12 easy and natural breaths in the bag covering the nose and mouth. The patient should continue abdominal breathing after removing the bag. The technique may be repeated as necessary.

van den Hout et al. (1988) suggested that some people may "show marked post-rebreathing hypocapnia overshoots" (p. 308). These occur after using the rebreathing technique with a fully closed system. As noted above, this study used normal subjects. However, this is consistent with their earlier work (van den Hout & Griez, 1985) on posthypercapnic overshoots leading to hypocapnia in some panic patients. The authors speculated that the mechanism is a hypersensitive chemoreceptory system, at least in panic patients. They argued for caution in using rebreathing, at least with panic patients. Readers should note that the Compernolle et al. (1979) technique involves placing a few fingers "inside the bag to provide some air and prevent hypoxemia which can cause hyperventilation" (p. 621).

The rebreathing technique with a paper bag has value for some patients. The value of the research from the Netherlands group is in providing some cautions and supporting the role of cognitive factors. As long as the CO_2 levels theory remains prominent as an explanation for the cause of symptoms in many patients, then a rebreathing technique is logical. The role of cognitive factors at least for some people is not surprising. It does not negate the role of CO_2. Both physiological and cognitive factors are operative with many applied psychophysiological and behavioral therapies for physical symptoms among many patients. Holloway (1994) cautions against using this method "as an easy way out" (p. 171). Also, he cautions practitioners to avoid plastic bags!

Pursed-Lip Breathing

PLB is a commonly used respiratory therapy indicated for patients with "advanced COPD [chronic obstructive pulmonary disease] who hyperinflate their lungs during attacks of bronchospasm, panic, or exercise; and as an adjunctive measure in patients undergoing exercise rehabilitation or respiratory muscle training" (Berkow & Fletcher, 1992, p. 632). The patient exhales very slowly with lips partially closed "as if ready to whistle" (p. 632). Patients with advanced COPD take small inhaled breaths to avoid and decrease hyperinflation. Tiep and colleagues (Tiep, Branum, & Burns, 1992; Tiep, Burns, Kao, Madison, & Herrera, 1986) used this technique successfully with oxygen feedback for patients with COPD. The mechanisms by which they felt this could help patients included increased oxygen saturation, breathing at higher lung volumes, slower breathing rate, and increased expiratory volumes.

Patients without COPD can use PLB with deeper breaths. It makes good sense to consider this technique with patients who have other disorders. Ideally, one would use oxygen monitoring/feedback instruments, although they are probably not needed for all patients. We could find no research on the use of PLB with patients other than those with COPD.

INSTRUMENTATION-BASED BREATHING FEEDBACK

There are several instrumentation-based breathing feedback systems available to enhance relaxed breathing. All are logical and in use by practitioners. There is no research showing any differential outcomes among them. Practitioners use those systems that are available and with which they feel most comfortable.

Nasal Airflow Temperatures[7]

A thermistor (an electrical resistor that measures temperature) taped below a nostril detects the changes in temperature of air inhaled and exhaled. Inhaled air is cooler, and exhaled air is warmer. With a computer-based visual display set sensitively, a therapist and patient can clearly see the rapid changes in temperature. The temperature falls during inhalation, and then rises during exhalation. One sees hills and valleys in the curve on the screen. One goal is to make the hills and valleys about the same size and duration. The patient watches the curve and, with this feedback, regulates the size and timing of breaths to create a regular rhythm of hills and valleys in the curve.

The clinician should set the display screen width to a time reflecting a few inhalations and exhalations. The temperature should be centered in the middle of the screen, and the range of temperature (sensitivity) should be set to create hills and valleys that are easy to see. The temperatures should not extend beyond the limits of the screen. The range depends partly on the patient. Therapists starting to use this technique will often try it with themselves first. They should consider starting with a display in which the range is at or less than about 5°F and tailor it for the individual.

This is a simple technique, requiring only one temperature feedback unit and a simple computer-based software display. However, it does not give any other information, such as that about muscles used and CO_2. Therefore, practitioners often use it in conjunction with other feedback instruments.

One caution is that to avoid transmission of infections from the nose, therapists must be very careful to disinfect the thermistor between sessions for all patients (see note 7).

Strain Gauges

Many practitioners use stretchable devices wrapped around the abdomen, chest, or both. These allow monitoring and feedback about abnormal breathing patterns, such as irregularity, breath holding, and apneas. Therapists also use this to help teach new breathing patterns. It is better than observation alone (Timmons & Ley, 1994). The device has sensors that convey the degree of expansion. These are connected to a computer-based feedback system that allows viewing the signals on a computer monitor. The purpose of this type of system is that it allows one to see the expansions in each body area, as well as the difference between the abdominal area and the chest area during each breath. The specific numbers are unimportant and may be different for each person. The numbers depend on the tightness of the bands and the sensitivity setting. The feedback signal provides hills and valleys that depend on the size of the breath and body area used. This is similar to the nasal airflow temperature measure; however, the advantage over the latter measure is that it gives information about abdominal versus chest breathing. The reader should note the use of a strain gauge in the DeGuire et al. (1992) study of breathing therapy for HV for patients with functional chest or cardiac symptoms. Like the nasal airflow temperature measure, this method provides no information about other muscles or CO_2. There are technical limitations to this type of measurement. Movement artifact is one problem. Recalibration after movements and position changes may be necessary (Timmons & Ley, 1994). The reader is directed to Fried (1993b, p. 40), Timmons & Ley, (1994, pp. 281–282), and Timmons and Meldrum (1993) for more discussion and references for using strain gauges.

Many of the newer biofeedback systems now have sophisticated breathing pattern guides. These allow the practitioner to set the pattern to vary inspiration–expiration ratio, respiration rate, and pauses. Although no systematic research exists as yet on these feedback devices, initial patient response has been very positive in anecdotal reports.

EMG from Accessory Breathing Muscles

Practitioners also use EMG from accessory breathing muscles. They should consider using the sternomastoids, upper back muscles (including the rhomboids and levator scapulae), and upper chest muscles (including the pectoralis and/or scalene muscles). The selection of muscles depends on therapist preference and practical considerations. The purpose is to show whether there are EMG increases from these muscles during each inhalation, to indicate the degree of any increases, and to give feedback to help the patient reduce these increases.

The Capnometer and Oximeter Method

The capnometer and oximeter method allows measurement and feedback of $ETCO_2$ and good estimates of arterial blood oxygen saturation (P_aO_2). One inserts a narrow plastic tube about 0.25 inches into either nostril (Fried, 1987a, 1993b; R. Fried, personal communication, March 13, 1994).[8] The tube's outer width is about 4 millimeters. One tapes the tube to the skin near the upper lip.

This method allows continuous sampling of end-tidal breath conducted to an infrared gas analyzer. The signal then goes to a computer that feeds back the wave of rising and falling $PetCO_2$ on a video monitor. It provides a hard-copy output of the pattern and gives statistics for specified periods. The therapist can place a goal wave for size and rate of the breaths. Fried (1993b) uses a capnograph and a J & J physiological monitoring and feedback system. One needs a system that recognizes and displays analyzed blood gas data. Others have used a standard nasal cannula. These plastic tubes are readily available and can be used one per patient.

Spirometry

For therapists without access to a capnometer, Lum (1991, cited in Timmons & Ley, 1994) recommends "spirometry." This is a measure of the amount of air moved. Nonphysicians and nonphysiologists should consider the smaller, less expensive, and relatively accurate Wright spirometer (Timmons & Ley, 1994). This allows an estimate of overbreathing by providing an estimate of minute volume. Normal resting minute volume is about 6 liters (Naifeh, 1994). An example of a criterion for overbreathing is 30 liters per minute (Lum, 1991, cited in Timmons & Ley, 1994).

Arterial Blood Oxyhemoglobin Saturation: Oximetry

Fried (1993b) uses and recommends a measure of arterial blood oxyhemoglobin saturation, in which one uses an oximeter attached to the index finger. One also could use an ear lobe, a practice commonly employed by sleep laboratories for overnight oximetry for assessing decreased oxygen saturations in patients with obstructive sleep apnea. The output from the oximeter connects to a physiological monitoring system (e.g., J & J I-430 System I-801 module). The oximeter shows percentage of saturated hemoglobin, and the biofeedback display shows the saturation of arterial blood oxygen over each breath cycle.

This display shows variations of oxygen. It gives an index of the oxygen delivery to tissues during monitoring of PetCO$_2$. For example, normal pCO$_2$ and elevated oxygen perfusion in the blood (SaO_2) reflect oxygen perfusion expected with deep diaphragmatic breathing. Some experts wonder about the accuracy of this index. Contrast this to the reduced oxygen in the tissues associated with hypocapnia.

Skin Temperatures: Hand and Head Apex

Skin temperature is an indirect measure of breathing, according to Fried (1993b). He attaches a temperature sensor to the fifth digit of the nondominant hand. Other practitioners may use other digits. By itself, skin temperature is not a good index; however, it is a common index of relaxation and is often monitored during breathing therapy procedures.

Fried's (1993b) unique contribution is a temperature sensor attached to the scalp apex. Normal levels of CO$_2$ increase cerebral blood flow. Fried asserts that this placement gives an index of blood flow in the brain. This procedure and its value as an indirect index of normalized and relaxed breathing await research.

Plethysmography: Pulse Rate and Sinus Rhythm

Another indirect measure is pulse information (Fried, 1993b). A common sensor placement is the second digit of the right hand. A biofeedback interface allows for measurement of variation of beat-to-beat pulse. This is an index of vagal tone and respiratory sinus arrhythmia (RSA) during the breath cycles, and provides an indirect index of cardiopulmonary status.

Cardiopulmonary techniques such as RSA biofeedback are now becoming popular method for breathing therapy. These are discussed in detail by Gevirtz and Lehrer in Chapter 11 of this volume.

CONCLUSIONS AND TREATMENT IMPLICATIONS

This chapter assumes that abnormal breathing styles such as HV are major factors resulting in or aggravating an array of symptoms. These include HVS, panic episodes in many patients (both while awake and during sleep), RIA, and noncardiac chest pain and related chest symptoms. Another assumption is that respiration therapies are logical and proper for these symptoms. Relaxed breathing methods often rapidly result in physiological relaxation. These methods can reduce or stop emotional distress, even for patients not treated with other relaxation methods.

There are multiple explanations for how relaxation therapies in general work. Similarly, there are multiple explanations for how breathing therapies work. There is no universal agreement among practitioners and researchers about how these therapies work. Possible explanations include altered CO$_2$ and oxygen levels, cognitive changes, and cortical and subcortical changes.

This chapter assumes that these therapies often alter biochemical mechanisms crucial to causing symptoms and crucial for stopping them. A very common assumption and particularly promising explanation is that altered partial pressure of CO$_2$ (pCO$_2$) is often crucial.

Slow diaphragmatic (abdominal) breathing is the most common breathing method. Deeper-than-usual breathing is a common part of this method. However, slow breathing and abdominal breathing also characterize other relaxation techniques. Furthermore, breathing therapy procedures require voluntary actions and thus provide a diversion from other cognitive activity, such as anxious and angry thoughts.

Another assumption is that many people who often experience HV are more prone to RIA and panic symptoms. A vulnerable situation arises when one abruptly stops vigorous exercise without voluntarily reducing the volume of air breathed each minute. For people who chronically experience HV, there may be more risk of symptoms during sedentary activities after hyperpneic breathing (increased depth and rate of respiration; panting) (Ley, 1988a). Such occasions might include driving or watching television or movies. Minute volume remains constant and greater than normal, or may increase in heavy traffic or when the patient is watching violence. One expects low metabolic production of CO_2 because of low physical energy needs during these activities. Panic attacks may result, however, from this combination of events.

Therapy Implications

Respiration therapy should be included in the treatment of a variety of symptoms and disorders. These include the symptoms of many patients with panic disorders or other anxiety disorders, functional chest and cardiac symptoms, some tachycardia conditions, RIA, HVS, and asthma.

1. *Qualifications and cautions.* There are signs on the ski lift poles of a Colorado ski resort that read "Know your limit; ski within it." This saying applies to many aspects of life. In this context, "know your limit; *practice* within it." Understanding breathing physiology and measurement, and using this knowledge in treatment, are complex. Employing this method requires both considerable knowledge and proper training. Several authorities emphasize the importance of practitioners' having proper understanding of anatomy, physiology, disorders, and breathing techniques and cautions. For example, Timmons and Ley emphasize that "faulty technique or inexperience may lead to complications in treatment" (p. 276). Discussing the importance of proper qualifications for practitioners and therapists, she refers to Bass (1994) and states that "it is possible to make some hyperventilators worse with breathing exercises, at least in the early stages of training" (p. 278).

Close collaboration with properly trained and credentialed professionals is prudent. Practitioners should collaborate with physicians who treat patients with chronic lung diseases. This is especially important for nonphysician practitioners. They should also consider learning and using techniques used by properly credentialed respiratory and physical therapists experienced with chronic lung diseases; they should consider collaboration with these therapists as well. Referral of selected patients is sometimes prudent.

2. *Matters concerning intake, patient education, and starting therapy.* Credible patient education is an important component in treating breathing-related symptoms and disorders. Holloway (1994) emphasizes and discusses patient education and demonstrations for patients. The therapist should consider using a printed patient-education booklet. For example, Holloway (1994) suggests a patient education book on HVS by Bradley (1991), published in New Zeland and now available in the United States.

Some patients should consider having a spouse/partner or close friend present to help reinforce the procedures at home and remind the patient of the procedures. This may be especially useful for patients with impaired concentration and memory (Holloway, 1994, p. 164).

Therapists should consider using the HVPT and stressful tasks to provoke symptoms in the office. Stressful tasks include time-pressured difficult tasks and thinking about personal events associated with naturally occurring symptoms. Proper safeguards must be employed when one is using HVPT.

Some clinicians suggest that some patients become "obsessed" with their breathing (Timmons & Ley, 1994). Timmons and Ley agree, but add that this is rare. It is not a contraindication to using breathing therapy for most patients. Experienced and prudent practitioners can assess this tendency and manage it early. For example, Timmons and Ley (1994) suggest helping these patients focus on general relaxation.

Many patients are using tranquilizers and/or sleeping medications when they present for relaxation and breathing therapies. Timmons and Ley (1994) state that "many psychotherapists consider it unethical to accept clients who are on tranquilizers or sleeping medications" (p. 279). The reason given is they are "unlikely to learn while their feelings are blunted [and] the ability to learn new breathing patterns may be diminished as well" (p. 279). However, many patients need to continue these medications, at least for a while. Examples are patients with severe anxiety. They may need the medications to lower their arousal level enough to cooperate with other treatments. Furthermore, we know of no research showing that these patients cannot or do not benefit from breathing therapies. Nevertheless, some patients probably should withdraw from the medications before breathing therapy. For example, reduction or cessation of some medications may allow HV symptoms to emerge that were suppressed by the drug.

3. *Therapy without instrumentation.* Practitioners can provide successful breathing therapy without physiological instrumentation-based feedback. For example, many therapists use a light sandbag (a few pounds) or an open, large city telephone directory or other large book placed on the abdomen. This provides sensory feedback from the pressure of the weight. It helps maintain the patient's awareness of the body area and thus provides continuous feedback. Also, therapists can place one hand over the sternum or chest and the other hand over the abdominal wall. At first, some therapists may place their hands over or under their patients' hands.

van Dixhoorn and colleagues (e.g., van Dixhoorn & Duivenvoorden, 1999) have been strong advocates of techniques that draw from European health movements of the past. Within this context, patients are encouraged to increase awareness of all aspects of breathing and find an effortless breathing pattern that functions for them.

4. *Therapy with instrumentation.* Feedback instrumentation is often useful for many patients. This chapter describes several such instruments. The usefulness of such instruments is increasingly recognized in research and clinical practice (see N. M. Schwartz & M. S. Schwartz, Chapter 3, this volume, for part of the rationale for instrumentation-based feedback).

Physiological measures, such as CO_2, can be useful in therapy and are often necessary in research. Furthermore, physiological monitoring of breathing probably has value for the practitioner even when it has less value for the patient. It provides much information and more accurate information for both the practitioner and the patient. It quantifies breathing parameters so that the therapist can sometimes treat the patient more efficiently. For example, instrumentation provides information about respiration rate, the magnitude and volume of breaths, the areas of the body used in the breaths, the pattern and regularity of breaths, blood chemistries, and changes within and between sessions.

However, the absence of physiological measures does not mean that patients cannot be treated successfully. Physiological changes are probably only part of the reasons for improvement in symptoms of HV. Distraction and other cognitive techniques affecting attributions and expectations are probably important for many patients.

5. *Techniques.* A common relaxed breathing method consists of slow, deep, abdominal inhalations for a few to several seconds and slow exhalations. The respiration cycles are typically at least 50% less than typical breathing rates. Holloway (1994) encourages patients "to count slowly and silently while practicing breathing exercises, aiming for a rate of 6–8 breaths per minute" (p. 166). Inhalations last from 4 to 8 seconds. Some techniques include brief pauses

for a few to several seconds after the inhalation. This increases blood CO_2. However, contrary to some other methods of breathing therapy, some therapists caution against pausing after the inhalation and recommend pausing after the exhalation:

> There must be no holding of inspired air. . . . [It] exacerbates some symptoms, particularly cardiac arrhythmias and chest pains. . . . The inspiration phases should flow naturally into the relaxed expiratory phase. . . . A pause is encouraged after the expiration. [Also], contrary to many methods of breathing exercise, inspiration is the active phase. Expiration is passive and relaxed, and a pause should occur at the end of expiration. (Holloway, 1994, p. 165)

However, we found no data supporting either this caution or this recommendation.

Patients should be instructed to feel themselves becoming more relaxed as they slowly exhale. Therapists should consider saying cue words with the exhalation. This cycle should be repeated a few times for about 1 minute and usually longer. Practice periods are often at least once per day for 5–20 minutes each. Application is often for briefer periods many times per day to reduce the frequency of HV throughout waking hours. Patients do this with eyes open or closed. The use of a pacing method or device comparable to a metronome (this is sometimes called "paced respiration," as described earlier) may help some patients.

Therapists should use structured tasks that distract patients from their anxiety and other symptoms. The goal is to increase the perception of control and increase thoughts of self-efficacy. Techniques including general relaxation, breathing therapies, cognitive distraction, and cognitive reattribution can serve this purpose.

Practitioners might also consider brief periods of breath holding up to 5–10 seconds or PLB to increase the CO_2 level. They should consider suggesting these methods to avoid hypocapnia for selected patients.

A mirror may be used to help a patient "observe areas of movement while breathing. Attention may be drawn to sternomastoid tensing and movement of the sternum and clavicles" (Holloway, 1994, p. 166).

After the patient has demonstrated ability to maintain a desired breathing pattern in a relaxed posture, the therapist might suggest changing to other positions to help transfer of training. For example, he or she can switch the patient to sitting upright, standing and leaning against a wall, standing, slow walking, and fast walking (Holloway, 1994). There is less abdominal excursion while standing. The therapist should discourage tightening of the abdominal muscles, carefully note breathing rhythms, and correct patients when he or she observes abdominal tensing and noisy breathing. The toning of abdominal muscles should be encouraged, with abdominal exercises tailored to the patient. Age, general condition, and back problems must all be considered.

6. *Daily practice and application.* Therapists should correct faulty breathing patterns during daily activities. They should discourage patients from "talking continuously in a steady stream, using long sentences, and then gasping and talking a sudden inhalation before setting off again! . . . [and, instead,] encourage short, concise sentences in a low register most of the time" (Holloway, 1994, p. 169).

Patients should also avoid "tight trousers or jeans, corsets, panty girdles, and belts" (Holloway, 1994, p. 170; see also MacHose & Peper, 1991). These encourage upper chest movements and inhibit abdominal movement. Weaning patients away from tight clothing can be difficult in many cases.

Patients should be encouraged to reduce breathing rate and volume when starting relaxation, They should reduce inhalation volume very soon after stopping exercise, or should gradually slow down near the end of exercising. For example, patients can walk and cool off until breathing is slower. They can get up often while watching television or otherwise move around, which might reduce the frequency of the symptoms. They can also do isometric exercises.

Therapists can encourage patients to suppress coughs, sighs, sniffs, and yawns. Patients can control sighs and yawns by either "swallowing or hold[ing] the breath to a count of five, breathing out slowly, holding to five again, and then resuming easy abdominal breathing" (Holloway, 1994, p. 166).

Therapists should consider instructions for the paper bag technique as an emergency maneuver, and patients should practice this first with supervision.

Closing Remark

"It is better not to change a patient's breathing unless you know what you're doing" (Lum, 1991, cited in Timmons & Ley, 1994, p. 276).

GLOSSARY

ACIDOSIS. A condition stemming from a buildup of acid or depletion of the alkaline reserve (bicarbonate content) in blood and body tissues. There is an increased concentration of hydrogen ions (i.e., decreased pH). "Hypercapnic acidosis," also called "respiratory acidosis," results from excessive retention of CO_2. "Compensated respiratory acidosis" occurs when the kidneys compensate and raise the low pH toward normal. There also are other causes. Compare with *alkalosis* (see below).

ALKALOSIS. A condition stemming from a buildup of base or alkali or from a loss of acid without comparable loss of base in body fluids. There is a decreased hydrogen ion concentration (i.e., increased pH). "Respiratory alkalosis" results from excess loss of CO_2 from the body. "Compensated respiratory alkalosis" occurs when the blood pH returns toward normal by acid retention or kidney mechanisms that excrete base (bicarbonate). There are also other causes. Compare with *acidosis* (see above).

BASE. In chemistry, the nonacid part of a salt. It produces hydroxide ions in liquids such as blood.

BICARBONATE. A type of salt (HCO_3-). "Blood bicarbonate" is an index of the alkaline reserve level.

BUFFER AND BICARBONATE BUFFERING SYSTEM. In biochemistry, a *buffer* is any chemical system preventing change in concentration of another chemical substance such as hydrogen ion concentration (pH). The kidneys release bicarbonate as part of the *bicarbonate buffering system* of the body.

-CAPNIA. A suffix referring to CO_2. "Hypocapnia" is low or below-normal CO_2. "Hypercapnia" is high or above-normal CO_2.

DYSPNEA. Labored or difficult breathing. "Functional dyspnea" is dyspnea not related to exercise and without an organic cause. "Sighing intermittent dyspnea" is very deep sighing respirations without a significant change in rate, without wheezing. It has functional or emotional causes rather than organic causes.

HYPERPNEA. Breathing large volumes of air in each breath. Compare with *tachypnea* (see below).

HYPERVENTILATION (HV). Hyperventilation may be defined as more tidal volume (or total air flow) than is needed for metabolic demands. Alveolar carbon dioxide falls below normal.

HYPERVENTILATION SYNDROME (HVS). A condition where prolonged hyperventilation leads to systemic compensation and the loss of the alkaline buffering system. There is some controversy surrounding this concept.

HYPOVENTILATION. A condition occurring when there is too little air entering the pulmonary alveoli.

HYPOXIA. A deficiency of oxygen in tissues. This can occur despite sufficient blood in the tissues. It can occur if not enough oxygen enters the blood, as with decreased barometric pressures at high altitudes. It can also result from decreased oxyhemoglobin in the blood, which is partly a function of the pH of the blood and is affected by fluctuations of CO_2 and other gases. There are other causes.

ISOCAPNIC OVERVENTILATION TEST (IOT). A technique that artificially prevents lowered percentage of end-tidal CO_2 ($PetCO_2$; see below) during hyperventilation by using a mixture of air enriched with CO_2.

PARESTHESIA. An abnormal sensation, such as burning or prickling.

pH. The concentration level and ratio of alkalinity to acidity. A pH of 7.35 to 7.45 is neutral for blood. A pH above 7.45 means more alkalinity, and one below 7.35 means more acidity. The symbol *pH* refers to the hydrogen ion concentration or activity of a solution, such as blood.

PULMONARY ALVEOLI (OR VESICLES). Tiny sacs at the ends of the bronchial tree through which gas is exchanged with the pulmonary capillaries.

TACHYPNEA. Rapid cycles of inhaling and exhaling. Compare with *hyperpnea* (see above).

TORR. A unit of pressure equal to 1 millimeter of mercury (1 mm Hg). It is used in the measurement of ETCO$_2$ (see below).

Volumes

MINUTE VOLUME (MV). (1) "Quantity of gas (air) expelled from the lungs per minute" (*Dorland's Illustrated Medical Dictionary*, 1988, p. 1847); (2) "volume of air expelled from the lungs per minute" (Dox et al., 1979, p. 521); (3) "sum of tidal volumes breathed per minute" (Ley, 1988a, p. 253); (4) "volume of air inspired per minute" (Kaufman & Schneiderman, 1986, p. 112).

RESIDUAL VOLUME (RV). Amount of gas remaining in the lungs at the end of a maximal expiration.

TIDAL VOLUME (V_T). Amount of gas inspired and expired (i.e., ventilation) during one respiratory cycle of a normal breath.

Abbreviations Involving Oxygen

PAO$_2$. Partial pressure of alveolar oxygen.

PaO$_2$. Arterial partial pressure of oxygen.

SaO$_2$. Arterial blood saturation.

Abbreviations Involving Carbon Dioxide

ETCO$_2$. Partial pressure of CO$_2$ in end-tidal breath. Values usually in torr but can be in percent. A valid estimate of arterial pCO$_2$ in normal lungs.

pCO$_2$. Partial pressure of CO$_2$ in alveolar (lung) air. Values in torr or percent. High positive correlation between ETCO$_2$ and pCO$_2$ often makes them interchangeable. When ETCO$_2$ is in percent, it is percent of end-tidal CO$_2$ or PetCO$_2$ (e.g., 38 torr = 5% PetCO$_2$).

PaCO$_2$, PCO$_2$, pCO$_2$. All three abbreviations, found in the literature, mean partial pressure of carbon dioxide. The first is arterial CO$_2$, and the others are options for the generic version.

PetCO$_2$. Percentage end-tidal CO$_2$.

P$_{TC}$CO$_2$. Transcutaneous estimate of pCO$_2$. It is closely related to arterial pCO$_2$, but with some delay from blood changes to transcutaneous values (Pilsbury & Hibbert, 1987).

ACKNOWLEDGMENTS

We are very thankful to Ronald Ley, PhD, Robert Fried, PhD, Eric Peper, PhD, and Charles D. Burger, MD, for their reviews of the 2nd edition drafts, many aspects of which are still reflected in the 3rd edition. Their many comments, suggestions, and corrections helped considerably. This appreciation in no way implies their endorsement of any of the content of this chapter.

NOTES

1. This chapter uses the terms "breathing therapy" and "relaxed breathing therapy" instead of "breathing retraining." This is for consistency with our general preference for using "therapy" instead of "training." The term "training" has an educational and instructional denotation. It is acceptable in many settings. We do educate and instruct patients, but "therapy" is more consistent with activities of therapists.

2. As noted earlier, pCO$_2$ is the partial pressure of CO$_2$ in alveolar (or atmospheric) air. It is not a partial-pressure measure of arterial blood CO$_2$, which is p$_a$CO$_2$.

3. The Valsalva maneuver is forced exhalation effort with the glottis closed. It substantially increases intrathoracic pressure and disrupts venous blood returning to the heart. Eastern breathing advocates avoid it because of its risks (Chandra, 1994).

4. This rate of 4–5 seconds per inhalation–exhalation cycle is faster than often recommended and instructed in relaxed breathing therapy. Note that nearly all patients reduced their breathing to 8–9 b/min (*SD* = 2–3)—much less than 14 b/min. This is slightly faster than the goal of 6 cycles per minute or 10 seconds per cycle that many practitioners recommend. This finding supports the robust nature of the treatment.

5. A problem develops when we consider the use of the term *minute volume* (MV) (see the glossary). Ley (1988a) refers to MV as the sum of tidal volumes breathed per minute. A tidal volume (V_t) is the amount of air inspired and expired during one normal respiratory cycle. Ley's definition of MV suggests the *total volume* of air. However, readers familiar with other definitions of MV may view MV as something slightly different. For example, two medical dictionaries define MV as the volume or quantity of air *expelled* from the lungs per minute (*Dorland's Illustrated Medical Dictionary*, 1988; *Melloni's Illustrated Medical Dictionary* [Dox, Melloni, & Eisner, 1979]). A third wording of the definition, "volume of air *inspired* per minute" in the classic book *Psychophysiology* (Kaufman & Schneiderman, 1986, p. 112), could lead some readers to slightly different conclusions. Some readers may be bewildered and initially frustrated with seemingly different definitions.

We offer the following resolution, which we trust is satisfactory. Despite the different wordings and potential implications, all these definitions mean the same thing. The dictionary definitions refer to "expelled air." Another definition refers to "inspired air." Since what comes in typically goes out, they include the volume of air inhaled. Thus they all imply that MV refers to the *total volume of inhaled or exhaled air in a minute*. Also, the term "expelled" eliminates breath holding during measurements. Holding one's breath for 1 minute means an MV of zero. Naifeh (1994) has said it clearly: "*Minute ventilation* refers to the total volume of air inspired (or expired) in a minute and is expressed in liters per minute. The normal value at rest is 6 liters per minute" (p. 26).

6. As noted in the glossary, normal pH is about 7.4. A pH lower than 7.35 is acid, and a pH above 7.45 is alkaline (*base*). The terms *acidosis* and *alkalosis* are relative terms in human tissue.

7. Dr. Fried (personal communication, March 13, 1994) believes that he was the first to use a thermistor to monitor nasal airflow. However, he expressed some embarrassment, as it was only a demonstration! His concern was related to the potential for transmitting infections (e.g., staphylococcus). We add the caution for careful disinfecting of the thermistor between all sessions.

8. Fried (1993b) specified the right nostril but did not indicate why. He tells us that either nostril is acceptable. He uses the right nostril for convenience because he sits to the right of the patient.

REFERENCES

Allen, J. P., Imbus, C. E., Powars, D. R., & Haywood, L. J. (1976). Neurologic impairment induced by hyperventilation in children with sickle cell anemia. *Pediatrics, 58*, 124–126.

Backon, J. (1989). Nasal breathing as a treatment for hyperventilation: Relevance of hemispheric activation. *British Journal of Clinical Practice, 43*, 161–162.

Barlow, D. H. (2002). *Anxiety and its disorders: The nature and treatment of anxiety and panic* (2nd ed.). New York: Guilford Press.

Baretti, P. A. (1994). Nasopulmonary physiology. In B. H. Timmons & R. Ley (Eds.), *Behavioral and psychological approaches to breathing disorders*. New York: Plenum Press.

Bass, C. (1994). Management of patients with hyperventilation-related disorders. In B. H. Timmons & R. Ley (Eds.), *Behavioral and psychological approaches to breathing disorders*. New York Plenum Press.

Bass, C., & Gardner W. N. (1985). Respiratory and psychiatric abnormalities in chronic symptomatic hyperventilation. *British Medical Journal (Clinical Research Edition), 290*, 1387–1390.

Bass C , Gardner W. N., & Jackson, G. (1994). Psychiatric and respiratory aspects of functional cardiovascular syndromes. In B. H. Timmons & R. Ley (Eds.), *Behavioral and psychological approaches to breathing disorders*. New York: Plenum Press.

Beck, J. G., Berisford, M. A., Taegtmeyer, H., & Bennitt, A. (1990). Panic symptoms in chest pain without coronary artery disease: A comparison with panic disorder. *Behavior Therapy, 21*, 241–252.

Beitman, B. D. (1992). Panic disorder in patients with angiographically normal coronary arteries. *American Journal of Medicine, 92*(Suppl. 5A), 33–40.

Berger, B. C., & Gevirtz, R. N. (2001). The treatment of pain disorder: A comparison between breathing retraining and cognitive-behavioral therapy [Abstract]. *Applied Psychophysiology and Biofeedback, 26*, 232–233.

Berkow, R., & Fletcher, A. J. (Eds.). (1992). *The Merck manual of diagnosis and therapy* (16th ed.). Rahway, NJ: Merck.

Biber, B., & Alkin T. (1999). Panic disorder subtypes: Differential responses to CO_2 challenge. *American Journal of Psychiatry, 156*(5), 739–744.

Blumenthal, J. A., Jiang W., Babyak, M. A., Krantz, D. S., Frid, D. J., Coleman, R. E., Waugh, R., Hanson, M., Appelbaum, M., O'Connor, C., & Morris, J. J. (1997). Stress management and exercise training in cardiac patients with myocardial ischemia: Effects on prognosis and evaluation of mechanisms. *Archives of Internal Medicine, 157*(19), 2213–2223.

Bonn, J. A., Readhead, C. P. A., & Timmons, B. H. (1984). Enhanced adaptive behavioural response in agoraphobic patients pretreated with breathing retraining. *Lancet, ii,* 665–669.

Bradley, D. (1991). *Hyperventilation syndrome.* Auckland, New Zealand: Tandem.

Bradley, L. A., Richter, J. E., Scarinci, I. C., Haile, J. M., & Schan, C. A. (1992). Psychosocial and psychophysiological assessments of patients with unexplained chest pain. *American Journal of Medicine, 92*(Suppl. 5A), 65–73.

Carter, C., Maddock, R., Amsterdam, E., McCormick, S., Waters, C., & Billett, J. (1992). Panic disorder and chest pain in the coronary care unit. *Psychosomatics, 33*(3), 302–309.

Chandra, F. A. (1994). Respiratory practices in yoga. In B. H. Timmons & R. Ley (Eds.), *Behavioral and psychological approaches to breathing disorders.* New York: Plenum Press.

Clark, D. M., & Hemsley, D. R. (1982). The effects of hyperventilation: Individual variability and itss relation to personality. *Journal of Behavior Therapy and Experimental Psychiatry, 13*(1), 41–47.

Clark, D. M., Salkovskis, P. M., & Chalkley, A. J. (1985). Respiratory control as a treatment for panic attacks. *Journal of Behavior Therapy and Experimental Psychiatry, 16*(1), 23–30.

Clark, M. E., & Hirschman, R. (1990). Effects of paced respiration on anxiety reduction in a clinical population. *Biofeedback and Self-Regulation, 15*(3), 273–284.

Clouse, R. E. (1992). Psychopharmacologic approaches to therapy for chest pain of presumed esophageal origin. *American Journal of Medicine, 92*(Suppl. 5A), 106–113.

Compernolle, T., Hoogduin, K., & Joele, L. (1979). Diagnosis and treatment of the hyperventilation syndrome. *Psychomatics, 19,* 612–625.

Craig, A. B. (1976). 58 cases of loss of consciousness during underwater swimming and diving. *Medical Science and Sports, 8*(3), 171–175.

Craske, M. G., & Barlow, D. H. (1990). Nocturnal panic: Response to hyperventilation and carbon dioxide challenges. *Journal of Abnormal Psychology, 99*(3), 302–307.

DeGuire, S., Gevirtz, R., Hawkinson, D., & Dixon, K. (1996). Breathing retraining: A three-year follow-up study of treatment for hyperventilation syndrome and associated functional cardiac symptoms. *Biofeedback and Self-Regulation 21*(2), 191–198.

DeGuire, S., Gevirtz, R., Kawahara, Y., & Maguire, W. (1992). Hyperventilation syndrome and the assessment of treatment for functional cardiac symptoms. *American Journal of Cardiology, 70,* 673–677.

Dorland's illustrated medical dictionary (27th ed.). (1988). Philadelphia: Saunders.

Dox, I., Melloni, B. J., & Eisner, G. M. (1979). *Melloni's illustrated medical dictionary.* Baltimore: Williams & Wilkins.

Drossman, D. A., Thompson, W. G., Talley, N. J., Funch-Jensen, P., Janssens, J., & Whitehead, W. E. (1990). Identification of subgroups of functional gastrointestinal disorders. *Gastroenterology International, 3*(4), 159–172.

Duivenvoorden, H. J., & van Dixhoorn, J. (1991). Predictability of psychic outcome for exercise training and exercise training including relation therapy after myocardial infarction. *Journal of Psychosomatic Research, 35,* 569–578.

Fensterheim, H. (1994). Hyperventilation and psychopathology: A clinical perspective. In B. H. Timmons & R. Ley (Eds.), *Behavioral and psychological approaches to breathing disorders.* New York: Plenum Press.

Folgering, H., & Colla, P. (1978). Some anomalies in the control of paCO2 in patients with a hyperventilation syndrome. *Bulletin Européen de Physiopathologie Respiratoire, 14,* 503–512.

Fried, R. (1987a). Relaxation with biofeedback-assisted guided imagery: The importance of breathing rate as an index of hypoarousal. *Biefeedback and Self-Regulation, 12*(4), 273–279.

Fried, R. (1987b). *The hyperventilation syndrome.* Baltimore: Johns Hopkins University Press.

Fried, R. (1993a). Respiration in stress and stress control. In P. Lehrer & R. L. Woolfolk (Eds.), *Principles and practice of stress management* (2nd ed.). New York: Guilford Press.

Fried, R. (1993b). *The psychology and physiology of breathing: In behavioral medicine, clinical psychology, and psychiatry.* New York: Plenum Press.

Gardner, W. N. (1994). Diagnosis and organic causes of symptomatic hyperventilation. In B. H. Timmons & R. Ley (Eds.), *Behavioral and psychological approaches to breathing disorders.* New York: Plenum Press.

Garssen, B., de Ruiter, C., & van Dyck, R. (1992). Breathing retraining: A rationale placebo? *Clinical Psychology Review, 12,* 141–153.

Grossman, P., De Swart, J. C. G., & Defares, P. B. (1985). A controlled study of a breathing therapy for treatment of hyperventilation syndrome. *Journal of Psychosomatic Research, 29*(1), 49–58.

Guthrie, D., Moeller, T., & Guthrie, R. (1983). Biofeedback and its application to the stabilization and control of diabetes mellitus. *American Journal of Clinical Biofeedback, 6,* 82–87.

Guyton, A. C., & Hall, J. E. (1996). *Textbook of medical physiology* (9th ed.). Philadelphia: Saunders.

Hegel, M. T., Abel, G. G., Etscheidt, M., Cohen-Cole, S., & Wilmer, C. I. (1989). Behavioral treatment of angina-like chest pain in patients with hyperventilation syndrome. *Journal of Behavior Therapy and Experimental Psychiatry, 20*(1), 31–39.

Hibbert, G. A., & Chan, M. (1989). Respiratory control: Its contribution to the treatment of panic attacks. *British Journal of Psychiatry*, *154*, 232–236.

Hibbert, G. A., & Pilsbury, D. (1989). Hyperventilation: Is it a cause of panic attacks? *British Journal of Psychiatry*, *155*, 805–809.

Hill, P. M. (1973). Hyperventilation, breath holding and alveolar oxygen tensions at the breaking point. *Respiratory Physiology*, *19*, 201–203.

Holloway, E. A. (1994). The role of the physiotherapist in the treatment of hyperventilation. In B. H. Timmons & R. Ley (Eds.), *Behavioral and psychological approaches to breathing disorders*. New York: Plenum Press.

Hornsveld, H., & Garssen, B. (1997). Hyperventilation syndrome: An elegant but scientifically untenable concept. *Netherlands Journal of Medicine*, *50*(1), 13–20.

Howell, J. B. L. (1990). Behavioral breathlessness. *Thorax*, *45*, 287–292.

Huey, S. R., & West, S. G. (1983). Hyperventilation: Its relation to symptom experience and to anxiety. *Journal of Abnormal Psychology*, *92*, 422–432.

Janis, I. L., Defares, P., & Grossman, P. (1983). Hypervigilant reactions to threat. In H. Selye (Ed.), *Selye guide to stress research* (Vol. 3). New York: Scientific and Academic Editions.

Kaufman, M. P., & Schneiderman, N. (1986). Physiological bases of respiratory psychophysiology. In M. G. H. Coles, E. Donchin, & S. W. Porges (Eds.), *Psychophysiology: Systems, processes, and applications*. New York: Guilford Press.

Lewis, R. A., & Howell, J. B. L. (1986). Definition of the hyperventilation syndrome. *Clinical Respiratory Physiology (Bulletin of European Physiopathologic Respiration)*, *22*, 201–205.

Ley, R. (1987). Panic disorder and agoraphobia: Fear of fear or fear of the symptoms produced by hyperventilation? *Journal of Behavior Therapy and Experimental Psychiatry*, *18*(4), 305–316.

Ley, R. (1988a). Panic attacks during relaxation and relaxation-induced anxiety: A hyperventilation interpretation. *Journal of Behavior Therapy and Experimental Psychiatry*, *19*(4), 253–259.

Ley, R. (1988b). Panic attacks during sleep: A hyperventilation-probability model. *Journal of Behavior Therapy and Experimental Psychiatry*, *19*(3), 181–192.

Ley, R. (1991). *Hyperventilation and panic attacks during sleep: A critical commentary on a study by Craske and Barlow*. Unpublished manuscript.

Ley, R. (1992). The many faces of Pan: Psychological and physiological differences among three types of panic attacks. *Behavior Research and Therapy*, *30*(4), 347–357.

Ley, R. (1993). Breathing retraining in the treatment of hyperventilatory complaints and panic disorder: A reply to Garssen, DeRuiter, and Van Dyck. *Clinical Psychology Review*, *13*, 393–408.

Ley, R. (1994). Breathing and the psychology of emotion, cognition, and behavior. In B. H. Timmons & R. Ley (Eds.), *Behavioral and psychological approaches to breathing disorders*. New York: Plenum Press.

Lichstein, K. L. (1988). *Clinical relaxation strategies*. New York: Wiley-Interscience.

Lum, L. C. (1994). Hyperventilation syndromes: Physiological considerations in clinical management. In B. H. Timmons & R. Ley (Eds.), *Behavioral and psychological approaches to breathing disorders*. New York: Plenum Press.

Lum, L. C. (1995). Hyperventilation: The tip and the iceberg. *Journal of Psychosomatic Research*, *19*, 375–383.

MacHose, M., & Peper, E. (1991). The effects of clothing on inhalation volume. *Biofeedback and Self-Regulation*, *16*(3), 261–265.

Missri, J. E., & Alexander, S. (1978). Hyperventilation syndrome: A brief review. *Journal of the American Medical Association*, *240*(19), 2093–2096.

Moynihan, J. E., & Gevirtz, R. N. (2001). Respiratory and cognitive subtypes of panic: Preliminary validation of Ley's model. *Behavior Modification*, *25*(4), 555–583.

Naifeh, K. H. (1994). Basic anatomy and physiology of the respiratory system and the autonomic nervous system. In B. H. Timmons & R. Ley (Eds.), *Behavioral and psychological approaches to breathing disorders*. New York: Plenum Press.

Naifeh, K. H., Kamiya, J., & Sweet, D. M. (1982). Biofeedback of alveolar carbon dioxide tension and levels of arousal. *Biofeedback and Self-Regulation*, *7*(3), 283–299.

Nixon, P. G. (1989). Human functions and the heart. In D. Seedhouse & A. Cribb (Eds.), *Changing ideas in health care*. Chichester, UK: Wiley.

Nixon, P. G., & Freeman, L. J. (1988). The 'think test': A further technique to elicit hyperventilation. *Journal of the Royal Society of Medicine*, *81*(5), 277–279.

Patel, C., Marmot, M. G., et al. (1985). Trial of relaxation in reducing coronary risk: Four year follow up. *British Medical Journal*, *(Clinical Research Edition)* *290*(6475): 1103–1106.

Pilsbury, D., & Hibbert, G. (1987). An ambulatory system for long-term continuous monitoring of transcutaneous pCO2. *Clinical Respiratory Physiology*, *23*, 9–13.

Rapee, R. M. (1985). A case of panic disorder treated with breathing retraining. *Journal of Behavior Therapy and Experimental Psychiatry*, *16*(1), 63–65.

Rosenthal, T. L. (1980). Social cueing processes. In M. Hersen, R. M. Eisler, & P. M. Miller (Eds.), *Progress in behavior modification* (Vol. 10). New York: Academic Press.

Roth, W. T., Wilhelm, F. H., & Trabert, W. (1998a). Autonomic instability during relaxation in panic disorder. *Psychiatry Research, 80*(2), 155–164.

Roth, W. T., Wilhelm, F. H., & Trabert, W. (1998b). Voluntary breath holding in panic and generalized anxiety disorders. *Psychosomatic Medicine, 60*(6), 671–679.

Salkovskis, P. M. (1992). Psychological treatment of noncardiac chest pain: The cognitive approach. *American Journal of Medicine, 92*(Suppl. 5A), 114–121.

Salkovskis, P. M., & Clark, D. M. (1990). Affective responses to hyperventilation: A test of the cognitive model of panic. *Behaviour Research and Therapy, 28*(1), 51–61.

Sartory, G., & Olajide, D. (1988). Vagal innervation techniques in the treatment of panic disorder. *Behaviour Research and Therapy, 26*(5), 431–434.

Schmidt, N. B., Woolaway-Bickel, K., Trakowski, J., Santiago, H., Storey, J., Koselka, H., & Cook, J. (2000). Dismantling cognitive-behavioral treatment for panic disorder: Questioning the utility of breathing retraining. *Journal of Consulting and Clinical Psychology, 68*(3), 417–424.

Third International Society for the Advancement of Respiratory Psychophysiology (ISARP) Congress, Nijmegen, The Netherlands, August 26–27, 1996: Abstracts. (1997). *Biological Psychology, 46*(1), 73–97.

Tiep, B., Branum, N., & Burns, M. (1992, March). Biofeedback breathing retraining reduces dyspnea and improves gas exchange. In *Proceedings of the 23rd Annual Meeting of the Association for Applied Psychophysiology and Biofeedback, Colorado Springs.* Wheat Ridge, CO: Association for Applied Psychophysiology and Biofeedback.

Tiep, B., Burns, M., Kao, D., Madison, R., & Herrera, J. (1986). Pursed lips breathing training using ear oximetry. *Chest, 90*, 218–221.

Timmons, B. H., & Ley, R. (Eds.). (1994). *Behavioral and psychological approaches to breathing disorders.* New York: Plenum Press.

Timmons, B. H., & Meldrum, S. J. (1993). *Behavioral applications of respiratory measurements.* Unpublished manuscript.

Tobin, M. J., Mador, M. J. Guenther, S. M., Lodato, R. F., & Sackner, M. A. (1988). Variability of resting respiratory drive and timing in healthy subjects *Journal of Applied Physiology, 65*(1), 309–317.

van den Hout, M. A., Boek, C., van der Molen, G. M., & Griez, E. (1988). Rebreathing to cope with hyperventilation: Experimental tests of the paper bag method. *Journal of Behavioral Medicine, 11*(3), 303–310.

van den Hout, M. A., De Jong, P., Zandbergen, J., & Merckelbach, H. (1990). Waning of panic sensations during prolonged hyperventilation. *Behavior Research and Therapy, 28*(5), 445–448.

van den Hout, M. A., & Griez, E., (1985). Peripheral panic symptoms occur during changes in alveolar carbon dioxide. *Comprehensive Psychiatry, 26*, 381–387.

van Dixhoorn, J. (1992). *Cardiac events after myocardial infarction: Four year follow-up of exercise training and relaxation.* Paper presented at the Fifth World Congress of Cardiac Rehabilitation, Bordeaux, France.

van Dixhoorn, J. (1993, September). *Breath relaxation–stress management in East and West.* Paper presented at the 3rd International Conference on Biobehavioral Self-Regulation and Health, Tokyo.

van Dixhoorn, J. (1994, March). *Breath relaxation.* Workshop presented at the 25th Annual Meeting of the Association for Applied Psychophysiology and Biofeedback, Atlanta, GA.

van Dixhoorn, J., & Duivenvoorden, H. J. (1989). Breathing awareness as a relaxation method in cardiac rehabilitation. In F. J. McGuigan, W. E. Sime, & J. M. Wallace (Eds.), *Stress and tension control 3.* New York: Plenum Press.

van Dixhoorn, J., & Duivenvoorden H. J. (1999). Effect of relaxation therapy on cardiac events after myocardial infarction: A 5-year follow-up study. *Journal of Cardiopulmonary Rehabilitation, 19*(3), 178–185.

van Dixhoorn, J., Duivenvoorden, H. J., Staal, J. A., Pool, J., & Verhage, F. (1987). Cardiac events after myocardial infarction: Possible effect of relaxation therapy. *European Heart Journal, 8*,1210–1214.

Wilhelm, F. H., Gevirtz, R. N. & Roth, W. T. (2001). Respiratory dysregulation in anxiety, functional cardiac, and pain disorders: Assessment, phenomenology, and treatment. *Behavior Modification, 25*(4), 513–545.

Wilhelm, F. H., Trabert, W., & Roth, W. T. (2001a). Characteristics of sighing in panic disorder. *Biological Psychiatry, 49*(7), 606–614.

Wilhelm, F. H., Trabert, W., & Roth, W. T. (2001b). Physiologic instability in panic disorder and generalized anxiety disorder. *Biological Psychiatry, 49*(7), 596–605.

CHAPTER 11

Resonant Frequency Heart Rate Biofeedback

RICHARD N. GEVIRTZ

PAUL LEHRER

RHYTHMS IN THE CARDIAC SYSTEM

The cardiac system, like most biological systems, demonstrates constant variation when in a healthy (or homeostatically balanced) state. It has long been postulated that heart rates that are "chaotic" or unpredictable are healthier than very steady rates. In recent years, we have acquired more understanding of the nature of variation in the human heart rate (or, more technically, in the interbeat interval [IBI]). Giardino, Lehrer, and Feldman (2000) and Berntson, Cacioppo, and Quigley (1993) present a detailed discussion of the meaning of *oscillators* and oscillations in biological systems. (In this chapter, as in several others, italics on first use of a term indicate that the term is included in the glossary at the chapter's end.) A technical review of variability in heart rate is presented by Berntson, Cacioppo, Quigley, and Fabro (1994) and Berntson et al. (1997).

In the last 10 years, due to improved technology in physiological measurement, there has been much interest in the relationship of heart rate variation and health outcomes. Decreased heart rate variability has been associated with increased cardiac mortality and morbidity (Bigger, Fleiss, Rolnitzky, & Steinman, 1993a, 1993b; Bigger, Rolnitzky, Steinman, & Fleiss, 1994; Bigger et al., 1995; Bigger, Steinman, Rolnitzky, Fleiss, & Albrecht, 1996) and a host of other poor health outcomes (Kleiger, Miller, Bigger, & Moss, 1987; Kristal-Boneh, Raifel, Harari, Malik, & Ribak, 1995; Katz, Liberty, Porath, Ovsyshcher, & Prystowsky, 1999; Kristal-Boneh, Froom, Raifel, Froom, & Ribak, 2000).

A measure of variability, usually the standard deviation of the *R-wave* to R-wave IBI, is indicative of autonomic control of the heart and perhaps also the lungs, the gut, and certain facial muscles. There are two pathways within the autonomic nervous system controlling the pacing of the heart rhythm: the sympathetic and parasympathetic.

The two systems interact in a complex synergistic relationship that is sometimes reciprocal, sometimes additive, and sometimes subtractive. Particular rhythms characteristic of each of them operate through these pathways. Porges (1995a, 1995b, 1997) has postulated that the vagus nerve in humans evolved to two pathways, originating from two medullary nuclei called the *vagal nuclei*. The first pathway, more primitive and older in evolutionary terms, originates in the dorsal motor nucleus (DMNX). The second, more recently evolved in higher mammals, originates in the nucleus ambiguus (NA). The DMNX system is best characterized as a primitive cardiac braking system, the best-known example of which is the "diving reflex." This system may be excited when the organism experiences cold water in the face or chest and greatly reduces cardiac speed and output. The NA system is of greater interest within applied psychophysiology, because it seems to be involved in heart rate pacing in nonthreatening, social situations. This is seen by observing a rhythmic braking and speeding of the heart rate (or IBI) associated with respiration. With inhalation, the vagal braking is removed, and thus heart rate speeds up. Upon exhalation, the vagal brake is reapplied and slows the rate down again. Heart rate increases during inhalation and decreases during exhalation This heart rate/respiration rhythm is often called "respiratory sinus arrhythmia (RSA)" or "high-frequency (HF) activity." If the vagus nerve is intact, during normal breathing (10–16 breaths per minute) one can observe a characteristic peak-and-valley pattern in heart rate, with differences of 15–30 beats per minute in younger people. This amplitude diminishes with age, so that one might see a peak-to-valley difference of 11 beats in a 65-year-old person. Many studies have shown that blockade of the vagal system eliminates this RSA or HF rhythm (Berntson et al., 1993).

The various rhythms are often reported in hertz (cycles per second; abbreviated Hz with specific numerals). The oscillators of interest are between 0.003 and 0.4 Hz. HF rhythms are between 0.15 and 0.4 Hz. With a cardiotachometer, one can see the HF rhythms, but other, slower oscillators are more difficult to see. To observe them, a *spectral analysis* is often used. A low-frequency (LF) rhythm occurs within the range of 0.08–0.14 Hz, usually at about six times per minute (0.1 Hz, with a period of 10 seconds). On a cardiotachometer, this would be difficult to see, but on the spectral analysis it is clearly visible. This oscillator correlates with measures of a reflex that plays an important role in the regulation of blood pressure. Small pressure sensors in the major arteries ("baroreceptors") send information back to the sinus node of the heart to maintain homeostasis in the blood pressure system. When blood pressure rises, the baroreceptors stimulate the vagus brake to slow down the heart so as to reduce pressure. Similarly, with blood pressure decreases, the baroreceptors send a signal to the sympathetic cardioaccelerator to speed up the heart and increase blood pressure. A delay in the baroreflex system of approximately 5 seconds causes the 10-second (0.1-Hz) waves in heart rate. Baroreflex gain is currently of interest to cardiologists, because it may be an early detector of cardiac disease. It is quantified as the change in IBI (in milliseconds) that co-occurs with changes in blood pressure (in millimeters of mercury).

A third oscillator, more difficult to see in the cardiotachometer record, is the very-low-frequency (VLF) rhythm. It is defined as oscillations from 0.003 to 0.08 Hz. It is thought to be driven by a slow rhythm mediated by the sympathetic nervous system, possibly related to thermoregulation or gastrointestinal regulation. A recent study by Vaschillo, Lehrer, Rishe, and Konstantinov (2002) suggests that this wave reflects baroreflex effects on smooth muscle tone in the blood vessels (vascular tone). Oscillations in vascular tone and blood pressure tend to show particularly large frequency peaks in the VLF range, centering at approximately 0.05 Hz (i.e., three times per minute, or having a period of 20 seconds). This oscillation thus suggests a delay in the vascular tone limb of the baroreflex system of about 10 seconds, perhaps due to plasticity of the blood vessels. This rhythm is also found in heart rate.

By using an ongoing spectral display that is sensitive to minute-by-minute changes in the autonomic nervous system, we can obtain a much richer picture of potential pathways for "mind–body" interaction. Together with traditional measures, such as skin conductance, temperature, or muscle activity, the heart rate variability measures can help us build a mediational model for such disorders as noncardiac chest pain. For example, the spectral display will provide an online assessment of sympathetic–parasympathetic balance [the ratio between HF and LF or VLF activity] (Berntson et al., 1997); it will provide a rough index of baroreflex gain (Bernardi et al., 1994); and it will reveal the occurrence of resonance between respiratory and baroreflex activity.

MEASUREMENT ISSUES

To observe the oscillators, one must perform a fast Fourier transform (FFT) (or differential Fourier transform [DFT]) on the IBI data. The IBI must be accurately measured with sampling rates at least at 256 samples per second. This is best done with an electrocardiogram (ECG), but is sometimes accomplished with a pulse plethysmograph (PPG). The PPG has the disadvantage of not having a clear cardiac spike to trigger the timer and calculate the IBI. However, some recent advances in calculating heart rate variability from the PPG have produced frequency calculations that closely parallel those obtained from the ECG (Giardino, Lehrer, & Edelberg, 2002).

INFLUENCE OF RESPIRATION RATE ON MEASURES OF HEART RATE VARIABILITY

A complication of the spectral band measures is that HF activity is influenced by respiration rate. For this reason, the HF measurement metric is dependent on a person's maintaining breathing rates in the designated range of 0.15–0.4 Hz. Grossman and others (Grossman, van Beek, & Wientjes, 1990; Grossman & Kollai, 1993; Wilhelm, Gevirtz, & Roth, 2001) have shown that HF values can be greatly affected by manipulation in respiratory rate. Therefore, when the practitioner trains the client to breathe slowly (usually about 6 breaths per minute), the HF activity moves down into the LF band. This means, not that the vagal braking system is not operating as might be perceived with the reduction of HF activity, but that the vagal oscillations are now showing up in the LF range.

RESONANT FREQUENCY BIOFEEDBACK THERAPY

The overlapping of respiratory and baroreflex effects on heart rate variability during slow respiratory rates may present some treatment opportunities. Lehrer, Vaschillo, and Vaschillo (2000b) have theorized that when an individual learns a breathing technique guided by heart rate variability biofeedback, resonance is created in the cardiorespiratory system between the effects of respiration and those of the baroreflex. Recent data from Lehrer's laboratory (Lehrer, Smetankin, & Potapova, 2000a) have shown that daily practice of this "resonant frequency biofeedback therapy" increases the total amount of heart rate variability, with almost all of the oscillations occurring at a single frequency. This method was also found to increase baroreflex gain and to improve pulmonary function while lowering blood pressure, even among healthy people.

In this vein, many groups around the world have been reporting that "RSA" biofeedback is a viable feedback modality. The client is instructed to maximize the peak–valley amplitude based on a cardiotachometer line graph. Over time, almost all participants achieve this by slowing and deepening breath, and entering a "mindful" mental state. Although this method may affect vagal activity, it appears to do much more. It provides high-amplitude heart rate oscillations that stimulate the baroreflexes about six times per minute. These oscillations provide much greater regular stimulation of the baroreflexes than generally occurs on a regular basis. They are, as described above, produced by resonance between biofeedback effects (or respiration) and baroreflex activity. This increased "exercise" of the baroreflexes is hypothesized to increase the efficiency of the reflex (Vaschillo, 1984). Lehrer et al. (1997) and Lehrer et al. (2000a) have shown the procedure to improve lung function in patients with asthmas, and Herbs, Gevirtz, and Jacobs (1994) have shown it to reduce blood pressure in patients with hypertension. Anecdotal preports from Russia suggest that it may be helpful in treating a variety of psychosomatic and stress-related physical disorders (Chernigovskaya, Vaschillo, Petrash, & Rusanovsky, 1990).

Studies evaluating this feedback mode are underway and, if successful, may offer a powerful new tool in the field of mind–body medicine.

PROCEDURE FOR PERFORMING RESONANT FREQUENCY BIOFEEDBACK THERAPY

Although the method is still too new for a codified procedure, a suggested procedural method has been outlined by Lehrer et al. (2000b). The first session is usually devoted to determining the person's resonant frequency. This is accomplished by having the individual breathe at various frequencies near 0.1 Hz, and finding the frequency that yields the highest amplitude of heart rate oscillations. The person is then advised to practice breathing at this frequency daily until the next session (approximately a week later). In subsequent sessions, biofeedback is provided in the form of a cardiotachometer display or an online Fourier analysis of heart rate, updated every few seconds. The person is instructed to maximize the amplitude of heart rate variability at his or her resonant frequency, and to fine-tune the estimation of his or her resonant frequency by observing the respiration rate that continues to yield the highest amplitude of heart rate variability. To enhance the effect, the individual is sometimes instructed to breathe abdominally and to exhale through pursed lips. The person is also advised to breathe shallowly in order to avoid hyperventilating during practice of this method. Although most people are able to produce high amplitudes of heart rate variability within just a few minutes of training, it usually takes several sessions to learn to stabilize heart rate variability at the resonant frequency. The number of sessions required to maximize effects is not yet known. Data from both of our laboratories suggest that the curve representing physiological effects has not yet leveled off after 10 sessions of training.

AREAS FOR FUTURE RESEARCH

The reader is cautioned that there are few clinical studies of this method. Hyperventilation has been documented as a potential side effect of the technique that must be managed during treatment (Lehrer et al., 1997). Other side effects may yet be documented, particularly among vulnerable individuals (e.g., people with heart failure, severe hypertension, etc.). However, initial findings in Gevirtz's clinic when the technique was used in cardiac rehabilitation have been promising, in that increases in heart rate variability were produced with no serious side effects. Further research using this method is necessary in order to understand both its potential benefits and any possible harm it may cause. Also, in view of Vaschillo's findings of large baroreflex effects on blood pressure oscillations at 0.05 Hz (Vaschillo et al., 2002), it is possible that training to produce large-amplitude oscillations within the VLF range may also have power effects on the baroreflex system and on autonomic control.

GLOSSARY

OSCILLATORS. Devices or physiological systems that produce to-and-fro, rhythmic activity.

R-WAVE. Electrocardioigraphic (ECG) wave that is represented by the peak during electrical stimulation of the ventricles. It is used in biofeedback settings to trigger a timer to measure "interbeat interval" (IBI; the time between R-wave peaks).

SPECTRAL ANALYSIS. A mathematical and graphical technique used to decompose complex waveforms into their constituent components (frequency bins). The mathematical formulae to do this were first worked out by Fourier, and thus the analysis is often called a "fast Fourier transform."

VAGAL NUCLEI. The two medullary nuclei from which the vagus nerve of the parasympathetic nervous system is thought to originate: the dorsal motor nucleus (DMNX), responsible for primitive cardiac braking, and the nucleus ambiguus (NA), responsible for subtle rhythmic braking in coordination with respiration.

REFERENCES

Bernardi, L., Leuzzi, S., Radaelli, A., Passino, C., Johnston, J. A., & Sleight, P. (1994). Low-frequency spontaneous fluctuations of R-R interval and blood pressure in conscious humans: A baroreceptor or central phenomenon? *Clinical Science, 87*(6), 649–654.

Berntson, G. G., Bigger, J. T., Jr., Eckberg, D. L., Grossman, P., Kaufmann, P. G., Malik, M., Nagaraja, H. N., Porges, S. W., Saul, J. P., Stone, P. H., & van Molen, M. W. (1997). Heart rate variability: Origins, methods, and interpretative caveats. *Psychophysiology, 34*, 623–648.

Berntson, G. G., Cacioppo, J. T., & Quigley, K. S. (1993). Cardiac psychophysiology and autonomic space in humans: Empirical perspectives and conceptual implications. *Psychological Bulletin, 114*(2), 296–322.

Berntson, G. G., Cacioppo, J. T., Quigley, K. S., & Fabro, V. T. (1994). Autonomic space and psychophysiological response. *Psychophysiology, 31*(1), 44–61.

Bigger, J. T., Jr., Fleiss, J. L., Rolnitzky, L. M., & Steinman, R. C. (1993a). The ability of several short-term measures of RR variability to predict mortality after myocardial infarction. *Circulation, 88*(3), 927–934.

Bigger, J. T., Jr., Fleiss, J. L., Rolnitzky, L. M., & Steinman, R. C. (1993b). Frequency domain measures of heart period variability to assess risk late after myocardial infarction. *Journal of the American College of Cardiology, 21*(3), 729–736.

Bigger, J. T., Jr., Fleiss, J. L., Steinman, R. C., Rolnitzky, L. M., Schneider, W. J., & Stein, P. K. (1995). RR variability in healthy, middle-aged persons compared with patients with chronic coronary heart disease or recent acute myocardial infarction. *Circulation, 91*(7), 1936–1943.

Bigger, J. T., Jr., Rolnitzky, L. M., Steinman, R. C., & Fleiss, J. L. (1994). Predicting mortality after myocardial infarction from the response of RR variability to antiarrhythmic drug therapy. *Journal of the American College of Cardiology, 23*(3), 733–740.

Bigger, J. T., Jr., Steinman, R. C., Rolnitzky, L. M., Fleiss, J. L., & Albrecht, P. (1996). Power law behavior of RR-interval variability in healthy middle-aged persons, patients with recent acute myocardial infarction, and patients with heart transplants. *Circulation, 93*(12), 2142–2151.

Chernigovskaya, N. V., Vaschillo, E. G., Petrash, V. V., & Rusanovsky, V. V. (1990). Voluntary regulation of the heart rate as a method of functional condition correction in neurotics. *Human Physiology, 16*, 58–64.

Giardino, N., Lehrer, P., & Edelberg, R. (2002). Comparison of finger plethysmograph to ECG in the measurement of heart rate variability. *Psychophysiology, 39*(2), 246–253.

Giardino, A., Lehrer, P., & Feldman, J. M. (2000). The role of oscillations in self-regulation: A revision of the classical model of homeostasis. In J. G. C. D. Kenney, F. J. McGuigan, & J. L. Sheppard (Eds.), *Stress and health: Research and clinical applications*. Amsterdam: Harwood.

Grossman, P., & Kollai, M. (1993). Respiratory sinus arrhythmia, cardiac vagal tone, and respiration: Within- and between-individual relations. *Psychophysiology, 30*(5), 486–495.

Grossman, P., van Beek, J., & Wientjes, C. (1990). A comparison of three quantification methods for estimation of respiratory sinus arrhythmia. *Psychophysiology, 27*(6), 702–714.

Herbs, D., Gevirtz, R. N., & Jacobs, D. (1994). The effect of heart rate pattern biofeedback for the treatment of essential hypertension. [Abstract]. *Biofeedback and Self-Regulation, 19*(3), 281.

Katz, A., Liberty, I. F., Porath, A., Ovsyshcher, I., & Prystowsky, E. N. (1999). A simple bedside test of 1-minute heart rate variability during deep breathing as a prognostic index after myocardial infarction. *American Heart Journal, 138*(1, Pt. 1), 32–38.

Kleiger, R. E., Miller, J. P., Bigger, J. T., Jr., & Moss, A. J. (1987). Decreased heart rate variability and its association with increased mortality after acute myocardial infarction. *American Jourrnal of Cardiology, 59*(4),
256–262.

Kristal-Boneh, E., Froom, P., Raifel, M., Froom, P., & Ribak, J. (2000). Summer–winter differences in 24 h variability of heart rate. *Journal of Cardiovascular Risk, 7*(2), 141–146.

Kristal-Boneh, E., Raifel, M., Harari, G., Malik, M., & Ribak, J. (1995). Heart rate variability in health and
disease. *Scandanavian Journal of Work and Environmental Health, 21*(2), 85–95.

Lehrer, P. M., Carr, R. E., Smetankine, A.,Vaschillo, E., Peper, E., Porges, S., Edelberg, R., Hamer, R., & Hochron, S.
(1997). Respiratory sinus arrhythmia versus neck/trapezius EMG and incentive inspirometry biofeedback
for asthma: A pilot study. *Applied Psychophysiology and Biofeedback, 22*(2), 95–109.

Lehrer, P. M., Smetankin, A., & Potapova, T. (2000a). Respiratory sinus arrhythmia biofeedback therapy for
asthma: A report of 20 unmedicated pediatric cases using the Smetankin method. *Applied Psychophysiology and Biofeedback, 25,* 193–200.

Lehrer, P. M., Vaschillo, E., & Vaschillo, B. (2000b). Resonant frequency biofeedback training to increase cardiac variability: Rationale and manual for training. *Applied Psychophysiology and Biofeedback, 25*(3), 177–
191.

Porges, S. W. (1995a). Cardiac vagal tone: A physiological index of stress. *Neuroscience and Biobehavioral Reviews, 19*(2), 225–233.

Porges, S. W. (1995b). Orienting in a defensive world: Mammalian modifications of our evolutionary heritage: A
polyvagal theory. *Psychophysiology, 32*(4), 301–318.

Porges, S. W. (1997). Emotion: An evolutionary by-product of the neural regulation of the autonomic nervous
system. *Annals of the New York Academy of Sciences, 807,* 62–77.

Vaschillo, E. G. (1984). *Dynamics of slow-wave cardiac rhythm structure as an index of the functional state of an
operant.* Unpublished doctoral dissertation, Leningrad State University, Leningrad, USSR.

Vaschillo, E. G., Lehrer, P., Rishe, N., & Konstantinov, M. (2002). Heart rate variability biofeedback as a method
of assessing baroreflex function: A preliminary study of resonance in the cardiovascular system. *Applied
Psychophysiology and Biofeedback, 27*(1), 1–27.

Wilhelm, F. H., Gevirtz, R., & Roth, W. T. (2001). Respiratory dysregulation in anxiety, functional cardiac, and
pain disorders: Assessment, phenomenology, and treatment. *Behavior Modification, 25*(4), 513–545.

Problems with Relaxation and Biofeedback-Assisted Relaxation, and Guidelines for Management

MARK S. SCHWARTZ
NANCY M. SCHWARTZ
VINCENT J. MONASTRA

Relaxation therapies and biofeedback-assisted relaxation procedures commonly lead to positive therapeutic results. Most people use these therapies without problems. Nevertheless, a few people do experience strong negative reactions and other problems. These difficulties can alarm both patients and therapists unnecessarily, and can result in stopping potentially useful therapy. Even if a patient experiencing such difficulties remains in therapy, they can reduce compliance with recommended relaxation and thus can reduce the patient's chances for improvement (Borkovec et al., 1987).

Fortunately, significant negative reactions are uncommon and can usually be avoided. Practitioners who are aware of these and other potential difficulties and their possible causes can often prevent or lessen these effects. Bernstein and Borkovec (1973), Bernstein and Carlson (1993), and McGuigan (1993) identified several possible problems and negative side effects of progressive muscle relaxation. Schultz and Luthe (1969) and Linden (1993) discussed potential problems and negative side effects associated with autogenic therapy. Poppen (1998) discussed potential problems associated with Behavioral Relaxation Training. The reader is referred to these excellent discussions and their suggested solutions.

NEGATIVE REACTIONS

A partial list of the potential negative reactions reported includes the following:

1. *Musculoskeletal activity.* Examples of such activities are tics, cramps, myoclonic jerks, spasms, and restlessness.

2. *Disturbing sensory experiences.* These experiences include sensations of heaviness, warmth, or cooling; feelings of depersonalization, misperceived body size, or floating; and a variety of visual, auditory, gustatory, and olfactory experiences.

3. *Sympathetic nervous system activity.* These reactions include increased heart rate and increased electrodermal activity.

4. *Distrubing cognitive and/or emotional reactions.* Examples include feelings of sadness, anger, depression, disturbing thoughts, intrusive thoughts or mind wandering, tearfulness, increased anxiety, and fears (such as fear of losing control).

5. *Other possible negative side effects.* These include hypotensive reactions, headache, sexual arousal, and psychotic symptoms.

A subset of these negative reactions has acquired the name of "relaxation-induced anxiety" (RIA) and is discussed below under that rubric. This is followed by a discussion of several other negative reactions to relaxation and biofeedback-induced relaxation, together with other problems that are not specific reactions to relaxation or biofeedback per se, but may cause patients to terminate therapy prematurely or to derive less than full benefit from therapy. The topic of adverse effects of electroencephalographic (EEG) biofeedback, which has not heretofore received much attention, is considered in a separate section. The chapter concludes with discussions of the paucity of research in this area as a whole, and of major cautions and contraindications for the use of physiological self-regulatory therapies.

RELAXATION-INDUCED ANXIETY

RIA is the term used to denote a variety of negative reactions associated with relaxation procedures. Heide and Borkovec (1983) defined RIA as "paradoxical increases in cognitive, physiological, or behavioral components of anxiety as a consequence of engaging in systematic relaxation training" (p. 171). Carrington (1977) described intense restlessness, profuse perspiration, shivering, trembling, pounding heart, and rapid breathing associated with a type of meditation. In essence, RIA is increased anxiety associated with attempts at relaxation.[1]

As the full term *"relaxation-*induced anxiety" indicates, most such negative reactions reported are reactions to relaxation procedures rather than to biofeedback alone. Indeed, we have found no reports of these reactions occurring with biofeedback alone. Thus one cannot determine the incidence or prevalence of "BIA" from any of the published reports. We believe that very few people have undesirable or negative reactions to biofeedback instruments and feedback signals alone. The few who do are probably anxious either about biomedical instruments and the process of recording internal body activity, or about various types of evaluations and seeing doctors.

Incidence of Relaxation-Induced Negative Reactions

Until the 1980s, little attention was given in the clinical and research literature to these problems. There are very few studies and almost none with medical patients. What studies do exist involve very few subjects. Available reports are mostly anecdotal surveys of mental health professionals, observations of subjects or patients in studies, and small samples of patients with anxiety disorders. Survey studies are helpful but fraught with methodological problems.

Papers by Jacobson and Edinger (1982) and Edinger and Jacobson (1982) were among the early reports of negative side effects associated with relaxation therapies. They conducted a brief mail survey of behavior therapists who used relaxation therapies. The 116 clinicians who responded reported a total of 17,542 patients and clients. An estimated 3.5% of patients had experienced negative reactions that interfered with relaxation therapy. These investigators partially defined "interference" as "noncompliance or client-initiated termination of treatment" (Edinger & Jacobson, 1982, p. 137). The professionals surveyed reported "discontinuing relaxation" because negative side effects confounded treatment in another 3.8% of their patients and clients.

The data from Edinger and Jacobson (1982, p. 138) indicated that the more commonly reported negative reactions were "intrusive thoughts" in 15% and "fears of 'losing control'" in 9.3%. The less commonly reported reactions were "disturbing sensory experience" in 3.6%, "sexual arousal" when the client and the therapist were of different sexes in 2.3%, "muscle cramps" in 2.1%, "spasms/tics" in 1.7%, "sexual arousal" when the client and the therapist were of the same sex in 0.85%, "emergence of psychotic symptoms" in 0.4%, and "other" or "miscellaneous" such as "sleep, increased anxiety, and depersonalization" reported by no more than two clinicians or 2.5%.

The investigators acknowledged that there are problems with survey research, and that "no attempt was made to examine client population(s) being treated and exact relaxation procedure(s) . . . being used by respondents" (Edinger & Jacobson, 1982, p. 138). They concluded, however, that "side-effects are generally infrequent and inconsequential" and that "very few . . . appear sufficient to stop therapy by an experienced and knowledgeable therapist except perhaps the sexual arousal and emergence of psychotic symptoms," the latter of which occurred in only about "1 out of every 263 cases treated" (p. 138).

In the one study of medical patients (Blanchard, Cornish, Wittrock, & Fahrion, 1990), 73 patients with hypertension received temperature biofeedback and relaxation. Of these, 4–9% reported negative sensations or experiences in any one session, but all were minor and none were RIA. Among a group of 30 undergraduates reporting chronic anxiety, 5 (17%) "reported increased anxiety" during a taped session of progressive relaxation (Braith, McCullough, & Bush, 1988, p. 193).

Heide and Borkovec (1983, 1984) provided a very thoughtful review of RIA. They conceded that although the evidence for RIA at that time was mostly anecdotal, it was present often enough to be of concern. They reviewed the mechanisms presumed to underlie the phenomenon, and suggested procedures for relieving some problems.

Also, they found physiological correlates of anxiety in some subjects who did not report anxiety. In some subjects who did report anxiety, physiological measures were lower—although not as low as in subjects reporting reduced tension. Thus RIA is a difficult phenomenon to understand in general terms. It is often a subjective experience, possibly more clearly understood through in-depth study of individual cases. This was discussed by Lehrer and Woolfolk (1993a, 1993b) in their chapter and elsewhere in their book.

Proposed Causes of RIA and Risk Factors

There are several hypothesized causes of RIA. Any one or a combination could apply to a specific individual. The first five were suggested by Heide and Borkovec (1984).

1. *Cognitive fear of unfamiliar sensations.* Some people may have a cognitive fear of the sensations associated with relaxation, such as tingling, heaviness, warmth, and muscle jerks. Patients may view these physiological–behavioral reactions and the related cognitive–affective reactions as uncomfortable or unfamiliar, rather than as positive signs that relaxation is occurring. This may be more common in people who rarely or never attend to body sensations, or among those who interpret these sensations as negative.

A related hypothesis (Denny, 1976) suggests that stimuli produced by relaxation may become conditioned to fear when paired with a history of punishment during relaxation or safety times. Another idea is that some chronically anxious people may be frightened by the unfamiliar sensations of deep relaxation. These thoughts may then trigger chemical changes in the body.

2. *Fear of losing control.* Some people are preoccupied with maintaining control over their physical and psychological processes (Braith et al., 1988; Lehrer, 1982). Furthermore, some people fear losing control and may use active, effortful relaxation strategies. Western culture assumes that exercising control requires active effort. Seligman (1975) defined "control" as being able to change outcomes by voluntary actions. Such patients may display a pattern of trying too hard. They maintain a high degree of activity out of fear that without it they will waste time and accomplish nothing. This fear of inactivity may lead to more anxiety.

The fear of losing control may be more common among people who avoid rest and reflection, and among those intent on maintaining control with active and effortful activity. For people with generalized anxiety, "daily maintenance of higher-then-normal tension may be a learned avoidance response to relaxation" (Borkovec et al., 1987, p. 887).

Associated with the loss of control is the perception that relaxation "signifies vulnerability, lack of control over anger and sexual desire, overpassivity, etc." (Lehrer, 1982, p. 424). This may have been the cause of the angry feelings evoked in five patients who were asked to relax, as reported by Abromowitz and Wieselberg (1978).

3. *Fear of experiencing anxiety.* RIA is more common in persons who are chronically anxious. Relaxation methods often direct people to focus away from external stimuli and to focus on body sensations or thoughts. This may increase their awareness of current internal cues, which are often associated with higher levels of anxiety. In the past, these cues were distressing: The person viewed them as meaning "out of my control," or associated the cues with heightened anxiety or even panic. For example, specific thoughts about anxiety may result in cognitive anxiety (Norton, Rhodes, Hauch, & Kaprowy, 1985).

4. *Fear of encountering oneself.* This is the hypothesized fear of attending to the heightened awareness of internal experience in general. Some professionals view this phenomenon as one resulting from dissatisfaction with oneself or from fearing the increased awareness of inner conflicts.

5. *Situation-produced worry, or intrusive thoughts and worries.* Patients may find, as they reduce their focus on external stimuli, that their own thoughts and worries arise and become more dominant. This phenomenon is similar to cognitive intrusions' interference with sleep onset. Note that these thoughts do not relate to relaxation but become associated with the relaxation, experience (see also Lichstein, 1988, p. 138).

6. *Breathing-related physical changes.* Another interesting and logical hypothesis with support is that of Ley (1988). Physical changes from breathing occur during relaxation and could cause or increase the chance of having RIA. Chronic hyperventilation alters the amount of carbon dioxide and other body chemicals in the blood. This could lead to RIA as the person shifts from activity to inactivity without changing breathing pattern to match the inactive state. (The reader is referred to Gevirtz & Schwartz, Chapter 10, this volume, for a more detailed discussion of breathing.)

7. *Parasympathetic or trophotropic responses.* An old hypothesis is the parasympathetic or trophotropic response hypothesis. According to this view, some people tend to have more parasympathetic responses. RIA is a compensatory ergotropic sympathetic nervous system response. This is similar to theories such as the one proposed by Stampler (1982), suggesting that relaxation may directly stimulate a "complex interplay of psychological and physiological factors" (Cohen, Barlow, & Blanchard, 1985, p. 99) that can lead to RIA in susceptible people.

For example, DeGood and Williams (1982) reported a case of a 40-year-old female patient treated with autogenic training and electromyographic biofeedback for low back pain and leg pain. They monitored her finger temperature and skin conductance. She developed acute headaches with nausea soon after each of the first two sessions. Revising the training procedure to having the patient sit upright with her eyes open helped to stop the postsession symptoms. DeGood and Williams speculated that the negative symptoms were caused by "vagal rebound" or "parasympathetic overcompensation" (p. 464) after physiological deactivation during the relaxation.

This explanation focuses on the possible role of the anterior hypothalamus (Gellhorn, 1965, 1967; Mefford, 1979). According to this view, "lowered somatic activity . . . tends to be accompanied by increased activation of the trophotropically dominant anterior hypothalamus and related structures (DeGood & Williams, 1982, p. 464).

8. *Switching from passive to active coping.* Another possible cause for RIA involves switching from a passive, immobilized, nonpreparatory, and relaxed state to the anticipation of or preparation for action (Elliott, 1974; Obrist, 1976, 1981; Cohen et al., 1985). Heart rate is slower during passive coping. The person switching from a passive to an active coping method could experience large accelerations of heart rate, according to this explanation (Cohen et al., 1985). Such accelerated heart rate is presumably not because of increased anxiety, but because of cardiac–somatic coupling. This is the close relationship between heart rate and striate muscle activity. Thus preparation for action may produce increased somatic arousal and increased heart rate.

9. *Other explanations.* Some patients who experience RIA are people who are competitive with themselves and who fear failure. In other individuals, relaxation may arouse thoughts and feelings of sexual arousal. Still other people take certain medications, and may confuse the side effects or interactions with the feelings induced by relaxation; this confusion may result in RIA.

Guidelines for Avoiding, Minimizing, and Managing RIA

People who experience RIA are among those who often most need psychophysiological self-regulation. The implication for practitioners is not to avoid relaxation, but to be aware of and anticipate reactions. Practitioners should provide understandable and realistic patient education, and should select types of relaxation that are less likely to result in these reactions with particular patients. A positive therapy alliance can help practitioners manage these reactions.

Patient preparation for relaxation should include an explanation that patients may experience certain sensations and thoughts during relaxation; these are normal signs that relaxation is taking place. This explanation is especially important for patients with chronic anxiety. Moreover, patients should be cautioned to expect intrusive thoughts in early sessions of relaxation; these should diminish as the patient's skills and confidence increase. In addition, the clinician should explain relaxation as increased control rather than as diminished control. He or she can explain that people often achieve relaxation proficiency and increased autonomic nervous system control through less rather than more effort.

The therapist can also consider a switch to a different type of relaxation. People rarely experience RIA with two different types of relaxation. If a patient is having difficulty with a bodily focus type, a switch to a more cognitive approach might achieve desired results. If a patient is having trouble with a cognitive method, a switch to an active, external attentional focus or to a bodily focus type might be tried. An example of this would be focusing on external sounds in or outside the office, rather than a mental focus on body awareness (Wells, 1990; see also the discussion of distraction and intrusive thoughts below).

OTHER REACTIONS AND PROBLEMS, AND GUIDELINES FOR AVOIDING, REDUCING, AND MANAGING THEM

1. *Embarrassment.* Some patients feel embarrassed or self-conscious about tensing certain muscles, such as those of the face. Others feel embarrassed about closing eyes or engaging in other relaxation procedures.

Solutions: Modeling the procedures and offering reassurance and supportive statements can sometimes help. In earlier trials, the therapist can look away from the patient and look at the visual display while the patient tenses muscles.

2. *Gender-related or sexual problems.* Some patients may feel sexually aroused, self-conscious, or threatened during relaxation. Reclining in a darkened room and using suggestive or other relaxation terms with double meanings can add to such patients' subjective discomfort. Self-consciousness and similar discomfort can also occur with patients (especially males) who are unaccustomed to the passive role in any situation. Now they find themselves asked to recline passively. This can be psychologically uncomfortable for them. We suspect that very few patients will explain these reasons for their discomfort, and indeed that many are not aware of the reasons.

Solutions: Practitioners should consider starting patients with these types of discomfort in a comfortable upright posture, to which they are more accustomed. Professionals should be sensitive to sexual and gender-related factors, and should adjust their language and procedures accordingly. Professionals should be certain to maintain boundaries and be careful about touching patients.

3. *Script content problems.* The contents of relaxation scripts are comfortable for many patients but uncomfortable for others. This depends on the patients' perceptions, attitudes, and fantasies. For example, the therapist might consider the potential effect of using the term "feelings of heaviness" with patients who have actual or perceived weight problems.

Solutions: Professionals should provide sufficient patient education and tailor their scripts as needed.

4. *Distraction and intrusive thoughts.* There are many sources of distraction from the concentration needed during relaxation and body awareness procedures. These can include associations to the contents of the relaxation script. Some people think about their life and responsibilities at these times.

Solutions: The therapist should discuss this problem with patients and reassure them that these distracting thoughts and images are normal. Then he or she can assist patients in ways to lessen them. To achieve such a goal, the therapist might consider shorter sessions, more breaks, or having the patients start with eyes open or partially open. Practitioners should also consider using active sensory awareness exercises, such as the example by Wells (1990) of external attentional focus on sounds in the environment.

One can expand this to training patients to focus on sensory awareness of the environment, rather than having them strive for internal awareness and a self-attentive focus. For example, the therapist can guide or direct a patient to attend to the texture of the armchair, sounds in the office, and the color of a wall. He or she can then guide the patient through switching from one to another to increase the patient's ability to choose and control his or her mental focus. The therapist should do these slowly, but for only a few seconds of focus on each, as in this example:

> "Right now, think about the color of the wall. Right now, think about the texture of the chair. Right now, think about the sound of _____. Now, switch your attention from one to another."

Another suggestion is for patients to think of the distracting thoughts as words or pictures on a television or movie screen. The patients can then imagine the screen becoming smaller and smaller until it becomes tiny and distant or disappears entirely. Patients can imagine that they are moving farther away or the screen is moving farther away. Sitting close to a big color screen is more distressing than seeing the same words and images on a 3-inch black-and-white screen several feet away.

5. *Restlessness and related problems.* Being silent and being motionless are paradoxically uncomfortable for some people. These people become restless with longer sessions. Some may have features of the syndrome sometimes known as adult attention-deficit/hyperactivity disorder (ADHD). Problems with laughing, talking, coughing, sneezing, and other body movements are related.

Solutions: Practitioners should assess and prepare for restleness early for all patients. They should ask whether a patient has any concern about sitting quietly for the planned amount of time. If a practitioner anticipates patient discomfort, he or she should discuss this early, reassure the patient, and suggest adjusted body positions and durations as indicated. Patients should be given choices about physical positions, lighting, and time to make adjustments. Sessions can be shortened or interspersed with breaks. All patients may keep eyes open or partially open. Therapists should also avoid long silences without verbal instructions, discussion, changes in feedback displays and tasks, or physiological changes that are obvious to patients.

6. *Low self-efficacy and fear of failure.* Patients often do not have the needed self-confidence in their abilities to develop effective relaxation skills. The theme in their self-statements is "I cannot do it." They also may not have realistic goals; they may expect the goal of therapy to be mastery. Similarly, fear of failure is a common problem. Such patients say to themselves, "Am I doing this right?", "Am I doing this better than the last time?", or "I will never get the feelings and benefits I need!"

Solutions: The therapist should explain and remind patients that learning any new physical or mental skill is a process with peaks, valleys, and plateaus. Moreover, developing or cultivating low or lower tension and arousal is often a gradual process. Using examples from the acquisition of athletic, musical, or other skills is often helpful. Patients should be encouraged and reminded to avoid hurrying and to apply the "three P's"—patience, practice, and persistence.

Discussing fear of failure early and periodically can help patients replace negative thoughts with positive ones. Therapists should remind patients that most people can make progress, and guide patients away from viewing physiological self-regulation as something that they "pass or fail." In addition, patients should be encouraged to allow relaxation to happen or to let go, rather than trying to make it happen. They should focus on increasing their awareness of feelings associated with physiological self-regulation. Finally, therapists should change the goals away from specific numbers; patients need not become Olympic competitors.

7. *Increased awareness of tension.* A few patients report increased symptoms during the early stages of relaxation therapies. Because general relaxation permits more awareness of tension of selected body areas, patients may perceive themselves as more tense than they were before. This does not mean that the patients are actually more tense, but simply that they are more body-aware. An increased awareness of tension can also result from increased focus on symptoms through the use of self-report symptom logs. Some relaxation procedures, such as tensing muscles, can increase some symptoms as well. Some body areas remain tense during some relaxation procedures, including tense–release procedures.

Solutions: Therapists should discuss this phenomenon and reassure patients that such perceptions are common and normal. By noticing tension earlier, one can reduce the tension and prevent symptoms. Patients can reframe the belief in increased tension as increased awareness.

8. *Problems with significant others.* Family members and other significant people in a patient's life who are around him or her during relaxation therapy may not be understanding and cooperative.

Solutions: If such people are not present during office sessions, a therapist should provide the patient with patient education materials explaining the rationale, procedures, and need for cooperation from others. Practitioners may need to counsel some patients on how to discuss this with others and how to increase cooperation from family members.

9. *Factors not related to starting therapy.* Factors other than starting relaxation therapy can increase symptoms. If a patient is not cognitively prepared for the therapy, he or she can experience increased concern, emotional arousal, and tension, and therefore increased symptoms. Another factor is the presence of continuing or even increasing stress in the patient's life, thereby adding to the symptoms.

Solutions: Discussion of current life events and counseling, adjustments, and reassurance are appropriate. A therapist must obviously rule out other causes, such as an incorrect diagnosis and treatment strategy.

10. *Viewing treatment as stressful.* Some patients view some aspects of treatment as stressful, and this can add to symptoms. Therapists should consider the time allotments and other arrangements required for patients to attend office sessions. These include time away from other duties and responsibilities, explanations to employers and supervisors, and often extra work when patients get back from appointments. Patients also invest time and effort in carrying out homework assignments, maintaining self-report records, and completing questionnaires. All of these pressures are stressful, and added to them are the expenses for therapy. Thoughts about any or all of these added sources of stress can intrude.

Solutions: Sensitivity and flexibility on the practitioner's part about scheduling and assignments can help decrease the effects of this stress.

11. *Disregarding instructions.* Patients sometimes disregard instructions during biofeedback and other relaxation procedures, in the practitioner's office and elsewhere. For example, they may not imagine the stress stimuli the practitioner presents, or may imagine the stress stimuli for only part of the time. In addition, some patients intentionally think of topics other than the biofeedback signal or verbal relaxation instructions. Patients are unlikely to admit such diversions without careful questioning. The therapist must be careful in discussing this, to avoid giving the impression of being critical.

Solutions: Sensitivity and flexibility on the practitioner's part about assignments and instructions can help. Once again, adequate patient education should be provided. A therapist can change the content of the relaxation script and procedures, or can consider saying something like the following:

> "Sometimes you might be thinking about other topics during relaxation and biofeedback. It is normal for that to occur at times, and I understand. However, I need to know if you shift away from the instructions here or in your practice at home. Please understand when I ask you about that. Please share it with me when it is happening, so we can discuss it."

12. *Not focusing on physiology.* Some people listen to relaxation audiotapes but do not focus on their physiology. Similarly, some patients just listen to or watch feedback signals, but with minimal or no focusing on their physiology. It is as if they are expecting or hoping that the relaxation instructions and biofeedback signals will induce the desired outcome by itself.

Solutions: The therapist can anticipate this potential problem and discuss it. He or she can guide patients away from a scenario of passively expecting the audiotape or feedback signal to be therapeutic by itself. Biofeedback gives patients information, suggestions, guidelines, and samples to use, but the patients themselves are responsible for the changes.

13. *Falling asleep.* Some patients fall asleep during relaxation procedures.

Solutions: Therapists should be aware of potential sleepers. Patients can make special efforts to keep their eyes open, can schedule sessions earlier in the day, or can avoid relaxation after meals unless it is needed for postprandial symptoms. In persistent cases, a therapist should consider a sleep disorder evaluation to check for sleep apnea, psychophysiological insomnia, sleep–wake schedule disorders, and narcolepsy.

14. *Misuse of relaxation audiotapes.* Some patients are dependent on audiotapes and use them too often and too long. They rely on them and do not learn to relax without them.

Solutions: Patient education should include clarifying the proper role of tapes and encouraging patients to avoid dependence on them. If patients do become dependent, they can be tapered from tapes via fading and related behavioral techniques. A therapist can consider using tapes with progressively briefer scripts. Patients can turn the tape player off progressively earlier in the script, or can lower the volume gradually and continue the relaxation.

15. *Not having or taking enough time to practice and apply relaxation.* This is a very common problem. Many patients who particularly need to develop and apply relaxation therapies also have substantial time use problems. They do not know how to or have not applied effective time use management in their lives.

Solutions: The therapist should conduct, or refer such patients for, an evaluation of and education about time use management. For example, practitioners can help such patients learn to set goals and priorities. Other valuable lessons for patients include learning to delegate responsibility appropriately, avoiding or reducing activities that waste time, reducing perfectionism, and managing procrastination. Patients should be encouraged to schedule relaxation and to make practice and application a high priority.

16. *Specific problems with biofeedback procedures.* In addition to more general problems with relaxation, problems can occur during biofeedback-assisted relaxation sessions that are specific to the biofeedback (Gaarder & Montgomery, 1981, p. 94). These remain relevant, although with the technological advantages of microcomputer-based biofeedback, there is a broader array of solutions. We include some of these problems here and suggest a few solutions for consideration. Experienced and very competent therapists can develop their own repertoire.

A. *Very small changes in a physiological parameter, or no patient perception the feedback signal is changing.*

Solutions: Therapists can use the threshold or change it to ease the task. The gain can be increased, so that the visual display feedback or audio feedback changes are more obvious with smaller physiological changes. Therapists can encourage shifting attention to other sites or cognitions, as well as switching to a different task or feedback site. They can use varied verbal relaxation instructions or change the visual display as well.

A therapist can ask a patient to close his or her eyes for a few moments and then freeze the visual display if it changes in the desired direction. Then the therapist can ask the patient to open his or her eyes gently to see the change. This should be repeated as needed.

B. *Movement of the feedback signal in the undesired direction.*

Solutions: The therapist can stop instrumentation-based feedback to the patient. He or she can discuss "trying too hard" and provide quiet, brief, and clear verbal feedback when the therapist sees the signal moving in the desired direction. The therapist should observe the patient's posture, breathing, and movements and suggest adjustments as needed. Focus can be shifted to other sites, tasks, or techniques. The therapist should use varied verbal relaxation instructions, ask about patients' cognitions, and discuss and suggest changes as needed. Increased control is the ability to move the signal in either direction. The experienced practi tioner will notice what makes it go in the wrong direction, as this can give clues for moving it in the desired direction.

C. *Patient fatigue with the feedback signal or task.*

Solutions: The therapist should change feedback displays. With computer-based systems, there are a wide variety of feedback options. The therapist can also conduct shorter sessions, or adjust the goals of a session to increase the chance of obvious successes and reinforce changes.

17. *Unable to exhibit a relaxation posture due to physical limitations.* Poppen (1998) discusses the specialized procedures he developed and calls Behavioral Relaxation Training (BRT)[2]. Physical limitations include scoliosis, arthritis, or unequal leg length that can interfere with the patient's ability to implement BRT.

Solutions: The therapist should be alert to these limitations and tailor adjustments in the relaxation process and criteria.

18. *Complaints that specific relaxation behaviors are uncomfortable.* These do not feel right to the patient and are typically due to habitual tension or asymmetrical positions (Poppen, 1998). Examples are the head and shoulders at midline feel out of line compared to the head turned slightly.

Solutions: Assure the patient that the newness of the relaxation behaviors are causing the discomfort and that it will feel natural after more practice.

19. *Breathing with open mouth while relaxing results in dry oral cavity.*

Solutions: Remind patient to breathe nasally and close mouth.

20. *Frustration from feeling that performing specific procedures are impossible.* Examples are being unable to keep eyes closed without twitching eyelids, breathing at a slower rate, or swallowing less often.

Solutions: Reassure patient that 100 percent perfection is not expected. Also provide positive feedback anytime the relaxed behavior occurs.

ADVERSE EFFECTS OF EEG BIOFEEDBACK[3]

Although clinical applications of EEG biofeedback have been reported for three decades, evidence of adverse reactions has not been frequently documented. As reviewed by Monastra in Chapter 19 of this text, clinical researchers have focused on examining issues of efficacy. Outcome studies reported in the scientific literature contain an abundance of information about treatment protocols and indicators of change in clinical status. In addition, the lack of treatment response has been documented. However, there is limited information provided about exacerbation of clinical status following EEG biofeedback.

Three published studies provide illustrations of the types of adverse clinical reactions that can occur as a result of EEG biofeedback. One study (Peniston & Kulkosky, 1989) reported the emergence of "spontaneously occurring images" during applications of their treatment protocol with patients diagnosed with alcoholism. In the Peniston and Kulkosky paradigm, EEG biofeedback is used to reinforce production of alpha and theta at O_1. According to these researchers, this process was used to promote a "relaxed state." However, it was evident from their report that certain patients experienced recollection of traumatic events, which required treatment with other types of behavioral therapy ("flooding"). Consequently, clinicians utilizing alpha or theta enhancement protocols need to be mindful of the possibility that patients with a history of abuse or psychological trauma may experience increased anxiety during this type of treatment.

A study by Monastra, Monastra, and George (2002) illustrates certain adverse side effects associated with combining EEG biofeedback with medication. In their study of 100 patients diagnosed with ADHD, stimulant therapy (Ritalin) was administered to all patients, and a titrated dose was maintained for a 1-year period. During that time, 51 of the patients received EEG biofeedback; the other 49 did not. Electrophysiological indicators revealed that only patients receiving the biofeedback developed increased cortical arousal over the central midline region, which was associated with sustained improvement on behavioral and neuropsychological measures. However, by the conclusion of the first year, evidence of increased irritability was noted in approximately 20% of the patients who had received EEG biofeedback. This irritability was eliminated once stimulant therapy was reduced or discontinued. Consequently, clinicians treating patients diagnosed with ADHD with a combination of stimulant therapy and EEG biofeedback may find it useful to monitor patient mood as treatment progresses, and to consider a reduction of stimulant dose should irritability emerge.

A third study, described by Lubar (1991), highlights the importance of adherence to researched treatment protocols in clinical applications of EEG biofeedback. In treating patients with ADHD, Lubar and his colleagues experimented with a reversal of training conditions. Initially, these researchers trained patients with ADHD to suppress "theta" activity (4–8 hertz) and increase "beta" activity (16–20 hertz). After establishing a training effect, they reversed the reinforcement protocol, reinforcing production of theta and inhibiting beta. In contrast to a desired improvement in attention and behavioral, patients became *more* disorganized, inattentive, and hyperactive during this phase of the study. Although resumption of the initial training protocol resulted in a return to improved functioning, Lubar's reversal of his training protocol illustrates the dramatic effect that operant conditioning of specified EEG frequency bands can exert on human functioning.

RESEARCH ON NEGATIVE REACTIONS AND OTHER PROBLEMS

Much more research is needed about the incidence and mechanisms of negative reactions and other problems associated with relaxation therapies, including biofeedback-assisted relaxation (Poppen, 1984; Edinger, 1984). Practitioners also need much more research on patient variables associated with these difficulties and on preventive and management procedures. We trust that those conducting such research will consider and incorporate most or all of the following suggestions.

Retrospective survey research is fraught with enough methodological problems to preclude its value for estimating the incidence of these difficulties. Imagine a practitioner receiving a survey with questions about how often each of several negative reactions and other problems occurred in his or her practice. Such recall is of doubtful accuracy. Some of the more common problems are these:

1. One has to recall such events among hundreds of patients.
2. One has to recall such events over years of practice.
3. Practitioners do not systematically inquire about such events among their patients.
4. Practitioners often supervise others who provide the relaxation and biofeedback therapies.
5. Retrospective surveys lack control over varied relaxation and biofeedback procedures, audiotapes, types of patients, therapist characteristics, patient education, durations of sessions, and environments.

One recommendation is that a major professional organization develop comprehensive and carefully constructed questionnaires and make these available for clinicians and researchers to use prospectively. Cooperative efforts between the organization gathering the prospective data and a national data bank would provide useful data.

Such a clinical research questionnaire would probably include questions and controls for many variables. Examples are varied relaxation procedures; presence or absence of therapist; patient education; duration of sessions; locations of negative physiological or sensory reactions; eyes open or closed; postural and lighting information; therapist characteristics; types of symptoms and disorders; patients' experience with these and other therapies; and names, doses, and side effects of medications.

CAUTIONS AND CONTRAINDICATIONS

There are other, more serious factors to consider when practitioners are providing physiological self-regulatory therapies. These constitute the cautions and contraindications (see M. S. Schwartz, Chapter 6, this volume, for a discussion of these). Therapists can expect potentially serious problems to occur if they provide these therapies to patients for whom such cautions and contraindications apply. However, they can use special approaches for carefully selected patients with some of these disorders and conditions, if the practitioners are knowledgeable about and experienced with these disorders.

CONCLUSION

Various problems can occur during relaxation therapies and biofeedback-assisted relaxation. The experience of significant negative reactions, such as RIA, can reduce compliance with recommended relaxation. However, very few patients are at risk, and very few experience negative reactions. Prudent practitioners use available information, wisdom from experience, skills, precautions, patient education, and good judgment in patient selection and implementing treatments. It is proper here to remind readers that

> Every patient should be treated with biofeedback by a professional with the appropriate credentials who is qualified to understand and treat both the illness and the patient without biofeedback, or by someone under the direct and personal supervision of a professional so qualified. (Adler & Adler, 1984, p. 612)

NOTES

1. Poppen (1998) questioned the accuracy of the term "relaxation-induced anxiety" for describing the phenomenon. He suggested considering a more general and descriptive term such as "training-induced arousal." The rationale he gives involves the implication of RIA implying "that the trainee first engages in relaxed behavior and that this, in turn, evokes unrelaxed behavior [but] studies of the phenomenon have not indicated that any degree of relaxation occurs prior to the trainee's upset; instead arousal occurs before training or right at the beginning" (p. 86).

The second reason is that the term "anxiety" implies a specific set of behaviors, but that term does not always accurately describe the discomfort experienced by some persons. The examples given by Poppen (1998) involve nausea or falling sensations, which he described as "not properly labeled anxiety."

2. BRT is useful for various populations but is particularly useful for special populations such as those with intellectual disabilities, including severe retardation, acquired brain injury, hyperactivity disorder, and schizophrenia. Poppen (1998) uses the terms trainee and client rather than patient. Items 17 through 20 are gleaned from Poppen (1998).

3. Vincent J. Monastra wrote the section "Adverse Effects of EEG Biofeedback."

REFERENCES

Abromowitz, S. I., & Wieselberg, N. (1978). Reaction to relaxation and desensitization outcome: Five angry treatment failures. *American Journal of Psychiatry, 135,* 1418–1419.

Adler, C. S., & Adler, S. M. (1984). Biofeedback. In T. B. Karasu (Ed.), *The psychiatric therapies: The American Psychiatric Association Commission on Psychiatric Therapies.* Washington, DC: American Psychiatric Association.

Bernstein, D. A., & Borkovec, T. D. (1973). *Progressive relaxation training.* Champaign, IL: Research Press.

Bernstein, D. A., & Carlson, C. R. (1993). Progressive relaxation: Abbreviated methods. In P. M. Lehrer & R. L. Woolfolk (Eds.), *Principles and practice of stress management* (2nd ed.). New York: Guilford Press.

Blanchard, E. B., Cornish, P. J., Wittrock, D. A., & Fahrion, S. (1990). Subjective experiences associated with thermal biofeedback treatment of hypertension. *Biofeedback and Self-Regulation, 15*(2), 145–159.

Borkovec, T. D., Mathews, A. M., Chambers, A., Ebrahimi, S., Lytle, R., & Nelson, R. (1987). The effects of relaxation training with cognitive or nondirective therapy and the role of relaxation-induced anxiety in the treatment of generalized anxiety. *Journal of Consulting and Clinical Psychology, 55*(6), 883–888.

Braith, J. A., McCullough, J. P., & Bush, J. P. (1988). Relaxation-induced anxiety in a subclinical sample of chronically anxious subjects. *Journal of Behavior Therapy and Experimental Psychiatry, 19*(3), 193–198.

Carrington, P. (1977). *Freedom in meditation.* Garden City, NY: Doubleday/Anchor.

Cohen, A. S., Barlow, D. H., & Blanchard, E. B. (1985). Psychophysiology of relaxation-associated panic attacks. *Journal of Abnormal Psychology, 94*(1), 96–101.

DeGood, D. E., & Williams, E. M. (1982). Parasympathetic rebound following EMG biofeedback training: A case study. *Biofeedback and Self-Regulation, 7*(4), 461–465.

Denny, M. R. (1976). Post-aversive relief and relaxation and their implications for behavior therapy. *Journal of Behavior Therapy and Experimental Psychiatry, 7,* 315–322.

Edinger, J. D. (1984). Re: Adverse reactions to relaxation training [Response to Poppen, 1984]. *The Behavior Therapist, 7,* 138.

Edinger, J. D., & Jacobson, R. (1982). Incidence and significance of relaxation treatment side-effects. *The Behavior Therapist, 5,* 137–138.

Elliott, R. (1974). The motivational significance of heart rate. In P. A. Obrist, A. H. Black, J. Brener, & L. V. DiCara (Eds.), *Cardiovascular psychophysiology: Current issues in response mechanisms, biofeedback, and methodology.* Chicago: Aldine.

Gaarder, K. R., & Montgomery, P. S. (1981). *Clinical biofeedback: A procedural manual for behavioral medicine* (2nd ed.). Baltimore: Williams & Wilkins.

Gellhorn, E. (1965). The neurophysiological basis of anxiety: A hypothesis. *Perspectives in Biology and Medicine, 8,* 488–515.

Gellhorn, E. (1967). *Principles of autonomic–somatic integrations: Physiological basis and psychological and clinical implications.* Minneapolis: University of Minnesota Press.

Heide, F. J., & Borkovec, T. D. (1983). Relaxation-induced anxiety: Paradoxical anxiety enhancement due to relaxation training. *Journal of Consulting and Clinical Psychology, 51,* 171–182.

Heide, F. J., & Borkovec, T. D. (1984). Relaxation-induced anxiety: Mechanisms and theoretical implications. *Behaviour Research and Therapy, 22,* 1–12.

Jacobson, R., & Edinger, J. D. (1982). Side effects of relaxation treatment. *American Journal of Psychiatry, 139*(7), 952–953.

Lehrer, P. M. (1982). How to relax and how not to relax: A reevaluation of the work of Edmund Jacobson—I. *Behaviour Research and Therapy, 20,* 417–428.

Lehrer, P. M., & Woolfolk, R. L. (1993a). *Principles and practice of stress management* (2nd ed.). New York: Guilford Press.

Lehrer, P. M., & Woolfolk, R. L. (1993b). Specific effects of stress management techniques. In P. M. Lehrer & R. L. Woolfolk (Eds.), *Principles and practice of stress management* (2nd ed.). New York: Guilford Press.

Ley, R. (1988). Panic attacks during relaxation and relaxation-induced anxiety: A hyperventilation interpretation. *Journal of Behavior Therapy and Experimental Psychiatry, 19*(4), 253–259.

Lichstein, K. L. (1988). *Clinical relaxation strategies.* New York: Wiley.

Linden, W. (1993). The autogenic training method of J. H. Schultz. In P. M. Lehrer & R. L. Woolfolk (Eds.), *Principles and practice of stress management* (2nd ed.). New York: Guilford Press.

Lubar, J. F. (1991). Discourse on the development of EEG diagnostics and biofeedback treatment for attention-deficit/hyperactivity disorders. *Biofeedback and Self-Regulation, 16,* 201–225.

McGuigan, F. J. (1993). Progressive relaxation: Origins, principles, and clinical applications. In P. M. Lehrer & R. L. Woolfolk (Eds.), *Principles and practice of stress management* (2nd ed.). New York: Guilford Press.

Mefford, R. B. (1979). The developing biological concept of anxiety. In W. E. Fann, I. Karacan, A. D. Pokorny, & R. L. Williams (Eds.), *Phenomenology and treatment of anxiety.* New York: Spectrum.

Monastra, V. J., Monastra, D. M., & George, S. (2002). The effects of stimulant therapy, EEG biofeedback and parenting style on the primary symptoms of attention-deficit/hyperactivity disorder. *Applied Psychophysiology and Biofeedback, 27,* 231–249.

Norton, G. R., Rhodes, L., Hauch, J., & Kaprowy, E. A. (1985). Characteristics of subjects experiencing relaxation and relaxation-induced anxiety. *Journal of Behavior Therapy and Experimental Psychiatry, 16*(3), 211–216.

Obrist, P. A. (1976). The cardiovascular-behavioral interaction as it appears today. *Psychophysiology, 13,* 95–107.

Obrist, P. A. (1981). *Cardiovascular psychophysiology: A perspective.* New York: Plenum Press.

Peniston, E. G., & Kulkosky, P. J. (1989). Alpha–theta brainwave training and beta endorphin levels in alcoholics. *Alcoholism: Clinical and Experimental Research, 13,* 271–279.

Poppen, R. (1984). Adverse reaction to relaxation training [Letter to the editor]. *The Behavior Therapist, 7*(1), 18.

Poppen, R. (1998). *Behavioral relaxation training and assessment* (2nd ed.). Thousand Oaks, CA: Sage Publications.

Schultz, J. H., & Luthe, W. (1969). *Autogenic therapy: Vol. 1. Autogenic methods.* New York: Grune & Stratton.

Seligman, M. E. P. (1975). *Helplessness: On depression, development and death.* San Francisco: Freeman.

Stampler, F. M. (1982). Panic disorder: Description, conceptualization, and implications for treatment. *Clinical Psychology Review, 2,* 469–486.

Wells, A. (1990). Panic disorder in association with relaxation induced anxiety: An attentional training approach to treatment. *Behavior Therapy, 21,* 273–280.

The Use of Audiotapes for Patient Education and Relaxation

MARK S. SCHWARTZ

Audiotapes have a legitimate place in applied psychophysiology, biofeedback, behavior therapy, and behavioral medicine. This chapter focuses on the advantages of using audiotapes for patient education and relaxation, and considerations in the use of such tapes. The dimensions of relaxation tapes, making one's own tapes versus getting commercially available ones, and the issue of taped versus live relaxation therapy are topics explored here.

ADVANTAGES OF USING AUDIOTAPES

Some advantages of audiotapes for patient education are part of the extensive discussions of audiotapes and patient education by Doak, Doak, and Root (1985). This section includes aspects of their cogent discussions, which conclude that tapes can be very useful. They have advantages for care providers, practical benefits, and advantages for patients and their families.

Professional Advantages

1. *Conservation of time.* Using tapes can conserve a practitioner's time. Carefully prepared tapes can be combined with face-to-face presentations and printed materials.

2. *Increased flexibility.* Printed patient education booklets have a place in helping to inform and prepare patients. However, these are impractical and/or insufficient for some patients. Audiotapes can increase the flexibility of patient education and relaxation training.

3. *Reduced "burnout" from repetition.* Because providers repeat the same or similar information to many patients, face-to-face presentations of patient education and relaxation procedures often become tedious. Frequent repetition of the same information can result in practitioners' losing interest. The use of well-developed audiotapes can ease routine instructions (Doak et al., 1985), as well as help to maintain quality control over the information provided.

4. *Language advantages.* Audiotapes often have language advantages (Doak et al., 1985). For example, they can be informal, use colloquial and natural language, and allow more variability. Furthermore, accents can enhance comprehension for some patients. However, Doak et al. (1985) note that accents can detract from other patients' comprehension.

Practical Considerations

1. *Lower costs.* The costs of providing face-to-face patient education and relaxation therapies have increased substantially. Providing all relaxation therapy with office-based interactions costs much more than supplementing these interactions with tapes. Costs partly depend on whether practitioners make their own tapes or buy them and on the quantities purchased. The proper use of audiotapes is important for achieving cost containment.

2. *Increased credibility and enthusiasm.* A well-prepared audiotape is often better organized, more complete, more credible, more professional, and more enthusiastic than presentations made in face-to-face situations.

3. *Reduced learning time.* Reduced learning time is a potential advantage of audiotapes for some patient education (Doak et al., 1985). Presumably, for most patients faster learning can result from increased patient satisfaction, better comprehension and knowledge, and increased interest and motivation (see below).

Patient Considerations

1. *Increased comprehension and retention.* A large percentage of patients display poor comprehension of printed instructions (Doak et al., 1985), and some patients do not understand or remember live, spoken instructions. Tapes can improve comprehension, and hence knowledge, for many such patients. Doak et al. (1985) particularly recommend considering tapes for patients who learn better by listening, those who are visually impaired, and those with low literacy. Other patients who can benefit are those who need variety to overcome attention span problems and those who prefer repetition of taped learning. Moreover, for patients whose first language differs from that of their care providers, tapes in the patients' language have obvious advantages.

Another consideration is that there is often not enough time in face-to-face sessions for practitioners to present all or most of the information needed. In addition, some information presented to patients in sessions will not reach family members. Furthermore, practitioners probably present the same topics differently to different patients; some of these presentations may be less clear and less complete at certain times.

Finally, many patients forget most new information after face-to-face communications. Tape-recorded information, which permits patients to listen to the material more than once, probably increases retention of such information.

2. *Increased patient satisfaction.* Many patients prefer face-to-face presentations, but this depends partly on the practitioner's verbal skills and personality. Properly developed audiotaped presentations can be as satisfactory as, or more satisfactory than, face-to-face presentations. I know of no published research comparing taped patient education presentations with face-to-face presentations. However, many years ago, in a pilot study (Schwartz, 1979) of 50 consecutive patients, I found that nearly all were very satisfied with a taped patient education presentation supplementing a face-to-face presentation.

3. *Increased motivation and compliance.* Well-developed and well-presented audiotaped patient education and relaxation procedures may enhance patients' understanding of and interest in the recommendations and therapy procedures. This in turn may increase patients' motivation and compliance. There is no research for this assumption; however, the alterna-

tive (i.e., assumption that face-to-face presentations are better for increasing patient motivation and compliance) also has no supporting data. Until there are adequate studies, the less costly approach is justified.

4. *Greater consistency of information and therapy procedures.* Well-developed audiotapes increase the consistency of the information given and standardize the presentation. Patients who receive such tapes at least receive the same information and procedures.

5. *Provision of information to family members.* Family members of patients often need education about the therapy rationale and procedures, but patients usually come alone to sessions. Involvement of family members can help increase compliance with relaxation procedures for some patients. In addition, it is very often difficult for patients to communicate adequately to family members, and audiotapes give such patients added ways to share information with their families.

6. *Reduction of distractions.* Distractions occur often when patients are learning relaxation, especially in early phases. Clinical experience suggests that the taped voice helps to keep patients focused on the procedures. This assumption deserves formal study.

7. *Assistance in pacing and timing of relaxation.* Some patients rush through relaxation. Some lose track of a good pace. Tapes can help to reduce this problem, because they provide instructions over fixed times and use standard pacing.

In tertiary professional practices, audiotapes are useful for all the reasons given above. Providers in tertiary practices see many patients who live long distances away, and/or see some patients only once. The responsibilities in the first (and often only) session include patient education and the answering of questions. These providers need to give the patients much useful and necessary information and explain many therapy procedures in the short time available. They must conserve time, be flexible, and contain costs.

When it is practical, tertiary practitioners usually try to refer patients who live at a distance to practitioners much closer to the patients' homes. The referral will probably result in more evaluative and explanatory interview time, and thus unnecessary duplication of effort should be avoided. Audiotapes allow presentations of useful information and procedures in a cost-efficient manner. Since professionals also have face-to-face discussions with all patients, the use of tapes allows a professional to review and select patient education topics specifically indicated by a particular patient's situation.

There are some potential *disadvantages* of using tapes. There are the risks of relying too much on them, or of using tapes with poorly developed scripts, inadequate recording style, and technically inadequate recordings. These factors can reduce both the efficiency and value of the tapes. Moreover, the use of too many tapes for a given patient may overburden that patient. Practitioners need to be flexible and use good clinical judgment concerning when, how, and with whom to use tapes. The following section addresses several considerations in using and making audiotapes, especially relaxation tapes. There are many useful ideas for making patient education tapes in Doak et al. (1985).

CONSIDERATIONS IN THE USE OF AUDIOTAPES

Practitioners disagree about whether or not to use tapes, and many practitioners sometimes do not know how to make good tapes. There is only limited research on these topics for relaxation, and the use of tapes for patient education has an even more limited literature. (The emphasis in the following discussion is henceforth on relaxation tapes, although patient education tapes are also considered somewhat further.)

Awareness of considerations in selecting, recording, and using relaxation audiotapes is useful. Again, for emphasis, it is not my intention to promote substitution of tapes for all live relaxation therapies. Instead, my intent is to recommend careful, prudent, cost-efficient, and effective use.

Dimensions of Relaxation Tapes

Several dimensions of relaxation tapes are important for patients' preference, comfort, compliance, and effectiveness. Gaarder and Montgomery (1981) have published the best listing and discussion of these dimensions; the interested reader should refer to their discussion of each dimension (pp. 149–154). The dimensions are as follows: length, source of voice, tonal quality of voice, hypnotic quality of voice, pace, voice quality, authoritarian suggestion, authoritativeness, suggestiveness, gender, dialect and vocabulary, and background sounds. The script can focus on breathing, muscle relaxation, muscle tensing, body parts, sensations, body imagery, mental imagery, and/or subjective cues.

Patients differ in their preference for at least some of these dimensions. These preferences will probably influence their use of the tapes and their psychological and physiological responses. In turn, these responses affect the results from the use of tapes. The practitioner should consider these dimensions when purchasing commercially available tapes, when recording tapes, and when recommending tapes to patients and colleagues.

There are no official guidelines or research to help professionals decide about which tapes to use and when they should record scripts themselves. There are no guidelines or research to help in matching patients with dimensions of tapes. Practitioner preferences may not match patient preferences.

A later section discusses research comparing taped versus live relaxation therapies. However, these studies usually provide no information about any of the dimensions of the tapes. The studies also do not include evaluations or ratings by practitioners or by the patients or subjects.

These studies often assume that a single tape is satisfactory for all or most subjects. This is usually a tape developed by the investigator. The implicit assumption is that a tape is a tape is a tape. This is as erroneous as assuming that biofeedback is biofeedback is biofeedback. Assessing the physiological and psychological responses of patients to different tapes is an important area that at present has not been adequately researched.

In conclusion, many practitioners use a variety of relaxation tapes. Careful practitioners listen to and try to relax with each tape they plan to give to their patients—including those tapes made by the practitioners themselves. Therapists should also recognize and respect the fact that some patients may want choices and may benefit from selecting their own tapes.

Making One's Own Tapes

This section focuses on making both patient education and relaxation tapes. Doak et al. (1985) provide many useful ideas for making patient education tapes, some of which apply to relaxation tapes as well. Advantages for practitioners making their own tapes include the fact that patients hear their own doctors' or therapists' voices. However, this is not always an advantage. Many providers do not have the voice quality needed for such recordings; their voices may be distracting or disturbing to some patients. I doubt that most patients expect personalized taped instructions.

Tapes made by professionals themselves do permit the use of informal, natural, and colloquial language. Such tapes also permit the use of local or regional language, as well as dialects and accents that can enhance comprehension and acceptance.

Making Patient Education Tapes

Practitioners should consider the many similarities between reading printed information and listening to patient education tapes that are noted by Doak et al. (1985). Both call for the same language-decoding process, and both provide cues via their structure, grammar, sequence, and tempo. Both demand attention and memory to increase comprehension, and both require patients to rely on prior knowledge to integrate new information.

Therapists should also consider the differences noted by Doak et al. (1985). The rate of information flow is usually not controllable by the person listening to tapes. There are no visual stimuli or graphics, unless these are presented in an accompanying book or with slides.

As with printed materials, in devising patient education audiotapes, practitioners should define the purpose and scope of the message explicitly. What new behaviors do the therapists want patients to engage in? What are the main points? The following guidelines for patient education scripts are presented by Doak et al. (1985), who suggest that practitioners do these things:

- Use conversational language.
- Use short, common-usage words.
- Vary sentence lengths.
- Use a predictable, repetitive format, such as instructions followed by examples.
- Maintain consistency in terms.
- Draw attention to key points, in several ways:
  - Change tone of voice.
  - Use repetition.
  - Give emphasis in the summary and ask questions.
- Use a rate of speech, between 100 and 150 words per minute. The average normal talking rate is 180 words per minute (http//www.audiobriefings.com/tipsbooklet.html).
- Consider combining tapes with worksheets or a workbook.

The duration of patient education tapes can be as brief as 5–10 minutes. Shorter tapes are better for those with low literacy skills and patients with very short attention spans. When making longer tapes, the clinician should consider inserting breaks about every 5 minutes. These intervals permit reviews, questions, and interactions with printed materials. The breaks also help to maintain patients' attention.

Prudent practitioners who make their own patient education tapes ask colleagues and patients to listen to drafts, get reactions, and make comments and criticisms. They then revise the tapes a few times as needed.

Making Relaxation Tapes

Practitioners can review Gaarder and Montgomery (1981), Gevirtz (1987), and Smith (1989) for further ideas about relaxation tapes. Consider the following suggestions gleaned and adapted from these sources, as well as my own experience.

- Consider tapes lasting 10–20 minutes, or less for some applications.
- Read several sample scripts aloud.
- Listen to several samples of relaxation tapes for ideas about scripting and other aspects.
- Specify all details in your script.

- Use a colloquial style, as if you were talking to someone.
- Before starting, decide whether to use one relaxation method or to combine methods.
- If you do separate scripts for each method on the same tape, select a sequence.
- Decide between directive and permissive instructions. For example, "My arms are feeling heavier" is more directive, and "Feelings of heaviness are developing in my arms" is more permissive.
- Consider including words, phrases, and mental pictures to help deepen the relaxation and relaxed feelings. See Smith (1989) for ideas.
- Consider including statements to permit acceptance of relaxing beliefs—for instance, "I am becoming more accepting of the relaxing powers within me."
- Consider writing brief pauses and quiet periods into the script. These can be as brief as 2–5 seconds, or longer if the patient will be repeating phrases.
- Type out the script with a word processor.
- Read it aloud several times. Jot down places for emphasis.
- Assess the script with the help of others. Check the length. Be sure the instructions are specific, and avoid instructions that are vague or uncertain. Avoid statements that patients will view as unrealistic and will not believe even with repetition (Smith, 1989, p. 214).
- Ask someone else to read it to you in the manner intended.
- Read the final script several times for familiarity.
- Record your script and listen to yourself a few times while trying to relax with it. Revise the script and rerecord as needed.
- Assess patients' physiological responses to the tape, and revise further as necessary.

Taped versus Live Relaxation

A basic and very important question is whether live relaxation therapy is more effective than taped relaxation procedures. Some professionals in this field are very critical of the use of any relaxation tapes. Others are critical of commercially available relaxation tapes, compared to those made by practitioners for their own patients.

One of the arguments against commercially available tapes (and, by implication, many provider-made standard tapes) is that they provide noncontingent reinforcement and poor pacing of the procedures. One contention is that contingent reinforcement and optimal pacing require looking at patients and carefully examining their musculature, facial expressions, and emotional responses. The research supporting the superiority of live over taped relaxation typically focuses on the tensing-and-releasing portion of progressive muscle relaxation. Face-to-face therapy may be more useful for this early stage of progressive muscle relaxation. Lichstein (1988) noted that there are "no data on the question of live versus taped presentations of other relaxation methods" (p. 98), and this situation has not changed since then.

I am expressing no disagreement here with the value of office-based live relaxation therapies provided by practitioners who are competent in their use. Nor am I disagreeing with the assumption that such therapy can provide better learning of relaxation than some taped procedures for many patients. My disagreement is with blanket assumptions that one approach is superior to the other in all or even most respects for all or even most patients. There are simply too many factors and circumstances preventing us from adopting such an assumption. For example, we can consider the many characteristics of taped procedures, the many procedures other than tensing and releasing, the cost–benefit ratio, and the feasibility of office-based sessions for many patients. We may also consider the advantages of audiotapes for other reasons discussed earlier in the chapter.

Reviews of studies comparing the physiological differences between taped relaxation therapy and live relaxation therapy in the office report statistically significant differences in favor of live relaxation therapy (Borkovec & Sides, 1979; Lehrer, 1982; Lichstein, 1988). However, as noted earlier, these studies have included no assessment and specifications of the tapes used. The published studies also typically do not provide much or any description of the many dimensions of tapes that can influence patient or subject acceptance and comfort. Studies concluding that live therapy is better have typically used tapes only in the office and only for a few sessions. There is also no indication of the researchers' biases. For all these reasons, the research results are incomplete and inconclusive.

Consider the study by Craw, Newton, and Newman (1993), who concluded that "taped and live procedures are equivalent when differences in cognitive preparation and expectancy inherent in these procedures are controlled for between groups" (p. 62). In this study, cognitive preparation was live for all 40 treated male Veterans Administration inpatients in a substance abuse program. Treated patients reduced their heart rate and galvanic skin reaction, increased their finger temperature, and decreased their state anxiety over four sessions. Live presentation of relaxation or taped presentation with the therapist present did not affect the results. A combined audio–video format was not better than audio alone. This study needs replication and extension, but it does illustrate one way in which audiotaped relaxation can be as effective as live presentation.

One cannot conclude that live relaxation is always or usually better than taped relaxation. Limiting relaxation therapies to live and office-based procedures limits the flexibility of a clinical practice. It creates unnecessary constraints on researchers of relaxation therapies. It increases costs to the professional, the patient, the health care institution, and third-party payers. In addition to ignoring the cost differential between these two methods, it disregards other advantages of tapes discussed elsewhere in this chapter. For example, are the clinical differences always or usually worth the greater costs associated with live presentations? Can taped relaxation therapy result in clinically meaningful and patient acceptable therapeutic gains for some patients? Within a stepped-care model of treatment, can practitioners reserve live relaxation therapy for those patients having trouble or obtaining insufficient results with taped procedures?

Another concern is that practitioners should not use relaxation tapes to provide instructions to patients during office-based sessions with the therapists absent. Some professionals go so far as to consider this bordering on unethical professional behavior. The issue of therapist presence or absence during biofeedback sessions is discussed in a later chapter of this volume (see Striefel, Whitehouse, & Schwartz, Chapter 37). Many of the same professional concerns and considerations about leaving patients alone without professional observation apply here.

There may be some circumstances in which leaving a patient alone for a few minutes listening to a relaxation tape is appropriate. However, most professionals frown on doing so in clinical practice. Until adequate data are available, it is prudent and sensible to avoid or at least limit such practices. When they are used at all, practitioners would be wise to provide clear and defensible justifications to the patient, referral source, and third-party payers, and to adjust fees for such sessions. I am personally unaware of any such justifications.

CONCLUSIONS

The criticism of audiotapes, especially relaxation tapes, is an unresolved empirical issue. The issue is far more complex than choosing either one approach or another. All tapes should receive critical evaluation and be used prudently. This chapter has discussed considerations for selecting tapes and guidelines for their use.

Live patient education and relaxation can be more expensive than the proper use of well-prepared tapes for many patients. Unanswered is the question of whether the repetitive use of taped relaxation therapy outside the practitioner's office yields results similar to those of office-based live relaxation therapy.

Practitioners are urged to consider audiotapes for patient education. Cost–benefit considerations have become increasingly important in the changing health care financial environment. Well-developed and prudently used audiotapes probably often result in more effective and cost-efficient patient education and relaxation therapies than does avoiding their use. However, research needs in this area remain substantial.

REFERENCES

Borkovec, T. D., & Sides, J. K. (1979). Critical procedural variables to the physiological effects of progressive relaxation: A review. *Behaviour Research and Therapy, 17,* 119–125.

Craw, M. J., Newton, F. A., & Newman, R. G. (1993, March). Biofeedback assisted relaxation training within a substance abuse program: A comparison of taped versus live instructions. In *Proceedings of the 24th Annual Meeting of the Association for Applied Psychophysiology and Biofeedback, Los Angeles.* Wheat Ridge, CO: Association for Applied Psychophysiology and Biofeedback.

Doak, C. C., Doak, L. G., & Root, J. H. (1985). *Teaching patients with low literacy skills.* Philadelphia: Lippincott.

Gaarder, K. R., & Montgomery, P. S. (1981). *Clinical biofeedback: A procedural manual for behavioral medicine* (2nd ed.). Baltimore: Williams & Wilkins.

Gevirtz, R. (1987). Appendix: How to make a personalized relaxation tape. In E. M. Catalano (Ed.), *The chronic pain control workbook.* Oakland, CA: New Harbinger.

Lehrer, P. M. (1982). How to relax and not to relax: A re-evaluation of the work of Edmund Jacobson—I. *Behaviour Research and Therapy, 20,* 417–428.

Lichstein, K. L. (1988). *Clinical relaxation strategies.* New York: Wiley-Interscience.

Schwartz, M. S. (1979, February). *Introducing patients to relaxation and biofeedback.* Paper presented at the 10th annual meeting of the Biofeedback Society of America, San Diego, CA.

Smith, J. C. (1989). *Relaxation dynamics: A cognitive-behavioral approach to relaxation.* Champaign, IL: Research Press.

Sticht, T. G. (Ed.). (1975). *Reading for working: A functional literacy anthology.* Alexandria, VA: Human Research Resources Organization.

PART V

Disorders Needing Lower Tension and Arousal

Headache

MARK S. SCHWARTZ
FRANK ANDRASIK

Applied psychophysiological treatments, including relaxation and biofeedback,[1] are commonly accepted treatments for tension-type and migraine headaches. We estimate that over the past 30 years, relaxation and biofeedback therapies have been used in the treatment of hundreds of thousands of people with these types of headaches. Hundreds of studies over the past 30 years have used relaxation and biofeedback for treating people with headaches termed "muscle tension," "psychogenic," "vascular," "migraine," and "combination" or "mixed" headaches. Furthermore, these biofeedback studies have stimulated research about the causes of headaches, treatment effectiveness, and mechanisms of treatment.

Investigations of treatment effectiveness are now too numerous to review case by case. Reviewers have resorted to meta-analytic and evidence-based approaches, which have consistently supported the value of these therapies (see Andrasik & Walch, 2002, and Penzien, Rains, & Andrasik, 2002, for more complete discussions). Tables 14.1 and 14.2 summarize results from the meta-analyses conducted to date for tension-type and migraine headaches, respectively. In addition, various groups have completed evidence-based reviews, wherein rigorous methodological criteria have been used to evaluate every study under consideration. These types of analyses—which have been performed by the Society of Clinical Psychology (Division 12 of the American Psychological Association; http://www.apa.org/divisions/div12/ rev_est/health.shtml), the U.S. Headache Consortium (composed of the American Academy of Family Physicians, American Academy of Neurology, American Headache Society, American College of Emergency Physicians, American College of Physicians, American Society of Internal Medicine, American Osteopathic Association, and National Headache Foundation) (Campbell, Penzien, & Wall, 2000), and the National Institutes of Health—are similarly supportive. There is also a fair amount of evidence demonstrating that treatment effects endure over time (see Andrasik & Walch, 2002).

The reader is referred to other chapters within this text that bear on topics addressed here (M. S. Schwartz, Chapter 6, for more on intake and cognitive preparation of patients; M. S. Schwartz, Chapter 8, for compliance; N. M. Schwartz & Schwartz, Chapter 3, for definitions; M. S. Schwartz, Chapter 13, for use of audiotapes; and Block, Schwartz, & Gyllenhaal, Chapter 9, for dietary considerations).

Some providers rely primarily on biofeedback and relaxation therapies, and others incorporate these approaches with other behavioral and stress management therapies. Research has helped provide useful information and answers to many questions and issues. Prudent

TABLE 14.1. Average Improvement Rates (%) for Tension-Type Headache in Separate Meta-Analyses

Study	EMG	REL	EMG + REL	BFCT	COG	PHARM	OTHER	PTCT	MDCT	WTLT
Blanchard, Andrasik, Ahles, Teders, & O'Keefe (1980)	61	59	59					35	35	−5
Holroyd & Penzien (1986)	46	45	57	15						−4
Bogaards & ter Kuile (1994)	47	36	56		53	39	38	20		−5
McCrory, Penzien, Hasselblad, & Gray (2001)	48	38	51		40	35[a]		17		3

Note. EMG, electromyographic biofeedback, generally provided from the frontal/forehead muscles; REL, relaxation therapy, generally of the muscle-tensing and -relaxing variety; BFCT, biofeedback control procedure, generally false or noncontingent biofeedback; COG, cognitive therapy, stress coping training, or problem-solving therapy; PHARM, various medications, ranging from aspirin and nonsteroidal anti-inflammatories to prophylactics to narcotics; OTHER, various approaches, other than biofeedback, REL, or COG; PTCT, psychological or pseudotherapy control procedure; MDCT, medication control procedure (results taken from double-blind placebo-controlled medication trials); WTLT, waiting-list control procedure (no treatment).
[a]Amitriptyline alone.

practitioners should be mindful of at least the questions and issues below. This chapter discusses several of these questions and issues:

- When should one use biofeedback versus other nonpharmacological therapies?
- Which procedures are more effective than others?
- What placements of surface electromyographic (EMG) electrodes should one use?
- Is treating to specified physiological criteria needed? How much skill do patients need?
- To what degree does patient education affect results?
- Who should provide biofeedback therapies?
- What are the mechanisms of therapeutic success?
- What are the most cost-effective ways for providing biofeedback and related therapies?
- How much assessment, and what types of assessment, are needed?
- What are the effects of medications on headaches and biofeedback?

TABLE 14.2. Average Improvement Rates (%) for Migraine Headache in Separate Meta-Analyses

Study	ATFB	THBF	REL	VMBF	THBF + REL	EMG	COG	COG + BF	PTCT	MDCT	WTLT
Blanchard et al. (1980)	65	52	53						17		
Holroyd, Penzien, Holm, & Hursey (1984a)		28	44	31	57						11
Blanchard & Andrasik (1987)	49	27	48	43		29			26		13
Goslin et al. (1999)		37	32	33	40	49	35	9			5

Note. See Table 14.1 footnote for abbreviations. In addition, ATFB, thermal biofeedback augmented by components of autogenic training, as developed at the Menninger Clinic; THBF, thermal biofeedback by itself; VMBF, vasomotor biofeedback provided from the temporal artery; BF, EMG or thermal biofeedback.

- What other therapies should one consider?
- Can biofeedback and related therapies be useful with elderly patients?
- Can biofeedback and related therapies be useful with menstrual-related headaches and migraines during pregnancy?
- What is the role of dietary changes in treating headaches?
- What is the role of sleep and treating sleep disorders for treating headaches?
- How close to research procedures do clinical applications need to be?

These questions require credible responses. However, their existence is not enough to interfere with clinical applications and reimbursement of biofeedback and related therapies for headaches.

Clinical biofeedback is justifiable and cost-efficient for treating many patients with headaches. Published research and clinical experience are sufficient to support reimbursement. However, some third-party reimbursement companies are unaware that reimbursing for biofeedback, relaxation, and other applied psychophysiological therapies can reduce costs to them. Practitioners need to remain aware of and sensitive to the questions and concerns of the very cautious critics, as well as of those providing payments. In particular, practitioners need to be careful about who provides the services, how, for whom, and when. Procedures need to be tailored to individual patients and provided in cost-effective and efficient ways. Before discussing these and other questions and issues, however, this chapter presents a selected review of headache diagnosis. (Note that throughout the chapter, terms given in italics are ones defined in the glossary at the chapter's end.)

DIAGNOSIS

The revision of classification and diagnostic criteria for headache disorders, *cranial neuralgias*, and facial pain (Olesen, 1988) offers some advances over the 1962 system.[2] The focus here is on the proposed groups of "tension-type headaches" and "migraines with and without aura" (Andrasik, 2001a; Olesen, 1988; Saper, Silberstein, Gordon, & Hamel, 1993). A listing of the diagnostic criteria is beyond the scope of this chapter, but they may be found in Olesen (1988).

With the 1988 system, practitioners make a diagnosis for each distinct headache form (utilizing a *Diagnostic and Statistical Manual of Mental Disorders* [DSM]-type approach). The new system acknowledges a possible continuum between pure migraines and pure tension-type headaches. The proponents have dropped the diagnoses of "mixed," "combination," or "tension–vascular" headache. If a patient has both types of symptoms, one now uses both a migraine and a tension-type diagnosis. Some professionals propose combining separate diagnoses into a unitary diagnosis, such as "recurrent benign headache." Part of the rationale for this proposed merger is the considerable overlap in the symptoms and treatments for headaches within the existing diagnoses. If the practitioner adopts the view of an amalgam diagnosis, then he or she should consider specifying the predominant features. In clinical practice, systems with separate diagnoses remain in use. Relaxation and biofeedback are often part of the treatment plan, regardless of the specific diagnostic name.

A major revision concerns what are now termed "tension-type" headaches. Four subtypes have been proposed to help clinicians and researchers sort out the role of various causative factors. Tension-type headaches are now grouped on the basis of chronicity (episodic vs. chronic), as this has been found to bear on outcome, and the presence of identifiable muscle involvement (evidence of pericranial muscle tenderness upon palpation or elevated surface EMG readings vs. the absence of such). The latter aspect is problematic, because no specific criteria are offered for muscle tenderness or surface EMG (hereafter referred to simply as EMG) microvolt levels. The system acknowledges the difficulty with this distinction, but has proposed this subdivision to stimulate further studies. The proposed system notes that the subdivision is optional "in view of the poor scientific basis for the subdivision." Specifically, the document states:

> There is not yet sufficient evidence available regarding the limits of normality of pericranial muscle tenderness. Neither has sufficient attention been given to the methodology of pericranial palpation. Evidence concerning normal EMG levels of pericranial muscles is similarly deficient. Until evidence accumulates concerning tenderness on palpation and pericranial EMG, each investigator must judge as best he (she) can on the basis of experience with non-headache sufferers and by comparing symmetrical sites. . . . (Olesen, 1988, p. 30)

The new system specifies that one assumes or suspects a "psychogenic" etiology if one cannot find evidence of muscle involvement based on tenderness or EMG. However, this assumption fails to consider the problem of lack of criteria. It also ignores patients whose headaches suggest a muscle and postural contribution, but for whom muscle involvement does not show in the office—for example, patients whose daily activities involve probable or clear excess muscle tension, but who relax well in a practitioner's office.

We also need to make a brief comment about "cluster headaches," a most painful and debilitating form of headache. We know of only one published attempt to treat this headache type by biofeedback and relaxation alone. This small trial met with limited success at best (Blanchard, Andrasik, Jurish, & Teders, 1982a). So caution is in order when dealing with this headache type. Nonpharmacological approaches may still be of value to some patients with cluster headaches, however, in helping them cope more effectively with the sometimes overwhelming distress that may result from having to endure repeated, intense attacks.

Selected implications of this diagnostic scheme include the following:

1. Practitioners should consider using the new terms "tension-type headaches" and "migraine with or without aura." They should also consider using multiple diagnoses instead of "mixed headache" or "combination headache."
2. Multiple criteria for assessing muscle tension should be considered. Practitioners can use multiple muscle sites, multiple postures (including sitting and standing), and multiple conditions of recording (including resting, stressors, eyes open, eyes closed, sitting, and standing) (see Flor, 2001, for further discussion).
3. Multiple methods should be used for assessing stress and other potential causes or aggravating factors. Practitioners should include a careful history and consider self-report measures.
4. If there are no signs of excess muscle tension in the office during baselines, practitioners should apply relaxation treatments to daily life before additional office-based biofeedback.

MECHANISMS OF HEADACHE CAUSES AND TREATMENT EFFICACY

Different models and explanations exist for explaining the etiology and progression of tension-type and migraine headaches. There are also different views about the mechanisms of successful therapies. Challenges even continue for the assumption that muscle contraction causes all tension-type headaches, as well as for the view that vascular changes triggered by biochemical agents are the primary or sole causative factors for migraine headaches. Questions about the role of stress and emotion also remain. This section summarizes several of the major models of etiology and treatment mechanisms. We offer selected comments, conclusions, and implications.

Resting EMG of People with and without Headache Diagnoses

Most earlier studies did not show a consistent difference between resting EMG levels in the frontal and/or neck regions of subjects with tension-type headaches versus subjects without such headaches (Andrasik, Blanchard, Arena, Saunders, & Barron, 1982a; Marcus, 1992; Flor & Turk, 1989). A meta-analysis of all studies published between 1974 and 1995 came to the same conclusion (Wittrock, 1997). One implication is that muscle activity during rest is not a good differential factor. Another implication is that more than muscle activity is involved in the etiology of tension headaches. Third, resting muscle activity may not be the best source of data upon which to base the decision for providing biofeedback.

Most prior comparisons involved only the frontal area, reclining or partially reclining postures, and eyes closed. Subsequent studies support a difference (Ahles et al., 1988; Schoenen, Gerard, De Pasqua, & Juprelle, 1991; Hatch et al., 1992). In Ahles et al. (1988), the difference was between a small group of subjects without headache (*n* = 21) compared to those with tension, migraine, or mixed headaches. There were no meaningful differences among the headache types. The difference from the no-headache group was for three different body positions. The positions were reclining, sitting without back supported, and standing with hands at sides. All conditions were with subjects' eyes closed. The sitting and standing positions had higher bilateral trapezius tension than the reclining. Also note that 40–50% of Ahles et al.'s sample did not show abnormal EMG activity in any positions. The authors logically speculated that their patients might represent a group with more severe and refractory headaches. The clinical setting in which this study took place was a *tertiary* headache clinic.

The study by Schoenen et al. (1991) compared patients with tension-type headaches and healthy controls in reclining and standing postures and with a math stressor. They recorded the left frontalis, temporalis, and trapezius muscles. The EMG activity was higher in the patients than the controls. This occurred for both postures, with the math stress, and for all sites. Most patients (62.5%) showed EMG levels exceeding those of the control groups by two standard deviations for all three muscles and recording conditions. Only 2 of the 32 patients showed EMG activity outside the defined normal range during all recordings.

Hatch et al. (1992) reported that "headache subjects showed significantly greater EMG activity than controls during baseline and stressful task performance" (p. 89). A study by Lichstein et al. (1991) also showed statistically higher frontal EMG activity during sitting resting baselines than in normal controls. This occurred during a headache-free session and with an even greater difference during the active headache period.

There were methodological limits in all of these studies. However, the conclusions are that differences can and do exist between patients and headache-free controls, and that placements and postures can be important. It is speculative yet logical to conclude also that the differences may be more likely in clinical settings in which practitioners see patients with more severe and refractory headaches. Nevertheless, EMG recordings are still not of clear diagnostic use. Using multiple recording sites and multiple conditions might eventually be a more useful procedure, but this too is speculative. Furthermore, these studies are not contrary to the possibility that more than muscle activity is involved in the etiology of tension-type and migraine headaches. Most data indicate that resting muscle activity in reclined postures does not differentiate between patients and headache-free controls.

The EMG during Headache-Active and Headache-Free States

People with tension-type headaches often do not show a difference in EMG activity between periods of headache and times when no headache is present. The Hatch et al. (1992) review noted "conflicting results" (p. 901). Some studies showed:

greater EMG activity during a headache and another larger group showing no difference . . . [and] one study . . . [reported] frontal EMG levels . . . significantly lower during the headache state than when they were headache free. (Hatch et al., 1992, p. 90)

An example of research on this topic is Lichstein et al.'s (1991) investigation of 13 people who had migraines with *prodromal symptoms*, and 8 who had both episodic and chronic tension-type headaches. They found no reliable difference in frontal muscle tension between headache-active and headache-free sessions, with subjects sitting quietly in a recliner chair. Again, one can assert that limited body positions (Ruff, Sturgis, & St. Lawrence, 1986) and recording sites obscured the difference. Furthermore, more than muscle activity may be involved in tension-type headaches, and the muscle sites that were monitored may not be the ones involved. For some subjects, the muscle activity might have been greater before and after the monitoring.

The lack of difference in EMG activity between headache-active and headache-free times is not enough to enable us to conclude that muscle tension does not cause these headaches. Consider a person carrying something heavy for a long enough time to produce pain in the arms and shoulders. We may observe no excess tension during recordings after the individual puts the burden down, even if the pain continues. This does not need further explanation.

Relationship between EMG Changes and Pain across Sessions

Some patients treated for tension-type headaches show a relationship between changes in office-recorded EMG activity across sessions and reduced headaches. Other patients do not show this relationship. This seldom and inadequately researched question "remains an area of controversy" (Blanchard, 1992, p. 539).

Most published reports do not show a consistent relationship. This suggests that something other than muscle tension may be involved in decreased tension-type headaches. There is some support for the idea that cognitive factors may play an important role in these changes (Holroyd et al., 1984b; Blanchard, 1992). This is probably true for some patients. Changes in patients' daily activities, including their use and misuse of various muscles, are probably more closely related to symptom changes than office-recorded muscle activity is. Furthermore, recording other muscle sites may be more appropriate than the ones commonly chosen in research.

Relationship between EMG Activity and Pain in Tension-Type Headaches

Practitioners often observe patients starting a relaxation session with a headache. Many of these patients clearly lower their *cephalic* and neck muscle tension, and report decreased intensities or elimination of the headache during the session. However, research shows no clear or consistent relationship between EMG activity and pain intensity or pain frequency in patients experiencing tension-type headaches (Lichstein et al., 1991; Hatch et al., 1992). Showing that variations of EMG activity result in changes in pain intensity and frequency has been elusive, although the logic is still valid.

One study, however, did support the relationship (Hatch et al., 1992). The researchers noted that "pain ratings and EMG activity increased during task performance and then showed a parallel decline during recovery periods" (p. 110). All their subjects denied a headache when they arrived at the laboratory, but some reported head or neck pain during the procedures.

Other factors besides decreased muscle tension could account for the clinical observations. These include reduced sympathetic nervous system (SNS) arousal and cognitive factors. Most patients want to feel better, and these sessions also provide distraction from their stressful daily activities. Nevertheless, reduced and resting muscle tension are likely factors for many of these patients as well. Practitioners should consider other monitoring sites and consider that muscle activity may be higher before the office monitoring starts.

Relationship between EMG and Site of Headache

Research on the relationship between EMG activity and pain sites is sparse. During rest or stress, there is sometimes more EMG activity from nonpain sites and sometimes more activity from pain sites. We may consider three possible explanations: (1) Referred pain from one site to another could produce this effect; (2) the muscle activity at the pain site may have been greater before the recordings; or (3) some or most of the muscle activity was outside the range of the EMG bandpass.[3]

The EMG of People with Tension-Type versus Migraine Headaches

Patients with tension-type headaches do not show more resting EMG activity than patients with migraines. Studies find similarities between muscle tension levels in patients diagnosed with tension-type or migraine headaches. Lichstein et al. (1991) showed this, using small groups of headache-free and headache-present patients with either diagnosis. Thus muscle tension may play a role in the etiology of migraines. Furthermore, muscle tension is probably not the differentiating factor between the two diagnoses. This type of finding has led some to assert that headaches with these diagnoses are more likely to be different degrees on a continuum than to constitute two distinct and separate diagnoses (Marcus, 1992).

Involvement of Head and Neck Muscles in Tension-Type Headaches

Although excess tension in the frontal, temporal, *occipital*, upper trapezii, and posterior neck muscles contributes to tension-type headaches, most research and some clinical practice still focus on the frontal area chiefly. However, Hudzinski and Lawrence (1988, 1990) and Hatch et al. (1992) looked at more than the frontal area. Hudzinski and Lawrence (1988, 1990) studied the *frontal–posterior neck* (*FpN*) placement. Hatch et al. (1992) studied the left and right temporalis and cervical neck sites.

Hudzinski and Lawrence (1990) noted that "conventional frontal surface EMG does not appear to reliably discriminate between muscle contraction headache sufferers or to be a means by which to distinguish the headache from nonheadache subject" (p. 24). The FpN placement encompasses multiple cephalic and neck muscles. Referring to their research on this placement, the authors reported that it is "the most discriminating" between headache and nonheadache activity (p. 24). (See the later "Placement of Electrodes" section, and Appendix 14.1, for more discussion of this electrode placement.) Hatch et al. (1992) reported that the temporalis muscles, the frontal area, and the posterior neck muscles reacted significantly to laboratory stress for both patients and controls.

Continued Excess Muscle Activity versus Level of Activity

Continued excess muscle tension may be more important for causing pain than the specific intensity or level of muscle tension may be. However, no research yet exists that supports this theory (Hovanitz, Chin, & Warm, 1989; Hatch et al., 1992). As Hatch et al. (1992) stated, "at the present time, it is not known how much muscle activity over what time interval is necessary or sufficient to elicit the pain experience" (p. 108). Nevertheless, practitioners often assume that sustained excess muscle activity is a causative or aggravating factor. An implication for practitioners who adopt this concept is to recommend that patients need to release excess muscle activity often. That is, practitioners recommend reducing the intensity, frequency, and duration of excess tension to patients, rather than only improving the depth of the relaxation.

Flor (2001) speculates that inadequate abilities for perceiving bodily states may contribute to the maintenance of chronic pain. In her research, patients with chronic pain were notoriously poor at discriminating muscle tension states, overestimated physical symptoms during tension production tasks, rated such tasks as more aversive, and reported more pain upon muscle tensing. The poor discrimination abilities may result in muscle tension levels remaining high even after stress has subsided. The intense or overfocus on bodily states may lead to the perception of pain even at low levels of stimulation.

The EMG Reactivity of People with Headaches Who Are Prone to Stress Reactions

The relationship between EMG reactivity to stress for patients with tension-type headaches compared to those without headaches appears inconsistent in the available research. This inconsistency implies that not all patients with tension-type headaches respond to stress with increased muscle tension. However, the stressors used in some research may be too weak in content and for duration. Again, the muscle sites monitored may not be the most reactive. Furthermore, it may be that individuals with tension-type headache are more sensitive to and have a lower threshold for pain (Wittrock & Myers, 1998). It is also possible that some people with tension-type and migraine headaches show changes in autonomic nervous system (ANS) reactivity, biochemical changes, and *cephalic blood flow* (*CBF*). That idea is congruent with the CBF studies of Gannon, Haynes, Cuevas, and Chavez (1987) and Haynes, Gannon, Bank, Shelton, and Goodwin (1990), discussed next. The reader should also see Hatch et al. (1992).

CBF and ANS Reactivity in People with Headaches

According to Haynes et al. (1990),

> Changes in extracranial cephalic blood flow in response to stressors has long been suggested as a possible mechanism to account for migraine pain and associated symptoms . . . [*and*] . . . suggested as a possible causal factor for muscle-contraction headache. . . . (p. 468)

The very important research of Haynes et al. (1990) and Gannon et al. (1987) demonstrated experimentally, rather than only with correlations, that environmental psychological stress can induce headaches. They also showed the involvement of CBF in both types of headaches. The first demonstration relates to the proposed mechanism of stress and headaches; the second relates to the present topic.

These respected researchers demonstrated that CBF patterns occurred in an analogue situation with recruited volunteers. Their studies with somewhat limited sample sizes improved on cross-sectional and correlational studies of stress and headaches; they helped clarify the uncertainty of whether observed psychophysiological changes follow or precede headaches. Their method used a 1-hour cognitive stressor with subjects without headaches at the start of the procedure. The subjects reported histories of frequent headaches diagnosed as muscle contraction, migraine, or mixed. Their earlier study showed that this stressor leads to "significant increases in multiple psychophysiological indices, subjective reports of stress, and headache reports by about 80% of subjects" (Haynes et al., 1990, p. 471). We include their description of the stressor:

[Subjects were told that] "we are attempting to see how accurately and quickly you can think." They were exposed to . . . arithmetic problems (e.g., 237 – 349) every 15 sec. for 1 hr. . . . [and] were informed that if their performance fell below the average for college sophomores, they would hear a buzzer. Buzzes (. . . 50 dB) were presented 22 times throughout the hour on a set variable-interval schedule. (Haynes et al., 1990, p. 471)

The results with stressor were impressive. Sixteen of 17 subjects diagnosed with tension headaches reported headaches, as did 2 of 5 subjects with migraines and 13 of 14 with mixed headaches. Average headache severity increased over the hour.

The researchers continuously measured *blood volume pulse amplitude* (*BVPA*) from six sites: two *supratrochlear* sites, two superficial temporal sites at the *bifurcation of the temporal artery*, and two cervical vertebrae at the *spinalis–semispinalis* site. The analyses indicated BVPA changes over the hour. Most of the subjects showed a significant relationship between CBF patterns and the induced headaches. The authors admitted that they did not know whether the changes represented a primary cause of headache or a correlate of other processes in the central nervous system (CNS), ANS, or neurotransmitter system. Furthermore, individual differences in BVPA pattern occurred. The pathophysiological mechanism might be different for headache types, as there was vasoconstriction in those subjects with migraines and vasodilation in those subjects with tension-type features.

The authors conservatively noted that BVPA patterns might vary with different stressors. They also noted that other blood vessels might play a role, and noted no confirmation of the factors regulating the vasomotor responses. The relationship between the vasomotor responses in the analogue situation and natural situations is also unknown.

One mechanism that may explain the relationship of CBF and headache is the sustained contraction of cephalic and neck muscles, such as from sustained psychosocial stress. This may restrict blood flow or create *ischemia*, resulting in *anoxia* and increased concentration of *lactic acid*. Ischemia at other local sites also might result in compensatory distension of the cephalic arteries and other changes. Examples are increased circulatory *neurokinins*, *catecholamines*, *vasopressin*, and platelet *serotonin*. These two explanations are not mutually exclusive. Another idea is that the cessation of stress might result in a rebound distension of some cephalic blood vessels.

The proposed role of CBF is consistent with the vascular and neurogenic theories of migraines. Either the CBF leads to headaches, or a central neurogenic dysfunction leads to CBF and headache. A CBF link is also consistent with the theory that sustained muscle contraction results in vascular and CBF changes among persons with tension-type headaches.

This research helps support the justification for treating psychosocial stress and reactivity. The CBF research helps explain the inconsistent findings of research using weaker office stressful stimuli. It suggests the use of both stronger stressors and longer durations of stressors than are now typical in clinical practice. It supports the potential use of the CBF modality for monitoring and feedback. It supports the evidence that different types of treatment can result in decreased headaches. It also implies that the use of each type or treatment does not preclude the role of the others. Thus, one can intervene with the psychosocial stressor, with the muscle tension, and/or at the biochemical and blood vessel stage.

Influence of Psychological, Emotional, Stress, and Other Factors

Examining an Age-Old Assumption

The common and usually accepted hypothesis that psychological, emotional, and stress factors can cause and/or worsen headaches is an age-old assumption and another complex topic.

There is considerable support for the relationship, although it is very difficult methodologically for research to demonstrate a clear, unequivocal, and strong causal relationship. More complex are the clear demonstration and full elucidation of the mechanisms.

Practitioners, many researchers, and many patients assume that many factors can affect the likelihood of developing or worsening a headache. Examples include the following:

- Major stressors and high-density minor daily stressors.
- Negative cognitive perceptions and appraisal of stress events.
- Excess or prolonged emotional reactions to stress.
- Inadequate stress management skills and behaviors.
- Personality features (e.g., obsessive–compulsive characteristics, avoidance of expressing anger).
- Lack of stress-moderating factors (e.g., social support).

See Adler, Adler, and Packard (1987) for more examples and discussions of the literature about these factors. This belief and assumption does not preclude other "risk factors" or triggers." The research below does not suggest or support the existence of migraine or tension headache "personalities."

Many practitioners may wonder why this long-held assumption even needs research support. "Everyone already knows it," some may say. However, consider that at least for many people with migraines and perhaps for many people with tension-type headaches, many very different types of factors are thought to act as "triggers" and contributing factors to these headaches when present either alone or in combination. Consider, for example, the list below of assumed and patient-reported factors in migraines[4] and some tension-type headaches:

- Lack of food, as in fasting, delayed meals, or missed meals.
- Specific foods and drinks.
- Sleep abnormalities (both excess and insufficient sleep).
- Hormones associated with menstruation, menopause, and pregnancy.
- Posture, head and neck positions, other ergonomic factors, sleeping positions, and incorrect pillows.
- Temporomandibular behaviors and other factors.
- Visual factors (e.g., eye strain, glare, and staring at a video display terminal screen).
- Environmental factors (e.g., barometric pressure, heat, and cold).
- Environmental irritants (e.g., noise, odors, smoke, and allergens).
- Activities such as exercise and automobile travel.
- A "let-down" phenomenon called "weekend headache," "Sunday headache," or "relaxation headache."

Further complicating the understanding of and demonstration of a relationship is the following: Many people with these types of headaches and a few or several of the assumed "psychological–affective–behavioral–physiological" risk factors probably also have other major, exclusive, or sufficient causes for their headaches (e.g., postures, muscle tension habits, sleep problems, dietary problems). Even assuming that the relationship in question exists (and we do make that assumption), and assuming the presence of these "risk factors" in a given person, do not automatically justify the conclusion that the risk factors are causing the headaches for that person. Furthermore, these assumptions do not necessarily mean that one must treat these cognitive and psychophysiological factors in order to obtain therapeutic effectiveness.

Although some research addresses either migraines or tension-type headaches, this discussion combines both for these reasons:

1. Many studies addressed both headache types.
2. There is disagreement about the distinction between the types.
3. Some studies do not make a distinction between migraines and tension-type headaches.
4. Frequently, both types exist in the same person.
5. Even when the two types are distinct, they often interact with each other.
6. Psychological and emotional factors influence both types.

Evidence from studies on psychological, emotional, and stress factors support their role for contributing directly or indirectly to headaches (Hovanitz et al., 1989; Blanchard, Kirsch, Appelbaum, & Jaccard, 1989; Nattero, De Lorenzo, Biale, Torrie, & Ancona, 1986; Holm, Holroyd, Hursey, & Penzien, 1986; Levor, Cohen, Naliboff, McArthur, & Heuser, 1986; Nattero et al., 1989; Kohler & Haimerl, 1990; Rugh et al., 1990; Leijdekkers & Passchier, 1990; deBenedittis, Lorenzetti, & Pieri, 1990; Hatch et al., 1991b; Passchier, Schouten, van der Donk, & van Romunde, 1991; Hatch et al., 1992; deBenedittis & Lorenzetti, 1992; Martin & Theunissen, 1993). A summary of these studies is beyond the space constraints of this chapter; interested readers are directed to the references for their own reviews.

Nevertheless, we offer a brief review of a few of the studies as illustrations. To start, we know that laboratory stress can induce headaches (Gannon et al., 1987; Haynes et al., 1990). In addition, we know there is support for ratings of stress being higher during periods before and on the day of migraine headaches (Levor et al., 1986). Support for the effect of stress on migraines also comes from a careful, prospective 6-month study showing that stress increased the day before the clear-cut migraine occurred for 6 of 7 subjects, and during the headache day for 3 more of 13 German postal employees (Kohler & Haimerl, 1990). Of these 13, 11 had "common migraine," 2 had "classic migraine," and some also had so-called "mixed" headaches. On the day before 109 of 192 migraines, patients scored in the upper third of the distributions on a 10-item ipsative stress questionnaire. This led the researchers to conclude that "the effects of stress on the occurrence of migraine attacks are considerable" (Kohler & Haimerl, 1990, p. 871). There was no significant relationship between low air pressure on the day of the migraines for any of the individuals. However, that factor was significant for the group and occurred on the days of 81 of 192 migraines. Compared with stress the day before, low air pressure had a weaker effect.

An interesting and clinically useful discussion of "weekend headaches" in Nattero et al. (1989) provides insights into potential psychological explanations for this phenomenon. People with "weekend headaches" tend to have headaches (usually diagnosed as migraines) during a "let-down" period rather than in the midst of stress. These investigators compared patients with only weekend headaches to those with common migraines without reference to day. The investigators explain their speculations about these patients:

> The . . . headache with 'a loss in his structure of the week' . . . might be generated by that feeling of emptiness experienced . . . in view of drab weekend days, where the patient has no real interests outside of work. . . . Some upsetting situations in patients' private lives, such as marital conflicts, can also be considered as precipitants especially during weekends. (Nattero et al., 1989, p. 97)

The Minnesota Multiphasic Personality Inventory (MMPI), the Beck Depression Inventory (BDI), and the State–Trait Anxiety Inventory (STAI) suggest that, compared to the patients with common migraines, the patients with weekend headaches reported more of a "lack of a real interest in sexual life, poor family and social life, dissatisfaction with what they have accomplished and low self esteem" (Nattero et al., 1989, p. 98). They had higher elevations on MMPI scales 1, 2, 3, 7, and 8 for females and scales 1, 2, 3, 4, and 7 for males. The authors acknowledged, "Whether the stress burden is greater in these weekend headache patients than in the others, or whether these patients have a lesser capacity to cope with stress, is still an open field of research" (p. 98).

The physiological disregulation model of G. E. Schwartz (1977, 1978) provides useful concepts to explain factors affecting the risk of developing a headache. Briefly,

> Physiological disregulation may occur when an individual does not or cannot attend to his/her physiological state and does not take corrective action to return to normal functioning. Failure to attend to or act upon physiological status may result from any of a number of causes, including (1) environmental demands that preempt attention or action, (2) CNS information processing (genetic or learned, such as life-style or personality) that results in inappropriate attention or response to external stimuli, (3) physiology that responds in a hyper- or hypoactive manner to CNS stimulation, and (4) absent or inappropriate sensory feedback to the CNS from a peripheral organ. (Hovanitz et al., 1989, p. 56)

For detailed discussions of the role of psychological and cognitive factors in the genesis of and worsening of headaches, and a discussion of the role of cognitive and psychotherapy treatments for headaches, see Martin (1993) and Adler et al. (1987).

Inclusion of studies in our listing above does not imply a demonstration of a clear and direct relationship or a lack of methodological limitations with the studies. However, the sheer number of supportive studies and the aggregate conclusions are consistent with aspects of these traditional views. At least for people prone to developing headaches, for some people not so prone, and for those already with headaches, there are psychophysiological (in the broadest sense of that term) "triggers" and "risk factors" that can increase the risk of developing and/or worsening a headache. This presumably occurs through increased muscle activity, biochemical changes associated with ANS changes, or both (Gannon et al., 1987; Haynes et al., 1990). Therapy often needs to address both these contributions. Marcus (1993) proposes a "combined biochemical–vascular–muscular" or "neurovascular" model (p. 165). For an excellent review and graphic illustrations of the role of triggers and risk factors resulting in changes in serotonin and other neurotransmitters and resulting in headaches, see Marcus (1993).

The present assumed relationship and research support are fundamental and essential for those practitioners engaged in providing cognitive-behavioral and other forms of psychotherapy for patients with these headaches. Despite this long-held belief among practitioners, further research support is needed to bolster these types of intentions and to support improvements in selection of patients for these types of therapies.

This assumption is also useful for practitioners using stressors in psychophysiological assessments ("stress profiling"; see Arena & Schwartz, Chapter 7, this volume). For example, if one can induce "sufficient" psychophysiological reactivity and assess this and the recovery from the stimulations, and if these psychophysiological measures are useful for patient education, fostering cognitive changes, and treatment planning (including biofeedback procedures), then supporting and demonstrating the hypothesized relationships achieve practical importance.

Furthermore, research support in this area helps identify possible precursors of the muscle tension and/or biochemical changes that are the presumed physiological correlates and assumed necessary contributing factors to causing or worsening headaches. (See M. S. Schwartz, Chapter 6, this volume, for measures of relevant variables, such as alexithymia, anger, perfectionism, obsessive–compulsiveness, depression, and anxiety.)

Conclusions and Implications for Clinical Practice

It is reasonable to assume that many risk factors and triggers exist for headaches. These include excess and/or sustained muscle tension and habits that increase and result in this tension; major and daily stress; anger, anxiety, depression, and other personality and mood factors; psychological/cognitive and psychophysiological effects of exposure to stressors; and inadequate social support. In addition to these, putting psychological and stress factors in proper perspective requires that practitioners be aware of and assess other potential risk factors and triggers—including eating habits, dietary chemicals, drugs, hormonal status, postures and related factors, sleep schedules and abnormalities, visual factors, and other potentially relevant factors (including the days on which and conditions in which the headaches occur).

Individual differences abound for both people prone to headaches and those not so prone. For a headache-prone person, one or a few risk factors or triggers may be enough to cause a headache. For other people, several more risk factors and triggers within a relatively short time may be needed to result in a headache. Furthermore, headaches are often "time-lagged," occurring several hours or days after the obvious exposure to the risk factors and triggers. Prudent and knowledgeable practitioners realize that the risk factors are triggers of the moment and often not just those that immediately precede a headache.

Assessment of patients with headaches usually requires multidimensional assessment and multicomponent treatment options and planning tailored to the individual. If one assumes the importance of the roles of serotonin and other neurotransmitters in at least many patients with headaches (e.g., the neurovascular model), the treatment options include avoidance of triggers and/or providing therapies that affect these neurotransmitters in desired directions. The latter are often medications, but the explanation for the mechanism of relaxation therapies, biofeedback, and cognitive therapies probably involves alterations of serotonin and other neurotransmitters. After all, beliefs do have biological correlates and effects. Our treatments are on a rather molar level, but there must be molecular changes that occur.

Type of Stress Events versus Cognitive Appraisals

Is it that stressful events themselves often lead to headaches, or is it that the perceptions of stressful events result in headaches? Implicated in the answer to this question is the role of cognitions in the development of headaches. Other implications are the roles of cognitive-behavioral therapy and patient education in the treatment of headaches. "Recurrent tension headaches are not typically triggered by major life changes but rather occur in conjunction with the chronic everyday stresses experienced by . . . people" who tend "to perceive stressful events as more distressing and disturbing occurrences than do controls" (Holm et al., 1986, p. 165).

One might propose that people with chronic benign headaches are not necessarily exposed to more stress, but rather are prone to a "tendency to interpret any life event, within his cognitive and emotional framework, as being more arousing or impactful than those people who remain healthy or develop less serious illness" (deBenedit025 et al., 1990, p. 66). This is the "cognitive appraisal" hypothesis. The study by deBeneditis et al. was a cross-sectional and retrospective investigation of people with chronic headaches (29 with chronic tension-type, 21 with migraine, and 6 with mixed headaches) who were compared to a matched headache-free sample. Personal negative ratings of stressful life events in the year before onset of headaches were predictive of headaches. There were many more such events in the groups with headaches than in the control group. Another retrospective study (Nattero et al., 1986) reported more prolonged stress in the 10 years before onset of tension-type and mixed head-aches, but not before the onset of vascular headaches. However, the differences were not in the year before onset of the headaches. Upon completing an extensive review of the litera-ture, Wittrock and Myers (1998) arrived at a similar conclusion—that people with tension-type headaches may use different coping strategies for dealing with stress and pain.

Another unique study used ambulatory EMG recordings of the posterior neck (Hovanitz et al., 1989). This study showed more EMG activity on days with stress than on days without stress. This was true both for patients with tension-type headaches and for headache-free control subjects. Elevated muscle activity was not associated with pain. However, even with the very small sample, the patients reported more subjective negative affect than the controls did. This is one of the more interesting and important studies in the literature. Among the conclusions is the "strong support for the role of disregulation in the etiology of tension head-aches" (p. 68).

Psychopathology

Another basic question is whether people with headaches develop more psychopathology. There was not much support for headaches' resulting in psychopathology in the cross-sectional and retrospective study of tension-type headaches and migraines by Blanchard et al. (1989). However, patients with headaches did show more psychological distress on sev-eral self-report measures than did no-headache control patients. Those with tension head-aches showed more distress than those with migraines. Those with mixed headaches were between the other two groups but closer to the migraine group. The study controlled for life stress differences in the prior year.

There was more psychopathology, as *operationally defined* in this study, associated with headache severity for persons with tension-type headaches than for those with migraines. Partial correlations showed that duration did not moderate this relationship. However, the type of headache did moderate the association. Furthermore, there was no association be-tween longer durations of headaches and psychopathology. In fact, there was less psychopa-thology for patients with 2 years of headaches than for those with 1 year. Those with 1–3 years of headaches reported the most distress on measures of somatic concern, but not much depression. However, distress was less for groups with 4–14 years and for those with 14–22 years of headaches. There was only slightly more distress among those with 23 or more years of headaches.

For patients aged 19–30 and headaches for 3 years or less, there was a higher correlation with somatization on the MMPI. We should note that several of the MMPI items involve head-ache-related content. For persons aged 31–41 years, this same relationship existed, with more recent onset of headaches associated with more depression on the BDI. For the group aged 42 and older, more recent onset of headaches was associated with more depression. Thus this study argues against chronic headaches' increasing long-term psychopathology. It indicates, as ex-pected, more distress with very recent onset but not increasing with more years of headaches.

More recent work, by Merikangas and colleagues (see Merikangas & Rasmussen, 2000, for a review), has critically examined the comorbidity of migraine and other conditions. "Comorbidity" refers to the coexistence of two conditions within the same person. In studies conducted to date, odds ratios have ranged from 2.1 to 3.6 for the association between mi-graine and depression, and from 1.9 to 5.3 for that between migraine and anxiety. Merikangas and Rasmussen speculate that migraine, anxiety, and depression may occur from a partially shared diathesis, consequently producing one syndrome, as opposed to three separate enti-ties. From this work and that of others (Holroyd, Lipchik, & Penzien, 1998; Lake, 2001; Merikangas & Stevens, 1997; Radat et al., 1999), the following conclusions emerge:

- The risk for major depression and anxiety disorders is higher for patients with migraines than for no-migraine controls.
- This influence is bidirectional. Migraine increases the risk of a subsequent episode of major depression (adjusted relative risk = 4.8), and major depression increases the risk of subsequent migraine (adjusted relative risk = 3.3).
- Comorbid anxiety and depression lead to increases in disability and contribute to headaches' becoming intractable.
- Psychological distress is greater in patients with more frequent and chronic headaches.
- Depression is implicated in transformation of episodic to chronic tension-type headaches.
- Certain personality disorders reveal a higher incidence of headache than otherwise would be expected.

Methodological Notes

This section notes a few observations about the methodologies of the above-described studies. We include it for students and those planning research on these topics.

Conclusions based on studies with college subjects and recruited subjects may be different from studies with patients in primary care and tertiary care institutions. The conclusions based on patients with less refractory headaches may be different from conclusions based on patients with more refractory headaches. Retrospective and cross-sectional studies may reach different conclusions from those of prospective, longitudinal studies. We should also consider that the accuracy and completeness of recall of life events and perceptions diminish with time.

We can use multiple measures to measure daily stress, and we should consider including both normative measures comparing subjects to others and *ipsative* measures within each person. For example, Kohler and Haimerl (1990) defined a "stress day" as the top 33% or the top 20% of an individual's (ipsative) distribution, based on selected items. One such item was "time urgency, strain, or overburdening during the past day." Subjects responded with ratings from 1 or "very much less than usual" to 5 signifying "very much more than usual." Ipsative measures are legitimate, in that each person defines his or her subjective stress.

Physiological monitoring in the office and laboratory permits more control and fewer sources of signal variability and confounding factors. It is less expensive than ambulatory monitoring. However, ambulatory monitoring (Arena, Bruno, & Brucks, 1993a; Arena, Hannah, Bruno, Smith, & Meador, 1991b; Arena, Sherman, Bruno, & Young, 1989, 1991c; Sherman & Arena, 1992; Sherman, Evans, & Arena, 1993; Hatch et al., 1991a; Schlote, 1989; Arena et al., 1994a, 1994b; Arena, Bruno, Bruck, Meador, & Sherman, 1993b; Sherman, Arena, Searle, & Ginther, 1991) will probably advance our knowledge more than relying solely on studies with office and laboratory measures.

ASSESSMENT

Assessment of headaches includes a description and history of the headaches and other potentially related symptoms and conditions. It also includes a medical and neurological physical examination, laboratory tests, and diagnosis. Often it includes psychological consultation, self-report measures, and sometimes psychiatric and sleep disorder consultations. Self-report measures include those of stress, emotions, and personality, as well as a daily self-report log. Assessment requires that practitioners understand the myriad of etiological factors that can cause, emit, maintain, and aggravate headaches. It requires knowing the myths and facts about headaches.

This chapter discusses selected assessment topics. Excellent sources of information and guidelines for assessing patients with headaches include Andrasik (2001a), Andrasik and Baskin

(1987), Adler et al. (1987), Blau (1990), and Saper et al. (1993). (Also, see M. S. Schwartz, Chapter 6, for more discussion of intake considerations.)

Nonphysician practitioners using biofeedback wisely prefer referrals from and collaboration with physicians, especially those who have much expertise with headaches. Differential diagnosis is basic (e.g., Saper et al., 1993). Nonphysician practitioners need to know the danger signs that suggest immediate referral to a physician (Andrasik & Baskin, 1987; Andrasik, 2001a). A practitioner who does not know the diagnostic and danger signs should consult these sources or others.

Interview and/or Questionnaire

Practitioners should resist the temptation to rely on a self-report questionnaire for diagnosing headaches. The careful clinical interview remains the gold standard. Rasmussen, Jensen, and Olesen (1991) made a good effort to develop a self-administered questionnaire for studying large populations, but concluded that "a questionnaire is not a satisfactory tool in diagnosing headache disorders" (p. 290). Some questionnaires may be useful as adjuncts to the interview, but not as the primary method of data gathering. The following quote explains the complexity of assessing and treating patients with headaches. It implies the need for a careful clinical interview and continuing assessment.

> The biopsychosocial model of headache states that headache depends upon the specific pathophysiological mechanisms that are "triggered" by the interplay of the individual's physiological status (e.g., level of autonomic arousal), environmental factors (e.g., stressful circumstances, certain foods, alcohol, toxins, hormonal fluctuations), the individual's ability to cope with these factors (both cognitively and behaviorally), and consequential factors that may serve to reinforce, and thus increase, the individual's chance of reporting head pain. (Andrasik, 1992, p. 350)

Symptom Records: The Headache Diary

There are primarily two types of self-report measures for headaches. The most common measure is daily rating of headaches, typically hourly or four to six times a day. These measures typically use a 6-point (0 to 5) or 11-point (0 to 10) rating scale. Other information usually recorded includes frequency of relaxation; the use of medications, caffeine, and alcohol; and comments about the day. The second type of measure is the global rating by the patient. Patients do this periodically or at the end of therapy. Global ratings can be made either orally or in writing (on a printed rating scale). Such ratings are rarely acceptable for evaluating outcome in research, however. Daily ratings are the norm in research and in clinical practice.

Andrasik and Holroyd (1980) compared the use of a headache questionnaire at the beginning of treatment to the use of continuous daily hourly ratings over the next 2 weeks. The similarity between the two methods with 99 subjects was very poor, with very small and nonsignificant correlations. The questionnaire reports underestimated the frequency of headaches, overestimated intensity, and both overestimated and underestimated headache durations. The questionnaire test–retest reliability was high and significant. However, it did not correspond well to the data obtained with the daily ratings on an 11-point scale. The authors suggested that "questionnaire methods of assessing headache symptoms should be supplemented by daily headache recordings whenever possible" (p. 46).

The relationship between patients' ratings and those by "significant others" was the focus of the study by Blanchard, Andrasik, Neff, Jurish, and O'Keefe (1981). The relationship between patients' four-times-daily ratings and the ratings obtained from the "significant others" at the end of therapy was significant, although with only a modest correlation ($r = .44$, $p < .002$). The authors pointed out that the correlation "is comparable to correlations between other concurrent measures of change used in behavior therapy research and does indicate a significant degree of social validation for improvement detected from the diary" (p. 714). The correlation between the patients' daily ratings and global ratings on a *visual analogue scale* (*VAS*) was even more modest ($r = .36$, $p < .002$). Analyses between the two global ratings and daily ratings suggested that global ratings may "produce overestimates of patient improvement" (p. 714).

It is easier to ask a patient for a global estimate of change. For example, professionals ask these questions: Are patients' headaches any different than before therapy? Are they any different compared with the prior week or month? These estimates are made verbally or via standard measures such as a VAS. The problem is that patients often overestimate their improvement compared to their hourly and daily records. This is consistent with the results of Blanchard et al. (1981).

The accuracy of the time a patient makes a rating may be a problem as well. Many subjects often record their ratings retrospectively (Epstein & Abel, 1977; Hermann & Blanchard, 1993). We do not know whether this is crucial for accuracy, but it is of concern if one assumes that retrospective ratings depart from accurate ratings. This question begs for research.

Consider reasons why patients may overestimate their improvement. Perhaps a patient is responding only to the improvement of the last few days. Perhaps he or she desperately wants to be better and deceives him- or herself into believing the degree of improvement. Another reason for such self-deception may be a desire to end therapy. A patient may be uncomfortable with telling the therapist he or she wants to end therapy; the patient also may want to please the therapist. Thus the patient may tell the therapist what he or she thinks the therapist wants or needs to hear.

There are several methods for analyzing patient symptom data. Consider using multiple measures of change. Methods that have commonly been used are (1) headache index/activity (calculated by summing all intensity values during which a headache is present); (2) average headache intensity (dividing the sum derived via method 1 by the number of recorded hours); (3) number of hours of severe- and very-severe-intensity headaches; (4) number of headache-free hours; and (5) number of days that are completely or almost completely headache-free. Scales used for rating intensity have varied.

Committees charged by the International Headache Society (IHS) to develop guidelines for conducting and evaluating pharmacological agents have recommended that composite measures (such as methods 1 and 2 above) no longer be used (IHS Committee on Clinical Trials in Migraine, 1999; IHS Committee on Clinical Trials in Tension-Type Headache, 1999). Such indices are seen as weighting severity and duration in an arbitrary manner, rendering them of little value when data are compared across subjects. These committees have recommended the following serve as the primary diary-based measures:

- Number of days with headache in a 4-week period.
- Severity of attacks, rated on either (a) a 4-point scale, where 0 = "no headache," 1 = "mild headache" (allowing normal activity), 2 = "moderate headache" (disturbing but not prohibiting normal activity, bed rest is not necessary), and 3 = "severe headache" (normal activity has to be discontinued, bed rest may be necessary); or (b) a VAS, wherein one end is anchored as "none" and the other as "very severe."
- Headache duration in hours.
- Responder rate—the number or percentage of patients achieving a reduction in headache days or headache duration per day equal to or greater than 50%.

Reviewing pain records regularly, socially praising efforts to comply (yet refraining from punishing noncompliance), anticipating problem areas, and having patients mail records to the office when gaps between appointments are large may help emphasize the importance of and facilitate accurate recording keeping (Lake, 2001; see the section on compliance in this chapter, as well as M. S. Schwartz, Chapter 8.) However, compliance issues demand flexibility and options for some patients. Practitioners should consider ratings at regular preset times. For example, ratings can be made soon after morning awakening time, at noon, at the end of the workday, and again in the late evening. Another option is every 3–4 hours, such as 7 A.M., 11 A.M., 3 P.M., 7 P.M., and 11 P.M. These two options are useful for patients with pain during nearly all waking hours. However, both options have limitations. For example, when using them, one does not see patterns. One cannot obtain a complete measure of the hours with headache, the exact durations, and the frequency of discrete headaches.

Patients also record their medication usage in the log. This helps document medication changes and assesses whether symptom improvement is the result of medication or of nonpharmacological therapies. Some practitioners choose to rate the potency of each medication and derive a medication index (Andrasik, 1992). One multiplies the potency of each medication by the number taken and sums the total weekly.

There are alternative and supplementary headache measurement approaches used in some research and clinical practices (Andrasik, 2001a). These include separately measuring multiple features of pain (e.g., as with the McGill Pain Questionnaire; Melzack & Katz, 1992) and methods for separating sensory and affective features of pain (Jensen & Karoly, 1992). Some patients report improvements in their affective reactions to their pain even without pain reduction. Consider a checklist of behaviors such as avoidance, activities, complaints, and help-seeking behaviors (Philips & Jahanshahi, 1986). Finally, a current focus is assessment of impact on other important aspects of functioning, such as general health or overall quality of life, physical functioning, emotional functioning, cognitive functioning, role functioning, and social well-being (see Andrasik, 2001a, 2001b; Holroyd, 2002).

Getting a Headache History

Getting a headache history is well described in many references (Kunkel, 1987; Andrasik, 2001a; Blau, 1990; Swanson, 1987; Dalessio, 1986). Chapters in Adler et al. (1987) are among the best sources describing the psychological assessment of people with headaches. We could not do justice to this complex topic in the space available, or present it better than Adler et al.'s contributors.

All practitioners with the responsibility for assessment and treatment are wise to avoid relying entirely on history information from other health professionals. This is true even when the prior history has been taken by competent physicians. It is sometimes necessary to forgo this added history taking because of time and cost factors.

A practitioner who needs to know specific information should get it directly from the patient. The prior written reports can be reviewed aloud with the patient for confirmation. Patients sometimes give different professionals different answers to the same types of questions. Some practitioners misunderstand patients' statements; other practitioners often get only the information needed to make a diagnosis, to rule out serious pathology, and to prescribe medication. Patient reports of such information as onset, location, frequency, and duration are sometimes different when another practitioner asks the questions.

Discrepancies from Prior History

• *Lower-grade headaches versus the bad headaches.* One sometimes reads a history of a specified number of headaches per month, such as six headaches each for 1–2 days. Then one finds out that there are nearly daily lower-grade headaches, but the patient told the prior doctor only about the bad headaches. "I have about five to six headaches a month" can mean that the patient does not want to complain about the others of lesser intensity. A practitioner needs to ask specifically whether a patient believes he or she has more than one type of headache—and, if so, to inquire about each separately.

• *Long history of less frequent and less intense headaches versus recent onset of headaches.* Patients sometimes report the onset of their headaches as when they became more intense or more frequent. The recorded history might say 1 or 2 years, but the onset could have been many years earlier.

• *Less frequent headaches, but other sites of pain.* Some patients report the location of their headaches as the areas in which the pain is the worst or most frequent. Practitioners should ask about other areas that may be important for diagnosis and therapy.

• *Items overlooked in interviews.* Even experienced and competent professionals sometimes miss or overlook potentially important information. These items include dietary factors, gum chewing, sleep problems, work postures, driving habits, and bed pillows.

Headache Interview and History Questions

The following summarizes topics and questions for a headache history. Each item often requires more than one question. Many of the items and questions are mainly for diagnosis; however, most also have implications for assessment and therapy by providers of applied psychophysiological methods. The focus here is less on diagnosis and more on the other uses and implications. Diagnosis is not less important, but other published sources cover the diagnostic implications. We have based the items and questions on multiple sources, including Blau (1990), Swanson (1987), and Dalessio (1986). We encourage reading Blau's (1990) erudite, insightful, refined, and skilled commentary on history taking.

Number of Headache Types. Ascertain the number of headaches of different types occurring both recently and in past years.

Onset. This is Blau's first "time" question. The duration and age of the patient are important mostly for diagnosis. Here are sample questions: "How long have you had this type of headache? How old were you when this type of headache started? When did the headaches begin? How did they begin? Did you have headaches in grade school, in high school, or in college?"

One is more concerned with a headache beginning in an elderly patient, especially if it starts suddenly and is severe (i.e., is there *temporal arteritis* or an expanding intracranial lesion, such as from a hemorrhage or brain tumor?). A headache that changes very little over many years is most likely to be benign.

For a practitioner planning biofeedback for headaches, knowledge of onset information is helpful in understanding the patient's experience with headaches and the patient's expectations. A very long history of headaches suggests many treatments, many disappointments, and a lifestyle focused on headaches. These factors must be considered in making a treatment plan.

Frequency, Regularity, and Periodicity. If the headaches are episodic, what is their frequency and regularity? This information is necessary for diagnosis and baseline information. It is Blau's second "time" question. Questions such as these should be asked: "When do you get headaches? How often are the headaches? How many days a week or month do you have no headache at all? Do your headaches increase at certain times of the month or year? Have you ever thought that your headaches increased before or during certain times of the year or events?" Even research subjects in headache-free control groups underestimate or underreport the frequency of their headaches (Wittrock, Ficek, & Cook, 1996).

In searching for potential triggers, one is looking for emotional/stress, dietary, physical, environmental/meteorological, and hormonal factors. These have all been subjectively reported by patients as likely to precipitate headaches, regardless of whether the diagnosis is tension-type, migraine, or combination (Scharff, Turk, & Marcus, 1995). Stress includes holidays, birthdays, or the anniversaries of deaths, divorces, and marriages. Physical factors include sleep changes, exertion, and skipping meals. Environmental factors include glare or flicker, strong odors, loud noises, and weather changes. Most of the literature is based on subjective self-report. However, as reviewed by Martin (2001), there is support for experimental validation for triggers classified as negative affect (e.g., stress, anxiety, anger, and depression; Martin & Seneviratne, 1997) and visual disturbance (flicker, glare, and eyestrain; Martin & Teoh, 1999). There is much support for the role of daily hassles, negative mood, and/or sleep quality factors preceding headaches within the prior 2–3 days (Sorbi, Maassen, & Spierings, 1996; Spierings, Sorbi, Haimowitz, & Tellegen, 1996; Reynolds & Hovanitz, 2000; Marlowe, 1998).

Timing of Headaches. "Timing" refers to whether the headache starts while the patient is awake or during sleep and at the same or different times. The practitioner can ask, "When or at what time of day do they occur? Do they always or usually occur then?" In addition to diagnostic purposes, this information is useful for understanding precipitating events and timing of relaxation. For example, some tension-type headaches typically start or worsen on the way to work, at about the same time at work, or near the end of the work day; this information has implications for when to use relaxation.

Characteristics of the Pain.
• *Location.* It is helpful to ask, "Where does the pain begin? What is the location at onset of pain, and how does it evolve?" For example, it can be useful to know whether the headache starts in the posterior neck, the temples, or the occipital area. "Does the pain move around?" (Blau's [1990a] "site" questions 4 and 5). "Is the pain deep, as in a stomachache? Is it near the surface, like something digging into your skin?" (Blau's "site" question 6).
• *Description of pain and intensity* (Blau's questions 10 for "quality" and 11 for "quantity"). Ask about *quality.* What is the pain like? Is it aching, burning, throbbing, or stabbing? Practitioners often offer choices from which patients can select; this is usually done orally. Also, questionnaires such as the McGill Pain Questionnaire can be used.

These questions are more useful for diagnosis than for treatment. For example, a short and stabbing pain occurring up to several times per minute and sometimes occurring in waves suggests trigeminal neuralgia. Band-like sensations or general feelings of tightness, like a tight cap, suggest a tension-type headache.

A severity-type question asks about quantity of pain—the intensity. "How bad is the pain?" One can verbally or visually present a rating scale. A related question is "How do the headaches affect your life?" This often unveils signs and discussion of depression and anxiety that may require separate evaluation.

Duration of Pain. "Duration" here refers to how long it takes for the headache to reach the maximum intensity (Blau's "time" question 3). Sample questions are these: "How long do most of your headaches last? Do they last for minutes, an hour or so, a few hours, a half day, a whole day, or more than a day? If the lengths vary, what are the shortest, longest, and usual lengths?"

The value of this information is mostly for diagnosis. However, it is also useful for understanding the impact of the headaches on the person, for treatment, and for assessing progress. For example, are the headaches disabling enough to justify treatment beyond the earliest steps of stepped care? Are the headaches briefer as treatment progresses?

Psychological Evaluation

Whether to evaluate psychological factors, where to begin, and how soon to introduce questions all depend on the patient, circumstances, and the practitioner's judgment. In many professional settings, such as medical clinics, even mental health practitioners are often wise to begin with a headache history or a review of the available recorded history. However, exceptions abound. For example, there are psychologically minded patients who can describe psychological factors clearly from the beginning. All or most of the headache history information is already available in the recorded history for many patients.

Not all or even most patients need a psychological evaluation. There are often practical constraints that result from a patient's schedule and distance from home. Many patients also show a limited or total lack of psychological-mindedness, or display resistance to such inquiries and evaluation. However, a brief psychological evaluation is often better than none. Asking even a few psychosocial questions can help with rapport, and can reveal a patient's receptiveness or resistance to this type of question and treatment. The practitioner can then determine whether a more detailed evaluation is needed then, or whether it can be deferred or eliminated. At the very least, the practitioner should infer the patient's mental status from the interview unless there is an obvious need for a more direct examination.

At a minimum, the practitioner should ask about the pressures and frustrations in the patient's life. In some way, he or she should convey to the patient that it is all right to talk about such matters—and, indeed, that this might be important for evaluation and treatment. This patient can be told that even if these matters are not evaluated fully now, they might become more important later. Patient education booklets can help convey this message.

We have based the following list of psychological factors on one by Adler and Adler (1987, pp. 70–83). Their chapter represents another erudite, insightful, refined, and skilled commentary on history taking. One must read the original to appreciate fully the authors' clinical wisdom and style. They suggest considering evaluation of many factors, including the following:

- Patients' expectations of themselves.
- Perceived expectations by others.
- Existence of past or present family conflicts.
- Sensitivity to criticism and to emotional expressions.
- Comfort with and skills at assertiveness.
- Illnesses and hospitalizations.
- Past or present grief or anticipated grief.
- Medication misuse.
- Experience, perception, and misperception of health care professionals.
- Perceived emotional triggers or factors that increase risk of a headache.

Personality and Psychopathology as Cause or Effect of Headaches

This section focuses on evaluation of personality and psychopathology, including depression, as a cause or an effect of headaches. The implications of this topic for assessment and treatment include the following:

- Should the practitioner assess psychopathology?
- Should the practitioner treat the psychopathology?
- What can one expect during and after nondrug treatment?
- What could account for changes or lack of changes in headaches?

Clinical lore is that psychopathology predisposes people to, contributes to, or causes tension and vascular headaches. A different view is that personality changes, depression, anxiety, and other psychopathology result from living with headaches. Both views have proponents, and both have support. Practitioners and researchers know that the two views represent extremes, and both have practical and heuristic value. Both are probably true for some persons.

A third view is probably also true for many people: Their anxiety, depression, and personality features probably enhance the chance of developing frequent headaches; in turn, the headaches have effects on their moods, lifestyle, personality, behaviors, and reactions to stress.

Measures of anxiety and depression may show slight positive changes during and after relaxation and biofeedback treatments for headaches, even without changes in headaches. Practitioners and investigators speculate on the explanations. Analyses of the measures need to look closely at the aspects of depression and anxiety that change. For example, some measures like the BDI and STAI deal with varied elements of each emotional construct. Reduction of a total score does not tell us what specific aspects changed. One also must note the changes of specific items and sets of items. For example, the BDI pretreatment scores of 6–11 reported in Blanchard, Steffek, Jaccard, and Nicholson (1991c) are not higher than scores of nondepressed or mildly depressed patients. Among nondepressed medical patients, such scores and even slightly higher scores do not reliably mean that a depression diagnosis is warranted. One can respond to these items and get slightly to mildly elevated scores for a variety of reasons. Practitioners who use the BDI know this and inspect individual items. However, we agree that some patients who do not show clinically significant improvements in their headaches do report improvements in mood.

A notable example of mood and anxiety improvement without changes in the target physical symptom is found among patients with tinnitus (see Flor & Schwartz, Chapter 33, this volume). These patients often report improved mood, reduced anxiety, and better adjustment despite no objective improvements in the tinnitus. "The ringing in my ears is the same, but I am sleeping much better and feel much better," some patients say. Such a report could be a response to implied demands of the clinical interview. It could be a way for a patient to reduce *cognitive dissonance* and justify his or her investment in treatment. It could also reflect nonsynchronous changes in varied dimensions—the affective or reactive dimension versus the intensity or sensory dimension. Patients who report sleeping better and experiencing less anxiety and depression may be referring to the affective/reactive dimension.

One reasonable speculation about implicated reduction of depression and anxiety without changes in physical symptoms comes from Blanchard et al. (1991c). They propose that depression reduction occurs because "most patients 'learn' a greater sense of being in control of their headaches as a function of receiving treatment . . . [and] . . . for many patients who achieve little actual reduction in headache activity, there is nevertheless a consistent inclination to perceive positive change" (p. 253). These investigators further speculate that anxiety reduction may occur because of reduced unpredictability rather than controllability. Anxiety decreases "may . . . be attributed to increased awareness of, knowledge about, and sensitivity to biopsychosocial factors mediating headache activity" (p. 253). Both speculations are credible and deserve more research attention.

Practitioners know that depression and other psychological factors can play a role in headache development and maintenance. Antidepressant medications are a major part of treatment programs for headaches. However, the antidepressant effects of the medications are not what account for the improvements. The doses often used for headaches are much less than those used for depression. Changes in sleep and changes in brain biochemistry are two other explanations. Packard and Andrasik (1989) note that "the exact mechanism by which depression causes headache has not been determined" (p. 17).

For discussions of the role of depression and other psychological factors in headache, and treatments, readers should see Adler et al. (1987, Chs. 8, 12, 13, 24, 30, and 31). Practitioners should not underestimate the potential value of pharmacotherapy and nonbehavioral psychotherapy in the treatment of many persons with headaches. Assessment of psychosocial behaviors and emotions becomes increasingly important as one accepts the potential role of these factors in causing and maintaining headaches and in interfering with successful treatments.

Measures: The MMPI

The inclusion of the MMPI reflects its prominence in the headache literature. It is a complex topic, requiring more space and time than it receives here. Some practitioners and researchers use it to classify persons, predict treatment outcome, and monitor progress. The gist of this discussion is that the MMPI has some value for assessing some patients with headaches, but less value than some professionals assert. The MMPI can help alert practitioners to special problems and needs of selected patients. However, the MMPI or other inventories should not be used as the criteria for avoiding applied psychophysiological therapies for a specific patient or group of patients.

Several attempts to find MMPI types associated with different headache types have usually met with meager results (Andrasik, Blanchard, Arena, Teders, & Rodichok, 1982b; Dieter & Swerdlow, 1988). Patients with headaches show elevations on scales 1 and 3.[5] These elevations, as expected, decrease with relaxation and biofeedback treatment. At least some of this reduction probably comes from headache-specific items.

Another classification approach looks at MMPI scale scores of people with different types of headaches. Most MMPI differences among headache diagnostic groups are below the elevations and differences that professionals usually consider clinically important. Nevertheless, the MMPIs of people with migraines and cluster headaches are often close to or indistinguishable from normal control subjects without headaches. In contrast, those with tension-type headaches show higher elevations than most other headache groups. Those with posttraumatic headaches sometimes show the highest elevations.

A paper on this topic by Williams, Raczynski, Domino, and Davig (1993) reported that patients with tension headaches had higher elevations on several scales than those with migraines.[6] The patients with migraines had higher elevations on scales 1, 2, 3, and 7 than nonpatient control subjects. A study using the MMPI-2 also showed significant elevations on scales 3, 1, and 2 for patients with posttraumatic headaches, and no differences from those patients with the diagnosis of *status migraine* with or without analgesic rebound (Kurman, Hursey, & Mathew, 1992).

After headache-related items were removed, a group with mixed headaches became the lowest-scoring group on scales 1 and 3 in the Dieter and Swerdlow (1988) data. The order of the other groups differed from that reported by other studies. The posttraumatic group continued to have the highest elevations, with *T scores* of 70 and 71 for scales 1 and 3, respectively. This probably reflects the damage and symptoms resulting from trauma. (Similar findings have been reported for the Symptom Checklist 90—Revised; Ham, Andrasik, Packard, & Bundrick, 1994).

The *pain density* concept of Sternbach, Dalessio, Kunzel, and Bowman (1980) refers to the overall time with pain. It might explain some of the headache group differences. Thus patients with the diagnoses of posttraumatic headaches often experience the most time with pain each year. Patients with tension-type headaches and mixed headaches often experience less time with pain than those with posttraumatic headaches. Patients with posttraumatic headaches experience more time with headache than most patients with migraines. This hypothesis awaits more research.

There are thus significant limits to using the MMPI with patients with headaches and using it to classify patients. There is much variability in MMPI responses among persons with headaches, and their responses vary to items on scales 1 and 3, including the headache-related items. Dieter and Swerdlow (1988) refer to this as the *disconnection between the MMPI and headaches*, in that some patients with chronic headaches do not endorse the obvious headache items.

Medical and Neurological Consultation and Laboratory Tests

All nonphysicians should know that nearly all patients with headaches need competent medical and/or neurological consultation. There are exceptions, but the prudent nonphysician practitioner errs on the side of caution. One example of a patient who might not need another medical or neurological examination is a patient in the 30s with a history of many years of clearly unchanging headaches diagnosed as tension-type headaches. In this example, the patient has had multiple medical and/or neurological examinations over the past few years. He or she has had appropriate and thorough laboratory studies over these years. In this scenario, the person goes to an independently licensed practitioner who is highly experienced in assessing and treating headaches. Perhaps a phone call or other brief contact with the patient's physician (duly noted in the patient's file) might be sufficient, without the necessity to repeat more medical or neurological examinations. There is a potential risk here, but it is small.

The reason for discussing this scenario is not to encourage this practice. However, in reality, it occurs. Sometimes patients ask for nonpharmacological treatments and want or need to avoid the added expense and time for medical or neurological examination. Such situations might improve cost containment and lessen financial hardships for many people obtaining medical and neurological services.

A practitioner who wants to treat such a patient, but feels uncomfortable with even the low risk and with the perceived ethical problems, can sometimes do the following:

1. Discuss the issue candidly with the patient.
2. Suggest and offer to arrange for the medical and/or neurological services.
3. Allow the patient to refuse those services for a specified period while starting treatment.

A prudent practitioner will clearly document this interchange in the official session notes; a more cautious practitioner will ask the patient to sign a document.

Morrill, Blanchard, Barron, and Dentinger (1990) found, among 278 carefully selected patients with headaches, that "the majority of clients with abnormal laboratory tests (most of which were mildly abnormal) still saw substantial headache reduction with self-regulatory treatment for chronic headache" (p. 27). Only 1 or 2 of the 278 patients had a serious structural abnormality. Of 112 patients getting a routine electroencephalogram (EEG), 14 (12.5%) had some abnormality, with most only being mildly abnormal. Of these, 12 completed treatment, with 3 improving 64–100% and 1 improving 30%. The others showed slight or no improvement. Of 166 patients not getting routine tests, 57 had one or more tests with 13 abnormal. The only abnormalities were for 1 of 29 with skull films, 6 of 45 with EEGs, 5 of

14 with computed tomography (CT) scans, and the 1 with a sinus X-ray. The overall abnormal rate was 22.8% among those selected for tests. Ten of the 13 patients completed treatment, with 6 showing clinically meaningful improvement of 48–81% and 2 others of 37%. "For those . . . with abnormal test findings who completed treatment, 29 percent of [those with] tension headache . . . and 40 percent of [those with] vascular headache . . . showed clinically significant . . . reduction in headache activity" (p. 34).

The selection of tests for each patient depends on the individual case and the physician's experience and opinion. This chapter is not the place to discuss the decision-making process and criteria for selecting laboratory tests. A brief discussion of medical and neurological assessments serves as a review for some readers and a source of basic knowledge for others. Practitioners should look for such items as a *complete blood count,* biochemical profile, *electrolytes, sedimentation rate,* and *total thyroxine.* These are often routine and easy-to-get tests for screening for possible systemic diseases. The sedimentation rate is a test for temporal arteritis; it is especially important for elderly patients with a recent onset of headaches in the distribution of these blood vessels.

Some headache specialists argue for skull X-rays, a CT or magnetic resonance imaging (MRI) scan, and an EEG for selected symptoms. Other specialists recommend the CT scan as the best clinical neurological test for detecting structural brain lesions. These specialists deemphasize the value of skull films and an EEG. "The yield for plane skull films and EEGs [is] very low and infrequently of value" (Swanson, 1987, p. 20). The appropriateness of the CT or MRI is especially important in ascertaining the etiology of a headache that differs from a patient's prior headaches, or one that is getting progressively worse. The value of routine CT or MRI scans for patients presenting with headaches is the subject of disagreement. Mitchell, Osborn, and Grosskreutz (1993) reviewed several studies and added their own data. They emphasize the strong preference for a careful history and neurological examination. From a statistical view, they argue persuasively against the value and cost–benefit ratio of routine brain CT scans for patients with headaches who have normal neurological exams and physical exams without focal findings or unusual clinical symptoms. However, they note that the value of the CT scan may vary in different patient populations.

Another logical and necessary view is that of Campbell (1993). His contrasting view departs from the "cold statistics" and takes into account the realities of the individual patient and the physician in clinical practice. In summary, he asks, "What if it [were] your head?" and "Now tell the jury, doctor . . ." (p. 52). The current care environment is heavy with the need for cost containment, government and other third-party payer involvement in medical practice, and no restrictions on our litigious society. Somewhere between the extremes of many expensive routine tests and very few of these tests exists the choice that constitutes the correct compromise.

Nonphysicians treating patients with headaches need to be aware that the yield from routine CTs is low for many populations of patients with headaches, and therefore their patients may not have had CT or MRI scans. Part of the rationale for discussing this topic is that it heightens the importance of being sure that a patient does have a very competent neurological history and examination, and that there are no unusual clinical symptoms. Being alert to changing symptoms and danger signs of nonbenign headaches will become more important for some practitioners. Working very closely with competent physicians, including neurologists, will become increasingly important.

If trauma has been involved, then cervical spine X-rays are appropriate. This is especially valid if the pain is mainly occipital or if the pain comes with splinting of neck muscles. See Swanson (1987), Saper et al. (1993), and other references for more discussions of this topic.

TREATMENT OF SPECIAL POPULATIONS

The populations discussed in this section are elderly patients, pregnant women, and women with menstrual-related headaches. (See Andrasik, Chapter 30, this volume, for a discussion of pediatric patients with headaches.) Obviously, each of these categories could involve a separate section or an entire chapter. The purposes here are to call the reader's attention to special considerations for each group, summarize selected conclusions, and provide selected references.

Elderly Patients with Benign Headaches

Tension-type and migraine headaches are very common among elderly individuals. Further development of nonpharmacological treatments for these benign headaches in elderly patients is important. The percentage of our population that is elderly is steadily growing (Williams, 1991). In one medical center outpatient sample (Solomon, Kunkel, & Frame, 1990), 4.3% (359/82,893 of those with a diagnosis of headache, excluding temporal arteritis) were aged 65 or older. Of these, 31.7% had tension, 17.8% had migraine, and 15.9% had mixed headaches. Hence two-thirds had diagnoses for which practitioners consider treatment with relaxation, biofeedback, and other applied psychophysiological methods.

Prevalence, Gender Links, and Coexisting Diagnoses

Very few data exist on the prevalence of these diagnoses among elderly individuals. People of various ages with headaches very often do not seek treatment. During a routine office visit in a well-studied elderly population in Dunedin, Florida (Hale, May, Marks, Moore, & Stewart, 1987), 9.1% (117/1284) reported frequent headaches. Female patients reported headaches more than twice as often as male patients (1–1.2% of 819 versus 5.4% of 465). However, we do not know the specific diagnosis of each group. We note this to give a sense of the prevalence of headache among elderly persons. The average age was 78 for those reporting headaches.

In a Japanese sample of 288 elderly patients with various types and degrees of dementia, 75 reported headaches. Of these, 43 (58.9%) had tension-type headaches, 15 (20.5%) had migraines without aura, and 2 had both types (Takeshima, Taniguchi, Kitagawa, & Takahashi, 1990). Of those with tension-type headaches, 12 had chronic and 31 had episodic headaches. Among the 59 patients with dementia of the Alzheimer type, 15 (25.4%) had headaches, including 11 with tension-type headaches. Among the 160 with cerebrovascular disease (CVD), 135 had vascular dementia, and 34 (21.3%) of the 160 had headaches without a direct relationship to their old CVD episodes. Among 160 with cerebrovascular disease, 135 had vascular dementia. Of the 160, 34 (21.3%) had headaches without a direct relation to their old CVD episodes. Twenty of these had tension-type headaches, and seven had migraines without aura. Others had combinations or uncertain diagnoses.

One conclusion is that tension-type and migraine headaches are common among elderly persons, including those with various degrees of dementia. Age and neurocognitive impairments compromise the quality of life among many of these people. They are often unlikely to complain about their headaches for many reasons; these include impaired memory, impaired verbal expressive abilities, depression, and lack of opportunity. We should note that the Takeshima et al. (1990) study excluded those patients "who did not have the ability to complain of headaches" (p. 735).

Practitioners expect more coexisting symptoms, diseases, and use of medications among their elderly patients. This potentially affects and complicates diagnosis and treatment. Notable examples include hypertension and depression. It is worth noting that the Dunedin program (Hale et al., 1987) reported an association of headaches among male patients with *"paroxysmal nocturnal dyspnea*, feeling lonely, and feeling depressed" (p. 274; italics added). Female patients reported many symptoms with their headaches, including brief losses of speech and temporary losses of vision. These could have been caused by *transient ischemic attacks* or microinfarctions and/or by the migraines (Hale et al., 1987). Other symptoms included feeling depressed and perceptions that other people did not care about them.

The diagnoses significantly ($p < .0001$) related to frequent headaches included arthritis, peptic ulcers, angina, cataracts, and diverticulosis among female patients. Among men, the diagnoses were temporal arteritis and kidney stones. It makes sense to think of osteoarthritis linked to tension headaches among the elderly. However, most with this diagnosis did not have an association with headache. The authors suggest that the headaches for those with angina and ulcers were probably caused by drug-induced complications. Examples are those from nonsteroidal anti-inflammatory agents used by persons with headaches and from nitroglycerin taken for angina. Unexpectedly, there was no significant association between hypertension and headache in this study. The only medications associated with frequent headaches were nitroglycerin and aspirin among women, but none for men.

For many of these people, medications are not sufficient or contraindicated because of medical conditions. This supports the role of nonpharmacological treatments if these are efficacious.

Biofeedback and Self-Regulatory Treatment for Headaches in Elderly Patients

The limited literature until about 1988 was pessimistic about the effectiveness of relaxation and biofeedback for treating headaches in elderly patients. This literature was retrospective and based on single cases or anecdotal reports. The general belief was that these treatments were not successful for older patients, especially those with very long-term symptoms. However, some clinical practitioners observed success with elderly patients, but there was limited support for this treatment without a published literature. Fortunately, some determined investigators prospectively studied series of older patients and found successful use of these treatments for headaches in such patients (Arena, Hightower, & Chang, 1988; Kabela, Blanchard, Appelbaum, & Nicholson, 1989; Arena, Hannah, Bruno, & Meador, 1991a). Pessimism and poor expectations by investigators may have resulted in poor results before these studies. Now optimism and positive expectations exist.

The ages of the patients in the Kabela et al. (1989) study were 60–77 (mean = 65) for the 16 treated patients, while the ages were 62–71 (mean = 65) for the 8 patients reported by Arena et al. (1991a). Some practitioners, especially ourselves, do not consider patients in their early and mid-60s as elderly (see M. S. Schwartz & Andrasik, Chapter 35, this volume).

One can only commend Arena, his colleagues, and others for their sensitivity and efforts to tailor the instructions and treatment for older subjects. The therapists simplified instructions, spoke more slowly, and summarized information. They made extra efforts to be patient and to spend more time listening. We question whether asking subjects to "repeat verbally each session's instructions" (Arena et al., 1991a, p. 384) is necessary for most patients, especially those without signs of neurocognitive impairments. However, as an advocate for more efforts for patient education, we agree with the intent.

The outcome of these series, totaling 34 patients, showed 21 or 62% (21/34) with improvements of 50% or greater. Others showed improvements of lesser degrees. The number of treatment sessions varied from 3 to 19 sessions; most patients had between 8 and 12 sessions. This included patients treated only with limited portions of treatment, such as only frontal EMG, only relaxation instructions, or only three office visits. The authors encouraged daily practice. These series are encouraging, and the results open the door to improvements. Tailoring treatment to the individual and using good professional judgment are still advisable practices for treating elderly patients.

The authors correctly point out the limits of their studies. For example, we do not yet know the efficacy of these treatments for elderly patients of non-European descent. We do not know the efficacy with patients with major psychological problems and those with concomitant medical and neurological problems. Nevertheless, the results are encouraging and help to justify these treatments for this population.

Conclusions

1. Practitioners should consider treating older and elderly patients with relaxation and biofeedback, including some patients with dementia.
2. Patients should be interviewed carefully about their headaches, and caretakers should be encouraged to do the same.
3. Medical, neurological, and/or psychiatric evaluations should be performed. Symptoms that could affect accurate diagnosis and/or affect relaxation and biofeedback treatments should be monitored.
4. All medications that could affect treatment should be noted and monitored.
5. Practitioners should develop special patient education and cognitive preparation for treatment of elderly patients, to reassure them and to increase their understanding and compliance.
6. Depression and sleep disorders should be assessed and treated as needed, at least before and/or during applied psychophysiological treatments. Treating depression and/or sleep problems may help decrease headaches in some patients.
7. Elderly patients' spouses, other family members, or caretakers should be included in evaluation and treatment as necessary.
8. Treatment may require 10–19 office sessions with some elderly patients. However, fewer office sessions may be successful with some patients.

Pregnant Women

Among pregnant women, medications for headaches are often ill advised or contraindicated. During pregnancy, and especially for migraines, at least 50% of women report relief from headaches (particularly after the first trimester). Others report more headaches. Some women without a history of headaches report onset of migraines during pregnancy. Scharff, Marcus, and Turk (1997) reported on 30 women through their pregnancies and up to 12 weeks postpartum reporting their migraine, tension-type, or combined headaches. There was a tendency toward an increase in headaches in the third trimester among multiparous women. There were fewer headaches thoughout pregnancy and the postpartum period for primiparous women.

One uncontrolled report (Hickling, Silverman, & Loos, 1990) used a combination of applied psychophysiological treatments for vascular headaches during pregnancy. They reported elimination of headaches or significant improvement for all five women who were treated with a combination of muscle and autogenic-type relaxation, EMG and thermal biofeedback, and cognitive psychotherapy. Sessions ranged from 4 to 12. Improvement usually started in the second trimester and was maintained at follow-up of 4 to 17 months.

The first controlled study of nonpharmacological treatments for headaches was conducted by Marcus et al. (1995). They combined progressive relaxation and skin-warming biofeedback in 4 office sessions, and 4 office sessions of physical therapies involving instructions for neck stretching and strengthening, and use of heat and ice. In two studies, the second a controlled study against an attention control group, the combined treatment was very effective, with significant improvement maintained over 6 months. The immediate postpartum period is often associated with increased headaches, but not in these treated subjects. The authors discussed limitations of the study, including the small sample of 11 in combined treatment and 14 controls, and the somewhat atypical sample (a mean age of 30, over half with college degrees, and more of the control group developing headaches during pregnancy). The 1-year follow-up (Scharff, Marcus, & Turk, 1996) showed good maintenance of improvement, with two-thirds maintaining significant improvement; results were also independent of breastfeeding (thus independent of changing hormones).

Women with Menstrual-Related Migraines

For many women, migraine headaches worsen before, during, and/or at the end of menstruation. There are few studies of the efficacy of thermal biofeedback for menstrual-related migraines, and conclusions are not yet clear. Reports include those by Solbach, Sargent, and Coyne (1984a), Szekely et al. (1986), Gauthier, Fournier, and Roberge (1991), and Kim and Blanchard (1992). The most recent of these summarizes the methodological shortcomings of these studies. A discussion of biochemical and methodological factors related to this topic is beyond the scope of this chapter. However, a summary of selected information is presented here.

The use of thermal biofeedback may or may not be effective. This depends on the definition of menstrual-related migraine, the treatment components, the data one selects, and the interpretation one adopts. It is obvious why confusion surrounds the topic. As Kim and Blanchard (1992) have pointed out, there is a clear conflict in the literature. Solbach et al. (1984a) interpreted their study as showing no effect of nonpharmacological treatment on menstrual migraine (as did Szekely et al., 1986), whereas Gauthier et al. (1991) interpreted their data as showing that biofeedback treatments work equally well with menstrual and nonmenstrual migraine. There is some support, although weak, for the use of thermal biofeedback and relaxation procedures for menstrual-related migraine headaches. It is reasonable to introduce this type of treatment if medications are not enough and if the headaches are interfering with a woman's life. Practitioners should ask patients to keep clear symptom records and clearly define the criteria for menstrual-related versus other migraine headaches. Patients should try to note midcycle ovulation headaches and consider them to be another type of menstrual-related migraines.

Definitions of Menstrual Migraine

There is no consensus on the definition of menstrual-related headaches. Do we use a patient's subjective definition? Do we use specific time limits, such as 3 days before or after menses or 7 days before and after onset of menses? For Szekely et al. (1986), the definition was headache occurring regularly during the menstrual phase; they defined this phase as a constant 15 days, plus and minus 7 days, around the onset of menses. Solbach et al. (1984a) did not distinguish menstrual-related headaches from other migraines. They defined the menstrual phase as the 3 days before the onset of menses, during menses, and the 3 days following menses. Gauthier et al. (1991) defined the menstrual phase the same way.

Kim and Blanchard (1992) classified these migraines and nonmenstrual migraines from the subjects' subjective reports confirmed by their headache logs. Some women with menstrual migraines reported worsening during 1 week before onset of menses, during menses, during ovulation, or at both menses-related and other times. Subjects defined the time when they thought their menstrual migraines were most likely to occur. These were either during the week before the menses or during the menses. See Silberstein (1992) for a discussion of biochemical factors and definitions; he proposes a differentiation of menstrual migraine from premenstrual migraine.

Results and Conclusions

We focus on the Kim and Blanchard (1992) study as the most recent and one that controls for factors not previously addressed. They reported on various combinations of relaxation, temperature biofeedback, and cognitive therapy with extended or limited office-based programs. As a group, these treatments were similarly effective for both menstrual and nonmenstrual migraines; they were significantly more effective than nontreatment. Among the group of 38 women reporting menstrual migraines, 16 (42%) reported at least 50% improvement, compared with a similar 33/60 (55%) of those with nonmenstrual migraines. Other percentages of improvement were also similar. Those with menstrual migraines showed slightly less improvement in headaches and medication reduction; however, they did improve compared to pretreatment.

Because of possible limitations of the first study, the researchers studied another 15 subjects reporting both menstrual and nonmenstrual migraines. They used only temperature feedback, presumably with relaxation home practice. This group did not do as well as the previous cohort. However, four patients reduced their nonmenstrual migraines by at least 50% (average = 74%). Three of these also reduced their menstrual migraines by at least 50% (average = 88%). Another subject improved her menstrual migraines by nearly 81%. Note that four subjects worsened when the 4 weeks after treatment were compared to the pretreatment baseline.

In conclusion, these treatments can result in significant improvements for many women with menstrual-related migraines. One can certainly justify this treatment approach. Practitioners should consider using a subjective definition of menstrual-related migraines and should verify these with headache logs.

COST CONTAINMENT CONSIDERATIONS

This section focuses on the rationale for and factors involved in the stepped-care model for providing health care. This model starts with effective therapies that are less expensive and typically less complicated.

The major treatments for tension-type and migraine headaches often proceed with medication management, dietary changes, relaxation and biofeedback therapies, physical therapies and ergonomics, stress management, and psychotherapy. This order does not imply a preference or standard of practice; it is one logical order. The order also logically starts with relaxation with limited biofeedback and limited office visits, and then proceeds to extensive biofeedback. Different medications and different dietary changes could appear at both ends.

The cost-effectiveness of biofeedback for treating people with headaches was reported in O'Grady's (1987) impressive and noteworthy study, which illustrated how biofeedback can reduce medical utilization and medication usage among patients with chronic headaches. In a large health management organization setting, 63 patients with chronic headaches completed 6–20 sessions of biofeedback treatment. O'Grady compared these patients with 17 others completing 5 sessions or fewer. At 1-year follow-up, those with more sessions had 75% fewer physician office visits, used 56% less medication, had 19% fewer emergency room visits, and also made 16% fewer phone calls to their physicians at 1 year. Office visits for headache remained consistently low over 5 years after treatment. In the year before treatment, patients had made an average of more than six visits per year for headaches. Over the next 5 years, the average was under two visits per year.

A retrospective investigation of medical costs alone showed a considerable reduction when the 2 years prior to relaxation and biofeedback treatment were compared with the 2 years after treatment (Blanchard, Jaccard, Andrasik, Guarnieri, & Jurish, 1985b), thus complementing the findings of O'Grady.

Medication

Most people with headaches who seek treatment consult with physicians first, and physicians usually prescribe medications. This practice is logical and often effective; one may disagree with it, but it remains a standard approach. For this reason, we start with considerations for cost containment for pharmacological therapies, and we focus on migraines. We do this because of the potential for high costs for treating migraines with prophylactic and abortive medications, and the potential for misuse. However, we consider tension-type headaches briefly as well.

Pharmacological Treatment of Migraines: Prophylaxis

Holroyd and Penzien (1990) conducted a meta-analysis of 25 clinical studies of *propranolol* and 35 clinical studies of relaxation and thermal biofeedback, with a combined total of 2445 patients. The studies revealed no consistent advantage for either approach. In the studies using daily symptom ratings, the reduction of headaches was about 45% for short-term periods. With less conservative outcome measures, such as physician ratings or patient global reports, the improvement was about 20% better. Both treatments were much better than studies with placebo or untreated subjects, both of which typically produce little or no improvement. Other prophylactic medications, such as beta-blockers, *calcium channel blockers*, and antidepressants, are also useful for individual patients. However, none are consistently better than propranolol (Holroyd, Penzien, & Cordingley, 1991).

Therefore, one makes the choice between using prophylactic medication and using relaxation on grounds other than effectiveness. Such factors include patient convenience, contraindications, professional preferences and habit, and cost.

Pharmacological Treatment of Tension-Type Headache: Prophylaxis

For tension-type headache, the most commonly administered medications include tricyclic and newer-generation antidepressants, muscle relaxants, nonsteroidal anti-inflammatory agents, and miscellaneous drugs (Mathew & Bendtsen, 2000). A recent, large-scale randomized controlled trial (203 adults, mean age = 37 years, 76% females) found stress management (three sessions and two telephone contacts; relaxation plus cognitive coping training) and drug prophylaxis (either *amitriptyline* or nortriptyline) to be equivalent in effectiveness, although time to response was quicker for medication. The combination of the two treatments was more effective than either treatment by itself (Holroyd et al., 2001). Combined care is probably the most common treatment in clinical practice.

Unanswered Questions

Unanswered or incompletely answered questions involving pharmacological treatment therefore include the following:

- What is the comparative effectiveness over longer periods?
- What is the effect of various combinations of treatment?
- Are there differential effects on specific subgroups of patients?
- Are there differential effects on quality of life and disability?
- What are the differential iatrogenic effects of these treatments?

Until we know the answers to these questions, the decision to start with a prophylactic medication or a nonpharmacological treatment (e.g., relaxation and biofeedback) depends on these factors:

- Patient preference.
- Physician preference.
- Patient experience with medication.
- Negative side effects.
- Medical contraindications.
- Practical considerations, such as availability of relaxation and biofeedback, treatment costs, and reimbursement.

Pharmacological Treatment: Abortive

We found one study comparing long-term effects of abortive pharmacological therapy for migraines with those of relaxation and thermal biofeedback (Holroyd et al., 1989). Both treatments resulted in clinically significant improvements. The patients maintained most of their gains at the 3-year follow-up. However, among the eight patients treated with relaxation and biofeedback, six were still using these treatments; only two had added other treatments. Furthermore, none were using prophylactic or narcotic medications at follow-up. In contrast, only 2 of 11 patients who started with ergotamine were still using it, and 5 were using prophylactic medications or narcotics. Two of the seven who changed treatments did so because of side effects of the ergotamine.

One often needs good patient education to help assure compliance and, at the other end of the spectrum, to prevent overuse or abuse. Although abortive medications have a place in the treatment of migraines, compliance can be a problem. Long-term reliance on abortive medications may not be as good as relaxation and biofeedback.

Dietary Changes

Stopping selected dietary substances should be considered before any other treatments if a patient or practitioner strongly suspects that this could reduce the patient's migraines. This is often easy and does not involve extensive changes in dietary habits. However, extensive dietary changes and challenges are occasionally proper. Such a regimen should be tailored to the patient. (See Block et al., Chapter 9, this volume, for a discussion of dietary factors and migraines.)

Cognitive and Other Psychotherapies

Rationale

Cognitive therapies have a long history in the treatment of migraine and tension headaches. One can logically justify the use of cognitive therapies for many patients with headaches, and there is research to show their specific value. However, research results vary in support of cognitive therapies, with less-than-desired demonstration of their added value. The reasons for continued research on and clinical use of cognitive-behavioral therapies include the following:

1. Many clinical practitioners and researchers believe that cognitive factors and therapies are important.
2. Practitioners and researchers desire to improve treatment.
3. Cognitive therapies may be well suited for addressing concomitant psychological distress (such as anxiety or depression) that often accompanies headache.
4. Documenting the value of the added investment of time and expense for cognitive therapies.

The rationale for cognitive therapies for headaches is well summarized by Appelbaum et al. (1990). They propose that patients' perceptions and experiences of stressful situations account for the worsening and/or maintenance of headaches. The automatic thoughts that accompany these perceptions probably mediate stress reactivity and headache onset for many patients. In turn, one or both of two factors may mediate tension-type headaches. One is the individual's perception of a lack of control when facing these stressful situations. Another is the chronic muscular tension and sympathetic arousal that occurs in response to these situations.

Review of Studies

Tension-Type Headaches. Pure cognitive therapy was more successful than a self-regulatory approach with relaxation and bifrontal EMG auditory biofeedback for recruited subjects (Holroyd, Andrasik, & Westbrook, 1977). Results were maintained at a 2-year follow-up (Holroyd & Andrasik, 1980).

Adding cognitive therapy to muscle relaxation therapy improved the percentage of patients showing clinically significant improvement within a regular office contact model (Blanchard et al., 1990b); 10 (62.5%) of 16 patients in the combined condition showed at least 50% reduction of headaches, compared to 6 (31.6%) of 19 in the relaxation-only group. However, the overall magnitude of change in a headache index did not reveal a similar advantage for adding cognitive therapy. We should note that this study used progressive muscle relaxation without biofeedback. We can also note that the relaxation-only group did not fare as well as expected from other studies, and fared no better than a "pseudomeditation" group. The data support the addition of cognitive therapy. However, it is not clear that it always yields better results than the results of relaxation alone or of biofeedback.

Combining a tailored cognitive therapy and a relaxation procedure was more effective than relaxation alone in a limited-contact, self-administered format (Tobin, Holroyd, Baker, Reynolds, & Holm, 1988). Tailoring involved problem solving and cognitive restructuring for each patient. The relaxation therapy was progressive muscle relaxation. One limitation was the lack of a control group.

Another study showed cognitive therapy to be better than a combination of muscle and autogenic relaxation procedures without biofeedback (Murphy, Lehrer, & Jurish, 1990) for reducing headache frequency and severity of the worst headache for each week. The authors speculated that the reason might be the patients' improved ability to manage stressors. It should be noted, however, that the improvement for both groups was below that typically observed in other studies. For example, the headache index improvement was only about 30% for relaxation and 47% for the cognitive therapy. These were both lower than rates found in other studies using similar therapies. The authors admitted doubting whether their subjects in both groups actually used the specific techniques; thus this may be more a study of *exposure* to therapy than of the use of therapy. The authors also asked whether the difference from other studies could have resulted from the slightly older ages of their subjects. The mean age was about 40. Other studies (Appelbaum et al., 1990) do not suggest that patients of this age should do worse than younger patients.

A limited-contact study showed no advantage for combining a fixed set of cognitive procedures and relaxation therapies compared with relaxation alone (Appelbaum et al., 1990). In contrast to the Tobin et al. (1988) study, the patients were an average of 9 years older (37 vs. 28) and had suffered headaches 6 years longer. Furthermore, the cognitive therapy protocol was fixed instead of tailored. These factors could result in reducing the advantage of cognitive therapy. The authors considered whether more time and more cognitive therapy would help. It might take longer than 1 month for the effects of cognitive therapy to show. The authors also considered a possible *ceiling effect*. In such a situation, adding more strategies to an already valid therapy might prove to be counterproductive.

In conclusion, the potential advantage of adding cognitive therapy to relaxation alone or to a combination of relaxation and biofeedback is not entirely clear. There are conditions in which adding cognitive therapy to relaxation does not increase treatment effectiveness. We also do not know whether brief and tailored cognitive therapy for each patient would be sufficient. Nevertheless, many practitioners continue to believe that cognitive factors and therapies are valuable, at least for selected patients. The logic is too strong to ignore this in clinical practice. The vital questions are these: What types of cognitive therapy are useful, what specific procedures are most useful, for whom are they useful, and when should one introduce cognitive therapy? Prudent clinical judgment, the use of a stepped-care model, and cost containment must remain in the forefront of clinical practice until research answers these questions, and support for them arrives.

Migraines and Mixed Headaches. The focus here is on selected research with cognitive therapies for migraines and patients with both migraine and tension-type headaches (mixed headaches). One study combined cognitive therapy with temperature biofeedback and compared this combination to temperature biofeedback and relaxation without the cognitive therapy component (Blanchard et al., 1990a). The patients had vascular or mixed headaches. Treatment was administered within a limited-office-contact model. All treatment was better than a symptom-monitoring, waiting-list control group; however, cognitive therapy did not result in better results than without it.

Another study showed that in a regular office-contact model, combining cognitive therapy with temperature biofeedback had about the same results as such biofeedback alone for patients with vascular (migraine and mixed) headaches (Blanchard et al., 1990c). Treatment was better than no treatment. There was no advantage for providing a combination of relaxation and cognitive therapy for patients with migraines treated in a clinic-based model with eight sessions versus a limited-contact model with two sessions (Richardson & McGrath, 1989). Both treatment groups fared better than a waiting-list control.

Conclusions and Recommendations for Cognitive Therapies

1. Practitioners can justify combining cognitive therapies with relaxation and biofeedback for selected patients. However, the added value is not consistent for all patients. One should not routinely start with the combination when one is using a stepped-care model and seeking cost containment.

2. Practitioners should use multiple measures of improvement; any one measure may not be sufficient.

3. A questionnaire such as that of Murphy et al. (1990) allows assessments of patients' ability to prevent headaches and function with headaches. It also allows assessment of patients' perceived personal control over their headaches.

4. Patient education is probably very important, to explain the rationale for cognitive and other therapies and to provide therapy instructions (see Holroyd & Andrasik, 1982, for further discussion).

5. Practitioners should consider tailoring cognitive therapies.

6. Results and the ceiling effect from relaxation and biofeedback may depend on several factors. One should consider asking these questions:
   a. Is biofeedback used to change patients' cognitions about their sense of control?
   b. Is the feedback information adequate?
   c. Is the relaxation with biofeedback tailored to patients? For example, was it from different muscle areas such as the cervical neck, trapezii, and occipital muscles? Is the feedback with varied postures and activities?
   d. Are there other therapy changes during and after therapy?
   e. Is there sufficient patient education to teach the rationale, procedures, and expectations for relaxation and biofeedback?
   f. What is the frequency and timing of relaxation practice?

One can speculate that these factors can result in approaching or teaching maximum effectiveness. If so, then cognitive therapy might not add much. Each practitioner decides the role of cognitive therapies and tailors treatment for patients.

Prudent Limited Office Treatment

Using fewer office sessions is a valid cost containment approach and may have certain practical and theoretical advantages (Andrasik, 1996). The terms "minimal-therapist treatment," "home-based treatment," and "limited-contact treatment" are interchangeable in the literature. None of these terms is ideal. "Minimal" implies least or insignificant, and that is not the intent. The term "home" implies a specific place for treatment, rather than everywhere other than in the professional's office. Of these three descriptions, we prefer "limited-contact."

M. S. Schwartz (1995) has proposed the term *prudent limited office treatment* (PLOT). The word "prudent" is used in the sense of discerning, judicious, logical, careful, conscientious, and economical. It does not imply that using more office sessions is imprudent or excessive. There are cases in which it is proper to start with more sessions rather than fewer sessions; however, it is prudent to consider the least number of office sessions to accomplish therapeutic goals. This approach is often appropriate, sufficient, and cost-containing. Patients whose headaches respond to uncomplicated therapies do not need extensive office-based relaxation and biofeedback. Relaxation therapies and/or biofeedback-assisted relaxation need not involve a lengthy series of office sessions to be effective. Research supports the strategy of preceding biofeedback with relaxation therapy for some patients (Blanchard et al., 1982b).

Research on Various Forms of PLOT

There are several studies showing PLOT to be as effective as longer office-based programs, beginning with the early work of Jurish et al. (1983), Teders et al. (1984), and Blanchard et al. (1985a). The regimen by Blanchard et al. (1985a) is typical of these approaches; it involved a series of audiotapes and therapy manuals, three office visits spaced over 12 weeks, and two telephone contacts of 10–15 minutes. Therapist time totaled about 2 hours. These studies reported that PLOT programs were far more cost-effective for reducing vascular, mixed, or tension headaches than traditional office-based treatment. Cost-effectiveness of PLOT depends on the costs of delivering care, the specific treatment components, and the professional time needed in each approach. Qualitative (Rowan & Andrasik, 1996) and quantitative (Haddock et al., 1997) reviews support the utility of the PLOT approach.

Group treatment is another type of cost containment in models of care involving PLOT within a stepped-care approach. In some clinical settings one can consider a group approach, although it is not feasible in many such settings. The group approach has typically focused on psychological treatments including cognitive-behavioral therapies and relaxation. However, an example of a multidisciplinary approach has been described by Scharff and Marcus (1994). Although one could provide this approach before individual treatment, they provided it *after* the patients had been unsuccessful with individualized therapy. The individual treatments involved various medications and/or various nonmedication therapies, including relaxation/biofeedback in a few cases. The care providers for the multidisciplinary treatment included a neurologist, physical therapist, occupational therapist, and psychologist. The results were encouraging at an average of 7 months' follow-up, with "over 70% of patients with a variety of diagnoses experiencing a 50% or greater reduction in [headache index] . . . accompanied by a 70.9% reduction in . . . medications" (p. 76). These results were significantly better than those for a control group (25.8%) who did not attend the group sessions. Speculations about possible reasons why this approach was helpful include integration of multiple disciplines with new content, support of a group, more practice, the prior lack of success increasing compliance and focus on the treatment, and/or increased sense of control associated with having various options.

Napier, Miller, and Andrasik (1997) reviewed the limited number of other studies that have evaluated various group approaches (ranging from biofeedback in dyads for specified headache types to treatments for larger groups comprised of multiple headache types). One such investigation (by Andrasik and colleagues) examined the utility of the PLOT approach, but within a group format, and compared this to a typical group approach. At short-term follow-up, the PLOT group approach lagged behind in outcome, but it caught up to the traditional group approach at 1 year. Perhaps additional time was needed to consolidate gains in the PLOT group treatment.

Most recently, researchers have begun to explore the feasibility of administering behavioral treatments to large number of patients via mass media and the Internet. A pilot study conducted in the Netherlands (de Bruijn-Kofman, van de Wiel, Groenman, Sorbi, & Klip, 1997) used television and radio instruction to supplement home study material on headache management. Favorable results were obtained for the small sample ($n = 271$) that was available to participate in the outcome analysis; however, this was just a fraction of the people who purchased the self-help program (approximately 15,000). The study has significant limitations, including the absence of a control group and the great difficulty of extrapolating the findings on so few (approximately just 1% of the sample) to the many who started the program. The first Internet-based study was centered at the worksite and was implemented via computer kiosks (Schneider, Furth, Blalock, & Sherrill, 1999). In the second such study, patients accessed the Web from terminals at home (Ström, Petersson, & Andersson, 2000). Modest improvements occurred, but attrition was considerable (greater than 50%) in both investigations. Nevertheless, there is potential value in these approaches as part of cost-containing stepped-care treatment and PLOT.

Finally, the emerging field of "behavioral telehealth" (Folen, James, Earles, & Andrasik, 2001) may be another method of providing cost-containing PLOT-type interventions for headaches, including relaxation therapies with biofeedback. Preliminary findings suggest that telehealth biofeedback may be equivalent to *in vivo* treatment.

Implications

There are alternatives for many patients, and cost containment is possible. Practitioners should consider starting a treatment trial within a PLOT model for most patients and include a suitable patient education package. If clinically significant and patient-acceptable symptom improvement does not occur, then more office-based therapy can be added.

The following example contains steps for practitioners to consider in the treatment of many patients with headaches.

1. Before individualized intervention:
   • Consider mass media/Internet behavioral intervention, if feasible and available.
   • Consider group uni- or multidisciplinary treatment, if feasible.
2. In the first sessions, include some or all of the following:
   • Make necessary dietary changes.
   • Stop gum chewing, especially with temporalis headaches.
   • Consider instructions for posture improvement and for neck and shoulder exercises.
   • Change easy-to-modify life stressors.
   • Assess at least multiple muscle sites during baseline rest and response to stress.
   • Provide limited biofeedback (e.g., in one to three sessions).
   • Use audiotaped relaxation and printed instructions.
   • Use oral, printed, and/or taped patient education.
   • Provide brief live relaxation instructions.
   • Recommend reducing or stopping selected medications that might be contributing to headaches.
   • Have patients use a self-report log to record headaches, medication, relaxation, caffeine, and so forth.
   • Arrange for follow-up in a few weeks.
3. Provide more office-based therapy if headaches do not decrease significantly. Consider:
   • Face-to-face relaxation therapy.
   • Additional biofeedback-assisted sessions, if indicated.
   • Further evaluation and other treatments.
   • Behavioral telehealth (including biofeedback-assisted relaxation, if feasible).
4. If headaches still do not decrease to an acceptable degree, provide different office-based therapy, as indicated. Consider:
   • Additional biofeedback-assisted relaxation, as indicated.
   • Cognitive and other stress management therapies, as indicated.
   • A multidisciplinary group approach, if feasible.
   • Deferral of treatment if the patient expects a major life change in a few weeks, and the change will probably result in a reduction of stress and symptoms. For example, one can defer treatment for a teacher seen in May who reports that symptoms typically improve substantially in the summer.

A stepped-care approach is not the model of choice for all patients. Many patients show considerable excess physiological tension and/or considerable stress in their lives. At the outset of therapy, they often need intervention strategies such as those in steps 2 and 3.

OTHER SELECTED FACTORS AFFECTING HEADACHES AND INTERFERING WITH TREATMENTS

Medications

Patients with High Consumption of Headache Medication

Practitioners often encounter patients who regularly consume large amounts of medications, some of which (analgesics or *ergotamine*) may actually induce headaches. Practitioners often begin applied psychophysiological treatments while patients are permitted to continue their medications. Therapists monitor the medications and look for reductions of both headaches and medications. Many patients resist or fear stopping medications before another treatment begins; however, the drugs themselves may become part of the problem for many of these people and confound treatment and interpretation of results.

The first paper describing *analgesic rebound headache* induced by analgesics was written by Kudrow (1982). This topic became a focus of clinical and research attention by Rapoport and his colleagues (Rapoport, Sheftell, Weeks, & Baskin, 1983; Rapoport, Weeks, Sheftell, Baskin, & Verdi, 1985; Rapoport, 1988). Practitioners now often encourage withdrawal as a treatment. The proposed syndrome is defined as "almost daily use of relatively high levels of analgesic medication combined with chronic low-to-moderate levels of headache" (Blanchard, 1992, p. 543). Severe headaches for several days follow stopping or markedly reducing chronic use of analgesics. However, continued abstinence often results in substantial reductions of headaches. Starting other medications for headaches during and after withdrawal of analgesics confounded interpretation of results in early and many later studies. Similar effects have been reported for ergotamine (Diener & Wilkinson, 1988; Saper, 1987).

Within a stepped-care framework, practitioners can consider the following, as suggested and field-tested by Blanchard, Taylor, and Dentingers (1992):

1. Ask patients to withdraw on their own or with a physician-prescribed tapering schedule.
2. Add self-regulatory treatment to choice 1. Consider a few sessions of relaxation and psychological support during the withdrawal. Add more self-regulatory treatment after withdrawal.
3. Start a multicomponent self-regulation treatment and withdrawal of medication.

Mathew, Kurman, and Perez (1990) studied the value of EMG and temperature biofeedback, along with a low-caffeine and low-tyramine diet, for medication-induced headaches. Among those who stopped all medications, headaches initially rose during about the first 2 weeks and then dropped steadily over several weeks. Those patients who did not stop medications showed no change in headaches. The improvement of patients without any medications was about the same as among those patients in other medication groups. The latter included patients continuing prophylactic medications without symptomatic medications. This led Mathew et al. (1990) to conclude that "concomitant use of symptomatic medications nullifies the effects of prophylactic medications" and that "discontinuing daily symptomatic drugs enhances the beneficial effects of prophylactic medications" (p. 637). Details of the relaxation and biofeedback procedures are scant. One has a sense that this study used a very basic version of these procedures.

The 10 high-medication-user female patients reported by Blanchard et al. (1992) illustrate the complexity of addressing this problem. This report further shows the difficulty some patients have stopping medications even with help. However, applied psychophysiological treatment appeared to help some patients withdraw from medications. Treatment included relaxation, biofeedback, cognitive therapy, support, or combinations of these. For these patients, practitioners may properly care less about the element of the treatment package that is working; withdrawal and significant clinical improvement are far more important. The headaches worsened during a marked reduction or total withdrawal of medication in a few but not most patients. Thus rebound is not inevitable among these patients. Tailoring the approach to the patient and using good professional judgment are crucial.

Implications and recommendations include the following:

1. Some patients should stop medications before starting treatment.
2. Patient education and support are very important before and during withdrawal.
3. Some patients should receive combined withdrawal, support, and relaxation or adjunctive treatments.

Patient education should deemphasize dependency on medications. A practitioner should explain how medications can lead to lessened effectiveness and should focus on the medications as the culprit rather than the patient as the problem. However, the practitioner should support and emphasize the patient's responsibility for changing. Negative attitudes toward the physicians who prescribed the medications should not be encouraged; patients can be told that medications are standard treatments and often successful, despite the undesirable results in some people. This is a delicate line to walk. We do not see benefits from arousing or reinforcing patients' ire against other doctors. There may be exceptions when the patients' prior doctors misused medications, and mismanagement raises ethical and malpractice questions.

One question is this: Could relaxation and biofeedback play a role in withdrawal from analgesics, and, if so, in what ways? Based on available data, the results from relaxation and biofeedback treatments are much less satisfactory for patients who use analgesics heavily (Michultka, Blanchard, Appelbaum, Jaccard, & Dentinger, 1989). These patients are among the more refractory to behavioral treatments such as relaxation and biofeedback. This result does not appear related to personality differences among patients.

Hospital-based detoxification is proper for certain patients, but this can be very costly and otherwise impractical (see Freitag, 1999, for hospital admission criteria). Baumgartner, Wessely, Bingol, Maly, and Holzner (1989) reported that 60% of the tension-type and migraine patients "experienced a long lasting relief of headaches" and 76% "a significant reduction of analgesic abuse" (p. 513) following this treatment. The treatment package was multicomponent and the types of patients and variables were complex, which complicates straightforward interpretation.

Grazzi et al. (2002) attempted a more controlled investigation of inpatient treatment focusing on a group of patients carefully diagnosed as having "transformed" migraine due to analgesic overuse. All patients were first withdrawn from their offending medications and then started on an appropriate prophylactic course. Some patients received EMG biofeedback in addition to detoxification. At the first planned follow-up (1 year posttreatment), both groups revealed similar levels of improvement. However, at the 3-year follow-up, patients receiving the combined treatment showed significantly greater improvement on two of three measures collected prospectively, as well as lower rates of relapse. Thus the addition of biofeedback seemed to help the patients deal more effectively with future difficult situations and led to more durable effects over the long term. This points also to the importance of conducting long-term follow-up investigations with this population.

Comprehensive (multimodal) inpatient treatment (Lake, Saper, Madden, & Kreeger, 1993) is a consideration for certain other patients, wherein relaxation and biofeedback are components in the treatment program. Despite the nearly $5000 average cost per patient for an average of 8.5 days, the authors' logic and justification are persuasive. The more conservative data indicated a reduction of days with severe headache by at least 50% in about two-thirds of 91 patients. There was long-term maintenance of the substantial reduction of pain medications.

Description of Analgesic-Induced Headaches. Some describe analgesic-induced headaches as "rather uniform and independent of the initial headache type and of the pharmacological substance abused" (Baumgartner et al., 1989, p. 510). "Drug-induced headache features" can include a constant, dull, and daily occipital pressure that spreads along both parietal areas (Baumgartner et al., 1989). The headache can also feel like a helmet that fits too tightly. There may be other headache attacks superimposed on these. Accompanying symptoms include *asthenia*, nausea, irritability, memory problems, and sleep disturbances.

Most of the headaches experienced by the patients seen by Mathew et al. (1990) were described as bilateral and diffuse with scalp tenderness, including suboccipital tenderness. Severity and location of headaches varied. Nearly everyone had some daily headaches consistent with migraine, "even though they rarely show the typical and distinct pattern of migraine attacks" (p. 637). Furthermore, "Most of the time it is difficult to distinguish [the drug-induced headache] from the primary headache disorders" (p. 637). Accompanying features were asthenia, nausea, restlessness, irritability, memory problems, difficulty in intellectual concentration, and depression. Seventy-nine percent of the patients showed combinations of these. "One of the most striking features of drug-induced headache is the early morning awakening (2 A.M. to 6 A.M.)" (p. 638). This could be an effect from withdrawal.

Withdrawal features described by Baumgartner et al. (1989) included "increased headache intensity (rebound headache), sleep disturbances, vegetative symptoms (nausea, vomiting, hypotension), mood disturbance, and non-specific heart sensations" (p. 511). One patient had an epileptic seizure. Withdrawal symptoms were most severe on days 3 and 4 after stopping the drug, and symptoms lessened substantially after that.

The criteria used by Baumgartner et al. (1989) for their diagnosis of "analgesic abuse" were proposed by Diener (1988):

- More than 20 days a month with headaches.
- More than 10 hours of headache each day.
- More than 20 days a month ingesting analgesics.
- Regular use of analgesics and/or ergotamines combined with barbiturates, codeine, caffeine, antihistamines, or minor tranquilizers.
- Increased headache intensity and frequency after stopping analgesics.
- Irrelevance of initial headache types for developing this syndrome.

See Baumgartner et al. (1989), Mathew et al. (1990), Rapoport (1988), Askmark, Lundberg, and Olsson (1989), Blanchard et al. (1992), and Michultka et al. (1989) for information about analgesics and details of their studies.

Arguments against Analgesic Rebound Headaches. One proposed mechanism for rebound headache is that analgesics produce more brain serotonin, which paradoxically increases pain in patients with headaches. If this is true, a question arises: How does this mechanism account for the lack of increased headaches among patients with arthritis, who take larger doses of aspirin than do patients with headaches? The same question applies to people taking aspirin daily to help prevent arterial thrombosis (Fisher, 1988). Possible answers are that (1) this mechanism is incorrect, (2) patients with headaches are biologically different from other persons with chronic pain, or (3) there is some other factor beyond the "biochemical rebound effects" of chronic analgesic use that results in persistent headaches and improvement after withdrawal. Could analgesics mask some pain and some of the body's internal or natural biofeedback? Could this add to the physiological disregulation and/or the discrepancy between tension and awareness of tension? This analgesic masking of pain could add to increased tension without awareness and therefore to worse and maintained headaches.

Another concern raised by Fisher (1988) is whether "rebound" is the proper term. It implies that "as the medication wears off headache comes back even worse" (p. 666). However, there are suggestions of habituation to analgesics. This leads to the need for more medication that can interfere with the effects of other medications, such as amitriptyline. This suggests that pain gets worse with the use of the medication. Another question is this: How can tension-type headaches, presumably often caused and worsened by muscle contraction, worsen from a *central origin* without muscle contraction? This relates to the issue of whether these headaches are distinct or whether they exist on a continuum with other headaches.

Lance, Parkes, and Wilkinson (1988) reported in a letter to the editor that among 89 patients at a rheumatology clinic, 50 were taking more than 14 analgesic pills per week, typically for several years. (This letter preceded the paper by Rapoport, 1988.) Based on interview data, these patients did not have more headaches than those taking less than 14 pills. This letter discussed the issue for migraine headaches.

Lance et al. (1988) took issue with the assertion that the mechanism of analgesic abuse is a "suppression or down-regulation of a central anti-nociceptive system" (p. 61). If this were true, then patients with chronic pain but without migraines should experience increased headaches with the use of "high numbers of analgesics." For this proposed mechanism to be accurate, "the anti-nociceptive system of a migrainous population must be already partly suppressed, or set at a different level to the rest of the population, so that analgesics in the quantities described tip the migraineur over the threshold into daily headache" (p. 61). However, their data did not support this assumption.

There is another problem with some studies thought to support the concept that regular use of analgesics causes headaches and that improvement occurs after withdrawal. Other medications used could account for the improvements. However, some reports did not substitute other medications. Those data offer stronger support for the negative effects of chronic analgesics.

In conclusion, there is research support for the view that daily or almost daily use of analgesics can worsen and maintain headaches, although the mechanisms remain unclear. Strong advice to selected patients to withdraw from these medications is now common practice. This fits well within a stepped-care model.

Negative Effects of Nonheadache Medications on Headaches

Practitioners treating headaches need to know about nonheadache medications that can provoke headaches. It is beyond the scope of this chapter to discuss this topic in detail; a short list and brief discussion will suffice to alert readers. Askmark et al. (1989) summarized the "drugs most frequently associated with headache according to 10,506 reports to [the World Health Organization] from five countries." The countries were Australia, New Zealand, Sweden, United Kingdom, and the United States. "The ten drugs most frequently reported . . . were *indomethacin, nifedipine, cimetidine, atenolol, trimethoprim–sulfamethoxazole, zimeldine, glyceryl trinitrate, isosorbide dinitrate, zomepirac,* and *ranitidine*" (p. 441; italics added). Oral contraceptives also were among the most reported drugs. The most common mechanism proposed for drug-related headaches from some drugs is "vasodilatation and salt and water retention with subsequent redistribution of intracranial fluid" (p. 441). The mechanism is unknown for other drugs.

Implications for the Effects of Medications on Headaches

• *Assessment.* Patients should provide information about all medications and include this in their daily symptom and medication logs. Practitioners should consider self-report measures of self-efficacy to assess patients' beliefs and perceptions.

• *Stepped care.* The issues to be considered include these: Should one use outpatient or inpatient treatment? How much patient education and cognitive preparation are necessary before withdrawal? Should one use physiological self-regulation treatments before and/or during withdrawal? Does one continue or start prophylactic medications to cover the withdrawal?

Medication Effects on Biofeedback

Little research has been done on the topic of how medication used for a specific headache or pain problem physiologically affects biofeedback training. This type of research is very complex. We must infer the potential effects of medications on biofeedback.

Jay, Renelli, and Mead (1984) examined propranolol (Inderal) and amitriptyline (Elavil) during biofeedback for developing vascular and neuromuscular control. Patients started medication at least 4 days before starting eight sessions of relaxation and of EMG and thermal biofeedback. The results suggested that the beta-blocker led to a "markedly increased variability in the ability of patients to control" their hand temperature. This also occurred for patients taking amitriptyline alone and trying to master muscle control. The use of either or both "may make concurrent biofeedback . . . more difficult by increasing physiological variability" (p. 67). Baseline physiological functioning varied markedly early in the sessions and after several sessions. However, this did "not prevent biofeedback-enhanced relaxation . . . from occurring" (p. 67), although for some patients it was particularly difficult.

The physiological variability for patients using each medication alone was less than for patients using both medications. All patients reached the criteria of 92°F and less than 1 microvolt. The authors did not specify either the conditions in which this occurred or the duration of these. We also do not know whether these patients decreased their headaches. We are grateful to these authors for their pioneering work; however, practitioners need improved studies and understandable data presentations.

These two medications probably result in physiological variability that could make treatment more frustrating for some patients. There are no data showing that such patients do not do as well as those treated without the medications. Jay et al. asked, "Does the combination of both medications make biofeedback training easier by decreasing the physiological variance on the measures . . . ?" (1984, p. 69). Practitioners continue to use relaxation and biofeedback with patients taking medications known or thought to affect physiological activity, including muscle tension and ANS reactivity and recovery.

Dietary Vasoactive Chemicals

Despite our best efforts and those of our patients, some patients with migraines do not benefit from relaxation, biofeedback, cognitive therapies, and other forms of stress management. Thus some practitioners suggest dietary treatments after unsuccessful trials with these other treatments. Published studies report inconsistent outcomes, which are thought to result from methodological problems (Radnitz, 1990; Radnitz & Blanchard, 1991). The two proposed mechanisms for food-triggered migraines are allergic and vasoactive mechanisms. Enough data supporting one or both mechanisms exist to justify a trial of dietary changes. (See Block et al., Chapter 9, this volume, for a detailed discussion of dietary factors.)

Sleep

Primary sleep disorders are found among patients presenting primarily with headaches, and sleep problems can cause or worsen headaches. Migraines, cluster headaches, *chronic paroxysmal hemicrania*, and hypnic headaches can be triggered during sleep. Obstructive *sleep apnea* and heavy snoring very often result in headaches.

Of 288 patients at a headache clinic, 49 (17%) reported headaches during their sleep time or early morning at least 75% of the time (Paiva, Farinha, Martins, Batista, & Guilleminault, 1997). Of these 49, 26 (53%, or about 10% of the 288) were diagnosed with a primary sleep disorder. These sleep disorders were obstructive sleep apnea (*n* = 7), periodic limb movements (*n* = 8), fibromyalgia syndrome[7] (*n* = 7), and psychophysiological insomnia (*n* = 1). Treatment[8] of the specific sleep disorders (e.g., continuous positive air pressure for sleep apnea) resulted in total cessation of headaches in 17 of the 26, including all with sleep apnea, 3/8 with periodic limb movements, 7/10 with fibromyalgia.

Other reports also support the common presence of morning headaches among persons with sleep apnea and/or heavy snoring (Ulfberg, Carter, Talback, & Edling, 1996; Jennum, Hein, Suadicani, & Gyntelberg, 1994; Loh, Dinner, Foldvary, Skobieranda, & Yew, 1999). The headaches associated with sleep apnea are typically briefer than 30 minutes. Possible causes include oxygen desaturation with vasodilation, sleep fragmentation with microarousals, excess daytime sleepiness, and/or bruxism. Among more than 3000 middle-aged and elderly men in Denmark, snoring and headaches were found to be strongly related (Jennum et al., 1994).

Disturbed sleep in patients with headaches can result from anxiety and/or depression. For persons vulnerable to headaches, either excess sleep or limited sleep can worsen headaches; this may be associated with fluctuations of brain neurotransmitters, including serotonin. Some believe that frequent naps may be associated with morning headaches, in part due to reduced good sleep at night. In a prospective and detailed study, increased stress (defined in terms of the incidence and stressfulness of hassles, particularly in the prior 24 hours), increased mood disturbance in the prior 60 to 24 hours, and sharply decreased sleep quality the night before were associated with migraine headache attacks (Sorbi et al., 1996).

Hypnic or "alarm clock" headache is a benign, rare, sleep-related headache disorder (Dodick, Mosek, & Campbell, 1998; Dodick, Jones, & Capobianco, 2000; Gould & Silberstein, 1997; Raskin, 1997). Females with this condition far outnumber males. Affected individuals are usually about 60 and older, but sometimes younger. The headaches awaken them at consistent times, typically between 1 and 3 A.M., and sometimes during daytime naps. The headaches last typically from about 15 minutes to 2–3 hours. They can occur one to three times per night. Symptoms include pulsating, usually bilateral pain, and sometimes nausea but not other ANS features. The headaches are probably serotonergically mediated. Neurological examinations, brain imaging, and laboratory studies are unrevealing. Helpful medications include lithium, indomethacin, and caffeine. Our aim here is to alert readers to this sleep-related headache type.

In cases where sleep problems or disorders may be affecting headaches, practitioners should conduct a thorough clinical interview to help determine onset time of headaches related to the sleep–wake cycle (i.e., headache onset during sleep time or early morning). This is more useful than the location and frequency of the headaches. Assessment of patients with headaches should include information about their sleep and about excess daytime sleepiness in opportunistic situations (e.g., dozing or sleeping while sitting and reading, watching television, or sitting inactive in a car or a public place). Sleep onset, sleep maintenance, rested feelings in mornings, and snoring should also be covered. Referral to a sleep disorder specialist should be considered if there is an indication of a sleep disorder. If so, it may be better to defer relaxation and biofeedback until after the sleep disorder evaluation has been completed and treatment has significantly improved the sleep.

Pillows

In the second edition of this book, no studies of the use of pillows for neck and/or head symptoms were reported, because there were none. Now four studies have been located (Lavin, Pappagallo, & Kuhlemeier, 1997; Hagino, Boscariol, Dover, Letendre, & Wicks, 1998; Persson & Moritz, 1998; Palazzi et al., 1999). The most ambitious of these studies (Persson & Moritz, 1998) is discussed here. Fifty-five Swedish subjects (37 hospital employees, 12 outpatients with muscle-related neck pain, and 6 post-cervical neck surgery patients) tested each of six different pillows for three consecutive nights. Subjects graded each for comfort and effects on neck symptoms, sleep quality, neck tension, and pain. Of the 42 persons with periodic neck and shoulder pain, 27 reported reduced pain. Of the 27 persons with periodic sleep problems, 23 reported improved sleep. The following additional conclusions were drawn from this work:

- There were variations among people in preferences and apparent advantages.
- Males and females differed in their preferences.
- The pillow with the highest rating was made of soft polyurethane (a material with high elasticity that yields when supporting the head) and contained two firmer supporting cores in the low and high sides.
- Three other pillows were rated favorably and did not differ among themselves.
- Neither treatment outcome data, nor EMG or other physiological data, were reported.
- Manufacturers of each pillow were not provided, but presumably all pillows are easily acquired.

Obviously, further research is needed. Given the variable response and the wide range of available pillows, patients will need to try a number of different pillows to give this approach an adequate test.

Aerobic Exercise

The available literature often suggests that exercise can induce migraines. There are reports of headaches caused by or aggravated by varying degrees of exercise (see Darling, 1991). However, other reports suggest that exercise may not uniformly be a risk factor for migraines. In some persons, exercise may even help reduce migraines. One interesting case reported by Darling (1991) suggests that it is possible for aerobic exercise to abort classic migraines. However, the subject of that report presented an unusual combination of features: She was a professional dancer and had exercised with aerobics and running several times a week for many years. At age 43, she reported that the exercise aborted the migraines either during a visual aura or during the headache phase. Thus this case may be atypical.

In a group of volunteers with classic migraines, Lockett and Campbell (1992) reported no increase in migraines for 11 women engaging in low-impact aerobic dancing and calisthenics three times a week for 6 weeks. Each session lasted 45 minutes, including a 10-minute warm-up and a 10-minute cool-down period. In this small sample, there was a nonsignificant tendency toward improvement on multiple variables. For the purposes of this discussion, the important point is that the headaches did not worsen.

Caution in interpreting the role of exercise in causing migraines is wise. Some of the reported research involved very strenuous exercises, such as running, and often without a warm-up period. Another factor could be the wearing of tight swimming goggles. It would be misleading to consider aerobic exercise a treatment for most persons with migraines; however, practitioners need to keep their clinical antennae up for that possibility.

A related topic of potential relevance to the management of headaches is exercise-induced analgesia (EIA; Padawer & Levine, 1992). Anecdotal reports by dancers and athletes that they feel no pain during strenuous exercise may be linked to the idea that exercise releases endorphins and thus results in pain reduction. The proposal and acceptance by some of EIA stem from this linkage. However, research support for the proposed EIA confounds the effects of exercise with pain test reactivity. Thus it provides only weak support, according to Padawer and Levine (1992), whose study did not support EIA. The purpose here is only to introduce the EIA concept and suggest that it remains controversial. Practitioners can use this information when discussing exercise with those patients who ask about it. Practitioners should also consider recommending that many patients with headaches avoid strenuous exercise.

COGNITIVE PREPARATION OF PATIENTS: PATIENT EDUCATION

The practitioner should consider the following questions when reviewing cognitive preparation of a patient with headache for biofeedback and associated therapies:

1. Have the patient's concerns, questions, and misperceptions about therapy been covered?
2. Does the patient understand the rationale for therapy, the procedures, the goals, and his or her responsibilities?
3. Does the patient remember enough information for therapy to proceed effectively?
4. Is the content of presentations clear enough and within the patient's reading level and intellectual range?
5. Are the methods for patient education acceptable to the patient and cost-effective?
6. Is the content of the presentations complete enough to anticipate the questions and concerns that are likely to arise after therapy starts?

COMPLIANCE

Therapists make recommendations that require cooperation from patients. For example, a self-report log involves frequent ratings of headache intensity, and often also includes information about medications and caffeine usage. Maintaining a log for many weeks places great demands on patients. Practitioners need to consider the office visits, cognitive stress management assignments, and dietary changes requested as well. Patients need to practice and apply relaxation often, and at those times when it will be of benefit. In addition, there are often suggestions for lifestyle changes involving work, social, and family activities. Reminding oneself to think and act differently before and during stressful events requires much cooperation. Moreover, patients often need to change their sitting, standing, and working postures, as well as their sleeping positions and the type and placement of their pillow(s). These all require understanding, acceptance, and cooperation by patients.

Pain is often painfully inadequate (pun intended) as a sole motivator. Practitioners should never assume that pain is sufficient to provide all or even most of the incentive needed for adherence to the therapy recommendations.

Many therapists believe that some patients need comprehensive programs including many recommendations. This gives the term "therapeutic alliance" a new dimension. In such cases, professionals must ensure that patients are sufficiently involved in the alliance to follow rec-ommendations. Otherwise, the patients waste time, effort, and money, and their needs often remain unmet. It is not enough only to make recommendations to patients, and then expect them to take responsibility for complying with these recommendations. They are trying to apply the recommendations while they are also trying to develop confidence in their abilities and to carry out their daily lives.

Patient responsibility is very important, but we practitioners often must cultivate it; we cannot assume that it adequately exists from the onset of therapy. This is especially impor-tant for patients for whom we make many recommendations—as well as for patients who find compliance difficult even for a few recommendations. We can emphasize patient respon-sibility, but must be patient and persistent as we ask our patients to do the same. We also need to examine our professional behaviors and practices. (See M. S. Schwartz, Chapter 8, this volume, for more discussion of compliance.)

PLACEMENT OF ELECTRODES

Rationale

Multiple muscles contribute to tension-type and some other headaches. The common bifrontal site does not adequately measure or reflect the activity of some of the other muscles, such as the cervical neck, upper trapezii, and occipital muscles. Occipital activity is undetected or inadequately detected by bifrontal or posterior neck placements (Nevins & Schwartz, 1985). This is important to consider, as the occipital area is a site of headaches for some patients. Reduced frontal activity does not reflect reductions in most other head and neck muscles. Some patients who attend to their head muscles and relax them will also often relax the occipital muscles. Bifrontal feedback and relaxation may generalize to other muscle areas, including the occipital area for some patients. However, some patients do not relax the occipital area even with excellent relaxation of the frontal and cervical neck areas.

Nevertheless, therapy using bifrontal EMG feedback often leads to successful results in many patients with headaches (Blanchard & Andrasik, 1985). When one suspects or knows that other muscles are involved, it is logical to record and provide feedback from those areas. This chapter assumes that decreasing muscle tension is important for many or most patients with tension-type headaches, and that sensor placement makes a difference. This does not rule out cognitive factors. Research supports the value of recording from sites other than the bifrontal (Hart & Cichanski, 1981; Hudzinski, 1983; Hudzinski & Lawrence, 1988; Pritchard & Wood, 1983; Sanders & Collins, 1981). For example, Pritchard and Wood (1983) reported that patients with tension or migraine headaches showed significantly higher occipital activ-ity than frontal activity during an experimental stress. Hudzinski (1983), in a paper address-ing the importance of recording and feedback from the posterior neck muscles, reported that his patients thought that the "neck, rather than the frontalis musculature, was the more use-ful electrode placement site for reducing their muscle activity," and that "14 of the 16 pa-tients . . . reported that using both electrode placement sites was more effective for under-standing the muscle activity involved in their headaches" (p. 88).

The FpN Placement

The FpN placement, mentioned earlier in this chapter, involves one electrode on a frontalis muscle and another electrode on the same side of the posterior neck. This includes activity from multiple muscles, including occipitalis and temporalis muscles in addition to frontalis and posterior neck (Nevins & Schwartz, 1985). The rationale for developing this placement was to have placements of electrodes that would help detect and help assess occipital activity without routine direct recording on the occipital muscles, as that would be impractical in routine clinical practice.

Occipitalis Muscles and EMG Placement

The occipitalis muscles pull the scalp back. They are under less voluntary control than the frontalis muscles. Their function is more limited than that of the frontalis, and hence they have less internal or proprioceptive biofeedback. When patients are asked to tense only the occipitalis muscles, most have much difficulty. Very few people can tense only the occipitalis muscles on command. Directly recording from the occipital placement is preferable. One can record a bilateral occipital site with standard electrodes without shaving any hair. It requires extra care and a few more minutes to attach the electrodes properly, with the use of extra conductive gel, extra tape, and other aids (e.g., bobby pins to keep the hair away from the site).

Uses of the FpN Placement

The primary advantages of the FpN placement are that it provides a more comprehensive measure of muscle activity in the head and neck than other placements do (including the bifrontal), and that it also provides an indirect measure of possible occipital activity. Higher-than-expected FpN recordings raise the question of occipital tension. One must rule out other causes of the elevated FpN signal. See Appendix 14.1 for more discussion of this placement and interpretation.

When Is the FpN Needed or Not Needed?

A single bifrontal site may be sufficient for some patients if the frontal site shows elevated activity and the headaches are mostly frontal. However, when symptoms involve the back of the head, or when symptom reduction is inadequate with only the frontal placement, a practitioner should consider recording elsewhere and adding FpN placements.

Case Examples

A patient stated that her headaches were in her forehead. The referring physician's notes stated the same, and an added clinical interview did not reveal other headache sites. The psychophysiological assessment proceeded with recording from the left and right FpN placements, as well as the bifrontal and bilateral posterior neck placements. The FpN signal was elevated beyond that expected from observing the muscle tension at the frontal and neck sites. When asked again about the location of her headaches, the patient again pointed to her forehead. Undaunted, the practitioner asked whether she ever had headaches in the back of her head. She said, "Sometimes." When asked how often that meant, she responded, "About 20% of the time." She paused and added with emphasis, "But they are the worst ones." Recording directly from the occipital area revealed excess tension far beyond resting levels.

What are the lessons learned from such an experience? A patient's interpretation of interview questions is sometimes different from our intention and understanding of the interview questions. For this patient, the question of "Where are your headaches?" meant "Where are most of them?" She had focused on frequency. The FpN elevation and the pattern suggested by the recordings alerted the practitioner to conduct further inquiry and assessment.

Another case report (Schwartz, Craggs, & Capobianco, 2002) demonstrates the clinical usefulness of the FpN placement, as well as the use and specific value of direct occipital biofeedback in treatment. A 19-year-old male who had experienced head trauma was assessed for possible involvement of occipital muscles after partial but insufficient response to frontal and posterior neck EMG biofeedback and relaxation therapies for recurrent posttraumatic headaches in other areas of his head. Occipital tension was suspected from a four-channel EMG assessment of his head and neck, including two FpN channels. The FpN elevations were noted to be over 50% higher than bifrontal and posterior neck activity combined. The patient then reported bilateral occipital headache of mild to moderate intensity. This implicated excess occipital activity, and led to the direct measurement of the bilateral occipital area, resulting in observations of relatively high occipital activity, independent of activity from all other muscle sites recorded.

A total of six sessions involving EMG biofeedback were conducted over 9 weeks, with the last three sessions involving occipital feedback. Discrimination training with visual EMG feedback from direct occipital placement markedly reduced the occipital activity. The subject showed a consistent ability to reduce occipital averages to less than 1 microvolt. Symptom ratings showed a significant reduction in frequency and intensity of headache pain with the use of occipital feedback. Identifying elevated occipital activity and providing direct occipital feedback significantly increased the success of treatment for this patient. This subject actually reported sensations of headache when tensing (verified by EMG) the occipital region; conversely, he reported a decrease in headache symptoms when relaxing. His symptom ratings (Figure 14.1) show the effectiveness of this therapy. The patient also reported feeling less tense at night and achieving a significant reduction in sleep latency. The 9-month follow-up showed continued success.

Conclusions and Implications

History taking should include specific questions relating to *all* the locations of head pain and discomfort. These location questions should be repeated periodically, because answers can change as tension and pain in other areas diminish. Some patients with headaches have symptoms in the occipital area to which the occipital muscles contribute. The FpN placement is the best indirect measure of occipital activity when used with bifrontal and posterior neck placements. Ideally, both left and right FpN placements should be used. A practitioner who suspects occipital tension should consider occipital recording and feedback.

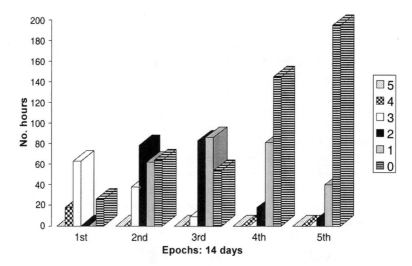

FIGURE 14.1. Symptom ratings for a 19-year-old male with posttraumatic occipital pain. From Schwartz, Craggs, & Capobianco (2002).

Some patients with headaches have symptoms in the posterior neck that contribute to their condition. Inclusion of EMG monitoring of that site can be useful. In patients with low frontal and/or posterior neck muscle activity, professionals might conclude that there is insufficient head and neck muscle activity to justify biofeedback. They also might conclude that there is sufficient relaxation of other cephalic muscles during the recording conditions. Both assumptions are sometimes incorrect. Frontal and/or posterior neck placements inadequately measure occipital tension. When only one EMG placement on the head or neck is used, the FpN is a more comprehensive index of muscle activity than other single placements. EMG recordings should always be used in conjunction with careful clinical interviews and observations during interviews and psychophysiological monitoring. A practitioner should watch a patient's face, ears, temples, neck, and scalp while talking to him or her, while the patient is talking, listening, and being exposed to stressors.

Additional research on the FpN and occipital placements and feedback would be valuable.

SELECTED TREATMENT PROCESS VARIABLES

Baseline Length

Multiple factors affect the decision to obtain a headache baseline and the desired duration. (See Arena & Schwartz, Chapter 7, this volume.) Blanchard, Hillhouse, Appelbaum, and Jaccard (1987) have also offered useful guidelines. They compared correlations between the total of 4 weeks after treatment with varying numbers of weeks selected from the baseline. They proposed that correlations must account for 75% of the variance (correlations of at least $r = .864$) for clinical purposes, and 90% for research purposes. For clinical purposes, they recommended baseline durations of 1 week for tension-type headaches, and 2 weeks for migraine and mixed headaches. For research purposes, the recommended baseline durations were 2 weeks for tension headaches, and 3 weeks for migraine and mixed headaches. Practical considerations suggest that a 1-week baseline would probably be acceptable in at least some clinical situations without doing an injustice to the 75% criterion. For follow-up, they suggested 1 week for migraine and tension-type headaches, and 2 weeks for mixed headaches. Blanchard et al.'s recommendations have practical use for practitioners and researchers. In particular, they support the acceptability of shorter baselines than were often thought needed prior to their study. These recommendations are based on group data; individual factors may dictate the need for baselines of different lengths.

Composition of Sessions and Conditions within Sessions

Many different session protocols are in use in both clinical and research settings. The type of clinical protocol selected for use depends upon available time, presence or absence of the therapist, type of instrumentation, number and type of modalities, patient's motivation, patient's learning ability, therapy stage, and practitioner preferences. No single protocol meets all needs and circumstances. However, the following are examples of basic stages in psychophysiological assessment and therapy protocols. (See Arena & Schwartz, Chapter 7, for more detailed discussion of basic stages.)

1. *Adaptation.*
2. *Baselines.* These periods last a few minutes each, often 3–5 or more minutes. They often include one and usually more conditions, such as eyes open, eyes closed, sitting, and standing.

3. *Self-regulation.* These periods also last a few minutes each, often 3–5 or more minutes. The therapist provides brief instructions to "relax" or "let go of tension" in the head, face, neck, and shoulders. This permits assessment of the patient's ability to relax without biofeedback.

4. *Stimulation.* Such stimulation may include cognitive stress; clenching fists; tensing shoulders, head, or face muscles; or all these. The duration of each stimulation is often 1–3 minutes.

5. *Biofeedback.* These periods last about 3–5 or more minutes in one or more conditions and positions.

6. *Reassessment of self-regulation.* This stage repeats the initial baseline and/or the self-regulation stage. The purpose is to assess recovery rate, degree, and duration of relaxation within the practical time limits of a session. (See Flor, 2001, for further discussion.)

Factors Potentially Affecting/Enhancing Treatment and Outcome

Determining Changes in Skin Temperature

There is no single or generally agreed-upon criterion for determining whether peripheral skin warming has occurred because of a person's own volitional efforts or is sufficient for a therapeutic effect. There are several possible criteria and comparisons (Morrill & Blanchard, 1989; Blanchard et al., 1997). One can compare baseline samples with a self-regulation and/or feedback sample. Therapists often start with a stable temperature near the end of a baseline of several minutes (see Arena & Schwartz, Chapter 7). They compare this with a stable temperature at or near the end of the self-regulation phase or a feedback phase.

One can use the highest skin temperature in the session as a criterion for change, especially if it is maintained for a few minutes. Reaching and maintaining a target temperature constitutes another criterion favored by some practitioners. (See the discussion of the dose–response model, below.) The number of sessions that the patient increased temperatures above a stable baseline is yet another criterion. The absolute temperature may not always be as important as the fact that the patient is making the changes. Smaller reductions in temperature during office stressors, and/or faster recovery to or near baseline temperatures, are other criteria used clinically.

Two problems are adaptation and baseline periods that are too short. In either case, one can mistakenly assume that the relaxation and/or biofeedback procedures are useful in the warming process. Natural warming often takes place with the stopping of activities and especially with rest. Natural warming takes place after longer periods following ingestion of caffeine, nicotine, and other chemicals. Body positions affect reduced SNS arousal and peripheral blood flow. Warming caused by these factors may be desirable to show patients how they affect physiology in a desired direction. Such demonstrations can also increase patient confidence and self-efficacy, especially early in treatment. However, this is not the same as volitional psychophysiological self-regulation. This type of therapy seeks to help people learn to use postures, breathing, images, and various cognitive changes to effect physiological changes. To demonstrate this credibly means adequate adaptation and stable baselines for comparison. It also means stable temperature changes within and across sessions and stress conditions.

A related problem is using integration periods that are too long. There is no generally agreed-upon duration. However, several trials of several seconds (e.g., 10–15) each will show trends and stability better than trials integrated over longer periods, such as a few minutes or longer.

The relationship of these criteria and others to improvement remains unresolved. This relates to the questions of mechanism of treatment and to dose–response relationships. Thus practitioners should consider using multiple criteria and should be cautious when interpreting any single criterion.

Temperature feedback sensitivity is yet another issue. Some practitioners and researchers recommend changes such as 0.01°F and even smaller. An exception is when the temperature lability and variability are large enough to be distracting and confusing for patients. Gradually increasing the sensitivity is an option in such situations. Feedback changes of 0.25°F or more are probably too large for many patients' and therapists' goals.

Possible Effects of EMG Filter Bandpass on Results

The commonly used bandpass of 100–200 hertz is above that for most muscle activity. There is a paucity of research on selecting the ideal bandpass for individual patients and recording conditions. Many practitioners also use a wide bandpass (e.g., 20–1000 hertz) that includes all muscle activity. Advances in instrumentation allow inspection of the *power spectrum* of EMG activity. This can help answer questions about the frequencies where the muscle activity is occurring for individual patients and recording conditions. Eventually, this may improve clinical practice.

Possible Role of Cognitive Factors in Symptom Changes

A "cognitive" model is another explanation for interpreting symptom changes occurring during and after biofeedback therapies (Holroyd et al., 1984b; Blanchard et al., 1997). The essence of this model is that reductions in headache symptoms are mediated by "the experience of success at an ostensibly relevant task of high credibility that leads to [headache] relief" (Blanchard et al., 1997, p. 243).

The study by Holroyd et al. (1984b) gave some subjects false verbal feedback indicating high success after a biofeedback session. These subjects reported significantly more symptom reduction than did subjects who received false postsession feedback suggesting moderate success. However, we should note that the study used undergraduate volunteers aged 18–19 who had recurrent headaches, but who were not seeking treatment. Generalization to more common clinical populations requires more research. Blanchard (1992) has reminded us that the Holroyd et al. study "needs to be replicated with the more prototypical tension headache patient, someone in his or her late 30s who has had headaches for 15–20 years" (p. 539). The Blanchard et al. (1997) study with vascular headaches used adult patients in their 20s to 50s, with an average age close to 40.

One should not take false feedback seriously as a therapeutic approach; it raises serious ethical questions. However, that caution does not detract from the value of the Holroyd et al. (1984b) study. The study supports the idea that cognitive factors may be important in explaining some individual differences in outcomes among patients, as well as differences among studies. Similarly, focusing treatment on cooling or stabilizing temperature (Blanchard et al., 1997) is probably not part of standard clinical practice, nor do they need to be as long as warming goals achieve at least the same results.

Other related theories and research support the importance of patients' perceptions of their own progress and of their self-efficacy (Bandura, 1977, 1982; Bandura, Taylor, Williams, Mefford, & Barchas, 1985). Beliefs cultivated in the cognitive preparation phase and during therapy probably do affect outcome. Gauthier, Côté, and French (1994) cited studies showing that treatment outcome may be mediated by cognitive changes, and that self-efficacy can affect physiology via various mechanisms such as endogenous opioids and nonopioids.

It is not surprising that a patient's belief that he or she is doing well is sometimes more closely related to reduction of headaches than is EMG activity. This should not be disappointing to anyone. The lack of EMG changes during some sessions or across sessions for some patients does not dismiss muscle tension reductions in daily life as important for successful results. However, support for cognitive factors does suggest the limitation of relying solely on EMG data and feedback as the only basis for a therapeutic strategy.

Consider this common clinical scenario. The patient feels helpless, has low self-efficacy about improvement, and has insufficient understanding of the causative role of muscle tension in his or her headaches. Furthermore, there are discrepancies between the patient's excess muscle tension and his or her awareness of the tension. The practitioner presents the patient with the rationale for relaxation, describes the need to relax often, and uses biofeedback to show the patient his or her own capacity to do so. The patient's self-efficacy and confidence change. The patient then changes his or her daily behaviors for reducing excess tonic muscle tension and frequency of phasic excess tension. Symptoms decrease. What was the role of biofeedback? It was not to teach relaxation! The therapist used it to show and convince the patient that he or she could do it. This therapeutic involvement could have been enough to motivate the patient to comply in daily life.

In this model, one may observe symptom changes even if EMG activity in the office remains unchanged. One assumes that the practitioner is persuasive. One further assumes that the patient understands the explanations and accepts them. This changes the patient's self-efficacy beliefs about therapy and reduces his or her sense of helplessness. A single biofeedback session may be sufficient in this model. One also assumes that the patient makes behavioral changes in his or her daily life. Practitioners should have no problems with such a model.

Conditions in which additional biofeedback is probably useful and necessary include (1) when a patient needs more convincing, and (2) when muscle tension levels are high in the office (and, by inference, also in daily life). One can make similar statements about SNS arousal and other feedback modalities.

The Peripheral Warming, Dose–Response, and Generalized ANS Models as Mechanisms for Thermal Biofeedback Treatment of Migraines

It is more than 30 years since the incidental finding of an association between hand warming and reduced migraines. Thermal biofeedback with regular home practice results in a significant reduction of headaches (Blanchard & Andrasik, 1987; Hatch, Fisher, & Rugh, 1987; Gauthier et al., 1994; Blanchard et al., 1997). However, we are still unsure of the mechanism(s) involved.

Is Warming Necessary? Some doubt the specific role or necessity of hand warming. Some researchers and practitioners point to data suggesting that temperature biofeedback warming is sometimes not better than general relaxation. Some also report that cooling or even stabilization is as effective as warming. The studies of the early 1980s had very small samples, did not control for practice, and had other methodological problems (Kewman & Roberts, 1980; Largen, Mathew, Dobbins, & Claghorn, 1981; Gauthier, Bois, Allair, & Drolet, 1981).

Home practice was the focus of a well-conducted study by Gauthier et al. (1994) that did not show a significant relationship between therapy outcome and thermal self-regulation or warming. Significant hand warming occurred in both the practice and no-practice groups, and there was no difference in warming between the two groups, who did differ significantly in improvement of migraines. About 90–95% of the total group of 17 subjects reached at least 94.5°F during the evaluation. Most subjects were able to achieve warming before and after treatment, with no difference between the practice and no-practice groups. The temperatures before and after biofeedback were similar, in the 80s and 90s. The authors speculate about the possible mechanism of practice for helping migraines. Practice may be prophylactic (preventing migraine episodes), abortive, and/or mediated by cognitive factors such as perceived self-efficacy and locus of control beliefs. Nevertheless, there are still pockets of data that support some focus on the temperatures achieved.

The best-controlled, most extensive, and most thoughtful research to date on direction of temperature control in thermal biofeedback for vascular headaches was reported by Blanchard et al. (1997). The original publication must be read to appreciate the study, especially the extensive and useful results and discussion. We present selected quotations here.

> Our results clearly showed no difference in [headache] relief between patients receiving thermal biofeedback for hand warming [the authors call this condition TBF-Warm] and the three control conditions (TBF-Cool, TBF-Stable, and EEG Alpha-Suppress). There was significant overall [headache] relief produced by the treatments. (p. 241)

> The data . . . seem to support that hand warming, hand cooling, or hand temperature stabilization, were, in fact, learned on a group basis. . . . For the three TBF Conditions we examined three different sets of criteria to indicate learning of the response in their respective conditions and found that from 69% to 94% met the least stringent criteria . . . less than half with the most stringent criteria. (p. 242).

> If one accepts . . . no difference among the four conditions . . . would seem to imply that any systematic, credible treatment during which the patient receives feedback . . . that he or she is gaining control of some aspect of the physiology will lead over time to a reduction of [headache] activity. . . . It may be the case that it is the experience of apparent success at an ostensibly relevant task of high credibility that leads to [headache] relief. (p. 243)

However, the authors then remind readers that they still face trying to explain how these cognitive variables work for headaches. The authors also point out the limitations of their study—especially that their "TBF-Warm" group was not very effective and was much less effective than they had shown in prior studies. They focus their explanation on the lack of home practice (a deviation from conventional clinical practice), and note the results of Gauthier et al. (1994). The speculation is that both a credible treatment and regular home practice are needed. This does not detract from the other results, but it leaves unanswered the question of a specific explanation for the direction of temperature control.

We can assume either that the explanation is entirely cognitive-related (i.e., attributable to cognitively focused psychophysiological factors), or that the treatment procedures and cognitive aspects are mediators of physiologically focused psychophysiological changes that have not yet been identified (hence the value of regular practice). If one assumes that warming is still better than other directions, then more questions need to be answered. We address these next.

How Warm Is Enough? Is There an Ideal Temperature Criterion? And Is This a Dose–Response Relationship? The dose–response relationship received no strong or clear support in a study by Blanchard et al. (1983). However, the more often there was hand warming, the more headache relief occurred overall. Some support for an ideal temperature criterion comes from Morrill and Blanchard (1989); this is the temperature threshold theory suggested years earlier by Fahrion (1977) and by Libo and Arnold (1983). Those patients who reached at least 96°F reported clinically significant headache relief more often than those reaching slightly lower temperatures (Blanchard et al., 1983). In their data, 63% (17/30) of subjects reaching temperatures above this level were successful in reducing migraines. However, this is not the same as a dose–response relationship. A dose–response relationship implies the degree of temperature change. This is the specific criterion or the threshold criterion.

Many practitioners were very skeptical about needing such a high temperature before the data of Morrill and Blanchard (1989). These data helped open the door, or kept the door open, to a temperature criterion or threshold model.

Do General ANS Changes Occur with Reduced Migraines? A related model is the generalized ANS conditioning model or conditioned adaptation–relaxation reflex theory developed by Dalessio, Sovak, and their colleagues in the late 1970s. Sovak, Kunzel, Sternbach, and Dalessio (1978) reported that in those patients who clinically improved, thermal biofeedback resulted in decreases of sympathetic tonic outflow. They determined this via multiple cardiovascular measures, including heart rate and vasomotor response of the supraorbital and temporal arteries. Morrill and Blanchard's (1989) data on heart rate are also consistent with this model; these authors noted that only "successful migraineurs had a strong and consistent reduction in heart rate after completing treatment" (p. 174). Unfortunately, there is a paucity of direct research on this model. Support for it would suggest and be consistent with using some types of relaxation and other biofeedback modalities and procedures with migraines.

Relaxation Practice: Is It Necessary? If So, What Amount Is Necessary?

Recommendations to practice daily, and repeated encouragements to do so, are basic parts of relaxation and biofeedback-assisted therapies. A few reports specifically examine this conventional wisdom for headaches (Hillenberg & Collins, 1983; Libo & Arnold, 1983; Solbach, Sargent, & Coyne, 1984b; Lake & Pingel, 1988; Blanchard, Nicholson, Radnitz, Steffek, Applebaum, & Dentiger, 1991; Blanchard et al., 1991a, 1991b; Allen & McKeen, 1991; Gauthier et al., 1994). Most reports support the value of practice. Practitioners continue to encourage applying relaxation in daily life, which is logical and prudent.

Definitions or criteria for practice differ and are sometimes unclear. Some reports describe practice as "regular" or "frequent," and define this as six or more times per week or one or more times per week. Others refer to patients' using relaxation "as needed," "when stressed," or "occasionally." Some report "practice" versus "no practice" (Hillenberg & Collins, 1983), and others report "more" versus "less" practice (Lake & Pingel, 1988). "Confirmation of practice" varies from self-report to more objective measurement (Hoelscher, Lichstein, & Rosenthal, 1984, 1986). Reports usually do not specify the "quality of practice," although some do (Solbach, Sargent, & Coyne, 1989). Research usually does not use rating scales for assessing "relaxation proficiency."

For patients with tension-type headaches, Blanchard et al. (1991b) supported the advantage of home practice. They relied on progressive muscle relaxation without biofeedback as the primary treatment. There were 10 sessions over 8 weeks, and they used audiotapes to help with home practice. Instructions for the no-practice group gently discouraged home practice. The practice group showed greater improvement in their headaches than those without practice. Their proficiency at relaxing in the office sessions was also better than that of the no-practice group. There was no symptom improvement among those monitoring their symptoms. The data indicated that expectation of improvement probably did not account for the effects, and medications did not change for any of the groups.

For vascular headaches, Blanchard et al. (1991a) found that home practice combined with thermal biofeedback and a brief introduction to autogenic phrases did not clearly result in more symptom improvement than no practice. However, the authors admit to limitations in the study. A crucial limitation was that 30% of the subjects in the no-practice group did practice, despite instructions to avoid practice. Inspection of their data suggests that home practice had some advantage for some subjects. Gauthier et al. (1994) extended and improved upon the Blanchard et al. (1991a) study. Contrary to the results of Blanchard and colleagues, they found that for females with migraines, regular home practice enhanced the efficacy of the biofeedback therapy. The group with no home practice instructions did not report any practice.

Lake and Pingel (1988) relied on a retrospective questionnaire from a large sample of patients diagnosed as having mixed headaches. The frequency of daily brief relaxations (as short as a few seconds) and extended relaxations was correlated with improvement of headaches, defined in several ways. The 102 fee-paying and mostly female (82%) patients reported brief relaxation as more useful than extended relaxation. Improvements included decreased headache intensity and duration, aborting of headaches, and lower medication usage. The authors concluded that "the analyses show a consistent and strong relationship between . . . frequency of brief relaxation and headache control" in these patients, "most of whom [had] chronic daily pain" (p. 126). The wide range of ages (13–73, with a mean and median of 33), was not related to outcome in the Lake and Pingel (1988) study. The number of biofeedback sessions, ranging from less than 5 to more than 16, also did not correlate significantly with the results.

Patients under age 36 were more compliant than older patients in the study of Solbach et al. (1989). For children aged 7–12 being treated for migraines, frequency of home practice was one significant factor related to treatment results (Allen & McKeen, 1991). The correlation between headache frequency and the average number of practices per day was significant ($r = .61$, $p < .01$). More frequent practice more often resulted in better patient ability to warm hands without biofeedback ($r = .50$, $p < .01$).

Toward Understanding Mechanisms of Practice. Reducing high levels of tension, rather than the practice of relaxation per se, could affect the relationship of practice to headache changes. Periods of high-intensity tension—such as that resulting from clenched teeth, raised shoulders, or a tilted head, as well as occipital tension—probably contribute significantly to onset and maintenance of symptoms. Consider the logic and potential for reducing such high-intensity tension, especially when it is also frequent and/or long-lasting.

One would not expect deep relaxation once or twice a day, or several brief relaxations each day, to be effective for counteracting such tension. For many patients, reducing high-intensity tension could be as important as (or more important than) increasing the frequency, duration, depth, and quality of their deeper relaxation. This could help explain why relaxation practice sometimes does not show a relationship to decreased headaches.

Many practitioners often seek to increase patients' awareness of excess tension. Some specifically instruct patients to attend to these episodes of high tension and stop or reduce them. However, research studies do not mention this latter type of instruction. We do not know whether research studies include this instruction. Studies of practice (and most other studies) also do not report changes in other behaviors that can affect headaches. These include sleep efficiency, sleep and daytime postures, type of pillow used, and dietary changes. Were they mentioned in any sessions? Did patients become aware of them from other sources and make these changes? In addition to including or controlling for these factors, using ambulatory multichannel EMG recordings might help clarify some factors involved in moderating the role of practice. These other factors may be about equal in groups who practice more and those who practice less or do not practice; however, in small samples, this might not be true even with random assignment.

For tension-type headaches, a measure of the "quality of relaxation" was more important than the quantity of relaxation in Solbach et al. (1989). Quality included awareness of muscle relaxation in the head and neck during practice, experiencing warmth sensations, and throbbing or fullness sensations in the hands. Thus, aside from quantity of practice, assessing quality may be useful.

Gauthier et al.'s (1994) discussion of mechanisms of practice for migraines includes useful speculation about possible prophylactic effects, abortive effects at the time procedures are applied, and/or cognitive factors such as self-efficacy. They remind readers of the speculation that treatment outcome may be mediated by cognitive changes; they also note that a physiological effect from self-efficacy increases may affect endogenous opioids and nonopioids.

Conclusions about Relaxation Practice.
- Research supports relaxation practice for tension-type and migraine headaches.
- There are logic and support for using many brief and extended relaxations daily.
- Practitioners and researchers need to continue evaluating and measuring quality and quantity of relaxation.
- Some patients may achieve good results with less practice.
- Mechanisms may include cognitive effects on physiology, prophylactic effects, and/or abortive effects.
- Practitioners should focus on reduction of frequency, intensity, and durations of excess tension and arousal.

SUMMARY

A major application of relaxation, biofeedback, and other applied psychophysiological therapies is in the treatment of tension-type and migraine headaches. An extensive research and clinical literature exists with good support for these treatments. There are still many unanswered questions about causes and their mechanisms, about evaluation and assessment, and about the treatment of special populations.

GLOSSARY

AMITRIPTYLINE. (Trade names Elavil and Endep.) A tricyclic antidepressant drug used in smaller doses for chronic daily headache, episodic tension-type headache, atypical face pain, neck pain, and pain syndromes with sleep disturbance or anxiety. Also used for intermittent migraines and related headaches. Proposed mechanisms include increased synaptic norepinephrine or serotonin (5-HT), inhibition of 5-HT and norepinephrine reuptake, effects on 5-HT_2 receptors, and decreased beta-receptor density.

ANALGESIC REBOUND HEADACHE. Almost continuous headache associated with regular daily use of high levels of analgesic medications (see text).

ANOXIA. Literally, total lack of oxygen. Often used interchangeably with "hypoxia" to mean a reduced supply of oxygen to the tissues.

ASTHENIA. Loss or lack of strength, especially weakness from cerebellar or muscular disease.

ATENOLOL. (Trade name Tenormin.) An antiadrenergic beta-selective adrenoreceptor-blocking agent. Used as an antihypertensive and heart drug.

BIFURCATION OF THE TEMPORAL ARTERY. Site where the temporal artery divides into two branches, one to the frontal region and the other to the parietal region.

BLOOD VOLUME PULSE AMPLITUDE (BVPA). Amount of blood in a pulse beat. Compare "finger pulse amplitude" (FPA), "finger pulse volume" (FPV), and "cephalic pulse amplitude" (CPA).

CALCIUM CHANNEL BLOCKERS. Drugs that decrease vascular resistance. Also called "calcium ion influx inhibitors" or "slow channel blockers." Verapamil (trade names Calan, Isoptin, Verelan, Verapamil HCl) is more commonly used for migraines than nifedipine (trade name Procardia), which may worsen headache in up to 30% of patients.

CATECHOLAMINES. Body compounds having a *sympathomimetic* (see below) action; they include epinephrine, norepinephrine, and dopamine. Epinephrine (also called adrenaline) is a hormone and neurotransmitter secreted by the adrenal medulla. Norepinephrine (also called noradrenaline) is a neurohormone and neurotransmitter released at sympathetic nerve endings.

CEILING EFFECT. The highest value a parameter (such as a physiological activity) can reach, thereby limiting changes depending on the starting point of the measurement.

CENTRAL ORIGIN. Starting in the central nervous system (CNS).

CEPHALIC. Referring to the head. Another term for headache is "cephalalgia."

CEPHALIC BLOOD FLOW (CBF). In the present chapter, extracranial cephalic blood flow. Also, cerebral blood flow.

CHRONIC PAROXYSMAL HEMICRANIA (CPH). A type of headache classified with cluster headaches. May be a variant form of cluster headache, and is often confused with it. Mostly in women and young girls. May be provoked by flexion and sometimes neck rotation; this latter finding distinguishes it from cluster headaches. Features include unilateral pain in the temple, forehead, ear, eye, or occipital areas. Attacks average 10–15 minutes and may last 5–30 minutes, in contrast to cluster headaches, which last longer (an average of 45 minutes). Sufferers average from 10 to 15 attacks per day, but may have up to 30. Attacks may awaken some from sleep. Autonomic symptoms are similar to cluster headaches. One must rule out intracranial diseases that can mimic CPH; these include ophthalmic artery aneurysm and pituitary tumor. Treatment includes indomethacin and sometimes corticosteroids.

CIMETIDINE. (Trade narne Tagamet.) A histamine H_2-receptor antagonist (blocker). Used in the treatment of duodenal and gastric ulcers and other gastrointestinal disorders.

COGNITIVE DISSONANCE. An unpleasant feeling arising when there is a lack of agreement (dissonance, discord, or disagreement) among one's ideas, beliefs, and/or behaviors.

COMPLETE BLOOD COUNT. Most common and basic blood test. "Involves counting the number of each type of blood cell in a given volume of . . . blood and examining the cells . . . under a microscope to check for any abnormalities in their size or shape" (Larson, 1990, p. 476).

CRANIAL NEURALGIA. Neuralgia (paroxysmal pain) along the course of a cranial nerve.

DISCONNECTION BETWEEN THE MMPI AND HEADACHES. Some patients with chronic headaches do not endorse obvious headache items on the MMPI.

ELECTROLYTES. Substances that dissociate into ions when fused or in solution, and thus become capable of conducting electricity. Examples are potassium, sodium, chloride, and phosphate. Blood chemistry group laboratory tests include electrolytes as a screen for possible systemic diseases.

ERGOTAMINE. Ergot alkaloid used in treating moderate to severe migraines and related headaches, such as cluster headaches, *status migraine* (see below), chronic daily headache, and menstrual migraine. Ergot is derived from a rye plant fungus. Available as ergotamine tartrate (Cafergot, Wigraine, Ergomar, Ergostat, Bellergal-S, Migrogot) and dihydroergotamine (DHE-45) injections (intravenous, intramuscular, or subcutaneous). DHE differs from ergotamine tartrate; it is a weaker arterial vasoconstrictor, has selective venoconstricting properties, substantially less emetic (nauseating) features, and fewer uterine effects. Both have agonist action on serotonin (5-HT_{1a} and 5-HT_{1d}) and alpha-adrenergic receptors. Both create vasoconstriction by stimulating arterial smooth muscle through 5-HT receptors. Both constrict venous capacitance. Both inhibit reuptake of norepinephrine at sympathetic nerve endings. Both reduce vasogenic/neurogenic inflammation (Saper et al., 1993). (See *sympathetic* in Chapter 17's glossary.)

FRONTAL–POSTERIOR NECK (FpN) PLACEMENT. One EMG electrode on one frontalis muscle, and another electrode on the *ipsilateral* side of cervical neck near the hairline. Proposed as a broader and better measure of cephalic muscle tension. Also provides an indirect indication of occipitalis tension when frontalis, posterior neck, and sternomastoid tension are ruled out as contributing to the EMG signal. Usually used with bilateral frontal and bilateral neck electrodes. Ideally, also used with matched set of FpN electrodes on the contralateral side; thus an ideal EMG montage is four channels.

GLYCERYL TRINITRATE (nitroglycerine). Dilates blood vessels. Used in treatment of angina.

INDOMETHACIN. An analgesic; a nonsteroidal anti-inflammatory drug.

IPSATIVE. Criterion-referenced as opposed to norm-referenced. Thus comparison is with a criterion rather than a normative group.

IPSILATERAL. Situated on, pertaining to, or affecting the same side, as opposed to contralateral (*Dorland's Illustrated Medical Dictionary*, 1988).

ISCHEMIA. Deficiency of blood flow in a body part from functional constriction or actual obstruction of a blood vessel.

ISOSORBIDE DINITRATE. (Trade names Isordil and Sorbitrate.) A vasodilator.

LACTIC ACID. Formed in muscle cells during intense muscular tension (as in heavy exercise or tense muscles) by the breakdown of glucose (glycolysis), the hydrolysis of sugar by enzymes in the body. This provides energy anaerobically, without inspired oxygen.

NEUROKININS, CIRCULATORY. A "kinin" is one of a group of peptides that cause contraction of smooth muscle and have other physiological effects. A "peptide" is one of many compounds that yield two or more amino acids on hydrolysis.

NIFEDIPINE. (Trade name Procardia, Adalat.) A calcium channel blocker that reduces and prevents coronary artery spasm and dilates peripheral arterioles.

OCCIPITAL. Pertaining to or situated near the occiput or occipital bone (back part of the head or skull). Occipitalis muscles are above the posterior neck hairline, and are connected to the frontalis muscles by tendonous tissue. Their function is to pull the scalp back. They are under voluntary control, but very difficult for nearly all people to control.

OPERATIONALLY DEFINED. Situation in which the meaning of a term or concept consists of the operations (method) performed to demonstrate it. For example, anxiety or any emotion may be operationally defined as the score on specific self-report questionnaires. Pain intensity, such as headache intensity, may be operationally defined by specified ratings.

PAIN DENSITY. Concept of Sternbach et al. (1980). Refers to the overall time with pain. For example, people with tension-type headaches usually have a greater pain density than those with migraines—that is, more time with pain.

PAROXYSMAL NOCTURNAL DYSPNEA. Respiratory distress usually thought to result from congestive heart failure with pulmonary edema. Sudden attacks of air hunger and difficult breathing during sleep or reclining. Patients awaken gasping and must sit or stand to catch their breath.

POWER SPECTRUM. Advanced method of analyzing electrical signals. Provides all frequency and amplitude components, including dominant and subdominant, of a waveform.

PRODROMAL SYMPTOMS. Visual (most common), motor, sensory, brainstem, or psychological signs indicating the onset of a *migraine with* aura. Less often, it occurs with or after onset of headache phase. Common visual auras are fortification "spectra" or "scotomata"—that is, zig-zag or scintillating (sparkling) images. Motor aura (much less common) includes hemiparesis or aphasia. Sensory aura includes hypersensitivity to feel and touch or reduced sensation. Other disturbances include ataxia (irregular muscle control/unsteadiness); vertigo (sensation of the external world revolving around patient or patient revolving in space—not the same as dizziness); tinnitus (ear ringing); hearing loss; diplopia (double vision); loss or change in level of consciousness; paresthesia (e.g., prickling sensation); and dysarthria (imperfect speech articulation from disturbed muscular control). Psychological prodromal symptoms can include depression, anger, euphoria, or hypomania. Other prodromal features associated with migraines include stiff neck (this must be distinguished from that in tension-type headaches), chilled feeling and peripheral vasoconstriction, fatigue, increased urination frequency, anorexia, fluid retention, and food cravings.

PROPRANOLOL. (Trade name Inderal.) A heart drug also used for migraines. It is a nonselective beta-adrenergic blocking agent that competes with beta-adrenergic receptor stimulant agents for available receptor sites.

PRUDENT LIMITED OFFICE TREATMENT (PLOT). Term proposed to replace "home-based treatment," "minimal-therapist treatment," and "limited-contact treatment."

RANITIDINE. A histamine-blocking ulcer drug.

SEDIMENTATION RATE. "Blood test [that] determines the rate at which red blood cells settle. . . . If the cells settle faster than normal, this can suggest an infection, anemia, inflammation, rheumatoid arthritis, rheumatic fever, or one of several types of cancer" (Larson, 1990, p. 1283). Also called "erythrocyte sedimentation rate."

SEMISPINALIS CERVICUS. Muscle that rotates vertebral column.

SEROTONIN. (Also called "5-hydroxytryptamine" or "5-HT.") Vasoconstrictor. Synthesized in humans in certain intestinal cells or in central or peripheral neurons. Found in high concentrations in many tissues, including the intestinal mucosa, pineal body, and CNS. Synthesis starts with uptake of tryptophan into serotonergic neurons. Tryptophan is hydroxylated by an enzyme to become 5-hydroxytryptophan, then decarboxylated by another enzyme to serotonin or 5-HT. There are three types of receptors (5-HT_1, 5-HT_2, 5-HT_3), and four subtypes of 5-HT_1 receptors. Serotonin has many physiological properties, including inhibiting gastric secretions, stimulating smooth muscle, and serving as a central neurotransmitter. It is a major factor in several medical/neurological and psychiatric conditions, such as migraines and depression. About 90% occurs in the gastrointestinal tract, about 8% in blood platelets, and the rest in the brain. The 8% found in blood platelets, known as platelet serotonin, falls at the onset of a migraine attack and is normal between attacks (Saper et al., 1993).

SLEEP APNEA. An obstructive sleep disorder. Recurrent episodes of stopping breathing during sleep, caused by obstruction of air in the upper respiratory passages. The person moves rapidly to a lighter level of sleep after several seconds (up to 20–30 seconds). The condition prevents reaching restorative sleep. Signs and symptoms include excessive daytime sleepiness despite suitable sleeping time, loud snoring, and episodes of breath stopping during sleep observed by another person. Morning headaches can occur. Many people successfully use a continuous positive air pressure device, a special machine that delivers air through a mask at a pressure above ambient air.

SPINALIS. Muscle that extends vertebral column.

STATUS MIGRAINE. Severe, debilitating migraine attacks that last for weeks. Also known as "status migrainosus" or "intractable migraine."

SUPRATROCHLEAR. In this context, above the trochlear nerve (fourth cranial nerve)—the motor nerve for the superior oblique muscles of the eyeball, which rotate the eyeball downward and outward.

SYMPATHOMIMETIC. "Mimicking the effects of impulses conveyed by adrenergic postganglionic fibers of the sympathetic nervous system" *(Dorland's Illustrated Medical Dictionary,* 1988). Also called "adrenergic."

T SCORE. Common statistical transformation of raw scores to allow comparison among different scales and psychological tests. *T* scores have a mean of 50 and a standard deviation of 10. Thus about 68% of a population have *T* scores between 40 and 59, and about 95.4% between 30 and 69.

TEMPORAL ARTERITIS. Also known as "cranial arteritis" and "giant-cell arteritis." Inflammation of an artery in the head, often near the temple. Probably a form of disordered immune reaction. Can thicken the lining of the affected artery, blocking blood flow, most commonly to the eyes. Can cause partial or total blindness if untreated. Condition of older people, usually between ages 60 and 75 and almost exclusively over age 50. Symptoms may be vague (e.g., feeling "run down"). Usual symptoms include throbbing headaches, loss of vision, temple area pain, jaw pain when chewing, and sore scalp. Only sure diagnostic test is biopsy of a piece of the artery, an outpatient procedure done with a local anesthetic. Treatment is usually with oral corticosteroid drugs, usually daily, often for 1 year or more (Larson, 1990).

TERTIARY. Third in order. Often used to refer to very large medical centers that provide a variety of health care services, including resolution of medical and/or psychological diagnoses and treatment questions unresolved by first and second opinions.

TOTAL THYROXINE (TOTAL SERUM THYROXINE or T4). A rapid, simple, direct, and inexpensive blood test of the thyroid hormone thyroxine.

TRANSIENT ISCHEMIC ATTACK. Temporary deficiency in blood supply to part(s) of the brain, usually lasting a few minutes. Signs and symptoms include sudden weakness, tingling, or numbness, typically on one side. Vision and speech difficulty, vertigo, double vision, imbalance, or incoordination of limbs are other signs and symptoms. These are similar to an ischemic stroke but disappear within 24 hours. May occur repeatedly in the same day or later. Should be regarded as a warning of possible stroke later (Larson, 1990).

TRIMETHOPRIM-SULFAMETHOXAZOLE. (Trades names include Bactrim and Septra.) An antibacterial used in the treatment of PCP pneumonia, urinary tract infections, and other bacterial infections.

VASOPRESSIN. One of two hormones formed by neuronal cells of the hypothalamic nuclei. Stored in the posterior lobe of the pituitary gland. Stimulates contraction of muscular tissue of capillaries and arterioles. Raises blood pressure. Also promotes contraction of intestinal muscles, increases peristalsis, and has some contractile effect on uterus. Used mainly as an antidiuretic, especially for treating diabetes insipidus. Also called "antidiuretic hormone."

VISUAL ANALOGUE SCALE (VAS). A straight line, usually 10 centimeters long, with ends labeled as the extremes of pain intensity (e.g, "no pain" to "pain as bad as it could be") or pain affect (e.g., "not bad at all" to "the most unpleasant feeling possible for me"). When scales have specific points along the line labeled with intensity-denoting adjectives or numbers, they are callcd "graphic rating scales." Patients indicate which point along the line best represents their pain intensity (and/or pain affect). The distance from the "no pain" (or "not bad at all") end to the mark made by the patient is the pain intensity (or pain affect) score (Jensen & Karoly, 1992).

ZIMELDINE. An antidepressant withdrawn from the market by the U.S. Food and Drug Administration (FDA).

ZOMEPIREC. An analgesic and anti-inflammatory withdrawn from the market by the FDA.

NOTES

1. For convenience, this chapter generally uses the term "biofeedback" instead of specifying "surface electromyographic (EMG) biofeedback" or "temperature biofeedback," and instead of such terms as "biofeedback-assisted physiological self-regulatory therapies," "augmented proprioception," or "applied clinical biofeedback." (The modality of biofeedback—EMG, temperature, etc.—is noted only when necessary.)

2. This system is once again undergoing revision, with the date of publication expected to be 2003.

3. Many practitioners and some researchers customarily record EMG activity within a 100- to 200-hertz bandpass. However, much muscle activity occurs below and some above this range. Power spectrum displays of muscle activity will allow research to answer this question and permit practitioners to tailor bandpass filters to each patient.

4. Based on a similar list in Blau and Thavapalan (1988).

5. We encourage the shift from using MMPI scale letters and names to using only the MMPI scale numbers. This practice has been common for many years among many professionals. The rationale is to stop using outmoded and ill-advised concepts and names for these scales. Also, each scale measures multiple concepts, and elevations often do not imply the designated entity embodied in the name. The use of the old names is confusing and misleading, and can be very troublesome, especially with patients. One exception is scale 2 for depression.

6. Note that these authors referred to "occipital EMG" recorded from "just below the hairline of the neck adjacent to the spinal column" (p. 150). We assume that they meant "neck EMG." This is not important for the MMPI results; we mention it here only to help readers avoid using this placement to assess occipital activity. See the "Placement of Electrodes" section, later in this chapter.

7. Fibromyalgia is associated with and perhaps partly due to nonrestorative sleep. (For more details, see M. S. Schwartz & Thompson, Chapter 34, this volume.)

8. Some of these treatments vary in clinical practice and have changed.

REFERENCES

Adler, C. S., & Adler, S. M. (1987). Evaluating the psychological factors in headache. In C. S. Adler, S. M. Adler, & R. C. Packard (Eds.), *Psychiatric aspects of headache.* Baltimore: Williams & Wilkins.

Adler, C. S., Adler, S. M., & Packard, R. C. (Eds.) (1987). *Psychiatric aspects of headache.* Baltimore: Williams & Wilkins.

Ahles, T. A., Martin, J. B., Gaulier, B., Cassens, H. L., Andres, M. L., & Shariff, M. (1988). Electromyographic and vasomotor activity in tension, migraine, and combined headache patients: The influence of postural variation. *Behaviour Research and Therapy, 26*(6), 519–525.

Allen, K. D., & McKeen, L. R. (1991). Home-based multicomponent treatment of pediatric migraine. *Headache, 31,* 467–472.

Andrasik, F. (1992). Assessment of patients with headache. In D. C. Turk & R. Melzack (Eds.), *Handbook of pain assessment.* New York: Guilford Press.

Andrasik, F. (1996). Behavioral management of migraine. *Biomedicine and Pharmacotherapy, 50,* 52–57.

Andrasik, F. (2001a). Assessment of patients with headaches. In D. C. Turk & R. Melzack (Eds.), *Handbook of pain assessment* (2nd ed.). New York: Guilford Press.

Andrasik, F. (2001b). Migraine and quality of life: Psychological considerations. *Journal of Headache and Pain*, 2, S1–S9.

Andrasik, F., & Baskin, S. (1987). Headache. In R. L. Morrison & A. A. Bellack (Eds.), *Medical factors and psychological disorders: A handbook for psychologists*. New York: Plenum Press.

Andrasik, F., Blanchard, E. B., Arena, J. G., Saunders, N. L., & Barron, K. D. (1982a). Psychophysiology of recurrent headache: Methodological issues and new empirical findings. *Behavior Therapy, 13*(4), 407–429.

Andrasik, F. A., Blanchard, E. B., Arena, J. G., Teders, S. J., & Rodichok, L. D. (1982b). Cross-validation of the Kudrow–Sutkus MMPI classification system for diagnosing headache type. *Headache, 22,* 2–5.

Andrasik, F., & Holroyd, K. A. (1980). Reliability and concurrent validity of headache questionnaire data. *Headache, 20,* 44–46.

Andrasik, F., & Walch, S. E. (2002). Biobehavioral assessment and treatment of recurrent headaches. In A. M. Nezu, C. M. Nezu, & P. A. Geller (Eds.), *Comprehensive handbook of psychology: Vol. 9. Health psychology*. New York: Wiley.

Appelbaum, K. A., Blanchard, E. B., Nicholson, N. L., Radnitz, C., Michultka, D., Attanasio, V., Andrasik, F., & Dentinger, M. P. (1990). Controlled evaluation of the addition of cognitive strategies to a home-based relaxation protocol for tension headache. *Behavior Therapy, 21,* 293–303.

Arena, J. G., Bruno, G. M., & Brucks, A. (1993a). *Biofeedback treatment of the chronic headache sufferer*. Toronto: Thought Technologies Press.

Arena, J. G., Bruno, G. M., Brucks, A. G., Meador, K., & Sherman, R. A. (1993b). Ambulatory monitoring of bilaterial upper trapezius surface EMG in tension and vascular headache sufferers. In *Proceedings of the 24th Annual Meeting of the Association for Applied Psychophysiology and Biofeedback, Los Angeles*. Wheat Ridge, CO: Association for Applied Psychophysiology and Biofeedback.

Arena, J. G., Bruno, G. M., Brucks, A. G., Searle, J. R., Meador, K., & Sherman, R. A. (1994a). Preliminary results in tension headache sufferers of pre- to post-treatment ambulatory neck EMG monitoring: Generalization of EMG biofeedback training and EMG changes as a function of treatment outcome. In *Proceedings of the 25th Annual Meeting of the Association for Applied Psychophysiology and Biofeedback, Atlanta*. Wheat Ridge, CO: Association for Applied Psychophysiology and Biofeedback.

Arena, J. G., Bruno, G. M., Brucks, A. G., Searle, J. R., Sherman, R. A., & Meador, K. J. (1994b). Reliability of an ambulatory electromyographic activity device for musculoskeletal pain disorders. *International Journal of Psychophysiology, 17,* 153–157.

Arena, J. G., Hannah, S. L., Bruno, G. M., & Meador, K. J. (1991a). Electromyographic biofeedback training for tension headache in the elderly: A prospective study. *Biofeedback and Self-Regulation, 16*(4), 379–390.

Arena, J. G., Hannah, S. L., Bruno, G. M., Smith, J. D., & Meador, K. J. (1991b). Effect of movement and position on muscle activity in tension headache sufferers during and between headaches. *Journal of Psychosomatic Research, 35,* 187–195.

Arena, J. G., Hightower, N. E., & Chang, G. C. (1988). Relaxation therapy for tension headache in the elderly: A prospective study. *Psychology and Aging, 3*(1), 96–98.

Arena, J. G., Sherman, R. A., Bruno, G. M., & Young, T. R. (1989). Electromyographic recordings of five types of low back pain subjects and non-pain controls in different positions. *Pain, 37,* 57–65.

Arena, J. G., Sherman, R. A., Bruno, G. M., & Young, T. R. (1991c). Electromyographic recordings of five types of low back pain subjects and non-pain controls in different positions: Effect of pain state. *Pain, 45,* 23–28.

Askmark, H., Lundberg, P. O., & Olsson, S. (1989). Drug-related headache. *Headache, 29,* 441–444.

Bandura, A. (1977). Self-efficacy: Toward a unifying theory of behavioral change. *Psychological Review, 84,* 191–215.

Bandura, A. (1982). Self-efficacy mechanism in human agency. *American Psychologist, 37,* 122–147.

Bandura, A., Taylor, C. B., Williams, S. L., Mefford, I. N., & Barchas, J. D. (1985). Catecholamine secretion as a function of perceived coping self-efficacy. *Journal of Consulting and Clinical Psychology, 53*(3), 406–414.

Baumgartner, C., Wessely, P., Bingol, C., Maly, J., & Holzner, F. (1989). Long term prognosis of analgesic withdrawal in patients with drug-induced headaches. *Headache, 29,* 510–514.

Blanchard, E. B. (1992). Psychological treatment of benign headache disorders. *Journal of Consulting and Clinical Psychology, 60*(4), 537–551.

Blanchard, E. B., & Andrasik, F. (1985). *Management of chronic headaches: A psychological approach*. New York: Pergamon Press.

Blanchard, E. B., & Andrasik, F. (1987). Biofeedback treatment of vascular headache. In J. P. Hatch, J. G. Fisher, & J. D. Rugh (Eds.), *Biofeedback: Studies in clinical efficacy*. New York: Plenum Press.

Blanchard, E. B., Andrasik, F. A., Ahles, T. A., Teders, S. J., & O'Keefe, D. M. (1980). Migraine and tension headache: A meta-analytic review. *Behavior Therapy, 11,* 613–631.

Blanchard, E. B., Andrasik, F., Appelbaum, K. A., Evans, D. D., Jurish, S. E., Teders, S. J., Rodichok, L. D., & Barron, K. D. (1985a). The efficacy and cost-effectiveness of minimal-therapist-contact, nondrug treatment of chronic migraine and tension headache. *Headache, 25,* 214–220.

Blanchard, E. B., Andrasik, F., Jurish, S. E., & Teders, S. J. (1982a). The treatment of cluster headache with relaxation and thermal biofeedback. *Biofeedback and Self-Regulation, 7*, 185–191.

Blanchard, E. B., Andrasik, F., Neff, D. F., Arena, J. G., Ahles, T. A., Jurish, S. E., Pallmeyer, T. P., Saunders, N. L., Teders, S. J., Barron, K. D., & Rodichok, L. D. (1982b). Biofeedback and relaxation training with three kinds of headache: Treatment effects and their prediction. *Journal of Consulting and Clinical Psychology, 50*, 562–575.

Blanchard, E. B., Andrasik, F., Neff, D. F., Jurish, S. E., & O'Keefe, D. M. (1981). Social validation of the headache diary. *Behavior Therapy, 12*, 711–715.

Blanchard, E. B., Andrasik, F., Neff, D. R., Saunders, N. L., Arena, J. G., Pallmeyer, T. P., Teders, S. J., Jerish, S. E., & Rodichok, L. D. (1983). Four process studies in the behavioral treatment of chronic headache. *Behaviour Research and Therapy, 21*(3), 209–220.

Blanchard, E. B., Appelbaum, K. A., Nicholson, N. L., Radnitz, C. L., Morrill, B., Michultka, D., Kirsch, C., Hillhouse, J., & Dentinger, M. P. (1990a). A controlled evaluation of the addition of cognitive therapy to a home-based biofeedback and relaxation treatment of vascular headache. *Headache, 30*, 371–376.

Blanchard, E. B., Appelbaum, K. A., Radnitz, C. L., Michultka, D., Morrill, B., Kirsch, C. L., Hillhouse, J., Evans, D. D., Guarnieri, P., Attanasio, V., Andrasik, F., Jaccard, J., & Dentinger, M. P. (1990b). Placebo-controlled evaluation of abbreviated progressive muscle relaxation and of relaxation combined with cognitive therapy in the treatment of tension headache. *Journal of Consulting and Clinical Psychology, 58*(2), 210–215.

Blanchard, E. B., Appelbaum, K. A., Radnitz, C. L., Morrill, B., Michultka, D., Kirsch, C. L., Guarnieri, P., Hillhouse, J., Evans, D. D., Jaccard, J., & Barron, K. D. (1990c). A controlled evaluation of thermal biofeedback and thermal biofeedback with cognitive therapy in the treatment of vascular headache. *Journal of Consulting and Clinical Psychology, 58*(2), 216–224.

Blanchard, E. B., Hillhouse, J., Appelbaum, K. A., & Jaccard, J. (1987). What is an adequate length of baseline in research and clinical practice with chronic headache? *Biofeedback and Self-Regulation, 12*(4), 323–329.

Blanchard, E. B., Jaccard, J., Andrasik, F., Guarnieri, P., & Jurish, S. E. (1985b). Reduction in headache patients' medical expenses associated with biofeedback and relaxation treatments. *Biofeedback and Self-Regulation, 10*(1), 63–68.

Blanchard, E. B., Kirsch, C. A., Appelbaum, K. A., & Jaccard, J. (1989). The role of psychopathology in chronic headache: Cause or effect? *Headache, 29*(5), 295–301.

Blanchard, E. B., Nicholson, N. L., Radnitz, C. L., Steffek, B. D., Appelbaum, K. A., & Dentinger, M. P. (1991a). The role of home practice in thermal biofeedback. *Journal of Consulting and Clinical Psychology, 59*(4), 507–512.

Blanchard, E. B., Nicholson, N. L., Taylor, A. E., Steffek, B. D., Radnitz, C. L., & Appelbaum, K. A. (1991b). The role of regular home practice in the relaxation treatment of tension headache. *Journal of Consulting and Clinical Psychology, 59*(3), 467–470.

Blanchard, E. B., Peters, M. L., Hermann, C., Turner, S. M., Buckley, T. C., Barton, K., & Dentinger, M. P. (1997). Direction of temperature control in the thermal biofeedback treatment of vascular headache. *Applied Psychophysiology and Biofeedback, 22*(4), 227–245.

Blanchard, E. B., Steffek, B. D., Jaccard, J., & Nicholson, N. L. (1991c). Psychological changes accompanying non-pharmacological treatment of chronic headache: The effects of outcome. *Headache, 31*, 249–253.

Blanchard, E. B., Taylor, A. E., & Dentinger, M. P. (1992). Preliminary results from the self-regulatory treatment of high-medication-consumption headache. *Biofeedback and Self-Regulation, 17*(3), 179–202.

Blau, J. N. (1990). Headache history: Its importance and idiosyncrasies. *Headache Quarterly: Current Treatment and Research, 1*(2), 129–135.

Blau, J. N., & Thavapalan, M. (1988). Preventing migraine: A study of precipitating factors. *Headache, 28*, 481–483.

Bogaards, M. C., & ter Kuile, M. M. (1994). Treatment of recurrent tension headache: A meta-analytic review. *Clinical Journal of Pain, 10*, 174–190.

Campbell, J. K. (1993). CT or not CT—that is the question [Editorial]. *Headache, 33*, 52.

Campbell, J. K., Penzien, D. B., & Wall, E. M. (2000). *Evidence-based guidelines for migraine headaches: Behavioral and physical treatments* [Online]. Available: http://www.aan.com/public/practiceguidelines/headache_g1.htm.

Dalessio, D. J. (1986). Headache, history, physical examination and laboratory tests. In *Headache: Theory, diagnosis, psychological aspects and therapy. Proceedings of the Annual Meeting of the American Association for the Study of Headache, Scottsdale, AZ*. Scottsdale: American Association for the Study of Headache.

Darling, M. (1991). The use of exercise as a method of aborting migraine. *Headache, 31*, 616–618.

deBenedittis, G., & Lorenzetti, A. (1992). Minor stressful life events (daily hassles) in chronic primary headache: Relationship with MMPI personality patterns. *Headache, 32*, 330–332.

deBenedittis, G., Lorenzetti, A., & Pieri, A. (1990). The role of stressful life events in the onset of chronic primary headache. *Pain, 40*, 65–75.

de Bruijn-Kofman, A. T., van de Wiel, H., Groenman, N. H., Sorbi, M. J., & Klip, E. (1997). Effects of a mass media behavioral treatment for chronic headache: A pilot study. *Headache, 37,* 415–420.

Diener, H. C. (1988). Clinical features of analgesic-induced chronic headache [German]. *Deutsche Medizinische Wochenschrift, 113*(12), 472–474.

Diener, H. C., & Wilkinson, M. (Eds.). (1988). *Drug-induced headache.* Berlin: Springer-Verlag.

Dieter, J. N., & Swerdlow, B. (1988). A replicative investigation of the reliability of the MMPI in the classification of chronic headaches. *Headache, 28,* 212–222.

Dodick, D. W., Jones, J. M., & Capobianco, D. J. (2000). Hypnic headache: Another indomethacin-responsive headache syndrome? *Headache: The Journal of Head and Face Pain, 40*(10), 830–835.

Dodick, D. W., Mosek, A. C., & Campbell, J. K. (1998). The hypnic ("alarm clock") headache syndrome. *Cephalalgia, 18,* 152–156.

Dorland's illustrated medical dictionary (27th ed.). (1988). Philadelphia: Saunders.

Epstein, L. H., & Abel, G. G. (1977). An analysis of biofeedback training effects for tension headache patients. *Behavior Therapy, 8,* 37–47.

Fahrion, S. L. (1977). Autogenic biofeedback treatment for migraine. *Mayo Clinic Proceedings, 52,* 776–784.

Fisher, C. N. (1988). Analgesic rebound headache refuted. *Headache, 28,* 666.

Flor, H. (2001). Psychophysiological assessment of the patient with chronic pain. In D. C. Turk & R. Melzack (Eds.), *Handbook of pain assessment* (2nd ed.) New York: Guilford Press.

Flor, H., & Turk, D. C. (1989). Psychophysiology of chronic pain: Do chronic pain patients exhibit symptom-specific psychophysiological responses? *Psychological Bulletin, 105,* 215–259.

Folen, R. A., James, L. C., Earles, J. E., & Andrasik, F. (2001). Biofeedback via telehealth: A new frontier for applied psychophysiology. *Applied Psychophysiology and Biofeedback, 26,* 195–204.

Freitag, F. G. (1999). Headache clinics and inpatient treatment units for headache. In M. L. Diamond & G. D. Solomon (Eds.), *Diamond and Dalessio's the practicing physicians' approach to headache.* Philadelphia: Saunders.

Gannon, L. R., Haynes, S. N., Cuevas, J., & Chavez, R. (1987). Psychophysiological correlates of induced headaches. *Journal of Behavioral Medicine, 4,* 411–423.

Gauthier, J. G., Bois, R., Allaire, D., & Drolet, M. (1981). Evaluation of skin temperature biofeedback training at two different sites for migraine. *Journal of Behavioral Medicine, 4,* 407–419.

Gauthier, J. G., Côté, G., & French, D. (1994). The role of home practice in the thermal biofeedback treatment of migraine headache. *Journal of Consulting and Clinical Psychology, 62*(1), 180–184.

Gauthier, J. G., Fournier, A. L., & Roberge, C. (1991). The differential effects of biofeedback in the treatment of menstrual and nonmenstrual migraine. *Headache, 31,* 82–90.

Goslin, R. E., Gray, R. N., McCrory, D. C., Penzien, D. B., Rains, J. C., & Hasselblad, V. (1999, February). *Behavioral physical treatments for migraine headache: Technical review 2.2.* (Prepared for the Agency for Health Care Policy and Research under Contract No. 290-94-2025. Available from the National Technical Information Service; NTIS Accession No. 127946.)

Gould, J. D., & Silberstein, S. D. (1997). Unilateral hypnic headache: A case study. *Neurology, 49*(6), 1749–1751.

Grazzi, L., Andrasik, F., D'Amico, D., Leone, M., Usai, S., Kass, S. J., & Bussone, G. (2002). Behavioral and pharmacologic treatment of transformed migraine with analgesic overuse: Outcome at 3 years. *Headache, 42,* 483–490.

Haddock, C. K., Rowan, A. B., Andrasik, F., Wilson, P. G., Talcott, G. W., & Stein, R. J. (1997). Home-based behavioral treatments for chronic benign headache: A meta-analysis of controlled trials. *Cephalalgia, 17,* 113–118.

Hagino, C., Boscariol, J., Dover, L., Letendre, R., & Wicks, M. (1998). Before/after study to determine the effects of the align-right cylindrical cervical pillow in reducing chronic neck pain severity. *Journal of Manipulative and Physiological Therapeutics, 21*(2), 89–93.

Hale, W. E., May, F. E., Marks, R. G., Moore, M. T., & Stewart, R. B. (1987). Headache in the elderly: An evaluation of risk factors. *Headache, 27,* 272–276.

Ham, L. P., Andrasik, F., Packard, R. C., & Bundrick, C. M. (1994). Psychopathology in individuals with post-traumatic headaches and other pain types. *Cephalalgia, 14,* 118–126.

Hart, J. D., & Cichanski, K. A. (1981). Comparison of frontal EMG biofeedback and neck EMG biofeedback in the treatment of muscle-contraction headache. *Biofeedback and Self-Regulation, 6,* 63–74.

Hatch, J. P., Fisher, J. G., & Rugh, J. D. (Eds.). (1987). *Biofeedback: Studies in clinical efficacy.* New York: Plenum Press.

Hatch, J. P., Moore, P. J., Borcherding, S., Cyr-Provost, M., Boutros, N. N., & Seleshi, E. (1992). Electromyographic and affective responses of episodic tension-type headache patients and headache-free controls during stress task performance. *Journal of Behavioral Medicine, 15*(1), 89–112.

Hatch, J. P., Prihoda, T. J., Moore, P. J., Cyr-Porvost, M., Borcherding, S., Boutros, N. N., & Seleshi, E. (1991a). A naturalistic study of the relationship among electromyographic activity, psychological stress and pain in ambulatory tension-type headache patients and headache-free controls. *Psychosomatic Medicine, 53,* 576–584.

Hatch, J. P., Schoefeld, L. S., Boueros, N. N., Seleshi, E., Moore, P. J., & Cyr-Provose, M. (1991b). Anger and hostility in tension-type headache. *Headache, 31,* 302–304.

Haynes, S. N., Gannon, L. R, Bank, J., Shelton, D., & Goodwin, J. (1990). Cephalic blood flow correlates of induced headaches. *Journal of Behavioral Medicine, 13*(5), 467–480.

Hermann, C. U., & Blanchard, E. B. (1993, March). *The role of the hand held computer in headache treatment and research.* Paper presented at the 24th Annual Meeting of the Association for Applied Psychophysiology and Biofeedback, Los Angeles.

Hickling, E. J., Silverman, D. J., & Loos, W. (1990). A nonpharmacological treatment of vascular headache during pregnancy. *Headache, 30,* 407–410.

Hillenberg, J. B., & Collins, F. L., Jr. (1983). The importance of home practice for progressive relaxation training. *Behaviour Research and Therapy, 21*(6), 633–642.

Hoelscher, T. J., Lichstein, K. L., & Rosenthal, T. L. (1984). Objective vs. subjective assessment of relaxation compliance among anxious individuals. *Behaviour Research and Therapy, 22,* 187–193.

Hoelscher, T. J., Lichstein, K. L., & Rosenthal, T. L. (1986). Home relaxation practice in hypertension treatment: Objective assessment and compliance induction. *Journal of Consulting and Clinical Psychology, 54,* 217–221.

Holm, J. E., Holroyd, K. A., Hursey, K. G., & Penzien, D. B. (1986). The role of stress in recurrent tension headache. *Headache, 26,* 160–167.

Holroyd, K. A. (2002). Assessment and psychological management of recurrent headache disorders. *Journal of Consulting and Clinical Psychology, 70,* 656–677.

Holroyd, K. A., & Andrasik, F. (1980). Do the effects of cognitive therapy endure?: A two-year follow-up of tension headache sufferers treated with cognitive therapy or biofeedback. *Cognitive Therapy and Research, 6,* 325–333.

Holroyd, K. A., & Andrasik, F. (1982). A cognitive-behavioral approach to recurrent tension and migraine headache. In P. C. Kendall (Ed.), *Advances in cognitive-behavioral research and therapy* (Vol. 1). New York: Academic Press.

Holroyd, K. A., Andrasik, F., & Westbrook, T. (1977). Cognitive control of tension headache. *Cognitive Therapy and Research, 1*(2), 121–133.

Holroyd, K. A., Holm, J. F., Penzien, D. B., Cordingley, G. E., Hursey, K. G., Marein, N. J., & Theofanous, A. (1989). Long-term maintenance of improvements achieved with (abortive) pharmacological and nonpharmacological treatments for migraine: Preliminary findings. *Biofeedback and Self-Regulation, 14*(4), 301–308.

Holroyd, K. A., Lipchik, G. L., & Penzien, D. B. (1998). Psychological management of recurrent headache disorders: Empirical basis for clinical practice. In K. S. Dobson & K. D. Craig (Eds.), *Empirically supported therapies.* Thousand Oaks, CA: Sage.

Holroyd, K. A., O'Donnell, F. J., Stensland, M., Lipchik, G. L., Cordingley, G. E., & Carlson, B. W. (2001). Management of chronic tension-type headache with tricyclic antidepressant medication, stress management therapy, and their combination. *Journal of the American Medical Association, 285,* 2208–2215.

Holroyd, K. A., & Penzien, D. (1986). Client variables and the behavioral treatment of recurrent tension headache: A meta-analytic review. *Journal of Behavioral Medicine, 9,* 515–536.

Holroyd, K. A., & Penzien, D. B. (1990). Pharmacological versus nonpharmacological prophylaxis of recurrent migraine headache: A meta-analytic review of clinical trials. *Pain, 42,* 1–13.

Holroyd, K. A., Penzien, D. B., & Cordingley, G. E. (1991). Propranolol in the management of recurrent migraine: A meta-analytic review. *Headache, 31,* 333–340.

Holroyd, K. A., Penzien, D. B., Holm, J. E., & Hursey, K. G. (1984a, June). *Behavioral treatment of recurrent headache: What does the literature say?* Paper presented at the meeting of the American Association for the Study of Headache, San Francisco.

Holroyd, K. A., Penzien, D. B., Hursey, K. G., Tobin, D. L., Rogers, L., Holm, J. E., Marcille, P. J., Hall, J. R., & Chila, A. G. (1984b). Change mechanisms in EMG biofeedback training: Cognitive changes underlying improvements in tension headache. *Journal of Consulting and Clinical Psychology, 52*(6), 1039–1053.

Hovanitz, C. A., Chin, K., & Warm, J. S. (1989). Complexities in life-stress–dysfunction relationships: A case in point—tension headache. *Journal of Behavioral Medicine, 12*(1), 55–75.

Hudzinski, L. G. (1983). Neck musculature and EMG biofeedback in treatment of muscle contraction headache. *Headache, 23,* 86–90.

Hudzinski, L. G., & Lawrence, G. S. (1988). Significance of EMG surface electrode placement models and headache findings. *Headache, 28,* 30–35.

Hudzinski, L. G., & Lawrence, G. S. (1990). EMG surface electrode normative data for muscle contraction headache and biofeedback therapy. *Headache Quarterly: Current Treatment and Research, 1*(3), 23–28.

International Headache Society (IHS) Committee on Clinical Trials in Migraine. (1999). Guidelines for controlled trials of drugs in migraine. In IHS (Ed.), *Members' handbook 2000.* Oslo: Scandinavian University Press.

International Headache Society (IHS) Committee on Clinical Trials in Tension-Type Headache. (1999). Guidelines for trials of drug treatments in tension-type headache. In IHS (Ed.), *Members' handbook 2000*. Oslo: Scandinavian University Press.

Jay, G. W., Renelli, D., & Mead, T. (1984). The effects of propranolol and amitriptyline on vascular and EMG biofeedback training. *Headache, 24,* 59–69.

Jennum, P., Hein, H. O., Suadicani, P., & Gyntelberg, F. (1994). Headache and cognitive dysfunctions in snorers. *Archives of Neurology, 51,* 937–942.

Jensen, M. P., & Karoly, P. (1992). Self-report scales and procedures for assessing pain in adults. In D. C. Turk & R. Melzack (Eds.), *Handbook of pain assessment*. New York: Guilford Press.

Jurish, S. E., Blanchard, E. B. Andrasik, F., Teders, S. J., Neff, D. F., & Arena, J. G. (1983). Home- versus clinic-based treatment of vascular headache. *Journal of Consulting and Clinical Psychology, 51*(5), 743–751.

Kabela, E., Blanchard, E. B., Appelbaum, K. A., & Nicholson, N. (1989). Self-regulatory treatment of headache in the elderly. *Biofeedback and Self-Regulation, 14*(3), 219–228.

Kewman, D., & Roberts, A. H. (1980). Skin temperature biofeedback and migraine headache: A double-blind study. *Biofeedback and Self-Regulation, 5,* 327–345.

Kim, M., & Blanchard, E. B. (1992). Two studies of the nonpharmacological treatment of menstrually-related migraine headaches. *Headache, 32,* 197–202.

Kohler, T., & Haimerl, C. (1990). Daily stress as a trigger of migraine attacks: Results of thirteen single-subject studies. *Journal of Consulting and Clinical Psychology, 58*(6), 870–872.

Kudrow, L. (1982). Parodoxical effects of frequent analgesic use. *Advances in Neurology, 33,* 335–341.

Kunkel, R. S. (1987). First things first: The physical workup. In C. S. Adler, S. M. Adler, & R. C. Packard (Eds.), *Psychiatric aspects of headache*. Baltimore: Williams & Wilkins.

Kurman, R. G., Hursey, K. G., & Mathew, N. T. (1992). Assessment of chronic refractory headache: The role of the MMPI-2. *Headache, 32*(9), 432–435.

Lake, A. E., III. (2001). Behavioral and nonpharmacological treatments of headache. *Medical Clinics of North America, 85,* 1055–1075.

Lake, A. E., III, & Pingel, J. D. (1988). Brief versus extended relaxation: Relationship to improvement at follow-up in mixed headache patients. *Medical Psychotherapy, 1,* 119–129.

Lake, A. E., III, Saper, J. R., Madden, S. F., & Kreeger, C. (1993). Comprehensive inpatient treatment for intractable migraine: A prospective long-term outcome study. *Headache, 33,* 55–62.

Lance, F., Parkes, C., & Wilkinson, M. (1988). Does analgesic abuse cause headache *de novo?* [Letter to the editor]. *Headache, 28,* 61–62.

Largen, J. W., Mathew, R J., Dobbins, K., & Claghorn, J. L. (1981). Specific and non-specific effects of skin temperature control in migraine management. *Headache, 21*(2), 36–44.

Larson, D. E. (1990). *Mayo Clinic family health book*. New York: Morrow.

Lavin, R. A., Pappagallo, M., & Kuhlemeier, K. V. (1997). Cervical pain: A comparison of three pillows. *Archives of Physical Medicine and Rehabilitation, 78*(2), 193–198.

Leijdekkers, M. L. A., & Passchier, J. (1990). Prediction of migraine using psychophysiological and personality measures, *Headache, 30,* 445–453.

Levor, R. M., Cohen, M. J., Naliboff, B. D., McArthur, D., & Heuser, G. (1986). Psychosocial precursors and correlates of migraine headache. *Journal of Consulting and Clinical Psychology, 54,* 347–353.

Libo, L. M., & Arnold, G. E. (1983). Relaxation practice after biofeedback therapy: A long-term follow-up study of utilization and effectiveness. *Biofeedback and Self-Regulation, 8*(2), 217–227.

Lichstein, K. L., Fischer, S. M., Eakin, T. L., Amberson, J. I., Bertorini, T., & Hoon, P. W. (1991). Psychophysiological paramerers of migraine and muscle-contraction headaches. *Headache, 31,* 27–34.

Lockett, D. M., & Campbell, J. F. (1992). The effects of aerobic exercise on migraine. *Headache, 32,* 50–54.

Loh, N. K., Dinner, D. S., Foldvary, N., Skobieranda, F., & Yew, W. W. (1999). Do patients with obstructive sleep apnea wake up with headaches? *Archives of Internal Medicine, 159,* 1765–1768.

Marcus, D. A. (1992). Migraine and tension-type headaches: The questionable validity of current classification systems. *Clinical Journal of Pain, 8,* 28–36.

Marcus, D. A. (1993). Serotonin and its role in headache pathogenesis and treatment. *Clinical Journal of Pain, 9,* 159–167.

Marcus, D. A., Scharff, L., & Turk, D. C. (1995). Nonpharmacological management of headaches during pregnancy. *Psychosomatic Medicine, 57*(6), 527–535.

Marlowe, N. (1998). Stressful events, appraisal, coping and recurrent headache. *Journal of Clinical Psychology, 54*(2), 247–256.

Martin, P. R. (1993). *Psychological management of chronic headaches*. New York: Guilford Press.

Martin, P. R. (2001). How do trigger factors acquire the capacity to precipitate headaches? *Behaviour Research and Therapy, 39*(5), 545–554.

Martin, P. R., & Seneviratne, H. M. (1997). Effects of food deprivation and a stressor on head pain. *Health Psychology, 16*(4), 310–318.

Martin, P. R., & Teoh, H. J. (1999). Effects of visual stimuli and a stressor on head pain. *Headache, 39*(10), 705–715.

Martin, P. R., & Theunissen, C. (1993). The role of life event stress, coping and social support in chronic headaches. *Headache, 33*, 301–306.

Mathew, N. T., & Bendtsen, L. (2000). Prophylactic pharmacotherapy of tension-type headache. In J. Olesen, P. Tfelt-Hansen, & K. M. A. Welch (Eds.), *The headaches* (2nd ed.). Philadelphia: Lippincott Williams & Wilkins.

Mathew, N. T., Kurman, R., & Perez, F. (1990). Drug induced refractory headache: Clinical features and management. *Headache, 30*, 634–638.

McCrory, D. C., Penzien, D. B., Hasselblad, V., & Gray, R. N. (2001). *Evidence report: Behavioral and physical treatments for tension-type and cervicogenic headache.* Des Moines, IA: Foundation for Chiropractic Education and Research (Product No. 2085).

Melzack, R., & Katz, J. (1992). The McGill Pain Questionnaire: Appraisal and current status. In D. C. Turk & R Melzack (Eds.), *Handbook of pain assessment.* New York: Guilford Press.

Merikangas, K. R., & Rasmussen, B. K. (2000). Migraine comorbidity. In J. Olesen, P. Tfelt-Hansen, & K. M. A. Welch (Eds.), *The headaches* (2nd ed.). Philadelphia: Lippincott Williams & Wilkins.

Merikangas, K. R., & Stevens, D. E. (1997). Comorbidity of migraine and psychiatric disorders. *Neurologic Clinics, 15*, 115–123.

Michultka, D. M., Blanchard, E. B., Appelbaum, K. A., Jaccard, J., & Dentinger, M. P. (1989). The refractory headache patient: II. High medication consumption (analgesic rebound) headache. *Behaviour Research and Therapy, 27*(4), 411–420.

Mitchell, C. S., Osborn, R. E., & Grosskreutz, S. R. (1993). Computed tomography in the headache patient: Is routine evaluation really necessary? *Headache, 33*, 82–86.

Morrill, B., & Blanchard, E. B. (1989). Two studies of the potential mechanisms of action in the thermal biofeedback treatment of vascular headache. *Headache, 29*, 169–176.

Morrill, B., Blanchard, E. B., Barron, K. D., & Dentinger, M. P. (1990). Neurological evaluation of chronic headache patients: Is laboratory testing always necessary? *Biofeedback and Self-Regulation, 15*(1), 27–35.

Murphy, A. I., Lehrer, P. M., & Jurish, S. (1990). Cognitive coping skills training and relaxation training as treatments for tension headaches. *Behavior Therapy, 21*, 89–98.

Napier, D., Miller, C., & Andrasik, F. (1997). Group treatment for recurrent headache. *Advances in Medical Psychotherapy, 9*, 21–31.

Nattero, G., De Lorenzo, C., Biale, L., Allais, G., Torre, E., & Ancona, M. (1989). Psychological aspects of weekend headache sufferers in comparison with migraine patients. *Headache, 29*, 93–99.

Nattero, G., De Lorenzo, C., Biale, L., Torrie, E., & Ancona, M. (1986). Idiopathic headaches: Relationship to life events. *Headache, 26*, 503–508.

Nevins, B. G., & Schwartz, M. S. (1985, April). An alternative placement for EMG electrodes in the study and biofeedback treatment of tension headaches. In *Proceedings of the 16th Annual Meeting of the Biofeedback Society of America, New Orleans.* Wheat Ridge, CO: Association for Applied Psychophysiology and Biofeedback.

O'Grady, S. J. (1987). Changes in medical utilization after biofeedback treatment for headache: Long-term follow-up (Doctoral dissertation, Pacific Graduate School of Psychology, Menlo Park, CA). *Dissertation Abstracts International, 49*, 49-01B (University Microfilms, No. 88-03939).

Olesen, J. (1988). Classification and diagnostic criteria for headache disorders, cranial neuralgias, and facial pain (lst ed.). *Cephalalgia, 8*(Suppl. 7), 1–96.

Packard, R., & Andrasik, F. (1989, March). *Psychological aspects of headache in adults and children.* Manual for workshop presented at the 20th Annual Meeting of the Association for Applied Psychophysiology and Biofeedback, San Diego, CA.

Padawer, W. J., & Levine, F. M. (1992). Exercise-induced analgesia: Fact or artifact? *Pain, 48*, 131–135.

Paiva, T., Farinha, A., Martins, A., Batista, A., & Guilleminault, C. (1997). Chronic headaches and sleep disorders. *Archives of Internal Medicine, 157*, 1701–1705.

Palazzi, C., Miralles, R., Miranda, C., Valenzuela, S., Casassus, R., Santander, H., & Ormeño, G. (1999). Effects of two types of pillows on bilateral sternocleidomastoid EMG activity in healthy subjects and in patients with myogenic cranio-cervical-mandibular dysfunction. *Journal of Craniomandibular Practice, 17*(3), 202–212.

Passchier, J., Schouten, J., van der Donk, J., & van Romunde, L. K. J. (1991). The association of frequent headaches with personality and life events. *Headache, 31*, 116–121.

Penzien, D. B., Rains, J. C., & Andrasik, F. (2002). Behavioral management of recurrent headache: Three decades of experience and empiricism. *Applied Psychophysiology and Biofeedback, 27*, 163–181.

Persson, L., & Moritz, U. (1998). Neck support pillows: A comparative study. *Journal of Manipulative and Physiological Therapies, 21*(4), 237–240.

Philips, H. C., & Jahanshahi, M. (1986). The components of pain behavior report. *Behaviour Research and Therapy*, 24, 117–125.

Pritchard, D. W., & Wood, M. M. (1983). EMG levels in the occipitofrontalis muscles under an experimental stress condition. *Biofeedback and Self-Regulation*, 8(1), 165–175.

Radat, F., Sakh, D., Lutz, G., El Amrani, M., Ferreri, M., & Bousser, M.-G. (1999). Psychiatric comorbidity is related to headache induced by chronic substance use in migraineurs. *Headache*, 39, 477–480.

Radnitz, C. L. (1990). Food-triggered migraine: A critical review. *Annals of Behaviaral Medicine*, 12(2), 51–71.

Radnitz, C. L., & Blanchard, E. B. (1991). Assessment and treatment of dietary factors in refractory vascular headache. *Headache Quarterly: Current Treatment and Research*, 2(3), 214–220.

Rapoport, A. M. (1988). Analgesic rebound headache. *Headache*, 28, 662–665.

Rapoport, A. M., Sheftell, F. D., Weeks, R. E., & Baskin, S. M. (1983). Analgesic-rebound headache. In *Proceedings of the 12th Meeting of the Scandinavian Migraine Society*.

Rapoport, A. M., Weeks, R. E., Sheftell, F. D., Baskin, S. M., & Verdi, J. (1985). Analgesic rebound headache: Theoretical and practical implications. *Cephalalgia*, 5(Suppl. 3), 448–449.

Raskin, N. H. (1997). Short-lived head pains. *Neurologic Clinics*, 15(1), 143–152.

Rasmussen, B. K., Jensen, R., & Olesen, J. (1991). Questionnaire versus clinical interview in the diagnosis of headache. *Headache*, 31, 290–295.

Reynolds, D. J., & Hovanitz, C. A. (2000). Life event stress and headache frequency revisited. *Headache*, 40, 111–118.

Richardson, G. M., & McGrath, P. J. (1989). Cognitive-behavioral therapy for migraine headaches: A minimal-therapist-contact approach versus a clinic-based approach. *Headache*, 29, 352–357.

Rowan, A. B., & Andrasik, F. (1996). Efficacy and cost-effectiveness of minimal therapist contact treatments of chronic headaches: A review. *Behavior Therapy*, 27, 207–234.

Ruff, M., Sturgis, E. T., & St. Lawrence, J. S. (1986, November). *EMG levels in tension headache sufferers: Does position make a difference?* Paper presented at the annual meeting of the Association for Advancement of Behavior Therapy, Chicago.

Rugh, J. D., Hatch, J. P., Moore, P. J., Cyr-Provost, M., Boutros, N. N., & Pellegrino, C. S. (1990). The effect of psychological stress on electromyographic activity and negative affect in ambulatory tension-type headache patients. *Headache*, 30, 216–219.

Sanders, S. H., & Collins, F. (1981). The effect of electrode placement on frontalis EMG measurement in headache patients. *Biofeedback and Self-Regulation*, 6, 473–482.

Saper, J.R. (1987). Ergotamine dependency: A review. *Headache*, 27, 435–438.

Saper, J. R., Silberstein, S., Gordon, C. D., & Hamel, R L. (1993). *Handbook of headache management*. Baltimore: Williams & Wilkins.

Scharff, L., & Marcus, D. A. (1994). Interdisciplinary outpatient group treatment of intractable headache. *Headache*, 34, 73–78.

Scharff, L., Marcus, D. A., & Turk, D. C. (1996). Maintenance of effects in the nonmedical treatment of headaches during pregnancy. *Headache*, 36, 285–290.

Scharff, L., Marcus, D. A., & Turk, D. C. (1997). Headache during pregnancy and in the postpartum: A prospective study. *Headache*, 37(4), 203–210.

Scharff, L., Turk, D. C., & Marcus, D. A. (1995). Triggers of headache episodes and coping responses of headache diagnostic groups. *Headache*, 35, 397–403.

Schlote, B. (1989). Long term registration of muscle tension among office workers suffering from tension headache. In C. Bischoff, H. Traue, & H. Zenz (Eds.), *Clinical perspectives on headache and low back pain*. New York: Hogrefe.

Schneider, W. J., Furth, P. A., Blalock, T. H., & Sherrill, T. A. (1999). A pilot study of a headache program in the workplace. *Journal of Occupational and Environmental Medicine*, 41, 202–209.

Schoenen, J., Gerard, P., De Pasqua, V., & Juprelle, M. (1991). EMG activity in pericranial muscles during postural variation and mental activity in healthy volunteers and patients with chronic tension-type headache. *Headache*, 31, 321–324.

Schwartz, G. E. (1977). Psychosomatic disorders and biofeedback: A psychobiological model of disregulation. In J. D. Maser & M. E. P. Seligman (Eds.), *Psychopathology: Experimental models*. San Francisco: Freeman.

Schwartz, G. E. (1978). Psychobiological foundations of psychotherapy and behavior change. In S. L. Garfield & A. E. Bergin (Eds.), *Handbook of psychotherapy and behavior change: An empirical analysis* (2nd ed.). New York: Wiley.

Schwartz, M. S. (1995). Headache: Selected issues and considerations in evaluation and treatment. Part B: Treatment. In M. S. Schwartz & Associates, *Biofeedback: A practitioner's guide*. New York: Guilford Press.

Schwartz, M. S., Craggs, J. H., & Capobianco, D. J. (2002). Case study of the value of direct occipital sEMG biofeedback in the treatment of occipital headaches. In *Proceedings of the 33rd Annual Meeting of the*

Association for Applied Psychophysiology and Biofeedback, Las Vegas. Wheat Ridge, CO: Association for Applied Psychophysiology and Biofeedback.

Sherman, R. A., & Arena, J. G. (1992). Biofeedback in the assessment and treatment of low back pain. In J. Basmajian & R. Nyberg (Eds.), *Spinal manipulative therapies*. Baltimore: Williams & Wilkins.

Sherman, R. A., Arena, J. G., Searle, J. R., & Ginther, J. R. (1991). Development of an ambulatory recorder for evaluation of muscle-tension related low back pain and fatigue in soldiers' normal environments. *Military Medicine, 150*(5), 245–248.

Sherman, R. A., Evans, C., & Arena, J. G. (1993). Environmental–temporal relationships between pain and muscle tension: Ramifications for the future of biofeedback treatment. [Russian with English abstract]. In M. Shtark & T. Sokhadze (Eds.), *Biofeedback: Theory and practice*. Moscow, Russia: Nauka.

Silberstein, S. D. (1992). Menstrual migraine [Guest editorial]. *Headache, 30*(6), 312–313.

Solbach, P., Sargent, J., & Coyne, L. (1984a). Menstrual migraine headache: Results of a controlled, experimental outcome study of nondrug treatments. *Headache, 24*, 75–78.

Solbach, P., Sargent, J., & Coyne, L. (1984b). An analysis of home practice patterns for non-drug headache treatments. *Headache, 29*, 528–531.

Solbach, P., Sargent, J., & Coyne, L. (1989). An analysis of home practice patterns for non-drug headache treatments. *Headache, 29*, 528–531.

Solomon, G. D., Kunkel, R. S., & Frame, J. (1990). Demographics of headache in elderly patients. *Headache, 30*, 273–276.

Sorbi, M. J., Maassen, G. H., & Spierings, E. L. H. (1996). A time series analysis of daily hassles and mood changes in the three days before the migraine attack. *Behavioral Medicine, 22*, 103–113.

Sovak, M., Kunzel, M., Sternbach, R. A., & Dalessio, D. J. (1978). Is volitional manipulation of hemodynamics a valid rationale for biofeedback therapy of migraine? *Headache, 18*, 197–202.

Spierings, E. L. H., Sorbi, M., Haimowitz, B. R., & Tellegen, B. (1996). Changes in daily hassles, mood, and sleep in the 2 days before a migraine headache. *Clinical Journal of Pain, 12*, 38–42.

Sternbach, R. A., Dalessio, D. J., Kunzel, M., & Bowman, G. E. (1980). MMPI patterns in common headache disorders. *Headache, 20*, 311–315.

Ström, L., Petersson, R., & Andersson, G. (2000). A controlled trial of self-help treatment of recurrent headache conducted via the Internet. *Journal of Consulting and Clinical Psychology, 68*, 722–727.

Swanson, J. W. (1987). History, examination, and laboratory tests for headache. *Journal of Craniomandibular Disorders: Facial and Oral Pain, 1*, 17–20.

Szekely, B., Botwin, D., Eidelman, B. H., Becker, M., Elman, N., & Schemm, R. (1986). Non-pharmacological treatment of menstrual headache: Relaxation–biofeedback behavior therapy and person-centered insight therapy. *Headache, 26*, 86–92.

Takeshima, T., Taniguchi, R., Kitagawa, R., & Takahashi, K. (1990). Headaches in dementia. *Headache, 30*, 735–738.

Teders, S. J., Blanchard, E. B., Andrasik, F., Jurish, S. E., Neff, D. F., & Arena, J. G. (1984). Relaxation training for tension headache: Comparative efficacy and cost-effectiveness of a minimal therapist contact versus a therapist-delivered procedure. *Behavior Therapy, 15*, 59–70.

Tobin, D. L., Holroyd, K. A., Baker, A., Reynolds, R. V. C., & Holm, J. E. (1988). Development and clinical trial of a minimal contact, cognitive-behavioral treatment for tension headaches. *Cognitive Therapy and Research, 12*, 325–339.

Ulfberg, J., Carter, N., Talback, M., & Edling, C. (1996). Headache, snoring and sleep apnea. *Journal of Neurology, 243*, 621–625.

Williams, D. E., Raczynski, J. M., Domino, J., & Davig, J. P. (1993). Psychophysiological and MMPI personality assessment of headaches: An integrative approach. *Headache, 33*, 149–154.

Williams, T. F. (1991). Health care trends for older people. *Biofeedback and Self-Regulation, 16*(4), 337–347.

Wittrock, D. A. (1997). The comparison of individuals with tension-type headache and headache-free controls on frontal EMG levels: A meta-analysis. *Headache, 37*, 424–432.

Wittrock, D. A., Ficek, S. K., & Cook, T. M. (1996). Headache-free controls? Evidence of headaches in individuals who deny having headaches during diagnostic screening. *Headache, 36*(7), 416–418.

Wittrock, D. A., & Myers, T. C. (1998). The comparison of individuals with recurrent tension-type headache and headache-free controls in physiological response, appraisal, and coping with stressors: A review of the literature. *Annals of Behavioral Medicine, 20*, 118–134.

APPENDIX 14.1. THE 5:4 AND 10:10 ELECTRODE-TO-CHANNEL MAYO EMG MONTAGES: TECHNICAL APPENDIX AND FPN PLACEMENT

James H. Craggs, Mark S. Schwartz, and Michael J. Burke[a]

FpN Placement

An FpN EMG placement includes activity from all muscles of the head and neck, including occipital and temporalis muscles in addition to frontalis and posterior neck (Nevins & Schwartz, 1985). Hudzinski and Lawrence (1988, 1990) published the first studies of this electrode placement.[b] Figure 14A.1 shows a single-channel bilateral occipital placement and the posterior neck placement portion of the montage described in this appendix.

Nevins and Schwartz (1985) demonstrated the following:

1. The frontalis, posterior neck, and occipitalis muscles can contract independently; one can substantially tense the occipitalis muscles independently of the frontalis muscles and the posterior neck muscles (see Figure 14A.2).
2. There is a relationship between muscle activity recorded from the FpN placement and the activity recorded directly from an occipital placement (see Figure 14A.2).
3. There is a greater relationship between occipital activity and the FpN placement than between occipital activity and frontal activity.

Figure 14A.2 shows, in a normal subject, the very high-intensity muscle tension that can be produced from the occipitalis muscles, and the minimal reflection of this muscle activity in the bifrontal and bilateral posterior neck channels. The rises and falls of the two FpN channels occur simultaneously with the changes in occipital tension.

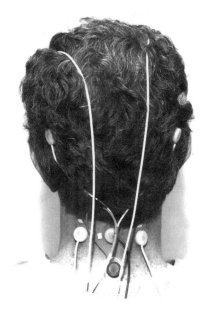

FIGURE 14A.1. Photograph of a single channel bilateral occipital placement and the posterior neck placement for electrodes number 3 and number 4 of the 5-electrode/4-channel FpN montage. The two frontal electrodes are on the forehead in the standard sites.

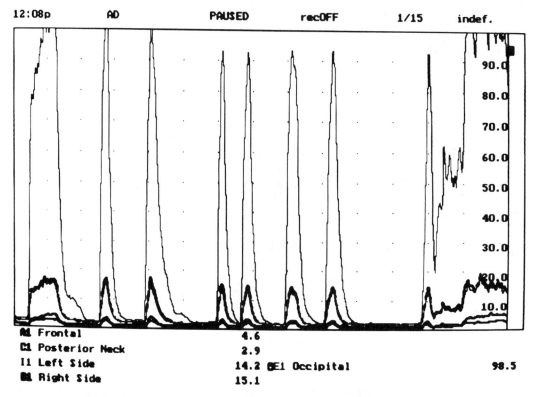

FIGURE 14A.2. This figure demonstrates, in a normal subject, the very high intensity of muscle tension that can be produced from the occipitalis muscles, and the minimal reflection of this muscle activity in the bifrontal and bilateral posterior neck channels.

The occipitalis channel is the one with the highest peaks up to and exceeding 100 microvolts. The bifrontal and bilateral posterior neck channels are the lowest two, and the two FpN channels are above those. Note the rises and falls of the two FpN channels occurring simultaneously with the changes in occipital tension.

Note that the scale is 0–100 root mean square microvolts (a bandpass of 100–200 hertz). This scale is used here for demonstration purposes only and is necessary because of the amount of occipital tension used in the demonstration. All channels are on the same 0–100 scale.

Hudzinski and Lawrence (1988, 1990) published their rationale and normative data on the FpN placement. They showed that this placement "was able to significantly discriminate headache from nonheadache activity" (p. 32). It also discriminated between sessions when patients with chronic headaches reported a headache and sessions when the same patients did not report a headache. There was increased microvolt activity with the headaches.

Uses of the FpN Placement

Higher-than-expected FpN recordings raise the question of occipital tension. One must rule out other causes of the elevated FpN signal. Thus, to interpret FpN activity, one needs to know from where the muscle tension emanates. One needs at least simultaneous recordings from the frontal area and from the posterior neck area. This helps determine the extent to which tension in those areas contributes to the microvolts shown on the FpN channel. For example, some people swallow without touching their upper and lower teeth together. They tense other muscles, including the sternomastoids. This muscle activity shows on the FpN channels. Muscle activity often remains low or unchanged in the frontal channel during these swallows.

An FpN elevation may indicate possible excess tension in muscles other than frontal and posterior neck areas when FpN microvolts exceed the sum of the bifrontal and bilateral posterior neck. The patient's headache description and reported location, as well as clinical judgment, indicate when to record the occipital area directly rather than rely on the FpN placement. Careful observation and instructions to patients should minimize other sources of muscle activity.

Technical Background

In the commonly used bipolar electrode configuration, each EMG channel consists of three wires independently attached to two detection electrodes and a ground or common-mode reference electrode (Soderberg, 1992). Therefore, for every EMG channel, there will be three electrodes attached to the body and a 3:1 electrode-to-channel ratio. Multiple EMG channels are desirable under many circumstances, but they necessitate having to apply numerous electrodes, which can be clinically challenging for many reasons.

The Mayo 5:4 EMG Montage

To utilize more EMG channels conveniently and efficiently, the five-electrode/four-channel (5:4) EMG montage was developed at the Mayo Clinic (see Figure 14A.3). Use of this montage reduces electrode usage from 12 to 5 electrodes for four channels.

This 5:4 electrode-to-channel montage was initially referred to (and, by us, still is) as the *FpN Placement*, since it involves a bilateral configuration of electrode on the frontalis muscle and another electrode on the same side on the posterior neck (see Figures 14A.4, sections A and C). It may be used to measure activity from muscles such as occipital, temporalis, frontalis, and posterior neck (Nevins & Schwartz, 1985). As noted earlier, Hudzinski and Lawrence (1988, 1990) published the first studies of this electrode placement. Of course, this electrode montage may also be applied to other muscle groups as well.

The Mayo 10:10 EMG Montage

Four EMG channels may be sufficient for some applications, but more channels are useful when one is concurrently monitoring, for example, the head, neck, and upper back areas (see Figure 14A.4, section C). For this reason, an electrode montage assembly was developed consisting of 10 electrodes for 10

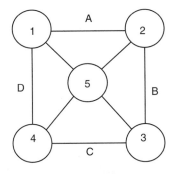

Channel	Electrode(s)
A	1-2
B	2-3
C	3-4
D	4-1
Ground	5

FIGURE 14A.3. The Mayo 5:4 electrode montage consists of a 5:4 electrode-to-channel ratio. Channels A-B-C-D are created out of a configuration where sharing occurs from electrodes 1 through 4, and all have a common ground electrode. Note that the Mayo EMG montages are used with a proprietary EMG biofeedback apparatus; adaptations of a system such as this should be made only with the equipment manufacturer's approval.

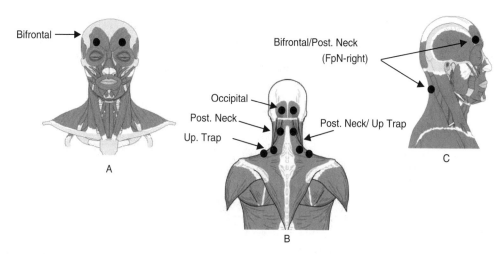

FIGURE 14A.4. Multiple EMG placements are illustrated. A four-channel (Mayo 5:4 EMG montage) configuration may consist of bifrontal (A), posterior neck (B), and bilateral frontal–posterior neck (C) placements. Occipital activity (B) may be directly measured, but, more conveniently, it can be inferred from the frontal–posterior neck placement (C). Other locations, such as the posterior neck–upper trapezius and bilateral upper trapezius (B), allow a more complete view of the head–neck–upper back region and are examples of Mayo 10:10 EMG montage applications. Illustrations from LifeArt Medical Clip Art: Super Anatomy Collections. (1998). Copyright 1998 by Lippincott Williams & Wilkins. Reprinted by permission.

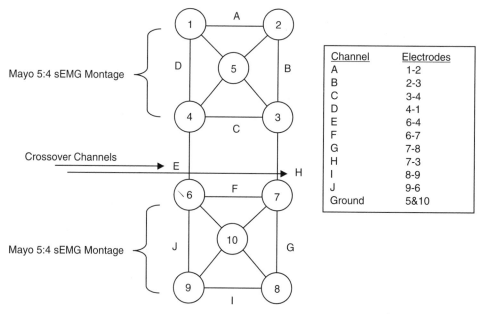

FIGURE 14A.5. The Mayo 10:10 EMG electrode montage is an amalgamation of two Mayo 5:4 EMG montages by use of a crossover design. It is possible to monitor up to 10 EMG channels utilizing only 10 electrodes. The 5:4 EMG montage consists of channels A-B-C-D. A second 5:4 montage consisting of channels F-G-I-J is tied in to the first montage by crossover channels E and H. Again, note that the Mayo EMG montages are used with a proprietary EMG biofeedback apparatus. Adaptations of a system such as this should be made *only* with the equipment manufacturer's approval.

EMG channels. The 10:10 electrode-to-channel montage was created on the same basis as the 5:4 montage in terms of electrode relationships. It broadens the application of EMG evaluation and treatment, while minimizing problems related to space and artifact. Figure 14A.5 illustrates the montage assembly.

The FpN EMG Placement

The ideal FpN EMG placement is the 5:4 electrode montage. The FpN placement is a more comprehensive measure of muscle activity in the head and neck than other single EMG placements. It is a more useful indicator of resting muscle tension of patients with tension-type headaches (Hudzinski & Lawrence, 1988). It is an indirect measure of possible occipital activity, and a more sensitive indirect measure of temporalis activity, than the bifrontal placement. The availability of four channels of muscle activity provides assessment of the right and left sides of the head and neck.

The two temporalis muscles contribute to FpN microvolts. However, temporalis tension is usually unlikely, given the resting posture of the head and jaw during recording sessions. There is no activity in the temporalis muscles unless the patient moves his or her jaw (Travell & Simons, 1983, p. 239). Unusual jaw and teeth positions sometimes occur, but are uncommon during recording sessions. They are easily observed and modifiable. Again, careful observation and instructions to patients should minimize this potential source of muscle activity.

NOTES

[a]Much appreciation is expressed to Michael J. Burke, of the Division of Engineering and Technology Services, for his development of the original electrode assembly at the Mayo Clinic, Rochester (Burke & Schwartz, 1995).

[b]Hudzinski and Lawrence (1988, 1990) thoughtfully referred to the FpN placement as the "Schwartz–Mayo method." Mark S. Schwartz is very grateful to them for providing the first published studies of this electrode placement, and for their thoughtfulness. He was unaware of their name choice for this placement until he read their publications. He is still more comfortable with calling it the FpN placement, and that is what it is called elsewhere in this chapter.

REFERENCES

Burke, M. J., & Schwartz, M. S. (1995). Technical appendix: Four-channel electrode assembly from five electrodes. In M. S. Schwartz & Associates, *Biofeedback: A practitioner's guide* (2nd ed.). New York: Guilford Press.

Hudzinski, L. G., & Lawrence, G. S. (1988). Significance of EMG surface electrode placement models and headache findings. *Headache, 28,* 30–35.

Hudzinski, L. G., & Lawrence, G. S. (1990). EMG surface electrode normative data for muscle contraction headache and biofeedback therapy. *Headache Quarterly: Current Treatment and Research, 1*(3), 23–28.

LifeArt Medical Clip Art: Super Anatomy Collections. (1998). Collection No. 1, p. 8. Baltimore, MD: Lippincott Williams & Wilkins.

Nevins, B. G., & Schwartz, M. S. (1985, April). An alternative placement for EMG electrodes in the study and biofeedback treatment of tension headaches. In *Proceedings of the 16th Annual Meeting of the Biofeedback Society of America, New Orleans.* Wheat Ridge, CO: Association for Applied Psychophysiology and Biofeedback.

Soderberg, G. L. (Ed.). (1992). *Selected topics in surface electromyography for use in the occupational setting: Expert perspectives* (National Institute for Occupational Safety and Health Publication No. 91-100). Washington, DC: U.S. Government Printing Office.

Travell, J. G., & Simons, D. G. (1983). *Myofascial pain and dysfunction: The trigger point manual.* Baltimore: Williams & Wilkins.

RESOURCES

Useful Web sites for information (and other information for relevant organizations) about headaches include the following:

http://www.mayoclinic.com/findinformation/diseasesandconditions/list.cfm?alpha=h (Mayo Clinic) http://www.mhni.com (Michigan Head Pain and Neurological Institute; address: 3120 Professional Drive, Ann Arbor, MI 48104; phone: 734-677-6000)

http://www.headaches.org (National Headache Foundation; address: 428 West St. James Place, 2nd Floor, Chicago, IL 60614-2750; phone: 773-388-6399 or 888-NHF-5552 [643-5552]; fax: 773-525-7357)

http://www.achenet.org (American Council for Headache Education, created in 1990 through an initiative of the American Headache Society; address: 19 Mantua Road, Mt. Royal, NJ 08061; phone: 856-423-0258 or 800-255-ACHE [255-2243]; fax: 856-423-0082)

CHAPTER 15

Temporomandibular Disorders

ALAN G. GLAROS
LEONARD LAUSTEN

Temporomandibular disorders (TMDs) are important disorders for dentistry, medicine, and psychology. TMDs are a heterogeneous collection of disorders involving the muscles of mastication and the hard and soft tissues of the temporomandibular joint (TMJ), and are sometimes called TMJ disorders. Dental professionals and other health care professionals recognize psychological and emotional factors as playing key roles in the etiology, maintenance, and treatment of TMDs (Dworkin & LeResche, 1992). This biopsychosocial approach (Greene & Laskin, 2000) creates an increasing role for clinicians using biofeedback in the treatment team for TMDs.

Many fine, comprehensive reviews of TMDs are available (Fricton & Dubner, 1995; Glaros & Glass, 1993; Sessle, Bryant, & Dionne, 1995), and excellent patient education is available from the National Institute of Dental and Craniofacial Research (http://www.nidcr.nih.gov/news/pubs/tmd/menu.htm). This chapter presents data on TMDs that can help practitioners using biofeedback understand the relationship between psychological, behavioral, or emotional factors and TMD symptoms. This understanding should then serve as a basis for treatment appropriate to the underlying pathogenesis. (Throughout the chapter, italics on first use of a term in text indicate that the term is included in the glossary at the chapter's end.)

ANATOMY AND PHYSIOLOGY OF THE TMJ AND ASSOCIATED MUSCULATURE

The TMJ is a dynamic complex that includes the mandibular *condyle*, the *articular disc*, the *articular fossa* of the temporal bone, and the associated membranes, fluids, and ligaments (Figure 15.1). The condyles arise as vertical projections of the U-shaped mandible, and they articulate with the cranium in the concave mandibular fossae of the temporal bones. The disc consists of dense fibrous connective tissue; it lacks nerves and blood supply. These structures and the associated nerves and vasculature provide for normal functions of the teeth and jaw.

Normal function of the TMJ is complex, involving two separate components to its movement. Upon initial opening, the joint works on a ball-and-socket or hinge principle in which the condyle rotates within the fossa. The disc remains in the fossa between the condyle and the temporal bone. As the jaw continues to open, the condyle translates ("dislocates") over a bony, articular eminence in the upper jaw. The articular disc slides between the eminence

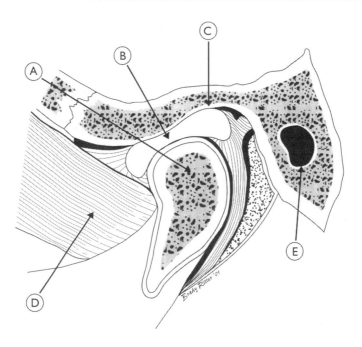

A. HEAD OF THE CONDYLE

B. ARTICULAR DISC

C. ARTICULAR FOSSA

D. LATERAL PTERYGOID MUSCLE

E. EXTERNAL AUDITORY MEATUS

FIGURE 15.1. Anatomy of the temporomandibular joint (TMJ).

and the condyle throughout the opening movement, and may act as a biological "Teflon" that facilitates smooth, pain-free translation of the condyles past the eminences.

Many conditions can adversely affect the joint. Degenerative disorders can lead to erosion and flattening of the condyle, or can form undesirable growths called "bone spurs." Both conditions may result in decreased function, pain, or both. The articular disc itself can function abnormally. Temporary displacement of the disc from its normal position during movement can cause clicking or popping noises. Difficulty in opening or closing may be caused by an abnormal position of the disc. A large portion of the population experiences TMJ noises. Although annoying to the affected individuals, joint noises in the absence of pain, limitation of movement, or changes in opening pattern do not warrant treatment (Glaros & Glass, 1993; Okeson, 1998).

The jaw functions are controlled by the muscles of mastication. The most important muscles for jaw function are the *masseter*, *temporalis*, and medial and lateral *pterygoid muscles*. The masseter and temporalis muscles elevate the mandible during mastication, and the temporalis muscles also retract the mandible. The masseter and temporalis muscles can be palpated by placing the fingers directly above the angle of the mandible and on the temples, respectively, while the patient clenches.

The lateral (external) pterygoid muscles protrude and depress the mandible. They also aid lateral jaw movement. The medial (internal) pterygoids close the jaw, produce lateral movements to the opposite side, and aid in protrusion. Both these muscles can be palpated intraorally, although distinguishing them may be difficult (Dworkin & LeResche, 1992). The *sternocleidomastoid*, *hyoid*, and *digastric muscles* also aid in the opening, closing and positioning of the TMJ.

Many cases of TMDs involve myalgia (muscle pain) not involving any disturbance or pathological deformation of the TMJ (Fricton & Schiffman, 1995). Travell and Simons (1983) propose that some or most chronic muscle pain is a result of "trigger points." These are palpable taut bands of muscle tissue that are tender to palpation. There is a characteristic pattern of pain associated with active trigger points. Research shows that careful needle electrode techniques can detect high levels of electromyographic (EMG) activity in a trigger point itself, where the adjacent nontender muscle is silent (Hubbard & Berkoff, 1993). In addition, data recorded from the trigger point needle EMG electrodes show responses to psychological stress, while the adjacent nontender muscle is silent during this stress (McNulty, Gevirtz, Hubbard, & Berkoff, 1994).

Work by several investigators (e.g., Passatore, Grassi, & Filippi, 1985) shows that sympathetic pathways innervate the muscle spindle, which is a proprioceptive component of muscle. However, little evidence exists for autonomic control of *extrafusal muscle fibers* (i.e., ordinary muscle fibers). These findings suggest that trigger points may be an important link between the muscle pain of TMDs and psychological stressors (Carlson, Okeson, Falace, Nitz, & Lindroth, 1993). Sympathetically mediated trigger points associated with the muscle spindles may develop because of stress. Prolonged emotional factors such as anger may maintain them.

This may help us to explain the link between behavioral or emotional factors and mechanisms of muscle pain. Research is underway to determine the exact process in the musculature responsible for muscle pain related to trigger points. However, it now appears that the sympathetic nervous system is involved in the innervation of trigger points, and that emotions play a role through this pathway.

SYMPTOMS AND ETIOLOGY OF TMDS

The primary symptoms of TMDs are as follows:

1. Pain in the muscles of mastication, in the preauricular area (i.e., immediately in front of the ear), or in the TMJ.
2. Clicking, popping, or grating sounds in the joint.
3. Difficulty in opening the mouth wide.
4. Patient's perception that his or her occlusion ("bite") is "off."
5. Jaw locking in the open or closed position.

In addition to masticatory muscle pain and other TMJ-related symptoms, a patient with a TMD may report a wide variety of other conditions, including headache; other facial pains; earache; dizziness; tinnitus; neck, shoulder, and upper and lower back pain; and tooth pain, accelerated wear on the dentition, fractured or mobile teeth, or defective and broken restorations ("fillings") without other known causes (Okeson, 1998).

In addition to dentists, it is not surprising that physicians and other health care professionals also evaluate and treat people who present with TMD symptoms. Glaros, Glass, and

Hayden (1995), for example, reported that approximately 40% of patients evaluated at a dental-school-based tertiary care clinic for patients with TMDs had also been seen by physicians. Patients reported contacts with primary care physicians and various specialists, including otolaryngologists, neurologists, and rheumatologists.

The complicated nature of TMDs requires that practitioners maintain a good working relationship with a dentist competent in TMDs and with other properly trained health professionals. The symptoms of TMDs can mimic a variety of physical conditions (e.g., headache, dizziness, tinnitus). Thus proper assessment and early intervention for TMDs may reduce individual and societal costs associated with the care of these patients.

Our coverage of the etiologies of TMDs addresses the roles of *parafunctional activity*, *occlusion*, psychological variables, psychophysiological variables, trauma, and abuse.

Parafunctional Activity

Clenching and grinding are parafunctional behaviors, and both are important causes and aggravating factors for TMD symptoms. Parafunctional oral activities, such as the chewing of pencils, erasers, gum, ice, cheeks, and lips, may also be related to TMDs (Moss, Sult, & Garrett, 1984). To examine the role of parafunctional tooth contact, Haggerty, Glaros, and Glass (2000) examined a group of patients with TMDs and a control group without pain or TMDs, using experience-sampling methodology. Figure 15.2 presents the data from this study. For the patients, the proportion of time that they reported tooth contact ranged from 23% to 93% (mean = 60%). For controls, the values for tooth contact ranged from 0% to 47%, with one clear outlier at 98%. For the entire control group, including the outlier, the mean tooth contact time was 27%. These mean values for tooth contact time differed significantly, t (19) = 2.78, $p < .01$. With the outlier removed, the proportion of time that the control group reported tooth contact reduced to 21%.[1] A replication of this study with a larger sample of participants reported similar results (Glaros & Lausten, 2002).

Glaros and colleagues have also conducted a series of studies examining the effect of low-level parafunctional clenching on pain. In these studies, healthy, normal individuals with no evidence or history of TMDs participated in biofeedback training to increase and/or decrease the activity of the temporalis and masseter muscles. In the increase condition, subjects could

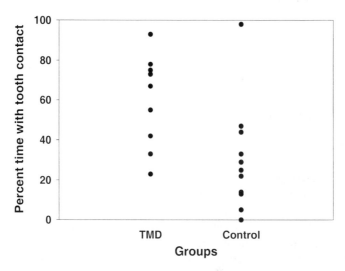

FIGURE 15.2. Proportion of time in which parafunctional tooth contact occurred. Data from Haggerty, Glaros, and Glass (2000).

attain the target level for biofeedback training by touching the posterior teeth together or engaging in light clenching. In the decrease condition, subjects could attain the target level by deeply relaxing the masticatory muscles and allowing the posterior teeth to separate approximately 8–12 millimeters (Rugh & Drago, 1981). Self-reported pain and the results of post-training screening examinations were used as the main dependent measures. The experimental procedures included A-B-A (Glaros, Tabacchi, & Glass, 1998b), crossover (Glaros, Baharloo, & Glass, 1998a), and between-group designs (Glaros, Forbes, Shanker, & Glass, 2000; Glaros & Burton, 2001). Sessions lasted 17–20 minutes and were carried out once a day for up to 8 days.

In each study, the results were similar: Laboratory-based experimental clenching increased pain (Figure 15.3) and could produce TMDs. The protocol used in these four studies caused about one-fourth of the participants to develop symptoms sufficiently intense to warrant the diagnosis of myofascial pain and/or arthralgia by trained examiners unaware of the research conditions. In all of the studies, the correlation between mean EMG activity and pain was significant and accounted for a significant proportion of the variance in self-reported pain ($r = .60$ to $.80$). These findings provide clear, replicated evidence that parafunctional clenching increases pain and can cause symptoms of TMDs.

The role of nocturnal parafunctional activity ("bruxism"), which can include both clenching and grinding, is less clear (Lobbezoo & Lavigne, 1997). Within an individual, the level of parafunctional activity from night to night varies considerably. Dental evidence of nocturnal grinding—accelerated wear on the teeth—may be misleading. The grinding behaviors that caused the wear may have occurred in the past, but may not be occurring at the present time. For these reasons, practitioners must conduct very careful and thorough evaluations of individuals who engage in nocturnal grinding.

Occlusion

Malocclusion is the relative failure of the *maxillary teeth* and *mandibular teeth* to fit together properly. Occlusal theories of the cause of TMDs remain popular among many dentists. The

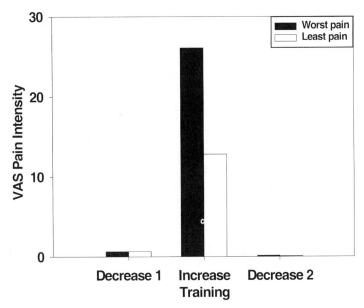

FIGURE 15.3. Effect of parafunctional clenching on self-reported pain. Data from Glaros, Tabacchi, and Glass (1998b).

dental literature contains a variety of clinical reports indicating the importance of malocclusion. However, more recent reviews strongly suggest that occlusion plays a minor role at best (Clark, Tsukiyama, Baba, & Watanabe, 1999; Okeson, 1998; Seligman & Pullinger, 1991). Epidemiological studies suggest that deviations from ideal occlusion are statistically normal in both child and adult populations (Kirveskari, Alanen, & Jamsa, 1992; Ramfjord & Ash, 1983). For example, over 95% of 5- and 10-year-old children showed occlusal interferences in one study (Kirveskari et al., 1992). Furthermore, there is no compelling experimental evidence to support the hypothesis that occlusal disharmony causes teeth clenching and grinding behaviors (Bell, 1986).

Psychological Variables

As a chronic, painful disorder, the psychological correlates of TMDs are similar to those reported for other chronic pain conditions. For example, Gatchel, Garofalo, Ellis, and Holt (1996) have shown that patients with chronic TMDs have significantly higher levels of somatoform disorders (particularly pain disorder) and mood disorders (typically involving depression) than newly diagnosed patients with TMDs. In contrast, newly diagnosed patients with TMDs are significantly more likely to report symptoms consistent with one or more anxiety disorders. Morris, Benjamin, Gray, and Bennett (1997) evaluated 97 patients with TMDs, using seven different psychiatric instruments, and determined that 33% had a mental disorder. Korszun, Hinderstein, and Wong (1996) evaluated 72 consecutive patients with chronic facial pain and reported that 28% met the criteria for major depressive disorder, 25% met the criteria for minor depression, and 22% reported subsyndromal symptoms of depression. Kinney, Gatchel, Ellis, and Holt (1992) reported that 30% of patients with TMDs showed evidence of major depression, based on a structured clinical interview. Wright, Deary, and Geissler (1991) reported that 13.5% of their patients with TMDs had clinically elevated depression scores on the Beck Depression Inventory. These data indicate that TMDs are often associated with psychological conditions as well.

However, the distribution of emotional distress may not be equal across all types of TMDs. Dahlström, Widmark, and Carlsson (1997), for example, classified patients with TMDs as "dysfunctional," "interpersonally distressed," and "adaptive" copers, based on their responses to the Multidimensional Pain Inventory. They further categorized the TMDs of these patients as either myofascial pain or disc displacement. Patients diagnosed with myofascial pain were much more likely to fall within the interpersonally distressed coping category than patients diagnosed with disc displacement. Similar findings with the Minnesota Multiphasic Personality Inventory have been reported by Michelotti, Martina, Russo, and Romeo (1998).

These findings show that psychological problems are more likely to be present in patients diagnosed with myofascial pain than in those with disc displacement. Since epidemiological studies have suggested that patients with muscle disorders outnumber those with joint-only problems (Fricton & Schiffman, 1995), practitioners should be prepared to consider the possibility that a patient with a TMD, particularly one with myofascial pain, may have a concomitant psychological disorder as well (Kight, Gatchel, & Wesley, 1999).

Psychophysiological Variables

Laskin's (1969) psychophysiological model of TMDs has been the focus of considerable research. Laskin's model integrates both biological and psychological findings. According to this model, people react to stress with different bodily systems. Some react via the head and neck muscles, and some of these develop TMDs (Kapel, Glaros, & McGlynn, 1989; Laskin, 1969; Zarb & Carlsson, 1979). The consistency of responding within individuals is often attributed to Lacey's (1950, 1967) concept of "individual response stereotypy."

A number of studies exploring the psychophysiological model proposed by Laskin have found that patients with TMDs (typically those with myalgia or myofascial pain dysfunction) show facial muscle activity responses to experimental stressors (Kapel et al., 1989; Flor, Birbaumer, Schulte, & Roos, 1991; Mercuri, Olson, & Laskin, 1979; Moss & Adams, 1984; Rao & Glaros, 1979). However, not all studies have reported such psychophysiological responsiveness to experimental stressors (e.g., Montgomery & Rugh, 1987; Intrieri, Jones, & Alcorn, 1994). Ohrbach, Blascovich, Gale, McCall, and Dworkin (1998) have suggested that these differing outcomes are related to methodological factors, especially the relevance of the stressor to the subject.

Several studies have also documented a relationship between stress and nocturnal clenching and grinding (Clark, Rugh, & Handelman, 1980; Clark, Rugh, Handelman, & Beemsterboer, 1977; Funch & Gale, 1980; Hopper, Gevirtz, Nigl, & Taddey, 1992; Rugh, 1975). Funch and Gale (1980) were among the first researchers to point out the importance of anticipatory anxiety rather than stressful life events in clenching and grinding. Hopper et al. (1992) found that the degree to which subjects worried or were anxious about the next day's stressors predicted the amount of masticatory muscle activity each night.

Trauma and Abuse

Work-related behaviors can contribute to TMDs. For example, the repeated raising of a shoulder to hold a telephone receiver to an ear puts pressure on the TMJ and increases tension in the neck and shoulder. This repeated behavior can create abnormal muscle tension in the neck and shoulder, and can produce pain or can exacerbate a preexisting problem. Poor positioning of a computer keyboard or monitor can increase or maintain pain in patients with TMDs.

Physical trauma to the TMJ, whether by accident or deliberate abuse, is an important etiological factor in TMDs. Emotional or sexual abuse during childhood may also be an etiological factor in TMDs (Harness & Donlon, 1988; Harness, Donlon, & Eversole, 1990). Studies suggest that patients with histories of abuse are likely to present with a variety of physical and psychological problems (Browne & Finkelhor, 1986; Cunningham, Pearce, & Pearce, 1988). The patient with a TMD who repeatedly seeks care or who complains of a wide spectrum of symptoms, despite lack of clear pathophysiology, may have a complex, undiagnosed medical condition (Aaron, Burke, & Buchwald, 2000). Alternatively, these behaviors may represent a disguised form of help seeking (Drossman et al., 1990).

The important point for our discussion is that practitioners must be alert to the possibility that a patient is not going to respond to a dental or behavioral treatment in the ways outlined below. Instead, biofeedback may serve as a "Trojan horse" (Wickramsekera, 1988). Many patients view biofeedback as a medical treatment and not strictly a psychological treatment. Therefore, it may attract those patients who would otherwise reject psychological interpretations for their symptoms. However, once such a patient is in the office, the rapport established between provider and patient may allow the patient an opportunity to discuss his or her traumatic past. Prudent clinicians need training to evaluate and treat such problems, or need to refer such patients to someone who can.

ASSESSMENT

The comprehensive assessment of a patient with a suspected TMD has several elements (Jagger, Bates, & Kopp, 1994):

- A history of current complaints and symptoms, including medical and dental history. The impact of the symptoms on activities of daily living and emotional functioning should also be assessed.
- Physical examination consisting of measures of range of motion of the mandible, palpation of the TMJ and masticatory muscles, auscultation of the TMJ for joint sounds, and observation of opening and closing patterns. The examination should also rule out ongoing dental disease, periodontal disease, or other diseases and disorders of the oral cavity.
- Imaging of the TMJ to rule out gross pathology in the joint.
- Identification of psychosocial stressors and other psychological factors that influence the current problem and can affect a patient's response to treatment.

Self-report measures for pain are both useful and inexpensive (Karoly & Jensen, 1987). Self-report measures of symptoms specific to TMDs (e.g., the TMJ Scale; Levitt, Lundeen, & McKinney, 1987) may also be useful. TMD-related behaviors and symptoms (such as clenching, grinding, joint mobility, and noise) should be assessed cautiously, because patients are often initially unaware of their parafunctional behaviors (Glaros & Glass, 1993). As patients become more aware of their parafunctional behaviors, they may report more of these behaviors. This increase may reflect greater awareness of the behaviors, but not unsuccessful treatment. In addition, the definitions of some behaviors may differ from patient to patient. For example, the level of activity that qualifies as "clenching" for one patient may be different in another patient. Definitions of parafunctional activities that are less open to interpretation should be used whenever possible (e.g., "tooth contact" rather than "clenching").

Psychophysiological devices that detect EMG activity relevant to parafunctional clenching and grinding are increasingly available to biofeedback practitioners. Some devices will store cumulative data over several hours, and others will provide ongoing feedback without data storage. Unfortunately, most devices for monitoring EMG activity are visually obvious and frequently difficult to use. The social consequences of wearing such devices may limit their acceptability for use during the day, although patients may be more willing to use them during sleep. Thus checking the effects of treatment for daytime clenching typically involves only self-report measures.

TREATMENT

Treatments for TMDs typically involve one or more elements, including home care, dental techniques, medications, and behavioral interventions. The selection from among and within these elements depends on the information obtained during the comprehensive assessment and should be individualized for each patient (Fricton, 1995).

Patients increasingly obtain information on TMDs from Internet-based sites, but the quality of the information obtained can vary widely (Glaros, Raamah, & Edlavitch, 2001). Patients can therefore benefit from authoritative information on the different types of TMDs (Table 15.1) and the relationship of proposed treatments to their conditions. This information can also increase the willingness of patients to participate actively in effective behaviorally based treatments.

Home Care

Patients with TMDs benefit from instruction in the biomechanics of the TMJ and from encouragement to avoid parafunctional behaviors, such as clenching, grinding, gum chew-

TABLE 15.1. Main Diagnostic Categories for TMDs

Diagnostic category	Major symptoms
Myofascial pain (with/without limited opening)	Pain to palpation in three or more of 20 muscle sites; limited movement and stiffness in the muscles
Disc displacement (with reduction; without reduction and with/without limited opening)	Clicking/popping sounds in the TMJ on opening and closing; difficulty opening/closing now or in the past
Arthralgia; Arthritis/arthrosis	Pain in the TMJ; evidence of degenerative change in the TMJ as assessed by auscultation or imaging, with/without pain

Data from Dworkin and LeResche (1992).

ing, fingernail biting, or chewing ice. Patients, especially those with myofascial pain or arthralgia, may be encouraged to use hot packs, cold packs, over-the-counter analgesics, massage, and stretching exercises to relieve their pain. There is little scientific evidence that these latter techniques are effective, and there is little evidence that patients with TMDs are compliant with suggestions to use these techniques.

Dental Techniques

The most common dental treatment for TMDs is a hard *interocclusal appliance* or mouth guard called an "intraoral splint" that covers the maxillary or mandibular teeth. The device prevents grinding behavior from causing additional damage to the teeth, but does not always reduce the amount of grinding. Theoretically, splints reduce masticatory muscle activity (Clark, Beemsterboer, Solberg, & Rugh, 1979) and spread the forces associated with the remaining activity over a larger area of the teeth. However, more recent EMG studies suggest that deliberate contact with a splint can increase masticatory muscle activity (Lobbezoo, Van der Glas, Van Kampen, & Bosman, 1993; Roark, Glaros, & O'Mahony, in press). Perhaps the purported efficacy of interocclusal appliances is based on their "cueing" function. That is, these splints may remind patients with TMDs to relax the masticatory muscles and avoid parafunctional activity.

Occlusal adjustment treatment involves *equilibration*, or adjustment of the fit between the upper and lower teeth. Dentists accomplish this by selectively grinding the teeth to fit better. However, research indicates that occlusal factors do not typically contribute to the etiology of TMDs and occlusal adjustments are seldom needed (Clark et al., 1999). Since the effects of equilibration are not reversible, current recommendations strongly discourage its use (see the Web site of the National Institute of Dental and Craniofacial Research, given at the start of this chapter).

Medications

Both nonsteroidal antiinflammatory drugs (NSAIDs) and tricyclic antidepressants (in low doses) can be used to treat TMD-related pain (Dionne, 1995). However, the use of NSAIDs increases the risk of gastrointestinal disorders. Benzodiazepines and muscle relaxants are commonly used by practitioners (Glass, Glaros, & McGlynn, 1993), but research provides little evidence that they are effective in reducing TMD-related pain (DeNucci, Sobiski, & Dionne, 1998).

Behavioral Interventions

Behavioral treatments include biofeedback-based strategies for relaxation, alarm systems, cognitive-behavioral/stress management programs, and habit reversal. A few studies have showed that *massed practice*, which is deliberate and repeated jaw clenching, may reduce subsequent nocturnal, EMG-measured jaw activity (Rugh & Solberg, 1974). Unfortunately, the procedure also exposes patients to the risk of broken teeth, increased pain, and more severe TMDs. We cannot recommend this procedure, considering the limited evidence for it and its aversive nature.

Biofeedback-Based Strategies for Relaxation

A meta-analysis of biofeedback-based treatments for TMDs shows that the treatments are effective and that the effects are long-lasting (Crider & Glaros, 1999). Crider and Glaros (1999) also reported that for each of the measures reported in Table 15.2, follow-up data showed maintenance of gains or a continued improvement. For the studies reviewed by Crider and Glaros (1999), follow-up periods lasted as long as 2 years.

The most common sites for biofeedback involve the masseter, temporalis, or frontal areas, combined with other relaxation procedures or stress management (Glass et al., 1993). Treatment typically ranges from 6 to 12 sessions. Many patients need to learn to position the jaw and teeth properly. They also need to learn how mild, sustained tooth contact increases EMG activity in the temporalis and masseter muscles. Learning these skills helps patients progress quickly.

Another view focuses on the lateral pterygoids as the muscles of interest. Scott and Lundeen (1980) showed that overuse of these muscles through excessive protrusion can produce pain patterns identical to those often reported by patients with TMDs. Furthermore, during physical examination with these patients, these muscles are often highly sensitive to palpation. Gevirtz (1990) has described an intraoral EMG device for recording from these hard-to-reach muscles.

The mechanism by which biofeedback works is not clearly understood. Studies show that patients with TMDs receiving biofeedback typically show decreases in facial muscle activity and decreases in self-reported pain (e.g., Burdette & Gale, 1988). One hypothesis suggests that biofeedback works directly by promoting decreased EMG activity, which in turn is responsible for the reduction in self-reported pain. The assumption of high baseline levels of EMG activity has mixed experimental support (Dahlström, Carlsson, Gale, & Jansson, 1985; Glaros, 1996; Kapel et al., 1989; Rao & Glaros, 1979). Similarly, some studies have found that patients with TMDs are more responsive to stressors in the facial and masticatory muscles, than in other physiological response systems (Kapel et al., 1989; Flor, Birbaumer, Schugens, & Lutzenberger, 1992); other studies have not obtained such findings (Intrieri et al., 1994). Although the evidence strongly indicates that biofeedback reduces the EMG activity in tar-

TABLE 15.2. Summary of Meta-Analysis of Biofeedback-Based
Treatments for TMDs

	Experimental groups	Control groups
Measures of pain (effect size)	1.04	0.47
Percent improved	68.6%	34.7%
Examination results (effect size)	1.33	0.26

Note. Data from Crider and Glaros (1999).

geted muscles, pre- to posttreatment changes in EMG activity are not correlated with the degree of clinical improvement (Burdette & Gale, 1988; Dahlström, Carlsson, Gale, & Jansson, 1984).

A second hypothesis states that EMG biofeedback is effective because it enhances awareness of facial and masticatory muscle activity and thereby improves patients' ability to detect, label, and voluntarily reduce muscle tension before it reaches uncomfortably high levels. Reduction of masseter and temporalis activity is typically accompanied by separation of the posterior teeth (Rugh & Drago, 1981). If patients acquire better awareness and control of these muscles and keep their teeth separated, they may avoid low-level parafunctional activity that can, by itself, produce myofascial pain and arthralgia (Glaros et al., 1998a, 1998b, 2000).

A third hypothesis proposes that EMG biofeedback is effective because it alters patients' perceptions of control over their symptoms (Hijzen, Slangen, & Van Houweligen, 1986; Stenn, Mothersill, & Brooke, 1979). Success in learning to regulate EMG activity helps patients adopt a more generalized belief in their ability to manage their psychophysiological states, which in turn leads patients to initiate and persist in efforts to cope with stressors, and with subsequent psychophysiological reactions that may be associated with TMDs. Unfortunately, direct tests of this hypothesis have not been reported, although studies of patients with headache (Rokicki et al., 1997) provide indirect support for this approach.

Alarm Systems

A *nocturnal alarm system* may help patients who clench and/or grind during sleep. A nocturnal alarm monitors EMG activity from a masseter or temporalis muscle as the patient sleeps. An alarm sounds when EMG activity exceeds a threshold (frequently set at 20 microvolts) for a specified time, or when a certain number of suprathreshold EMG events occur within a brief period. During treatment with nocturnal alarms, patients typically show reductions in nocturnal EMG events, particularly when sounding of the alarm is associated with a task that requires wakefulness (Cassisi, McGlynn, & Belles, 1987). Follow-up data suggest that the efficacy of nocturnal alarms may be limited to the active treatment period (see also Hudzinski & Walters, 1986; Cassisi & McGlynn, 1988; Hudzinski & Lawrence, 1992). An intermittent schedule for biofeedback may produce more enduring results (Hudzinski & Walters, 1986).

The use of alarm systems may result in sleep disturbance, at least until the procedures significantly suppress the nocturnal bruxing activity. Some patients may experience rebound effects. Thus, after stopping the use of the alarm system, patients may experience higher levels of clenching or grinding (Cassisi et al., 1987). Practitioners need to be aware that most commercially available devices for nocturnal monitoring of TMD-relevant EMG activity cannot discriminate parafunctional clenching and grinding from normal swallowing or gross motor activities that may occur during sleep (e.g., turning over in bed). One can usually monitor from only one EMG site with a single device, and it is difficult to assess the meaningfulness of the data obtained by such devices (Biedermann, 1984; Burdette & Gale, 1990; Hatch, Prihoda, & Moore, 1992).

Clark, Koyano, and Browne (1993) reported on the use of mild electrical shock to the upper lip as the contingent feedback. When this system was used during sleep, heart rate and respiration did not change, but there was considerable reduction of activity of masticatory muscles. Data on the endurance of the effect are not available.

Cognitive-Behavioral / Stress Management Programs

Cognitive-behavioral and stress management programs utilize a variety of techniques to help patients identify cognitive, behavioral, and environmental triggers for pain, to develop strategies for coping more effectively with pain and its consequences, and to reduce the number and impact of the triggers for pain. Several studies have examined the utility of cognitive-behavioral and stress management programs for TMDs. Crider and Glaros (1999) found little evidence that combining stress management techniques with EMG biofeedback training was superior to biofeedback alone (cf. Olson & Malow, 1987). Cognitive-behavioral techniques alone can reduce TMD pain, but they do not appear to be superior to biofeedback alone (Mishra, Gatchel, & Gardea, 2000). Since TMDs can be chronic disorders, some patients may have high levels of psychological disturbance. The addition of cognitive components to their treatment regimen may be especially helpful to these distressed individuals (Turk, Rudy, Kubinski, Zaki, & Greco, 1996).

Habit Reversal

Habit reversal (Azrin & Nunn, 1973; Miltenberger, Fuqua, & McKinley, 1985) may be a useful technique for managing daytime clenching. Habit reversal training consists of three main steps:

1. *Making patients more aware of the unwanted behavior.* In the case of TMDs, frequent contact via pagers, possibly supplemented by diary keeping, could be used to increase the patients' awareness of parafunctions.
2. *Developing an alternative to the unwanted behavior.* For patients with TMDs, the alternative to parafunctional tooth contact would be relaxation of the masticatory muscles and subsequent elimination of contact. A variety of techniques could be used to teach such skills, including relaxation training and biofeedback.
3. *Substituting the alternative behavior for the unwanted behavior.* Each time patients are paged or become aware that their muscles are becoming tight or their teeth are touching unnecessarily, they can substitute masticatory muscle relaxation as needed. As patients improve in their ability to detect and avoid episodes of parafunctional tooth contact, their pain and discomfort should diminish.

Preliminary work using this technique suggests that habit reversal techniques can effectively reduce facial pain at potentially low cost (Gramling, Neblett, Grayson, & Townsend, 1996; Kim, Glaros, & Lausten, 2002; Peterson, Dixon, Talcott, & Kelleher, 1993).

A STRATEGY FOR TREATING THE PATIENT WITH A TMD

Our approach to treating the patient with a TMD involves stepped care, beginning with assessment and moving to various treatment modalities. Available data show that biofeedback-based treatments are effective in the management of TMD-related pain that is not related to another medical or dental condition. There is no evidence that biofeedback-based treatments are effective with patients who complain only of disc displacement or degenerative joint disease. Accordingly, our discussion focuses on the myofascial pain and arthralgia of TMD. The following outline serves as a guide for each segment of assessment and treatment. We emphasize biofeedback-based treatments below, but there is evidence that combined behavioral and dental treatments may be more effective than either type individually (Turk, Zaki, & Rudy, 1993). We again urge biofeedback practitioners to develop effective professional collaborations with dentists, so that patients can benefit from their combined efforts.

   I. General assessment.
      A. Rule out other medical factors (Glaros & Glass, 1993).
      B. Obtain dental consultation to assess the condition of the TMJ and masticatory musculature. If information from the dentist does not include information about

the patient's response to muscle and TMJ palpation, ask the dentist to perform this evaluation, or consider performing palpation yourself if you have proper credentials and training. See Dworkin and LeResche (1992) for specific directions for performing such palpations.

    C. Obtain a detailed history of the condition, including prior treatments.

    D. Assess psychological, psychophysiological, and behavioral patterns that might be salient.

    E. Obtain relevant self-monitoring data, including daytime logs of clenching or presleep cognitive logs that target worrying, *ruminative thinking*, and dysfunctional cognitions.

II. Psychosocial and behavioral assessment.

    Assess and determine the amount of:

    A. Depression.

    B. Sleep disturbance, including sleep-onset and sleep-maintenance insomnia.

    C. Obsessive worrying or ruminative thinking.

    D. Anxiety.

    E. Daily/weekly life stressors.

    F. Parafunctional clenching and grinding.

    G. Other parafunctional oral habits, such as chewing ice, biting fingernails, chewing gum, biting on the inside of the cheek, and chewing pencil tip erasers.

    H. Adequacy of skills to cope with situational stressors.

    I. Reinforcers for pain.

    J. The patient's attributions about symptoms and motivation for treatment. Patients may hold the belief that their symptoms are best treated by a dentist or physician. Some such patients may view a referral to a biofeedback provider as evidence that their dentist or physician does not take their complaints seriously, and they may be poorly motivated to participate in a biofeedback treatment program. The assessment techniques (see below) may help shape their beliefs about TMJ dysfunction versus occlusion versus psychophysiological muscle habits and reactivity to stress.

    K. Other relevant factors.

III. Psychophysiological assessment.

    The goal of psychophysiological assessment is to detect salient modalities for treatment and to demonstrate to patients their physiological reactions to individual stressors. Psychophysiological reactivity may be greater to situations and cognitions identified by the patient as stressful (Ohrbach et al., 1998). Thus appropriate individual stressors should be incorporated into an assessment protocol, and sole reliance on a standardized protocol should be avoided.

    A. Recording from at least two muscle placement sites, preferably the masticatory muscles.

    B. Resting baseline assessment of facial and head muscles while reclining, sitting up, during manual tasks, and so on.

    C. Assessment of reactivity and recovery of facial and head muscles during office stress simulation.

    D. If appropriate, sleep-time assessment, including nocturnal activity frequency, amplitudes, durations, and time of night.

IV. Patient education: Setting the stage for treatment.

    Confirm that the patient understands the basics of the explanation for the pain syndrome. Assure that the patient has an accurate understanding, based on the role of muscle hyperactivity and/or trigger point models. Patients often benefit from a demonstration of the impact of relaxation, tooth contact, and moderate clenching on the activity of the masticatory muscles. A patient must "think muscle"! Assess understanding by asking the patient to repeat the rationale for treatment. There will be limited or no treatment success if the patient continues to believe inaccurately that the pain is caused by a deteriorating jaw joint or poor occlusion rather than muscle activity.

   A. Describe the normal anatomy and physiology of the TMJ and associated muscles.

   B. Describe the patient's data about the physical state of the TMJ and muscles.

   C. Describe the effects of stress and parafunctional activities on the TMJ and muscles.

   D. Describe the relationship between the assessment data and the proposed treatment.

   E. Describe proposed treatment, and provide take-home pamphlets and other informational sources. Patient education brochures are available in both print and electronic versions from the National Institute of Dental and Craniofacial Research.

   F. Assess the patient's understanding of the disorder at the start of treatment and periodically during treatment. The patient should have a working model in mind for each treatment phase.

V. Initial treatment.

   A. Have dentist fabricate intraoral splint, if appropriate. Emphasize the utility of the splint as a device to remind the patient not to touch his or her teeth and to relax the masticatory musculature.

   B. Use analgesics (primarily for arthralgia) and/or tricyclic antidepressants (primarily for muscle pain), if appropriate (Pettengill & Reisner-Keller, 1997).

   C. Demonstrate effects of parafunctional activities on masticatory muscles. Demonstrate that tooth contact, even at very low levels, increases the activity of the masticatory muscles.

   D. Begin office-based EMG feedback from masseter and/or temporalis placements. Include resting, stressor, and activity reactivity and recovery. Include relaxation procedures for daily use. Consider the use of relaxation tapes.

      Standard electrode placements for the temporalis and masseter have been described by Kawazoe, Kotani, and Hamada (1979) and Fridlund and Cacioppo (1986), respectively. Use the anterior portion of a temporalis muscle. If asymmetry is suspected, consider two channels with one set of electrodes on each side. Teach the patient to find jaw positions that maximize relaxation of the masticatory muscles. Instruct the patient to slowly open his or her mouth, as if to eat a small piece of food. This usually produces the lowest EMG readings. Then use other maneuvers until the patient can easily relax the jaw.

      Use feedback thresholds to help the patient achieve very low levels of muscle activity in this region. For patients who have considerable difficulty identifying muscle tension, instruct them to use tooth contact as a surrogate for increased activity in the masticatory muscles (i.e., inform patients that tooth contact or "setting" of the jaw is the same as increased muscle activity). As patients learn to identify tooth contact episodes, ask patients to increase their focus directly on muscle sensations.

VI. Second-stage treatment if the first stage is not adequate.

   A. Cognitive therapies focusing on coping strategies for pain and on anger management.

   B. More EMG feedback sessions, incorporating additional facial and cervical muscles.

Cognitive therapies are often used for selected patients for whom the preceding treatments were not satisfactory. Focusing on issues of anger management, assertion, and avoiding confrontation is often critical in treating people with muscle tension disorders. Help patients become aware of and change dysfunctional beliefs about not being assertive or angry. This can allow for gradual changes in behavior and reduce chronic self-deprecating rumination. The use of these procedures requires proper professional credentials and training.

Patients are often seeing other treating professionals at the same time you are treating them. For example, patients are often in treatment with chiropractors or physical therapists when they come for biofeedback. However, other therapies may minimize or negate the effects of biofeedback-based treatments. Discussions with the other treating professionals and coordination of treatment are often prudent.

VII. Third-stage treatment if the second stage is not adequate.
   A. More extensive cognitive therapy.
   B. Alarm system, if appropriate.
   C. Reevaluation of presenting complaints.

When the treatments above are insufficient, seriously reconsider the initial diagnosis of TMD or reconsider the treatments. For example, patients with TMDs may also have concurrent medical conditions such as fibromyalgia. Referral to a physician for further evaluation may be warranted. Alternatively, examine more closely the possible roles of dysfunctional family or couple relationships, prior sexual and physical abuse, and *secondary gain*.

CONCLUSION

Biofeedback and other applied psychophysiological therapies have a place in the treatment of TMDs. Working closely with dentists and other health care professionals is critical to increase treatment effectiveness. This chapter emphasizes the importance of identifying proposed mechanisms that play an important role in the etiology of TMD symptoms, and of matching treatments to these mechanisms. Research suggests that the behavioral and psychological interventions presented in this chapter can be effective in treating these patients. Most patients will experience considerable relief from their symptoms if they conscientiously use these techniques.

GLOSSARY

ARTICULAR DISC. A dense fibrous connective tissue located between the *articular fossa* and the *condyle* of the mandible. Intermittent displacement of the disc can produce clicking or popping sounds when the jaw opens or closes, and a permanent displacement can make it impossible for the jaw to open fully or to close fully.

ARTICULAR FOSSA. The TMJ "socket" part of the temporal bone.

CONDYLES. Bony structures arising from the U-shaped mandible. The "ball" part of the TMJ. Located directly in front of the ears.

DIGASTRIC MUSCLES. Raise hyoid bone and base of tongue, and lower mandible.

EQUILIBRATION. Adjustment of the *occlusion* ("bite") between the upper and lower teeth by selective grinding of the teeth.

EXTRAFUSAL MUSCLE FIBERS. Ordinary muscle fibers.

HABIT REVERSAL. A behavioral therapy in which the person detects the preclench state, substitutes an incompatible behavior in place of clenching, and overlearns this response in every situation where clenching might occur. It is a useful technique for managing daytime clenching.

HYOID MUSCLES. Muscles that control the hyoid bone—the horseshoe-shaped bone at the base of the tongue. These muscles include the stylohyoid, thryrohyoid, and geniohyoid. These muscles draw the hyoid bone upward and backward, depress the hyoid bone and elevate the larynx, and elevate the hyoid bone, respectively.

INTEROCCLUSAL APPLIANCE. An orthotic device or mouth guard called an "intraoral splint" covering the *maxillary* or *mandibular teeth*. Intended to protect the teeth from wear from grinding ("bruxism"), and/or to reduce TMJ and masticatory muscle pain.

MANDIBULAR TEETH. Teeth of the lower jaw (mandible).

MASSED PRACTICE (or MASSED NEGATIVE PRACTICE). A behavioral therapy involving intentionally engaging in the undesired behavior under voluntary control (e.g., clenching) to increase awareness and help eliminate it. An aversive and risky procedure, not recommended here.

MASSETER MUSCLES. Square or rectangular shaped muscles that originate on the zygomatic arches (i.e., cheekbones) and extend downward and slightly backward to insert on the inferior border of the mandible, just ahead of the mandibular angles. These muscles lift the mandible.

MAXILLARY TEETH. Teeth of the upper jaw (maxilla).

NOCTURNAL ALARM SYSTEMS. A system providing sleep interruption biofeedback from a masseter and/or temporalis muscle, with a loud auditory stimulus contingent on clenching and grinding of teeth when it exceeds a preset threshold of intensity, duration, and/or frequency. Potentially useful, but with limitations.

OCCLUSION. Dental bite or alignment of maxillary and mandibular teeth when one closes the jaw or makes functional contact. "Occlusal disharmony" or "malocclusion" means improper or bad bite.

PARAFUNCTIONAL ACTIVITY. Clenching and grinding of teeth, or chewing of materials other than food. Nonfunctional.

PTERYGOID MUSCLES. Two pairs of muscles (medial or internal pterygoid and lateral or external pterygoid) controlling jaw movements. Accessible intraorally to palpation. The lateral pterygoid muscles assist in opening the mandible (jaw) by pulling the head of the mandible forward. They also protrude the mandible and move it to either side. The medial pterygoid muscles close the jaw and assist in lateral movements.

RUMINATIVE THINKING. Cognitive preoccupation with one or more ideas or thoughts, and difficulty dismissing or stopping them.

SECONDARY GAIN. Advantages that a person gets from being ill. Examples are attention from others, being cared for, and avoiding responsibilities. People are often unaware of this as a potential contributing factor in maintaining their symptoms and disorders. Should not be confused with malingering.

STERNOCLEIDOMASTOID MUSCLES. Muscles connecting the sternum (breastbone) and the clavicle (collar bone) to the mastoid process of the temporal bone at the nuchal line of the occipital bone (back of the lower part of the ear). These rotate and extend the head, and flex the vertebral column.

TEMPORALIS MUSCLES. Large flat muscles that originate on the lateral surfaces of the skull at the temporal bones. These muscles extend downward under the zygomatic arches (i.e., cheekbones) and taper to narrow bands where they insert into the coronoid processes of the mandible. These muscles lift the mandible upward.

NOTE

1. The outlier in the control group was contacted several months after her participation in the study. She reported noticing sensations of soreness and tightness in the face and head about a month after she completed the study. A change to a less stressful working environment was reportedly completely successful in eliminating her pain.

REFERENCES

Aaron, L. A., Burke, M. M., & Buchwald, D. (2000). Overlapping conditions among patients with chronic fatigue syndrome, fibromyalgia, and temporomandibular disorder. *Archives of Internal Medicine, 160,* 221–227.

Azrin, N. H., & Nunn, R. G. (1973). Habit reversal: A method of eliminating nervous habits and tic. *Behaviour Research and Therapy, 11,* 619–628.

Bell, W. (1986). *Temporomandibular disorders: Classification, diagnosis, management.* Chicago: Year Book Medical.

Biedermann, H.-J. (1984). Comments on the reliability of muscle activity comparisons in EMG biofeedback research with back pain patients. *Biofeedback and Self-Regulation, 9,* 451–458.

Browne, A., & Finkelhor, D. (1986). Impact of child sexual abuse: A review of the research. *Psychological Bulletin, 99,* 66–77.

Burdette, B. H., & Gale, E. N. (1988). The effects of treatment on masticatory muscle activity and mandibular posture in myofascial pain-dysfunction patients. *Journal of Dental Research, 67,* 112–130.

Burdette, B. H., & Gale, E. N. (1990). Reliability of surface electromyography of the masseteric and anterior temporal areas. *Archives of Oral Biology, 35,* 747–751.

Carlson, C., Okeson, J., Falace, D., Nitz, A., & Lindroth, J. (1993). Reduction of pain and EMG activity in the masseter region by trapezius trigger point injection. *Pain, 55,* 397–400.

Cassisi, J. E., & McGlynn, F. D. (1988). Effects of EMG-activated nocturnal alarms on nocturnal bruxing. *Behavior Therapy, 19,* 133–142.

Cassisi, J. E., McGlynn, F. D., & Belles, D. R. (1987). EMG-activated feedback alarms for the treatment of nocturnal bruxism: Current status and future directions. *Biofeedback and Self-Regulation, 12,* 13–30.

Clark, G. T., Beemsterboer, P. L., Solberg, W. K., & Rugh, J. D. (1979). Nocturnal electromyofascial evaluation of myofascial pain dysfunction in patients undergoing occlusal therapy. *Journal of the American Dental Association, 99,* 607–611.

Clark, G. T., Koyano, K., & Browne, P. (1993). Oral motor disorder in humans. *California Dentistry Association, 21*(1), 19–30.

Clark, G. T., Rugh, J. D., & Handelman, S. L. (1980). Nocturnal masseter muscle activity and urinary catecholamine levels in bruxers. *Journal of Dental Research, 59,* 1571–1576.

Clark, G. T., Rugh, J. D., Handelman, S. L., & Beemsterboer, P. L. (1977). Stress perception and nocturnal muscle activity. *Journal of Dental Research, 56*(Special Issue B), B161.

Clark, G. T., Tsukiyama, Y., Baba, K., & Watanabe, T. (1999). Sixty-years of experimental occlusal interference studies: What have we learned? *Journal of Prosthetic Dentistry, 82,* 704–713.

Crider, A. B., & Glaros, A. G. (1999). A meta-analysis of EMG biofeedback treatment of temporomandibular disorders. *Journal of Orofacial Pain, 13,* 29–37.

Cunningham, J., Pearce, T., & Pearce, P. (1988). Childhood sexual abuse and medical complaints in adult women. *Journal of Interpersonal Violence, 3*(2), 131–134.

Dahlström, L., Carlsson, S. G., Gale, E. M., & Jansson, T. G. (1984). Clinical and electromyographic effects of biofeedback training in mandibular dysfunction. *Biofeedback and Self-Regulation, 9,* 37–47.

Dahlström, L., Carlsson, S. G., Gale, E. M., & Jansson, T. G. (1985). Stress-induced muscular activity in mandibular dysfunction: Effects of biofeedback training. *Journal of Behavioral Medicine, 8,* 191–200.

Dahlström, L., Widmark, G., & Carlsson, S. G. (1997). Cognitive-behavioral profiles among different categories of orofacial pain patients: Diagnostic and treatment implications. *European Journal of Oral Science, 105,* 377–383.

DeNucci, D. J., Sobiski, C., & Dionne, R.A. (1998). Triazolam improves sleep but fails to alter pain in TMD patients. *Journal of Orofacial Pain, 12,* 116–123.

Dionne, R. A. (1995). Pharmacologic treatments for temporomandibular disorders. In B. Sessle, P. S. Bryant, & R. A. Dionne (Eds.), *Progress in pain research and management: Vol. 4. Temporomandibular disorders and related pain conditions.* Seattle, WA: IASP Press.

Drossman, D., Leserman, J., Nachman, G., Li, Z., Gluck, H., Toomey, T., & Mitchell, C. (1990). Sexual and physical abuse among women with functional and organic gastrointestinal disorders. *Annals of Behavioral Medicine, 113,* 828–833.

Dworkin, S. F., & LeResche, L. (Eds.). (1992). Research diagnostic criteria for temporomandibular disorders: Review, criteria, examinations and specifications, critique. *Journal of Craniomandibular Disorders: Facial and Oral Pain, 6,* 301–355.

Flor, H., Birbaumer, N., Schugens, M., & Lutzenberger, W. (1992). Symptom specific psychophysiological responses in chronic pain patients. *Psychophysiology, 29,* 452–460.

Flor, H., Birbaumer, N., Schulte, W., & Roos, R. (1991). Stress-related electromyographic responses in patients with chronic temporomandibular pain. *Pain, 46,* 145–152.

Fricton, J. R. (1995). Prevention and risk–benefit of early treatment for temporomandibular disorders. In B. Sessle, P. S. Bryant, & R. A. Dionne (Eds.), *Progress in pain research and management: Vol. 4. Temporomandibular disorders and related pain conditions*. Seattle, WA: IASP Press.

Fricton, J. R., & Dubner, R. (Eds.). (1995). *Advances in pain research and therapy: Vol. 21. Orofacial pain and temporomandibular disorders*. New York: Raven Press.

Fricton, J. R., & Schiffman, E. L. (1995). Epidemiology of temporomandibular disorders. In J. R. Fricton & R. Dubner (Eds.), *Advances in pain research and therapy: Vol. 21. Orofacial pain and temporomandibular disorders*. New York: Raven Press.

Fridlund, A. J., & Cacioppo, J. T. (1986). Guidelines for human electromyographic research. *Psychophysiology*, 23, 567–589.

Funch, D. P., & Gale, E. N. (1980). Factors associated with nocturnal bruxism and its treatment. *Journal of Behavioral Medicine*, 3, 385–397.

Gatchel, R. J., Garofalo, J. P., Ellis, E., & Holt, C. (1996). Major psychological disorders in acute and chronic TMD: An initial examination. *Journal of the American Dental Association*, 127, 1365–1374.

Gevirtz, R. (1990). Recording the lateral pterygoid in MPD patients. *Biofeedback*, 18(1), 45–47.

Glaros, A. G. (1996). Awareness of physiological responding under stress and non-stress conditions in temporomandibular disorders. *Biofeedback and Self-Regulation*, 12, 261–272.

Glaros, A. G., Baharloo, L., & Glass, E. G. (1998a). Effect of parafunctional clenching and estrogen on temporomandibular disorder pain. *Journal of Craniomandibular Practice*, 16, 78–83.

Glaros, A. G., & Burton, E. (2001). Relationship of effort in parafunctional activity to self-reported pain in temporomandibular disorder. *Journal of Dental Research*, 80, 1200.

Glaros, A. G., Forbes, M., Shanker, J., & Glass, E. G. (2000). Effect of parafunctional clenching on temporomandibular disorder pain and proprioceptive awareness. *Journal of Craniomandibular Practice*, 18, 198–204.

Glaros, A. G., & Glass, E. G. (1993). Temporomandibular disorders. In R. Gatchel & E. Blanchard (Eds.), *Psychophysiological disorders*. Washington, DC: American Psychological Association.

Glaros, A. G., Glass, E. G., & Hayden, W. J. (1995). History of treatment received by TMD patients: A preliminary investigation. *Journal of Orofacial Pain*, 9, 147–151.

Glaros, A. G., & Lausten, L. (2002). Prospective assessment of parafunctional activity in temporomandibular disorder patients. *Journal of Dental Research*, 81, A-458.

Glaros, A. G., Raamah, D., & Edlavitch, S. A. (2001). Searching the Internet for information on temporomandibular disorders. *Journal of Dental Research*, 80, 156.

Glaros, A. G., Tabacchi, K. N., & Glass, E. G. (1998b). Effect of parafunctional clenching on temporomandibular disorder pain. *Journal of Orofacial Pain*, 12, 145–152.

Glass, E. G., Glaros, A. G., & McGlynn, F. D. (1993). Myofascial pain dysfunction: Treatments used by ADA members. *Journal of Craniomandibular Practice*, 11, 25–29.

Gramling, S. E., Neblett, J., Grayson, R., & Townsend, D. (1996). Temporomandibular disorder: Efficacy of an oral habit reversal treatment program. *Journal of Behavior Therapy and Experimental Psychiatry*, 27, 245–255.

Greene, C. S., & Laskin, D. M. (2000). Temporomandibular disorders: Moving from a dentally based to a medically based model. *Journal of Dental Research*, 79, 1736–1739.

Haggerty, C., Glaros, A. G., & Glass, E. G. (2000). Ecological momentary assessment of parafunctional clenching in temporomandibular disorder. *Journal of Dental Research*, 79, 605.

Harness, D., & Donlon, W. (1988). Cryptotrauma: The hidden wound. *Clinical Journal of Pain*, 4, 257–260.

Harness, D., Donlon, W., & Eversole, L. (1990). Comparison of clinical characteristics in myogenic, TMJ internal derangement, and atypical facial pain patients. *Clinical Journal of Pain*, 6, 4–17.

Hatch, J. P., Prihoda, T. J., & Moore, P. J. (1992). The application of generalizability theory to surface electromyographic measurements during psychophysiological stress testing: How many measurements are needed? *Biofeedback and Self-Regulation*, 17, 17–39.

Hijzen, T. H., Slangen, J. L., & Van Houweligen, H. C. (1986). Subjective, clinical and EMG effects of biofeedback and splint treatment. *Journal of Oral Rehabilitation*, 13, 529–539.

Hopper, D., Gevirtz, R., Nigl, A., & Taddey, J. (1992). Relationship between daily stress and nocturnal bruxism. *Biofeedback and Self-Regulation*, 17, 309.

Hubbard, D., & Berkoff, G. (1993). Myofascial trigger points show spontaneous needle EMG activity. *Spine*, 18, 1803–1807.

Hudzinski, L., & Lawrence, G. (1992). Effectiveness of EMG biofeedback in the treatment of nocturnal bruxism: A three-year retrospective follow-up. *Biofeedback and Self-Regulation*, 17, 312.

Hudzinski, L., & Walters, P. (1986). Use of portable electromyograms in determining and treating chronic nocturnal bruxism. *Psychophysiology*, 23, 442–443.

Intrieri, R. C., Jones, G. E., & Alcorn, J. D. (1994). Masseter muscle hyperactivity and myofascial pain dysfunction syndrome: A relationship under stress. *Journal of Behavioral Medicine*, 17, 479–500.

Jagger, R. G., Bates, J. F., & Kopp, S. (1994). *Temporomandibular joint dysfunction: The essentials.* Boston: Wright.

Kapel, L., Glaros, A. G., & McGlynn, F. D. (1989). Psychophysiological responses to stress in patients with myofascial pain dysfunction syndrome. *Journal of Behavioral Medicine, 12,* 397–406.

Karoly, P., & Jensen, M. P. (1987). *Multimethod assessment of chronic pain.* Oxford: Pergamon Press.

Kawazoe, Y., Kotani, H., & Hamada, T. (1979). Relation between integrated electromyographic activity and biting force during voluntary isometric contraction in human masticatory muscles. *Journal of Dental Research, 58,* 1440–1449.

Kight, M., Gatchel, R. J., & Wesley, L. (1999). Temporomandibular disorders: Evidence for significant overlap with psychopathology. *Health Psychology, 18,* 177–182.

Kim, N., Glaros, A. G., & Lausten, L. (2002). Effectiveness of habit awareness training for temporomandibular disorder pain. *Journal of Dental Research, 81,* A-458.

Kinney, R. K., Gatchel, R. J., Ellis, E., & Holt, C. (1992). Major psychological disorders in chronic TMD patients: Implications for successful management. *Journal of the American Dental Association, 123*(10), 49–54.

Kirveskari, P., Alanen, P., & Jamsa, T. (1992). Association between craniomandibular disorders and occlusal interferences in children. *Journal of Prosthetic Dentistry, 67,* 692–696.

Korszun, A., Hinderstein, B., & Wong, M. (1996). Comorbidity of depression with chronic facial pain and temporomandibular disorders. *Oral Surgery, Oral Medicine, Oral Pathology, Oral Radiology, and Endodontics, 82,* 496–500.

Lacey, B. C. (1950). Individual differences in somatic response patterns. *Journal of Comparative and Physiological Psychology, 43,* 338–350.

Lacey, B. C. (1967). Somatic response patterning and stress: Some revisions in activation theory. In M. H. Appley & R. Trumbull (Eds.), *Psychological stress: Issues in research.* New York: Appleton-Century-Crofts.

Laskin, D. M. (1969). Etiology of the pain–dysfunction syndrome. *Journal of the American Dental Association, 79,* 147–153.

Levitt, S. R., Lundeen, T. F., & McKinney, M. W. (1987). *The TMJ Scale manual.* Durham, NC: Pain Resource Center.

Lobbezoo, F., & Lavigne, G. J. (1997). Do bruxism and temporomandibular disorders have a cause–effect relationship? *Journal of Orofacial Pain, 11,* 15–23.

Lobbezoo, F., Van der Glas, H. W., Van Kampen, F. M. C., & Bosman, F. (1993). The effect of an occlusal stabilization splint and the mode of visual feedback on the activity balance between jaw-elevator muscles during isometric contraction. *Journal of Dental Research, 72,* 876–882.

McNulty, W., Gevirtz, R., Hubbard, D., & Berkoff, G. (1994). Needle electromyographic evaluation of trigger point response to a psychological stressor. *Psychophysiology, 31,* 313–316.

Mercuri, L. G., Olson, R. E., & Laskin, D. M. (1979). The specificity of response to experimental stress inpatients with myofascial pain dysfunction syndrome. *Journal of Dental Research, 58,* 1866–1871.

Michelotti, A., Martina, R., Russo, M., & Romeo, R. (1998). Personality characteristics of temporomandibular disorder patients using M.M.P.I. *Journal of Craniomandibular Disorders, 16,* 119–125.

Miltenberger, R. G., Fuqua, R. W., & McKinley, T. (1985). Habit reversal: Replication and component analysis. *Behavior Therapy, 16,* 39–50.

Mishra, K. D., Gatchel, R. J., & Gardea, M. A. (2000). The relative efficacy of three cognitive-behavioral treatment approaches to temporomandibular disorders. *Journal of Behavioral Medicine, 23,* 293–309.

Montgomery, G. T., & Rugh, J. D. (1987). Physiological reactions of patients with TM disorders vs. symptom-free controls on a physical stress task. *Journal of Craniomandibular Disorders: Facial and Oral Pain, 1,* 243–250.

Morris, S., Benjamin, S., Gray, R., & Bennett, D. (1997). Physical, psychiatric and social characteristics of the temporomandibular disorder pain dysfunction syndrome: The relationship of mental disorders to presentation. *British Dental Journal, 182,* 255–260.

Moss, R. A., & Adams, H. E. (1984). Physiological reactions to stress in subjects with and without myofascial pain dysfunction symptoms. *Journal of Oral Rehabilitation, 11,* 219–232.

Moss, R. A., Sult, S., & Garrett, J. C. (1984). Questionnaire evaluation of craniomandibular pain factors among college students. *Journal of Craniomandibular Practice, 2,* 364–368.

Ohrbach, R., Blascovich, J., Gale, E. N., McCall, W. D., Jr., & Dworkin, S. E. (1998). Psychophysiological assessment of stress in chronic pain: Comparisons of stressful stimuli and of response systems. *Journal of Dental Research, 77,* 1840–1850.

Okeson, J. P. (1998). *Management of temporomandibular disorders and occlusion* (4th ed.). St. Louis, MO: Mosby.

Olson, R. E., & Malow, R. M. (1987). Effects of biofeedback and psychotherapy on patients with myofascial pain dysfunction who are nonresponsive to conventional treatments. *Rehabilitation Psychology, 32,* 195–204.

Passatore, M., Grassi, C., & Filippi, G. (1985). Sympathetically-induced development of tension in jaw muscles: The possible contraction of intrafusal muscle fibers. *Pfluegers Archiv, 405,* 297–304.

Peterson, A. L., Dixon, D. C., Talcott, G. W., & Kelleher, W. J. (1993). Habit reversal treatment of temporomandibular disorders: A pilot investigation. *Journal of Behavior Therapy and Experimental Psychiatry, 24,* 49–55.

Pettengill, C. A., & Reisner-Keller, L. (1997). The use of tricyclic antidepressants for the control of orofacial pain. *Journal of Craniomandibular Practice, 15,* 53–56.

Ramfjord, S. P., & Ash, M. M. (Eds.). (1983). *Occlusion* (3rd ed.). Philadelphia: Saunders.

Rao, S. M., & Glaros, A. G. (1979). Electromyographic correlates of experimentally induced stress in diurnal bruxists and normals. *Journal of Dental Research, 58,* 1872–1878.

Roark, A. L., Glaros, A. G., & O'Mahony, A. (in press). Effects of interocclusal appliances on EMG activity during parafunctional tooth contact. *Journal of Oral Rehabilitation.*

Rokicki, L. A., Holroyd, K. A., France, C. R., Lipchik, G. L., France, J. L., & Kvaal, S. A. (1997). Change mechanisms associated with combined relaxation/EMG biofeedback training for chronic tension headache. *Applied Psychophysiology and Biofeedback, 22,* 21–41.

Rugh, J. D. (1975). *Variables involved in extinction through repeated practice therapy.* Unpublished doctoral dissertation, University of California–Santa Barbara.

Rugh, J. D., & Drago, C. J. (1981). Vertical dimension: A study of clinical rest position and jaw muscle activity. *Journal of Prosthetic Dentistry, 45,* 670–675.

Rugh, J. D., & Solberg, W. K. (1974). Identification of stressful stimuli in the natural environments using a portable biofeedback unit. In *Proceedings of the 5th Annual Meeting of the Biofeedback Research Society, Colorado Springs.* Wheat Ridge, CO: Biofeedback Research Society.

Scott, D. S., & Lundeen, T. F. (1980). Myofascial pain involving the masticatory muscles: An experimental model. *Pain, 8,* 207–215.

Seligman, D., & Pullinger, A. (1991). The role of functional occlusal relationships in temporomandibular disorders: A review. *Journal of Craniomandibular Disorders: Facial and Oral Pain, 5,* 265–276.

Sessle, B. J., Bryant, P. S., & Dionne, R. A. (Eds.). (1995). *Progress in pain research and management: Vol. 4. Temporomandibular disorders and related pain conditions.* Seattle, WA: IASP Press.

Stenn, P. G., Mothersill, K. J., & Brooke, R. I. (1979). Biofeedback and a cognitive behavioral approach to treatment of myofascial pain dysfunction syndrome. *Behavior Therapy, 10,* 29–36.

Travell, J. G., & Simons, D. G. (1983). *Myofascial pain and dysfunction: The trigger point manual.* Baltimore: Williams & Wilkins.

Turk, D. C., Rudy, T. E., Kubinski, J. A., Zaki, H. S., & Greco, C. M. (1996). Dysfunctional patients with temporomandibular disorders: Evaluating the efficacy of a tailored treatment protocol. *Journal of Consulting and Clinical Psychology, 64,* 136–146.

Turk, D., Zaki, H., & Rudy, T. (1993). Effects of intraoral appliance and biofeedback/stress management alone and in combination in treating pain and depression in patients with temporomandibular disorders. *Journal of Prosthetic Dentistry, 70,* 158–164.

Wickramasekera, I. (1988). *Clinical behavioral medicine.* New York: Plenum Press.

Wright, J., Deary, I. J., & Geissler, P. R. (1991). Depression, hassles and somatic symptoms in mandibular dysfunction syndrome patients. *Journal of Dentistry, 19,* 352–356.

Zarb, G. A., & Carlsson, G. E. (1979). *Temporomandibular joint function and dysfunction.* Copenhagen: Munksgaard.

CHAPTER 16

Raynaud's Disease and Raynaud's Phenomenon

MARK S. SCHWARTZ
KEITH SEDLACEK

DEFINITIONS, SYMPTOMS, DIAGNOSIS, AND CAUSES

Raynaud's symptoms involve spasms of arterioles and small arteries in the digits of the hands and feet. Triphasic skin color changes are classic: They involve whiteness (*blanching* or *pallor*), blueness (*cyanosis*), and redness (*rubor* or reactive *hyperemia*). (As in other chapters, italics on first use of a term indicate that the term is included in the chapter's glossary.) Some people show biphasic skin color changes involving the cyanosis and then reactive hyperemia. Occasionally, symptoms include the nose and tongue. They rarely involve the thumb. The duration of spasms ranges from minutes to hours. Cold exposure is the usual stimulus for the spasms; however, emotional and other psychological events can also provoke an attack in many patients. Estimates vary widely for the incidence of this type of stimulus.

An important distinction is between "primary Raynaud's" or "idiopathic Raynaud's" (Raynaud's disease), which has no known cause, and Raynaud's symptoms secondary to another condition, sometimes called "secondary Raynaud's" or "Raynaud's phenomenon" (RP). Examples of such conditions are *connective tissue disorders*, such as *rheumatoid arthritis* (*RA*), *systemic lupus erythematosus* (*SLE*), and most commonly *scleroderma* (*progressive systemic sclerosis*, or *PSS*). Nearly all patients with PSS experience these vasospastic episodes. Others include *mixed connective tissue disease* (*MCTD*), *Sjögren's syndrome*, *polymyositis*, and *dermatomyositis* (Coffman, 1991).

Other conditions that cause Raynaud's symptoms include *obstructive arterial diseases*, such as *thromboangitis obliterans* and *arteriosclerosis obliterans* (Coffman, 1991). Trauma, as from *traumatic vasospastic disease* (vibration-induced), is another secondary cause. *Carpal tunnel syndrome* and *thoracic outlet obstruction syndromes* are other common causes (Coffman, 1991). *Reflex sympathetic dystrophy* (*RSD*), dysproteinemias, *polycythemia*, *myxedema* or *adult hypothyroidism*, *primary pulmonary hypertension* (*PPH*), and *renal* diseases add to the list (Coffman, 1991).

Drugs can also result in the spasms and are secondary causes. Notable examples are *ergot preparations*, *methysergide*, *beta-adrenergic blocking agents* (*beta-blockers*), and *imipramine* (Coffman, 1991). Prudent nonmedical practitioners understand the necessity of proper medical examination and testing so that any underlying disorder may be found.

Raynaud's disease usually affects females from preadolescence to early middle age. The estimated ratio of females to males is about 4:1. It is characterized by (1) bilateral involvement, and (2) the presence of symptoms for at least 2 years without progression and without evidence of another cause. Occasionally, it takes longer for the underlying disease to become manifest. Some patients initially diagnosed as having idiopathic Raynaud's disease later learn that their symptoms are secondary to another disorder, which went unrecognized earlier in the history of the symptoms. *Trophic changes* in the skin and gangrene, if present at all, are minimal in persons with the primary type.

In 1862, Maurice Raynaud first defined this clinical syndrome as episodic digital ischemia provoked by cold, cyanosis, and emotion. Raynaud (1888) suggested that hyperactivity of the sympathetic nervous system (SNS) caused the increased vasoconstrictive response to cold. Current theories still include increased activity of the SNS and local faults in the digital arteries, and there is supportive evidence for each position or the combination (Coffman, 1991). Other theories of pathophysiology include *serotonin*, *platelets*, and *blood viscosity*. The theories of a general vascular abnormality cannot account for the differences in drug responses and neurogenic controls among the different circulatory beds. In conclusion, many factors may contribute to the vasospasms in digits.

TREATMENTS

There are no universally accepted medical treatments for Raynaud's disease. Stepped-care treatment and sensible first treatments involve protecting the body and extremities from cold, stopping smoking, and stopping the use of caffeine.

Advances in pharmacotherapy show promise and are part of current medical practice (Berkow & Fletcher, 1992). However, the drugs are nonspecific, and negative side effects are problematic; thus medication treatments have their limitations. A discussion of pharmacotherapy is beyond the scope of this chapter. However, we include a brief mention of several medications for interested readers. One notable example is *nifedipine*, a *calcium entry blocker* (Coffman, 1991). Others include other calcium entry blockers, *sympatholetic* agents such as *reserpine* and *guanethidine*, and *prazosin* and *thymoxamine*. Again, these drugs often have bothersome side effects that cause poor compliance or discontinuation. Others in this class have mixed or poor results, and/or intolerable side effects. See Coffman (1991) for a discussion of all these drugs and others.

We note certain types of medications because they are contraindicated for their use with Raynaud's. They induce digital vasoconstriction and may actually worsen the condition. Notable examples are beta blockers, clonidine, and ergot preparations (Berkow & Fletcher, 1992; Coffman, 1991).

Regional sympathectomy often has major drawbacks and complications. There is limited long-term success, especially for the hands. When considered at all, regional sympathectomy is usually a last resort for patients with Raynaud's disease who are suffering from progressive disability. It is contraindicated for secondary RP (Coffman, 1991), and is of "doubtful value in the primary disease" (Coffman, 1991, p. 600). However, relief may last from 1 to 2 years for the upper extremities, and there are reports of considerable and lasting benefit for *lumbar sympathectomy* to relieve the spasms in the toes (Coffman, 1991).

Well-controlled research supports the use of thermal-biofeedback-assisted treatment for idiopathic Raynaud's disease. Combining thermal biofeedback with cold stress challenges can improve both initial and long-term results. See the studies by Freedman and his colleagues (Freedman, 1987; Freedman, Ianni, & Wenig, 1983) for thermal biofeedback without and with cold stress challenges. However, including cold stress challenges is not yet a standard or common clinical practice, because of very limited access to such equipment to create the cold challenges.

To a much smaller degree than for Raynaud's disease, a few case studies and limited research support biofeedback as part of the clinical management for RP that is secondary to connective tissue disorders (Stambrook, Hamel, & Carter, 1988).

THE USEFULNESS OF THERMAL BIOFEEDBACK IN TREATING RAYNAUD'S DISEASE AND SECONDARY RP

The reduction of peripheral vasoconstriction and vasospastic attacks often lessens significantly with various forms of physiological self-regulation. Some practitioners and researchers still believe that autogenic therapy and similar relaxation techniques can be effective without biofeedback. In our view, however, biofeedback appears to result in improved greater acquisition of hand-warming skills (Freedman, Ianni, & Wenig, 1983, 1987; Freedman et al., 1983; Sedlacek & Taub, 1996).

There are several publications describing the use of thermal biofeedback and other biobehavioral therapies for Raynaud's disease (Grove & Belanger, 1983; Sedlacek, 1984, 1989; Rose & Carlson, 1987). The most convincing and best-controlled between-groups experimental study is still that by Freedman et al. (1983). This study and the follow-up reports (Freedman, 1987) over 3 years strongly support the advantage of thermal biofeedback over autogenic relaxation for treating Raynaud's disease. The ambitious treatment study employed a focal cold stimulus as part of the therapy with biofeedback. The authors reported a 32.6% reduction of vasospastic episodes in the group receiving autogenic therapy. However, there was a 66.8% reduction in the group receiving thermal biofeedback, and a 92.5% reduction in the group receiving thermal biofeedback plus the cold stress challenge. Major methodological advantages of this study included ambulatory monitoring and a 1-year initial follow-up during the same cold months in which therapy began. The results lasted at least 3 years following treatment (Freedman et al., 1983; Freedman, 1987).

By contrast, in the Raynaud's Treatment Study (RTS)—a comparison of sustained-release nifedipine and temperature biofeedback—the investigators (Thompson & RTS Investigators, 2000) concluded that the biofeedback was inferior to the sustained-release medication in treating RP. Previously, with regular nifedipine for RP, from 30% to 100% of patients had had adverse side effects (e.g., tachycardia, headache, dizziness, flushing, and edema). Because of these side effects, many of the patients had stopped using nifedipine. However, the new sustained-release formulation of nifedipine in this double-blind study of RP, 24% reported edema, 17% reported headache, and a small percentage reported flushing (8%) and tachycardia. Only 57% of participants continued to take the full 60-milligram dosage. Thus 24%, 8%, and 3%, respectively using the new sustained-release nifedipine reported edema, flushing, and tachycardia, compared with 56%, 30%, and 23%, respectively, when regular nifedipine was used in previous studies.

The RTS showed that the "new" nifedipine resulted in a 60% reduction in RP symptoms, while the biofeedback temperature feedback did not. This study showed that 67% of normal participants learned to increase finger temperature, while only 35% of participants with RP were able to satisfy successful learning criteria. (The criterion for improvement of RP was greater than a 60% reduction in RP attacks at the end of the first and second winters.) The RTS results thus differ from the successful learning seen in studies of primary and secondary Raynaud's in the laboratory (Freedman et al., 1983; Freedman, 1987) and in clinical practice (Freedman, 1987, 1991; Sedlacek & Taub, 1996).

Some qualifications of the RTS results should be noted, however. Among the causes for the disparate learning rates in the healthy normal controls versus the participants with RP were inexperienced therapists for the latter; a primitive training protocol, in which evidently only eight sessions using temperature feedback were provided; and instructions to participants with RP basically to try their own ideas on how to increase their finger temperature. There were no home charts or home temperature feedback devices, and only with the second group (cohort 2) was "coaching" allowed, because successful learning in the first cohort was less than expected. (Home temperature devices are available at a cost of from $.10 to $10–20). In addition to these problems, it appears that the biofeedback "providers" evidently had little or no clinical experience.

A second report, by Middaugh et al. (2001), has discussed some of the learning that did and did not take place in the RTS. Middaugh et al. point out that research and clinical studies (Freedman, 1987; Sedlacek & Taub, 1996) show that about two-thirds of patients with Raynaud's disease or RP learn finger temperature biofeedback skills. This is similar to the learning rate for the healthy subjects in the RTS. Furthermore, Middaugh's group notes that RTS participants with RP were instructed to use the feedback display to "increase hand temperature using mental strategies of their own choosing. No adjunctive relaxing techniques were taught" (2001, pp. 255–256).

Middaugh et al. (2001) also look at the five different RTS training sites, in which learning rates varied from 12.5% to 75%, despite use of the same research protocol. They conclude that successful learning of hand-warming skills was associated with clinic sites and coping strategies, as well as with anxiety and gender, but not with RP severity. Since the two clinics with lowest learning rates for hand warming also had the lowest success rate for electromyographic (EMG) frontalis relaxation, this suggests the laboratory environment as a major factor in the lack of learning for the participants with RP. Middaugh et al. (2001) cite Taub and School (1978), whose work showed that a "friendly" versus "impersonal" approach to teaching finger warming may be a large factor, along with the use of adjunctive techniques. The Taub and School (1978) paper discusses many of the relevant clinical training issues for biofeedback treatment of Raynaud's disease or RP.

The RTS thus apparently compared a "new" sustained-release nifedipine with a primitive temperature protocol dating from the 1980s, with little learning taking place at most biofeedback sites. As discussed in this chapter, treatment for Raynaud's needs experienced clinicians, good protocols, home practice with inexpensive thermal units, homework twice a day with reports of home finger temperature, and perhaps as many as 20–30 sessions.

In general, relevant issues and questions include the following:

1. What are the mechanisms involved in successful therapy with thermal biofeedback and other physiological self-regulatory therapies?
2. What are the mechanisms involved in focal cold stimulus challenges?
3. For which patients are thermal biofeedback therapies and other procedures needed to achieve the best therapeutic results?
4. When should a practitioner include thermal biofeedback and focal cold challenge stimuli for patients with Raynaud's disease or RP?
5. What therapeutic procedures in thermal biofeedback are more appropriate and useful than others?
6. Are there preferred therapist characteristics and skills needed to provide effective thermal biofeedback for Raynaud's disease or RP?
7. Would combinations of selected medications and biobehavioral therapies attain better results than either does alone?

GUIDELINES FOR TREATING RAYNAUD'S DISEASE OR RP

1. Practitioners should be sure that a very careful clinical interview, medical examination, and tests establish a patient's diagnosis as either Raynaud's disease or RP. They should look for environmental, physiological, and psychological factors that contribute to the vasospastic episodes. The patient should avoid vasospastic-inducing medications and other vasospastic chemicals during evaluation. Cold stimuli, environmental cold, emotional stressors, and other stressors are the common triggers of vasospastic episodes. See Table 16.1 for an outline adapted from Freedman, Lynn, and Ianni (1982).

TABLE 16.1. Interview Protocol for Raynaud's Disease/RP

1. When did your symptoms begin?
2. Please describe your symptoms.
   A. Where do they occur? Do they occur in your hands? Do they occur in one or both hands? Do they occur in your feet? Do they occur in one or both feet? Do the symptoms occur in your face? You may want to use a hand and/or foot drawing to show which digits are affected.
   B. What sequence of color changes occurs? Do they get white, blue, and red?
   C. Are these changes always the same?
   D. What do your hands, feet, or face feel like during each color change? Do they feel cold, numb, burning, tingling, and/or painful?
3. How long does a typical attack last? How long does a mild attack last? How long does your worst attack last?
4. How frequent are your attacks?
   A. In what month do you usually get most attacks? How many do you get in that month?
   B. In what month do you tend to get the fewest attacks? How many attacks occur in that month?
   C. When your problem was the worst, how often did you get attacks?
   D. When your problem was the least troublesome, how often did you get attacks?
   E. What is the longest period you recall without an attack?
   F. What is the longest period in cold weather you recall without an attack?
5. Do you wear special clothing to prevent attacks?
6. Do you regulate the room temperature to decrease attacks? At what room temperature do you feel most comfortable?
7. Assuming that you are not wearing protective clothing, what outside temperature would begin to create problems for you?
8. When you are wearing protective clothing, at what temperature do you begin to have problems?
9. In what circumstances are you likely to get attacks?
10. What do you do when you get an attack? Do you do anything *to* reduce it?
11. What kinds of events, thoughts, or feelings seem to cause an attack? Try to be specific.
12. How do you feel when you get an attack? What do you think about when you get an attack? Try to be specific.
13. Do your attacks prevent you from doing anything?
14. If you did not have these attacks, how would your life change?
15. Are you taking any medication? Are you in any treatment? Tell me about it.
16. How helpful is your treatment?
17. How helpful do you think this treatment will be?

Note. Adapted from Freedman, Lynn, and Ianni (1982). Copyright 1982 by Grune & Stratton. Adapted by permission.

2. The gender, anxiety level, and denial of clients should be considered (Middaugh et al., 2001).

3. Peripheral vascular activity and reactivity should be assessed in response to temperature, cognitive, and other stressors. Standard "stressful" cognitive tasks, such as mental arithmetic, are not stressful for all patients.

4. To evaluate results faster, a practitioner should start treatment in the late summer or early fall if cold is the main precipitating factor. This is especially important if symptoms are infrequent, are easily managed in warm weather, and respond to nonphysiological self-regulatory procedures. What if a patient requests treatment in the late winter or early spring? Should treatment be deferred for several months? Several choices are acceptable.

a. The patient can be told that treatment can begin now, but it will probably require several office visits over 1–3 months and considerable practice. The therapist should explain that the motivation to practice may be less because the patient's symptoms are much less frequent. The patient and therapist may choose to delay office visits until such time that motivation to practice is stronger. However, this is a good time to have the patient keep a self-report log for a few weeks. Such a log includes the frequency and intensity of the vasospastic episodes and precipitating factors. For example, the patient can provide to the practitioner information about cold exposure, emotional stress, nicotine use, caffeine use, and other dietary contributions to vasoconstriction. The therapist and patient can then plan for thermal biofeedback in late summer or early fall.

b. A reasonable second alternative is to have the patient begin keeping a self-report log for a few weeks, and then to introduce nonbiofeedback physiological self-regulation procedures (and cognitive stress management, if indicated). The need for practice, self-regulation, and a self-report log during these warmer months must be emphasized . The therapist should explain that the expected reduction of vasospastic episodes is probably no more than about one-third with this approach, should clarify the difficulty in evaluating progress during this period, and should discuss the possibility or probability of needing to add thermal biofeedback in the upcoming fall or winter. This compromise allows the professional to start therapy in a realistic context.

c. Third, treatment can begin with a self-report baseline, thermal biofeedback with or without a cold stress challenge, and other indicated therapies (such as stress management). Realistic explanations and expectations, as described in paragraphs a and b above, should be provided.

Professionals must be realistic with patients and with themselves that the season of the year will probably influence motivation and symptoms. Effective treatment is more than learning to warm one's extremities in the office and elsewhere. It must also be effective in response to precipitating stimuli. If emotional and stressful events precipitate many attacks, the season will be a less important factor. In this case, the third option (with emotional stimuli incorporated into the therapy program) will be the most realistic at any time of year.

5. Practitioners should gather adequate self-report data on vasospastic attacks outside the office in comparable ambient temperatures. The self-report symptom log is the major method for getting symptom data. Some experts believe that the most useful datum is the frequency of vasospastic attacks (Freedman et al., 1982). Patients must be carefully educated as to what constitutes a vasospastic episode. Many patients are surprisingly unaware of the criteria for such episodes.

6. Therapists should have the requisite personal characteristics and skills to foster comfort in the therapy procedures.

7. Practitioners should provide advice and recommendations to reduce or stop the use of caffeine, nicotine, and other vasoconstrictive substances whenever applicable (see Block, Schwartz, & Gyllenhaal, Chapter 9, this volume).

8. Ambient room temperature and humidity need to be proper and constant. Ideally, 72–74°F should be suitable. Significant fluctuations in temperature and moisture are likely to cause artifacts and other problems.

9. Drafts of all kinds should be prevented, as should any varying airflow (from vents, air conditioning, fans, or heaters) that selectively warms or cools the patient.

10. Adequate adaptation and baseline periods are required for proper assessment of thermal biofeedback. Warming occurs while a person is sitting quietly in a warmer environment after coming in from cooler outside temperatures, especially with eyes closed. Also, warming occurs after hurrying to make the appointment while sitting quietly in a calmer environment. If the adaptation and baseline periods are too short, one may observe warming during feedback that is unrelated to the feedback.

It is common for patients to show little or no warming in the first several minutes of sitting quietly. Then many patients show rapid warming, without physiological feedback or any specific relaxation procedures taught by the therapist. Without adequate adaptation and baseline periods, therapists may mistakenly think that the biofeedback experience is important for this warming. Sometimes therapists want their patients to know that such sitting and relaxing often result in warming. In such cases, providing physiological feedback after a shorter-than-ideal baseline is reasonable once or even a few times. However, an adequate adaptation period is still needed (Taub, 1977). Furthermore, this is separate from the physiological feedback that occurs after clear plateaus of skin temperature.

The duration of the adaptation and baseline periods is partly a matter of professional choice and practicality. Where was the patient before the session, and what was he or she doing? For example, a period of sitting quietly in the waiting room for 15 minutes, and a 10-minute baseline after being attached to the instruments, are often sufficient. (See Arena & Schwartz, Chapter 7, this volume, for discussion of adaptation and baseline periods.)

11. A thermal biofeedback training phase of about 15 minutes or slightly longer is probably sufficient. Much longer phases, such as 20 minutes or longer, may result in frustration and impatience. The duration should be tailored to the patient, therapist, and situation.

12. The therapist should remember that even minute amounts of perspiration on or near the thermistor site(s) may affect the temperature. Also, physiological measurement of blood flow should be considered, to control for perspiration and *thermal lag* (Freedman et al., 1982).

13. Practitioners should plan for several office sessions with, some or most employing thermal biofeedback. A total of 15–20 sessions, or even more, may be needed.

14. Practitioners should consider *bidirectional thermal biofeedback*.

15. If therapists use guided imagery to enhance relaxation and warming, they should tailor it to each patient and should monitor the patient to evaluate its usefulness.

16. Practitioners should assess the transfer of training and generalization of reduced vasoconstriction to daily-life situations.

17. Therapists should do as much as necessary and possible to increase both short-term and long-term compliance. Patients need ample motivation to comply with the many therapeutic recommendations and the duration of therapy and follow-up. Skeptical patients require more cognitive preparation to maintain compliance. Patients who are too enthusiastic and have unrealistic expectations also require special attention, to give them a realistic context for treatment.

18. Therapists should remind patients that despite the potential success of treatment, they need to continue using reasonable protective measures to minimize or avoid cold exposure. For example, they need adequate clothing and hand protection, and must avoid unnecessary direct cold exposure.

19. Therapists should get adequate self-reports of vasospastic episodes during the next cold season, comparable to the symptom baseline.

20. During the redness phase (the reactive hyperemia phase), patients can experience much pain and burning. The prudent practitioner must be aware that many patients are very hesitant about learning hand-warming skills because of the fear of exacerbating the hyperemia. This is a difficult problem. Until more research is done in this area, clinical sensitivity and careful observations are recommended.

RECENTLY PROPOSED PHYSIOLOGICAL MECHANISMS IN RAYNAUD'S DISEASE/RP AND THERMAL BIOFEEDBACK

Research by Robert Freedman and his colleagues has shed light on the physiological mechanisms involved in digital temperature changes (Freedman, 1991, 1994; Freedman et al., 1988a, 1988b; Freedman, Mayes, & Sabharwal, 1989; Freedman et al., 1991; Freedman, Keegan, Rodriguez, & Galloway, 1993). There are important implications for treatment, including with biofeedback.

The palmar surface and tips of the fingers are replete with *arteriovenous shunts* that function with the capillaries. These shunts can rapidly change their size and blood flow rate in response to external temperature, mainly as a result of activity in the sympathetic adrenergic vasoconstrictor nerves. *Circulating vasoactive substances* interact with sympathetic *alpha-* and *beta-adrenergic receptors* and affect finger blood flow circulation. Sympathetic vasoconstricting nerves also affect circulation in fingers.

Freedman and his colleagues showed that feedback-assisted vasodilation operates at least partly via a non-neural, beta-adrenergic mechanism. It does not require activity of *efferent digital nerves*; even when these nerves are blocked, a person can still get vasospastic attacks. This research challenges the previously assumed sole and primary role of general decreased sympathetic activity for feedback-assisted vasodilation. Finger temperature increases can and do occur with thermal biofeedback, but without other signs of decreased sympathetic activation. These researchers showed this with normal subjects (Freedman et al., 1993) and with patients with Raynaud's disease (Freedman et al., 1991). Measures of SNS activation included heart rate, blood pressure, and the circulating *catecholamines epinephrine* and *norepinephrine*. This research supports a local or focal role of blood flow and finger temperature biofeedback at least for Raynaud's disease.

Furthermore, these investigators supported the idea that different mechanisms mediate feedback-assisted vasoconstriction and vasodilation (Freedman et al., 1988a, 1988b). Thus the mechanism is probably different when patients engage in bidirectional temperature feedback.

What are the implications for practitioners? One implication is that thermal biofeedback is preferable to other physiological self-regulation therapies, which focus only on general reductions of sympathetic arousal.

Other research with clinical implications focuses on possible differences in ease of hand warming between the sexes and races. These studies compared beta-adrenergic activity in blacks and whites (McGrady & Roberts, 1991) and in female and male patients (Freedman, Sabharwal, & Desai, 1987). Whites and male patients could warm their hands with thermal biofeedback more easily than blacks and female patients could.

CONDITIONING PROCEDURES AND THE USE OF BIOFEEDBACK THERAPY

Hand warming under conditions of induced cold directly to the fingers resulted in the best short-term and long-term effects with thermal biofeedback using the paradigm employed by

Freedman and his colleagues. Jobe et al. (1985) used a different paradigm to create vasodilation and hand warming during a cold challenge. They formulated their rationale and procedures within a classical or Pavlovian counterconditioning model. The cold stressor was cold ambient air viewed as the conditioned stimulus. The conditioned response was rapid hand warming via immersing the hands (or feet) in hot tap water. Their subjects with Raynaud's disease showed significantly higher digital temperatures when exposed to cold after this treatment. The results also suggested that this procedure had an enduring effect at the 1-year follow-up (as assessed via survey data).

One can speculate that the Freedman paradigm and the Jobe paradigm may have something in common. Both involve hand warming during induced cold challenges. However, there are not enough data yet with the Jobe procedures. We look forward to research that replicates the Jobe procedures, compares these techniques, and studies possible common biochemical, physiological, and conditioning mechanisms. Both are practical for clinical application.

CONCLUSIONS

Raynaud's disease and RP are not uncommon. However, Raynaud's symptoms rarely occur naturally or fully in the research laboratory or practitioner's office. This is true both for spontaneous symptoms and for those induced with cold challenges. Causes of and mechanisms of Raynaud's disease involve multiple factors and combinations. These include physiological, biochemical, environmental, and local cold stimuli, as well as emotional and psychological factors. Although RP is secondary to other conditions, it too can be influenced by such factors.

Biofeedback-assisted therapy has a place in the treatment of Raynaud's disease and RP. The interfaces between and among biofeedback, psychology, psychophysiology, biochemistry, and pharmacology will help to further our understanding of these conditions and their treatment.

GLOSSARY

ALPHA-ADRENERGIC RECEPTORS. Receptors that respond to epinephrine and specific blocking agents. Includes sites that produce vasoconstriction.

ARTERIOSCLEOSIS OBLITERANS. Peripheral atherosclerotic disease. Occlusion of blood to the extremities by atherosclerotic plaques (atheromas).

ARTERIOVENOUS SHUNTS. Direct passages of blood from arteries to veins. These can rapidly change their size and blood flow rate in reaction to external temperature, primarily through activity in the sympathetic adrenergic vasoconstrictor nerves.

BETA-ADRENERGIC BLOCKING AGENTS (BETA-BLOCKERS). Drugs that block adrenergic transmission. Examples are propranolol (Inderal) and atenolol (Tenormin).

BETA-ADRENERGIC RECEPTORS. Adrenergic receptors that respond to norepinephrine and certain blocking agents.

BIDIRECTIONAL THERMAL BIOFEEDBACK. Thermal biofeedback procedures to assist patients to warm and cool fingers alternately, in order to increase physiological self-regulation.

BLANCHING (OR PALLOR). Whiteness of skin that results from decreased blood supply.

CALCIUM ENTRY BLOCKERS (CALCIUM CHANNEL BLOCKERS). Drugs used to decrease vascular resistance. Also called "calcium ion influx inhibitors" or "slow channel blockers."

CARPAL TUNNEL SYNDROME. Swelling or inflamed tissues in the passageway through the wrist (carpal or wrist tunnel) that compresses the median nerve. Involves numbness and tingling sensations in fingers and hand, as well as wrist pain shooting into the forearm or into palm or surfaces of fingers. Common to keyboard operators, carpenters, grocery clerks, factory workers, meat cutters, violinists, mechanics, and some others, all of whom are subject to repeated stress and strain of the wrist, and who often pinch or grip instruments with a flexed wrist.

CATECHOLAMINES. Autonomic nervous system chemicals, such as *epinephrine* and *norepinephrine* (see below), as well as dopamine. Epinephrine and norepinephrine are hormones/neurotransmitters secreted by the adrenal medulla.

CIRCULATING VASOACTIVE SUBSTANCES. Substances that interact with biochemical alpha- and beta-adrenergic receptors and affect finger blood flow.

CONNECTIVE TISSUE DISORDERS. Group of diseases of connective tissue with similar anatomical and pathological features. These include *rheumatoid arthritis (RA)*, *systemic lupus erythematosus (SLE)*, *scleroderma (progressive systemic sclerosis or PSS)*, *polymyositis* and *dermatomyositis*, vasculitis, and *Sjögren's syndrome*. Many believe that these are autoimmune diseases—in which the immune system malfunctions and attacks itself, resulting in damaged skin, muscles, and other parts of the body. The common clinical sign is inflammation, of unknown cause, of the connective tissue and often blood vessels.

CYANOSIS. Blueness of skin caused by slow blood flow (reduced oxyhemoglobin, usually less than arterial blood saturation of oxygen) in blood vessels.

DERMATOMYOSITIS. Similar to *polymyositis* (see below) that also involves the skin.

DYSPROTEINEMIAS. "Derangement of protein content of the blood" (*Dorland's Illustrated Medical Dictionary*, 1988, p. 521).

EFFERENT DIGITAL NERVES. A nerve, such as a motor nerve, carrying impulses from the central nervous system to the digits (fingers or toes). Contrast with afferent nerves.

EPINEPHRINE. Also called "adrenaline." Hormone/neurotransmitter secreted by the adrenal medulla.

ERGOT PREPARATIONS. Alkaloids used in treating moderate to severe migraine and related headaches. Ergot is derived from rye plant fungus. Available as ergotamine tartrate (e.g., Cafergot, Wigraine, Ergomar) and dihydroergotamine (DHE-45) injections (intravenous, intramuscular, or subcutaneous).

GUANETHIDINE. A drug that depresses postganglionic adrenergic nerves, inhibiting sympathetic nervous system (SNS) activity.

HYPEREMIA. Excess of blood in a part. Two causes are local or general relaxation of arterioles or blocked outflow from the area. Reactive hyperemia involves temporarily arrested flow and restoration, such as in Raynaud's.

HYPOTHYROIDISM, ADULT. Caused by an underactive thyroid gland. A shortage of thyroid hormone slows the basal metabolic rate. It usually develops slowly over months or years, and when long untreated it is known as *myxedema* (see below). It afflicts men and women of any age, but most commonly middle-aged women. The person feels physically and mentally sluggish. Symptoms include constant tiredness, muscle aches, slowed heart rate, constipation, dry and lusterless skin, thickened skin, hoarse voice, hearing loss, puffy face, dry hair, goiter in some people, heavy and prolonged menstrual periods, decreased interest in sex, and/or an inability to stay warm in cool or cold ambient temperatures. Increased weight, if present, is slight. Treatment is usually successful.

IMIPRAMINE HYDROCHLORIDE (TOFRANIL). The first tricyclic antidepressant. Blocks uptake of norepinephrine at nerve endings, and thus potentiates adrenergic synapses.

LUMBAR SYMPATHECTOMY. Cutting of the sympathetic nerves from the lumbar spine.

METHYSERGIDE. Potent serotonin antagonist having vasoconstrictor effects. Inhibits or blocks serotonin.

MIXED CONNECTIVE TISSUE DISEASE (MCTD). A rheumatic disease with overlapping features similar to three other connective tissue diseases: SLE, scleroderma (PSS), and polymyositis/dermatomyositis. Most patients with MCTD respond to corticosteroids if treated early, and long-term remissions do occur.

MYXEDEMA. Untreated hypothyroidism for several years. Myxedema coma involves drowsiness and a sensation of intense intolerance for cold. Profound lethargy and unconsciousness follow this. Sedatives may precipitate this. Requires emergency medical treatment.

NIFEDIPINE (PROCARDIA). One type of *calcium entry blocker* (see above). Now available in sustained-release form.

NOREPINEPHRINE. Also called "noradrenaline." A natural neurohormone. One type of *catecholamine* (see above), a body compound having a sympathomimetic action. A powerful vasopressor (constrictor of capillaries and arteries). Norepinephrine is released by postganglionic adrenergic nerves and the adrenal medulla. Has mostly alpha-adrenergic activity and some beta-adrenergic activity.

OBSTRUCTIVE ARTERIAL DISEASES. Examples include *thromboangitis obliterans* (see below) and *arteriosclerosis obliterans* (see above).

PLATELETS (THROMBOCYTES). Round or oval discs in blood that adhere to each other and the edges of an injured small vessel, and thus clot or plug it.

POLYCYTHEMIA VERA (TRUE). Caused by bone marrow producing too many red blood cells. There are also increased white blood cells and platelets. Usually develops gradually and appears in late middle age. Differentiated from secondary polycythemia, which is caused by heavy smoking of cigarettes, severe lung disease, abnormal hemoglobin, or living at high altitudes. The secondary form is the body's overcompensating for low concentration of oxygen and making too many red blood cells. Treatment is necessary to avoid thicker (more viscous) blood, increasing the risk of stroke or a heart attack.

POLYMYOSITIS. A rare disorder of inflamed muscles. The presence of skin and muscle inflammation is called *dermatomyositis* (see above). Women are twice as likely to have these disorders, and they occur at any age. Both disorders can disappear within a few months. However, when they affect the throat muscles and swallowing, death can occur.

PRAZOSIN. It causes decreased total peripheral resistance in part by blocking postsynaptic alpha-adrenoceptors. Used for hypertension with most effect on diastolic blood pressure.

PRIMARY PULMONARY HYPERTENSION (PPH). Very uncommon obliterative disease involving small and medium pulmonary arteries. Narrowing of the vessels lumen always occurs. Females have this five times more often than males. Raynaud's phenomenon (RP) and arthralgias are often present and often precede, by years, the apparent onset of PPH.

REFLEX SYMPATHETIC DYSTROPHY (RSD). Burning sensation or pain and tenderness, usually in a hand or foot. Other symptoms are thin or shiny skin, along with increased sweating and hair growth. It can develop weeks or months after an injury, heart attack, or stroke. RSD can affect a kneecap or hip. In the second phase, which usually develops over months, the skin becomes cool and shiny. Contracture may occur. If not treated promptly, irreversible damage can occur.

REGIONAL SYMPATHECTOMY. An interruption of some portion of the sympathetic nervous pathway by transection, resection, or other means.

RENAL. Pertaining to the kidneys.

RESERPINE. An alkaloid derived from Rauwolfia root. Depletes catecholamines. Has antihypertensive, bradycariac, and tranquilizing properties. May cause mental depression.

RHEUMATOID ARTHRITIS (RA). An autoimmune, systemic disease (unlike osteoarthritis, which is caused by wear and tear in normal use, and affects only the musculoskeletal system).

RUBOR. Redness of skin caused by excess blood. Often accompanied by painful, throbbing, or burning sensations. Reactive hyperemia. In Raynaud's, the third stage when there are three color changes (triphasic).

SCLERODERMA (PROGRESSIVE SYSTEMIC SCLEROSIS, or PSS). Means "hard skin." This connective tissue disorder leads to a permanent tightness and shiny skin in affected areas. Common areas are arms, face, or hands. Other symptoms are puffy hands and feet, especially in the morning, and joint pain and stiffness. Women are about four times as likely as men to get it. Management depends on the severity and body systems affected.

SEROTONIN. A vasoconstrictor. It has many physiological properties, including inhibiting gastric secretions, stimulating smooth muscle, and serving as a central neurotransmitter. Also often called "5-hydroxytryptamine" or "5-HT." A major factor in certain medical/neurological and psychiatric conditions, such as migraines and depression. About 90% occurs in the gastrointestinal tract, about 8% in blood platelets, and the rest in the brain.

SJÖGREN'S SYNDROME. A connective tissue disease. Symptoms are dryness of the eyes, with a sandy or gritty feeling, and dry mouth. Often occurs with RA or other disorders, such as SLE, scleroderma (PSS), or polymyositis. Mostly found in middle-aged women.

SYMPATHOLETIC AGENTS. Agents that oppose the effects of adrenergic postganglionic fibers of the SNS (hence, "antiadrenergic").

SYSTEMIC LUPUS ERYTHEMATOSUS (SLE). A lifelong and usually episodic disease affecting 10 times more women than men and usually starting between ages 15 and 35. Frequently affects the synovial membrane in joints and produces inflammation, swelling, and pain, usually in the fingers and wrists. Other symptoms include rashes, especially on the nose and cheeks; localized chest pain and coughing; sunlight sensitivity causing rash and fever; and baffling fatigue. It is a serious disease that can affect all organ systems. Patients with Raynaud's disease need to have this disorder ruled out.

THERMAL LAG. Lag between change in the amount of peripheral blood flow regulated by the diameter of peripheral blood vessel and the change in skin surface temperature, as detected by the thermistor.

THORACIC OUTLET OBSTRUCTION SYNDROMES. Group of ill-defined syndromes with symptoms of arm pain and paresthesias in the hand, neck, shoulder, or arms; vasomotor symptoms including RP. Several causes are proposed.

THROMBOANGITIS OBLITERANS (BUERGER'S DISEASE). A rare disorder. An obstructive or occlusive disease with ischemia and superficial phlebitis and inflammation in small and medium-sized veins and arteries of the hands and feet. Early symptoms include coldness, numbness, tingling, or burning (RP). Pain from severe ischemia then develops, and ulcers or gangrene appear later. Usually (about 95%) occurs in young and middle-aged men who smoke cigarettes. Unless one stops smoking early and avoids other factors (e.g., trauma from tight shoes, therrnal injury), amputation is typical.

THYMOXAMINE. A sympatholytic agent that is mainly an alpha-adrenergic receptor antagonist, also with some alpha$_2$-adrenergic receptor blocking effects. Not available in the United States.

TRAUMATIC VASOSPASTIC DISEASE (VIBRATION DISEASE). A disorder caused by the continual use of vibratory tools. It can include diminished flexion of the fingers; loss of cold, heat, and pain perception; blanching; and osteoarthritic changes in the arm joints.

TROPHIC CHANGES. Changes (e.g., in skin) caused by nutritional changes.

VISCOSITY. "A physical property of fluids (e.g., blood) that determines the internal resistance to shear forces (*Dorland's Illustrated Medical Dictionary*, 1988, p. 1843).

REFERENCES

Berkow, R., & Fletcher, A. J. (1992). *The Merck manual of diagnosis and therapy* (16th ed.). Rahway, NJ: Merck.
Coffman, J. D. (1991). Raynaud's phenomenon: An update. *Hypertension, 17,* 593–602.
Dorland's illustrated medical dictionary (27th ed.). (1988). Philadelphia: Saunders.
Freedman, R. R. (1987). Long-term effectiveness of behavioral treatments for Raynaud's disease. *Behavior Therapy, 18,* 387–399.
Freedman, R. R. (1991). Physiological mechanisms of temperature biofeedback. *Biofeedback and Self-Regulation, 16*(2), 95–115.
Freedman, R. R. (1994, March). *Mechanisms of temperature biofeedback: Invited Citation Lecture presented at the 25th Annual Meeting of the Association for Applied Psychophysiology and Biofeedback, Atlanta, GA* [Audiotape]. Aurora, CO: Sound Images.
Freedman, R. R., Ianni, P., & Wenig, P. (1983). Behavioral treatment of Raynaud's disease. *Journal of Consulting and Clinical Psychology, 51,* 539–549.
Freedman, R. R, Keegan, D., Migaly, P., Vining, S., Mayes, M., & Galloway, M. P. (1991, March). Plasma catecholamines during behavioral treatments for Raynaud's disease. In *Proceedings of the 22nd Annual Meeting of the Association for Applied Psychophysiology and Biofeedback, Dallas.* Wheat Ridge, CO: Association for Applied Psychophysiology and Biofeedback.
Freedman, R. R., Keegan, D., Rodriguez, J., & Galloway, M. P. (1993, March). Plasma catecholamine levels during temperature biofeedback training in normal subjects. In *Proceedings of the 24th Annual Meeting of the Association for Applied Psychophysiology and Biofeedback, Los Angeles, CA.* Wheat Ridge, CO: Association for Applied Psychophysiology and Biofeedback.
Freedman, R. R., Lynn, S. J., & Ianni, P. (1982). Behavioral assessment of Raynaud's disease. In F. J. Keefe & J. A. Blumenthal (Eds.), *Assessment strategies in behavioral medicine.* New York: Grune & Stratton.
Freedman, R. R., Mayes, M. D., & Sabharwal, S. C. (1989). Induction of vasospastic attacks despite digital nerve block in Raynaud's disease and phenomenon. *Circulation, 80*(4), 859–862.
Freedman, R. R., Morris, M., Norton, D. A., Masselink, D., Sabharwal, S. C., & Mayes, M. D. (1988a). Physiological mechanism of digital vasoconstriction training. *Biofeedback and Self-Regulation, 13*(4), 299–305.
Freedman, R. R., Sabharwal, S. C., Ianni, P., Desai, N., Wenig, P., & Mayes, M. (1988b). Nonneural beta-adrenergic vasodilating mechanism in temperature biofeedback. *Psychosomatic Medicine, 50,* 394–401.

Freedman, R. R., Sabharwal, S. C., & Desai, N. (1987). Sex differences in peripheral vascular adrenergic receptors. *Circulation Research*, 61(4), 581–585.

Grove, R. N., & Belanger, M. T. (1983). Biofeedback and Raynaud's diathesis. In W. H. Rickles, J. H. Sandweiss, D. W. Jacobs, R. N. Grove, & E. Criswell (Eds.), *Biofeedback and family practice medicine*. New York: Plenum Press.

Jobe, J. B., Beetham, W. P., Roberts, D. E., Silver, G. R., Larsen, R. F., Hamlet, M. P., & Sampson, J. B. (1985). Induced vasodilation as a home treatment for Raynaud's disease. *Journal of Rheumatology*, 12(5), 953–956.

McGrady, A., & Roberts, G. (1991). Racial differences in the relaxation response of hypertensives. *Psychosomatic Medicine*, 54, 71–78.

Middaugh, S. J., Haythornthwaite, J. A., Thompson, B., Hill, R., Brown, K. M., Freedman, R. R., Attanasio, V., Jacob, R. G., Scheier, M., & Smith, E. A. (2001). The Raynaud's Treatment Study: Biofeedback protocols and acquisition of temperature biofeedback skills. *Applied Psychophysiology and Biofeedback*, 26, 251–278.

Raynaud, M. (1862). *De l'asphyxie locale et de la gangrène symétique des extremités*. Paris: Rigoux.

Raynaud, M. (1888). *New research on the nature and treatment of local asphyxia of the extremities* (T. Barlow, Trans.). London: New Sydenham Society.

Rose, G. D., & Carlson. J. G. (1987). The behavioral treatment of Raynaud's disease: A review. *Biofeedback and Self-Regulation*, 12(4), 257–272.

Sedlacek, K. (1984). Biofeedback treatment of primary Raynaud's. In F. J. McGuigan, W. E. Sime, & J. M. Wallace (Eds.), *Stress and tension control*. New York: Plenum Press.

Sedlacek, K. (1989). Biofeedback treatment of primary Raynaud's disease. In J. V. Basmajian (Ed.), *Biofeedback: Principles and practice for clinicians* (3rd ed.). Baltimore: Williams & Wilkins.

Sedlacek, K., & Taub, E. (1996). Biofeedback treatment of Raynaud's disease. *Professional Psychology: Research and Practice*, 27(6), 548–553.

Stambrook, M., Hamel, E. R., & Carter, S. A. (1988). Training to vasodilate in a cooling environment: A valid treatment for Raynaud's phenomenon. *Biofeedback and Self-Regulation*, 13(1), 9–23.

Taub, E. (1977). Self-regulation of human tissue temperature. In G. E. Schwartz & J. Beatty (Eds.), *Biofeedback: Theory and research*. New York: Academic Press.

Taub, E., & School, P. J. (1978). Some methodological considerations in thermal biofeedback training. *Behavioral Research Methods and Instrumentation*, 10, 617–622.

Thompson, B., & Raynaud's Treatment Study (RTS) Investigators. (2000). Comparison of sustained-release nifedipine and temperature biofeedback for treatment of primary Raynaud phenomenon: Results from a randomized clinical trial with 1-year follow-up. *Archives of Internal Medicne*, 160, 1101–1108.

Biobehavioral Treatment of Essential Hypertension

ANGELE MCGRADY

WOLFGANG LINDEN

This chapter begins with a summary of the basic physiology of blood pressure (BP) regulation. It proceeds to the classification of BP, the definition of hypertension, and finally the characteristics of hypertensive disease. The chapter reviews traditional pharmacotherapy for hypertension according to the revised stepped-care approach, and briefly discusses non-pharmacological therapies other than biofeedback and relaxation. For the most part, the chapter comprises a detailed description of a composite treatment plan for essential hypertension. This plan utilizes and references key research from several biofeedback treatment centers and psychophysiological laboratories. We develop characteristics of baseline, treatment, and follow-up; discuss patient education; and list evaluation criteria for outcome. The chapter also suggests ways of preselecting patients to enhance their chances for success in lowering BP. It ends with suggestions for further research. (Throughout the chapter, as in other chapters, italics on first use of a term in text indicate that the term is included in the glossary at the end.)

Also germane to the behavioral treatment of patients with essential hypertension are (1) the general principles of biofeedback measurement, (2) considerations in developing low physiological arousal, (3) the intake process, (4) cognitive preparation of patients, (5) adherence, and (6) generalization. In this chapter, however, we discuss only those topics that are specific to treatment of essential hypertension.

NORMAL REGULATION OF BP

A basic understanding of the physiology of BP (Vander, Sherman, & Luciano, 2001; Ganong, 1997) is necessary before the biofeedback practitioner can implement a treatment plan to reduce high BP. Appreciation of the complexities of *neural* and endocrine influences is not essential. However, the practitioner must (1) understand the variables that determine BP and the elements of BP regulation, (2) have a working knowledge of common antihypertensive medications, and (3) be able to explain to patients in lay terms the potential effects of biofeedback and relaxation on BP.

BP values are expressed as systolic/diastolic values in millimeters of mercury (abbreviated mm *Hg* with specific measurements). *Systolic BP (SBP)* is the maximum pressure during ejection of blood from the heart in the *cardiac cycle*, and *diastolic BP (DBP)* is the minimum pressure that occurs during cardiac relaxation. *Mean arterial pressure (MAP)* is the average BP driving blood through tissues.

Cardiac output and *total peripheral resistance (TPR)* determine BP (see Figure 17.1). One calculates cardiac output by multiplying heart rate (beats per minute) by *stroke volume* output. The latter is the amount of blood ejected during each beat of the heart. Factors controlling heart rate and stroke volume include *sympathetic* and *parasympathetic* nerve activity. TPR is the resistance or impediment to the flow of blood in the arteries, the arterioles, and (to a minor extent) the veins. Sympathetic activity, circulating substances in the blood, and local conditions in the tissues all influence TPR. For example, if sympathetic activity increases, arterioles constrict and present a larger resistance to the flow of blood, raising BP (Vander et al., 2001).

Neural, renal, and hormonal factors all exert an influence on BP. The nervous system is very important in the moment-to-moment control of arterial pressure. Special stretch receptors (*baroreceptors*) are located in the walls of the heart and blood vessels, and constantly monitor BP. The baroreceptors respond to distention caused by increased pressure by sending an electrical signal through nerves to the vasomotor center in the medulla of the brain. Here, groups of neurons exert modulating effects on BP. Nerve responses begin within a few seconds and can decrease pressure significantly within 5–10 seconds. So the baroreceptor system is most important for short-term regulation of arterial pressure, whereas long-term regulation requires mechanisms based in the kidney (renal system) and the endocrine system (Ganong, 1997).

Blood volume is a critical determinant of long-term BP level. For example, when the circulatory system contains too much fluid, arterial pressure rises. Increased BP in turn signals the kidneys to excrete the excess fluid (pressure diuresis). Loss of fluid through the urine subsequently returns fluid balance to normal and decreases BP. The hormone *aldosterone*, re-

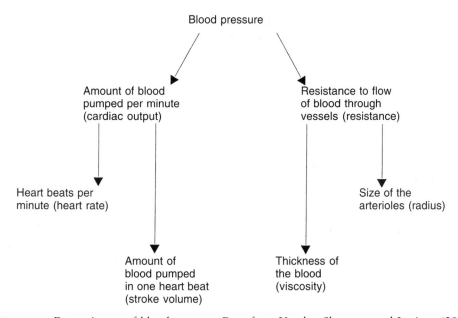

FIGURE 17.1. Determinants of blood pressure. Data from Vander, Sherman, and Luciano (2001).

leased from the *adrenal cortex* by the *renin–angiotensin II* system, is also important in BP regulation because it facilitates reabsorption of sodium by the kidneys. In turn, the renin–angiotensin II hormonal complex releases aldosterone. For example, decreased *plasma* volume instigates a neural and endocrine reflex response that consists of increased renin–angiotensin II and aldosterone, resulting in increased sodium reabsorption. Since sodium draws water with it, fluid loss will decrease, and balance is restored.

Maintenance of blood flow to the *vascular* beds, such as those in skin and muscle, requires a certain level of BP. If BP is too low, the tissues will not receive enough blood. The variation in the proportion of blood flow to different tissues depends on the metabolic needs of those tissues. The end products of *metabolism* build up in active tissues; then dilation of blood vessels occurs to ensure delivery of more oxygenated blood. This is local regulation. On the other hand, some substances circulate within the blood and affect tissues distant from where the substance was originally produced and secreted. For example, the *adrenal medulla* releases epinephrine, which dilates the vessels in skeletal muscles. The *atrial natriuretic factor (ANF)*, secreted by the heart, antagonizes the actions of various vasoconstrictor chemicals. Other vasoactive compounds, released by the walls of blood vessels (e.g., endothelium-derived relaxing factor), affect tone and diameter, and therefore affect resistance and BP.

In summary, receptors (monitoring structures, in this case) keep track of BP. Change in BP alerts the nerve cells in the vasomotor center. Response to the change in BP involves modulation of the two basic determinants of BP—cardiac output and TPR—by neural, renal, or hormonal action.

Assessment of BP

Practitioners must recognize the many possible errors in routine BP assessment. The patient him- or herself, the professionals, the devices, and the entire measurement situation merit consideration. Mercury *sphygmomanometers* and properly calibrated aneroid sphygmomanometers are standard choices. Practitioners should recalibrate an aneroid sphygmomanometer every 3–12 months, depending on the frequency of its use. For office professional use, relatively inexpensive automatic BP monitors can provide reliable measures of SBP, DBP, and heart rate. Before purchase, however, the monitor should be carefully evaluated, because even devices with similar measurement methodologies can differ substantially in their accuracy. It is very important to remember that office readings may falsely lead to a positive diagnosis because of measurement apprehension (the so-called "white-coat hypertension") (Selenta, Hogan, & Linden, 2000). Furthermore, the patients who have high BP all day but present with normal readings in the clinic ("white-coat normotension") may be missed with only clinic readings (Liu et al., 1999). These diagnostic errors can be minimized when a 24-hour ambulatory monitor is used. These devices, however, are costly and noticeably more inconvenient for patients (Yucha, 2001), so may be more appropriate for clinical research.

Practitioners should help patients select good-quality, easy-to-use instruments and train them in their use. Given recent progress in device development and validation, practitioners should recommend electronic BP instruments that provide a digital readout; such instruments can avoid measurement errors due to poor training. These may also be preferable for home use by individuals with poor hearing. All BP instruments need to be recalibrated at regular intervals, according to the manufacturers' instructions. Medical supply stores stock several types of monitors, and store staff members are able to help patients with assembly and calibration of their instruments.

Both standardized and repeated BP measurements are critical to establish a patient's actual pretreatment BP and to evaluate therapy effects. BP measurements taken under very similar conditions are also more similar than such measurements obtained under different conditions.

Many factors, including those listed below, can either artificially increase or decrease the values obtained. The four categories that subsume these factors are patient, practitioner, setting, and equipment. The following list is based on Kaplan (1998) and Joint National Committee (JNC, 1997).

Patient

1. The position and level of the patient's arm. The arm and back should be supported; the arm should be at heart level. One should initially measure BP in both arms.
2. The position of the patient: sitting, standing, supine. Measurements should begin after the patient has been sitting for 5 minutes. The patient should be quiet during measurements (Linden, Herbert, Jenkins, & Raffle, 1989).
3. The emotional state of the patient shortly before or at the time one obtains the BP. Slow breathing should be encouraged. The patient's attitudes toward both BP measurement and the professional doing the measuring should be considered.
4. The length of time since the patient has eaten, exercised, or used nicotine, caffeine, or other chemicals. Patients should not have had caffeine or smoked within 30 minutes of BP measurement.
5. Type and dosage of antihypertensive medications, other prescription drugs, and over-the-counter medications, and when the medicines were last taken.

Practitioner

6. The person (health care provider) measuring the BP. This should be recorded and should remain the same for repeated measures.
7. The interval between BP measurements in the same session. The average should be at least two measurements separated by 2 minutes.

Setting

8. The site and setting of BP measurement (e.g., work, home, professional's office).
9. The patient's familiarity with the environment in which one measures the BP.
10. The date (day of the week) and time of day.

Equipment

11. The instrument used, whether it be a manual sphygmomanometer or an electronic model. The same instrument should be used each time. Proper calibration is important.
12. The placement of the cuff on the arm, appropriate cuff size, and the rate of deflation of the cuff.

An incorrect cuff size may significantly alter BP readings. A cuff that is too small produces a falsely high BP reading. As a result, one could incorrectly classify obese patients as having hypertension. For arm circumferences of less than 33 centimeters, we recommend a regular-size adult cuff (12 × 23 centimeters). The recommendation for arm circumferences between 33 and 41 centimeters is a large size (15 × 33 centimeters). A thigh-size cuff (18 × 36 centimeters) should be used for those arms larger than 41 centimeters. Practitioners often purchase cuffs of different sizes for the clinical setting, so a properly sized cuff will be available when needed.

Classification of BP

The Joint National Committee (JNC) on Detection, Evaluation, and Treatment of High Blood Pressure is a group of experts in the diagnosis and treatment of hypertension. They meet approximately every 4 years to study and discuss results of epidemiological studies and therapeutic trials. Their published reports guide practitioners who care for patients with hypertension. The sixth report presents the classification of BP shown in Table 17.1 (JNC, 1997). The terminology for levels of BP above normal, formerly termed "mild," "moderate," "severe," and "very severe," is currently indicated by "stages 1–4." The report discusses recommendations for treatment using lifestyle modification and antihypertensive medications. The World Health Organization prefers the terms "grades 1–3," because the terminology of "stages" assumes a progression over time that does not always occur (Guidelines Subcommittee, 1999).

HYPERTENSION

Definition and Characteristics

"Hypertension" is a complex disease characterized by sustained elevations of SBP, DBP, or both. "Essential" or "primary" hypertension is elevated BP of unknown etiology and is the diagnosis for more than 90% of people with chronically elevated BP (Julius, 2000). Central to the development of essential hypertension is "autonomic imbalance" (i.e., sympathetic overactivity and underactivity of the parasympathetic system) (Brook & Julius, 2000).

"Secondary" hypertension results from a specific disease or pathological abnormality in the body. Some examples are diseases of the kidney, tumors of the *adrenal gland, Cushing's disease*, primary *aldosteronism*, and diseases of the thyroid gland (*hyperthyroidism*) (Kaplan, 1998). Medical and surgical management of secondary hypertensive disorders must supersede psychophysiological therapy. Thus it is unlikely that physicians would refer these individuals for biofeedback for their hypertension.

The detrimental effects of hypertension are well documented. Sustained elevations of BP can damage the brain, kidneys, heart, and blood vessels. Untreated hypertension contributes to premature death through stroke, heart attack, or kidney failure. The presence of certain laboratory values outside the normal range, in addition to elevated BP, increases the incidence of complications of hypertensive disease. The presence and the type of organ damage are also part of classifying hypertension and determining its severity.

TABLE 17.1. Classification of Blood Pressure in Adults Aged 18 or Older

Category	Systolic (mm Hg)	Diastolic (mm Hg)
Normal	<130	<85
High-normal	130–139	85–89
Hypertension		
Stage 1	140–159	90–99
Stage 2	160–179	100–109
Stage 3	180–209	110–119
Stage 4	>210	>120

Note. Adapted from Joint National Committee (JNC, 1997). Copyright 1997 by the American Medical Association. Adapted by permission.

Epidemiological studies illustrate that 4% of adults aged 18–34 years have BP greater than 140/90 mm Hg, and in the age group 18–74 years, the percentage is 20% (Joffres, Hamet, MacLean, L'italien, & Fodor, 2001). The risk factors associated with the development of essential hypertension include increasing age, obesity, presence of comorbidities (particularly type 2 diabetes and hyperlipidemia), lifestyle factors (alcohol use, high-sodium diet, inactivity), chronic psychological stress, sociocultural variables, and personality (Kaplan, 1998). In general, BP increases with age; men have higher BP than women until the mid-60s, and African Americans' BP is higher than that of European Americans (M'Buyamaba-Kabangu, Amery, & Lijnen, 1994; Reckelhoff, 2001). African Americans are much more likely to have elevated BP and more severe hypertension than European Americans (Winkleby, Kraemer, Ahn, & Warady, 1998). Socioeconomic status is correlated inversely with incidence and severity of primary hypertension (Shakoor-Abdullah, Kotchen, Walker, Chelius, & Hoffmann, 1997). Anxiety, anger, and depression are the primary personality factors that have been investigated (Byrne, 1992; Jonas, Franks, & Ingram, 1997; Jorgensen, Johnson, & Kolodziej, 1996). About 25% of children with one hypertensive parent will have sustained elevated BP. If both parents have hypertension, then about 50% of their children will develop the disease. Hypertension develops about 10 times more often in persons whose body weight is 20% or more over normal than in those maintaining normal body weight (JNC, 1997).

In summary, scientists cannot reliably identify a single characteristic or risk factor as the causal factor in the development or maintenance of elevated BP. For example, in the 30% of hypertensive individuals who are sensitive to sodium, BP (MAP) can decrease 10 mm Hg or more when sodium and fluid become depleted (Chobanian & Hill, 2000; Weinberger, 1993). Both sodium and volume are important factors, but not all persons with hypertension are salt-sensitive. The Dietary Approaches to Stop Hypertension (DASH) diet (high in fruits and vegetables and low in fat) also significantly reduced BP (Conlin et al., 2000). Attempts have been made to describe the pathophysiology of hypertension in terms of disordered cardiac output, TPR, or both. The hypersympathetic state of initial BP elevation depends on high cardiac output. In time, high resistance predominates due to increased arteriolar constriction and hypertrophy of the vessels' muscular walls (Julius, 1991). BP, particularly DBP, is maintained at elevated levels. In addition, the baroreceptor system resets and maintains the higher BP. It is clear that the diagnosis of essential hypertension alone tells us very little about causes and psychophysiological characteristics of this heterogeneous condition. Rather, a mosaic of behavioral, psychological, and physiological factors contributes to the development of chronically elevated BP, and the presence of multiple risk factors is correspondingly associated with a higher likelihood of developing hypertension over time (Light et al., 1999).

Lifestyle Modifications

In addition to classifying hypertension, the JNC (1997) has recommended preferred treatment strategies based on a stepped-care model. The JNC recommends the following "lifestyle modifications" (formerly called "nonpharmacological therapies") as step 1 in the treatment algorithm:

Lose weight if overweight.
Limit alcohol intake to <1 ounce per day of ethanol (24 ounces of beer, 8 ounces of wine, or 2 ounces of 100-proof whiskey).
Exercise aerobically on a regular basis.
Reduce sodium intake to less than 100 millimol per day (<2.3 grams of sodium, or approximately <6 grams of sodium chloride).

Maintain adequate dietary potassium, calcium, and magnesium intake.

Stop smoking.

Reduce dietary saturated fat and cholesterol intake for overall cardiovascular health; reducing fat intake also helps reduce caloric intake, which is important for control of weight and type 2 diabetes.

Health care professionals who offer psychophysiological therapies, including biofeedback, should question patients about their lifestyle during the initial interview and then consider recommending changes in behavior. Providers of biofeedback and associated therapies, however, would do well to enlist the services of dietitians, smoking cessation experts, and established exercise programs to complement the biofeedback and relaxation therapies. From a research perspective, combining other therapies with relaxation and biofeedback makes it more difficult to determine the relative contributions of each to lowered BP. In the clinical setting, the analysis of separate efficacy of each treatment is often less important, because the overall objective is to lower patients' BP to normal levels and to decrease their medication requirements if possible. However, knowing the relative contribution of each therapy can sometimes be used to foster compliance, and make it easier to justify the cost and time commitment necessary for each therapy. The recommendation for lifestyle changes should be part of all hypertension management, but is indicated as monotherapy only after careful assessment of BP level and other risk factors.

The introduction of lifestyle changes should include an explanation to those patients being asked to change their behaviors and habits. Practitioners should explain to patients that because sodium causes retention of fluid, the increased blood volume increases BP. Moreover, caffeine and nicotine are nervous system stimulants that acutely increase heart rate, and therefore cardiac output and BP. Patients should be reminded that risk factors are additive; for example, excess caffeine consumption during high-stress conditions can exacerbate BP increases (Shepard, al'Absi, Whitsett, Passey, & Lovallo, 2000). An exercise program (especially aerobic exercise) should be encouraged, because of the conditioning effect of exercise on the muscles. For example, because active muscles need more blood, dilation of blood vessels decreases the resistance to blood flow and thereby lowers BP. A sedentary patient should get proper medical screening and approval before beginning a program of moderate or strenuous aerobic exercise. A contract can be set with the patient: "Let's try lifestyle changes first. We'll recheck monthly for 4–6 months, then discuss alternatives."

Pharmacological Therapies

Pharmacotherapy is the core of treatment for persons with stage 2, 3, or 4 hypertension, particularly those persons with other risk factors for cardiovascular complications. For patients with high-normal or mild hypertension, one may delay medication with careful monitoring, while the persons attempt to implement lifestyle changes (JNC, 1997). Adherence to taking medication may be poor in individuals who do not have noticeable symptoms, as is the case with most patients with hypertension. The practitioner is then challenged to design a multicomponent treatment plan, engage the patient in appropriate self-care and monitor adherence. Many patients do not understand the importance of therapy and the necessity of implementing lifestyle changes as well as taking medication. However, the rewards of effective management are great, because it is clear that aggressive treatment of high BP decreases the incidence of morbidity and mortality from cardiovascular events (Cushman, 2001; Weber, 2000). Many physicians use a standardized pharmacological stepped-care approach to treating hypertension. However, the design of a multicomponent treatment plan should consider the following factors:

1. Patients' present quality of life and motivation for change.
2. Desire of many patients to be involved in their own self-care.
3. Research that supports matching one class of drug with a subset of the hypertensive population.
4. Any significant comorbidity, such as diabetes or hyperlipidemia.
5. Gender and ethnicity of patients.
6. Presence of psychiatric illness.

The major classes of antihypertensive drugs include *diuretics*, *beta-blockers*, *angiotensin-converting enzyme (ACE) inhibitors*, angiotensin receptor antagonists, and *calcium channel blockers*. Diuretics increase sodium and water excretion by the kidney, and also decrease TPR. Beta-blockers decrease cardiac output and indirectly decrease blood volume. The ACE inhibitors lower vascular resistance and decrease sodium retention via aldosterone reduction. The calcium channel blockers inhibit blood vessel wall contraction, thus decreasing TPR (Mycek, Gertner, & Perper, 1992). The JNC (1997) recommends beginning pharmacological therapy in most cases with diuretics or beta-blockers, because of demonstrated reduction in morbidity and mortality. Interestingly, a recent review concluded that a thiazide diuretic is superior to beta-blockers as a drug of first choice (ALLHAT Officers and Coordinators, 2000; Wright, 2000). There are other differences in first-line therapy and target BP, however, based on a patient's comorbidities. ACE inhibitors, for example, are preferred in patients with diabetes mellitus, and target BP is lower (Luke, 1996). If BP response is inadequate, further therapy can include an increase in drug dose, substitution of a drug from another class (ACE inhibitors, calcium channel blockers, alpha-blockers, alpha- and beta-blockers), or the addition of a second agent (JNC, 1997). Because any of a number of pharmacotherapies or combinations can be effective, pharmacological treatment of hypertension remains highly complex.

PSYCHOPHYSIOLOGICAL THERAPY: A MULTICOMPONENT APPROACH INCORPORATING BIOFEEDBACK

The biobehavioral therapies, including biofeedback, are typically used as adjuncts to pharmacological treatments, as part of lifestyle change, or as monotherapy in a patient with high-normal or stage 1 hypertension and without other risk factors. Early reports (Patel, 1973; Benson, Shapiro, Tursky, & Schwartz, 1971; Kristt & Engel, 1975; McGrady, Yonker, Tan, Fine, & Woerner, 1981) demonstrated the effectiveness of biofeedback alone or combined with relaxation in lowering BP in individuals with essential hypertension. The JNC (1997) report stated that relaxation and biofeedback therapies have not been sufficiently tested to lead to firm conclusions. The Canadian consensus group (Spence, Barnett, Linden, Ramsden, & Tanezer, 1999) concluded that individualized stress management may be an effective intervention after all. This conclusion was partly based on the argument of Linden and Chambers (1994) that the classification of biofeedback and relaxation as "mere" adjuncts may be unfairly based on research protocol peculiarities. In particular, nondrug studies typically include patients with much lower baseline BP than those included in drug studies. This is important, because Jacob, Chesney, Williams, Ding, and Shapiro (1991) showed a high positive correlation between BP at entry and subsequent degree of BP change. When Linden and Chambers (1994) adjusted for different BP levels at baseline in their meta-analysis, the best nondrug treatments were as efficacious as a variety of different drug regimens. In a recent trial, using a combination of techniques (including temperature biofeedback and autogenic training), stress management therapy reduced 24-hour means for SBP and DBP; the results were even stronger at follow-up, and the findings could be cleanly replicated (Linden, Lenz, & Con, 2001).

There are valid criticisms of many of the published biofeedback studies because of deficiencies in design and methodology. These critiques include the absence or inadequacy of pretreatment BP monitoring, medication changes during treatment, lack of clearly defined outcome measures, questionable generalization of the decreased BP to the home or work setting, and poorly designed or absent long-term follow-up (Jacob et al., 1991). However, close inspection of the results of even the criticized studies reveals that a percentage of participants do lower BP and/or medication significantly. The benefits of maintaining BP in the normal range with reduced or no medication are noteworthy. Therefore, we conclude that one can justify the psychophysiological therapies in the treatment of all levels of elevated BP.

Therapy Rationale and Justification

The psychophysiological therapies are indicated as part of the treatment plan when:

1. Lifestyle changes such as weight loss and exercise are not enough to lower BP to the normotensive range.
2. The patient has a specific interest in self-regulation and has realistic expectations.
3. The patient has high-normal BP but wishes to pursue a preventive measure to decrease risk, because the family history is positive for hypertension and cardiovascular disease.
4. The patient has a stressful lifestyle and notices a slow increase in BP over time.
5. The patient understands the relationship between chronic stress and elevated BP.

The cost-effectiveness of psychophysiological therapy and the possible use of alternative, less expensive methods (such as losing weight, stopping smoking, reducing sodium intake, moderating alcohol intake, increasing physical activity, or combinations of these) should be considered. Altering these risk factors is a less costly alternative than medication for both patients and third-party payers. Nonetheless, design of the treatment plan must include risk calculation, optimal BP, and patient psychosocial characteristics.

Pharmacotherapy and Psychophysiological Therapy

Biofeedback has been studied as an adjunct to diuretics (Jurek, Higgins, & McGrady, 1992), beta-blockers, and other medications (Blanchard et al., 1986; Hatch et al., 1985; Glasgow, Engel, & D'Lugoff, 1989). Patients provided with adjunctive biofeedback and/or relaxation therapy are often able to decrease BP more than patients on medication alone. These two treatment modalities can be advantageously combined in the care of patients with essential hypertension. In fact, Brody (1981) suggested that the extent of a patient's psychological distress is directly proportional to the amount of medication required to control his or her BP.

If BP decreases to 120/80 mm Hg or lower than 120/75 mm Hg for certain subgroups, and remains at that level, then reduction in medication is a possibility. The therapist should consult with the patient's physician and ask for a withdrawal schedule for reducing medication. Whereas some antihypertensive drugs can be stopped abruptly, others must be tapered. If the physician does not approve a medication dose reduction prior to treatment, or if patients enter treatment with poorly controlled BP despite medication, then, following biofeedback treatment, medication withdrawal should again be considered. Other possibilities are to reduce the dosage of medication or, if the patient is medicated with more than one type of antihypertensive medication, to withdraw one type while maintaining the other one. Throughout therapy and follow-up, regular monitoring of BP must continue.

Stages of Treatment

Patient Education

Health care professionals provide various types of patient education throughout all the stages of treatment. During baseline, one may describe the basic facts about hypertension, instruct patients in the accurate measurement of BP, and give a simple explanation of the major factors affecting BP. During treatment, one can provide the rationale for psychophysiological therapies as each procedure is introduced. One should also provide detailed information about each intervention in lay terms. Most patients can comprehend the basic biology of BP and the ways specific biological, chemical, and psychological factors affect their BP. Written materials and videos are helpful adjuncts to oral explanations, particularly in teaching groups of patients. An excellent source of educational materials is Krames, Health and Safety Education, 1100 Grundy Lane, San Bruno, CA 94066; www.krames.com.

The first treatment stage consists of a baseline period during which the therapist repeatedly monitors and records BP. Multiple measurements of BP can, in a portion of the hypertensive population, result in BP decreases that are statistically and clinically significant (Engel, Gaarder, & Glasgow, 1981; McGrady & Higgins, 1990). Decreases in office BP to normal levels with only monitoring do not always coincide with equal declines in home BP, so both office and home BP data should be available to the practitioner. Twenty-four-hour ambulatory monitoring should also be considered. Although the mechanism underlying the reduction in BP with monitoring is unknown, decreased anxiety or *desensitization* to BP measurements may be relevant factors.

Patients should receive careful instructions in how to take their own BP. They can be loaned a BP device or encouraged to purchase one. The practitioner should calibrate instruments and recheck them against the clinic instruments. For simplicity of learning and daily use, a properly validated electronic monitor is preferable. Training patients to take their own BP is quite important. The practitioner should demonstrate positioning of the arm and the rest of the body, provide step-by-step procedures, and model the correct techniques in the clinic setting. A standard rest period should be allotted before measuring the BP; usually 3–5 minutes of sitting quietly are sufficient, as are 1–2 minutes between two or three measurements. Patients should receive a written set of instructions along with their log sheets.

The BP log sheets should contain space for recording date, time of day, caffeine/alcohol consumption, smoking, exercise, and all medications taken. In this way, the patient and practitioner can identify variations in BP coincident with time of day and activities. During the baseline period, patients should also have their BP taken professionally each week in the health care provider's office. Baselines are necessarily flexible and variable in length. In a research setting, 3 weeks of BP monitoring allows the BP to stabilize. In clinical practice, however, a lengthy pretreatment period is impractical. The practitioner must reach the best compromise. A patient who already owns a BP monitoring device can be asked to log BP and bring the recordings to the first appointment. Otherwise, monitoring should begin at the first appointment. If appointments are 1 week apart, the interview, initial psychophysiological measurements, and beginning therapy will still give the practitioner 10–14 days (20–28 values) of patient BP readings.

Biofeedback

Researchers and practitioners use several different types of biofeedback in treating essential hypertension. These include thermal, direct BP, surface electromyographic (EMG), electrodermal, and respiratory sinus arrhythmia (RSA) feedback. Direct BP feedback (Glasgow,

Gaarder, & Engel, 1982) is a technique that presents to the patient the information from an SBP or DBP monitoring device. The procedure was introduced by Tursky, Shapiro, and Schwartz (1972) and revised by Kristt and Engel (1975).

> In this procedure [focusing on SBP], the patient is trained to inflate the BP cuff to about the systolic pressure and to try to inhibit brachial artery sounds. Patients . . . attempt to control brachial artery sounds for about 25–30 seconds, after which they . . . deflate the cuff for about 15 seconds. If successful in inhibiting 25% of sounds on the previous trial, the patient . . . inflates the cuff to a pressure level 2 mm Hg less than that of the previous trial. The procedure was repeated until the patient could no longer lower SBP on two consecutive trials. . . . Patients were urged to practice . . . several times daily, but were especially encouraged to practice at the time of day when their pressures were likely to be highest as indicated by the findings during baseline. For most patients this was the afternoon. (Glasgow et al., 1982, p. 158)

Patients learn the procedure over a 3-month period. They develop the ability to identify the sensations that accompany reductions in SBP and devise personalized techniques to lower BP. Generalization is also explained to patients, so they may continue to apply the techniques without the sphygmomanometer many times each day and in many places and situations.

Thermal biofeedback has been studied by Fahrion, Norris, Green, Green, and Snarr (1986) and Blanchard et al. (1986, 1988), and reviewed in Blanchard (1990). With thermal biofeedback, the practitioner instructs the individual to pay attention to the information indicating the temperature of his or her finger or toe. Patients attempt to warm their hands or feet using this feedback. Foot warming is more difficult to achieve and should be approached in temperature approximations.

In an uncontrolled study (Fahrion et al., 1986), 77 patients monitored BP and received thermal biofeedback, muscle feedback, instructions in diaphragmatic breathing, and relaxation techniques. The training criterion was 95°F for the hands and 93°F for the feet. Fifty-eight percent of the medicated patients eliminated medication; an additional 35% of the medicated patients reduced medications by half. The decreases in BP and medications were stable at 33 months.

The results of the controlled studies by Blanchard and colleagues favored monotherapy with thermal biofeedback over progressive relaxation in a group of medicated patients. Specific temperature training criteria were not set. Supine and standing norepinephrine levels decreased concomitant with thermal-biofeedback-mediated reduction in BP (McCoy et al., 1988).

McGrady (1994) utilized thermal biofeedback and relaxation therapy in a group format for 100 hypertensive patients, some of whom were medicated and some who were not. Forty-nine percent of the sample met the criterion for success—a decrease in MAP of 5 mm Hg. Significant decreases in measures of anxiety and plasma aldosterone also occurred in the treated patients, but not in the untreated controls. European Americans, African Americans, and Hispanics did equally well in lowering BP, although the physiological mechanisms underlying the BP decrease may be different (McGrady & Roberts, 1992).

The physiological rationale for the use of thermal biofeedback is that increased sympathetic activity commonly observed during stress constricts the blood vessels in the skin. The decreased blood flow results in cooler temperature. In contrast, decreased sympathetic activation results in less vasoconstriction. As individuals warm their hands, they are actually learning how to decrease neurally mediated vasoconstriction and subsequently to decrease TPR. A criticism of this explanation is that the skin vasculature actually contributes only a small percentage to the overall TPR. Furthermore, Freedman (1991) showed in his laboratory that the small but statistically significant increases in temperature mediated by thermal feedback in normotensive individuals depend on nonneural factors. Others have argued that a generalized reduction in arousal occurs with thermal biofeedback, particularly when it is combined with relaxation therapies (Fahrion et al., 1986). The decreases in anxiety reported in the McGrady (1994) study tended to support this opinion.

EMG feedback was the modality used by McGrady et al. (1981), Goebel, Viol, and Orebaugh (1993), Jurek et al. (1992), and McGrady and Higgins (1989). The theoretical framework underlying the use of EMG feedback in hypertension is that EMG feedback mediates general relaxation, and therefore decreases in autonomic arousal. Changes in blood flow to skeletal muscle occur during contraction and relaxation of muscles. Control of circulation to skeletal muscles, the largest vascular area, is brought about by both neural and local factors. Strong contractions of skeletal muscles impede blood flow within those muscles. Fatigue and pain can occur during prolonged skeletal muscle activity, and *ischemia* (reduced blood supply) can result from a chronic contracted state. Thus sustained contraction is associated with increased BP. On the other hand, one can maintain weaker or intermittent contractions for prolonged periods. With weak muscular contractions, the muscle receives more blood flow than the blood flow sent to that muscle during a strong contraction. Vasodilation in muscle can decrease TPR and BP (Vander et al., 2001).

McGrady et al. (1981) and McGrady and Higgins (1989) showed that decreases in SBP and DBP occurred in both medicated and unmedicated patients receiving EMG biofeedback and relaxation therapy. In the earlier study of medicated patients, significant SBP and DBP decreases were observed only in the treated patients and not in the controls. Concomitant decreases were also demonstrated in *cortisol* and aldosterone in the treated patients. In the later study, 39 unmedicated hypertensive patients monitored BP for 6 weeks. This was followed by 16 sessions of EMG and temperature biofeedback combined with autogenic or progressive relaxation. Patients practiced relaxation at home twice daily for 15 minutes. A 6-week BP monitoring period followed therapy. Twenty-three patients reduced their BP by at least 5 mm Hg MAP; seven reduced their MAP by less than 5 mm Hg, whereas the remaining nine showed no change or an increase (McGrady & Higgins, 1989).

Goebel et al. (1993) reported on 12 years of research in 117 hypertensive patients. Simple relaxation, relaxation plus EMG feedback, relaxation plus direct BP feedback, and BP feedback alone each produced small, consistent decreases in BP and in medication use. Patients in the active and believable control condition did not show similar BP decreases.

Electrodermal feedback depends on the amount of sweating, a sympathetically mediated response to change in ambient temperature or stressful conditions. Electrodermal activity is directly proportional to the amount of sweat (see Peek, Chapter 4, this volume). Galvanic skin response (GSR) is the form of electrodermal feedback that was used by Patel (1973) and Patel and Marmot (1988). GSR combined with EMG feedback was provided in group format to hypertensive patients as part of a multimodal treatment program. In the report by Patel and Marmot (1988), groups of patients participated in 1-hour weekly sessions provided by general practitioners for 10 weeks. Education took place in the first half-hour, and the second half-hour included relaxation training, breathing exercises, and GSR feedback. Patients practiced at home daily. The net drop in SBP was 7.3 mm Hg (statistically significant); DBP decreased 2.2 mm Hg (not significant). This cost-effective way of providing treatment to hypertensive patients should be explored further. A meta-analysis of the effect of biofeedback in hypertension identifed electrodermal feedback as an effective modality in reducing both SBP and DBP, in comparison to an inactive control (Yucha et al., 2001).

RSA feedback has been compared to thermal biofeedback (Herbs, 1994). Both types of feedback have been found to be effective in lowering BP. However, the underlying mechanisms mediating the decrease are probably different. It has been suggested that RSA is effective through an increase in parasympathetic activity, whereas thermal feedback facilitates decreased sympathetic hyperactivity, as described above.

Relaxation

Practitioners use relaxation therapies as a sole treatment or in combination with biofeedback modalities in stepped psychophysiological approaches for treatment of essential hypertension. Although the relaxation therapies differ in instructions and processes, each shares a common goal of enhanced calmness and reduced sympathetic arousal. The most common types of relaxation used to treat elevated BP include the following:

- Progressive relaxation (Bernstein & Borkovec, 1973; Jacobson, 1977; Bernstein & Carlson, 1993).
- Autogenic therapy (Linden, 1990, 1994; Luthe, 1969) and modified autogenic therapy (Green, Green, & Norris, 1980).
- Hypnotic relaxation (Deabler, Fidel, Dillenkoffer, & Elder, 1973).
- Transcendental Meditation (TM) (Schneider, Alexander, & Wallace, 1992; Wallace, 1970).
- Benson's "relaxation response" (Benson, Beary, & Carol, 1974).
- Yogic meditation, including deep breathing (Patel, 1973; Patel & North, 1975).

TM has been utilized in several studies of individuals with hypertension. Alexander et al. (1996) compared TM to education and to progressive relaxation in a group of elderly blacks. TM was associated with a decrease in both SBP and DBP in the group reporting high stress, while the progressive relaxation group decreased SBP only. TM was tested against lifestyle modification in 100 African Americans with mild hypertension. The results favored the TM group, with decreases in SBP of 10.7 mm Hg and DBP of 6.4 mm Hg (Schneider et al., 1995).

No one type of relaxation has been proven to be more efficacious than other types in treatment of hypertension (Linden & Chambers, 1994). However, the incorrect use of progressive relaxation may be problematical for patients with hypertension, for the following reasons. The first is that the muscle contraction component of progressive relaxation may produce breath holding and a *Valsalva response* (Herman, 1989). The Valsalva response results in an increase in cardiac output, and thereby increased SBP and DBP. Second, holding the breath initiates an increase in sympathetic neural activity that will increase BP. Third, the type of tensing done during progressive relaxation is of the isometric variety, in contrast with the isotonic or aerobic type. Isometric exercises produce increases in SBP and DBP; tensing muscles very tightly or for too long impedes blood flow to the muscles, as described earlier.

Yet progressive relaxation is too valuable a therapeutic modality to be eliminated completely from the treatment of hypertension. The practitioner can use progressive relaxation to help patients to discriminate tension and relaxation. However, it is important to do these things:

- Attend to the breathing pattern of patients who are using this technique.
- Encourage patients to monitor their breathing and to make sure that they do not hold their breath during the muscle tension phase.
- Instruct patients to use the minimal amount of tension that allows them to learn to discriminate between the tension and the relaxation state. Shorten the time for tensing, compared to the time for the relaxation phase.
- Remember to include passive relaxation procedures after ending progressive relaxation practice.

Glasgow et al. (1989) have suggested sequencing relaxation and biofeedback as follows. After a 1-month BP monitoring phase, patients start the SBP feedback procedure. If BP falls to acceptable levels, patients may not need further treatment, but only a check of BP at 6 months or yearly. If SBP feedback does not lower BP sufficiently, the relaxation procedures should be implemented and should include both progressive and passive relaxation. Patients are instructed to use the relaxation procedures multiple times each day, especially if they find their BP elevated. If BP is sufficiently low after relaxation therapy, then patients should start the follow-up protocol. If BP still is too high, consultation with a physician and appropriate pharmacological intervention should be recommended.

The number of clinic sessions varies, depending on the severity of the hypertension and patient adherence. In one study, patients who received biofeedback first and relaxation second did slightly better than those who received the therapies in reverse order. Furthermore, patients who received both treatments were better at long-term follow-up than patients who received only one (Engel, Glasgow, & Gaarder, 1983).

Although the designs of most experimental protocols emphasize a standardized treatment package, Linden et al. (2001) used a combination of techniques (including temperature biofeedback, autogenic therapy, and coping skills instruction) with some individualization. Average 24-hour means for SBP and DBP were reduced significantly at posttest and were more striking at the 6-month follow-up.

It is likely that biofeedback and relaxation operate through different physiological mechanisms. Relaxation may have a generalized effect in reducing sympathetic nerve activity that affects heart rate and decreases stroke volume. On the other hand, biofeedback may work primarily through vasomotor control, because BP increases and decreases (with biofeedback) without a concomitant change in heart rate. Thus biofeedback and relaxation may be complementary rather than alternative methods in BP control (Engel & Baile, 1989).

Cognitive strategies are also included in psychophysiological therapies. Development of coping skills assists patients in managing their anxiety and their reactions to stress (Davis, Eshelman, & McKay, 1995). Sometimes significant anxiety occurs when a patient hears the diagnosis of essential hypertension. Practitioners should consider evaluation of anxiety and cognitive strategies before the biofeedback component begins. Then they can integrate new coping skills into the biofeedback and relaxation therapies, as was done by Linden et al. (2001).

Because primary hypertension is a complex, multidimensional illness, it is logical to expect that people with it will respond with varying degrees of success to relaxation and biofeedback. As with pharmacological agents, each modality helps some individuals. The psychophysiological profile can be used to tailor the treatment program to the individual; for example, individuals with cold hands and feet, but slightly elevated facial tension may benefit more from thermal feedback than from EMG feedback. Psychological testing for anxiety or anger can also be used to guide treatment (Linden et al., 2001).

Home Practice

Steptoe, Patel, Marmot, and Hunt (1987) demonstrated a significant association between relaxation practice and reduced BP. However, in research by Wittrock, Blanchard, and McCoy (1988), patients succeeding and failing to reduce their BP reported a similar frequency of practice and sensations of relaxation. Nonetheless, researchers and clinicians usually agree that relaxation practice is essential if a patient is to transfer or generalize what he or she has learned in the clinical setting to home or work.

It is commonly recommended that home practice occur at least twice a day for 15–20 minutes. Practice encompasses relaxation with or without simple biofeedback devices. Consideration should be given to having patients maintain a daily record of practice and a more detailed diary of thoughts and feelings during practice. The patients should be instructed in the procedures, and then provided with written scripts and relaxation tapes. Practitioners should emphasize the importance of learning the relaxation procedures well enough that lowering of BP occurs without scripts or tapes. Home practice using the direct SBP feedback techniques has been explained above. Patients can incorporate thermal biofeedback into home relaxation practice by using small, inexpensive temperature devices.

Patients should be instructed to measure the temperature of their hands, feet, or both before and after relaxation practice. They also may use continuous visual feedback during relaxation practice. Patients should keep their bodies warm by covering themselves (excluding the hands and feet) if necessary, because it is more difficult to elicit a hand- or foot-warming response in a room that is cold. This may be particularly significant for elderly individuals and for economically challenged persons who may be keeping their thermostats set at lower levels. Elderly persons often have some difficulty maintaining adequate blood supply to the extremities, so they may start their practice with colder hands.

Long-term follow-up is very important for patients who complete a clinical program for reducing their BP. Hypertension is a progressive disease; thus one expects BP increases over time as part of the aging process. Long-term maintenance of reductions in BP resulting from relaxation and/or biofeedback therapies were reported by Taylor, Farquhar, Nelson, and Agras (1977), Agras, Southam, and Taylor (1983), Engel et al. (1983), Blanchard et al. (1986, 1988), Fahrion et al. (1986), Leserman et al. (1989), McGrady, Nadsady, and Schumann-Brzezinski (1991), and Goebel et al. (1993). Although the percentage of patients retaining the treatment effects varies, some patients maintain criterion BP for 1–3 years, and in one study of stress management therapy the BP continued to decrease during the 6-month follow-up period (Linden et al., 2001).

The necessity of continuing to practice relaxation to maintain BP at lower levels lacks consensus. Some research supports the use of relaxation practice as an essential component of maintaining lowered BP. However, other studies have not been able to demonstrate conclusively the necessity for continued relaxation practice. It seems logical for practitioners to suggest, nonetheless, continued practice of relaxation. The improved cognitive processing of stressful stimuli initiated during treatment should be emphasized. If research confirms the necessity of consistent practice, then the psychophysiological therapies can be viewed in the same context as aerobic exercise. Although exercise may lower BP during a short-term program, it too requires continued adherence to maintain the gains achieved during conditioning. If one stops exercising, the cardiovascular and skeletal muscle systems decondition faster than the training period necessary to build them up. It is wise, therefore, in a clinical practice, to make clear and organized arrangements for follow-up with patients before they end treatment.

The design of an efficacious follow-up program for patients is challenging. Here are several options:

- Mail BP log sheets to patients, and ask them to return the log in a preaddressed stamped envelope.
- Contact patients by phone at regular intervals, and ask for recent blood pressures.
- Schedule periodic follow-up booster or refresher sessions with relaxation and biofeedback. For example, patients may receive one refresher therapy session every other week for 6 weeks, followed by monthly sessions for 6 months, and then follow-up sessions at 6-month intervals (progressing to yearly intervals).
- In a physician-based or collaborative setting, obtain the BP values from the physician's office at the time of the patient's regular checkups.

SPECIAL POPULATIONS

Pregnant Women

The efficacy of biofeedback-based and relaxation-based interventions in pregnancy-induced hypertension (PIH) has been investigated. PIH is a condition where previously normotensive pregnant women develop high BP after the 20th week of gestation. If BP is left untreated, prospective mothers can develop serious complications, including edema of the hands or face, protein in the urine, and damage to organs (kidneys, liver, heart, brain, and eyes). PIH can become life-threatening for both a mother and baby. Traditional treatment for PIH consists of bed rest and obstetrical monitoring. Frequently, women find adherence difficult, particularly if they have other family obligations.

Somers, Gevirtz, Jasin, and Chin (1989) divided women with PIH into three groups. One group received standard medical care. The second group was provided an additional 4 hours of education to increase compliance to bed rest. The third or active-intervention group received treatment consisting of self-monitoring of BP, thermal-biofeedback-assisted relaxation, hand and foot warming, and diaphragmatic breathing. Total therapy time was also 4 hours. Subjects were instructed to practice the techniques twice daily at home in bed. Subjects in the biobehavioral group maintained their BP at a significantly lower level than did the group on bed rest alone or the group with enhanced compliance to bed rest. Although these findings were encouraging, no systematic replication of this study has been reported.

Elderly Persons

Isolated systolic hypertension is a relatively common problem in elderly persons. These individuals have an abnormal SBP, but their DBP is below 90 mm Hg. Pearce, Engel, and Burton (1989) instructed 15 individuals over the age of 60 with SBP feedback to lower SBP, using their own sphygmomanometers. Relaxation therapy followed the biofeedback period. Significant decreases averaging 13 mm Hg SBP were recorded in the 15 hypertensive patients. As mentioned above, TM has also been applied successfully to elderly persons with essential hypertension in whom both SBP and DBP are elevated.

The positive results from preliminary studies of these special populations are promising and indicate a need for larger clinical trials.

TREATMENT OUTCOME MEASURES AND ASSESSMENT OF SUCCESS

An evaluation of the effects of biobehavioral interventions for essential hypertension in individual patients includes the following specific questions:

- Did the patient succeed in reducing BP to the target level?
- Is the reduction of BP clinically significant and statistically significant?
- Has the patient reduced his or her medication? Has the BP remained in the normal range while the patient decreased medication?
- If the BP is normal, did the patient alter his or her lifestyle or dietary habits (e.g., sodium intake, weight loss, exercise) after treatment? If so, could these changes account for the reductions of BP?

- Has the patient shown positive transfer of physiological self-regulation? That is, can he or she lower BP and maintain lower BP at work, at home, and in the physician's office, as well as in the biofeedback practitioner's office? Is 24-hour ambulatory BP also significantly decreased?
- For how long after completion of therapy is the BP in the normal range?
- Has the patient achieved specified and credible criteria for physiological self-regulation? For example, if peripheral skin temperature of 95°F is the established criterion, is the patient consistently able to raise the temperature to that level for specified durations?

Evaluation of clinical applications of biofeedback in "group outcome studies" should include the following considerations:

- The clinical significance of the decreases in SBP and DBP, based on calculation of the change in risk for stroke and coronary artery disease. Even relatively small decreases of DBP of 5–6 mm Hg are associated with a 35% decrease in incidence of stroke (Schneider et al., 1995).
- The statistical significance of the decreases in SBP and DBP.
- The stability of the lower BP.
- The proportion of treated patients who improved significantly.
- The degree of transfer of BP changes obtained in the clinic to the patients' environments (home and work).
- Sufficient length of baseline period to separate treatment effects from monitoring or habituation effects.
- Documentation of learning of the relaxation response or biofeedback technique.
- Adequate controls for medication changes.
- Adequate controls for changes in weight, dietary sodium, and physical exercise.
- An attempt to identify which patient or therapy process characteristics account for differential therapy outcome. Such information can later be used to refine clinical decision-making processes (see below for more discussion).

PREDICTION OF TREATMENT RESPONSE

It is cost-effective and efficient to attempt to describe characteristics of patients that enhance their ability to lower their BP. Before a practitioner accepts a hypertensive patient for biobehavioral treatment, he or she should ensure that a physician has ruled out secondary hypertension. Determination of the pretreatment BP and medication history is also important. Furthermore, if an individual's diagnosis is primary hypertension and the BP is already controlled, then psychophysiological therapies may not produce any further lowering of BP. Under these circumstances, the clinical goal can be reduction in medication.

Adherence to the therapist's recommendations is also part of the patient selection process. If a person resists the BP monitoring recommendations and misses appointments during the baseline period, then that person's adherence to biofeedback and relaxation instructions is in doubt. If a patient shows poor adherence (missed appointments, sporadic monitoring, unwillingness to learn the measurement technique), then adherence to relaxation instructions is also apt to be problematic. However, poor adherence to antihypertensive medication does not automatically translate into poor adherence to relaxation instructions. Some people oppose beginning antihypertensive medication in the early stages of treatment. A better test of a patient's willingness to adhere to psychophysiological therapy is the baseline period. At that time, the practitioner should discuss potential adherence problems with the patient. In all professional biobehavioral therapy settings, patients should demonstrate a high level of involvement and motivation. Patients must understand clearly their own responsibilities and the need to self-manage medication regimens, to obtain BPs according to instructions, to attend office sessions, and to apply therapy procedures consistently.

There have been several attempts at characterizing patients to assess their chances of success in biofeedback programs. Early work pointed to successful patients' having higher neurogenic tone (Cottier, Shapiro, & Julius, 1984), as well as higher anxiety, forehead muscle tension, and cortisol levels (McGrady, Utz, Woerner, Bernal, & Higgins, 1986). Later, McGrady and Higgins (1989) and Weaver and McGrady (1995) suggested a predictor profile potentially useful in recommending treatment to patients. The factors tested in this profile included indicators of the classical stress response and substances related to the pathophysiology of hypertension. Patients with the best chances for success in lowering BP had higher pretreatment anxiety scores, heart rate, cortisol, and plasma renin activity, as well as lower hand temperatures. Confirmation of this profile is currently underway. Interestingly, patient age did not correlate with treatment success, suggesting that older patents do not need to be excluded from research studies (Linden et al., 2001). In a controlled comparison between thermal biofeedback and progressive relaxation, the three variables investigated were expectancies, skill acquisition, and home practice. There were no significant differences in practice between treatment groups or between successful and unsuccessful patients; for thermal biofeedback, skill acquisition and expectancies were related to outcome; for the progressive relaxation group, perceptions of relaxation correlated with success (Wittrock et al., 1988). There is no evidence that success is limited to one ethnic group, although the mechanisms underlying decreases in BP may differ (McGrady & Roberts, 1992).

THE WELL-EQUIPPED OFFICE

The well-equipped office for treating patients with primary hypertension includes the following:

- An automated BP monitor (with digital readouts) that has a demonstrated high level of accuracy.
- Several different-sized BP monitoring cuffs.
- A *Physicians' Desk Reference*.
- A manual of drug interactions.
- Self-monitoring BP devices to lend to patients.
- Written instructions for the measurement and recording of BP by patients.
- A variety of written and visual aids for patient education.
- Log sheets for recording BP and home practice.

Ideally, 24-hour ambulatory monitors should be available to settle issues of proper diagnosis.

DIRECTIONS FOR FUTURE RESEARCH AND UNANSWERED QUESTIONS

We encourage professionals to use appropriate clinical research designs to test patients' responses to biofeedback and related therapies, and to help advance the basis for using these therapy procedures. The most effective biobehavioral therapy programs are treatment packages that include education, BP monitoring, positive expectancies, one or more relaxation therapies, and direct or indirect biofeedback modalities. Each of the individual components may contribute a unique or overlapping modulation of cardiac output or TPR.

Here are some of the unresolved questions in this field:

- How reliable and long-lasting are the BP decreases induced by biofeedback and relaxation?
- What is the role of home practice of relaxation in short-term and long-term outcome?
- Can one predict BP responses to biofeedback, relaxation, or the two combined?
- Can the efficacy of biofeedback and relaxation be demonstrated in special populations, such as pregnant women and elderly persons?
- Can one improve cost-effectiveness using a group format or a minimal-therapist-contact format instead of a series of individual therapy sessions?
- Is an individualized treatment package more effective than a standardized or manual-driven approach?
- Are the patients who respond to biofeedback and relaxation the same patients who respond to salt restriction and exercise? Should the lifestyle modifications be combined for greater effectiveness?
- Subject, therapist, and procedural variables all need investigation. Which therapies work better for different patients, provided by whom, how often, for how long, and under what conditions?

CONCLUSIONS

The final goal of health care practitioners is for their patients to have BP adequately controlled with a treatment regimen that the patients can maintain for a long time with the least amount of medication. There is considerable evidence that individuals can develop and retain effective self-regulation of their BP. Combined pharmacological and nonpharmacological therapies, including lifestyle changes, hold great promise in management of hypertension. Further research will clarify which persons can benefit most from biofeedback and relaxation therapy, as well as which therapies are preferentially efficacious.

GLOSSARY

ADRENAL CORTEX. Outer region of each adrenal gland, which secretes aldosterone, cortisol, and androgens.

ADRENAL GLANDS. A pair of endocrine glands located above each kidney. The outer portion of the gland is the adrenal cortex. The inner portion is the adrenal medulla.

ADRENAL MEDULLA. The medulla or inner core of each adrenal gland. Epinephrine (adrenaline) and a small amount of norepinephrine (noradrenaline) are secreted by the medulla.

ALDOSTERONE. Hormone secreted by the adrenal cortex that regulates balance of electrolytes.

ALDOSTERONISM. An abnormality of electrolyte metabolism caused by excessive secretion of aldosterone.

ANGIOTENSIN II. Hormone that stimulates secretion of aldosterone from adrenal cortex. Promotes smooth muscle contraction and arteriolar constriction.

ANGIOTENSIN-CONVERTING ENZYME INHIBITORS (ACE INHIBITORS). Drugs used to lower blood pressure (BP) by decreasing vascular resistance. Example: enalapril (Vasotec).

ATRIAL NATRIURETIC FACTOR (ANF). Hormone secreted by atrial cells that causes a decrease in reabsorption of sodium by the kidney. More sodium is excreted.

BARORECEPTORS. Stretch receptors in the carotid sinus or aortic arch. Sensitive to stretch induced by changes in arterial blood pressure.

BETA-BLOCKERS. Drugs used to lower BP by decreasing cardiac output by adrenergic blockade at either beta- or beta$_2$-adrenergic receptors or at both. Example: propranolol (Inderal).

CALCIUM CHANNEL BLOCKERS. Drugs used to lower BP by decreasing vascular resistance. Example: verapamil (Calan).

CARDIAC CYCLE. One contraction–relaxation cycle of the heart.

CARDIAC OUTPUT. Blood volume pumped by each ventricle per minute.

CORTISOL. The major natural glucocorticoid hormone released from the adrenal cortex. Influences many aspects of metabolism.

CUSHING'S DISEASE. Syndrome in which the pituitary secretes excessive adrenocorticotropic hormone, and the adrenal cortex secretes too much cortisol.

DESENSITIZATION (SYSTEMATIC DESENSITIZATION). A common type of behavior therapy to assist patients to decrease fear, phobias, and arousal responses associated with certain stimuli. There is gradual exposure for very limited periods from the least anxiety-producing to increasingly anxiety-producing activity. Exposure is imagined, with artificial stimuli (e.g. pictures, video—known as *in vitro*), and/or is actual, with real-life stimuli (known as *in vivo*). An example of *in vivo* exposure is gradually exposing a person with "white-coat hypertension" to BP instruments and procedures so the person can become accustomed to them.

DIASTOLIC BLOOD PRESSURE (DBP). Minimum BP during relaxation of the heart that occurs during the cardiac cycle.

DIURETICS. Drugs that increase the excretion of urine, thus decreasing plasma volume. Example: hydrochlorothiazide (Dyazide).

HG. Abbreviation for mercury. Millimeters of mercury (abbreviated mm Hg with specific measurements) are units of pressure.

HYPERTHYROIDISM. Excessive secretion of hormone by the thyroid gland; characterized by increased metabolic rate, goiter, and disturbances in the autonomic nervous system.

ISCHEMIA. Reduced blood supply to the heart.

MEAN ARTERIAL PRESSURE (MAP). The average pressure during the cardiac cycle. It is calculated by adding DBP to one-third pulse pressure.

METABOLISM. Total chemical reactions that occur in a living organism.

NEURAL. Having to do with nerve cells or nervous system. "Non-neural" means not related to nerve cells or nervous system.

PARASYMPATHETIC. A subdivision of the autonomic nervous system whose fibers originate from brainstem and the sacral region of spinal cord.

PLASMA. Liquid portion of the blood.

RENIN. Enzyme secreted by the kidney that, along with angiotensin-converting enzyme, catalyzes formation of angiotensin II; important in BP regulation.

SPHYGMOMANAMETER. Device that consists of a cuff, which can be inflated, and a pressure gauge used for measuring BP. In the aneroid type, the pressure gauge does not contain liquid. In the mercury type, the pressure gauge contains mercury.

STROKE VOLUME. Amount of blood ejected by a ventricle during one heartbeat.

SYMPATHETIC. Subdivision of the autonomic nervous system whose fibers originate in the thoracic and lumbar regions of the spinal cord.

SYSTOLIC BLOOD PRESSURE (SBP). Maximum arterial BP during the cardiac cycle.

TOTAL PERIPHERAL RESISTANCE (TPR). The sum of all resistances to blood flow in all the systemic blood vessels.

VALSALVA RESPONSE. Forcible exhalation effort against a closed glottis, or against occluded (pinched) nostrils and closed mouth. Increases intrathoracic pressure and interferes with venous return to the heart.

VASCULAR. Pertaining to blood vessels or indicative of a copious blood supply.

ACKNOWLEDGMENTS

We thank hypertension subspecialist William E. Haley, MD, of the Mayo Clinic in Jacksonville, Florida, for his review of a draft of this chapter. His comments and suggestions were very helpful. This does not imply his endorsement of the content of this chapter.

REFERENCES

Agras, W. S., Southam, M. A., & Taylor, C. B. (1983). Long-term persistence of relaxation induced blood pressure lowering during the working day. *Journal of Consulting and Clinical Psychology, 51*, 792–794.

Alexander, C. N. Schneider, R. H., Staggers, F., Sheppard, W. Clayborne, B. M., Rainforth, M. Salerno, J., Kondwani, K., Smith, S., Walton, K. G., & Egan, B. (1996). Trial of stress reduction for hypertension in older African Americans. *Hypertension, 28*, 228–237.

ALLHAT Officers and Coordinators for the ALLHAT Collaborative Research Group. (2000). Major cardiovascular events in hypertensive patients randomized to doxazosin versus chlorthalidone: The Antihypertensive and Lipid-Lowering Treatment to Prevent Heart Attack Trial (ALLHAT). *Journal of the American Medical Association, 283*, 1967–1975.

Benson, H., Beary, J. F., & Carol, M. P. (1974). The relaxation response. *Psychiatry, 37*, 37–46.

Benson, H., Shapiro, D., Tursky, B., & Schwartz, G. E. (1971). Decreased systolic blood pressure through operant conditioning techniques in patients with essential hypertension. *Science, 173*, 740–741.

Bernstein, D. A., & Borkovec, T. D. (1973). *Progressive relaxation training: A manual for helping professions.* Champaign, IL: Research Press.

Bernstein, D. A., & Carlson, C. R. (1993). Progressive relaxation: Abbreviated methods. In P. M. Lehrer & R. L. Woolfolk (Eds.), *Principles and practice of stress management.* New York: Guilford Press.

Blanchard, E. B. (1990). Biofeedback treatments of essential hypertension. *Biofeedback and Self-Regulation, 15*(3), 209–228.

Blanchard, E. B., Kharashvili, V. V., McCoy, G. C., Aivazyan, T. A., McCaffrey, R. J., Salenko, B. B., Musso, A., Wittrock, D. A., Bereger, M., Gerardi, M. A., & Pangburn, L. (1988). The USA–USSR collaborative cross-cultural comparison of autogenic training and thermal biofeedback in the treatment of mild hypertension. *Health Psychology, 7*, 175–192.

Blanchard, E. B., McCoy, G. C., Musso, A., Gerardi, M. A., Pallmeyer, T. P., Gerardi, R. J., Cotch, P. A., Siracusa, K., & Andrasik, F. (1986). A controlled comparison of thermal biofeedback and relaxation training in the treatment of essential hypertension: I. Short-term and long-term outcome. *Behavior Therapy, 17*, 563–579.

Brody, D. S. (1981). Psychological distress and hypertension control. *Journal of Human Stress, 6*(1), 2–6.

Brook, R. D., & Julius, S. (2000). Autonomic imbalance, hypertension, and cardiovascular risk. *American Journal of Hypertension, 13*(6), 112S-122S.

Byrne, D. G. (1992). Anxiety, neuroticism, depression, and hypertension. In E. H. Johnson, W. D. Gentry, & S. Julius (Eds.), *Personality, elevated blood pressure, and essential hypertension.* Washington, DC: Hemisphere.

Chobanian, A. Y., & Hill, M. (2000). The NHLBI workshop on sodium and blood pressure: A critical review of current scientific evidence. *Hypertension, 35*(4), 858–863.

Conlin, P. R., Chow, D., Miller, E. R. III, Svetkey, L. P., Lin, P-H, Harsha, D. W., Moore, T. J., Sacks, F. M., & Appel, L. J., for the DASH Research Group. (2000). The effect of dietary patterns on blood pressure control in hypertensive patients: Results from the Dietary Approaches to Stop Hypertension (DASH) trial. *American Journal of Hypertension, 13*, 949–955.

Cottier, C., Shapiro, K., & Julius, S. (1984). Treatment of mild hypertension with progressive muscle relaxation. *Archives of Internal Medicine, 144*, 1954–1958.

Cushman, W. C. (2001). Clinical overview of hypertension and emerging treatment considerations. *American Journal of Hypertension, 14*, 226S–230S.

Davis, M., Eshelman, E. R., & McKay, M. (1995). Coping skills training. In M. Davis, E. R. Eshelman, & M. McKay (Eds.), *The relaxation and stress reduction workbook* (4th ed.). Oakland, CA: New Harbinger.

Deabler, H. L., Fidel, E., Dillenkoffer, R. L., & Elder, S. T. (1973). The use of relaxation and hypnosis in lowering high blood pressure. *American Journal of Clinical Hypnosis, 16*, 75–83.

Engel, B. T., & Baile, W. S. (1989). Behavioral applications in the treatment of patients with cardiovascular disorders. In J. B. Basmajian (Ed.), *Biofeedback: Principles and practice for clinicians* (3rd ed.). Baltimore: Williams & Wilkins.

Engel, B. T., Gaarder, K. R, & Glasgow, M. S. (1981). Behavioral treatment of high blood pressure: I. Analyses of intra- and inter-daily variations of blood pressure during a one-month, baseline period, *Psychosomatic Medicine, 43*, 255–270.

Engel, B. T., Glasgow, M. S., & Gaarder, K. R. (1983). Behavioral treatment of high blood pressure: II. Follow-up results and treatment recommendations, *Psychosomatic Medicine, 45*(1), 23–29.

Fahrion, S., Norris, P., Green, A., Green, E., & Snarr, C. (1986). Behavioral treatment of essential hypertension: A group outcome study. *Biofeedback and Self-Regulation, 11*(4), 257–259.

Freedman, R. R. (1991). Physiological mechanisms of temperature biofeedback. *Biofeedback and Self-Regulation, 16,* 95–115.

Ganong, W. F. (1997). *Review of medical physiology* (18th ed.). Los Altos, CA: Lange Medical.

Glasgow, M. S., Engel, B. T., & D'Lugoff, B. C. (1989). A controlled study of a standardized behavioral stepped treatment for hypertension. *Psychosomatic Medicine, 51,* 10–26.

Glasgow, M. S., Gaarder, K. R., & Engel, B. T. (1982). Behavioral treatment of high blood pressure: II. Acute and sustained effects of relaxation and systolic blood pressure biofeedback. *Psychosomatic Medicine, 44*(2), 155–170.

Goebel, M., Viol, G. W., & Orebaugh, C. (1993). An incremental model to isolate specific effects of behavioral treatments in essential hypertension. *Biofeedback and Self-Regulation, 18*(4), 255–280.

Green, E. E., Green, A., & Norris, P. A. (1980). Self-regulation training for control of hypertension. *Primary Cardiology, 6,* 126–137.

Guidelines Subcommittee, World Health Organization—International Society of Hypertension. (1999). 1999 World Health Organization—International Society of Hypertension Guidelines for the Management of Hypertension. *Journal of Hypertension, 17,* 151–183.

Hatch, J. P., Klatt, K. D., Supik, J. D., Rios, N., Fisher, J. G., Bauer, R. L., & Shimotsu, G. W. (1985). Combined behavioral and pharmacological treatment of essential hypertension. *Biofeedback and Self-Regulation, 10*(2), 119–138.

Herbs, D. (1994). *The effects of heart rate pattern biofeedback versus skin temperature biofeedback for the treatment of essential hypertension.* Unpublished doctoral dissertation, California School of Professional Psychology, San Diego.

Herman, J. (1989). Valsalva response during progressive relaxation: An extension study. *Scholarly Inquiry for Nursing Practice, An International Journal, 3,* 217–225.

Jacob, R. G., Chesney, M. A., Williams, D. M., Ding, Y., & Shapiro, A. P. (1991). Relaxation therapy for hypertension: Design effects and treatment effects. *Annals of Behavioral Medicine, 13*(1), 5–17.

Jacobson, E. (1977). The origins and development of progressive relaxation. *Journal of Behavior Therapy and Experimental Psychiatry, 8,* 119–123.

Joffres, M. R., Hamet, P., MacLean, D. R., L'italien, G. J., & Fodor, G. (2001). Distribution of blood pressure and hypertension in Canada and the United States. *American Journal of Hypertension, 14,* 1099–1105.

Joint National Committee (JNC) on Detection, Evaluation, and Treatment of High Blood Pressure. (1997). The sixth report of the Joint National Committee on Detection, Evaluation and Treatment of High Blood Pressure: JNC VI. *Archives of Internal Medicine, 157,* 2413–2446.

Jonas, B. S., Franks, P., & Ingram, D. D. (1997). Are symptoms of anxiety and depression risk factors for hypertension? *Archives of Family Medicine, 6,* 43–49.

Jorgensen, R. S., Johnson, B. T., & Kolodziej, M. E. (1996). Elevated blood pressure and personality: A meta-analytic review. *Psychological Bulletin, 120,* 293–320.

Julius, S. (1991). Autonomic nervous dysfunction in essential hypertension. *Diabetes Care, 14*(3), 249–259.

Julius, S. (2000). Worldwide trends and shortcomings in the treatment of hypertension. *American Journal of Hypertension, 13*(5), 57S–61S.

Jurek, I. E., Higgins, J. T., Jr., & McGrady, A. (1992). Interaction of biofeedback-assisted relaxation and diuretic in treatment of essential hypertension. *Biofeedback and Self-Regulation, 17*(2), 125–141.

Kaplan, N. M. (1998). *Clinical hypertension.* Baltimore: Williams & Wilkins.

Kristt, D. A., & Engel, B. T. (1975). Learned control of blood pressure in patients with high blood pressure. *Circulation, 51,* 370–378.

Leserman, J., Stuart, E. M., Mamish, M. E., Deckro, J. P., Beckman, R. J., Friedman, R., & Benson, H. (1989). Nonpharmacologic intervention for hypertension: Long-term follow-up. *Journal of Cardiopulmonary Rehabilitation, 9,* 316–324.

Light, K. C., Girdler, S. S., Sherwood, A., Bragdon, E. E., Brownley, K. A., West, S. G., & Hinderliter, A. L. (1999). High stress responsivity predicts later blood pressure only in combination with positive family history and high life stress *Hypertension, 33,* 1458–1464.

Linden, W. (1990). *Autogenic training: A clinical guide.* New York: Guilford Press.

Linden, W. (1994). Autogenic training: A narrative and a quantitative review of clinical outcome. *Biofeedback and Self-Regulation, 19,* 227–264.

Linden, W., & Chambers, L. A. (1994). Clinical effectiveness of non-drug therapies for hypertension: A meta-analysis. *Annals of Behavioral Medicine, 16,* 35–45.

Linden, W., Herbert, C. P., Jenkins, A., & Raffle, V. (1989). Should we tell them when their blood pressure is high? *Canadian Medical Association Journal, 141,* 409–415.

Linden, W., Lenz, J. W., & Con, A. H. (2001). Individualized stress management for primary hypertension: A randomized trial. *Archives of Internal Medicine, 161,* 1071–1080.

Liu, J. E., Roman, M. J., Pini, R., Schwartz, J. E., Pickering, T. G., & Devereux, R. B. (1999). Elevated ambulatory with normal clinic blood pressure ("white coat normotension") is associated with cardiac and arterial target organ damage. *Annals of Internal Medicine, 131,* 564–572.

Luke, R. G. (1996). Evaluation of the patient with hypertension. In J. S. Alpert (Ed.), *Cardiology for the primary care physician.* St. Louis, MO: Mosby.

Luthe, W. (1969). *Autogenic therapy.* New York: Grune & Stratton.

M'Buyamaba-Kabangu, J. R., Amery, A., & Lijnen, P. (1994). Differences between black and white persons in blood pressure and related biological variables. *Journal of Human Hypertension, 8,* 163–170.

McCoy, G. C., Blanchard, E. B., Wittrock, D. A., Morrison, S., Pangburn, L., Siracusa, K., & Pallmeyer, T. P. (1988). Biochemical changes associated with thermal biofeedback treatment of hypertension. *Biofeedback and Self-Regulation, 13*(2), 139–150.

McGrady, A. V. (1994). Effects of group relaxation training and thermal biofeedback on blood pressure and related psychophysiological variables in essential hypertension. *Biofeedback and Self-Regulation, 19*(1), 51–66.

McGrady, A. V., & Higgins, J. T., Jr. (1989). Prediction of response to biofeedback-assisted relaxation in hypertensives: Development of a hypertensive predictor profile (HYPP). *Psychosomatic Medicine, 51,* 277–284.

McGrady, A. V., & Higgins, J. T., Jr. (1990). Effect of repeated measurements of blood pressure on blood pressure in essential hypertension: Role of anxiety. *Journal of Behavioral Medicine, 13*(1), 93–101.

McGrady, A. V., Nadsady, P. A., & Schumann-Brzezinski, C. (1991). Sustained effects of biofeedback-assisted relaxation therapy in essential hypertension. *Biofeedback and Self-Regulation, 16*(4), 399–413.

McGrady, A. V., & Roberts, G. (1992). Racial differences in the relaxation response of hypertensives. *Psychosomatic Medicine, 54*(1), 71–78

McGrady, A. V., Utz, S. W., Woerner, M., Bernal, G. A. A., & Higgins, J. T. (1986). Predictors of success in hypertensives treated with biofeedback-assisted relaxation. *Biofeedback and Self-Regulation, 11*(23), 95–103.

McGrady, A. V., Yonker, R, Tan, S. Y., Fine, T. H., & Woerner, M. (1981). The effect of biofeedback-assisted relaxation training on blood pressure and selected biochemical parameters in patients with essential hypertension. *Biofeedback and Self-Regulation, 6*(3), 343–353.

Mycek, M. J., Gertner, S. B., & Perper, M. M. (1992). Antihypertensive drugs. In R. Harvey & P. Champe (Eds.), *Lippincott's illustrated reviews: Pharmacology.* Philadelphia: Lippincott.

Patel, C. H. (1973). Yoga and biofeedback in the management of hypertension, *Lancet, ii,* 1053–1055.

Patel, C. H., & Marmot, M. (1988). Can general practitioners use training in relaxation and management of stress to reduce mild hypertension? *British Medical Journal, 296,* 21–24.

Patel, C. H., & North, S. (1975). Randomized controlled trial of yoga and biofeedback in management of hypertension. *Lancet, ii,* 93–99.

Pearce, K. L., Engel, B. T., & Burton, J. R. (1989). Behavioral treatment of isolated systolic hypertension in the elderly. *Biofeedback and Self-Regulation, 14*(3), 207–219.

Reckelhoff, J. F. (2001). Gender differences in the regulation of blood pressure. *Hypertension, 37,* 1199–1208.

Schneider, R. H., Alexander, C. N., & Wallace, R. K. (1992). In search of an optimal behavioral treatment for hypertension: A review and focus on transcendental meditation. In E. H. Johnson, W. D. Gentry, & S. Julius (Eds.), *Personality, elevated blood pressure, and essential hypertension.* Washington, DC: Hemisphere.

Schneider, R. H., Staggers, F., Alexander, C. N., Sheppard, W., Rainforth, M., Kondwani, K., Smith., S., & King, C. G. (1995). A randomized controlled trial of stress reduction for hypertension in older African Americans. *Hypertension, 26,* 820–827.

Selenta, C., Hogan, B., & Linden, W. (2000). How often do office blood pressure measurements fail to identify true hypertension? *Archives of Family Medicine, 9,* 533–540.

Shakoor-Abdullah, B., Kotchen, J. M., Walker, W. E., Chelius, T. H., & Hoffmann, R. G. (1997). Incorporating socio-economic and risk factor diversity into the development of an African-American community blood pressure control program. *Ethnicity and Disease, 7*(3),175–183.

Shepard, J. D., al'Absi, M., Whitsett, T. L., Passey, R. B., & Lovallo, W. R. (2000). Additive pressor effects of caffeine and stress in male medical students at risk for hypertension. *American Journal of Hypertension, 13,* 475–481.

Somers, P. J., Gevirtz, R. N., Jasin, S. E., & Chin, H. G. (1989). The efficacy of biobehavioral and compliance intentions in the adjunctive treatment of mild pregnancy-induced hypertension. *Biofeedback and Self-Regulation, 14*(4), 309–318.

Spence, J. D., Barnett, P. A., Linden, W., Ramsden, V., & Tanezer, P. (1999). Nonpharmacologic therapy to prevent and control hypertension: Recommendations on stress management. *Canadian Medical Association Journal, 160,* S46–S50.

Steptoe, A., Patel, C., Marmot, M., & Hunt, B. (1987). Frequency of relaxation practice, blood pressure reduction and the general effects of relaxation following a controlled trial of behavior modification for reducing coronary risk. *Stress Medicine, 3,* 101–107.

Taylor, C. B., Farquhar, J. W., Nelson, E., & Agras, W. S. (1977). Relaxation therapy and high blood pressure. *Archives of General Psychiatry, 34,* 339–343.

Tursky, B., Shapiro, D., & Schwartz, G. E. (1972). Automated constant cuff pressure system to measure average systolic and diastolic blood pressures in man. *IEEE Transactions on Biomedical Engineering, 19,* 271–276.

Vander, A. J., Sherman, J. H., & Luciano, D. S. (2001). *Human physiology* (8th ed.). New York: McGraw-Hill.

Wallace, R. K. (1970). Physiological effects of transcendental meditation. *Science, 167,* 1751–1754.

Weaver, M. T., & McGrady, A. (1995). A provisional model to predict blood pressure response to biofeedback-assisted relaxation. *Biofeedback and Self-Regulation, 20*(3), 229–240.

Weber, M.A. (2001). Rationalizing the treatment of hypertension. *American Journal of Hypertension, 14,* 3S–7S.

Weinberger, M. H. (1993). *Hypertension primer.* Dallas, TX: American Heart Association.

Winkleby, M. A., Kraemer, H. C., Ahn, D. K., & Warady, A. N. (1998). Ethnic and socioeconomic differences in cardiovascular disease risk factors. *Journal of the American Medical Association, 280,* 356–362.

Wittrock, D. A., Blanchard, E. B., & McCoy, G. C. (1988). Three studies on the relation of process to outcome in the treatment of essential hypertension with relaxation and thermal biofeedback. *Behaviour Research and Therapy, 26*(1), 53–66.

Wright, J. M. (2000). Choosing a first-line drug in the management of elevated blood pressure: What is the evidence? 1. Thiazide diuretics. *Canadian Medical Association Journal, 163,* 57–60.

Yucha, C. B. (2001). Ambulatory blood pressure monitoring: Measurement implications for research. *Journal of Nursing Measurement, 9,* 49–59.

Yucha, C. B., Clark, L., Smith, M., Uris, P., LaFleur, B., & Duval, S. (2001). The effect of biofeedback in hypertension. *Applied Nursing Research, 14,* 29–35.

PART VI

Electroencephalographic Biofeedback Applications

CHAPTER 18

Neurofeedback for the Management of Attention Deficit Disorders

JOEL F. LUBAR

Attention-deficit/hyperactivity disorder (ADHD) exists in all countries and in all cultures. Its recognition and characteristics became considerably clearer in the last two decades. It is a very significant neurobiological and genetically based disorder affecting a large number of children and many adults. Certainly ADHD can be debilitating in terms of achieving educational objectives, maintaining employment, and developing careers. It is also a disorder that can be extremely disruptive within family systems, and it affects most aspects of one's ability to function effectively in a complex society and to set and achieve important life goals.

In this chapter, I describe a relatively new, very promising, and powerful adjunctive procedure for treatment and long-term management of this disorder. My work in this area began in the mid-1970s. Later publications (Lubar, 1991; Lubar, Swartwood, Swartwood, & Timmermann, 1995; Lubar & Lubar, 1999) have described the details of the development of this treatment approach for ADHD. During the early development of this technique, the treatment involved what was commonly called "electroencephalographic (EEG) biofeedback." However, in the last few years, a new term emerged—*neurofeedback*. (Note that in this as in other chapters, terms in italics are included in the glossary at the end of the chapter.) This word specifically refers to feedback designed to alter a condition that displays evidence of being neurologically based.

However, *neurofeedback* in a broader sense is defined as biofeedback linked to a specific aspect of the electrical activity of the brain—such as the frequency, amplitude, or duration of activity such as theta (4–8 hertz), alpha (8–13 hertz), or beta (13 hertz or greater)—from certain scalp or brain locations. Neurofeedback can also be linked to components of auditory, visual, or somatosensory event-related potentials (ERPs) or slow direct-current shifts in cortical excitability, as shown by Schneider et al. (1992) and others in the research group in Tuebingen, Germany, in their work with schizophrenia and other conditions. (See Neumann, Strehl, & Birbaumer, Chapter 5, this volume, for an introduction to EEG instrumentation written by some of the Tuebingen group.)

Currently, there are over 1200 organizations in the United States and many in Australia, Israel, Europe, and Japan using EEG neurofeedback in the treatment of ADHD, based on information from manufacturers of neurofeedback equipment. These include private clinics, university-based groups, and individuals working within school systems. Neurofeedback is employed by a wide range of practitioners, including pediatricians, psychiatrists, clinical and counseling psychologists, clinical psychophysiologists, social workers, educational specialists, nurses, and other health care providers.

This chapter first provides a description of ADHD and its characteristics, a brief historical review, and a description of some of the existing therapies for this disorder. Next I present a detailed description of the EEG characteristics of ADHD, along with the rationale for new databases derived from EEG measures. I then discuss the rationale for neurofeedback, including the criteria for an effective intervention with specific individuals. I also describe the details of instrumentation and treatment protocols that are recommended for this type of training, and how they vary as a function of age, intelligence, and severity of the disorder. Pre- and post-treatment measurements used to determine the effectiveness of neurofeedback constitute the next topic. I then describe the results from our clinic, our university-based research, and those of others. The next section of this chapter focuses on the integration of neurofeedback with other therapies, including the use of medications, family therapy, individual therapy, and parent support groups. Finally, I outline future directions that need to be considered for the further development of neurofeedback therapy for ADHD.

Treatment of ADHD is complex and is guided by a number of considerations. It is important to determine which scalp locations and which amplitude and frequency characteristics of the EEG need to be enhanced or decreased, and what electrical parameters need to be incorporated into the instrumentation. Careful management of these specific variables will greatly determine whether the outcome of the treatment is a success in terms of decreased negative behaviors associated with ADHD, or whether little of significance occurs. In our early studies in the late 1970s, that employed double-blind crossover designs where we purposely trained children to increase slow activity in the EEG, there was a deterioration of behaviors observed in the classroom; that is, more ADHD behaviors emerged. When the children were trained to decrease the slow activity and increase faster activity, their behaviors improved (Lubar & Shouse, 1977). These data are described in more detail later on. They show that careful attention to what is being trained in the EEG is important if we are to obtain improvements in ADHD-related behaviors. No single treatment, no matter how powerful, can totally bring ADHD under control without long-term follow-up. This is because ADHD affects so many aspects of a person's life. The integration of neurofeedback with other modalities is crucial to obtain maximum results. It is imperative that individuals planning to use neurofeedback have proper training. New practitioners should receive intensive training that includes observing and being supervised working with patients with ADHD. It is my experience that regardless of a therapist's background, to become a seasoned neurofeedback practitioner often requires the equivalent of an internship of 1–2 years. One needs to understand the complexity of ADHD, its many components, and how they interact and affect the lifestyle and family systems of individuals with this disorder. The Biofeedback Certification Institute of America (BCIA) now has a separate certification in EEG biofeedback for healthcare and educational professionals.

DESCRIPTION OF ADHD

The description of ADHD in this chapter is not exhaustive. There are many excellent published reviews of this disorder. In 1991, a special supplement of the *Journal of Child Neurology* was devoted entirely to ADHD. The introduction to that special edition stated that even 10 years earlier more than 2000 papers had been published about this disorder, and that the number of publications had grown exponentially since then (Voeller, 1991). There is still considerable disagreement as to the best diagnostic and treatment approach. It is becoming clearer that attention deficit disorder (ADD) occurs in two main forms—with or without hyperactivity. The form with hyperactivity is sometimes referred to as ADHD or ADD+; the form without hyperactivity is sometimes referred to as ADD or ADD– (Barkley, 1998a). The *Diagnostic and Statistical Manual of Mental Disorders*, fourth edition (DSM-IV; American Psychiatric Association, 1994) refers only to ADHD, but classifies it into three subtypes: the "inattentive type," "hyperactive–compulsive type," and "combined type."

In the 1950s and 1960s, this disorder was referred to as "minimal brain dysfunction." At that time many believed that there was something structurally wrong within the central nervous system (CNS), with some type of brain injury or inadequate integration of perceptual mechanisms (Anderson, 1963). G. F. Still (1902), a British physician, published a very early description of this disorder in *The Lancet*. He referred to the complex of behaviors we now call ADHD as "abnormal deficits in moral control . . . and wanton mischievousness and destructiveness." We recognize this today as a combination of ADHD, conduct disorder (CD), and oppositional defiant disorder (ODD). Even as late as 1998, Barkley described one aspect of ADHD as a deficit in rule-governed behavior. In some ways, this refers to some of the same problems that Still recognized over 100 years ago.

Currently, in consistency with the DSM-IV, the term ADHD is the most common description. Lahey, Schaughency, Hynd, Carlson, and Nieves (1987), working with the DSM-IV committee, strongly suggested that ADD without hyperactivity be considered a separate entity from ADHD, even though they can overlap. This is partly because ADD has some characteristics that are different from ADHD. (From this point on, this chapter generally refers to "ADD or ADHD" to preserve this distinction, unless otherwise indicated.)

Figure 18.1 shows some relationships among ADHD (or ADD+), ADD (or ADD–), and other disorders. Regardless of the nosology, one underlying emerging fact seems very clear: ADHD and ADD have a strong biological basis. In many families, these may be genetic and are likely to be neurologically based. The neurological basis may be structural in some instances where there is overlap with severe specific learning disabilities, such as developmental dyslexia. Furthermore, there is a likely abnormality in neurometabolism, as shown by recent *positron emission tomography (PET) scan* studies. This provides the basis for the use of stimulant medication therapy for dealing with certain aspects of this disorder (Zametkin & Rapoport, 1987; Zametkin et al., 1990), particularly if individuals have ADHD. If they have ADD, they display inattentiveness as their main characteristic.

One view of ADHD is that there is a significant motivational component. In addition to rapidly losing interest in their toys, these children also lose interest in friendships and have difficulty developing good peer relationships. They have a decreased response to punishment that is related to their problems with rule-governed behaviors. They experience rapid extinction to new stimuli or satiate more rapidly to new situations (Barkley, 1998b). This is particularly relevant in any kind of behavioral intervention and has direct implications for how neurofeedback sessions have to be conducted in order to maintain motivation and interest.

Both ADD and ADHD are more common in the male population than in the female population, with ratios ranging anywhere from 3:1 to 6:1, depending on which review one reads (Barkley, 1998b; Whalen & Henckler, 1991). Whereas ADD does not go away as one matures, ADHD often changes in that the hyperkinetic component may decrease with age. Many professionals now believe that a significant proportion of both individuals with ADHD and individuals with ADD continue to experience this disorder throughout their life history (Barkley, 1998b). As far as inattentiveness and difficulty with rule-governed behavior are concerned, adolescents and adults continue to have difficulty maintaining or sustaining activity leading to completion of tasks. This is the case with completing homework in high school,

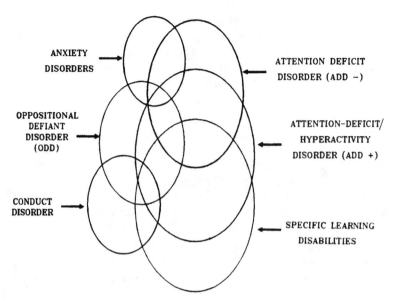

FIGURE 18.1. Schematic diagram illustrating relationship among ADHD (or ADD+), ADD (or ADD–), and other comorbid conditions. The circles are meant to be representations and are not drawn to a scale that represents the amount of overlap of the different disorders, but to show that there is a relationship between them.

meeting deadlines imposed in work situations, and maintaining commitments in social or marital/couple relationships later in life.

The differential diagnosis of ADHD/ADD from other disorders is often difficult and requires considerable skill. In order to develop a comprehensive treatment program, it is also necessary to determine the extent the individual is experiencing *comorbidity*, or other conditions together with the ADHD/ADD. This is especially the case if the program involves neurofeedback combined with medication, family and/or individual psychotherapy, and behavior therapy. Comorbid conditions may include ODD, CD, learning disabilities, anxiety and mood disorders, and various thought disorders.

Common tools for determining diagnoses and comorbidities involve extensive interviewing and family history; medical history; and in some cases detailed medical workups involving EEG, neurological scanning (*single-photon emission computerized tomography* [SPECT], magnetic resonance imaging [MRI], or PET) techniques, blood work, and even genetic studies. The use of psychodiagnostic tools such as the Minnesota Multiphasic Personality Inventory, and metrics designed specifically for children, can be useful as part of the assessment of possible thought and mood disorders.

Neuropsychological measures are particularly useful for assessing possible organic brain dysfunction and specific learning disabilities. These techniques include but are not limited to the Halstead–Reitan Battery, the Luria Neuropsychological Battery, the Wechsler Intelligence Scale for Children—Revised (WISC-R) or Third Edition (WISC-III), the Wechsler Adult Intelligence Scale—Revised, the Woodcock–Johnson Psychoeducational Evaluation—Revised, and other neuropsychological and achievement measures.

For the behavioral–observational assessment of ADD and ADHD, there are excellent rating scales available. These include the scales in Barkley (1997), the Conners Parent and Teacher Rating Scales (Conners, 1969), the Achenbach Child Behavior Checklist (Achenbach, 1991), the Child Activity/Attention Profile of Edelbrock, the Home and School Situation

Questionnaire (McCarney, 1995), and others in development. Many of these are checklists filled out by parents or teachers and often include items based on the DSM-IV categorization of ADHD. The same checklist should be employed before and after an intervention, to help determine the extent to which the treatment has affected the behaviors described. This is particularly important for neurofeedback, which is a treatment method that is still being established.

CURRENT THERAPIES

Most prevalent approaches for the treatment of ADHD/ADD currently involve the use of antihyperactive medications—primarily stimulants, occasionally supplemented by (1) tricyclic antidepressants, (2) alpha-blockers, and in rare cases (3) antipsychotic medications or (4) selective serotonin reuptake inhibitors (SSRIs). Other nonmedical therapies involve (1) the extensive use of behavior therapy involving complex schedules of rewards and punishments (Barkley, 1998b; Wolraich et al., 1990), (2) cognitive-behavioral therapy, (3) traditional individual psychotherapy, and (4) the family systems approach. Techniques such as visual–motor integration and dietary management have proved effective only in some cases and are not a part of the treatment mainstream at the present time.

The use of stimulant medications for the treatment of the hyperactive component of ADHD, and in many cases, the treatment of ADD without hyperactivity is represented by literature dating back at least to the 1940s. As early as 1937, Bradley reported that amphetamine sulfate significantly decreased the hyperkinetic behavior of children and allowed them to function better in social and academic settings. At that time, the reason for the positive results from using stimulants with hyperactivity was not understood. Very briefly, the two main hypotheses that have been developed to explain how stimulants may be useful for these children are (1) the low-arousal hypothesis, developed by Satterfield and Dawson in 1971 and further elaborated by Satterfield, Lesser, Saul, and Cantwell (1973); and (2) the noradrenergic hypothesis, developed over years and elegantly elaborated by Zametkin et al. (1990).

Essentially, these two hypotheses propose that children with ADHD/ADD experience low arousal. This low arousal comes about as the result of decreased impact of sensory stimuli, in all modalities, acting on the CNS mechanisms for sensory integration and resulting in these children's engaging in stimulus-seeking behavior. Self-stimulation and object play are primary features of the hyperactive (hyperkinetic) syndrome in particular (Lubar & Shouse, 1976, 1977; Shouse & Lubar, 1978). Children with hyperactivity often exhibit intense but brief interest in new stimuli. For example, they rub objects against their bodies, smell them, taste them if they can, and often engage in other stimulus-seeking behaviors (such as excessive movement, spinning around, running from place to place within a room, or picking up one object after another and examining it). If they are in a room where there is very little stimulation, they will very often fall asleep after a brief flurry of activity.

The basis for this stimulus-seeking behavior might lie in decreased *noradrenergic activity*, particularly in the *brainstem reticular formation* and perhaps in the *basal ganglia* as well. Heilman, Voeller, and Nadeau (1991) and Riccio et al. (1993) proposed that in many of these children, as well as adults with this disorder, there is a defect in *response inhibition*—particularly in the *nigrostriatal system*, more on the right side of the brain than the left side. Motor restlessness may reflect not only frontal lobe dysfunction, but possible impairment of the *dopaminergic system* as well. Basically, we think of arousal as being mediated by (1) connections from the brainstem reticular formation, which receives inputs from all of the sensory modalities except olfaction; (2) the transmission of this information to the diffuse thalamic (reticular) projection system; and (3) the *basal forebrain*, which does receive olfactory projections. These input systems, in conjunction with the basal ganglia and the *cerebellum* (which is involved in programming the output of the motor cortex), are all affected by decreased noradrenergic activity. Norepinephrine, a key transmitter in this system, is produced by a very important brainstem nucleus located in the midbrain, the *locus coeruleus*. This nucleus has extensive projections with these mesolimbic, striatal, and forebrain systems. Not only is the neuroanatomy of these systems complex, but the resulting neurochemical dysfunctions and/or neuropathologies associated with them are also complex. The latter include movement disorders and mood disorders. As we discuss below, these abnormalities in neurochemistry and neurophysiology are reflected in EEG measures, in ERP measures, and in regional brain metabolism.

Even more important than norepinephrine, the neuromodulator dopamine does play a very important role in attentional mechanisms. There are two dopaminergic systems in the human brain. One originates in the substantia nigra, and one of the extrapyramidal motor structures is involved through the basal ganglia in the modulation of motor activity via the motor cortex. The second originates in a region called the ventral tegmental area in the midbrain and is often referred to as the ventral dopaminergic system; it streams anteriorly through the subcallosal cortex under the anterior portion of the corpus callosum, and then is widely distributed to the prefrontal lobes and the anterior cingulate gyrus. This system has been identified as the attention-modulating system (Posner & Raichle, 1994). There is also evidence from the work of Kenneth Blum and his colleagues (Blum & Noble, 1997) that specific *alleles* associated with dopamine metabolism are abnormal in nearly 50% of individuals who experience ADHD (ADD+).

The picture becomes even more complex in terms of a general disorder referred to as the "reward deficiency syndrome" (RDS), which occurs when there are abnormalities in dopamine metabolism. Sometimes it is additionally associated with abnormalities in norepinephrine and serotonin metabolism. Serotonin is important in the modulation of mood states. Individuals experiencing RDS often have ADHD combined with substance use disorders. There are other forms of RDS: obsessive behavior, compulsive gambling, carbohydrate bingeing, excessive cigarette smoking, and other reward-seeking and thrill-seeking behaviors, all of which are linked to abnormal alleles associated with either dopamine production, dopamine transport across the synapse, or the breakdown of dopamine into metabolites that are eventually excreted. Evidence of dopamine dysfunction can even be seen in neuroimaging studies involving the SPECT scan as described by Amen and Carmichael (1997); these again confirm how pervasive attentional disorders are from a structural and neurochemical point of view from childhood to adulthood.

At the current time, several types of stimulants are used in trying to restore noradrenergic balance. In young children, dextroamphetamine (Dexedrine) is commonly used. In children from age 6 through adolescence and even adulthood, other medications are in common use: methylphenidate (Ritalin) and extended-release methylphenidate (Concerta); and newer combinations of stimulants (e.g., Adderall). Children and adults who either experience impulsive behavior or have extreme difficulty with organizational and planning skills may respond positively to small amounts of a tricyclic antidepressant, such as desipramine or imipramine. The latter has more anticholinergic side effects than the former. In some children when the impulsive behavior also becomes very aggressive, clonidine, an alpha-adrenergic blocker, is sometimes helpful. There is little doubt that between 60% and 80% of children with ADHD show varying degrees of positive response to these medications when properly administered (Barkley, 1997). In some cases, the response is ideal, in that the children no longer exhibit all components of the hyperactive syndrome or any significant attentional difficulties. Individuals who have this ideal response can remain on these medication regimens for a long time without any significant negative side effects. Other individuals show partial responses to the medications and may exhibit a variety of side effects. These can include anorexia, varying degrees of sleep disturbance, and mood changes. Some children respond to Ritalin with an almost totally flat affect; they are sometimes described as "zombie-like" by parents or others familiar with them. Such a response would warrant the use of either a different medication or a nonmedication alternative.

Of the 20–25% of children who do not respond well to medications, there may be a combination of reasons: (1) gastrointestinal disturbances; (2) increased tic disorders when tics are present (a possible problem with Ritalin); (3) seizure disorders; (4) headaches; (5) urinary problems; or (6) changes in mood that are unacceptable to the person or family. One of the main problems with medication is that its effects can be short-lived or state-dependent. Ritalin clears the system rapidly within 3–4 hours. (Dexedrine clears less rapidly, often within 8 hours of administration, and the newer Adderall and Concerta clear even more slowly.) The effects of the medication are then gone. For this reason, it is often necessary to give two or three doses of the medication a day, particularly for Ritalin. Ritalin is very commonly administered in a larger dose in the morning, a second dose at noon, and a very small dose after school to help the child complete homework assignments.

The administration of these medications is rarely based on body weight, and more appropriately based on response. An adult or a large child may respond very effectively to 5 milligrams of Ritalin, whereas a small child may require 40 milligrams or more to obtain an adequate response. The important factor is not how much Ritalin is administered per unit of body weight, but how much of it enters the CNS. As far as basic mechanisms are concerned, there is a sizable literature indicating that Ritalin does improve certain characteristics of the evoked response, such as the latency and amplitude of the P3 component associated with sensory discrimination (Klorman, 1991).

There is little present evidence that Ritalin has any effect on cortical EEG (Lubar et al., 1995; Lubar & Lubar, 1999). This may explain one of the reasons why there is a very limited carryover effect with the use of these medications. One of the major complaints of parents is that a child performs well with the medication, but the effect is medication-dependent. As soon as the medication is metabolized or when it is discontinued (during holiday periods or weekends), many of the undesirable behaviors return, and the child is still not able to complete work, especially in academic settings. Sometimes when medications are given for long periods of time (i.e., several years), there is a carryover effect for several months after administration is stopped, but many of the undesirable behaviors may eventually return.

With children who have a hyperkinetic component to their ADHD, I have observed the motor component to decrease with maturation and aging. It may even disappear or be replaced by fidgetiness and inability to sit still for long periods of time. However, the attention deficit associated with ADHD or ADD may actually become worse as children become older. The reason for the latter is that the demands of society, particularly in the academic realm, become greater. Many children who do well in grade school begin to experience decreased performance in junior high or middle school. They then begin to receive failing grades in many courses, because they cannot keep up with the work and do not complete long and tedious assignments.

Although this chapter takes the perspective that neurofeedback is a powerful adjunctive technique, treatment is usually integrated with medications in cases where medications are necessary or desirable. Medication is a powerful adjunct to other therapies. Medication is often combined with the use of behavior modification techniques based on Skinnerian principles of reinforcement, including withdrawal of rewards or punishment where appropriate. "Time out" as a primary technique, or cognitive-behavioral therapy techniques that try to change the child's perception of why certain behaviors are inappropriate, are often part of a behavioral regimen.

Cognitive-behavioral therapy often involves the use of self-induced messages to try to maintain behavioral control. This technique has not been used extensively, and the results are variable (Whalen & Henckler, 1991). The main criticism of the behavioral therapies is that they are effective in only 40–60% of cases. When they are effective, the techniques have to be used extensively on a moment-by-moment basis, every day for many months and years. The administration of these schedules of reinforcement is tedious and is often resented by parents, because it dominates their life circumstances and requires extensive parent training to maintain.

One of the biggest problems in treating ADHD or ADD is that there is often underlying prefrontal lobe dysfunction. The prefrontal lobes of the brain are the "executive" portions of the brain involved in planning and judgment. Although inappropriate behaviors occurring today can lead to very significant future consequences, children with ADHD/ADD often live for the present. It has very little meaning for them when they are told that they may get a bad grade at the end of a grading period if their assignments are not completed. This is especially true if the end of the grading period is several weeks or months away. One of the goals of behavior therapy is to make consequences more salient and immediate (e.g., rewarding the child for completing particular assignments, perhaps punishing the child by withdrawing rewards or by applying "time outs" when assignments are not completed). These techniques may work well for a particular circumstance, but the effects may not generalize well, and they may need to be repeated on a day-to-day basis. Children without ADHD/ADD have the cognitive structures to understand why not getting the assignment done will be important for them. They more readily stop engaging in nonproductive behaviors that lead to punishment or withdrawal of rewards, because they can plan for the future and understand the consequences of behaviors.

Many children with ADD/ADHD are adopted, often by families that do not have such a disorder, do not understand it, and do not know how to deal with it. Another unfortunate fact is that in many families where ADHD or ADD is present, the family system is markedly affected by the child's behaviors; as a result, separation or divorce is more likely. In situations where there are custody issues, severe conflicts between parents, or serious conflicts between the child and his or her biological parents and/or stepparents, family systems approaches are often much more important than the use of behavior therapy or medication alone. Individual psychotherapy is often integrated with family systems and other approaches for children experiencing depression or severe adjustment problems.

The main hypothesis underlying the use of neurofeedback is simply stated: If ADHD and ADD are associated with neurological/biological dysfunction, particularly at the cortical level and primarily involving prefrontal lobe function, and if the underlying neurological deficit can be corrected, a child with ADHD or ADD may be able to develop strategies and insights (paradigms) that children without ADHD/ADD already have. With the use of these paradigms, the abilities to organize, plan, and understand the consequences of inappropriate behavior are facilitated. As a result, there is a much stronger carryover of the effectiveness of rewards, time outs, and other behavioral approaches. The need for medication may actually diminish if we can show that changing cortical functioning also results in a change in brainstem functioning, such as brainstem or cortical ERPs or measures of sensory integration. The long-term effects of neurofeedback have already been documented (Tansey, 1990; Lubar, 1989, 1991, 1992; Lubar et al., 1995). Therefore, this technique, which leads to normalization of behavior, can lead to normalization of neurological dysfunction in the child with ADHD or ADD and can have long-term consequences for academic achievement, social integration, and overall life adjustment.

EEG CHARACTERISTICS OF ADHD/ADD

Abnormalities in EEG were reported in children who would now be classified as having ADD or ADHD as early as the 1930s (Jasper, Solomon, & Bradley, 1938). There is an extensive early literature, much of it reviewed in the supplement to the *Journal of Child Neurology* published in 1991. Basically, EEG studies show excessive slow activity in central and frontal regions of the brain. These studies are supported by recent PET and SPECT scan studies, which also indicate abnormalities in cerebral metabolism in these particular brain areas. More recent research by Amen and Paldi (1993) and Amen and Carmichael (1997) has uncovered several patterns of EEG abnormalities in children with ADHD/ADD. One pattern involves frontal lobe deactivation. These children experience decreased metabolism in prefrontal regions of the brain and, according to these investigators, are good candidates for the use of stimulant medications as well as neurofeedback. Other children show deficits in limbic system activity and are characterized as having oppositional behavior, emotional outbursts, and impulsiveness. These children also show significant decreased metabolism in their prefrontal lobes and the anterior cingulate gyrus. They are good candidates for the use of tricyclic antidepressants, such as imipramine or desipramine. The third subgroup comprises individuals who have increased activity in the medial superior frontal gyrus. Although these individuals experience ADD, they are often characterized as having an attention deficit with obsessive–compulsive disorder. They have a very short attention span and are often impulsive and oppositional. They take an excessive time to complete required work, because they become obsessed with sometimes irrelevant material and cannot seem to discriminate between what is essential and what is nonessential. These patients sometimes respond to clomipramine. By far the most common group of children with ADD consists of those with excessive slow activity in frontal and central brain regions (Chabot & Serfontein, 1996).

We (Mann, Lubar, Zimmerman, Miller, & Muenchen, 1992) examined the difference between a group of 25 children with ADD without hyperactivity or learning disability and 27 controls, carefully matched for IQ and socioeconomic status. They were all right-handed males. Differences between the groups during baseline studies and reading and drawing challenges were examined and displayed in topographic maps. During the academic challenges, there were significant increases in slow (~8-hertz) theta activity along the midline and in the frontal regions, and decreased beta activity, especially along the midline and posteriorly. This was the first quantitative, multichannel neurological study to show that children with pure ADD versus ADHD are statistically different in terms of their EEG characteristics.

Several large-scale studies have been published since our original work in 1992. Chabot and Serfontein (1996), for example, studied 407 children with ADD and 310 controls. Using discriminant analysis, they were able to distinguish the children with ADD from the control group, with a specificity of 88% and a sensitivity of 94%. They then showed that two major subtypes of ADD could be accounted for by 96% of the EEG profiles. These subtypes were distinguished either by slowing in frontal regions or by increased activity in the frontal areas. Hypoarousal associated increased slow activity in frontal and central areas is a primary marker for children with the inattentive type of ADD and for many of those who also have hyperactivity. Increased frontal activity is often seen in individuals with aggressive CD, although the picture is complicated by the fact that many individuals with ODD also have slowing in their EEG in extreme frontal locations. Lazarro, Gordon, Whitmont, Meares, and Clarke, (1998) replicated our original 1992 work by showing that theta activity is increased in adolescents with ADHD in the anterior regions and that beta activity was decreased in posterior areas.

Our research has also shown that it is not always necessary to evaluate activity in all 19 channels of the traditional *International 10-20 System* of EEG electrode localization. For example, in our multicenter study (Monastra et al., 1999), we evaluated 482 individuals between ages 6 and 30 during four conditions: an eyes-open baseline, and reading, listening, and drawing tasks. We measured the ratio of theta activity (4–8 hertz) to beta activity (13–21 hertz) in terms of percentage power (see below). We found for all groups (and now have data up to age 64) that there are significant differences between controls and individuals with DSM-IV-defined ADHD of both the inattentive and hyperactive–impulsive types. The importance of this latest study is that it provides a quick and easy screening method for making a first approximation in terms of evaluation. These results were cross-validated in a subsequent study we have conducted (Monastra, Lubar, & Linden, 2001). In this study, 129 individuals aged 6–20 (98 males and 31 females) were evaluated using rating scales, continuous-performance tasks, structured clinical interviews, and computerized power-spectral analysis of the EEG. The EEG measures employed were the same as in our previous study: power ratios of theta to beta at location C_z, *the vertex*. Participants were accurately classified as experiencing DSM-IV-defined ADHD of the inattentive type or of the hyperactive–impulsive or combined type. Ninety percent (90%) of the participants classified as having ADHD scored positively for ADHD on the quantitative EEG, and 94% of the participants classified as nonclinical controls scored negatively for ADHD on the quantitative EEG evaluation. A second study reported in that same publication involved 285 additional individuals aged 6–20, with a male-to-female ratio of 3:1. A test–retest correlation from the quantitative EEG analysis performed on two occasions indicated considerable stability in the measures. The correlation was .96, indicating that the one quantitative EEG channel-scanning procedure is very consistent over time.

During the past 12 years, we have collected data on the Lexicor NRS24 system (Boulder, CO) to develop a database examining one particular measure of EEG activity. This measure is the percentage power ratio of theta activity (4–8 hertz) divided by beta activity (13–21 hertz). This baseline study has involved the following protocol. A cap (Electro Cap, Inc.) containing all 19 of the electrodes according to the International 10-20 System of EEG electrode placement is fitted to the participant's head. There are different caps, depending on head size (see Figure 18.2). The cap is connected to a harness that holds it tightly in place and to a band that is placed around the chest. Electrode gel is placed into each of the electrode cups embedded in the cap, and impedances of less than 5 kohms are obtained before recording can be started. Linked ears are used as references for the 19 cortical channels. The subject is placed in front of an easel, which is used to present materials at different times during the test protocol. The test consists of six parts, each with an approximate duration of 3 minutes. It begins with an eyes-open baseline, which is followed by an eyes-closed baseline. The subject is then requested to read material silently that is grade- or age-level-appropriate. (Participants are first asked to read out loud, so that the experimenter can assess fluency before the material is presented silently.) The participant next reproduces figures from the Beery–Bender Visual–Motor Gestalt Test, and then completes the Raven's Progressive Color Matrices Test. The next task involves the experimenter's reading to the subject content that continues the material that the child has read silently before. Additional tasks sometimes follow the formal database testing. These may involve the Coding task from the WISC-R or WISC-III, or measures from the Halstead–Reitan Battery, to see whether there are unusual patterns of cognitive activity associated with these neuropsychological tasks.

The data from the 19 recording channels are analyzed by compressed power-spectral analysis and displayed as a multicolored topographic brain map showing the absolute activity in microvolts for each of the different bandpasses of interest. A second set of maps compares all of the bandpasses on the same numerical scale, so that it is possible to evaluate where the primary activity is occurring—that is, theta, beta, or some other bandpass.

Figure 18.3 shows the status of our database for three groups of individuals with ADD. These individuals consisted of children, adolescents, and adults not taking any medication. A small group of matched control subjects is compared to the 15-year and older group.

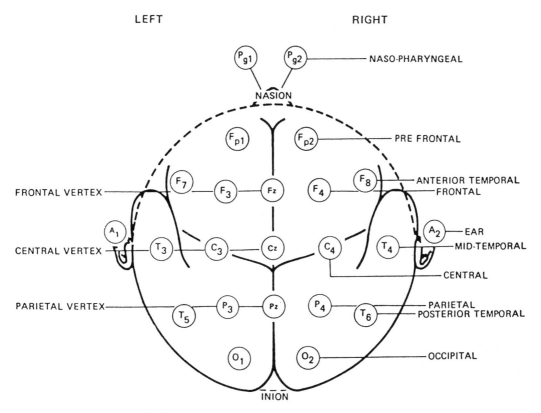

FIGURE 18.2. Locations of the standard 19 electrode placements, according to the International 10-20 System.

The database we originally developed (Mann et al. 1992) was based on 16 channels of information recorded with electrodes placed on the International 10-20 sites and attached with *Nihon Kohden Elefix paste*. The data from the Nihon Kohden EEG were analyzed by an offline analysis system called Stellate, developed by 1990. Some of those data were presented in a review paper (Lubar, 1991). Significant differences ($p < .05$ and $p < .001$) were obtained for many central and frontal locations. The current simple channel database replicates those findings and extends them to older groups (Monastra et al., 1999).

An important point in the development of an EEG database is that EEG is age-dependent. For example, there are many published studies (Gasser, Verleger, Bacher, & Sroka, 1988) that illustrate age-related differences in the distribution of EEG activity in different bands from low delta to high beta. Figure 18.3 illustrates that for children with ADD, the differences between 8- to 11-year-olds and 12- to 14-year-olds are relatively small. The difference between groups is probably somewhat larger for normal controls. Our current database includes both male and female subjects, with all being right-handed. The current database is heterogeneous for IQ and includes individuals with Full Scale IQs ranging from 85 to 140. In contrast, in our previous study (Mann et al., 1992), the IQ range was very restricted in the normal range (101–107). Both age and IQ differences may be important.

Figure 18.4 shows a raw EEG sample gathered from an adolescent male with ADD during a reading task. Normally we associate active processing tasks with blocking alpha and theta activity and increasing beta activity. However, it is clear from the figure that there is considerable slow activity in many of the frontal central and posterior channels. This consists

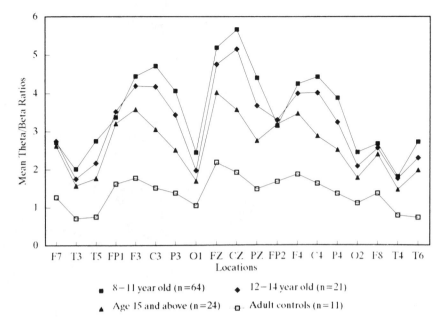

FIGURE 18.3. Current status of database for three groups of individuals with ADD and matched controls for the adult group. The measure illustrated is the ratio of theta activity (4–8 hertz) to beta activity (13–21 hertz), measured in terms of percentage total power. Note that the highest ratios are obtained in location C_z for children and at F_z for older adolescents and adults.

primarily of theta and some alpha activity, and characterizes the ADD/ADHD EEG. In many children as well as adolescents and even adults, the degree of slowing is very apparent without any numerical analysis. Another point is that alpha activity often occurs in adults with ADD or ADHD even more than theta, and alpha shows lack of blocking to complex stimuli. This may result from the normal evolution of the EEG, in that children reveal a greater amount of slow-wave activity than do adults. At approximately age 12–14, alpha finally reaches its adult frequency and stabilizes; in children below the age of 6, by contrast, alpha activity actually occurs in the range below 8 hertz, although it has different physical characteristics and is generated by different subcortical regions than theta activity. Alpha is very sinusoidal in its appearance, whereas theta is more irregular and sporadic in its appearance and rate of occurrence.

RATIONALE FOR NEUROFEEDBACK

This section discusses the rationale for neurofeedback and examines criteria for effective intervention. Subsequent sections discuss instrumentation specifications, treatment protocols for neurofeedback sessions, pre- and posttreatment measures, and some results from my group's clinic and other clinics currently using neurofeedback training.

Part of the rationale for neurofeedback treatment for ADD or ADHD relates directly to some of the characteristics of these children, described earlier. A primary problem that an individual with ADD or ADHD experiences is difficulty in completing tasks that are long, repetitive, and perceived as boring. This relates to much of the activity that occurs in the school setting, including homework. Another characteristic of the individual with ADD or ADHD is difficulty in accepting the reality that socially appropriate behavior is governed by rules, and that rule-following behavior is essential in order to progress through the various develop-

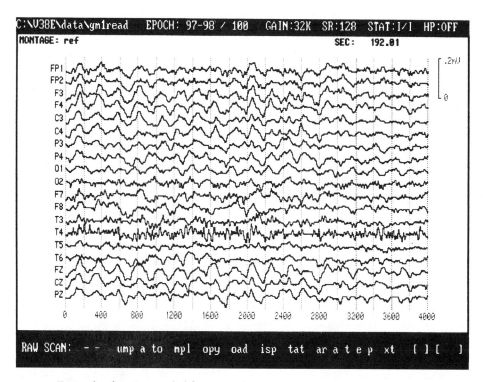

FIGURE 18.4. Example of EEG recorded from an adolescent (age 14) with ADHD, who was on Ritalin. The main features of this EEG recording are the large slow waves between 4 and 6 hertz in the theta range, seen in almost all channels except for temporal locations. Excessive theta activity and lack of beta activity are the primary neurological landmarks of ADHD. The fast (high-frequency) activity in temporal channels T_3 and T_4 is due to muscle tension in the massater and temporal muscles. This is a common non-EEG artifact found in recordings from these locations.

mental milestones necessary to achieve a functional adulthood. Individuals who are not able to follow these rules may ultimately experience ODD, CD, or (in the worst cases) antisocial personality disorder. This does not mean that all children with ADD or ADHD have this pathway as an inevitable consequence of their behaviors, but there is a higher incidence of such problems in this population (Barkley, 1998b).

Two other general characteristics of the ADD/ADHD population are poor motivation and rapid habituation to the reward properties of stimuli. Thus play activities and specific toys do not remain interesting very long for these children. There is also the thrill-seeking behavior sometimes seen in adolescents with ADD/ADHD. The use of stimulant medication, whether it be Ritalin (methylphenidate), Dexedrine (dextroamphetamine sulfate), or a newer formulation, are primarily directed toward increasing arousal or impact of stimulation. There is little clear evidence that these medications, particularly methylphenidate, change cortical function (Lubar & Lubar, 1999).

Parents commonly complain that although medication leads to improvements in school performance, concentration abilities, and motor behavior, their child still has difficulty completing required work, following rules, and understanding why inappropriate behaviors need to be corrected. These latter problems arise from altered cognitive functioning and, in large part, frontal lobe functioning. The frontal lobes are the executive portions of the brain—particularly the frontal pole, orbitofrontal cortex, and dorsal and lateral surface of the frontal lobe extending back centrally along the midline to the premotor cortex. These are the cortical areas that reveal decreased metabolism in adults with ADD, as well as probably in children with ADD and decreased fast EEG activity and excessive slow EEG activity.

Neurofeedback appears to work best with medication in children with ADD or ADHD if one can change cortical functioning as well as arousal functions. By changing cortical functioning, we are attempting to establish a "cortical template" that responds, in terms of its EEG signatures, similarly to that of individuals without ADD or ADHD in those circumstances and situations that cause problems for the individual with ADD or ADHD. Many groups working with these children report that once they learn the neurofeedback techniques, when they behave inappropriately and this behavior is pointed out to them, they can move readily to correct it. Inappropriate behaviors are not repeated as often, once they understand why the behaviors are considered inappropriate. In essence, children with ADD or ADHD who are provided with neurofeedback often experience long-term transfer of what they learn to school and home settings, because they begin to function cortically more like individuals without ADD. Hence rule-following behavior increases, impulsiveness decreases, inappropriate social behaviors decrease, motivation levels improve, and family interactions improve.

During the past 15 years, work carried out by my own and other groups working with children with ADD and ADHD has helped to clarify a number of matters that have led us to develop a position statement for the treatment of ADD/ADHD with neurofeedback. The position statement is as follows:

Previous and current results of the treatment of ADD/ADHD with neurofeedback are promising for those individuals demonstrating certain quantitative EEG and behavioral characteristics. Practitioners utilizing this treatment modality recognize that ADD and ADHD are complex disorders and have a wide range of symptoms, etiologies, and therapeutic interventions. Neurofeedback offers patients a psychophysiological treatment that, when combined with other traditional therapies, produces significant improvement for many patients. More research, currently being conducted, is needed to extend these results. To date, this treatment has been successfully applied for several thousand children treated by approximately 1500 health care organizations. Neurofeedback is neither a panacea nor a cure, but a powerful adjunctive technique.

1. *Who is a candidate for neurofeedback therapy?* Anyone with a *primary diagnosis* of ADD or ADHD, between the ages of 7 and 65 (perhaps older), with low-average, average, or above-average intelligence is a candidate. Neurofeedback treatment should not be offered as a primary treatment when any of the following is present:

- Mental retardation.
- Childhood psychosis.
- Severe depressive or bipolar illness.
- Significant seizure disorder where medications interfere with learning (i.e., sedating medications).
- Hyperkinesis, where multiple medications or high dosages with monotherapy have been ineffective.
- Learning disabilities *without* ADD or ADHD as a primary problem.
- Substance abuse or dependence.
- Dysfunctional families whose members refuse to participate in indicated therapy.

2. *What symptoms can be improved with neurofeedback?*

- Attention, focus, and concentration.
- Task completion and organizational skills.

- Impulsiveness.
- Mild hyperactivity.

3. *What are the results of treatment?*

- Improved behavior and learning.
- Improvement in school grades.
- Increased self-esteem.
- Better job performance.
- Greater realization of innate potential.
- Higher intelligence test scores.
- Improved scores on parent–teacher rating scales.

4. *How effective is this treatment approach?* When the criteria listed under point 1 above are used to select candidates for therapy and treatment, the majority of patients completing treatment show marked improvement in the areas listed under points 2 and 3—both as measured by independent observers and testing, and as reported by teachers, parents, and other involved health care professionals. This position statement is an evolving document. As more data are gathered on more patients, modifications will occur. Those using neurofeedback in their practice or in research can help refine this position statement through an interactive dialogue that will continue to develop among practitioners.

SPECIFICATION CRITERIA
FOR NEUROFEEDBACK INSTRUMENTATION

At the present time, there are nearly a dozen instruments designed and developed for the use of neurofeedback for ADD/ADHD. The main requirements for appropriate instrumentation include very accurate signal processing with the ability to discriminate changes as small as 0.1 microvolt for purposes of setting thresholds. The ideal instrumentation must allow the researcher/clinician to observe the raw signal and to see how it is processed in order to produce reward or inhibition of reward and to observe the relationship between changes in events in the raw EEG and the feedback. Excellent systems employ both analog and digital processing. Such systems have been described in detail previously (Lubar & Culver, 1978; Lubar, 1991; Lubar & Lubar, 1999).

Those persons engaged in neurofeedback treatment have to fulfill several well-defined physiological criteria simultaneously. They have to increase either (1) sensorimotor rhythm (SMR) (between 12 and 15 hertz), especially if they are hyperactive, or (2) beta activity (often defined as 16–20 hertz)—and they must do so without concurrently producing excessive theta, theta–alpha ("thalpha") movement, or surface electromyographic (EMG) activity. The task is to isolate the SMR or beta activity, and to increase its duration, its prevalence, and (if possible) its amplitude, while simultaneously decreasing the amplitude and percentage of theta, thalpha, EMG activity, or gross movement. To do this, the participant has to be very alert, but also relaxed. Children with ADD/ADHD have great difficulty staying on task (as measured by poor performance on continuous-performance tasks, such as the Gordon Diagnostic System, Integrated Auditory and Visual Test (IVA) or the *Test of Variables of Attention* [*TOVA*]). The essence of neurofeedback treatment involves engagement in a continuous-performance-type task under an altered EEG state for significant periods. However, children with ADD/ADHD are able to play other computer and arcade games for long periods of time, with no significant transfer to homework situations or other situations that are long, boring, and repetitive, such as school-related tasks. Similarly, it is unlikely that training children to perform continuous-performance tasks by themselves will have any significant carryover, but being able to perform these types of tasks in the altered but more normal EEG state *does* appear to work.

There are different explanations regarding the mechanism of how neurofeedback works. If one believes that individuals become aware of the different EEG states and can discriminate when they are producing alpha, SMR, theta, beta, or other frequencies, then the argument is quite simple. Individuals simply learn to produce the desired EEG pattern in the appropriate setting. They learn to produce beta when they need to concentrate, theta and/or low-frequency alpha when they want to relax and experience a considerable amount of visual imagery, and higher alpha when they want to relax in a more blank-mind, "open-focus" state. However, many individuals undergoing neurofeedback tell us that they do not know exactly how they produce the different EEG patterns; the important thing is that they are often able to do so upon request.

At one level, this is evidence that there are unconscious processes operating in this type of learning phenomenon, and that an individual can learn without direct awareness. Evidence to support learning without awareness has been discussed and debated (e.g., Kamiya, 1979) for more than a quarter of a century as the field of biofeedback has evolved. Individuals without ADD or ADHD are very aware of changes in their levels of alertness. If a person is reading a very exciting passage or engaged in listening to a particularly powerful audio presentation or speech, the person usually becomes very alert, fixates on the speaker or on the material being presented, and actively processes the content. If, after a while, the individual experiences fatigue, wandering of attention, or forgetting of the content, the EEG shows a shift toward lower frequencies. People can sometimes force themselves into an attentive state, and this is associated with higher-frequency EEG activity. Individuals with ADD or ADHD probably have greater difficulty making these discriminations. Therefore, they need the augmented information, in the form of feedback, presented for many sessions before they begin to develop in demand settings an almost reflexive normal response to shifts in attention. This allows them to increase their level of concentration and focusing.

Instrumentation appropriately designed for this type of treatment must provide very clear feedback stimuli indicating when different conditions have been met. Some of the instruments use game displays, such as color wheels that light up sequentially with different colors every time a burst of beta activity occurs with a specific duration and specific amplitude. Another example display is an airplane flying above a specified threshold level line and a tone that changes in frequency or intensity. Both signals correspond to the amplitude and duration of the rewarded activity. These instruments also provide warning lights, that are activated when the person produces theta (or, in some cases, alpha) above a set threshold or EMG activity above threshold. Gross body movement will usually activate the theta filter. In some cases, filters with lower bandpasses in the region of 0–2 or 0–4 hertz are also used to detect gross body movements. More recent systems employ complex animation or animated sequences and music from compact discs on synthesized wave tables.

High-quality instrumentation should also record and score data for each session. The most useful EEG parameters to record are (1) average microvolt levels of rewarded or inhibited activities; (2) percentage of rewarded or inhibited activities above or below their appropriate thresholds; (3) threshold settings; and perhaps (4) ratios of fast to slow activity, measured in either power units, percentage units, or amplitude units. The following session details need to be recorded as well: (5) session duration; (6) number of points achieved, if a point system is used; and (7) the activities taking place during the session. These data should be maintained on a session-to-session basis. They should also either be transportable into a database or graphing programs (such as Excel, SPSS, or SAS statistical programs), or have the capability to display the data graphically either within and/or over sessions. Such data can then be compiled in order to examine group difference in controlled studies. Ideally designed instruments will allow the therapist or researcher to access this graphical material and print it out in either black and white or multicolor, for purposes of reports to patients, schools, insurance companies, or referral sources, or for publication.

Instruments that have all of these capabilities—including computer systems containing Pentium III or IV chips capable of running at 1–25 gigahertz, with printers—range in price from about less than $1,000 to over $10,000. The more expensive instruments often have multichannel capacity; the additional channels are primarily used for assessment purposes or other feedback modalities. In clinical practice, feedback is typically based on either a *bipolar (sequential) electrode montage* with *ear reference*, or, in some cases, a *referential montage* with a forehead ground and ear references. At present, data are insufficient for determining which is the better montage. Each has its advantages and disadvantages.

Bipolar-Sequential and Referential Montages

The bipolar or sequential montage has the advantage that there is *common-mode rejection* of signals that occur simultaneously in phase at both of the electrode inputs. This will include 60-hertz activity, perhaps certain types of movement activities, and cardiac and other physiological artifacts. However, the signal that is processed represents the algebraic subtraction of the EEG activity at two different points. It does not tell us about the absolute activity at each individual electrode site. Referential recording uses a single electrode and covers a smaller area than bipolar sequential recording. However, the EEG that is being recorded represents the actual electrical activity at that point as compared with a reference (either a ground reference and/or ear references, which are supposedly electrically more neutral). Consequently, larger signals are obtained from referential recordings. However, these are much more prone to artifact because of the lack of common-mode rejection. Hence there may be more inhibit circuit activity, and therapy may be somewhat more difficult.

It would be instructive to conduct a controlled study in which one group receives monopolar recording and the other receives bipolar sequential recording to see whether there is any significant difference between the two. This has yet to be done.

One manufacturer has an instrument that has the capability of recording from up to five channels simultaneously and processing the summated activity from all of these channels together in order to provide feedback. This type of recording provides coverage over a larger area of the scalp, but at the present time, no published data are available using this multichannel montage. Thus it is not known whether this approach is more or less beneficial than the referential or bipolar sequential recordings currently in use. When a bipolar sequential montage is used, it is essential that the distance between the electrodes be carefully measured every session. For example, if the distance between the electrodes for a person is 4.5 centimeters, it should remain at that distance, plus or minus 1 millimeter, for all sessions. Otherwise, data relating to magnitude (amplitude in microvolt levels) will be inaccurate, and any conclusion based on these data about learning will be erroneous.

Electrode Materials

Electrodes usually are made of silver or tin or are plated with gold, and contain a hole in the middle for the extrusion of excess electrode paste. Impedances between the electrode and skin should be 5 kohms or less, and for some instruments, it is extremely important that there be no significant *offset voltage* between the electrodes and the skin. Offset voltages occur when electrodes act as batteries and impose a voltage in addition to that already imposed by the

EEG. This can cause a baseline shift of the entire signal that is sent to the amplifier, and sometimes actually distorts the waveforms. In some cases it is impossible for the signal to be processed, and only noise appears on the screen. Many manufacturers offer an impedance meter that measures both impedance between the electrodes and voltages offset. We have found that with offsets of less than plus or minus 50 millivolts and an impedance of less than 5 kohms, high quality, reliable recordings are obtained.

Electrode Locations

Electrode preparation is very simple. Electrode sites are shown in Figure 18.2. Measurements are taken as follows: For training the SMR, we place electrodes at International 10-20 locations C_3 or C_4. In order to locate these two points, it is necessary to locate C_z, the vertex. To do this, a tape measure is applied from the *nasion* (at the top of the bridge of the nose, where the forehead is indented) to the *inion* (just underneath the *occipital condyle*, the bump at the back of the head). Half this total distance is marked with a dry marker, the same type of marker that is often used on whiteboards. The tape is then placed from the *preauricular notch* of the left ear through this marked spot to the preauricular notch on the right ear. The midpoint is again located. The intersection of the two measurements locates C_z. When C_z is obtained, then 20% of that total distance from ear to ear is recalculated. That distance is then marked from the vertex toward the left ear and the right ear along the line between the two ears. These are the locations of C_3 and C_4. When working with beta training, we have found that the best location is a point 10% of the total distance from nasion to inion, in front of C_z and 10% behind C_z. These two points are halfway between C_z and F_z and halfway between C_z and P_z, and are called F_{cz} and C_{pz}. Once the appropriate locations are marked, the marking dot is removed with (Omniprep or Nuprep, a gel that contains a small amount of pumice. Omniprep or Nuprep can be obtained from D. O. Weaver Company, Aurora, CO 80033). Next, a small mound of electrode paste is placed over the cleansed spot. Nihon Kohden, 10-20, or Grass Instrument Co. conductive paste can be used. The electrode is then pushed down on the mound until the paste extrudes through the small hole in the middle of the electrode. Our preference has been to use Grass E5SH electrodes; in some cases, the smaller E6SH electrode works equally well. A small cotton ball or piece of cheesecloth is finally pushed down on top of the electrode in the mound of paste, and this completes the electrode application for the head. For the ear, a Grass Instrument Co. ear clip electrode is used. This involves two cup electrodes placed in a small plastic holder. The ear is simply cleaned by rubbing it with Omniprep or Nuprep, removing the preparation, and then placing some electrode paste in the cups of the electrode and placing the clip on the ear. Bipolar sequential placements for SMR training usually involve electrode positions C_1–C_5 in the left hemisphere, or sometimes corresponding locations in the right hemisphere. C_1 lies halfway between C_z and C_3, and C_5 halfway between C_3 and T_3.

Some neurofeedback systems require only three electrodes, two active electrodes for the scalp and one ear clip. Others require the active electrodes on the head, an ear clip, and a forehead ground. These requirements are outlined by the specific manufacturers. Once the electrodes are placed, the subject experiences no discomfort. There may be some discomfort on the scalp during the application of electrodes. It is usually not significant and might occur from rubbing the Omniprep or Nuprep, which is mildly abrasive, on the scalp before placing the electrode in its appropriate location. Since this procedure has been tolerated very well by children as young as age 6, it is not a major problem. In adolescents and adults, there is hardly any response at all to this preparation procedure. Typically, a well-trained therapist can perform the entire electrode connection in 2 minutes or less. At the end of the session, one simply removes the electrodes by lifting them from the head. The scalp location is cleansed either with mild soap and warm water or with isopropyl alcohol. Patients tolerate the removal of electrodes without difficulty. The term "sensor," is better to use than "electrodes," especially with children.

TREATMENT PROTOCOLS

Because our goal is to provide comprehensive treatment for persons with ADD/ADHD, it is important to do this in the context of the activities where they are having difficulty. Many children with ADD or ADHD score poorly on measures of reading, handwriting, auditory skills, spelling, or mathematical computational skills. This is one of the reasons why pretesting information is important before beginning neurofeedback. Once a therapist knows in which areas a child is experiencing the most difficulty, the neurofeedback can be designed to help the child overcome some of these problems. Pretesting involves psychoeducational measures, IQ determination, a continuous-performance test, and rating scales, as well as a thorough family, academic, and social adjustment evaluation.

The typical session, for example, might consist of a 2-minute baseline in which there is neither auditory nor visual feedback. The computer screen can be turned off, and the data gathered in order to determine the baseline measures. These measures include (1) microvolts of theta, (2) microvolts of beta, (3) percentage of theta below the theta threshold, (4) percentage of beta above the beta threshold, (5) perhaps ratios of theta to beta activity, and (6) threshold settings. If training involves SMR enhancement or suppression of thalpha or alpha, then these need to be recorded and graphed over sessions.

After a complete baseline, the child or adult might engage in a feedback component for about 5 minutes. During this portion of the session, the participant sits with eyes open in front of the screen in an upright chair, and tries to obtain as high a score as possible using the various feedback displays. The patient should be introduced to various display options in the first session and given the chance to choose those most preferred. Now the patient can receive auditory feedback during a reading task. The goal of this portion of the session is to read and, at the same time, produce the desired EEG activity.

If the person starts producing too much theta, the therapist can cue him or her to stop reading, try to restart the feedback, and then continue reading. The idea is for the individual to be able to perform the academic tasks while producing the desired EEG response. For a reading task, auditory feedback is the appropriate modality, as visual feedback would interfere with the task. Next, the therapist can present a 5-minute period in which the person uses both auditory and visual feedback alone without additional academic tasks. The therapist can then present another academic component, such as a listening task, in which the patient experiences the visual feedback while listening to a story. An option is a listening task with very-low-amplitude auditory feedback being provided in the background.

Other conditions can involve an initial baseline, several feedback components, and several academic components. These academic components might involve math problems, spelling, and handwriting, each combined with feedback. The type of feedback should be appropriate for each task—so as not to interfere with the task, but to give the person cues in the background linked to changing the EEG while the person performs the task. It is very important for the therapist to be involved in the feedback process. With all children and adolescents, the therapist should always be in the room; adults sometimes prefer to work alone.

Sometimes children become bored during a session. If this happens, the therapist can tell the child, "if you obtain a certain number of points, we will stop and play a game." The game can be a board game such as checkers, a thinking game such as Twenty Questions, a short card game, or something else familiar to both the therapist and the child. Games are used as rewards for good performance.

However, if the child does not meet feedback goals, the therapist should be understanding and make the criteria for the game rewards easier in the subsequent sessions. Often this treatment is taking place after school and at the time of day when children are most fatigued. If children are able to perform well under these conditions, the transfer into school settings is even better than if they complete all of their treatment in the early morning—the time of day when they are most alert.

I do not use reclining positions for this type of treatment, because in classrooms, children sit at desks and maintain upright postures. In this way, EEG neurofeedback for ADD/ADHD is very different from relaxation therapy for anxiety disorders or stress reduction. From time to time, a therapist should question a child or adult to determine whether the patient is aware of EEG changes, what is making the displays work, and what makes the displays stop—in other words, what is producing beta and SMR, and what is producing theta, thalpha, and EMG. This awareness is important, because the information gathered can be used in the classroom setting for teachers to cue the child when they see the child is not attending.

In research settings, one is interested in determining the most important factors in neurofeedback. Researchers asks questions such as these: Are the therapist variables important? Is the nature of the display important? To what extent does the neurofeedback have a positive effect, compared with neurofeedback integrated with academic skill instruction, therapy, or other techniques? Answers to these questions are best learned by research designs with carefully matched groups. Such a design should include a control group that receives no training, but for which all assessment measures are taken over the same time intervals as other groups receiving treatment. There should be (1) a group receiving only neurofeedback with a relatively neutral therapist in terms of therapist–patient interaction; (2) a group that might receive some other type of biofeedback, such as EMG or thermal and electrodermal feedback; (3) a group receiving some other treatment, such as behavior therapy or psychotherapy; and perhaps (4) a group receiving neurofeedback combined with some of these other approaches. The last condition would help determine whether the effects are additive or multiplicative.

There is a very critical need for controlled studies of this kind if neurofeedback for ADD/ADHD is to be accepted by those professionals who believe that only double-blind studies or studies with matched control groups are valid. Consider this important point about double-blind studies: They are excellent for determining whether short-acting drugs are effective, particularly in the context of Ritalin or Dexedrine. In this situation, one administers a drug that clears body systems within 6 hours. It is relatively easy to conduct double-blind studies when one group receives Ritalin, another group receives a placebo, and then a crossover is employed. It is also easy in an *A-B-A design*, when one group first receives Ritalin alone, then a placebo, and then Ritalin alone.

In our early laboratory-based work (Lubar & Shouse, 1976, 1977), we carried out double-blind studies of this type. However, one of the drawbacks is that children require treatment over many weeks and months, and part of that time, they receive bogus or irrelevant feedback (control condition) that may exacerbate their symptoms. For ethical reasons, one cannot do this in a fee-for-service setting. There also is the question of whether it is appropriate for children to receive a type of feedback that could make them worse or lead them to become disappointed and stop the treatment, possibly in worse condition than when they started. For this reason, I personally do not advocate double-blind crossover studies with this population. These children can be very fragile, and their families are very sensitive to negative outcomes. However, studies with accurately matched groups could be more convincing.

Clinical case outcome studies that have recently been carried out, some of which have been published, are extremely important (Thompson & Thompson, 1998). They help to define the groups that are appropriate for neurofeedback treatment. It is through our clinical work that my colleagues and I have been able to develop the position statement given earlier. Based on this statement, it is easier to design and carry out controlled outcome studies than it was before knowing the types of children, adolescents, or adults appropriate for this type of treatment. As in many other treatments for other disorders, the results with controlled outcome studies may not be as strong as those completed in clinical settings where feedback is integrated into a multi-component treatment program.

PRE- AND POSTTREATMENT MEASURES

I strongly recommend pre- and posttreatment measures for all patients whenever possible in order to document treatment effects and to help in supporting the validity of neurofeedback for ADD/ADHD. These measures can include measurements from intelligence tests, psycho-educational assessments, continuous performance tasks, and single-channel or multichannel EEG assessments. Behavior rating scales are also excellent, but are less reliable than other behavioral measures because of their subjectivity, especially when completed by each parent or by teachers. It is particularly important to obtain follow-up data from patients for as long as possible and to provide periodic "booster" sessions, if indicated.

OVERVIEW OF RESULTS OF RECENT RESEARCH

We were able to collect retrospective data from some of our clinic patients. Fifty-two patients seen over a 10-year period were contacted by telephone by an independent surveyor who had no contact with any of the patients during their treatment or evaluation. The criteria for inclusion in this study were that these patients completed treatment and were available. Many more patients completed treatment over the 10 years but could not be contacted. One of the problems was that some of the older persons reached adulthood, left the area, and were not available. Other families also moved from the area and were not available. The survey used 16 items from the Conners Parent and Teacher Rating Scales. The results are shown in Figures 18.5 and 18.6. The first graph (Figure 18.5) shows changes in behaviors 1–8, and the second (Figure 18.6) shows behaviors 9 through 16.

Note that the highest ratings were in the two categories "Very Much Improved" and "More Change." This was particularly the case for reductions in these behaviors: constant fidgeting, being demanding or easily frustrated, restlessness or overactivity, excitability, inattention, failure to finish things, and temper outbursts or moody behavior. Note the improvements in overall behavior, attitude, homework, grades, family interactions, and general relationships. The *greatest* changes were for completing homework and improved grades. In some cases, there were many "Not Applicable" (N/A) responses. This was particularly the case for fidgeting, being easily frustrated, crying often, disturbing others, relationship with friends, and general relationships. The reason for these N/A responses was that at least 50% of the subjects had finished treatment between 5 and 10 years ago. For those subjects who had moved into adolescence or adulthood, these categories no longer applied.

Perhaps the most important finding in our retrospective study was that the greatest improvements occurred in the areas with which parents and schools are most concerned—that is, behavior, attitude, homework, and grades. In each case, the parent providing the rating was asked specifically to what extent he or she felt the neurofeedback had played a significant role in the change, and to what extent this change was the result of maturation. Although this was a subjective question, virtually all parents and older patients felt that the changes

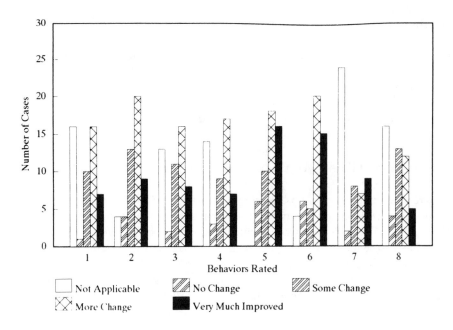

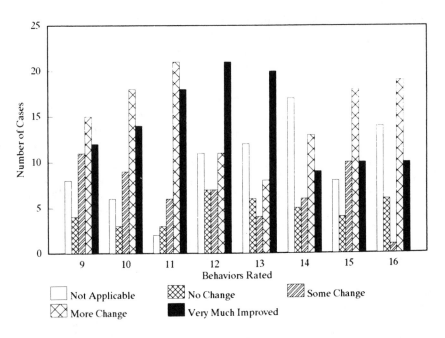

FIGURES 18.5 AND 18.6. Results from a retrospective study employing Conners Parent and Teacher Rating Scale items for 51 patients extending from less than 1 year to 10 years posttreatment. See text for detailed explanation.

were the result of the neurofeedback experience. In many cases, parents or older patients said that they believed that these changes would not have taken place without the neurofeedback. Again, it must be emphasized that retrospective data are highly subjective. Parents will often report positive results more readily than negative results, because they do not like to feel that their children failed at a particular task or treatment. It is very likely that some of the positive results obtained over long periods of time will be shown to have occurred as the result of other factors, such as maturation or possibly other treatments that may have been employed during the period over which the study was completed. To answer these criticisms would require essentially a series of controls followed for an equally long period of time, where either no treatments were employed or other treatments were employed and compared with groups where neurofeedback was the primary or only treatment.

It is important that all practitioners using neurofeedback for ADD/ADHD collect the type of data described above. Other behavioral rating scales may be as good as, or perhaps more appropriate than, the ones used in this example. The important point is that patients are not successful if they just complete treatment and only do better at that point. Success is best judged by significant long-term life changes and in individuals for whom such changes occur.

Another study was completed by Michael Linden in California (Linden, Habib, & Radojevic, 1996). It included a waiting-list control group given the WISC-R and behavior rating scales before and after the waiting period, and an active neurofeedback group that was given the theta–beta paradigm. The active neurofeedback group showed an increase of 10 WISC-R Full Scale IQ points and a significant decrease in inattentiveness. The waiting-list control group showed no changes in either of these measures.

Daniel Chartier and Ned Kelly (personal communication) in North Carolina followed their patients for more than 6 months posttreatment and used the Conners Rating Scales. They followed 16 patients and obtained results identical to ours. At present there have been approximately 75 studies regarding the effectiveness of neurofeedback for treating ADD/ADHD published in peer-reviewed journals or books. One recent source of information is a book, *Introduction to Quantitative EEG and Neurofeedback* (Evans & Abarbanel, 1999).

In a recent paper, Kaiser and Othmer (2000) found significant improvements in TOVA scores after treatment, as well as changes of more than 10 points in Verbal and Performance IQ, for more than 100 subjects with diagnosed ADD/ADHD and many others without a specific diagnosis. (Some individuals showed more than a 20-point change.) Unfortunately, that large study was flawed because no EEG data were presented; therefore, there was no evidence that the parameters that were trained actually changed as intended. Tansey (1990, 1991) reported increases of more than 15 points in the WISC-R Full Scale IQ score following neurofeedback. However, Tansey's population included primarily reading-disabled children rather than children with primarily ADD/ADHD.

At present, a number of insurance carriers and managed care plans consider this treatment as promising but still experimental, and are awaiting more published results before allowing more coverage for this type of treatment.

INTEGRATION OF NEUROFEEDBACK WITH OTHER THERAPEUTIC APPROACHES

Many children adolescents and some adults are treated with stimulant medications, especially if the diagnosis is ADHD. The main stimulant medications are dextroamphetamine sulfate (Dexedrine), methylphenidate (Ritalin and Concerta), and the newer combined formulations (e.g., Adderall and Atomoxetine). At present, it appears that at least for Ritalin, there is very little effect on cortical EEG activity (Swartwood et al., 1997; Lubar & Lubar, 1999).

We need more studies to determine whether in fact these and similar medications affect cortical functioning, ERPs, and specific behavioral measures related to ADD/ADHD. There is little evidence that these medications interfere with neurofeedback; still, many parents and children prefer to avoid them. My personal view is not to promise medication reduction or elimination as part of a neurofeedback-based treatment program. However, if a person responds very well to neurofeedback, and the individual (and parents, if the subject is a minor) feels that he or she would like to try a medication reduction trial, this should be undertaken in conjunction with an appropriate physician or specialist over time.

I find that the best regimen for Ritalin is to reduce it gradually, even though it clears the system very quickly. For example, if a child is on 20 milligrams of Ritalin in the morning, 10 milligrams at noon, and 5 milligrams in the late afternoon, the medication reduction might be as follows: 20, 10, 0; 20, 5; 10, 5; 5, 5; 5, 0; and finally 0. One should carry out this stepwise reduction at the rate of about one step every 7 days. If, in the process of medication reduction, the child or adolescent appears to be losing control over hyperkinesis or impulsiveness, one should stop the medication reduction at that point (or perhaps even increase the medication). More recently Concerta, an extended-release form of methylphenidate that has a more prolonged effect over the course of its daily administration, has been introduced.

One can reduce Dexedrine very much in the same manner as Ritalin. Sometimes medication reduction appears to work very well for a period of 1–2 months, and then the child begins to show signs of needing medication again. If this is the case, one can reintroduce the medication if requested by a physician, the parent, or the school. Many children with ADHD are able to completely eliminate medications with follow-up periods of up to 5 years or longer without reintroducing medication at any time. These are the most fortunate outcomes and probably represent one end of a continuum. If a child is on high doses of stimulant medication and still has poor control, that child is probably a poor candidate for neurofeedback, does not meet the requirements set forth in our position statement, and therefore should not be treated with neurofeedback.

There are other medications commonly used in treating ADD/ADHD comorbidity problems. These problems include impulsiveness, aggression, depression, seizure disorders, and tic disorders. Tricyclic antidepressants such as desipramine (Norpramin) and imipramine (Tofranil) are often prescribed, not only for depression but occasionally for impulsiveness. Clonidine (Catapres), an alpha-blocking agent, is also in use. Recently, SSRIs such as fluoxetine (Prozac) and paroxefine (Paxil); the antipsychotic risperidone (Risperdal); and other medications have been employed. These drugs, especially the tricyclics, take several weeks to reach maximum blood levels and a similar time period to clear the body. Medication reduction for these must be carried out much more slowly and under very careful medical supervision.

Many patients, particularly children and adolescents, in neurofeedback treatment and/or on medications may also need to participate in individual or family therapy. Many families with children with ADD/ADHD experience serious degrees of dysfunctionality. Adolescents with ADD/ADHD sometimes have children themselves and, because they are not emotionally and financially capable of raising a child, may place these children for adoption. These children are often adopted by families with no history or current evidence of ADD/ADHD, and the parents are unprepared to manage the children. Occasionally these children are physically or emotionally abused. These families need considerable counseling and parent education to understand the biological nature of ADD/ADHD and to accept that it is not their fault that a child has one of these disorders. Sometimes the children and adolescents have additional concerns, such as abuse and neglect, that merit attention. There are many parents who do not know how to manage children with ADD or ADHD, especially the latter. These parents benefit significantly from parenting groups.

I recommend that practitioners using neurofeedback for ADD/ADHD offer services to help parents develop skills for helping their children who (1) refuse to do their homework, (2) claim that the homework does not exist, (3) lose their school materials, (4) are continually teased, (5) are separated from other children by teachers, and/or (6) are left out of peer activities.

The majority of children with ADD or ADHD know that they have problems and that they are different from other children. They have enormous problems with feeling good about themselves. Some of them seek drugs and/or alcohol to boost their lowered self-esteem. The incidence of suicide is also higher among adolescents with ADD or ADHD than most other adolescents. The incidence of incarceration for crimes is much higher among adolescents and adults with ADD/ADHD (Miller & Blum, 1996).

The progression from ODD to CD to antisocial personality disorder is tragic and sometimes can be circumvented by appropriate family interventions. It is very important that practitioners and others not view neurofeedback as a cure-all or a single stand-alone approach for the treatment of these children. The best neurofeedback instrument does not replace a poor therapist who is not empathetic to the needs of the person and does not understand the complexity of the disorder. Similarly, an outstanding healthcare professional can only go so far in helping a person manage this disorder, unless that therapist can intervene either pharmacologically and/or neurologically to change the underlying neurophysiology of the system.

CONCLUSION AND FUTURE DIRECTIONS

The development of neurofeedback in the treatment of ADD/ADHD has progressed slowly and steadily since the late 1970s. During the past decade the development of this area has rapidly accelerated. Many more health care professionals now are being trained and are providing this type of treatment. There are some traditionalists who challenge neurofeedback. Their position usually focuses on the absence of controlled studies and the fact that most existing work is primarily clinical in nature. There is a need for multiple-group, controlled outcome studies, as well as for more and improved clinical studies. The position statement provided in this chapter needs modification as more is learned. The limits of neurofeedback and the integration of the technique with other traditional approaches need more thorough investigation. There are many parent support groups formed to promote understanding of and treatment for ADD/ADHD, and such groups may be instrumental in increasing the use of neurofeedback.

The evolution of this treatment will be a slow process. Third-party reimbursement for neurofeedback is necessary to treat most children appropriate for this treatment modality. The majority of children with ADD/ADHD live in family situations of modest income.

We can now anticipate future directions of instrumentation development. We need development of EEG pattern recognition programs that more accurately analyze the EEG and provide feedback that is more contingent and more precisely paired with specific EEG characteristics. The detection of activity in the EEG is presently either through active bandpass filters with the analog and/or digital processing imposed upon filter outputs or through Fourier spectral analyses of EEGs. This is not the approach taken by professional electroencephalographers when making a determination regarding abnormal or normal EEG activity. The human brain performs a pattern analysis. A trained expert can very clearly see complex patterns in the EEG consisting of the interweaving of slow, fast, normal, and abnormal activity. Development of such programs could help increase the rate of learning and make it possible to successfully treat more difficult cases, and perhaps show more clearly the power and the specificity of neurofeedback as a treatment modality. The use of quantitative EEG, whether few or many channels, is extremely important for accurate determination of proper training protocols for subtypes of ADD/ADHD and its comorbidities.

Long-term follow-up of patients is very important, not just for 1 year, but for 5–15 years. Only through longitudinal studies can we learn whether neurofeedback fulfills the promise of being able to offer a technique that changes cognitive functioning and produces long-term shifts in cerebral function.

Neurofeedback offers other possibilities now being seen on the horizon. One is the increase in human cognitive functioning. If we identify electrophysiological activity associated with special abilities and higher intellectual functioning, then perhaps we can enhance neurocognitive functioning. In a sense, neurofeedback holds promise for everyone if it can be shown to enhance human potential, creativity, and a better quality of life.

GLOSSARY

A-B-A DESIGN. An experimental design in which a baseline period (A) precedes an intervention or treatment (B), followed by another baseline (A). Often used in single-case research.

ALLELES. One of two or more different genes that occupy corresponding positions (loci) on paired chromosomes. They are usually indicated by a capital letter for the dominant gene and a lowercase letter for the recessive gene.

BASAL FOREBRAIN (FOREBRAIN, PROSENCEPHALON). One of three major subdivisions of the brain (the others are also midbrain and hindbrain)—the most forward part. It includes the telencephalon (front or end brain), containing the *basal ganglia* (see below), limbic system, olfactory bulb and tract, and lateral ventricles. Also includes the thalamus of the diencephalon (posterior portion of the forebrain).

BASAL GANGLIA. Collection of four masses of gray matter located deep in the cerebral hemisphere and mainly under the anterior region of the neocortex and to the side of the thalamus. Involves extrapyramidal regulation of motor activity and probably other functions, including sequencing complex movements into a smoothly executed response. Often referred to as the "*extrapyramidal system.*"

BIPOLAR (SEQUENTIAL) ELECTRODE MONTAGE. An electrode configuration where activity between two electrodes is subtracted and compared to a reference or neutral ground electrode.

BRAINSTEM RETICULAR FORMATION. The *brainstem* connects the cerebral hemispheres with the spinal cord. *Reticular* means "in the form of a network." The *reticular formation* is a diffuse network of groups of cells and fibers throughout the brainstem. They connect the ascending and descending tracts. They are important (essential) in their influence on and control of alertness, waking, sleeping, and several reflexes. The reticular formation includes the "reticular activating system" which initiates and maintains wakefulness and directs attention, and which extends to the entire cerebral cortex.

CEREBELLUM. A large structure behind and above the pons and medulla oblongata of the brainstem, which plays an important role in coordination and regulation of voluntary movements of skeletal muscles. It does not initiate movements, but interrelates with brainstem structures in execution of many movements, including posture, balance, walking, running, writing, dressing, eating, playing musical instruments, and eye movement tracking. It controls speed, acceleration, and trajectory of movements.

COMMON MODE REJECTION. The ability of a bipolar sequential recording to reject signals that are identical in both electrode leads simultaneously and are also in phase—for example, in-phase eye blinks, gross body movements, electrocardiographic activity, and other artifacts that might contaminate the electroencephalographic (EEG) signal. See also Neumann et al., Chapter 5, this volume.)

COMORBIDITY. The occurrence of other disorders at the same time as the target disorder. An example would be the co-occurrence of depression with the target disorder, ADHD.

C_z, THE VERTEX. EEG electrode placement on the top of the head.

C_3 and C_4. Specific sites for two of the EEG surface electrodes near and lateral to C_z. C stands for "central."

DOPAMINERGIC SYSTEM. The system of tissues influenced by dopamine, a catecholamine neurotransmitter that is the immediate precursor in norepinephrine synthesis.

EAR REFERENCE. Reference electrode placed on an ear. The point of reference against which the voltage from other active electrodes is gauged.

EVENT-RELATED POTENTIAL (ERP). A scalp surface measure of evoked cortical potential. ERPs are changes in electrical activity in response to physical stimuli, associated with psychophysiological processes, and/or in preparation for motor responses. Special computer analysis of the electroencephalogram (EEG) allows measurement of the latency, duration, and amplitude of selected cortical waveforms. (Again, see also Neumann et al., Chapter 5.)

INION. The most prominent point or center of the external protuberance of the occipital bone.

INTERNATIONAL 10-20 SYSTEM. Standard system of sites for surface EEG electrodes. (See Neumann et al., Chapter 5.)

LOCUS COERULEUS. Structure in the midbrain that produces most of the norepinephrine in the central nervous system (CNS).

NASION. Skull location or landmark immediately above the nose, roughly at the depression at the nose root, and just lower than the position of the eyebrows.

NEUROFEEDBACK. The term that typically refers to EEG feedback designed to alter a condition for which there is evidence that it has a neural basis. A form of EEG biofeedback training.

NIGROSTRIATAL SYSTEM. Projection from the substantia nigra to the corpus striatum (one of the parts of the basal ganglia). Substantia nigra ("black" or deep gray substance) is involved with extrapyramidal motor control. It is located from the upper edge of the pons into the subthalamic region. The neurotransmitter is dopamine. (See *basal ganglia*, above.)

NIHON KOHDEN ELEFIX PASTE. EEG electrode paste made by Nihon Kohden.

NORADRENERGIC ACTIVITY. Activated by or secreting norepinephrine. (See *norepinephrine* as defined in M. S. Schwartz & Sedlacek, Chapter 16, this volume.) The source in the CNS is the locus coeruleus.

OCCIPITAL CONDYLE. The bump at the back of the head.

OFFSET VOLTAGE. Voltage produced when electrodes act as batteries and impose a voltage.

POSITRON EMISSION TOMOGRAPHY (PET) SCAN. A technique based upon images created by the interaction of positrons and electrons. These subatomic particles annihilate each other, releasing photons that are collected and through appropriate analysis lead to a formation of brain images. PET scanning is particularly useful for visualizing glucose metabolism and oxygen utilization in different brain tissues.

PREAURICULAR NOTCH. A notch in front of the auricle of the ear. The "auricle" is the part of the external ear not within the head; also called the "flap" or "pinna." The notch (incisura antcrior auris) is the depression between the crus of the helix (upper end of outer hook-like structure) and the tragus (small knob-like protuberance lower and to the side of the opening to the ear canal (external acoustic meatus). The preauricular notch is just anterior to this ear location and posterior to the hair as at the top of a sideburn.

REFERENTIAL MONTAGE. A combination of EEG electrodes that obtain information about the electrical activity of specific areas of the brain, compared with a relatively neutral ground or reference.

RESPONSE INHIBITION. The ability to inhibit responding to inappropriate stimuli. Measured by computer-based continuous-performance tests. Used in the assessment of ADHD.

SINGLE-PHOTON EMISSION COMPUTERIZED TOMOGRAPHY (SPECT) SCAN. Similar to a *PET scan* (see above). A technique that allows for the evaluation of blood flow and metabolism in the living brain.

TEST OF VARIABLES OF ATTENTION (TOVA). A computer-based continuous-performance test for assessing very detailed information about sustained attention. Used in the assessment of ADHD.

REFERENCES

Achenbach, T. M. (1991). *Manual for the Child Behavior Checklist/4–18 and 1991 Profile*. Burlington: University of Vermont, Department of Psychiatry.

Amen, D. G., & Carmichael, B. (1997). Oppositional children similar to OCD on SPECT: Implications for treatment. *Journal of Neurotherapy*, 2(2), 1–7.

Amen, D. G., & Paldi, J. H. (1993, May). *Evaluating ADHD with brain SPECT imaging*. Paper presented at the annual meeting of the American Psychiatric Association, San Francisco.

American Psychiatric Association. (1994). *Diagnostic and statistical manual of mental disorders* (4th ed.). Washington, DC: Author.

Anderson, W. W. (1963). The hyperkinetic child: A neurological appraisal. *Neurology, 13*, 968–973.

Barkley, R. A. (1997). *Defiant children: A clinician's manual for parent training* (2nd ed.). New York: Guilford Press.

Barkley, R. A. (1998a). Attention-deficit hyperactivity disorder. In E. Mash & R. A. Barkley (Eds.), *Treatment of childhood disorders* (pp. 39–72). New York: Guilford Press.

Barkley, R. A. (1998b). *Attention-deficit hyperactivity disorder: A handbook for diagnosis and treatment.* New York: Guilford Press.

Bradley, C. (1937). The behavior of children receiving benzedrine. *American Journal of Psychiatry, 94*, 577–585.

Blum, K., & Noble, E. P. (Eds.). (1997). *Handbook of psychiatric genetics.* Boca Raton, FL: CRC Press.

Chabot, R. J., & Serfontein, G. (1996). Quantitative EEG profiles of children with attention deficit disorder. *Biological Psychiatry, 40*, 951–963.

Conners, C. K. (1969). A teacher rating scale for use with drug studies with children. *American Journal of Psychiatry, 127*, 884–888.

Evans, J. R., & Abarbanel, A. (Eds.). (1999). *Introduction to quantitative EEG and neurofeedback.* San Diego, CA: Academic Press.

Gasser, T., Verleger, R., Bacherj, P., & Sroka, L. (1988). Development of the EEG of school-age children and adolescents: I. Analysis of band power. *Electroencephalography and Clinical Neurophysiology, 69*, 91–99.

Heilman, M., Voeller, K. S., & Nadeau, S. (1991). A possible pathophysiologic substrate of attention deficit hyperactivity disorder. *Journal of Child Neurology, 6*, S76–S81.

Jasper, H. H., Solomon, P., & Bradley, C. (1938). Electroencephalographic analysis of behavior problems in children. *American Journal of Psychiatry, 95*, 641–658.

Kaiser, D. A., & Othmer, S. (2000). Effect of neurofeedback on variables of attention in a large multi-center trial. *Journal of Neurotherapy, 4*, 5–15.

Kamiya, J. (1979). Autoregulation of the EEG alpha rhythm: A program for the study of consciousness. In E. Peper, S. Ancoli, & M. Quinn (Eds.), *Mind/body integration: Essential readings in biofeedback.* New York: Plenum Press.

Klorman, R. (1991). Cognitive event-related potentials in attention deficit disorder. *Journal of Learning Disabilities, 24*(3), 130–140.

Lahey, B. B., Schaughency, E., Hynd, G., Carlson, G., & Nieves, N. (1987). Attention deficit disorder with and without hyperactivity: Comparison of behavioral characteristics of clinic-referred children. *Journal of the American Academy of Child Psychiatry, 26*, 718–723.

Lazzaro, I., Gordon, E., Whitmont, S., Meares, R., & Clarke, S. (2001). The modulation of late component event related potentials by pre-stimulus EEG theta activity in ADHD. *International Journal of Neuroscience, 107*, 247–264.

Linden, M., Habib, T., & Radojevic, V. (1996). A controlled study of the effects of EEG biofeedback on the cognition and behavior of children with attention deficit disorders and learning disabilities. *Biofeedback and Self Regulation, 21*(1), 35–49.

Lubar, J. F. (1989). Electroencephalographic biofeedback and neurological applications. In J. V. Basmajian (Ed.), *Biofeedback: Principles and practice for clinicians* (3rd ed.). Baltimore: Williams & Wilkins.

Lubar, J. F. (1991). Discourse on the development of EEG diagnostics and biofeedback treatment for attention-deficit/hyperactivity disorders. *Biofeedback and Self-Regulation, 16*, 201–225.

Lubar, J. F. (1992, October). *Point/counterpoint: Is EEG neurofeedback an effective treatment for ADHD?* Paper presented at the 5th Annual Meeting of CHADD, Chicago.

Lubar, J. F., & Culver, R. M. (1978). Automated signal-detection methodologies for biofeedback conditioning. *Behavioral Research Methods and Instrumentation, 10*, 607–617.

Lubar, J. F., & Lubar, J. O. (1999). Neurofeedback assessment and treatment for attention deficit/hyperactivity disorders (ADD/HD). In J. R. Evans & A. Abarbanel (Eds.), *Introduction to quantitative EEG and neurofeedback.* San Diego, CA: Academic Press.

Lubar, J. F., & Shouse, M. N. (1976). EEG and behavioral changes in a hyperkinetic child concurrent with training of the sensorimotor rhythm (SMR): A preliminary report. *Biofeedback and Self-Regulation, 3*, 293–306.

Lubar, J. F., & Shouse, M. N. (1977). Use of biofeedback in the treatment of seizure disorders and hyperactivity. In B. B. Lahey & A. E. Kazdin (Eds.), *Advances in clinical child psychology*, Vol. 1. New York: Plenum Press.

Lubar, J. F., Swartwood, M. O., Swartwood, J. N., & Timmermann, D. L. (1995). Quantitative EEG and auditory event-related potentials in the evaluation of attention-deficit disorder: Effects of methylphenidate and implications for neurofeedback training. *Journal of Psychoeducational Assessment Monographs, series, Special ADHD Issue)*, 143–160.

Mann, C., Lubar, J., Zimmerman, A., Miller, C., & Muenchen, R. (1992). Quantitative analysis of EEG in boys with attention-deficit/hyperactivity disorder: A controlled study with clinical implications. *Pediatric Neurology, 8*, 30–36.

McCarney, S. B. (1995). *Home and School Situation Questionnaire* (2nd ed.). Columbia, MO: Hawthorne Educational Services.

Miller, D., & Blum, K. (1996) *Overload: Attention deficit disorder and the addictive brain.* Kansas City, MO: Andrews & McMeel.

Monastra, V. J., Lubar, J. F., & Linden, M. K. (2001). The development of a quantitative electroencephalographic scanning process for attention deficit-hyperactivity disorder: Reliability and validity studies. *Neuropsychology, 15*(1), 136–144.

Monastra, V. J., Lubar, J. F., Linden, M., VanDeusen, P., Green, G., Wing, W., Phillips, A., & Fenger, T. N. (1999). Assessing attention deficit hyperactivity disorder via quantitative electroencephalography: An initial validation study. *Neuropsychology, 13*(3), 424–433.

Posner, M. I., & Raichle, M. E. (1994). *Images of mind.* New York: Scientific Books.

Riccio, C. A., Hynd, G. W., Cohen, M. J., Gonzalez, J. J., et al. (1993). Neurological basis of attention deficit hyperactivity disorder. *Exceptional Children, 60,* 118–124.

Satterfield, J. H., & Dawson, M. E. (1971). Electrodermal correlates of hyperactivity in children. *Psychophysiology, 8,* 191–197.

Satterfield, J. H., Lesser, R I., Saul, R. E., & Cantwell, D. P. (1973). EEG aspects in the diagnosis and treatment of minimal brain dysfunction. *Annals of the New York Academy of Sciences, 205,* 274–282.

Schneider, F., Rockstroh, B., Heimann, H., Lutzenberger, W., Mattes, R, Elbert, T., Birbaumer, N., & Bartels, M. (1992). Self-regulation of slow cortical potentials in psychiatric patients: Schizophrenia. *Biofeedback and Self-Regulation, 17*(4), 277–292.

Shouse, M. N., & Lubar, J. F. (1978). Physiological bases of hyperkinesis treated with methylphenidate. *Pediatrics, 62,* 343–351.

Still, G. F. (1902). The Coulstonian lectures on some abnormal psychological conditions in children. *Lancet, i,* 1008–1012, 1163–1168.

Swartwood, M. O., Swartwood, J. N., Lubar, J. F., Timmermann, D. L., Zimmerman, A. W., & Muenchen, R. A. (1998). Methylphenidate effects on EEG, behavior, and performance in boys with ADHD. *Pediatric Neurology, 18*(3), 244–250.

Tansey, M. A. (1990). Righting the rhythms of reason, EEG biofeedback training as a therapeutic modality in a clinical office setting. *Medical Psychotherapy, 3,* 57–68.

Tansey, M. A. (1991). Wechsler's (WISC-R) changes following treatment of learning disabilities via EEG biofeedback training in a private setting. *Australian Journal of Psychology, 43,* 147–153.

Thompson, L., & Thompson, M. (1998). Neurofeedback combined with training in metacognitive strategies: Effectiveness in students with ADD. *Applied Psychophysiology and Biofeedback, 23*(4), 243–263.

Voeller, K. K. S. (1991). Toward a neurobiologic nosology of attention deficit hyperactivity disorder. *Journal of Child Neurology, 6* (Suppl), S2–S8.

Whalen, C. K., & Henckler, B. (1991). Therapies for hyperactive children: Comparisons, combinations, and compromises. *Journal of Consulting and Clinical Psychology, 59,* 126–137.

Wolraich, M. L., Lindgren, S., Stromquist, A., Milich, R., Davis, C., & Watson, D. (1990). Stimulant medication use by primary care physicians in the treatment of attention-deficit hyperactivity disorder. *Pediatrics, 86,* 95–101.

Zametkin, A. J., Nordahl, T. E., Gross, M., King, A. C., Semple, W. E., Rumsey, J., Hamburger, S., & Cohen, R. M. (1990). Cerebral glucose metabolism in adults with hyperactivity of childhood onset. *New England Journal of Medicine, 323,* 1361–1366.

Zametkin, A. J., & Rapoport, J. L. (1987). Noradrenergic hypothesis of attention deficit disorder with hyperactivity: A critical review. In H. V. Metsler (Ed.), *Psychopharmacology: The third generation of progress.* New York: Raven Press.

CHAPTER 19

Clinical Applications of Electroencephalographic Biofeedback

VINCENT J. MONASTRA

The purposes of this chapter are to provide an overview of the primary types of electroencephalographic (EEG) biofeedback, describe the most common clinical applications of each of these treatment protocols, summarize research investigating the application of these treatment protocols in the context of American Psychological Association (APA) guidelines, and present a perspective on directions for future clinical research and practice. Although a substantial number of scientific papers examining the application of EEG biofeedback (neurofeedback) have been published (see Byers, 1995, for a comprehensive overview), a much more restricted number of papers are available for review via Medline and PsycSCAN searches. Overall, a sufficient number of positive outcomes have been noted in the treatment of attention-deficit/hyperactivity disorder (ADHD), anxiety disorders, mood disorders, seizure disorders, traumatic brain injury (TBI), and addictions to prompt reviewers like Duffy (2000) to comment that "if any medication had demonstrated such a wide spectrum of efficacy, it would be universally accepted and widely used" (p. v).

However, as noted by Duffy (2000), progress in the clinical application of EEG biofeedback appears to have been limited not so much by the lack of research as by the kind of scientific provincialism that is evident when new treatment paradigms are introduced. Duffy (2000) has summarized this issue as follows: "On one hand, some proponents may be overly and uncritically enthusiastic, whereas on the other hand many critics may be quite ignorant of the real data and/or theoretical underpinnings of EEG biofeedback therapy and overly sensitive to self-perpetuating common wisdom" (p. vi). My review of the literature indicates that certain essential questions remain unanswered with respect to neurophysiological models of psychopathology and the identification of specific biofeedback treatment protocols that optimize the therapeutic process and yield enduring improvement in health status. However, as will be illustrated in this chapter, several clinical applications of EEG biofeedback meet established scientific criteria to be considered at least "probably efficacious" in the treatment of a number of psychological and neurological conditions.

DETERMINING TREATMENT EFFECTIVENESS

Although certain types of individual, group, and family/couple therapies appear to be "empirically supported" for the treatment of psychiatric disorders in children/adolescents (Kazdin & Weisz, 1998) and adults (DeRubeis & Crits-Christoph, 1998; Baucom, Shoham, Mueser, Daiuto, & Stickle, 1998), there is little evidence that the effects of any of the psychological treatments endure beyond a brief follow-up period (Kazdin & Weisz, 1998). It is within this context that the clinical efficacy of EEG biofeedback is examined.

Because of the limited number of studies demonstrating efficacy in applied settings, several task forces have attempted to develop guidelines to assist in the identification of effective psychological treatments (APA Task Force on Psychological Intervention Guidelines, 1995; APA Task Force on Promotion and Dissemination of Psychological Procedures, 1995) and medical procedures for conditions caused by neuropathy (the American Academy of Neurology (AAN) and the American Clinical Neurophysiology Society (ACNS), as reported by Nuwer, 1997). In these guidelines, randomized clinical trials (RCTs), as well as other types of controlled case and group designs, are strongly encouraged.

Chambless and Hollon (1998) proposed a process for defining "empirically supported therapies" based on the results of the APA task forces, and concluded as follows: "Treatment efficacy must be demonstrated in controlled research in which it is reasonable to conclude that the benefits observed are due to the factors of the treatment and not to chance or confounding factors such as passage of time, the effects of psychological assessment, or the presence of different types of clients in the various treatment conditions" (p. 8). Although these authors expressed a preference for RCTs because they control for "nonspecific" treatment factors (e.g., patient variability; therapist "personality"; matching of patient, therapist, and technique based on patient preference), others (Luborsky, McLellan, Diguer, Woody, & Seligman, 1997; Garfield, 1998) have emphasized the need to systematically examine patient and therapist factors.

Based on their recognition of the importance of both specific and nonspecific factors in determining treatment outcome, Chambless and Hollon (1998) proposed the following classification scheme: "possibly efficacious," "probably efficacious," and "efficacious and specific." They concluded that RCTs and "carefully controlled single case experiments and their group analogues" (p. 7) were appropriate scientific procedures to be used in determining efficacy. Their classification system was defined as follows:

> "Possibly efficacious": The treatment was determined to yield a clinical outcome that was superior to no treatment (or a waiting-list control) in one study or in a series of studies conducted by the same research team.
> "Probably efficacious": The treatment was determined to yield a clinical outcome that was superior to no treatment (or a waiting-list control) in at least two studies conducted by independent research teams.
> "Efficacious and specific": The treatment was determined to yield a clinical outcome that was superior to a placebo that controls for nonspecific factors (e.g., the process of receiving attention from an interested person or the expectation of change) or comparable to another "bona fide" treatment in at least two studies conducted by independent research teams.

The AAN/ACNS guidelines (Nuwer, 1997) utilized an "A to E" rating system, based on the design of supporting studies (double-blind control vs. controlled case or group study vs. uncontrolled case reports/expert opinion). These guidelines emphasize the importance of independent replication by multiple research teams and recognize the contribution of various types of research designs. However, the primary emphasis of the AAN/ACNS on blinded, placebo-controlled studies fails to recognize certain ethical considerations in the conduct of psychological and psychophysiological research (LaVaque & Rossiter, 2001). Consequently, the APA guidelines (as revised by Chambless & Hollon, 1998) are utilized in the examination of the various EEG biofeedback applications reviewed in this chapter.

EEG BIOFEEDBACK TRAINING PROTOCOLS: AN OVERVIEW

Clinical researchers seeking to investigate a type of operant conditioning that would result in sustained symptom elimination began examining certain electrophysiological "behaviors" approximately three decades ago. Psychophysiologists initially defined target behaviors via EEG procedures, developed technologies to "reinforce" these behaviors, demonstrated that children and adults could increase or decrease these behaviors in response to systematic reinforcement or extinction procedures, and showed that modifications in these electrophysiological behaviors resulted in improvement in neurological and psychiatric conditions (see reviews by Sterman, 1996, and Lubar, 1997).

Historically, the most commonly examined electrophysiological behaviors have been descriptively defined as theta (3.5–8 hertz [Hz]), alpha (9–11 Hz), sensorimotor rhythm (SMR; 12–15 Hz), and beta (16–20 Hz). Most of the studies conducted to date have examined the effects of decreasing theta and increasing alpha, SMR, or beta. However, recent developments in the field have led to interest in slow cortical potentials (SCPs; Birbaumer, Elbert, Canavan, & Rockstroh, 1990) and in the examination of electrophysiological behaviors other than the frequency and amplitude of EEG waveforms over single or paired active electrode sites (e.g., coherence, Thatcher, 2000; asymmetry, Rosenfeld, 2000).

During the course of the past three decades, biofeedback instrumentation has been developed so that patients and their health care providers can view raw EEG data, as well as information converted via analog and digital processing. In addition, many of these instruments provide statistical information that can be useful in establishing initial training parameters, monitoring patient progress, adjusting training protocols, and evaluating treatment efficacy. Examples of useful statistical information are electrophysiological power within specified frequencies (absolute and relative); average amplitudes within specified frequency bands; percentage of time that the patient maintains cortical activity within specified thresholds; and the degree of symmetry and coherence in the activity patterns of cortical hemispheres and specific regions within hemispheres.

Based on the availability of instrumentation that is able to measure electrophysiological activity, provide "real-time" feedback, and permit statistical analysis of "neuronal behavior," applied psychophysiologists have examined the effects of EEG biofeedback in treating a wide range of psychiatric and medical disorders—including seizure disorder, anxiety disorders, ADHD, substance disorders, schizophrenia, mood disorders, Tourette's disorder, TBI, stroke, and learning disabilities. This chapter concentrates on examining those applications in which data have been published in peer-reviewed journals and are available for review via Medline and/or PsycSCAN literature searches.

ANXIETY DISORDERS

The *Diagnostic and Statistical Manual of Mental Disorders*, fourth edition (DSM-IV; American Psychiatric Association, 1994) classifies 11 different types of psychiatric diagnoses as anxiety disorders. EEG biofeedback researchers have reported positive outcomes in the treatment of college students presenting with anxiety but not diagnosed with an anxiety disorder (Sittenfield, Budzynski, & Stoyva, 1976; Hardt & Kamiya, 1978; Plotkin & Rice, 1981); patients diagnosed with generalized anxiety disorder (Rice, Blanchard, & Purcell, 1993; Vanathy, Sharma, & Kumar, 1998), students presenting with test anxiety (Garrett & Silver, 1976), adults diagnosed with obsessive–compulsive disorder (Mills & Solyom, 1974; Glueck & Stroebel, 1975), and Vietnam veterans with combat-related posttraumatic stress disorder (PTSD) (Peniston & Kulkosky, 1991).

Treatment Protocols

EEG biofeedback protocols for the treatment of anxiety disorders have included alpha enhancement (e.g., Hardt & Kamiya, 1978), theta enhancement (e.g., Sittenfield et al., 1976), and alpha–theta enhancement (Peniston & Kulkosky, 1991) paradigms. Information regarding location of sensors, frequency bands to be reinforced/inhibited, and type of feedback is provided below. For illustrations of the International 10-20 System of electrode placement please see Figure 5.3 (Neumann, Strehl, & Birbaumer, Chapter 5) and Figure 18.2 (Lubar, Chapter 18).

Alpha enhancement protocol

• Sensor location	O_1, O_z (most common); C_3, C_4 (less common).
• References	Ear and forehead references have both been used.
• Reinforced frequencies	8–13 Hz.
• Reinforced EEG pattern	Percentage of time patient produces alpha amplitudes above a threshold (e.g., 10 microvolts), or patient production of alpha amplitudes above a set-point (e.g., 19–21 microvolts).
• Feedback modality	Auditory (tones and/or verbal feedback); eyes are typically closed during training.
• Timing of sessions	Ranges from daily to weekly.

Theta enhancement protocol

• Sensor location	O_z or C_4.
• References	Ear and forehead references have both been used.
• Reinforced frequencies	3.5–7.5 Hz; inhibiting 8–12 Hz.
• Reinforced EEG pattern	Maintaining 3.5- to 7.5-Hz activity above a preset microvolt threshold, while suppressing 8- to 12-Hz production below a specified microvolt threshold.
• Feedback modality	Primarily auditory with eyes closed; visual feedback has been provided in instances where surface electromyographic (EMG) feedback is also provided.
• Timing of sessions	Daily to weekly.

In those studies that use alpha–theta enhancement, occipital sites (O_1, O_z) have been monitored, and feedback is contingent on the patient's achieving a combined voltage greater than a preset microvolt threshold.

Clinical Outcome Studies

Among the studies reported to date, only the research reported by Garrett and Silver (1976), Rice et al. (1993), Vanathy et al. (1998), and Peniston and Kulkosky (1991) are controlled experiments involving patients diagnosed with an anxiety disorder. Because guidelines for efficacy research require control for nonspecific factors, only these studies are reviewed here.

The Garrett and Silver (1976) paper reports the results of a randomized, controlled study of students with test anxiety. Fifty participants were assigned to one of the following five groups: alpha enhancement, EMG voltage reduction, alpha enhancement plus EMG voltage reduction ("combined" treatment), relaxation training, or no treatment. Treatment was conducted for 10 weekly sessions. Both the alpha enhancement and combined treatment groups increased alpha. The EMG and combined treatment groups demonstrated decrease in muscle tension. The relaxation training group showed mild increase in alpha and significant reduction in muscle tension. No changes were noted in the untreated group. Only participants in the three feedback groups reported significant reduction in test anxiety, suggesting that improvements were not due to the passage of time or nonspecific factors.

Two controlled studies have examined the effects of EEG biofeedback in the treatment of patients with generalized anxiety disorder. Initially, Rice et al. (1993) used a randomized design in which 45 patients were assigned to one of the following conditions: waiting-list control, pseudomeditation, EMG biofeedback, alpha enhancement biofeedback, or alpha suppression biofeedback. Treatment was conducted twice weekly for 4 weeks, and each session consisted of 5 minutes of baseline, 3 minutes of self-control, and 20 minutes of biofeedback. Outcome measures revealed significant improvement on the State–Trait Anxiety Inventory and the Psychosomatic Symptom Checklist in all of the treatment groups compared to the waiting-list control. In addition, the EMG and alpha enhancement groups showed improvements on the Welsh Anxiety Scale. Clinical improvements persisted 6 weeks posttreatment. However, the absence of a significant increase in alpha production in the alpha enhancement group precluded interpretation of results as due to change in alpha.

The Vanathy et al. (1998) study used random assignment to either a waiting list, an alpha enhancement/beta suppression protocol, or a theta enhancement/beta suppression protocol in order to assess the effects of EEG biofeedback on 18 patients diagnosed with generalized anxiety disorder. A total of 15 sessions were provided. Outcome measures (State–Trait Anxiety Inventory, Hamilton Anxiety Rating Scale) showed improvements in patient self-report of anxiety in both treatment groups relative to the untreated control group. However, similar to the Rice et al. (1993) study, pre- and posttreatment EEG spectral analysis did not show significant change in alpha or theta production.

EEG biofeedback treatment of PTSD was examined in a randomized, controlled study conducted by Peniston and Kulkosky (1991). In their study, 29 Vietnam veterans diagnosed with PTSD were assigned to either an alpha/theta enhancement protocol ($n = 15$) or traditional medical treatment ($n = 14$). Patients in both groups also received medications for PTSD symptoms. Participants assigned to the EEG biofeedback group initially received 8 sessions of temperature biofeedback, followed by 30 alpha/theta enhancement sessions (30 minutes per session, 5 sessions per week). Patients in the biofeedback group demonstrated significant improvements on all 10 of the clinical Minnesota Multiphasic Personality Inventory (MMPI) scales (compared to improvement on only 1 scale in the control group), were able to reduce medication dosage (compared to only 1 of the members in the control group), and at follow-up (30 months) showed significantly less recidivism (relapse rates: EEG biofeedback, 20%; control, 100%).

Analysis of Efficacy

Based on the criteria presented by Chambless and Hollon (1998), the application of EEG biofeedback in the treatment of certain anxiety disorders (specific phobia, generalized anxiety disorder, PTSD) is considered to be "possibly efficacious" in the treatment of specific phobia (test anxiety) and PTSD, and "probably efficacious" in the treatment of generalized anxiety disorder. These ratings are based on the presence of only one controlled group study demonstrating efficacy in the treatment of specific phobia and PTSD, and the absence of anticipated changes in electrophysiological measures in the two studies of generalized anxiety disorder.

Examination of the clinical application of EEG biofeedback in the treatment of anxiety disorders reveals the presence of well-defined treatment protocols and the availability of self-report scales to monitor patient progress. Outcome studies have repeatedly indicated clinical improvement on these measures in response to EEG biofeedback. However, no consistent pattern of electrophysiological change has been observed on the few EEG indicators examined in these studies. Clinical improvement has been noted in patients where there has been no increase in alpha voltage, as well as in patients who exhibited decline in alpha voltage.

As emphasized by Thatcher (1998), it seems essential to identify those quantitative EEG (QEEG) measures that reliably differentiate patients with an anxiety disorder from unaffected individuals. It is the identification of such "neurometric" markers that has guided successful clinical applications in the treatment of seizure disorders (Sterman, 2000), ADHD (Nash, 2000), and mood disorders (Rosenfeld, 2000), and that appears needed in this area. Although the absence of reliable electrophysiological indicators of anxiety disorders hinders our ability to define specific EEG protocols that could optimize the treatment process, the lack of an EEG-based dependent measure cannot be presumed to indicate that the effects of biofeedback are due to placebo effects alone. Controlled studies assessing the clinical effects of EEG biofeedback have revealed improvement in clinical symptoms on other dependent measures. EEG researchers now need to identify those electrophysiological abnormalities that are evident in patients with anxiety disorders, and to develop protocols that target those symptoms.

Consequently, in order for EEG biofeedback to be considered "efficacious and specific" for the treatment of anxiety disorders, randomized, controlled group studies that compare EEG biofeedback protocols with previously demonstrated efficacious treatments (e.g., selective serotonin reuptake inhibitors [SSRIs] such as Paxil) are needed. Although studies involving "sham" treatments or placebo controls have been advocated (Barkley, 1992) as necessary to identify efficacious treatments, these procedures are not considered essential by the APA (see APA Task Force references) and appear to be ethically unacceptable in the conduct of biomedical research with humans, since the use of such deceptive procedures would prevent individuals in the control group from receiving the "best proven diagnostic and therapeutic methods" (World Medical Association Declaration of Helsinki, 1997, p. 926). In addition (as will be asserted throughout this chapter), in order to be accepted as a viable treatment option, any EEG biofeedback application will need to demonstrate efficacy at least equal to existing medical treatments, or show that the biofeedback treatment results in sustained clinical improvement when medications are reduced or eliminated.

SEIZURE DISORDERS

In contrast to neurofeedback for anxiety disorders, EEG-based protocols for the treatment of seizure disorders are founded on numerous studies that examine the origin of the SMR (Sterman, 2000) and SCPs (Kotchoubey et al., 1999b), and explore the relationship between these EEG phenomena and the inhibition of cortical excitation from the focal region of a seizure to surrounding neurons. These treatment procedures emerged primarily for the treatment of refractory epilepsy, in which seizures were not being adequately controlled by medication.

Treatment Protocols

As noted by Sterman (2000), seizure disorders can be caused by genetic factors or can be secondary to other forms of pathology. Electrophysiological examination of patients with epilepsy reveals recurring patterns of abnormal, excessive synchronous discharge of neurons, presumably due to hyperexcitability or hyperexcitation of cortical regions (e.g., temporal lobes). EEG-based treatments target the reduction of neuronal excitability in affected tissues and seek to limit the impact of transient neuronal discharge. Two treatment protocols—one based on feedback of the SMR (Sterman & Friar, 1972), and one derived from research on SCPs (Rockstroh, Elbert, Canavan, Lutzenberger, & Birbaumer, 1989)—constitute the primary types of EEG biofeedback used in the treatment of seizure disorders.

The SMR protocol is based on an extensive body of scientific knowledge demonstrating that the 12- to 14-Hz rhythmic activity evident over the rolandic cortex (C_3, C_4) is associated with an alert, motionless state. It has been demonstrated that SMR is generated in the thalamic relay nuclei of the somatosensory pathway (see review by Sterman, 1996). Sterman and his colleagues demonstrated that cats could be trained to produce this rhythm (Wyricka & Sterman, 1968), that "SMR-trained" cats were resistant to convulsions produced by monomethylhydrazine (Sterman, LoPresti, & Fairchild, 1969), and that patients with seizure disorders could reduce their rate of seizures after learning this procedure (Sterman & Friar, 1972).

SMR treatment protocols seek to increase production of 12- to 14-Hz activity at C_3 or C_4, while suppressing 4- to 7-Hz activity. Bipolar montages are commonly used (C_3–T_3; C_4–T_4, ear reference). Reinforcement is given in the form of auditory or visual displays for patient production of brief bursts of 12- to 14-Hz activity (e.g., 6 waveforms in 0.5 seconds; Seifert & Lubar, 1975). Sessions are conducted two or three times per week. Average amplitude of SMR, percentage of SMR, and percentage of SMR above threshold are physiological measures that have been used in order to monitor patient progress. However, the primary indicator of patient progress is reduction in the frequency of seizures.

Scientific examination of the role of SCPs in the emergence and reduction of epileptiform activity has been conducted primarily at the Institute of Medical Psychology and Behavioral Neurobiology at the University of Tuebingen in Germany. Kotchoubey et al. (1999b) define SCPs as "electroencephalographic phenomena lasting several hundred milliseconds or several seconds (i.e. slower than usual EEG rhythms)" (p. 281). An extensive body of research (presented in Rockstroh et al., 1989, as well as by Strehl, Chapter 20, this volume) indicates that negative SCP shifts are related to heightened excitability of underlying cortical areas, whereas positive SCP shifts may reflect inhibition of cortical regions. These authors have also noted that epileptic seizures are often preceded and accompanied by sustained, high-amplitude superficial negative potential shifts, and have postulated that frequency of seizures can be reduced via learning to control SCPs.

Similar to SMR research, initial SCP investigations demonstrated that humans could learn to control SCPs (Birbaumer, Elbert, Rockstroh, & Lutzenberger, 1981), that a "defect" in this ability was evident in patients with seizure disorders (Birbaumer et al., 1991), and that reduction in frequency of seizures would occur as patients learned to decrease negative SCPs and/or increase positive SCPs (Birbaumer et al., 1991). EEG recordings were obtained at C_z with linked ear reference. Treatment was conducted in three phases and incorporated daily training sessions (15–20 sessions), a "practice" phase (8 weeks), and a second training phase (10 sessions). Visual feedback was provided that showed the averaged EEG amplitude over 0.5 seconds. Primary dependent measures of interest were the number of trials in which patients produced negative SCP amplitude values and the number in which positive SCP values were produced.

Clinical Outcome Studies

Examination of the efficacy of EEG biofeedback in the treatment of seizure disorders has been conducted primarily via controlled, multiple-case studies. Studies of the SMR protocol have used extended pretreatment baseline periods (Sterman & Friar, 1972; Seifert & Lubar, 1975), noncontingent feedback (Finley, Smith, & Etherton, 1975), A-B-A designs with crossover (Sterman & Macdonald, 1978; Lubar & Bahler, 1976), and use of relaxation training in which EEG electrodes were attached (Tozzo, Elfner, & May, 1988) in order to control for certain nonspecific factors. In addition, Lantz and Sterman (1988) report the use of yoked non-contingent and waiting-list controls. Examinations of the SCP protocol have similarly employed extended pretreatment baseline periods (Kotchoubey, Busch, Strehl, & Birbaumer, 1999a), as well as extended "nonfeedback" practice phases (Kotchoubey et al., 1999b). In all of these studies, patients were maintained on antiseizure medications.

The primary evidence of efficacy in each of these studies was patient report of number of seizures. In addition, the ability of patients to demonstrate reduction in targeted electrophysiological measures was examined in order to assess the importance of neuronal self-regulation. As summarized by Sterman (2000), a total of 174 patients have participated in the reported SMR biofeedback studies, with 82% showing significant reduction in the number of seizures (by at least 30%) and 66% showing significant improvement on EEG measures. No relationship between anticonvulsant drug levels and effects of EEG biofeedback was evident.

Among the studies examining SCPs, two studies (Kotchoubey et al., 1999a, 1999b) appear noteworthy, in that both experimental designs incorporated an extended "no-training" period and one (Kotchoubey et al., 1999b) attempted to assess the importance of patient "expectancy" of treatment success in determining outcome. The total number of patients in these studies was 53, and both focal and multifocal seizures were treated.

In the Kotchoubey et al. (1999a) study, significant improvement in patient ability to produce the desired directional SCP shift was noted. Six-month follow-up analysis of frequency of seizures was conducted in 28 of the 34 patients. Nine patients demonstrated a significant decrease in their seizure rates (average decrease was 72%). Eleven others showed a tendency toward reduced frequency (average decrease was 19%). None showed an increase in seizures. In the Kotchoubey et al. (1999b) study, patients also demonstrated significant improvement in their ability to produce directional SCP shifts. In this study, six patients showed an average reduction of 62% in the number of seizures; five showed a mean reduction of 28% (eight patients showed no clear pattern of improvement). Examination of patient belief that treatment would be "useful" in controlling seizures revealed no difference in clinical response among patients who had high versus low expectancy of improvement.

Analysis of Efficacy

Collectively, the research on both SMR and SCP biofeedback is impressive, in that significant reductions in the number of seizures were reported by patients who exhibited disorders that were refractory to "bona fide" pharmacological treatments. In essence, this treatment has been primarily field-tested in the treatment of a subset of patients with epilepsy who were not treated successfully with medications developed for the control of seizure activity. Although the number of controlled group studies is quite limited, the use of A-B-A designs, extended baseline measures, and follow-up monitoring of symptom reduction make it difficult to dismiss the results as merely placebo effects.

According to Chambless and Hollon's (1998) classification system, both SMR and SCP biofeedback would appear to meet criteria for a determination of "probably efficacious." However, the medical risks associated with the development of research designs in which epileptic patients are denied active treatment, provided with a placebo treatment, or placed on a waiting list are substantial, and clearly are in violation of ethical standards. EEG research in this area has identified electrophysiological symptoms of epilepsy, developed EEG-based interventions to control the kind of neuronal hyperexcitability that causes seizure activity, clarified the neural pathways underlying the production of these neurotherapeutic changes, and demonstrated that the SMR and SCP biofeedback protocols result in significant clinical improvement in patients who have not been successfully treated by medications. An additional randomized study, in which patients whose epilepsy has proven refractory to medication therapy are given medication maintenance or medication maintenance plus biofeedback, would appear needed in order to establish these biofeedback applications as "efficacious and specific." As has been done in prior studies, monitoring of targeted electrophysiological indicators (i.e., SMR, SCPs) in both groups is essential.

ATTENTION-DEFICIT/HYPERACTIVITY DISORDER

Considerable scientific interest has centered on examination of treatment for ADHD. DSM-IV (American Psychiatric Association, 1994) defines this disorder in terms of behavioral symptoms of inattention with or without evidence of hyperactivity–impulsivity. Prevalence is estimated to be approximately 3–5% of the U.S. population, although there is considerable variability in the occurrence of this disorder in other countries (Barkley, 1998). As reviewed by Barkley (1998), the most common type of treatment has been stimulant therapy (e.g., Ritalin, Concerta, Adderall, and Metadate). Antidepressant, antihypertensive, and antiseizure medications have also been utilized (e.g., Tofranil, Norpramin, Wellbutrin, Catapres, and Depakote). Other types of treatment include parent counseling (Anastopoulos, Smith, & Wien, 1998), social skills training (Pelham, Wheeler, & Chronis, 1998) and various types of cognitive therapies (Barkley, 1998).

Although Swanson, McBurnett, Christian, and Wigel (1995) summarized a number of well-controlled studies demonstrating short-term efficacy of stimulants for the core symptoms of ADHD, it is generally accepted that these medications provide no enduring change in the core symptoms. Moreover, a significant percentage of patients develop adverse side effects (approximately 50%; Barkley, 1998), and a substantial number fail to respond to stimulant therapy (20–40%; Barkley, 1998). In addition, as noted by the National Institutes of Health (1998), there is little evidence that cognitive therapies are efficacious, and although parent counseling and social skills training were included in a well-controlled, multicenter study examining treatments for ADHD (MTA Cooperative Group, 1999), there was no evidence that these types of treatment provided any significant clinical gains in the treatment of the core symptoms of ADHD beyond that provided by stimulant therapy. The absence of clinical improvement in a sizable percentage of patients with ADHD, the presence of adverse side effects, the potential medical risks associated with chronic use of any medication, the lack of enduring clinical change, and concerns about substance abuse among patients maintained on stimulant medication have all fostered the development of EEG-based treatments for ADHD.

Treatment Protocols

Therapeutic protocols for use in the treatment of ADHD are based on the clinical research of Lubar and his colleagues (e.g. Lubar & Shouse, 1976; Lubar & Lubar, 1984; Mann, Lubar, Zimmerman, Miller, & Muenchen, 1992; Lubar, Swartwood, Swartwood, & O'Donnell, 1995). Two primary protocols have emerged: SMR (12- to 15-Hz) enhancement over the rolandic cortex (C_3, C_4, C_z), and theta (4- to 8-Hz) suppression/beta (16- to 20-Hz) enhancement over midline regions (F_{cz}; P_{cz}; C_z). Both monopolar and bipolar montages are used, with ear reference(s). Sessions are conducted with eyes open. Both auditory feedback and visual feedback are provided. Positive feedback is provided when a patient produces desired EEG behaviors (either SMR or beta) above a specified microvolt threshold), while suppressing EEG (theta) or EMG (typically derived from eye, facial, or gross muscle movements) below specified microvolt thresholds. Since a detailed presentation of the history, neurological foundations, and therapeutic protocols for neurotherapeutic treatment of patients with ADHD is provided by Lubar in Chapter 18 of this book, this chapter focuses primarily on an evaluation of treatment efficacy.

Clinical Outcome Studies

Whereas A-B-A designs were utilized in the initial demonstration studies (Shouse & Lubar, 1979), and a number of multicase studies have been reported (e.g., Alhambra, Fowler, & Alhambra, 1995; Kaiser & Othner, Thompson & Thompson, 1998), controlled group studies supporting the use of EEG biofeedback in the treatment of ADHD have incorporated a waiting-list control group (Linden, Habib, & Radojevic, 1996) and "active treatment" control group comparisons (Rossiter & LaVaque, 1995; Monastra, Monastra, & George, 2002).

Linden et al. (1996) randomly assigned 18 children/adolescents (diagnosed with either ADHD or a learning disorder) to either a theta suppression/beta enhancement treatment (40 sessions, twice per week) or a waiting-list control group. No medications were used in the treatment of any of the participants. Statistical analysis of results indicated significant improvement in scores on a test of intelligence, and significant reduction in the frequency of inattentive behaviors, in the group treated with EEG biofeedback.

Rossiter and LaVaque (1995) conducted a study of 46 children/adolescents diagnosed with ADHD. Twenty-three of the patients received stimulant therapy, 18 received EEG biofeedback, and 5 received EEG biofeedback plus stimulant therapy. Assignment to groups was not randomized. EEG treatment protocols included both SMR and theta suppression/beta enhancement. Twenty sessions were conducted prior to posttreatment data collection. Analysis of results indicated no difference between patients treated with stimulant therapy and those receiving EEG biofeedback on behavioral or attentional measures (continuous-performance test).

We (Monastra et al., 2002) recently completed a study in which 100 patients with ADHD were treated in a clinic that provides a comprehensive range of treatments to patients with attentional disorders. The study incorporated a dismantling design in which all patients received the following active treatments: a carefully titrated dose of stimulant therapy, academic support in school via an individual education plan or a 504 accommodation plan, and parent training (derived from the model presented by Anastopoulos et al., 1998). Based on parental preference, 51 of the participants also received EEG biofeedback (theta suppression/beta enhancement); the other 49 did not. Although random assignment was not used in this clinical field study, analysis of pretreatment measures indicated that the groups were equivalent on behavioral, attentional, and electrophysiological measures, as well as on a variety of parental demographic characteristics. EEG biofeedback was continued until a patient demonstrated "normalization" of cortical arousal at C_z, based on a published database (Monastra et al., 1999; Monastra, Lubar, & Linden, 2001). The average number of sessions needed to achieve this training goal was 44.

One year after the initial evaluation, each patient was reassessed on behavioral, attentional (continuous-performance test), and electrophysiological measures (QEEG scanning process; Monastra et al., 1999). Two posttreatment assessments were conducted. One evaluation was conducted while patients were still being treated with stimulant therapy; the other session was conducted after a 1-week medication-free "washout" period. Statistical analysis indicated significant improvements on behavioral and attentional measures in both the group receiving comprehensive clinical care (CCC) and the group receiving CCC plus EEG biofeedback provided that medication was being administered. Only the group receiving EEG biofeedback showed improvement on EEG measures. When tested after the 1-week medication-free period, only patients treated with EEG biofeedback maintained improvements on behavioral, attentional, and EEG measures. All of the patients receiving CCC without EEG biofeedback relapsed, based on behavioral rating scales (home, school) and continuous-performance test results.

Analysis of Efficacy

Studies examining the effects of EEG biofeedback have consistently shown positive outcomes on a variety of behavioral, intellectual, academic, attentional, and electrophysiological measures. Well-defined treatment protocols, derived from research that has identified specific neurological pathways underlying the observed behavioral and cognitive symptoms, are utilized. Multiple-Clinical case studies, controlled case studies (A-B-A design), and controlled group studies using waiting-list and active treatment comparisons have been reported.

Based on Chambless and Hollon's (1998) criteria, both SMR protocols and theta suppression/beta enhancement protocols are considered to be at least "probably efficacious," since both protocols have been shown to be better than no treatment or a waiting-list control. In addition, both the Rossiter and LaVaque (1995) and the Monastra et al. (2002) studies demonstrate the efficacy of EEG biofeedback compared to the most commonly used type of active treatment for this disorder (stimulant therapy). Whereas the lack of random assignment of participants to groups in the Rossiter and LaVaque (1995) study makes it difficult to dismiss nonspecific factors, the Monastra et al. (2002) study's use of a medication-free washout period and of behavioral ratings from 100 teachers (who were unaffiliated with the study site and would not be expected to be positively biased to what has been reported to be an "experimental" treatment), as well as their analysis of computer-scored measures of attention and electrophysiological arousal, makes it difficult to dismiss their findings as a function of nonspecific factors.

Nevertheless, it seems likely that an additional study utilizing random assignment to EEG biofeedback and active treatment (e.g., stimulant therapy) groups will be needed before this type of treatment is considered "efficacious and specific" for the treatment of ADHD. Since patients with ADHD are legally entitled to school-based interventions (e.g., individual education plans, 504 accommodation plans), and other types of psychoeducational treatments are commonly provided in the course of biofeedback treatment (e.g., parent counseling), it would appear that efficacy studies need to incorporate experimental designs that control for these community-based interventions. The use of placebos or "sham" treatments is not recommended, due to ethical issues related to denying patients the best proven diagnostic and therapeutic methods. In studies of ADHD, active treatments with at least short-term efficacy have been identified and would appear to be mandatory for members of the control groups, according to standards developed by the World Medical Association (1997).

PSYCHOACTIVE SUBSTANCE ABUSE AND DEPENDENCE

Systematic reviews of the scientific literature (e.g., APA Task Force on Promotion and Dissemination of Psychological Procedures, 1995; Carroll, 1996; McCrady, 2000) have examined dozens of psychological and psychosocial treatments for the various types of psychoactive substance abuse and dependence, yet few of these treatments have met standards for efficacy for even a minimal 6-month follow-up period. As recently as 1995, the APA concluded that no psychological treatment for alcohol abuse or dependence was "efficacious." Although subsequent reviews have indicated that a limited number of brief interventions and relapse prevention interventions appear "efficacious" for alcohol abuse/dependence (McCrady, 2000), as well as other psychoactive substance use disorders (e.g., those related to nicotine, cocaine, and cannabis use; Carroll, 1996), these reviews utilize a narrow definition of treatment "success" (e.g., reducing the frequency and severity of relapse during a 6-month follow-up) rather than sustained remission of symptoms. EEG biofeedback has not been considered to be among the treatments considered "efficacious" by these reviewers.

Clinical research examining the efficacy of EEG biofeedback has primarily focused on the treatment of alcoholism (Twemlow & Bowen, 1976, 1977; Peniston & Kulkosky, 1989, 1990; Schneider et al., 1993). Less attention has been given to studies of EEG biofeedback in the treatment of other psychoactive substance use disorders (e.g., those related to cannabis and cocaine; Goslinga, 1975). Similar to other clinical applications, in which treatment protocols are not directly derived from research delineating the electrophysiological characteristics of psychopathology or the neurological pathways underlying symptom development and maintenance, EEG-based treatments for psychoactive substance abuse and dependence have not been demonstrated to be as successful as protocols developed for the treatment of other medical or psychiatric conditions (e.g., seizure disorders, ADHD).

Treatment Protocols

Two types of EEG biofeedback treatment for alcoholism and for cannabis and cocaine use disorders have been reported. The first type of treatment seeks to enhance production of both alpha (8–13 Hz) and theta (4–8 Hz). Recordings are obtained at O_1 and/or O_2, with ear reference(s). EEG outcome measures have included alpha amplitude, theta amplitude, and the percentage of time that alpha and theta exceed threshold values. This EEG protocol is based on the findings of Green, Green, and Walters (1974), who observed that skilled meditators produced high amplitudes of alpha and theta (followed by a decline in alpha amplitude) during meditative states. They further noted that showing individuals how to increase production of occipital alpha and theta led to a state of deep relaxation. The prophylactic effect of this type of treatment in facilitating abstinence in alcoholism has been the focus of multiple uncontrolled and controlled studies.

The other type of EEG biofeedback treatment protocol is derived from the efforts of Birbaumer et al. (1981), who examined SCPs. In this type of treatment, EEG activity is measured at C_z (ear references). Treatment includes periods in which patients attempts to decrease negative SCPs and/or increase positive SCPs. Patient success in producing periods of decreased negativity and increased positivity on demand is the primary outcome measure. This procedure has been shown to be helpful in reducing the frequency of seizures in epileptic patients (e.g., Birbaumer et al., 1991), as well as in promoting other types of clinical improvements (see review by Strehl, Chapter 20, this volume). The beneficial effects of teaching alcoholic individuals to control SCPs were initially reported by Schneider et al. (1993).

Clinical Outcome Studies

A number of clinical case studies have shown a variety of positive outcomes following use of alpha/theta enhancement protocols. These improvements include increase of verbal expressiveness in psychotherapy (Goslinga, 1975), increased "religiousness" (Twemlow & Bowen,

1977), improved ability to tolerate stress and a decline in craving for alcohol (Fahrion, Walters, Coyne, & Allen, 1992), and reduction in reports of depression and other psychiatric symptoms (Saxby & Peniston, 1995). In addition, the 21-month follow-up data reported by Saxby and Peniston (1995) indicated that 13 of 14 patients treated with a combination of temperature and alpha/theta biofeedback sustained their abstinence from alcohol. Similarly encouraging reports of sustained remission of alcohol use was reported by Schneider et al. (1993) following an SCP protocol. Six of seven patients, who were evaluated 4 months after hospitalization for alcohol dependence, were able to demonstrate control over SCPs. None of the six had relapsed. The patient who was unable to control SCPs had resumed use of alcohol.

Despite a variety of positive outcomes reported in case studies, the controlled group outcome studies that have been published have not provided strong support for the efficacy of EEG biofeedback. These studies have examined what has been termed the "Peniston protocol" (Peniston & Kulkosky, 1989). This protocol combines several different types of treatment, including temperature biofeedback "pretraining" (at least five sessions) and the use of a trance induction script that is read prior to the beginning of sessions. Following a pretreatment phase, patients receive a series of EEG biofeedback sessions to increase alpha/theta at O_1, typically with ear references. The number of sessions has ranged from 15 to 30 in reported studies. Sessions are conducted with eyes closed. One tone is heard when the patient produces amplitudes of alpha above a certain microvolt threshold; another tone sounds when theta amplitudes exceed a specified threshold. Finally, once the patient is in a "relaxed state" a therapy session is conducted in which the contents of spontaneously occurring images are discussed, and the anxiety associated with these images is "extinguished" via a type of flooding therapy.

The Peniston protocol was investigated in a randomized, controlled study in which 20 males with chronic alcoholism, who had been unable to develop sustained remission of alcohol consumption, were assigned to one of two treatment groups (Peniston & Kulkosky, 1989). One group received the traditional type of alcoholism treatment provided at a Veterans Adminstration Hospital at that time. The other group received temperature biofeedback, followed by 15 sessions of alpha/theta biofeedback lasting 30 minutes each. A nonalcoholic control group ($n = 10$) was used in assessing the results of blood tests that examined levels of beta-endorphins (an indicator of stress). The biofeedback group demonstrated a significant increase in the percentage of time above threshold for both alpha and theta, as well as increased alpha amplitudes. Psychological measures showed decreased scores on the Beck Depression Inventory among patients treated with biofeedback. Blood analysis showed increased beta-endorphins in the patients who did not receive biofeedback. Abstinence (defined as alcohol-free periods of at least 6 days) was higher in the biofeedback group.

Because the Peniston protocol incorporates a variety of treatment strategies, several controlled studies have been conducted in order to examine whether alpha/theta biofeedback was necessary in order to achieve positive clinical outcomes (e.g., a state of relaxation). Taub, Steiner, Smith, Weingarten, and Walton (1994) conducted a randomized, controlled study in which Transcendental Meditation and EMG biofeedback were compared to a "sham" neurotherapy (cranial electrical stimulation). Relapse prevention was the primary dependent measure. The results of this study indicated that both of the active treatments were effective in achieving a state of relaxation and promoting prevention of relapse (compared to the "sham" treatment control), leading the authors to question whether EEG biofeedback was a necessary treatment.

Moore and Trudeau (1998) randomly assigned participants to either alpha feedback, alpha/theta feedback, or EMG feedback (designed to promote suppression of 24- to 30-Hz activity recorded from EEG sensors at occipital sites). Participants were unaware of the type of feedback that they were receiving. Identical tones were used as feedback. Outcome measures indicated that brain wave parameters of deeply relaxed states occurred in both the EMG and alpha/theta groups, and that all three types of feedback yielded subjective reports of relaxation and imagery. Consequently, these authors also questioned whether alpha/theta training was essential to achieving a state of relaxation.

Analysis of Efficacy

Although a number of clinical case studies provide data to suggest that alpha/theta and SCP biofeedback can provide benefits for patients with substance use disorders, the absence of multiple, well-controlled studies demonstrating the necessity of EEG biofeedback in the treatment process makes it difficult to determine the efficacy of these applications. In addition, as noted by Graap and Friedes (1998), the Peniston protocol appears to combine a number of interventions (EMG biofeedback trance induction, flooding, and EEG biofeedback). This precludes a conclusion that the EEG biofeedback protocol is "efficacious and specific."

At this time, the scientific literature contains detailed descriptions of two protocols that utilize EEG biofeedback. However, the lack of controlled studies from independent teams, the reports of researchers who have observed that EEG treatment protocols do not provide benefit beyond that noted for EMG biofeedback or other active treatments, and the absence of research designs that permit examination of the benefits of the various treatment components incorporated in the Peniston protocol mean that it is most appropriate to term this application as "possibly efficacious," according to Chambless and Hollon's (1998) criteria. Additional RCTs, in which specific EEG biofeedback treatment components are examined in clinical studies that provide active treatments to the control group(s) (e.g., medical and nutritional interventions, relaxation training, systematic desensitization, education, counseling in relapse prevention, Alcoholics Anonymous, etc.) are needed. In addition, continued research efforts to define the electrophysiological characteristics of patients with psychoactive substance use disorders seems necessary in order to develop efficacious treatment protocols.

MOOD DISORDERS

As noted in the DSM-IV (American Psychiatric Association, 1994), mood disorders are among the most common types of psychiatric disorders in adults, causing significant adverse effects on vocational and social functioning. These conditions are frequently characterized by prolonged periods of depressed mood, loss of interest and diminished pleasure in vocational and avocational activities, and social withdrawal. Due to the marked functional impairment associated with these disorders, a variety of pharmacological and psychological treatments have been developed. Among the psychological treatments, cognitive therapy (Beck, Rush, Shaw, & Emery, 1979), behavior therapy (Lewinsohn, 1974), and interpersonal psychotherapy (Klerman, Weissman, Rounsaville, & Chevron, 1984) have been sufficiently examined in well-controlled group studies that they are considered to be efficacious for the treatment of depression (DeRubeis & Crits-Christoph, 1998).

The electrophysiological correlates of depressive symptoms have been investigated by Davidson (1995) and his colleagues. Davidson (1995) postulates that the right frontal lobe is essential for the organization and production of negative emotion and avoidance behaviors, and that the left frontal lobe is needed for the organization and production of positive affect and approach behavior. In their model, relative "deactivation" of the left frontal cortex (evidenced by the presence of a greater amount of power in 8- to 12-Hz "alpha" frequencies recorded at F_3 than at F_4) was considered likely to be associated with a preponderance of negative affective states.

Based on their review of existent literature on frontal lobe functioning, Davidson and his colleagues proposed that individuals who display a preponderance of negative affect are more likely to exhibit "asymmetry" in the activation of the frontal lobes. A neurometric termed the "asymmetry score" was developed. As defined by Davidson (1995), this score is the difference in alpha power recorded at F_3 and F_4 (referenced to C_z). Two mathematical formulas have been presented, wherein R equals the alpha power at F_4, and L equals the alpha power at F_3:

$$A_1 = \log R - \log L$$
$$A_2 = R - L/R + L$$

It was hypothesized that higher asymmetry scores are associated with positive affect, and lower scores with negative affect. Consistent with this model, Tomarken, Davidson, and Henriques (1990) demonstrated that individuals' affective responses to emotionally "positive" and "negative" film clips could be predicted from their asymmetry scores; Sobotka, Davidson, and Senulis (1992) showed change in asymmetry scores in response to reward and punishment; and Ekman, Davidson, and Friesen (1990) illustrated the association between asymmetry scores and facial expressions of emotions.

Examination of Davidson's (1995) asymmetry model in clinical populations has been reported by Henriques and Davidson (1990, 1991) and Gotlib, Ranganath, and Rosenfeld (1998). As anticipated, Henriques and Davidson (1990) reported lower asymmetry scores in depressed patients (compared to never-depressed persons); Henriques and Davidson (1991) found relative hypoactivation of the left frontal lobe in previously depressed patients (vs. never-depressed persons); and Gotlib et al. (1998) replicated both of these studies, finding relative hypoactivation in both currently depressed and previously depressed patients. This body of research serves as the foundation for the studies examining the efficacy of efforts to treat depression via modification of frontal asymmetry.

Treatment Protocols

Although the research of Davidson and his colleagues serves as the foundation for EEG biofeedback treatments for mood disorders, Rosenfeld and his associates are primarily responsible for the development of a potentially efficacious treatment protocol. Following their initial demonstration that nondepressed individuals could learn to increase asymmetry scores (Rosenfeld, Cha, Blair, & Gotlib, 1995), Rosenfeld and his colleagues observed the relationship between A_2 scores and affect during therapy sessions with depressed patients (Rosenfeld, Baehr, Baehr, Gotlib, & Ranganath (1996). They subsequently developed a biofeedback protocol, which has now been tested in several clinical case studies (Baehr, Rosenfeld, & Baehr, 1997; Earnest, 1999).

Similar to the Peniston protocol (Peniston & Kulkosky, 1989), the EEG biofeedback protocol developed by Rosenfeld and his colleagues begins with a type of relaxation therapy. As described by Rosenfeld (2000), patients learn to breathe diaphragmatically for 15–30 minutes (warming their hands to a 95° F criterion). During the EEG biofeedback, electrophysiological activity is recorded at F_3 and F_4 (C_z reference). A patient receives auditory feedback (a clarinet tone) for increasing the A_2 value $(F_4 - F_3)/(F_4 + F_3)$. When the value exceeds zero, the tone sounds. Pitch varies with the A_2 value, increasing as the value of A_2 increases. Patients are instructed to try to increase the pitch of the tone. Following the biofeedback portion of the session, patients participate in a psychotherapy session. Sessions are conducted twice per week. The number of sessions ranges from 30 to 60 sessions. The primary dependent measure is the asymmetry index, which is compared to changes in self-report of depression on an "objective" measure (e.g., the Depression scale of the MMPI).

Clinical Outcome Studies

Although the application of EEG biofeedback for the treatment of mood disorders proceeds from electrophysiological studies that associate frontal alpha asymmetry with negative affective states (e.g., depression), treatment protocols derived from these findings have only been recently developed and field-tested. To date, only case studies have been published. Baehr et al. (1997) reported an increase in the A_2 score, a decrease in the Depression scale of the MMPI, and clinical improvement in two depressed adult patients. In addition, one of the patients was able to discontinue pharmacological treatment for depression (Paxil) and maintain clinical improvement. Earnest (1999) replicated Baehr et al.'s (1997) study, demonstrating EEG change and clinical improvement in an adolescent diagnosed with depression.

Analysis of Efficacy

As summarized by Rosenfeld (2000, pp. 11–12), investigators seeking to examine the application of EEG biofeedback in the treatment of mood disorders "have a viable EEG protocol in need of further support via controlled studies." Based on Chambless and Hollon's (1998) criteria, this protocol lacks sufficient evidence to be judged as "possibly efficacious" at this time (empirical support consists only of uncontrolled case studies). Like the Peniston protocol, Rosenfeld's treatment for depression incorporates several types of clinical interventions. Consequently, experimental designs developed to test this treatment will need to examine the individual and combined effects of these various treatment components.

Patients diagnosed with depression are at significant risk for suicide if other treatments (e.g., antidepressant medications) are not provided during the experimental process. Given these considerations, EEG biofeedback should be examined in studies in which all participants are provided active treatment(s) (e.g., antidepressant medications and/or interpersonal and behavioral therapies) that have been shown to be efficacious. As noted in the Baehr et al. (1997), one of the more compelling dependent measures would be the demonstration of a reduction or elimination of medication use following successful biofeedback treatment.

SCHIZOPHRENIA

Schizophrenia is an enduring psychiatric disorder that significantly impairs psychosocial functioning. Psychological treatments for schizophrenia have primarily consisted of social skills training and family psychoeducational training. Both of these approaches are intended to teach interpersonal problem-solving skills, assist the patient in addressing sources of conflict and stress, and prevent relapse. As reviewed by DeRubeis and Crits-Christoph (1998), social skills training has typically been studied in combination with antipsychotic medications, using active treatment comparison groups. They conclude that these approaches appear "possibly efficacious," however, the effects have not been strong and robust. Similarly, Baucom et al. (1998) note that couple and family interventions appear to benefit schizophrenic patients; however, these treatments have not been demonstrated to be "efficacious and specific."

EEG biofeedback treatment of schizophrenia has also proceeded from a perspective that stress and anxiety may be significant factors in precipitating psychotic episodes (Gruzelier, 2000). Within this context, it is hypothesized that the failure of patients to regulate the cortical excitability triggered by such stressful events could be contributing to relapse. Hence efforts to promote the development of self-regulation of cortical excitability are considered to be a potentially useful application of EEG biofeedback.

Treatment Protocols

Although prior EEG research has provided evidence that schizophrenic patients consistently demonstrate an excess of theta that occurs in isolation, as well as in conjunction with excess beta activity (Itil, 1977; Morihisa, Duffy, & Wyatt, 1983; Sponheim, Clementz, Iacono, & Beiser, 1994), there are no published reports of the application of theta or beta suppression paradigms. However, two EEG biofeedback protocols for treating patients with schizophrenia have been published during the past decade. Both have been derived from the work of Birbaumer and his colleagues (e.g., Birbaumer et al., 1981), who have investigated the impact of excessive cortical excitability on various medical and psychiatric disorders. One treatment protocol (Schneider et al., 1992) attempts to teach regulation of SCPs to schizophrenic patients. The other protocol (Gruzelier et al., 1999) identified two patterns of lateral asymmetry in the production of negative SCPs among such patients. This treatment approach seeks to improve clinical symptoms by changing the pattern of cortical activity from the dominant to the nondominant hemisphere.

Gruzelier et al. (1999) described an adaptation of the SCP protocol, focusing on the symmetry of the distribution of negative SCPs. They noted that certain patients displayed a dominance of negative SCPs in the left hemisphere (at F_3 and C_3), compared to right frontal (F_4) and central (C_4) locations. These patients tended to have an active schizophrenic syndrome, characterized by "physical and mental overactivity" and delusions. Other patients showed the opposite pattern (R > L). They tended to display social withdrawal, motor retardation, and suppressed affect. In this treatment protocol, patients are taught to shift patterns of dominance. Those patients who show L > R dominance are taught to produce more negativity in the right hemisphere. Patients exhibiting R > L dominance are given feedback intended to promote increased negativity in the left hemisphere.

In the Gruzelier et al. (1999) protocol, patients are instructed to move a rocket ship up or down. Upward movements occur when a patient is able to produce a shift in dominance toward the left hemisphere; downward movements occur when the patient is able to produce a dominance shift toward the right hemisphere. Similar to the standard SCP protocol, all patients are cued to produced shifts to the left, as well as to the right. Multiple 8-second trials are administered, during which visual stimuli are displayed. EEG recordings are obtained at C_3 and C_4 with ear reference. Patients receive a small monetary reward for correct directional shifts. The number of correct shifts, and changes in psychiatric status, are the primary dependent measures.

Clinical Outcome Studies

Two studies are reported in the literature. Schneider et al. (1992) examined the ability of schizophrenic patients to learn regulation of SCPs and the effects of this skill acquisition on primary symptoms of schizophrenia. Twelve patients aged 20–30, who had been diagnosed with schizophrenia for an average of 3 years, hospitalized on 1–8 occasions, and treated with antipsychotic medications, were given 20 daily sessions. Control subjects (5 adults without psychiatric disorder) were also examined. The standard SCP protocol was used.

The control subjects learned to differentiate positive and negative SCPs within five sessions. The patients demonstrated learning during certain portions of sessions 1–5; however, they showed no evidence of learning during trials 6–17. Unexpectedly, they began to demonstrate ability to differentiate positive and negative potentials during sessions 18 to 20. Despite learning this differentiation during the latter sessions, no evidence of clinical improvement was noted.

Gruzelier et al. (1999) examined the effect of training shifts in lateral dominance of negative SCPs on core symptoms of schizophrenia. Twenty-four patients (mean age = 34.2 years), diagnosed with schizophrenia according to DSM-IV criteria, initially agreed to participate in the study. Subsequently, 4 of these patients refused to continue in the project, and 4 others withdrew after 1–2 sessions. The 16 remaining patients (11 males, 5 females) participated in at least 5 sessions (10 patients completed all 10 sessions). Unlike the standard SCP protocol, the asymmetry in distribution of negative SCPs (i.e., C_3 vs. C_4) was monitored. Patients were instructed to move the on-screen rocket up or down, in response to left- or right-hemispheric shifts. During each of the 10 sessions, patients participated in 60 training trials lasting 8 seconds each. The trials were administered in blocks of 20, with rests given between blocks and after every 5th trial.

The results of this study demonstrated that schizophrenic patients were able to learn interhemispheric control of negative SCPs. Those who initially showed L > R asymmetry learned to produce larger rightward than leftward shifts. Similarly, those who displayed R > L asymmetry showed larger leftward than rightward shifts. However, there was no significant relationship between learning to change asymmetry and the severity of global symptoms of schizophrenia (obtained from independent psychiatrist ratings on the Schizophrenia Syndrome Scale).

Analysis of Efficacy

This review of EEG biofeedback applications in the treatment of schizophrenia reveals the presence of two well-defined treatment protocols. However, neither has been shown to result in clinical improvement in schizophrenic patients. In one study, patients did not appear able to learn regulation of SCPs. In the other, the acquisition of an ability to shift lateralization of negative SCPs did not result in a change in psychiatric status. Consequently, according to Chambless and Hollon's (1998) criteria, these applications cannot be considered "possibly efficacious" at this time.

Despite the failure of these initial investigations to demonstrate clinical improvement in patients with this highly treatment-resistant disorder, the ability of patients to recognize and shift patterns of asymmetry of negative SCPs may prove clinically useful. In the study reported by Gruzelier et al. (1999), the number of sessions was approximately 25% of the number needed to produce clinical change in patients diagnosed with other psychiatric symptoms (e.g., ADHD, mood disorders). Consequently, before efforts to teach schizophrenic patients how to regulate the lateral distribution of SCPs are discontinued, controlled clinical studies in which the number of sessions more nearly matches those found necessary in the treatment of other neuropsychiatric disorders seem warranted. In addition, given the evidence associating schizophrenia and excess theta and/or beta output, controlled clinical studies examining theta suppression or "suppress all" paradigms may be useful in identifying self-regulatory strategies to reduce schizophrenic symptoms.

TRAUMATIC BRAIN INJURY

One of the more complex applications of EEG biofeedback has been the treatment of individuals who are recovering from TBI. Patients with TBI routinely suffer from a combination of attentional, cognitive, afffective, and behavioral symptoms. As summarized by Thatcher (2000), there is loss of consciousness, followed by impairments of memory, attention, and concentration. There is also loss of control over affective regulation, and periods of depression, anxiety, and anger are common. There can also be dramatic changes in personality and reduction in interpersonal sensitivity. However, unlike other medical and psychiatric disorders, TBI is associated with no "signature" EEG pattern (as in epileptiform activity) and no localized area in which EEG abnormalities are consistently observable (as in ADHD). Rather, patients with TBI are evaluated following traumatic events that have affected multiple cortical and subcortical regions. Identifying the specific affected regions via QEEG examination, and developing EEG biofeedback protocols to treat the affected regions, constitute the foundation of this application.

Treatment Protocols

Because of the variability and multiplicity of brain regions affected by TBI, protocols for use in clinical applications require the availability of comprehensive, integrative QEEG databases that permit determination of power, coherence, and phase, as advocated by Thatcher (1998, 1999). In this way, the impact of the varying sources of physical trauma on brain functioning can be specified for individual patients, and an individualized treatment protocol can be developed.

Thatcher (2000) proposes a model in which QEEG measures are obtained from multiple cortical locations prior to treatment. Subsequently, the patient's QEEG data are compared to a normative EEG database, and z-scores are computed for such variables as power, coherence, and phase. Based on this analysis, the therapist targets those cortical regions in which the most deviant results are noted. At a minimum, amplitude, phase and coherence are monitored. Primary emphasis is placed on treating regions that show the greatest degree of deviance on the coherence measure, because EEG coherence appears to be the most sensitive measure of TBI (Thatcher, Walker, Gerson, & Geisler, 1989). Deviations of amplitude are also treated. Both monopolar and bipolar montages are used with ear reference(s). Visual and auditory feedback are provided based on patient achievement of targeted EEG parameters. Sessions include 20–45 minutes of active feedback. The number of sessions is variable, with clinical improvement reported in as few as 10 sessions (Hoffman, Stockdale, & VanEgren, 1996) and as many as 40 sessions (Hoffman, Stockdale, & Hicks, 1995).

Clinical Outcome Studies

To date, no studies have systematically examined EEG biofeedback treatment for TBI via controlled group experimental designs. The published studies primarily consist of case studies in which multiple dependent measures are obtained pre- and posttreatment. Of the uncontrolled case studies that have been reported (e.g., Ayers, 1987; Hoffman et al., 1995; Ham & Packard, 1996), the investigation conducted by Hoffman and his colleagues constitutes the most comprehensive case study report.

Hoffman et al. (1995) used a QEEG-based therapy to treat 14 patients with TBI. Self-report and neuropsychological test results constituted the dependent measures. Individualized EEG biofeedback was provided, depending on the affected regions and a comparison of QEEG results with a reference database. Self-report of improvement and/or enhanced performance on neuropsychological measures were found in approximately 60% of patients following 40 biofeedback sessions. Significant normalization of the QEEG was also reported.

Analysis of Efficacy

The absence of a single controlled group study precludes a conclusion that EEG biofeedback has been shown to be even "possibly efficacious" for the treatment of TBI at this time. However, the treatment protocol described by Thatcher (2000) warrants systematic evaluation. At present, there is case study support for this treatment approach. Controlled studies, in which the recovery of patients with TBI who receive standard medical care is compared to others who receive EEG biofeedback in addition to this type of care, are needed. In the development of these research designs, random assignment to group and demonstrated equivalency of treated groups is essential. The use of a no-treatment control group would clearly violate ethical considerations, because ongoing medical care is necessary in the clinical management of these patients. However, the use of a "sham" feedback condition may be justifiable, as there is no generally accepted method of treatment that has been shown to be efficacious in the treatment of TBI. An alternate strategy to control for nonspecific factors associated with the use of EEG biofeedback could include the monitoring of EEG variables as participants are receiving another type of cognitive treatment (e.g., Captain's Log; Sanford, Brown, & Turner, 1996).

OTHER CLINICAL APPLICATIONS

The topics of the preceding sections do not constitute the only clinical applications of EEG biofeedback. Neurotherapy to increase SMR amplitude over the rolandic cortex has been associated with improved scores on tests of intelligence in children diagnosed with learning disabilities (e.g., Tansey, 1984), with reduction of simple motor tics and multiple motor and vocal tics associated with Tourette's disorder (Tansey, 1986), and with recovery from chronic fatigue syndrome (James & Folen, 1996). Photic stimulation followed by theta suppression and beta enhancement over sensorimotor and speech areas was used by Rozelle and Budzynski (1995) to treat functional impairments displayed by a patient recovering from a cardiovascular accident. Alpha training at P_4 was used by Tyson (1996) to "desensitize" women to infants' crying. Training in self-regulation of SCPs was used by Siniatchkin et al. (2000) to treat children suffering from migraine headaches. These and other specific clinical applications have not been extensively reviewed in this chapter, because of the lack of controlled group studies or the absence of published reports by multiple research centers.

A PERSPECTIVE ON THE FUTURE OF EEG BIOFEEDBACK

As I reflect on the future of EEG biofeedback, I am appreciative of the scientific progress that has occurred in this field during the past 40 years. In contrast to the status of applied psychophysiology circa 1965, current clinical researchers and practitioners are able to incorporate the knowledge gleaned from scientific advances in the fields of neuroanatomy, neurophysiology, neurochemistry, and computer science, and can utilize highly sensitive and reliable instrumentation for assessing and treating patients. For this, we owe the pioneers in applied psychophysiology our gratitude. Based on their efforts, we can proceed to investigate the efficacy of well-defined QEEG-based protocols for the assessment and treatment of a variety of psychiatric and medical disorders. Although critical examination of the scientific literature clearly indicates that additional controlled clinical studies are required in order to demonstrate that EEG biofeedback is an efficacious and specific treatment for any medical or psychiatric condition, it seems important to recognize that the need for additional validation studies is no greater for EEG biofeedback than it is for most other types of treatment currently used in psychotherapy.

Kazdin and Weisz (1998) have emphasized this point in their review of psychological treatments for psychiatric disorders of childhood and adolescence. While supporting the scientific view that mental health professionals need to identify and use effective treatment protocols, they acknowledge "that the vast majority of the well over 200 treatments for use with children and adolescents have not been investigated" (p. 31). Furthermore, they state that "as a general principle, there would probably be widespread agreement that applying treatments with some evidence in their behalf is to be preferred, even if all of the criteria are not met for a fairly well-established (e.g., possibly efficacious) or very well-established (e.g., efficacious) treatment" (p. 31). They conclude that "although it may be worth drawing distinctions between possibly efficacious and efficacious treatments, certainly the sharper contrast is between those treatments that have no evidence on their behalf and those that do" (p. 31).

My review of the literature reveals that EEG biofeedback meets scientific criteria to be considered at least "probably efficacious" in the treatment of generalized anxiety disorder, seizure disorders, and ADHD, and "possibly efficacious" in the treatment of specific phobias, PTSD, and psychoactive substance abuse/dependence. In addition, empirical findings support continued examination of this type of treatment in other applications (e.g., mood disorders, learning disorders, TBI, and schizophrenia). Similar to the type of clinical research that was conducted in order to identify the essential components of other forms of behavioral therapy, EEG biofeedback research is at a stage of development in which these types of investigations can be meaningfully conducted within a broad spectrum of clinical applications. As was needed in the refinement of other forms of behavioral therapy, the identification of the essential treatment components of specific EEG biofeedback applications and the development of treatment paradigms that may provide more rapid and substantial clinical response will require systematic analysis of well-defined treatment protocols. The availability of QEEG databases provides clinical researchers with a process both to guide the development of treatment protocols, and to monitor clinical progress in a manner that permits evaluation of the association between patient improvement and neurophysiological change.

Despite these advances, several factors seem likely to impede the development and clinical application of EEG biofeedback. Health care providers have a multitude of treatments to apply in their care of patients. Physicians have available a variety of medications, each of which has been demonstrated to be efficacious in the treatment of specific disorders in well-controlled, double-blind studies. Although health care professionals and the general public are concerned about the potential adverse long-term effects of these pharmacological agents, there has been no indication that any of the currently available pharmacological treatments pose a significant health risk. Moreover, in those cases where risk for the development of health problems has been identified (e.g., liver complications with the use of the stimulant Cylert), alternative medications are readily available. These medications can be administered without cost to the physician and monitored in brief, targeted office visits. Consequently, it seems unlikely that physicians will change their practice patterns, which rely extensively on pharmacological therapies.

Nonphysician health care providers can select from hundreds of different psychological treatments. To my knowledge, none has been shown to be more effective than EEG biofeedback. However, costs to the providers are substantially less in offering nonbiofeedback treatments. Hence this question is in order: Why would providers purchase the equipment and obtain the training in order to offer EEG biofeedback in their clinical practice? Although theoretical orientation with respect to psychopathology and the healing process seems relevant, my sense is that a practitioner's experience of personal effectiveness as a healer, and the ability of EEG biofeedback to demonstrate efficacy in the treatment of the kinds of cases that the therapist has previously been ineffectively treating, are what will determine the eventual acceptance of this form of treatment.

My recommendation to clinical researchers, therefore, is to investigate the clinical efficacy of EEG biofeedback in the treatment of patients who are unresponsive to medications, who are unable to tolerate pharmacological treatment due to adverse side effects, whose functional impairments persist to a significant degree despite medication, who experience symptom relapse when medications are withdrawn, who fail to profit from available interactional psychotherapies, or for whom there is no known efficacious and specific treatment. As with other types of outcome research, controlled studies in which patients are randomly assigned to EEG biofeedback, other active treatments, or waiting-list controls (in studies of disorders for which no type of effective treatment has been identified) appear needed. Monitoring of the primary clinical symptoms via multiple, standardized psychometric measures, and the use of database-referenced QEEG measures, seem essential in the assessment process. In addition, follow-up evaluation of patient progress seems significant, because it is hypothesized that EEG biofeedback will produce enduring improvement in a patient's clinical status.

At this time, there is considerable interest in conducting double-blind studies. As I present my biofeedback research and attend scientific meetings, there is a sense that such studies will prove "once and for all time" that EEG biofeedback "works." I am supportive of my colleagues who are seeking to examine the efficacy of EEG biofeedback in studies in which neither the therapist nor the patient is informed about what type of electrophysiological activity is being rewarded. These studies seem relevant for assessing the significance of the therapist–patient interaction and the importance of therapeutic verbal coaching of the patient during biofeedback sessions.

However, from my perspective, it seems important that we use our resources to investigate whether the EEG biofeedback protocols described in this chapter (and elsewhere) serve an essential role in clinical practice. Without this type of demonstration, it would seem that the results of double-blind studies are essentially pointless. Even if researchers can demonstrate through such studies that scientists have created a computerized "token-dispensing" system that does not require interaction with a trained therapist in order to produce a positive clinical outcome, we still miss the point. The issue is not whether we need a knowledgeable therapist in the room during EEG biofeedback sessions. Rather, the issue is whether EEG biofeedback is needed at all.

REFERENCES

Alhambra, M. A., Fowler, T. P., & Alhambra, A. A. (1995). EEG biofeedback: A new treatment option for ADD/ADHD. *Journal of Neurotherapy, 1*, 39–43.

American Psychiatric Association. (1994). *Diagnostic and statistical manual of mental disorders* (4th ed.). Washington, DC: Author.

American Psychological Association (APA) Task Force on Promotion and Dissemination of Psychological Procedures. (1995). Training in and dissemination of empirically-validated psychological treatments: Report and recommendations. *The Clinical Psychologist, 48*, 3–23.

American Psychological Association (APA) Task Force on Psychological Intervention Guidelines. (1995). *Template for developing guidelines: Interventions for mental disorders and psychological aspects of physical disorders.* Washington, DC: American Psychological Association.

Anastopoulos, A. D., Smith, J. M., & Wien, E. E. (1998). Counseling and training parents. In R. A. Barkley, *Attention-deficit hyperactivity disorder: A handbook for diagnosis and treatment* (2nd ed.). New York: Guilford Press.

Ayers, M. E. (1987). Electroencephalographic neurofeedback and closed head injury of 250 individuals. In *National head injury syllabus.* Washington, DC: Head Injury Foundation.

Baehr, E., Rosenfeld, J. P., & Baehr, R. (1997). The clinical use of an alpha asymmetry biofeedback protocol in treatment of depression disorders: Two case studies. *Journal of Neurotherapy, 2*, 12–27.

Barkley, R. A. (1992). Is EEG biofeedback treatment effective for ADHD children? *ChA.D.D.er Box, 1*, 5–11.

Barkley, R. A. (1998). *Attention-deficit hyperactivity disorder: A handbook for diagnosis* and treatment (2nd ed.). New York: Guilford Press.

Baucom, D. H., Shoham, V., Mueser, K. T., Daiuto, A. D., & Stickle, T. R. (1998). Empirically supported couple and family interventions for marital distress and adult mental health problems. *Journal of Consulting and Clinical Psychology, 66*, 53–88.

Beck, A. T., Rush, A. J., Shaw, B. F., & Emery, G. (1979). *Cognitive therapy of depression*. New York: Guilford Press.

Birbaumer, N., Elbert, T., Canavan, A. G. M., & Rockstroh, B. (1990). Slow potentials of the cerebral cortex and behavior. *Physiological Reviews, 70*, 1–41.

Birbaumer, N., Elbert, T., Rockstroh, B., Daum, I., Wolf, P., & Canavan, A. (1991). Clinical-psychological treatment of epileptic seizures: A controlled study. In A. Ehlers (Ed.), *Perspectives and promises of promises of clinical psychology*. New York: Plenum Press.

Birbaumer, N., Elbert, T., Rockstroh, B., & Lutzenberger, W. (1981). Biofeedback of event-related slow potentials of the brain. *International Journal of Psychology, 16*, 389–415.

Byers, A. P. (1995). *The Byers neurotherapy reference library*. Wheat Ridge, CO: Association for Applied Psychophysiology and Biofeedback.

Carroll, K. M. (1996). Relapse prevention as a psychosocial treatment: A review of controlled clinical trials. *Experimental and Clinical Psychopharmacology, 4*, 46–54.

Chambless, D. L., & Hollon, S. D. (1998). Defining empirically supported therapies. *Journal of Consulting and Clinical Psychology, 66*, 7–18.

Davidson, R. J. (1995). Cerebral asymmetry, emotion, and affective style. In R. J. Davidson & K. Hugdahl (Eds.). *Brain asymmetry*. Cambridge, MA: MIT Press.

DeRubeis, R. J., & Crits-Christoph, P. (1998). Empirically supported individual and group psychological treatments for adult mental disorders. *Journal of Consulting and Clinical Psychology, 66*, 37–52.

Duffy, F. H. (2000). The state of EEG biofeedback therapy (EEG operant conditioning) in 2000: An editor's opinion. *Clinical Electroencephalography, 31*, v–vii.

Earnest, C. (1999). Single case study of EEG asymmetry biofeedback for depression: An independent replication in an adolescent. *Journal of Neurotherapy, 3*, 28–35.

Ekman, P., Davidson, R. J., & Friesen, W. V. (1990). Duchenne's smile: Emotional expression and brain physiology. *Journal of Personality and Social Psychology, 58*, 342–353.

Fahrion, S. L., Walters, E. D., Coyne, L, & Allen, T. (1992). Alterations in EEG amplitude, personality factors, and brain electrical mapping after alpha–theta brainwave training: A controlled case study of an alcoholic in recovery. *Alcoholism: Clinical and Experimental Research, 16*, 547–552.

Finley, W. W., Smith, H. A., & Etherton, M. D. (1975). Reduction of seizures and normalization of the EEG in a severe epileptic following sensorimotor biofeedback training: Preliminary study. *Biological Psychiatry, 2*, 189–203.

Garfield, S. L. (1998). Some comments on empirically supported treatments. *Journal of Consulting and Clinical Psychology, 66*, 121–125.

Garrett, B. L., & Silver, M. P. (1976). The use of EMG and alpha biofeedback to relieve test anxiety in college students. In I. Wickramesekera (Ed.), *Biofeedback, behavior therapy, and hypnosis*. Chicago: Nelson-Hall.

Glueck, B. C., & Stroebel, C. F. (1975). Biofeedback and meditation in the treatment of psychiatric illness. *Comprehensive Psychiatry, 16*, 303–321.

Goslinga, J. J. (1975). Biofeedback for clinical problem patients: A developmental process. *Journal of Biofeedback, 2*, 17–27.

Gotlib, I. H., Ranganath, C., & Rosenfeld, J. P. (1998). Frontal EEG alpha asymmetry, depression, and cognitive functioning. *Cognition and Emotion, 12*, 449–478.

Graap, K., & Freides, D. (1998). Regarding the database for the Peniston alpha–theta EEG biofeedback protocol. *Applied Psychophysiology and Biofeedback, 23*, 265–272.

Green, E. E., Green, A. M., & Walters, E. D. (1974). Alpha–theta biofeedback training. *Journal of Biofeedback, 2*, 7–13.

Gruzelier, J. (2000). Self regulation of electrocortical activity in schizophrenia and schizotypy: A review. *Clinical Electroencephalography, 31*, 23–29.

Gruzelier, J., Hardman, E., Wild, J., Zaman, R., Nagy, A., & Hirsch, S. (1999). Learned control of interhemispheric slow potential negativity in schizophrenia. *International Journal of Psychophysiology, 34*, 341–348.

Ham, L. P., & Packard, R. C. (1996). A retrospective, follow-up study of biofeedback-assisted relaxation therapy in patients with posttraumatic headache. *Biofeedback and Self-Regulation, 21*, 93–104.

Hardt, J. V., & Kamiya, J. (1978). Anxiety change through electroencephalographic alpha feedback seen only in high anxiety subjects. *Science, 201*, 79–81.

Henriques, J. B., & Davidson, R. J. (1990). Regional brain electrical asymmetries discriminate between previously depressed and health control subjects. *Journal of Abnormal Psychology, 99*, 22–31.

Henriques, J. B., & Davidson, R. J. (1991). Left frontal hypoactivation in depression. *Journal of Abnormal Psychology, 100*, 535–545.

Hoffman, D. A., Stockdale, S., & Hicks, L. (1995). Diagnosis and treatment of head injury. *Journal of Neurotherapy, 1*, 14–21.

Hoffman, D. A., Stockdale, S., & VanEgren, L. (1996). Symptom changes in the treatment of mild traumatic brain injury using EEG neurofeedback. *Clinical Electroencephalography, 27*, 164.

Itil, T. M. (1977). Qualitative and quantitative EEG findings in schizophrenia. *Schizophrenia Bulletin, 3*, 61–79.

James, L. C., & Folen, R. A. (1996). EEG biofeedback as a treatment for chronic fatigue syndrome: A controlled case report. *Behavioral Medicine, 22*, 77–81.

Kaiser, D. A., & Othmer, S. (2000). Effect of neurofeedback on variables of attention in a large multi-center trial. *Journal of Neurotherapy, 4*, 5–15.

Kazdin, A. E., & Weisz, J. R. (1998). Identifying and developing empirically supported child and adolescent treatments. *Journal of Consulting and Clinical Psychology, 66*, 19–36.

Klerman, G. L., Weissman, M. M., Rounsaville, B. J., & Chevron, E. S. (1984). *Interpersonal psychotherapy of depression*. New York: Basic Books.

Kotchoubey, B., Busch, S., Strehl, U., & Birbaumer, N. (1999a). Changes in EEG power spectra during biofeedback of slow cortical potentials in epilepsy. *Applied Psychophysiology and Biofeedback, 24*, 213–233.

Kotchoubey, B., Strehl, U., Holzapfel, S., Schneider, D., Blankenhorn, V., & Birbaumer, N. (1999b). Control of cortical excitability in epilepsy. In H. Stefan, F. Andermann, P. Chauvel, & S. Shorvon (Eds.) *Advances in neurology* (Vol. 8). Philadelphia: Lippincott Williams & Wilkins.

Lantz, D., & Sterman, M. B. (1988). Neuropsychological assessment of subjects with uncontrolled epilepsy: Effects of EEG biofeedback training. *Epilepsia, 29*, 163–171.

LaVaque, T. J., & Rossiter, T. (2001). The ethical use of placebo controls in clinical research: The Declaration of Helsinki. *Applied Psychophysiology and Biofeedback, 26*, 23–37.

Lewinsohn, P. M. (1974). A behavioral approach to depression. In R. J. Friedman & M. M. Katz (Eds.), *The psychology of depression: Contemporary theory and research*. Washington, DC: Winston–Wiley.

Linden, M., Habib, T., & Radojevic, V. (1996). A controlled study of EEG biofeedback effects on cognitive and behavioral measures with attention-deficit disorder and learning disabled children. *Biofeedback and Self-Regulation, 21*, 35–49.

Lubar, J. F. (1997). Neocortical dynamics: Implications for understanding the role of neurofeedback and related techniques for the enhancement of attention. *Applied Psychophysiology and Biofeedback, 22*, 111–126.

Lubar, J. F., & Bahler, W.W. (1976). Behavioral management of epileptic seizures following EEG biofeedback training of the sensorimotor rhythm. *Biofeedback and Self-Regulation, 7*, 77–104.

Lubar, J. F., & Shouse, M. N. (1976). EEG and behavioral changes in a hyperactive child concurrent with training of the sensorimotor rhythm (SMR): A preliminary report. *Biofeedback and Self Regulation, 1*, 293–306.

Lubar, J. F., Swartwood, M. O., Swartwood, J. N., & O'Donnell, P. H. (1995). Evaluation of the effectiveness of EEG neurofeedback training for ADHD in a clinical setting as measured by changes in T.O.V.A. scores, behavioral ratings and WISC-R performance. *Biofeedback and Self Regulation, 20*, 83–99.

Lubar, J. O., & Lubar, J. F. (1984). Electroencephalographic biofeedback of SMR and beta for treatment of attention deficit disorders in a clinical setting. *Biofeedback and Self-Regulation, 9*, 1–23.

Luborsky, L., McLellan, A. T., Diguer, L., Woody, G., & Seligman, D. A. (1997). The psychotherapist matters: Comparison of outcomes across 22 therapists and 7 patient samples. *Clinical Psychology: Science and Practice, 4*, 53–65.

Mann, C. A., Lubar, J. F., Zimmerman, A. W., Miller, B. A., & Meunchen, R. A. (1992). Quantitative analysis of EEG in boys with attention-deficit/hyperactivity disorder (ADHD). A controlled study with clinical implications. *Pediatric Neurology, 8*, 30–36.

McCrady, B. S. (2000). Alcohol use disorders and the Division 12 Task Force of the American Psychological Association. *Psychology of Addictive Behaviors, 14*, 267–276.

Mills, G. K., & Solyom, L. (1974). Biofeedback of EEG alpha in the treatment of obsessive ruminations: An exploration. *Journal of Behavior Therapy and Experimental Psychiatry, 5*, 37–41.

Monastra, V. J., Lubar, J. F., & Linden, M. (2001). The development of a quantitative electroencephalographic scanning process for attention deficit-hyperactivity disorder: Reliability and validity studies. *Neuropsychology, 15*, 136–144.

Monastra, V. J., Lubar, J. F., Linden, M., VanDeusen, P., Green, G., Wing, W., Phillips, A., & Fenger, T. N. (1999). Assessing attention deficit hyperactivity disorder via quantitative electroencephalography: An initial validation study. *Neuropsychology, 13*, 424–433.

Monastra, V. J., Monastra, D. M., & George, S. (2002). The effects of stimulant therapy, EEG biofeedback, and parenting style on the primary symptoms of attention-deficit/hyperactivity disorder. *Applied Psychophysiology and Biofeedback, 27*, 231–249.

Moore, J. P., & Trudeau, D. L. (1998). Alpha–theta brainwave biofeedback is not specific to the production of theta/alpha crossover and visualizations. *Journal of Neurotherapy, 3*, 63.

Morihisa, J. M., Duffy, F. H., & Wyatt, R. J. (1983). Brain electrical activity mapping (BEAM) in schizophrenic patients. *Archives of General Psychiatry, 40*, 719–728.

MTA Cooperative Group. (1999). A 14–month randomized clinical trial of treatment strategies for attention-deficit/hyperactivity disorder. *Archives of General Psychiatry, 56*, 1073–1086.

Nash, J. K. (2000). Treatment of attention-deficit/hyperactivity disorder with neurotherapy. *Clinical Electroencephalography, 31,* 30–37.

National Institutes of Health. (1998). *Consensus statement on the diagnosis and treatment of attention-deficit/hyperactivity disorder.* Bethesda, MD: Author.

Nuwer, M. (1997). Assessment of digital EEG, quantitative EEG and EEG brain mapping: Report of the American Academy of Neurology and the American Clinical Neurophysiology Society. *Neurology, 49,* 277–292.

Pelham, W. E., Wheeler, T., & Chronis, A. (1998). Empirically supported psychosocial treatments for attention-deficit/hyperactivity disorder. *Journal of Clinical Child Psychology, 27,* 190–205.

Peniston, E. G., & Kulkosky, P. J. (1989). Alpha–theta brainwave training and beta endorphin levels in alcoholics. *Alcoholism: Clinical and Experimental Research, 13,* 271–279.

Peniston, E. G., & Kulkosky, P. J. (1990). Alcoholic personality and alpha-theta brainwave training. *Medical Psychotherapy, 2,* 37–55.

Peniston, E. G., & Kulkosky, P. J. (1991). Alpha–theta brainwave neuro-feedback therapy for Vietnam veterans with combat-related post-traumatic stress disorder. *Medical Psychotherapy, 4,* 47–60.

Plotkin, W. B., & Rice, K. M. (1981). Biofeedback as a placebo: Anxiety reduction facilitated by training in either suppression or enhancement of alpha brainwaves. *Journal of Consulting and Clinical Psychology, 49,* 590–596.

Rice, K. M., Blanchard, E. B., & Purcell, M. (1993). Biofeedback treatment of generalized anxiety disorder: Preliminary results. *Biofeedback and Self-Regulation, 18,* 93–105.

Rockstroh, B., Elbert, T., Canavan, A. G. M., Lutzenberger, W., & Birbaumer, N. (1989). *Slow cortical potentials and behavior* (2nd ed.). Baltimore: Urban & Schwarzenberg.

Rosenfeld, J. P. (2000). An EEG biofeedback protocol for affective disorders. *Clinical Electroencephalography, 31,* 7–12.

Rosenfeld, J. P., Baehr, E., Baehr, R., Gotlib, I. H., & Ranganath, C. (1996). Preliminary evidence that daily changes in frontal alpha asymmetry correlate with changes in affect in therapy sessions. *International Journal of Psychophysiology, 23,* 137–141.

Rosenfeld, J. P., Cha, G., Blair, T., & Gotlib, I. H. (1995). Operant (biofeedback) control of left–right frontal alpha power differences: Potential neurotherapy for affective disorders. *Biofeedback and Self-Regulation, 20,* 241–258.

Rossiter, T. R., & LaVaque, T. J. (1995). A comparison of EEG biofeedback and psychostimulants in treating attention deficit hyperactivity disorders. *Journal of Neurotherapy, 1,* 48–59.

Rozelle, G. R., & Budzynski, T. H. (1995). Neurotherapy for stroke rehabilitation: A single case study. *Biofeedback and Self Regulation, 20,* 211–228.

Sanford, J. A., Brown, R. J., & Turner, A. (1996). *The Captain's log cognitive training system.* Richmond, VA: Braintrain.

Saxby, E., & Peniston, E. G. (1995). Alpha–theta brainwave neurofeedback training: An effective treatment for male and female alcoholics with depressive symptoms. *Journal of Clinical Psychology, 51,* 685–693.

Schneider, F., Elbert, T., Heimann, H., Welker, A., Stetter, F., Mattes, R., Birbaumer, N. & Mann, K. (1993). Self-regulation of slow cortical potentials in psychiatric patients: Alcohol dependency. *Biofeedback and Self-Regulation, 18,* 23–32.

Schneider, F., Rockstroh, B., Heimann, H., Lutzenberger, W., Mattes, R., Elbert, T., Birbaumer, N., & Bartels, M. (1992). Self-regulation of slow cortical potentials in psychiatric patients: Schizophrenia. *Biofeedback and Self-Regulation, 17,* 277–292.

Seifert, A. R., & Lubar, J. F. (1975). Reduction of epileptic seizures through EEG biofeedback training. *Biological Psychology, 3,* 157–184.

Shouse, M. N., & Lubar, J. F. (1979). Operant conditioning of EEG rhythms and ritalin in treatment of hyperkinesis. *Biofeedback and Self-Regulation, 4,* 301–312.

Siniatchkin, M., Hierundar, A., Kropp, P., Khunert, R., Gerber, W. D., & Staphani, U. (2000). Self-regulation of slow cortical potentials in children with migraine: An exploratory study. *Applied Psychophysiology and Biofeedback, 25,* 13–32.

Sittenfield, P., Budzynski, T. H., & Stoyva, J. M. (1976). Differential shaping of EEG theta rhythms. *Biofeedback and Self-Regulation, 1,* 31–46.

Sobotka, S., Davidson, R. J., & Senulis, J. (1992). Anterior brain electrical asymmetries in response to reward and punishment. *Electroencephalography and Clinical Neurophysiology, 83,* 236–247.

Sponheim, S. R., Clementz, B. A., Iacono, W. G., & Beiser, M. (1994). Resting EEG is first episode and chronic schizophrenia. *Psychophysiology, 31,* 37–43.

Sterman, M. B. (1996). Physiological origins and functional correlates of EEG rhythmic activities: Implications for self-regulation. *Biofeedback and Self-Regulation, 21,* 3–33.

Sterman, M. B. (2000). Basic concepts and clinical findings in the treatment of seizure disorders with EEG operant conditioning. *Clinical Electroencephalography, 31,* 45–55.

Sterman, M. B., & Friar, L. (1972). Suppression of seizures in epileptics following sensorimotor EEG feedback training. *Electroencephalography and Clinical Neurophysiology, 33,* 89–95.

Sterman, M. B., LoPresti, R. W., & Fairchild, M. D. (1969). *Electroencephalographic and behavioral studies of monomethylhydrazine toxicity in the cat* (Technical Report No. AMRL-TR-69-3 [AD691474]. Dayton, OH: Wright–Patterson Air Force Base, Aerospace Medical Research Laboratory.

Sterman, M. B., & Macdonald, L. R. (1978). Effects of central cortical EEG feedback training on incidence of poorly controlled seizures. *Epilepsia, 19,* 207–222.

Swanson, J. M., McBurnett, K., Christian, D. L., & Wigal, T. (1995). Stimulant medications and the treatment of children with ADHD. In T. H. Ollendick & R. J. Prinz (Eds.), *Advances in clinical child psychology* (Vol. 17). New York: Plenum Press.

Tansey, M. A. (1984). EEG sensorimotor rhythm biofeedback training: Some effects on the neurologic precursors of learning disabilities. *International Journal of Psychophysiology, 1,* 163–177.

Tansey, M. A. (1986). A simple and a complex tic (Gilles de la Tourette's syndrome): Their response to EEG sensorimotor rhythm biofeedback training. *International Journal of Psychophysiology, 4,* 91–97.

Taub, E., Steiner, S. S., Smith, R. B., Weingarten, E. I., & Walton, K. G. (1994). Effectiveness of broad spectrum approaches to relapse prevention in severe alcoholism: A long term randomized controlled trial of transcendental meditation, EMG biofeedback, and electronic neurotherapy. *Alcoholism Treatment Quarterly, 11,* 187–220.

Thatcher, R. W. (1998). EEG normative databases and EEG biofeedback. *Journal of Neurotherapy, 2,* 8–39.

Thatcher, R. W. (1999). EEG database quided neurotherapy. In J. R. Evans & A. Arbarbanel (Eds.), *Introduction to quantitative EEG and neurofeedback.* San Diego, CA: Academic Press.

Thatcher, R. W. (2000). EEG operant conditioning (biofeedback) and traumatic brain injury. *Clinical Electroencephalography, 31,* 38–44.

Thatcher, R. W., Walker, R. A., Gerson, I., & Geisler, F. (1989). EEG discriminant analyses of mild head trauma. *Electroencephalography and Clinical Neurophysiology, 73,* 93–106.

Thompson, L., & Thompson, M. (1998). Neurofeedback combined with training in metacognitive strategies: Effectiveness in students with ADD. *Applied Psychophysiology and Biofeedback, 23,* 243–263.

Tomarken, A. J., Davidson, R. J., & Henriques, J. B. (1990). Resting frontal brain asymmetry predicts affective responses to films. *Journal of Personality and Social Psychology, 59,* 791–801.

Tozzo, C. A., Elfner, L. F., & May, J. G. (1988). EEG biofeedback and relaxation training in the control of epileptic seizures. *International Journal of Psychophysiology, 6,* 185–194.

Twemlow, S. W., & Bowen, W. T. (1976). EEG biofeedback induces self actualization in alcoholics. *Journal of Biofeedback, 3,* 20–25.

Twemlow, S. W., & Bowen, W. T. (1977). Sociocultural predictors of self actualization in EEG biofeedback treated alcoholics. *Psychological Reports, 40,* 591–598.

Tyson, P. D. (1996). Biodesensitization: Biofeedback-controlled systematic desensitization of the stress response to infant crying. *Biofeedback and Self-Regulation, 21,* 273–290.

Vanathy, S., Sharma, P. S. V. N., & Kumar, K. B. (1998). The efficacy of alpha and theta neurofeedback training in treatment of generalized anxiety disorder. *Indian Journal of Clinical Psychology, 25,* 136–143.

World Medical Association Declaration of Helsinki. (1997). Recommendations guiding physicians in biomedical research involving human subjects. *Journal of the American Medical Association, 277,* 925–926.

Wyricka, W., & Sterman, M. B. (1968). Instrumental conditioning of sensorimotor cortex EEG spindles in the waking cat. *Physiology and Behavior, 3,* 703–707.

Biofeedback of Slow Cortical Potentials in Epilepsy

UTE STREHL

OVERVIEW

Slow cortical potentials (SCPs) of the electroencephalogram (EEG) reflect cortical excitability. Negative SCPs appear in animals as well as in humans before and during epileptic *seizures*, which are followed by positive potential shifts after their abatement. This leads to the hypothesis that epilepsy involves a deficit in regulating cortical hyperactivation. Operant learning and behavioral principles have been used to develop a treatment program to control SCPs and to teach patients to cope with seizures. The program is described in this chapter, and predictors of outcome are reported. (As in other chapters, italics on first use of a term indicate that the term is included in the glossary at the chapter's end.)

EPILEPSY: EPIDEMIOLOGY, CLASSIFICATION, AND PROGNOSIS

Epilepsy is one of the most common neurological disorders. For every 1000 persons, there are 5 to 10 active cases. Epilepsy is most likely to occur at two periods: the first 10 years of life, and after the age of 60. The annual incidence of new cases is about 50 per 100,000 (Hauser & Hesdorffer, 1990).

The causes of epilepsy are diverse, but in most cases they are unknown. In young children, genetic factors, congenital defects, and developmental disturbances are the most common causes; in elderly patients, mostly cerebrovascular diseases are found.

Epilepsy can be described as a group of neurological conditions that are characterized by recurrent seizures. These seizures are the result of a disturbed balance between excitation and inhibition of neurons that are located predominantly in the cerebral cortex. Exclusively subcortical seizures, and disturbed corticothalamico and corticostriatal circuits, can be observed as well. Depending upon the specific underlying pathophysiological conditions and clinical signs, *partial seizures* are distinguished from *generalized seizures*. Partial seizures consist of initial activation of neurons limited to one area of the cortex, the "focus." Patients may have more than one focus. When consciousness is not impaired, the seizure is classified as a *simple partial seizure*. When consciousness is impaired, it is classified as a *complex partial seizure*. A simple partial seizure may progress to a complex partial seizure, and a complex partial seizure may progress to a generalized seizure. Clinical signs of a partial seizure may include motor symptoms, somatosensory or special sensory symptoms, autonomic symptoms, or psychological experiences. The very first signs of a (simple) partial seizure are called an *aura*.

In contrast, when the onset of a seizure involves both hemispheres, seizures are classified as generalized. Generalized seizure subtypes are *absence seizures, atypical absence seizures, myoclonic seizures, clonic seizures, tonic seizures, tonic–clonic* (grand mal) *seizures*, and *atonic seizures* (Commission on Classification and Terminology of the International League Against Epilepsy, 1981, 1989).

The degree of severity of the illness is extremely variable. Most patients are completely normal between their seizures, and in many cases friends, colleagues, and even relatives do not recognize that a person has epilepsy. Only 5% of epileptic patients are handicapped or mentally disabled and need special education. On the other hand, suffering from seizures is a frightening condition; for many patients, the seizures seem to be unpredictable and accompanied by a complete loss of control. In the public opinion, epilepsy is often misunderstood as mental illness, and patients are discriminated against.

TREATMENT

Medical treatment of epileptic seizures with antiepileptic drugs (AEDs) is specific for the seizure type. Treatment is normally initiated with one single drug type. If the patient does not become seizure-free, another drug suited for that seizure type will be prescribed. The treatment may be continued by gradually changing AEDs and/or combining different drugs. Patients who continue to have seizures after 2 years of treatment are considered to have drug-resistant epilepsy (Bourgeois, 1994). It is estimated from community and hospital-based studies that about one-quarter to one-third of newly diagnosed patients will have intractable epilepsy (Reynolds, 1994). For these patients, surgery becomes an option. Because of medical, psychological, and social reasons, only about 12% of patients with intractable epilepsy can be operated upon, and about 8% become seizure-free after a neurosurgical intervention. Thus at least 15–17% of all patients cannot be treated by standard medical interventions and are thus prime candidates for behavioral treatments, which are also applicable as adjunct methods to pharmacological and/or neurosurgical intervention.

Therefore, treatment strategies in a behavioral medicine framework have become an option for patients within the last several decades. Efron (1956) first reported classical conditioning of aura disruption. The most systematic behavioral training was developed by Dahl (1992), who integrated principles of identifying and controlling antecedents of seizures, teaching patients relaxation techniques, utilizing contingency management, and implementing other behaviors that are incompatible with seizures ("countermeasures").

Since the early 1970s, biofeedback of EEG rhythms (Lubar, 1977; Sterman, 2000) as well as respiration parameters (Fried, 1993) has been used in epilepsy therapy. Beginning in the late 1970s, Niels Birbaumer and colleagues have developed a physiological model wherein SCPs of the EEG are viewed as reflecting the level of cortical excitability. Negative SCPs can be observed in animals as well as in humans before and during *ictal discharges*, and positive SCP shifts follow the abatement of seizures. This model has led to the hypothesis that epilepsy is characterized by a problem in restraining the hyperactivation of neurons. Accordingly, suppression of cortical negativity should correspond to a state in which epileptic discharge is attenuated. Thus seizure frequency may be reduced by training epileptic patients in suppressing cortical negativities. Two multicenter studies to date have shown that patients are able to learn to regulate their SCPs, and this treatment has been found to yield a significant decrease in seizure rates (Rockstroh et al., 1993, Kotchoubey et al., 2001).

SCP SELF-REGULATION

Today, patients are taught SCP self-regulation with the so-called *Thought Translation Device (TTD)*. The SCPs are recorded at the vertex (Cz), referred to two mastoid electrodes shunted over a 10-kiloohm resistance. The time constant is set at 10 seconds. For detailed information about the TTD's arrangement, hardware requirements, software, signal processing, and artifact control, see Birbaumer et al. (1999) and Kübler, Winter, and Birbaumer (Chapter 21, this volume).

The patient sits in a comfortable armchair, with a notebook computer or personal computer in front of him or her. Depending on the discriminative stimulus (rectangle at the top or bottom on the screen), the patient has to produce SCP shifts in either a negative or positive direction. Feedback is given by a small (1-centimeter diameter) round graphic symbol (the "cursor" or "ball"), which moves during each feedback trial upward (negative shift) or downward (positive shift). Ball movements start on the left edge of the computer screen and end in a rectangle at the right edge. Trials with required negativity and required positivity are randomly distributed, with each occurring 50% of the time initially. During the second training phase, 67% of trials require positivity. In order to assess learning and generalization of SCP skills in everyday life, feedback trials are mixed with transfer trials in which no ball movement is shown. The length of each trial is 8 seconds; 100 trials constitute one session.

The patient is monitored by the therapist, who stays in an adjacent room. The therapist observes the patient's EEG data online on a separate screen and can intervene if necessary. After the end of a session, patients are invited to observe trial-by-trial data, in order to understand where they were successful and unsuccessful.

As shown in Figure 20.1, the whole treatment program is divided into three parts. The first phase includes at least 20 sessions over 3 weeks. Thereafter, patients are given an 8-week break from coming to the laboratory, so they can concentrate on practicing and applying the strategies they have learned in everyday life. Finally, in a second intensive phase (15 sessions within 2 weeks), emphasis on feedback is withdrawn in favor of transfer exercises.

Period		Behavior Therapy	
		SCP biofeedback (response-oriented method)	Behavioral analysis Antecedent-oriented methods Contingency management
3 weeks	Phase 1	20 sessions	One session per day
8 weeks	Practice phase at home	Homework and training under everyday life conditions	
2 weeks	Phase 2	15 sessions	One session per day
According to demand	Follow-up	Booster sessions	

FIGURE 20.1. Schedule of behavioral training for epilepsy.

Patients are instructed to continue doing exercises after completing the program. As they have no EEG equipment at home, they have to get used to doing the exercises in imagination. Returning for booster sessions in the lab helps to reassure patients that they are still able to control their SCPs.

SCP SELF-REGULATION IN A BEHAVIORAL MEDICINE FRAMEWORK

In a behavioral medicine paradigm for medical diseases, the symptoms (in this case, the epileptic seizures) are conceived as behaviors that are largely influenced by their antecedents as well as by their consequences. In addition to the neurological examination, a behavioral analysis concentrates on a careful description of internal (physiological states, emotions, cognitions, behaviors) and external (behaviors of other persons, changes of behavior plans) events. This analysis is based on a detailed seizure diary.

The aims of behavioral self control training are to increase knowledge and perceptual skills about antecedents and early signs of seizure behavior, to change reinforcing contingencies, and to transfer self-control skills to everyday life conditions.

Thus treatment includes behavioral change of seizure-eliciting and seizure-reinforcing behaviors, as well as the psychophysiological intervention to control the brain states that are thought to induce seizure activity. Depending upon the results of the behavior analysis, various other intervention strategies besides SCP training are incorporated for sensitizing self-perception. These may include relaxation training, stress management, cognitive restructuring, activity assignments, social skills training, education of patients and significant others, changes in reinforcement patterns, coping with illness, and addressing quality-of-life issues.

EVALUATION

Results of the evaluation of the program are reported in detail elsewhere (Kotchoubey et al., 2001). Progress in self-control of SCPs can be shown by the increase in differentiation between mean SCP amplitudes for positivity and negativity conditions, as depicted in Figure 20.2. This figure illustrates how patient AB made progress in the second phase of training in producing required positivity and negativity. In the new version of the TTD, additional measures can be evaluated by determining the percentage of hits, changes in power spectra, and so forth.

Changes in seizure frequency are documented by seizure diaries. A statistical decision about the significance of seizure decrement can be computed on the basis of a week-by-week sequence analysis (Künkel, 1979). With the probability of type I error at $a_1 = .05$ and a probability of type II error at $a_1 = .10$, the reliability of individual changes in seizure frequency during a 52-week follow-up period versus the baseline period was tested. The criterion of seizure decrement was set at 50%. Figure 20.3 shows the cumulative number of seizures following the therapy in the patient whose SCP amplitudes are presented in Figure 20.2. As can be seen in this figure, the decrease in the patient's seizure frequency became significant in week 32 of the follow-up period, and after week 42 there were no seizures.

THERAPISTS AND PATIENTS

In a behavioral medicine framework such as this, therapists should be licensed psychologists who are qualified to conduct psychophysiological procedures. Neurological consultation before

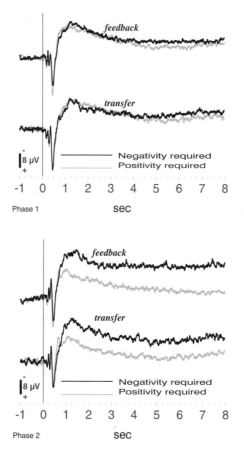

FIGURE 20.2. Slow cortical potentials (SCPs) of patient AB, averaged across 20 sessions of treatment phase 1 (upper panel) and 15 sessions of phase 2 (lower panel). From Strehl, Kotchoubey, & Birbaumer (2000b). Copyright 2000 by Schattauer GmbH. Reprinted by permission.

and after treatment is necessary. Criteria for the patients are less clear. Contrary to common sense, cognitive and personality variables have no predictive power. It was shown, for example, that a patient with mental retardation and organic brain disorder was able to follow the self control training and to reduce seizures considerably (Holzapfel, Strehl, Kotchoubey, & Birbaumer, 1998). In another study, patients with higher Depression and Hysteria scores on the Minnesota Multiphasic Personality Inventory were found to have a better outcome in seizure reduction. Instead, physiological features—such as the average SCP amplitude at the beginning of training, and the location of the epileptic focus—seem to be much more important. Larger negative amplitudes covary with less success, and patients with a left temporal focus profit less than patients with bilateral foci, multiple foci, or a right temporal focus (Strehl, Kotchoubey, & Birbaumer, 2000a). On the other hand, the two patients with the best training results had a left-side focus. Therefore, it cannot be concluded with certainty that all patients with a large SCP amplitude or a left-side focus should be excluded from the program. Rather, the therapist should try to adapt training conditions to maximize the potential for improvement (e.g., by extending the duration of active treatment phases and/or by placing more emphasis on cortical positivity tasks or using advanced shaping schedules). The TTD software (see Kübler et al., Chapter 21) allows these variations if the therapist is sensitive enough to the patient's needs.

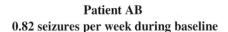

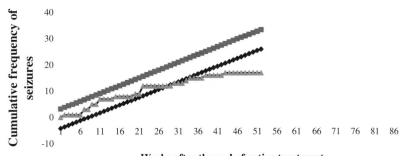

FIGURE 20.3. Sequence analysis of seizure frequency after the end of active treatment. The two straight lines indicate the limits of significance for the two types of errors. Specifically, the lower (dashed) line stands for the .05 significance limit for the type I error; if the actual cumulative number of a patient's seizures (shown by the gray line) drops under that limit, a 50% seizure reduction as compared with the baseline is regarded as significant. The upper (solid) line stands for the .10 significance limit for the type II error; if the actual cumulative number of seizures rises above that line, the lack of 50% improvement is regarded as significant. As long as the actual cumulative number of seizures remains inside the corridor created by the two straight lines, the outcome is uncertain. From Strehl, Kotchoubey, & Birbaumer (2000b). Copyright 2000 by Schattauer GmbH. Reprinted by permission.

GLOSSARY

AURA. Altered sensations at the very first sign of a *simple partial seizure* (see below), which allow patients to use self-control techniques in order to interrupt the spreading of neuronal discharge.

ICTAL DISCHARGE. An abnormal firing of neurons, producing electrophysiological activity that can be observed as seizure activity in the electroencephalogram (EEG).

SEIZURES. The results of a disturbed balance between excitation and inhibition of neurons. They are classified on the basis of clinical manifestations and EEG signs. For practical reasons, the EEG criteria are not mentioned here. For further information, see Commission on Classification and Terminology of the International League Against Epilepsy (1981, 1989). The following seizure types have been identified:

GENERALIZED SEIZURES. Seizures in which the first clinical signs (e.g., impaired consciousness, bilateral motor manifestations) indicate that both hemispheres are involved from the beginning. Neuronal discharge is widespread in both hemispheres. Subtypes of generalized seizures types are as follows:

ABSENCE SEIZURES. Seizures with sudden onset and interruption of ongoing activities.

ATONIC SEIZURES. Sudden diminution of muscle tone, which may lead to dropping of the head and slumping to the ground.

ATYPICAL ABSENCE SEIZURES. Seizures with more pronounced change in tone and/or onset, and in which cessation is not abrupt.

CLONIC SEIZURES. Generalized seizure with lack of the tonic component.

MYOCLONIC SEIZURES. Single or multiple jerks, generalized or confined to the face, trunk, extremities, or (groups of) muscles.

TONIC SEIZURES. Muscular contraction of the whole body, usually with a deviation of the eyes and of the head to one side.

TONIC–CLONIC SEIZURES. Often known as "grand mal seizures"; the most frequent type of generalized seizures. In most cases, onset is signaled with a cry or moan, caused by a sharp tonic contraction of muscles. The tonic stage is followed by clonic convulsive movements. At the end of the seizure, deep respiration occurs with relaxation of all muscles. The patient awakens slowly from unconsciousness.

PARTIAL (FOCAL) SEIZURES. Seizures in which the first clinical signs indicate that the initial activation of a group of neurons is limited to a part of one cerebral hemisphere. Subtypes of partial seizures are classified on the basis of whether or not consciousness is impaired during the attack.

COMPLEX PARTIAL SEIZURES. Partial seizures in which consciousness is impaired. These seizures may develop from simple partial seizures; patients may show "automatisms" (behavior performed without intent or conscious will, often without realization of occurrence). Both simple partial seizures and complex partial seizures may evolve to *secondary generalized seizures* with symptoms like generalized seizures (see above).

SIMPLE PARTIAL SEIZURES. Partial seizures in which consciousness is not impaired. Depending on the focus of the seizure, the patient may experience motor signs, autonomic symptoms, somatosensory or special sensory symptoms, or psychic symptoms.

SLOW CORTICAL POTENTIALS (SCPs). Negative or positive polarizations of the EEG that last from 0.3 seconds up to several seconds. They originate in depolarizations of the apical dendrites in cortical layers I and II that are caused by synchronous firing, mainly from thalamocortical afferents. Functionally, they constitute a threshold regulation mechanism for local excitatory mobilization (negative SCPs) or inhibition (positive SCPs) of cortical networks. SCPs are typically seen preceding either voluntary movement or an expected imperative event.

THOUGHT TRANSLATION DEVICE (TTD). Direct connection between the brain and a computer controlled by SCPs and used for communication.

REFERENCES

Birbaumer, N., Flor, H., Ghanayim, N., Hinterberberger, T., Iversen, I., Taub, E., Kotchoubey, B., Kübler, A., & Perelmouter, J. (1999). A spelling device for the paralyzed. *Nature, 398,* 297–298.

Bourgeois, B. F. K. (1994). Establishment of pharmacoresistance. In P. Wolf (Ed.), *Epileptic seizures and syndromes.* London: Libbey.

Commission on Classification and Terminology of the International League Against Epilepsy. (1981). Proposal for the revised clinical and electroencephalographic classification of epileptic seizures. *Epilepsia, 22,* 489–501.

Commission on Classification and Terminology of the International League Against Epilepsy. (1989). Proposal for the revised classification of epilepsies and epileptic syndromes. *Epilepsia, 30,* 389–399.

Dahl, J. (1992). *Epilepsy.* Toronto: Hogrefe & Huber.

Efron, R. (1956). Effect of olfactoric stimuli in arresting uncinate fits. *Brain, 79,* 267–281.

Fried, R. (1993). Breathing training for self regulation of alveolar CO2 in the behavioral control of idiopathic epileptic seizures. In D. I. Mostovsky (Ed.), *The neurobehavioral treatment of epilepsy.* Hillsdale, NJ: Erlbaum.

Hauser, W. A., & Hesdorffer, D. C. (1990). *Epilepsy: Frequencies, causes, and consequences.* New York: Demos.

Holzapfel, S., Strehl, U., Kotchoubey, B., & Birbaumer, N. (1998). Behavioral psychophysiological intervention in a mentally retarded epileptic patient with brain lesion. *Applied Psychophysiology and Biofeedback, 23,* 189–202.

Kotchoubey, B., Strehl, U., Uhlmann, C., Holzapfel, S., König, M., Fröscher, W., Blankenhorn, V., & Birbaumer, N. (2001). Modification of slow cortical potentials in patients with refractory epilepsy. *Epilepsia, 42*(3), 406–416.

Künkel, H. (1979). Zur Kontrolle des Behandlungserfolges bei Epilepsien. *Aktuelle Neurologie, 6,* 215–225.

Lubar, J. F. (1977). Electroencephalographic biofeedback methodology and the management of epilepsy. *Pavlovian Journal of Biological Science, 12*(3), 147–185.

Reynolds, E. H. (1994). Mechanisms of intractability. In P. Wolf (Ed.), *Epileptic seizures and syndromes.* London: Libbey.

Rockstroh, B., Elbert, T., Birbaumer, N., Wolf, P., Düchting-Röth, A., Reker, M., Lutzenberger, W., & Dichgans, J. (1993). Cortical self-regulation in patients with epilepsies. *Epilepsy Research, 14,* 63–72.

Sterman, M. B. (2000). Basic concepts and clinical findings in the treatment of seizure disorders with EEG operant conditioning. *Clinical Electroencephalography, 31,* 45–55.

Strehl, U., Kotchoubey, B., & Birbaumer, N. (2000a). A behavioral medicine treatment for patients with medically intractable epilepsies: Prediction of outcome. *International Journal of Behavioral Medicine, 7*(Suppl. 1), 27.

Strehl, U., Kotchoubey, B., & Birbaumer, N. (2000b). Biofeedback von Hirnaktivität bei epileptischen Anfällen: ein verhaltensmedizinisches Behandlungsprogramm. In W. Rief & N. Birbaumer (Eds.), *Biofeedback-Therapie.* Stuttgart, Germany: Schattauer.

The Thought Translation Device

Slow Cortical Potential Biofeedback for Verbal Communication in Paralyzed Patients

ANDREA KÜBLER

SUSANNE WINTER

NIELS BIRBAUMER

The *Thought Translation Device* (TTD) is a direct connection between the brain and a computer. This interface can be used to communicate—a process referred to as "brain–computer communication" (Kübler, Kotchoubey, Kaiser, Wolpaw, & Birbaumer, 2001). Self-regulation of *slow cortical potentials* (SCPs) (see Neuman, Strehl, & Birbaumer, Chapter 5, and Strehl, Chapter 20, this volume) is used to control a cursor on a computer screen. Cursor movement occurs according to the alterations of the SCP amplitude. SCPs are used to control cursor movement for three reasons: First, their physiological origin is well understood; second, they are universally present in cortical cell assemblies; and, third, self-regulation of SCPs can be acquired by means of biofeedback and operant learning principles. The TTD is described in detail in this chapter. (Italics on first use of a term indicate, as in other chapters, that the term is included in the glossary at the chapter's end.)

THE LOCKED-IN SYNDROME

Patients who have diseases that lead to severe or total motor paralysis are unable to communicate their needs and feelings (either orally or by keyboard) to the environment. Such patients are said to have the *locked-in syndrome*, a condition described impressively by Jean-Dominique Bauby in his famous book *The Diving Bell and the Butterfly* (Bauby, 1997); Bauby developed the syndrome after a *stroke* in the *brainstem*. Usually sensory and cognitive functions remain intact. Hemorrhage in the anterior brainstem (mainly in the ventral parts of *pons cerebri*) or nonhemorrhagic stroke in the ventral pons can cause the locked-in syndrome, which includes *tetraplegia* and paralysis of cranial nerves (Allen, 1993; Chia, 1991; Patterson & Grabois, 1986).

In the "classic" locked-in syndrome, vertical eye movements as well as eye blinks remain intact, whereas in the "total" locked-in syndrome, patients lose all abilities to move and communicate (Bauer, Gerstenbrand, & Rumpl, 1979; Hayashi & Kato, 1989). Although locked-in syndrome is usually caused by pontine lesions, it has also been observed after lesions in other brain regions (Chia, 1984). Tumors, *encephalitis*, and brain injuries localized in the *ventral* midbrain may also result in locked-in syndrome (Patterson & Grabois, 1986). Other causes of total motor paralysis are degenerative neuromuscular diseases, the most frequent being *amyotrophic lateral sclerosis (ALS)*. This disease involves a continuously progressive degeneration of central and peripheral motor neurons. Most often, paresis begins with the lower extremities and then moves to the hands and arms, finally paralyzing breathing and swallowing as well as facial muscles. At the final stage, patients can stay alive only with artificial feeding and ventilation.

Quality of life and the will to live in paralyzed patients depend essentially on the maintenance of communication (Bach, 1993). To provide these patients with a means of communication independent of voluntary muscle control, the TTD has been developed (Kübler et al., 1998, 1999).

ARRANGEMENT AND HARDWARE OF THE TTD

Figure 21.1A depicts schematically the arrangement of the TTD; Figure 21.1B shows a patient using the system. SCPs are recorded from the vertex (C_z in the International 10-20 system) against two mastoids (A_1 and A_2) and then averaged online to obtain a single mastoid-referenced channel ($\frac{1}{2} [(C_z - A_1) + (C_z - A_2)]$). Silver/silver chloride electrodes are used for recording and are filled with Elefix (Nihon Coden). Abrasive cream is applied to the skin underneath the electrodes to ensure that electrode impedances remain below 5 kiloohms. The brain signals are amplified with an electroencephalographic (EEG) amplifier (EEG 8, Contact Precision Instruments), set to a low-pass filter of 40 hertz and a time constant of 16 seconds, and then digitized with a sampling rate of 256 hertz. Note that the time constant of most commercially available amplifiers is much lower.

Patients sit in armchairs or wheelchairs, viewing a notebook computer's screen on which two rectangles—one at the top and one at the bottom of the screen—and a small (1-centimeter diameter) moving round graphic symbol (referred to as the "cursor") are displayed (see Figure 21.2). Patients are taught to use the TTD at home or in nursing homes. Two to three sessions are conducted per week. A session consists of 10–20 runs, dependent on the patient's attention and motivation, and a run comprises about 100 trials (see next section).

SIGNAL PROCESSING

Rhythmic acoustic signals set the time for generation of an SCP amplitude shift. A high-pitched tone marks the start of a trial, which begins with a 2-second "passive phase," during which the cursor cannot be moved. A low-pitched tone introduces the "active feedback phase," signaling that the cursor can now be moved. The feedback phase lasts for 2–4 seconds, depending on the individual patient's performance. During the last 500 milliseconds (ms) of the passive phase, an online baseline for the SCP feedback calculation is recorded; the mean EEG amplitude within this 500-ms window is set to zero. During the following feedback phase, the current SCP amplitude is calculated every 62.5 ms as an average of the preceding 500 ms (sliding time window). The current position of the cursor corresponds to the amplitude difference between every 500-ms time window in the feedback phase and the 500-ms baseline. At the beginning of every trial, horizontal cursor movement starts at the left margin of the screen

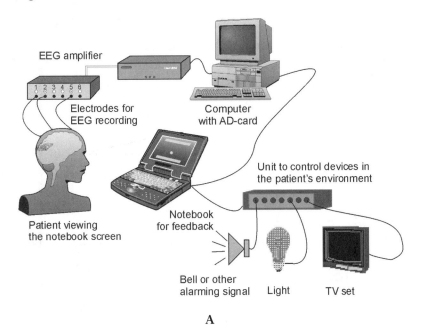

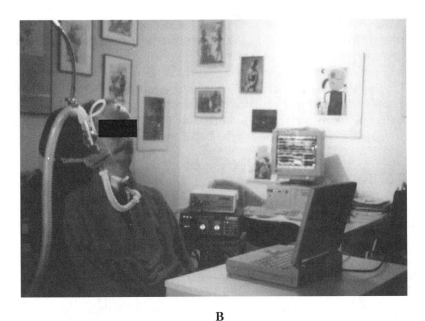

FIGURE 21.1. The Thought Translation Device (TTD). (A) Schematic presentation of the setup. Patients who use the system sit or rest in front of a notebook computer, which provides them with visual feedback of the slow cortical potential (SCP) amplitude. The electroencephalogram (EEG) is recorded with silver/silver chloride electrodes at the vertex. An EEG amplifier transfers the signal to a personal computer with an analog-digital (AD) card. The output signal of the notebook can be used to control external devices (e.g., to ring a bell, to turn a light or TV set on or off), or to communicate verbally with the Language Support Program (LSP). (B) A patient using the TTD at home.

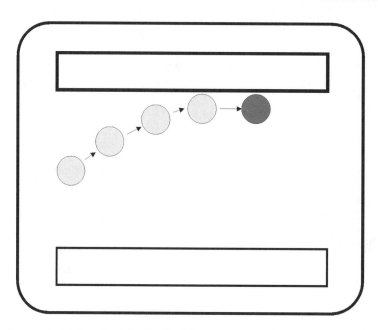

FIGURE 21.2. Screen design for visual feedback of SCPs. Horizontal cursor movement starts at the left margin of the screen. The rectangle toward which the cursor has to be moved is highlighted—in this case, the top rectangle. Vertical cursor movement occurs in proportion to the SCP amplitude.

(see Figure 21.2); vertical cursor movement occurs according to the changes of the SCP amplitude and polarity. If a negative SCP shift (cortical negativity) is produced in the active phase compared to baseline, the cursor moves upward; conversely, when the SCP is more negative during baseline than during the feedback phase (cortical positivity), the cursor moves downward. The SCP amplitude is integrated over the entire feedback phase. If the average SCP amplitude is negative, the trial is regarded as "negativity performed," and if it is positive, the trial is regarded as "positivity performed." The trial is considered invalid and is repeated when the SCP amplitude is on average in the range of –0.5 to 0.5 microvolts.

ARTIFACT CORRECTION

As described by Neumann et al. in Chapter 5, eye movements cause strong artifacts in SCP feedback. For this reason, the *vertical electrooculogram* (*vEOG*) is recorded. The algorithm used for online EOG-correction is based on the fact that the C_z-linked mastoid channel cannot be affected by horizontal eye movements (Kübler et al., 1999). The maximum vEOG influence on the EEG signal at the vertex is assumed to be in the range of 10% (Lutzenberger, Elbert, Rockstroh, & Birbaumer, 1985); therefore, the vEOG is multiplied by 0.1, and this product is then subtracted from the EEG at the vertex. For feedback of SCPs, the correction is calculated for averages of EEG (A_{EEG}) and EOG (A_{EOG}) in a sliding time window of 500 ms. To calculate the vEOG-corrected cursor position at a given time (t), the averaged EEG signal A_{EEG} (t) and the averaged vEOG signal A_{EOG} (t) in the feedback phase are compared to the EEG and vEOG values during baseline (referred to as B_{EEG} and B_{EOG}). Thus the current EEG signal at a given time, or D_{EEG} (t), is calculated as D_{EEG} (t) = $k \cdot$ (B_{EEG} – A_{EEG} (t)), where k is the transformation coefficient of microvolts into screen amplitude values. The current EOG signal at a given time D_{EOG} (t) is calculated as D_{EOG} (t) = $k \cdot$ (B_{EOG} – A_{EOG} (t)). For the EOG correction, three cases need to be distinguished and calculated according to the formulas in Table 21.1.

TABLE 21.1. Artifact Correction for Eye Movement in Three Different Cases

If D_{EEG} (t) and D_{EOG} (t) (averaged EEG and vEOG signals in the feedback phase subtracted from baseline; see text) . . .	Formula	Consequence
(1) have a different sign (amplitudes of different polarity),		No correction necessary.
(2) have the same sign and the EEG amplitude is larger than 10% of the vEOG amplitude—that is, $\lvert D_{EEG}$ $(t)\rvert >$ $\lvert 0.1 \cdot D_{EOG}$ (t) $\rvert$,	D_{EEG_corr} $(t) =$ D_{EEG} $(t) - 0.1 \cdot D_{EOG}$ $(t) =$ $k \cdot [(B_{EEG} - A_{EEG}$ $(t)) -$ $0.1 \cdot (B_{EOG} - A_{EOG}$ $(t))]$	Artifact-corrected EEG signal.
(3) have the same sign and the EEG amplitude is smaller than or equal to 10% of the vEOG amplitude—that is, $\lvert D_{EEG}$ $(t)\rvert \leq \lvert 0.1 \cdot D_{EOG}$ (t) $\rvert$,	A_{EEG} $(t) \leq 0.1 \cdot (B_{EOG} - A_{EOG}$ $(t))$ D_{EEG} $(t) =$ $k \cdot [(B_{EEG} - 0.1 \cdot (B_{EOG} - A_{EOG}$ $(t))) -$ $0.1 \cdot (B_{EOG} - A_{EOG}$ $(t))] =$ $k \cdot B_{EEG}$	No cursor movement; the trial is invalid.

With this correction procedure, cursor control with the aid of eye movement is excluded. The algorithm corrects only those EOG changes with a polarity that coincides with the EEG shift; opposite-direction EOG potentials are not corrected. It implies further that the value subtracted from the current EEG amplitude cannot be larger than the EEG amplitude itself (in case 3 in Table 21.1), the cursor remains in the center of the screen); this prevents over-correction.

THE LANGUAGE SUPPORT PROGRAM

To enable verbal communication mediated by self-regulation of SCPs, patients are provided with the *Language Support Program* (*LSP*; Perelmouter, Kotchoubey, Kübler, Taub, & Birbaumer, 1999). The rectangles on the notebook screen are now used for letter presentation. The German alphabet (including ä, ö, and ü), a space mark, a comma, and a period are split into two subsets, each containing 16 symbols. These two subsets are presented one after another until the patient selects the subset that contains the target letter or mark he or she wants to select. After selection this subset is again split in two, and this is continued until a single symbol is presented for selection. With the "return" and "delete" function keys, patients can correct erroneous selection of a subset or symbol (see Figure 21.3).

The LSP comprises two different versions: *copy spelling* and *free spelling*. In the copy-spelling mode, patients are required to copy symbols or words presented in the top rectangle by the practitioner. In the free-spelling mode, patients can write whatever they want to communicate. The transient phase with the copy-spelling mode is necessary to train the patients to use the acquired skill to self-regulate the SCP amplitude for symbol selection.

STEPS FOR MASTERING THE TTD

With the following steps, patients are enabled to master communication by means of self-regulation of SCPs (Kübler et al., 2001).

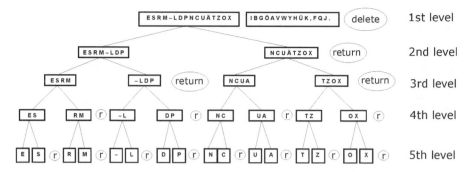

FIGURE 21.3. In the LSP, symbols are presented in a dichotomous manner. At the first level, the whole set of 32 LSP symbols (29 letters, a space mark, a period, and a comma) is subdivided into two letter banks, each containing 16 symbols. The figure shows the division of the first symbol bank up to the 5th level. Letters are arranged according to their incidence in the German language. If the patients select the first symbol bank (E to X), it is again split in two. In the following trial the patients are presented with a symbol bank containing 8 symbols (E to P and N to X). If the patients select a symbol bank erroneously, they have the option to reject the two symbol banks presented at this level and to select the "return" function to return to the previous level. Symbol banks are split in two after selection up to the 5th level, where the symbol bank contains only one symbol for selection. The second symbol bank at the 1st level (I to period) is split in the same way as the E to X symbol bank. At the first level, a "delete" function to erase the last selected symbol is presented. (r, return.)

Step 1: Acquaintance

When patients are confronted with the TTD for the first time, they are advised just to observe the movement of the cursor on the screen in relation to their thoughts. They are encouraged to "play" with the cursor, for example, to try to keep it in the midline of the screen. No particular task has to be performed in each trial during this first step. Patients thus have the opportunity to become familiar with the system, with the electrodes on the scalp, and with cursor movement. Step 1 comprises 2 or 3 runs only and is completed within the first session.

Step 2: Basic Training

In this second step, patients have to learn the self-regulation of their SCP amplitude at the vertex (C_z). For this purpose, the cursor has to be moved toward either the top or bottom rectangle. At the beginning of every trial, one of the rectangles is highlighted to indicate in which direction the cursor has to be moved. Whenever the cursor is moved successfully according to the task requirement, the corresponding rectangle flashes and a smiling face appears (see Figure 21.4), informing the patient that he or she has produced an SCP amplitude of correct polarity. Patients then try to repeat the successful strategy. We do not advise the patients how to move the cursor, because no optimal strategy exists, and strategies vary from subject to subject (Roberts, Birbaumer, Rockstroh, Lutzenberger, & Elbert, 1989). They have to find the most suitable strategy by watching the feedback signal on the screen. This step continues until the patients (1) achieve a percentage of correct responses above 70% in several consecutive runs, (2) increase correct responding to above 75% for a few additional runs, and (3) reveal an increasing trend in the percentage of correct responses throughout this step. A threshold of 70% correct responses is set because with this level of accuracy, verbal communication with the LSP is possible—albeit slowly.

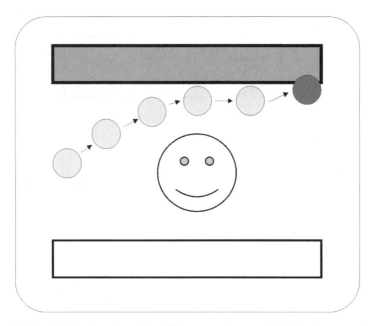

FIGURE 21.4. Feedback during basic training. The rectangle toward which the cursor has to be moved is highlighted. When the cursor is moved according to the task requirement, the rectangle blinks, and a smiling face appears to confirm that the behavior is correct and that the strategy should be followed.

Step 3: Error Ignoring

In order for patients to progress from basic training to verbal communication, the error sensitivity of the system is reduced temporarily. Therefore, this step is called "error ignoring." Symbols (letters or other marks) are presented in the bottom rectangle for selection. In the top rectangle, symbols or words are presented by the practitioner, and the patient is instructed to copy them (see Figure 21.5). Whenever the patient either fails to select a required symbol or selects a wrong one, the program does not react. Instead, the trial is repeated until the correct brain response is performed. Therefore, no false selections can occur; consequently, no wrong symbols appear in the top rectangle, and thus no punishment is given for erroneous brain responses. To introduce this new task slowly, the number of symbols with which patients are presented is increased step by step from 2^2 (4 symbols) to 2^3, 2^4, and finally 2^5 (the entire LSP set of letters and other marks). At first, single symbols have to be copied. As soon as the patient masters this task, the next level of symbols is introduced, and short words have to be copied. Finally, the patient is confronted with the whole set of 32 symbols. Along with an increasing number of symbols, longer words and afterwards short sentences have to be copied. The program records errors for an offline analysis, although this is not visible to the patient.

Step 4: Copy Spelling

The copy-spelling mode of the LSP is introduced when patients master error ignoring according to the criteria described in step 2. Again, patients are required to copy symbols or words presented by the practitioner, but in the copy-spelling mode errors have consequences. Miss-

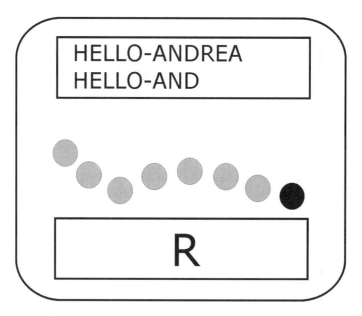

FIGURE 21.5. Copy spelling. Patients have to copy symbols, words, or sentences written in the top rectangle by the practitioner. Symbols are presented in the bottom rectangle for selection. Selected symbols appear in the bottom half of the top rectangle.

ing a subset or symbol means waiting until the subset containing the target symbol or the symbol itself is presented again. When a subset or symbol is selected erroneously, patients have to return to the previous level or to delete the selected symbol. As in error ignoring, the number of symbols with which the patients are presented increased step by step from 4 to the entire set of 32 symbols, and patients have to copy single symbols, then short words, longer words, and finally short sentences. The criteria to decide when to progress to the next level of symbols and to step 5 are the same as described in step 2.

Step 5: Free Spelling

Free spelling is the final step, the goal of the whole procedure. Patients are advised to begin with short words to become accustomed to the new task—not only to copy words, but to imagine which word to write and how to write this word correctly. As in steps 3 and 4, the number of symbols is increased gradually. In the end patients are presented with the whole set of 32 symbols, enabling them to communicate whatever they wish. An individually adapted dictionary is included in the LSP to accelerate the patients' communication speed. The program then suggests words after one letter is selected. The patient can either accept the word by selecting "Accept suggestion?" or select the next letter (see Figure 21.6). Then the dictionary suggests a new word.

LEARNING PROGRESS

The patient's learning progress over time is quantified as the percentage of correct responses per run. To calculate the percentage of correct responses, the patient's SCP amplitude in each trial is compared to the task requirement. Consider a run with 100 trials in which the

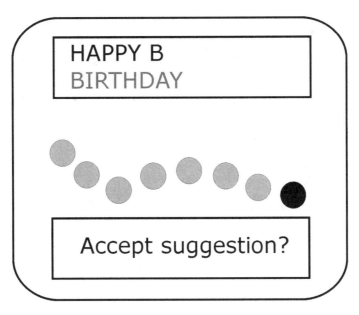

FIGURE 21.6. Free spelling. Patients can write whatever they wish. After selection of a letter, a dictionary suggests a word, which can either be accepted (by selecting the "Accept suggestion?" function) or rejected. In the case of rejection, another letter is selected by the patient, and the dictionary makes another suggestion.

cursor has to be moved upward 60 and downward 40 times, and the patient succeeds 45 times in the upward and 32 times in the downward condition. The correct response rate then would be 75% (45 divided by 60) for upward cursor movement, and 80% (32 divided by 40) for downward cursor movement. The overall percentage of correct responses would be 77% (45 plus 32, divided by 100). The percentage of correct responses has to be calculated for every run and charted continuously during all steps of the learning process (see Figure 21.7). A slowly increasing learning trend should be visible over time.

CONCLUSIONS AND RECOMMENDATIONS

In addition to the LSP, other applications can be controlled by the TTD. Examples include a menu with preset expressions, wishes, and commands, or an apparatus that enables the patients to control the equipment in their environment (see Figure 21.1). The application has to be adapted to the various needs, performance, and learning progress of the individual user.

Readers interested in finding out whether biofeedback of SCPs could serve as the basis for treatment a patient of theirs who is paralyzed, has epilepsy (see Strehl, Chapter 20), or has some other neurological condition, are strongly urged to contact one of the laboratories with widespread expertise and no commercial aims for assistance and supervision (e.g., Kübler or Strehl at the laboratory in Tuebingen). This may prevent both readers and patients from experiencing treatment failure with subsequent disappointment. Readers who are contemplating purchasing a commercial neurofeedback system are similarly advised to consult an internationally known laboratory (e.g., the Tuebingen lab for SCP biofeedback, or the New York State Department of Health in Albany, NY, if feedback of EEG spectral components is

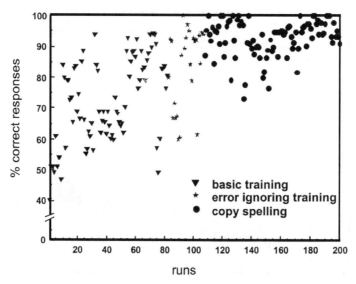

FIGURE 21.7. Learning progress of a patient with amyotrophic lateral sclerosis (ALS). The percentage of correct responses is depicted as a function of runs. At the beginning of basic training, the percentage of correct responses is about 50% (i.e., at the chance level). During step 2 (basic training), the percentage of correct responses increases, and in some runs the patient is better than 90%. At the beginning of step 3 (error ignoring), the patient's performance drops but increases again to above 90%. During step 4 (copy spelling), the patient's performance becomes more and more stable (compared to the high variation during basic training) and is 90% or better most of the time. An increasing linear trend indicates the learning progress over time.

of interest), because not all of these systems actually meet the standards necessary for biofeedback of electrocortical potentials.

GLOSSARY

AMYOTROPHIC LATERAL SCLEROSIS (ALS). A disorder causing progressive loss of control of voluntary muscles because of destruction of nerve cells in the brain and spinal cord. Most often, paresis begins with the lower extremities and then moves on to hands and arms, finally paralyzing breathing and swallowing as well as facial muscles. In the end stage, patients can stay alive only with artificial feeding and ventilation. In most patients with ALS, control of eye muscles, sphincters, and a few face muscles is retained up to the end stage of the disease.

BRAINSTEM. In the mature human brain, the medulla, pons, and midbrain.

ENCEPHALITIS. Inflammation of the brain. The condition is frequently associated with viral infections.

LANGUAGE SUPPORT PROGRAM (LSP). Menu presenting letters to the users of the *Thought Translation Device* (see below), enabling them to communicate verbally.

COPY SPELLING. Mode of the LSP in which letters given by the practitioner have to be copied.

FREE SPELLING. Mode of the LSP in which the users can communicate whatever they wish.

LOCKED-IN SYNDROME. The inability to communicate (i.e., the intact brain is locked in a paralyzed body). In the classic form, vertical eye movements as well as eye blinks remain intact. In the total form, no voluntary muscle movement is possible.

PONS CEREBRI. Part of the brainstem that lies between the medulla (caudal portion of the brainstem) and the midbrain; appears to constitute a bridge between the right and left halves of the cerebellum (large part of the brain with motor functions).

SLOW CORTICAL POTENTIALS (SCPs). Negative or positive polarizations of the EEG that last from 0.3 seconds up to several seconds. (For a full definition, see the glossary in Strehl, Chapter 20, this volume.)

STROKE. A group of brain disorders, involving loss of brain functions, that occur when the blood supply to any part of the brain is interrupted.

TETRAPLEGIA. Paralysis of both lower and upper limbs. Also called "quadriplegia."

THOUGHT TRANSLATION DEVICE (TTD). Direct connection between the brain and a computer controlled by SCPs and used for communication.

VENTRAL. Pertaining to the belly. Denoting a position closer to the belly surface than to some other object of reference.

VERTICAL ELECTROOCULOGRAM (vEOG). Measurement of electrical activity caused by vertical eye movement.

REFERENCES

Allen, C. M. C. (1993). Conscious but paralysed: Releasing the locked-in. *Lancet, 342,* 130–131.

Bach, J. R. (1993). Amyotrophic lateral sclerosis: Communication status and survival with ventilatory support. *American Journal of Physical Medicine and Rehabilitation, 72,* 343–349.

Bauby, J.-D. (1997). *Le scaphandre et le papillon.* Paris: Editions Robert Laffont.

Bauer, G., Gerstenbrand, F., & Rumpl, E. (1979). Variables of the locked-in syndrome. *Journal of Neurology, 221,* 77–91.

Chia, L. G. (1984). Locked-in state with bilateral internal capsule infarcts. *Neurology, 34,* 1365–1367.

Chia, L. G. (1991). Locked-in syndrome with bilateral ventral midbrain infarcts. *Neurology, 41,* 445–446.

Hayashi, H., & Kato, S. (1989). Total manifestations of amyotrophic lateral sclerosis: ALS in the totally locked-in state. *Journal of the Neurological Sciences, 93,* 19–35.

Kübler, A., Kotchoubey, B., Hinterberger, T., Ghanayim, N., Perelmouter, J., Schauer, M., Fritsch, C., Taub, E., & Birbaumer, N. (1999). The Thought Translation Device: A neurophysiological approach to communication in total motor paralysis. *Experimental Brain Research, 124,* 223–232.

Kübler, A., Kotchoubey, B., Kaiser, J., Wolpaw, J. R., & Birbaumer, N. (2001). Brain–computer communication: Unlocking the locked-in. *Psychological Bulletin, 127,* 358–375.

Kübler, A., Kotchoubey, B., Salzmann, H.-P., Ghanayim, N., Perelmouter, J., Hömberg, V., & Birbaumer, N. (1998). Self-regulation of slow cortical potentials in completely paralyzed human patients. *Neuroscience Letters, 252,* 171–174.

Kübler, A., Neumann, N., Kaiser, J., Kotchoubey, B., Hinterberger, T., & Birbaumer, N. (2001). Brain–computer communication: Self-regulation of slow cortical potentials for verbal communication. *Archives of Physical Medicine and Rehabilitation, 82,* 1533–1539.

Lutzenberger, W., Elbert, T., Rockstroh, B., & Birbaumer, N. (1985). *Das EEG.* Berlin: Springer-Verlag.

Patterson, J. R., & Grabois, M. (1986). Locked-in syndrome: A review of 139 cases. *Stroke, 17,* 758–764.

Perelmouter, J., Kotchoubey, B., Kübler, A., Taub, E., & Birbaumer, N. (1999). A Language Support Program for Thought-Translation-Devices. *Automedica, 18,* 67–84.

Roberts, L., Birbaumer, N., Rockstroh, B., Lutzenberger, W., & Elbert, T. (1989). Self-report during feedback regulation of slow cortical potentials. *Psychophysiology, 26*(4), 392–403.

PART VII

Neuromuscular Applications

CHAPTER 22

Biofeedback in Neuromuscular Reeducation and Gait Training

DAVID E. KREBS
TIMOTHY L. FAGERSON

Biofeedback is increasingly used in neuromuscular reeducation and gait training, largely because of the growing consensus in rehabilitation about the importance of motor learning. The two key ingredients in motor learning are practice and feedback (Schmidt, 1988). Properly understood and applied, biofeedback is an excellent tool for enhancing practice and performance of motor skills. The purpose of this chapter is to review the rationale and methods for using biofeedback to augment neuromuscular reeducation and gait training. (As in other chapters with glossaries, italics on first use of a term in this chapter indicate that the term is included in the glossary.)

REVIEW OF REQUIREMENTS FOR INFORMATION FEEDBACK

Some Motor Learning Considerations

Feedback must be relevant in order to enhance learning. Therapists are well aware that providing verbal cues can improve motor performance. This feedback may, for example, be in the form of verbal cues to focus attention on *agonist* muscles, praise for the patient who has just mastered straight-leg raising after *knee arthrotomy*, or congratulations to the child who has for the first time gained control of a prosthetic myoelectric hand.

Studies of specificity of information, in which, for example, subjects are asked to pitch a ball at a target, demonstrate that performance decrements can occur with each piece of lost information. However, the converse may not be true; that is, more feedback is not necessarily better. The timing and type of feedback, whether exogenous or endogenous, may be as important as the amount of feedback. General verbal encouragement is often a relatively nonspecific and inefficient means of aiding motor performance. In addition, there are the frequent long delays (i.e., latency) between completion of tasks by patients and the provision of verbal feedback by therapists. In some cases, however, these delays may actually be more effective than immediate biofeedback in motor performance enhancement (Gable, Shea, & Wright, 1991).

Although therapists may describe the location of agonist and *antagonist* muscles, and even make attempts to describe the "feelings" patients should experience if the proper muscles are used appropriately, there is still no way to communicate which motor units to activate. How should the motor units be recruited? Should they be activated synchronously or asynchronously? Surface electromyographic (EMG) biofeedback can provide some useful information regarding motor unit activity that patients do not otherwise have available.

Disagreement exists regarding the utility of providing EMG feedback, because most forms of feedback are tantamount to merely communicating "more" or "less" EMG activity. The information provided to patients via current technology is decidedly unsophisticated and incomplete, compared to that which intact nervous systems can provide during muscle contractions. Therefore, many therapists prefer to work with devices that directly measure and feed back force or joint range of motion (ROM). This preference is based on the assumption that EMG signals are not sufficiently informative or sophisticated to be true "process" feedback, and that EMG does not adequately reflect actual outcome (e.g., limb displacement or torque) to provide accurate knowledge of results. This is discussed further below.

In summary, feedback must be accurate and relevant in order to qualify as assistance in neuromuscular reeducation.

Speed of Information

Feedback must be timely with regard to therapy tasks. Several studies have demonstrated that the utility of feedback from the environment is greatest in unfamiliar tasks, and that feedback is nearly worthless or even counterproductive in well-learned, rapid movements (e.g., typing or playing the piano) (Mulder & Hulstyn, 1984). The fastest cortical feedback loops (i.e., those loops that could reflect changes in environmental conditions) have latencies of at least 100–200 milliseconds. For example, a pianist performing a fast "run" cannot possibly rely on visual or auditory feedback during the "run." If a mistake has occurred, several more notes will be played (i.e., about 0.2 seconds of music) before any adjustments to the motor plan can be made. At that point, the performer must make a decision to ignore the mistake or to back up and correct it. Either way, timely auditory feedback is critical.

Ambulation also requires a series of preplanned motor events. If a disruption occurs, feedback of the "mistake" must be acted upon and built into the plan for ensuing steps. Normal walking speed is about 1 cycle per second. *Ankle dorsiflexors*, for example, must resist foot slap from heel strike to foot flat for about 60 milliseconds. Therapists attempting to encourage normal gait in hemiplegic patients by using feedback from dorsiflexor EMG cannot possibly hope for correction of inadequate dorsiflexor motor unit activity during that gait cycle. The information is that EMG activity was inadequate during the past gait cycle, and patients must therefore figure out how to increase that activity before ensuing heel strikes.

In addition to endogenous latencies within patients, most EMG biofeedback instruments have built-in integrators or averages, which may slow the signal within the instruments. Furthermore, all EMG processors delay electrical events during amplification. A further latency results at the audio speaker and visual meter because of inherent mechanical delays from inertia. In short, most commercial EMG feedback instruments introduce delays of 50–100 milliseconds before the signal can even reach the ears and eyes of patients.

Summary of Requirements for Information Feedback

Information to be fed back to patients must be relevant and timely to be of therapeutic use. Therapists must choose, from a variety of modalities, the instrument or device that provides the most meaningful information to patients. Commercially available EMG instruments can provide timely feedback if the events being monitored are at least 0.5 seconds in duration. Thus, for feedback during 5-second isometric contractions, adequate time may be available for patients to adjust the motor program and change the number of motor units being activated during contractions. During most functional activities, however, the "feedback" acts as an error signal or knowledge of results, to be used in planning future skeletal movements. For amputees, prosthetic feedback during training may help compensate for severed sensory systems. The following sections examine some applications of biofeedback in the rehabilitation of patients with neuromotor dysfunction and amputation.

NEUROMUSCULAR REEDUCATION USING EMG FEEDBACK

In this section, the origins of the EMG signal are briefly reviewed, and its progress is traced on a hypothetical round trip from a patient's central nervous system (CNS)—starting with the intention to move, through monitoring instrumentation, and back to the CNS for the patient to reprocess (i.e., proprioception and *exteroception*). The astute reader will note that, as in any other journey, a potential problem lurks at every junction and intermediate step. This section should help therapists to avoid those hazards, or at least to recognize them.

Muscle Physiology: Where Does the EMG Signal Arise?

After the CNS causes the anterior horn cell to discharge, the motor nerve depolarizes, conducting its electrical current about 40–60 meters per second. Because a motor unit is, by definition, the anterior horn cell, its nerve, and all the muscle fibers it innervates, the amount of muscle to be excited depends upon the size of the motor field (i.e., the number of muscle fibers innervated by each anterior horn cell and its axon). In EMG feedback, we most often use surface electrodes that sum all potentials beneath their surfaces.

The size of a motor unit varies among muscles. Skeletal muscles that require very fine control, such as the extraocular or intrinsic hand muscles, have very few muscle fibers in one motor unit—often as few as four to five fibers per anterior horn cell. Conversely, large postural muscles need less fine control and may have as many as 1000 muscle fibers supplied by a single anterior horn cell.

Variations also exist within muscles. By differentially recruiting large and small motor units within a muscle, the CNS has the ability to activate the same motor units over and over again, to do so more quickly or slowly, and to apportion the amount of muscle firing to the tension generation requirements. That is, at least two recruitment methods can increase tension within a given muscle: activating more motor units, increasing the motor unit firing rate, or both.

Controversy exists regarding the preferred recruitment training method for use with patients having very low levels of muscle activation. Therefore, the patient with *paretic muscles* who is being trained to increase EMG signals may be learning to recruit more motor units or to activate the same motor units more quickly; most EMG biofeedback instruments cannot discriminate between these two methods, and in any case, it is unknown which recruitment method is more therapeutic. The rectified and smoothed EMG signal will increase whether these patients are developing increased activation of small motor units more rapidly and synchronously, or a greater number of units are being recruited. After the terminal branches of a motor nerve have discharged, the action potential hits the neuromuscular junction. The distal end of the nerve releases *acetylcholine*, which diffuses across the *synaptic cleft* to begin the *muscle action potential* (see Figure 22.1). The acetylcholine receptors cause the muscle action potential to occur, in the "sarcolemma," or jacket, surrounding the muscle (Greek, *sarcos* = "flesh," *lemma* = "sheath"). The sarcolemmal depolarization (action potential) is much slower than the nerve action potential propagation. It is this sarcolemmal electrical event that the EMG instrument records. After the electrical excitation travels through the muscle, the action potential reaches a storage area for calcium ions, the *sarcoplasmic reticulum*. Only after the electrical depolarization reaches this storage area and causes calcium to be released does the mechanical event—muscle contraction—occur. That is, the nerve action potential travels about 60 meters per second, reaches the muscle, and causes a chemical reaction that causes another electrical event, the muscle action potential, traveling at about 5 meters per second. The muscle electrical action potential normally results in calcium ion release, which in turn causes tension (force) production by the muscle.

The preceding paragraph indicates clearly that measuring a muscle's electrical production with EMG is *not* equivalent to measuring the muscle's tension production. A common example may help clarify the difference between a muscle's electrical and mechanical events. Most people have experienced a "charley horse." These painful muscle contractions are apparently the result of the spontaneous calcium liberation from the sarcoplasmic reticulum. They have no EMG activity associated with them, because no sarcolemmal discharge precedes the mechanical event. That probably explains why one cannot stop a charley horse by voluntarily contracting the muscle. Mechanically stretching the muscle, which dissociates the actomyosin and allows the calcium to return to the sarcoplasmic reticulum, however, promptly relieves the pain.

In short, measuring muscles' electrical activity with EMG is not synonymous with specifically measuring muscle activity. Some discussion of this is provided by Peek in Chapter 4 of this volume. A more detailed discussion of the biochemical and electrical activity is be-

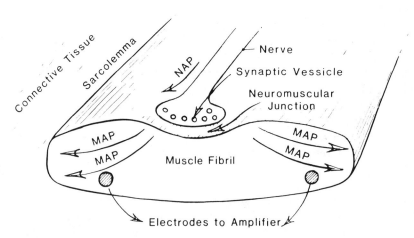

FIGURE 22.1. Schematic representation of neuromuscular electrical events. Following nerve depolarization, the nerve action potential (NAP) travels distally to the synaptic vesicles, which release acetylcholine across the synaptic cleft at the neuromuscular junction. The resulting muscle action potential (MAP) is the event recorded by the EMG, whether via intramuscular electrodes (shown) or surface electrodes.

yond the scope of this chapter. The important point for biofeedback is that the EMG signal arises before, and occasionally independently of, muscle mechanical activity, so the EMG device can indeed be misleading.

Relationship between the EMG Device's Signals and Normal Muscle Activity

The EMG biofeedback device is simply a very sensitive voltmeter. Like any voltmeter, EMG instruments can only measure electrical signals if one pole of an instrument is negative with respect to the other pole. After the electrical signal is measured, most biofeedback instruments "condition" EMG signals so that positive and negative impulses are "rectified" (the machine finds the signal's absolute amplitude); then the device "smooths" (filters) the signal prior to display, to decrease the normal, minor fluctuations present in the muscle's electrical output. Thus, although the electrical event within the patient occurs prior to the mechanical contraction, the mechanical event may be over by the time the EMG machine "conditions" the signal for feedback to patients. Of course, these delays are on the order of milliseconds; nonetheless, the type of signal processing affects the feedback delivered to the patient.

The primary features of an EMG biofeedback device that govern the fidelity of the signal produced are *input impedance, common-mode rejection ratio (CMRR),* bandwidth, noise, and electrode type.

Input Impedance

Any intervening tissue between the muscle and the electrode can resist (impede) the muscles' electrical signal. *Ohm's law* states that resistance (impedance) is inversely related to voltage. Because skin resistance varies but internal resistance from fat and other tissues probably remains constant within a given limb segment, only skin resistance is typically a concern. If a large resistance is found at the skin, the measured muscle signals will be reduced. If, on the other hand, the EMG machine's impedance is much greater than skin impedance, a more valid measure of the muscle's electrical activity will be obtained. The clinical relevance of Ohm's law is that EMG instruments should have at least 1000 times as much input impedance as that measured between the two active electrodes.

Common-Mode Rejection Ratio

Modern EMG instruments use differential amplifiers. The advantage of the differential recording system is its "rejection" of extraneous voltages. Although we may not be aware of it, patients' skin receives a great many voltages (such as from lights, motors, and other appliances), which produce currents that travel through the air and can affect the recordings on the skin. Muscles other than the ones of interest (e.g., the myocardium) also produce voltages within patients' bodies. If the electricity from these other sources reaches the two active electrodes simultaneously, the differential amplifier will "reject" those artifactual signals.

The voltage from lights and other exogenous generators nearly always reaches the two skin electrodes simultaneously, so room current (60 hertz) interference is often minimal if common-mode rejection ratio (CMRR) is high enough. Myocardial activity, however, is often a problem when recording near the heart, such as on the chest or upper back. Since the anatomical progression of the cardiac "R" wave is well known, therapists who perceive a regularly alternating signal unrelated to the skeletal muscle(s) of interest should refer to a vector cardiography map and place the electrodes perpendicular to the progression of the R wave, so that the electrocardiographic (EKG) signal arrives at both electrodes concurrently. In practice, it is usually sufficient simply to experiment with different electrode placements until the EKG artifact is minimized.

CMRR is not perfect. If a 60-hertz signal interferes with a therapy session, the therapist should turn off the room lights or look for a nearby whirlpool or diathermy machine as the culprit. An ungrounded appliance operating from the same electrical circuit as the EMG feedback instrument will occasionally interfere with EMG recordings. If the EMG instrument cannot operate on batteries, then the therapist should disconnect the ungrounded appliance. Electricians can install an outlet isolated from other appliances, thus eliminating feedback interference from power lines.

As with input impedance, higher is better. CMRRs should be at least 200,000:1. If the muscles being monitored are especially paretic and generate only a few microvolts, then large amplifier gains are required; large gains, unfortunately, also amplify the artifacts. Therefore, high CMRRs are especially important when therapists are recording the low myoelectric signals common in neuromuscular reeducation.

Frequency Response (Bandwidth)

"Bandwidth" is the range between the lowest and highest frequency detected by an EMG instrument. Consider the difference between the treble (high-frequency) and bass (low-frequency) pitch settings of a stereo player's tone control. Some stereos have a broader frequency range (more bass, usually) than others. Similarly, EMG amplifiers vary in their frequency bandwidth. Although most of the power at surface kinesiological EMG recordings is between 20 and 300 hertz, instrument responsiveness (bandwidth) relates not only to the frequency of the monitored signal, but also to how quickly the signal changes. Therefore, monitoring rapid, transient movements like piano "runs" requires a bandwidth of up to 500 hertz.

Noise Level of EMG Instruments

In information theory, "noise" is anything that interferes with the information being sampled. Noise intrinsic to the recorder is most problematic when one is amplifying signals from paretic muscles. The high gains necessary to amplify the electrical signal from a weak muscle contraction also amplify the noise of the instrument. In instruments with, for example, a noise level of 2 microvolts, trying to feed back a 0.8-microvolt contraction is impossible, because the signal-to-noise ratio is too low.

In general, the lower the noise, the better. Fortunately, most commercially available instruments have noise levels of less than 2 microvolts.

Electrode Type

Electrodes used with modern EMG biofeedback devices are usually active. Today, active electrodes are preferred to passive electrodes. An active electrode has, within its housing, the electronics needed to amplify the signal from the muscle. Amplifying the signal at the skin surface negates artifact picked up while the signal travels to the amplifier. In other words, the signal leaving the electrode now has a large voltage, so that any artifact picked up thereafter is relatively insignificant. This helps greatly in reducing the significance of movement artifact and *volume-conducted artifact*. Most authorities agree that a fixed interelectrode distance (e.g., 1 centimeter) is preferred. Fixed-distance active electrodes are usually 1-centimeter-diameter discs or 1-centimeter-long bars with a 2- or 3-centimeter interelectrode distance. If a wider interelectrode distance or larger electrode size is required, electrodes can be attached to the preamplifier via short leads; this will still allow one to reap the benefits of signal amplification close to the source (De Luca, 1994).

EMG as a Kinesiological Monitor during Movement

Even if artifacts are eliminated, a "clean" EMG signal must be interpreted with caution. Many researchers have shown that EMG amplitude is linearly related to force production only under isometric conditions. Since the 1950s, it has been known that once joint movement occurs, the EMG–force relationship depends upon the speed of contraction and the length of the associated muscle (Lenman, 1959; Lippold, 1952). It is well known that muscles exert greater or lesser force in a given joint at different points in the ROM because of biomechanical factors, such as changes in the joint's lever arm and the degree of sarcomere (i.e., actomyosin) overlap. Much less is known about neurophysiological influences governing muscle activity over different arcs of motion within the same joint (Basmajian, 1974).

To investigate the neurophysiological mechanisms of muscle control, one of us (Krebs) studied the effects of knee and hip joint positions on EMG amplitude of normal, maximally contracting *quadriceps muscles* and those of patients with joint mechanoreceptor deficits (Krebs, Stables, Cuttita, & Zickel, 1983). In normal subjects, maximum EMG activity occurred with the knees and hips at 0° flexion; less EMG amplitude was observed with knees and hips flexed, although all subjects were requested to give maximal effort in all positions.

Patients who had recent anterior joint capsule incisions following *meniscectomy* responded quite differently from normal subjects. Maximum EMG activity was found in the affected limb with the knee at 30° knee flexion and the hip at 15° flexion. Krebs and his colleagues concluded that motor unit activity depends not only on joint angle, but also upon the integrity of the joint structures. Therefore, the neurophysiological control and activation of muscles with disruption of their peripheral joint receptors may be very different from those of normal limbs, even during maximal effort and at equivalent joint angles.

Activation aside, what information does EMG amplitude contain regarding force output? Under isometric conditions and equivalent joint angles, force and EMG are at least approximately linearly related for an individual subject: An increase in EMG amplitude is accompanied by a proportional increase in force production. This relationship also appears to hold if only length is changed. Nelson (1976) at New York University (NYU) demonstrated that subjects performing constant-speed (isokinetic) exercise show a proportional increase in force output and in EMG amplitude.

Functional activities, however, rarely occur at either constant speed or constant muscle length, the only known conditions under which EMG amplitude is a valid predictor of force output. Nearly all biofeedback sessions include procedures with active, functional movements. During functional movement, force, muscle length, joint position, and movement velocity change freely (Keefe & Surwit, 1978). Under such conditions, therapists must not equate increases in EMG amplitude with functional gains or muscle force improvement. Some studies show a weak relationship between EMG amplitude increases and functional gains, but large numbers of subjects are required to show a statistically significant effect (Krebs, 1989). Even in laboratory settings with sophisticated equipment, the EMG output for a given activity in a given subject can be significantly variable (Shiavi, Champion, Freeman, & Griffin, 1981).

The comments above are not intended to suggest that no relationship exists between EMG and limb force output from muscles contracting at various speeds. Rather, the relationship is simply unknown. Krebs and colleagues have reported that maximum EMG amplitude, *Manual Muscle Test* (*MMT*) scores, and isokinetic scores are significantly correlated, at least in severely paretic quadriceps muscles following knee arthrotomy (Krebs, Stables, Cuttita, Chui, & Zickel, 1982). The relationship, however, is a moderate one ($r = .70$). That is, as patients recover following surgery, functional and muscle power improvements may in part result from improvements in recruitment of motor units.

Recruitment of motor units may be aided by EMG biofeedback. Much more research is needed before EMG biofeedback can provide valid information to patients under movement conditions. In the meantime, most of us will simply view the EMG amplitude "with a grain of salt," and will depend upon other objective means for validating the efficacy of biofeedback in motor learning.

Summary

Instruments used for neuromuscular reeducation biofeedback must be of the same quality as those used in kinesiological EMG measurement to obtain "clean" and useful signals. Surface electrodes summate the electrical muscle action potentials, which are filtered and attenuated as they pass through body tissues. Most biofeedback instruments then rectify and smooth the signal to provide an indication of the absolute amplitude of muscle activity. Skin resistance should be minimal (e.g., less than 1000 ohms), whereas the input impedance should be as large as feasible (i.e., at least 1 *megohm*), so the muscle voltage will be accurately conveyed to the amplifier and then to the patient. High CMRRs (e.g., 200,000:1 or more) should also be sought from EMG instruments to minimize artifacts present at both electrodes.

Therapists must be especially careful to eliminate electrocardiographic, power-line, movement, and volume-conducted artifacts. Some artifacts can be controlled electronically. Filters, such as for 60-hertz artifact, may be used to selectively suppress frequencies that commonly contain more noise than signal. For biofeedback with a notebook computer, noise reduction cables are available. However, surface EMG has most of its power in the bandwidth of 20–200 hertz, so instruments with restricted bandwidth (e.g., "60-hertz notch filters") generally should be avoided. A frequency response or bandwidth of 20–1000 hertz is adequate for kinesiological EMG feedback. Machine noise levels of less than 2 microvolts are necessary for use with paretic muscles.

Use of EMG Feedback in Clinical Settings

Having considered some limitations of the EMG signal, we can now turn to clinical applications. We must bear in mind the sources of contamination of EMG signals, because the unlearning of bad habits formed by inadvertently feeding back artifact or "unclean" EMG signals is not only of no benefit; it may actually make the condition worse. The following discussion assumes that the therapist has obtained a clean signal and now wants to proceed with treatment.

General Considerations

A behavioral paradigm of positive reinforcement is with the norm in biofeedback (Barton & Wolf, 1992). When patients generate appropriate motor behaviors, they are positively reinforced. Rewarding or positively reinforcing motor activity is frequently done verbally, with therapists commenting on the patients' progress in an effort to shape the motor responses toward normality. The audio and visual feedback, however, are usually much faster and more accurate than a therapist's comments. Even if a patient does not fully understand the feedback signals, the therapist's knowledge of that patient's kinesiology should be enhanced by the biofeedback signals. The therapist's increased access to the patient's physiological functions probably underlies much of the reported successes of biofeedback as a treatment (Krebs, 1989).

We most often use a "two-thirds success" criterion. That is, the "magnitude threshold" for hearing the audio feedback or turning on the visual feedback is set so that, on the average, patients achieve success on two-thirds of their attempts that are in the correct direction. We make no claim that this two-thirds ratio has been scientifically validated, but we find it a useful starting point for most neuromuscular reeducation applications. If the "success" criterion is achieved too often, the patients are not challenged; if "success" is achieved on fewer than 50% of the trials, the patients tend to become frustrated, hence diminishing their motivation.

Biofeedback is slower and less complete than natural proprioception. Therapists should relate patients' kinesthetic feelings during functional tasks to the EMG feedback during successful movements. After patients regularly attain the target criteria, they are requested to perform the activities without feedback. Then it becomes clear whether patients have learned the tasks and whether they can generalize the internal sensations achieved during activities performed with feedback to those performed without feedback (e.g., during home exercises). Thus merely learning to control the audio or visual feedback signals is functionally useless. The ability to call upon the internal correlates of useful movement without biofeedback is the hallmark of successful training.

Treatment Overview

In general, a therapist should start with easy tasks and progressively make the activities more difficult (i.e., more functional). One method is the following. First, the therapist explains the task to the patient, perhaps demonstrating with the therapist's own limbs. At this point, electrodes may be attached to the patient's contralateral limb, if it is uninjured, so the task may be understood and "normal" EMG levels established. If both a patient's limbs are affected, we often attach the electrodes to one of our own muscles and demonstrate exactly what the patient is expected to do. The therapist's familiarity with the instrument, and a simple explanation of what the EMG is measuring, can accelerate the patient's understanding and achievement of the motor task.

When feedback is obtained from a paretic muscle, the thresholds must initially be set very low (or the gains set very high), so any muscle activity results in audio or visual feedback. Establishing and recording a baseline are important, so that progress within the first session and during subsequent sessions can be compared (see Figure 22.2). To enhance the validity of the initial assessment, a maximum isometric contraction of the monitored muscle is requested, and the criterion thresholds and gains are adjusted accordingly.

After maximum activity is recorded, the therapist should set the instrument so that achievement of the criterion occurs on about two-thirds of the trials, as noted above. A period of 5–10 minutes of working with any one muscle group is usually the maximum desirable time, since longer periods seem to lead to fatigue, boredom, and thus less than optimal learning. After amplitude improvement occurs, the patient should be trained for temporal muscle activity control (ability to rapidly activate motor units) (see Figure 22.3, last two lines). One way of accomplishing this with EMG biofeedback instruments is to set a time limit and amplitude threshold, asking the patient to reach the threshold as many times as possible within the time limit. We use a microvolt level of about 60–80% maximum isometric activity, and count the number of times the threshold light comes on during a 10-second trial. For a valid trial to be scored, the muscle must relax completely between each repetition (i.e., the meter must return to the relaxation level before the next attempt is made to exceed the threshold). The relaxation requirement is especially difficult for patients

Patient   Hosp.   Date of

Name: _____   #: _____   Exam: _____

Birthdate: _____ Sex: _____ Duration/Onset Date: _____

See attached appendices for problem-specific evaluation forms, if any.

PROM:

MMT:

DTRs: <u>BJ</u> <u>TJ</u> <u>KJ</u> <u>AJ</u> <u>Clonus</u> <u>Babinski</u> <u>Hoffman</u>

Right:
Left:

Sensory and Proprioception:

ADL and Gait:

Other Therapies/Information:

Skin Condition: Atrophic?   Obesity?   Skin Preparation:

BF Device Used: Electrode Size: Separation Distance:

Electrode Placement:

Pretreatment: Resting Level: Maximum Isometric 12 sec.):

Treatment: Threshold Settings:

Posttreatment: Reseting: Max. lsometric

Electrode Placement, Size, and Preparation of Other Muscles:

Pretreatment: Resting Level: Max. Isometric:

Posttreatment: Resting Level: Max. Isometric:

Electrode Placement, Size, and Preparation of Other Muscles:

Pretreatment: Resting Level: Max. Isometric:

Posttreatment: Resting Level: Max. Isometric:

FIGURE 22.2. Initial evaluation form for neuromuscular reeducation via biofeedback. PROM, passive range of motion; DTRs, deep tendon reflexes; BJ, biceps jerk; TJ, triceps jerk; KJ, knee jerk; AJ, ankle jerk. Developed by David E. Krebs for use at St. Luke's Hospital Center Biofeedback Clinic, New York, NY; used by permission of St. Luke's Hospital.

Name: _____ Hosp. #: _____ Date: _____

Home Practice Regimen:

Functional Status:

Treatment Strategy:

    Muscle(s):   Skin Preparation: Device:

    Electrode Size: Separation Distance:

Pretreatment:

Threshold Settings (Best):

Posttreatment:

Rapid Alternating Activity Increase and Decrease:

Goals: Time:

FIGURE 22.3. Treatment record form for neuromuscular reeducation via biofeedback. Used by permission of St. Luke's Hospital, New York, NY.

with spasticity, so care should be taken not to frustrate a patient by performing this test too early in the course of treatment.

Sophisticated EMG instruments can calculate the rate of increase in EMG for each contraction. Higher rates of isometric EMG development mean faster tension development. This task may be made more functional, and more difficult, by making it contingent upon simultaneous relaxation of the antagonist and/or other muscles.

There is now good evidence that EMG biofeedback is an effective adjunct in restoring motor function to patients with hemiplegia (Schleenbaker & Mainous, 1993). In our experience, normalization of hemiplegic gait may require development of rapid dorsiflexor tension with concomitant relaxation of spastic plantar flexors. For example, requesting rapid alternating 0- to 60-microvolt relaxation and activation of the *anterior tibialis* muscle for 10 seconds, while maintaining electrical silence in the *triceps surae*, is a difficult task, but patients who improve their performance on this test seem to walk better. It seems especially helpful to have patients perform this test while standing, although this functional position makes the rapid EMG activity alternations more difficult.

At minimum, therapy must be functionally relevant. Attention to mobility and muscle power must not be neglected in favor of biofeedback therapy. Biofeedback is only a tool to aid therapeutic exercise. If the exercises are inappropriate, they will remain so even after feedback is added. If biofeedback-assisted skills cannot be generalized to functional situations, patients and therapists have wasted their time. Therefore, patients must always be asked to perform activities of daily living (ADLs) without feedback as tests of the efficacy of the treatment regimen by timing or rating the task in some way (e.g., see Figure 22.3, third line).

However, the clinical situation is rarely a sufficient test. The clinical environment may differ radically from a patient's normal surroundings (see Cataldo, Bird, & Cunningham, 1978). The clinical office setting may be quite different from the situation on the street outside, or on the subway or bus. Only after a patient can perform the activities without feedback in his or her normal, open environment should a therapist feel that treatment has been successful.

Summary

In summary, patients with neuromuscular impairments often need movement reeducation. Biofeedback does not reeducate; therapists and practice do. Used properly, biofeedback may be a useful adjunct to therapeutic exercise (Inglis, Campbell, & Donald, 1976; Schleenbaker & Mainous, 1993).

The critical elements of success with biofeedback-enhanced therapeutic exercise are as follows:

1. The task should be explained clearly, with a demonstration on the unimpaired side if possible.

2. As biofeedback success occurs, the tasks should be incremented toward function and no-feedback conditions.

3. The therapist must be sure to test the patient's progress on functional tasks. Therapy that teaches control of audio signals, meters, and lights may be seductive to the therapist, but it does not help the patient!

Clinical Example: EMG Feedback of Quadriceps Activity for Patients with Postmeniscectomy Quadricep Muscle Weakness

Patients with paretic muscles from lower motor neuropathy or with postsurgical muscle weakness appear to benefit greatly, at least in muscle performance, from biofeedback-assisted therapeutic exercises. It should be borne in mind that ROM, ambulation, and ADL instructions may be higher priorities than muscle power enhancement for some paretic patients. The message here, as throughout this chapter, is that therapists should not suspend their clinical judgment for this "magic" therapy; patients should be treated according to their functional needs, not according to what equipment is available.

We find EMG feedback helpful for muscles with MMT scores of "fair-plus" (F+) or below. Stronger muscles can and should be given resistive exercises rather than EMG feedback. Consider the typical patient referred following knee arthrotomy. The patient is unable to do a straight-leg raise, and ipsilateral quadriceps activity is barely palpable—certainly less than F+. The usual treatment regimen might include 20 minutes of "quad setting" (i.e., isometric contraction of quadriceps with the knee and hip at 0°), straight-leg raising, and gait training, if possible. Biofeedback can be very useful in such cases.

A study by one of us (Krebs) randomly assigned patients to two groups; he found that the "conventional" treatment group achieved only one-tenth as much improvement in EMG activity as, and significantly less improvement in MMT scores than, the group receiving the identical regimen using EMG feedback (Krebs, 1981). A later paper, however, showed that the usual "quad set" position (hip and knee at 0° is not optimal for developing maximum EMG activity in postmeniscectomy quadriceps (Krebs et al., 1983). Flexion of 0° apparently inhibits the quadriceps in postmeniscectomy limbs, whereas slight flexion enhances motor unit activity. A logical synthesis of currently available information is needed to optimize treatment regimens, since a definitive empirical study of postarthrotomy recovery has yet to be reported. The following treatment description incorporates elements from basic physical therapy procedures, from research, and from general biofeedback considerations.

Before treatment, a thorough history and a physical examination are conducted. The latter includes an assessment of upper-extremity muscle power and sitting–standing balance, to determine whether gait training can be accomplished with crutches or other assistive devices. The patient's motivation, psychological status, and discharge plans are also reviewed. Discharge planning should determine whether unusual barriers (such as carpets or stairs) that would impede independent function with assisting devices are present in patients' homes. Outpatient follow-up care may then be more adequately planned.

Because improvement of one muscle, the quadriceps femoris, is the primary goal of strengthening exercises, a one-channel (one-muscle) EMG feedback instrument may be used. The affected limb is placed on a "short-arc quad board" (see Figure 22.4), which positions the knee at 30° and the hip in enough flexion to accommodate the knee flexion.

The electrode sites are then chosen. Because the quadriceps muscles are multipennate (i.e., the fibers run in many directions), nearly any electrode placement on the skin is acceptable as long as the placement is as remote as possible from other superficial muscles, such as adductors and hamstrings. The location of the electrodes must be marked on the skin and noted in the patient's record for replication during ensuing therapy sessions (see Figure 22.5). It is most convenient simply to develop a consistent placement for each muscle, which is used for all treatment sessions. Such a standardized placement speeds application of electrodes and enhances comparability of between-session recordings of EMG activity without confounding the measures by variability of electrode placements.

The therapist should abrade the chosen electrode site, and then wipe the site with alcohol to prepare the skin. If unusually thick epithelium, skin atrophy, excessive oil, or dirt is present, a more extensive skin preparation is performed. Often merely wiping the skin vigorously with alcohol "prep" pads or cotton-soaked with alcohol will result in the pinkish hue indicative of hyperemia, and hence minimal skin resistance.

The patient is then asked, "Straighten your leg as hard as you can; make a muscle with your thigh." After several such efforts without feedback to the patient have been recorded for baseline assessment, the biofeedback training can begin. The patient is instructed in the use of EMG biofeedback during isometric exercise. The therapist may say,

"Use the instrument to help you know when the muscle is active. The higher the meter reading, the stronger your muscle contraction. Experiment with different speeds of tightening the muscle and other methods. Try to make the reading as high as possible, by straightening your knee."

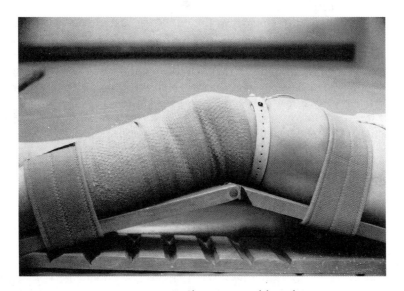

FIGURE 22.4. Short-arc quad board.

Patient: Date:

Meniscectomy type and location:

Age: Sex:

Tourniquet time:

Location of electrodes:

Spacing:

Date of operation:

		Day 1	Day 2	Day 3	Day 4
Resting microvolts	Pre				
	Post				
Maximum microvolts	Pre				
	Post				
Muscle grade or	Pre				
straight-leg raise	Post				
Crutch walking:					
Weight bearing?					

FIGURE 22.5. Treatment record form for biofeedback therapy for patients with postmeniscectomy paresis. Used by permission of St. Luke's Hospital, New York, NY.

After 10 minutes or a little longer, the patient may be reassessed, the results recorded on a form such as that shown in Figure 22.5, and the EMG instrument disconnected. Instructions in active knee extension and straight-leg raising then begin. Once the patient can do a straight-leg raise, gait instructions with weight bearing to tolerance usually follow.

After the patient can easily generate maximum motor unit activity and the MMT score is "good-minus" (G–) or greater, active resistive exercises replace EMG feedback.

Let us briefly consider the perceived disadvantages of EMG biofeedback. Therapists have complained that it is time-consuming to apply electrodes and teach patients how to use the instrument. Although the initial time investment is greater than that for nonfeedback therapy, patients usually can be left alone to exercise, hence freeing the therapists for other activities (Krebs, 1981). Indeed, portable instruments can be lent to very motivated and intelligent patients to use between therapist contacts; these permit practice to occur at other times and on other days.

Given an informational tool like biofeedback, many patients can improve upon the exercises provided to them by therapists. In fact, the idea to flex the knee during postmeniscectomy exercises came directly from watching patients struggle at 0° knee flexion, but masterfully control their quadriceps at 30°.

EMG Feedback Training for Myoelectric Prosthesis Control

Biofeedback as a therapeutic tool has grown out of several fields. One such field is prosthetics. Over 50 years ago, Berger and Huppert (1952) at NYU reported that EMG might be used to control motors to open and close prosthetic hands and to control other prosthetic functions. Battye, Nightingale, and Whillis (1955), from England, reported the first successful application of myoelectric signals in the control of a prosthetic hand. The concept was simple: As Berger and Huppert explained, "Since the electric motor supplies the power for the artificial arm movements, the amputee's only responsibility is the control of the motor" (1952, p. 110). Despite the early work in this area, clinical application of EMG-controlled prostheses remains of controversial efficacy. Until the late 1970s, poor energy sources for the motors and mechanical systems made electrically powered prostheses rather inefficient and subject to frequent repair (Wirta, Taylor, & Finley, 1978). A number of electric prosthetic control systems now exist, including switches and harnesses. This section focuses on training for myoelectrically controlled systems, without attempting to address the issue of which control system is more nearly optimal.

Two types of myoelectric control are generally available: *dichotomous* and proportional control. Dichotomous control is similar to threshold control of biofeedback (i.e., turning an audio or visual signal on and off). For example, the EMG signal from the forearm flexors of a patient with a below-elbow amputation or missing limb can control prosthetic hand closing. If the EMG exceeds a threshold value, the prosthetic hand "flexes." Similarly, EMG activity in the forearm extensors that exceeds a threshold value opens the hand.

Proportional control is analogous to biofeedback's continuous EMG amplitude feedback from a meter, or proportional audio tone or clicks; a large signal results in proportionally faster or more forceful prosthetic movement. Low-amplitude EMG signals result in slow movement for fine control. Krebs and his colleagues have added another prosthesis control variable: prosthetic joint stiffness. This "impedance controller" prosthesis appears to be a more natural use of the EMG signal in prosthetics (Popat et al., 1993).

General Considerations

Because EMG signal control is prerequisite to myoelectric prosthesis control, EMG biofeedback occurs prior to functional training with the prosthesis. Indeed, this is one of the few cases in which the acquisition of biofeedback skill is a prerequisite to other therapy. Until the patient can control the EMG signal from the control-site muscles, the myoelectric prosthesis is merely an expensive passive appliance.

Availability of a strong EMG signal from the proposed control site (see Figure 22.6) is the first factor to examine in the potential candidate. Most patients with missing limbs, whether the causes are congenital or surgical, are capable of generating currents from the residual limb. Patients with congenital missing limbs, having never had the opportunity to functionally use their truncated muscles, often meet with difficulty in the early stages of EMG biofeedback. After they learn to generate some signal, no matter how small, training usually proceeds apace.

Control sites are carefully chosen to meet three criteria: (1) The muscles must be superficial, so that surface electrodes may be employed; (2) EMG activity from the muscle must exceed the noise and movement artifacts, so that prosthetic activation does not inadvertently occur (the same EMG artifacts may be present in EMG amplifiers and electrode systems for prostheses as described for biofeedback systems); and (3) the patient must become capable, with training, of rapid, reliable, and repeated voluntary activation and relaxation of the EMG signal.

Frequently, the control muscle is chosen for its ontological function. For example, hand opening is usually controlled by forearm extensors in the patient with a below-elbow amputation or missing limb. However, no empirical evidence exists supporting the validity of such reasoning. Indeed, patients with above-elbow amputations/missing limbs must control apprehension with muscles that ontologically function at the elbow or shoulder. These patients

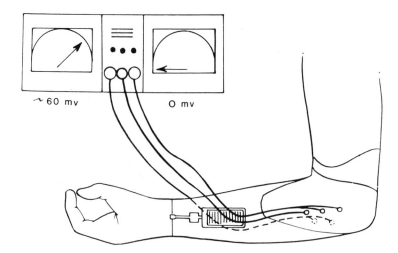

FIGURE 22.6. Myotestor biofeedback unit monitoring below-elbow residuum's flexor EMG. Note that extensors (dial on right) are quiescent.

apparently fare none the worse in their control of apprehension. In most cases, the control-site electrode placements are generally the same as those used in other upper-limb EMG feedback situations.

No matter what control muscles are selected, biofeedback therapy goals are as follows:

1. Facilitation of EMG output from the control muscle.
2. Rapid EMG generation to the threshold necessary for prosthetic activation.
3. Inhibition of EMG during antagonist activation.

Most often, therapy starts with conventional EMG biofeedback instruments. Several prosthetic manufacturers even supply their own EMG instruments for preprosthetic biofeedback therapy; although the amplifier specifications (e.g., input impedance, CMRR, bandwidth, and noise level) are frequently suboptimal, the obvious advantage of such machines is their compatibility with the EMG signal conditioning used in the prosthesis.

Many myoelectric prostheses are fitted to children. To maintain children's attention, various "myotoys" have been developed. For example, the Milton-Bradley Myotoy truck shown in Figure 22.7 moves forward and backward, contingent upon flexor or extensor muscle activation, respectively. Children often attend to toys more readily than to lights, clicks, or meters. Proportional speed control can be introduced, so that greater EMG activity moves the toy faster than less EMG activity.

For all patients, therapy with a bench-mounted or hand-held prosthesis, such as that shown in Figures 22.8 and 22.9, proceeds after initial EMG and control skills have been acquired. The patient with a unilateral amputation or missing limb should learn such manual skills as holding jars while screwing the top on or off with the unimpaired hand. Holding the prosthesis in his or her unimpaired hand, the patient may then learn crude prehension activities (see Figure 22.9).

It is important to pause and digress somewhat at this point. A prosthetic hand is a poor substitute for the natural member. A person with a unilateral amputation/missing limb will perform most ADLs with the unimpaired limb (Krebs, 1987). The prosthetic device is most often used for assistance, and then only when unilateral prehension is insufficient. Therefore,

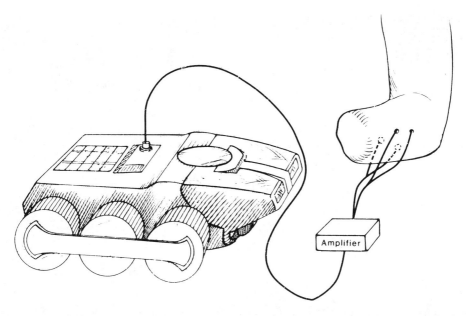

FIGURE 22.7. Myotoy (made by Milton-Bradley, Springfield, MA). EMG activity controls the toy's movement, such that agonist–antagonist EMG causes movement in opposite directions.

training in complex prosthetic prehension tasks (e.g., picking up jelly beans or holding an egg), although impressive to some clinicians, is largely irrelevant to functional prosthetic use. Just as frustration may result from training with the prosthetic hand prior to acquiring sufficient EMG control, so may ennui ensue from training for unrealistic prosthetic goals.

Prosthetic hands are less functional than hooks; their bulk and mechanical complexity limit visual feedback and fine prehension. Myoelectric hands, in addition, are much more costly, are heavier, and probably break down more frequently than body-powered ("conventional") hooks.

Summary

In summary, as electronic and prosthetic technologies improve, patients with amputations or missing limbs will be afforded more kinesiological control of their prosthetic devices. Therapists must design biofeedback programs that mimic the control system of the prosthesis. The design limitations of any artificial limb, however, define the maximum functional capacity of the user.

LOCOMOTOR TRAINING

The Gait Cycle

Human *locomotor* activity is normally a regular, rhythmical, and repeatable series of oscillating "stance" and "swing" phases. When the foot touches the floor, the limb is in stance phase, which constitutes about 60% of a normal gait cycle. Advancing the limb through the air is the swing phase. The joint motions (i.e., "kinematics") and the forces that produce the motions (i.e., "kinetics") have been studied extensively in normal populations. Much less is

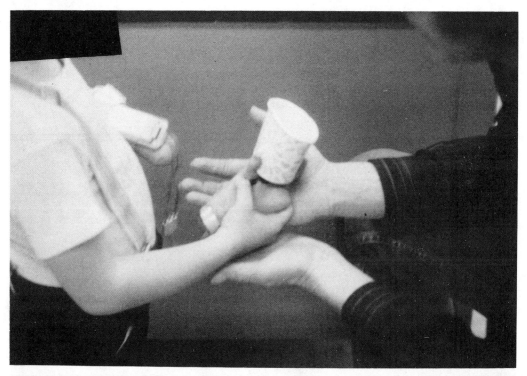

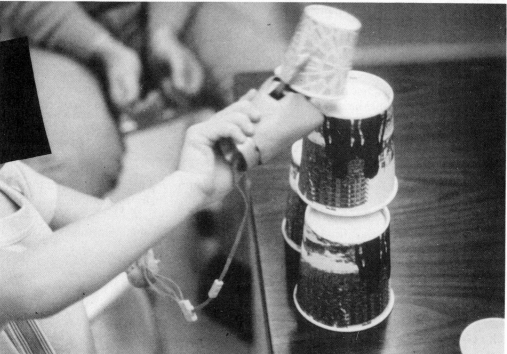

FIGURE 22.8. Two illustrations of therapy with a young patient after amputation, using a hand-held prosthesis.

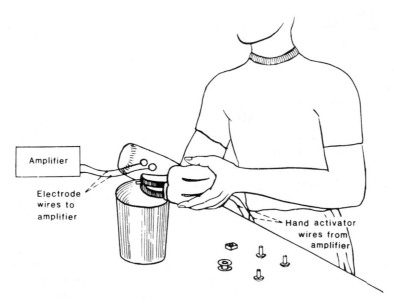

FIGURE 22.9. The patient in Figure 22.8 progresses to crude prehension activities with the hand-held prosthesis.

known regarding abnormal gait, the subject of most therapists' attention. A gait deviation such as a unilateral limp (i.e., decreased stance time) may result from a variety of kinematic or kinetic abnormalities, including loss of motor power, pain, fear, and/or poor neuromuscular coordination. Sherman and Arena (1992) provide a superb literature review on back pain biofeedback and its relationship to motor function.

Colborne, Olney, and Griffin (1993) have reported significant advances in the gait of patients with hemiplegia treated with *both* soleus EMG and ankle joint electrogoniometric biofeedback; EMG is often used to estimate muscle contribution to locomotion. However, muscle force is just one of many biomechanical determinants of locomotion. Gravity, inertia, and the floor reactions are at least as important as the forces generated by superficial lower-extremity muscles that are accessible to surface EMG feedback (Krebs, 1992). Joint motion electrogoniometry captures the limb motions resulting from all these force sources.

Although EMG feedback attempts to provide information and answers to patients, we practitioners do not fully understand the questions. We encourage subjects to activate their muscles in a prescribed sequence, but we do not yet know the correct sequence for normal muscle activity, let alone the complex compensations required by pathomechanics or patho-physiology (e.g., lower-limb amputation or CNS disorders).

Several authors have reported that EMG activity for a given muscle varies widely even within the same subject under identical walking conditions. Indeed, even Basmajian (1974) has suggested that EMG amplitude should only be classified as "none," "minimal," "moderate," or "marked," and not given numerical values. Of course, we do not mean to imply that EMG feedback for gait training is de facto useless; rather, therapists should be cautious about attaching too much importance to the EMG signal. Winter (1984) and Yang and Winter (1984) have provided insight into the reliability of various EMG-averaging methods; as such work progresses, therapists will have a more meaningful scientific basis for EMG-feedback-assisted gait training.

Neurophysiological control mechanisms aside, force resultants in gait have been fairly well documented. It is known, for example, that weight-bearing forces and stance times must be shared approximately equivalently by the lower extremities; otherwise, asymmetry and increased energy consumption result. Symmetric timing is achieved by moving right- and left-extremity and spinal joints through approximately equivalent arcs at similar speeds. Thus, although the impetus for the motions may derive from complex interactions of exogenous (e.g., gravity and inertia) and endogenous (i.e., muscle) locomotor forces, the resultant kinematics and kinetics are mechanically somewhat easier to measure and therefore may be more amenable to error detection and biofeedback therapy.

Several forms of kinematic and kinetic biofeedback are clinically available. Unlike EMG feedback, electronic processing of gait motions and forces is rather direct. The primary equipment consideration is linearity of output (i.e., feedback) to input (i.e., joint motion or force reaction). That is, the signal reaching the patient should closely track kinematic or kinetic activity. Although 100% linearity is never achieved, therapists should scrutinize technical specifications before purchasing any such instrument, to ensure that the feedback to patients is valid.

Most biofeedback gait therapy uses an audio signal, thus allowing the patient's visual system to attend to the walking environment. The most widely used devices are those providing electrogoniometric and floor reaction force feedback (i.e., limb load monitors). These therapy aids are designed to provide patients and therapists with indications of limb positions or applied loads (Binder, 1981; Gapsis, Grabois, Borrell, Menken, & Kelly, 1982). After a few sessions, most patients can use the devices without constant supervision.

Kinematic Feedback

An *electrogoniometer* (see Figure 22.10) is simply a potentiometer (i.e., variable-resistor rheostat). Potentiometers are common; they are used to control the volume of stereos and to dim room lights. Turning the potentiometer causes its resistance to electric currents to increase or decrease. Since voltage is inversely proportional to resistance, turning the potentiometer causes the stereo volume to change or the light's brightness to vary.

In gait measurement, two "arms" are attached to the potentiometer as in Figure 22.10—one to its base and the other to the movable rheostat. The arms are strapped to the limb segments, so joint rotation changes the potentiometer's resistance to current. Just as a 20° turn of the volume control knob on a stereo should always result in the same change of audio volume, so should a 20° knee flexion always result in the same change of voltage in an electrogoniometer. The voltage through the electrogoniometer is provided by a battery. Joint movement causes a pitch or buzz of known frequency from the audio feedback system (Gilbert, Maxwell, George, & McElhaney, 1982).

For example, a high pitch may indicate knee flexion, whereas a low pitch or no pitch tells the patient that the knee is extended and that it is therefore safe to accept weight for the ensuing stance phase. Frequently the signal is dichotomized, so that knee flexion of more than 10° results in a warning signal, and silence indicates knee extension (Wooldridge, Leiper, & Ogston, 1976). Applications of the electrogoniometer to the therapist's knee will demonstrate "normal" knee motions and feedback tones. The patient attempts to simulate the normal pitch with the involved knee (Koheil & Mandel, 1980).

An electrogoniometer is especially useful in training a patient with an above-knee amputation or missing limb how to control the prosthetic knee (Fernie, Holden, & Soto, 1978). Patients are instructed to load the prosthesis only when its knee is extended (i.e., only when the warning buzzer is not heard). After stance phase weight bearing is safely achieved during prosthetic knee extension, joint angle feedback may be employed to teach knee flexion during the swing phase.

Biofeedback of joint position, whether for patients with amputations/missing limbs, hemiplegia, or osteoarthritis, should proceed according to the same general guidelines as any biofeedback therapy to attain relative normality. Positive reinforcement is emphasized, and

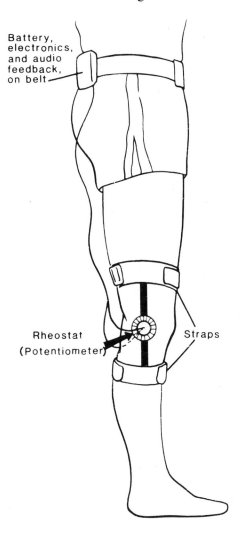

FIGURE 22.10. An electrogoniometer.

the "two-thirds" success rule may be applied. Thus patients must be given the opportunity to achieve successive approximations to normality, by setting the "error" warning range quite broadly during initial training and incrementing the tasks toward replication of normal (or safe!) kinematics as skill improves. Dichotomous feedback is often provided during initial training. We find that the introduction of continuous feedback is simply too much information for patients to act upon until a fairly normal gait is established.

It is also critical that therapists be fully familiar with normal gait kinematics (see Figure 22.11). We have seen patients valiantly struggling to comply with the admonishments of therapists to dorsiflex beyond neutral during the swing phase, despite the fact that the ankle reaches only 0° or so during the swing. If the therapists had only applied the electrogoniometer to their own ankles, the futility of the task would have been obvious.

Therapists must appreciate the differences between normal persons' gaits and those of patients with amputations/missing limbs, because prostheses move quite differently from normal limbs. The normal knee flexes just after heel strike, at the beginning of the stance phase (see Figure 22.11). The knee then extends to about 7° and begins to flex again in antici-

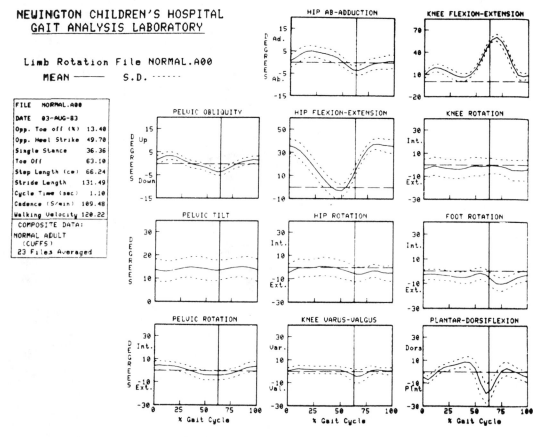

FIGURE 22.11. Gait kinematics of 14 healthy adults walking at their preferred rate on a smooth, level surface. Solid line indicates mean; dashed lines, ± 1 standard deviation. Reprinted by permission of Newington Children's Hospital, Newington, CT.

pation of the swing phase. No commercially available prosthetic knees (except the BRADU "bouncy" knee from Nuffield Labs, England) allow this "double-flexion wave" in stance. Most prosthetic knees must remain fully extended, or the prosthesis will buckle during weight bearing.

It is important to be cognizant of the major compensations for neuromotor abnormality. For example, patients with paretic quadriceps will often compensate by strongly plantarflexing the shank during midstance, thus extending the knee. Ankle–foot orthoses are frequently prescribed with the ankle set at 5° plantar flexion, in order to help provide this extension moment to the knee. Training such patients to mimic normal knee kinematics will obviously result in a poor gait.

West Park Hospital, in Toronto, has devised a device for training knee control that may be useful for patients who persist in knee flexion while that limb is loaded. A buzzer is silent only if knee extension occurs while the foot switch, indicating stance phase, is closed. Although the system was designed for above-knee prosthesis training, it should be useful in training wearers of above-knee orthoses. For example, arthritic patients could be trained to bear weight on an involved limb more normally while simulating normal stance kinematics.

The components of an electrogoniometer are quite inexpensive and may be fabricated by anyone with a rudimentary knowledge of electricity (Gilbert et al., 1982). The engineering or electrical maintenance shops of most hospitals can provide a usable feedback device, using components costing less than $15. As long as the potentiometer is of high quality (i.e., >90% linearity), it should be perfectly adequate for clinical purposes. Additional contingency or logic features, such as heel switches to indicate stance or swing phases, may be added, but are obviously "luxury" items.

Kinetic Feedback

A limb load monitor may be employed to provide patients with information regarding the amount or rate of loading on the lower limbs. Generally, an audio signal, linearly proportional to vertical load, warns patients of excessive or insufficient weight bearing.

The simplest type of limb load monitor is a foot switch (see Figure 22.12). This biofeedback device is readily fabricated by any clinician. A tone generator (e.g., a buzzer) and speaker are connected in series with a battery to metal strips. When the strips are approximated during the stance phase, the circuit is completed, and audible feedback results. Although no indication of the amount of weight bearing can be discerned from foot switch biofeedback, information regarding stance duration may help achieve symmetrical lower-limb timing.

One foot switch for each limb may be placed under the patient's heel, providing incentive to achieve heel strike at the beginning of each stance phase. Hemiplegic patients are asked to equalize duration of the audible tones from both foot strikes. This simple device can be used in the physical therapy department, or virtually anywhere. Switches attached to the heels of children with cerebral palsy (CP) have successfully decreased the frequency of "toe walking" by reinforcing heel contact. Heel switches can also be used to document the efficacy of EMG relaxation therapy for spastic calf muscles in improving the gait of patients with CP.

Most limb load monitors in clinical use have provision for feedback of the amount of weight borne on a limb. In essence, a strain gauge is inserted between the floor and the patient's limb, usually into the sole of a sandal attached to the patient's shoe (see Figure 22.13). The two plates shown are really a type of transducer, so that as more weight is applied, resistance through the transducer decreases (Wolf & Binder-MacLeod, 1982). Similar to the electro-

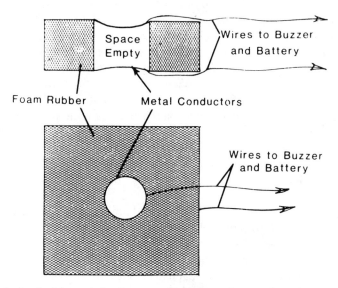

FIGURE 22.12. A simple foot switch. Contact of metal conductors during stance causes auditory or visual feedback.

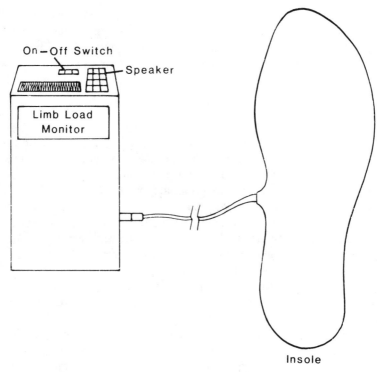

FIGURE 22.13. A more sophisticated limb load monitor.

goniometer described earlier that can be fashioned very easily and affordably, Batavia, Gianutsos, Vaccaro, and Gold (2001) describe a limb load monitor that can be constructed from materials costing approximately $12.

Limb load feedback is most often used to help patients attain partial weight bearing on a lower limb with a fracture or recent hip or knee *endoprosthesis*. A threshold level is set to indicate the maximum allowable weight to be applied on the limb. When weight bearing exceeds the threshold, an audible tone is emitted. Thus non- or partial-weight-bearing ambulation can be achieved by training, to keep the unit silent. In biofeedback with postfracture gait training, elimination of the guesswork regarding weight on the limb is a most attractive feature of limb load biofeedback (Craik & Wannstedt, 1985; Wannstedt & Herman, 1978). Winstein, Christensen, and Fitch (1993), however, report that delayed, or summary, knowledge of results rather than concurrent biofeedback enhances both acquisition and retention of the skills needed for successful partial-weight-bearing gait. But Winstein et al. used only normal, healthy subjects, so more research on impaired populations must precede firm conclusions on biofeedback versus knowledge of results.

Encouraging patients to increase the load on their limbs, by progressively increasing the threshold as therapy sessions proceed, is somewhat more complex (Warren & Lehmann, 1975). Successive approximation to the "normal" loading and time sequence, positive reinforcement, and the "two-thirds" success ratio incentive all remain operative.

Increasing limb stress can be accomplished by loading the limb horizontally as well as vertically. Limb load feedback is intended only to monitor the vertical component of the floor reaction force. Although fore–aft, torsional, and horizontal shear forces are well known from force plate gait studies, limb load biofeedback essentially ignores these components, because of complex problems of measurement and of patients' information processing. Clinically, this means that (especially during early and late stance, when shear stresses are great) limb load monitors may provide invalid information regarding the forces the limb is experiencing. The practical result of the kinetic limitations of limb load monitors is often an artifactually high feedback at heel strike and toe off, especially during fast walking.

For any patient wearing a lower extremity prosthesis, the ability to bear full weight on the prosthetic limb is critical, and vertical force kinetic feedback can be profitably employed for such patients (Kegel & Moore, 1977). Reports of technicians attempting to use force plate readouts during gait to train patients with above-knee amputations have appeared. These were apparently designed to include the nonvertical components of kinetic biofeedback. Although laudable in theory, training of patients to simulate all components of normal gait kinetics is practically impossible. Practicing therapists must again recall that patients who wear lower extremity prostheses use complex adaptations to attain energy-efficient gait. No prosthetic knee (nor, indeed, any severely arthritic knee) can perform exactly like a normal knee, simply because it is physically quite unlike a normal knee. Thus therapists are again cautioned against expecting biofeedback to cure all gait ills. The "errors" fed back to patients may, in fact, be normal compensations of the patients' seeking to walk as efficiently as possible, given their mechanical limitations.

More recently, standing posture and kinetic biofeedback to reduce falls in elderly patients have gained favor (Krebs, 1990; Hu & Woollacott, 1992). For example, Jobst (1989) randomly assigned 72 subjects with postural ataxia, primarily from encephalitis and cerebellar disease, to center-of-pressure biofeedback or physical training alone. Following treatment, the biofeedback group performed significantly better than the controls in locomotion and other ADL tasks.

Moore and Woollacott (1992) provide an excellent literature review describing the usefulness of biofeedback in patient treatment. Patients are encouraged to increase, reduce, or simply become aware of the normal postural sway experienced during quiet standing. There is at present no evidence that such feedback is helpful; there are several reports that such feedback is detrimental (Sheldon, 1963) or at best not helpful (Winstein, Gardner, McNeal, Barto, & Nicholson, 1989). Perhaps part of the problem is that the wrong variable is fed back to patients (Benda, Riley, & Krebs, 1994)! Although most commercially available "posture and balance" feedback devices claim to monitor a subject's center of gravity, instead all monitor the center of pressure beneath the feet. In normal quiet standing, the center of pressure and center of gravity do move together, but in subjects with poor balance or during locomotion, the center of pressure must be decoupled from the center of gravity (Zachazewski, Riley, & Krebs, 1993; Benda et al., 1994).

In summary, it would appear that clinical application of limb load feedback should be limited at present to informing patients of gross errors in timing and weight bearing.

Kinematic and Kinetic Biofeedback in a Clinical Setting

Therapists using both joint position and force feedback should begin sessions by familiarizing patients with the equipment and the desired outcomes of therapy. Because biofeedback is essentially a learning process, we generally begin therapy sessions with gait training. Therapeutic exercise is tiring, and fatigue seems to interfere with skill acquisition. Most frequently, following an overview of the goals of therapy (including a gait demonstration from a normal subject, usually the therapist), the first session is devoted to static standing activities.

Biofeedback sessions should be brief, to avoid fatigue. With the patient in the parallel bars, training begins by practicing walking in place. Frequent rests should be interspersed with therapeutic trials of 30–60 seconds. If a patient does not quickly comprehend the idea of weight-bearing feedback, we often use two bathroom scales (Peper & Robertson, 1976).

For static biofeedback, these cheap and familiar devices are often overlooked in biofeedback's preoccupation with high technology!

After a patient can successfully perform the activity statically, weight shifting begins. The patient should be asked to advance the more involved limb while eliciting the appropriate biofeedback signal. By the second session, patients can usually shift their weight from limb to limb, and can practice stance phase and swing phase biofeedback. Once performance is error-free on over half (e.g., two-thirds or more) of the trials, ambulation for short distances can be attempted.

At this point, each patient should be reassessed. Questions that should be asked include these: (1) Are the therapy goals appropriate for this patient? (2) Is biofeedback enhancing or interfering with progress in other areas of therapy? Most sessions beyond the first two or three should include static weight shifting and dynamic gait activities, so the basic skills learned in the first sessions are not lost.

After the patient acquires ambulatory skills, it is imperative to check his or her performance without biofeedback. Gait should be a smooth, automatic, subconsciously controlled activity. In contrast, biofeedback requires voluntary attention to the tasks to be developed. Hesitation may develop if the patient attends excessively to the biofeedback instruments, thereby inhibiting normal gait.

While locomotor skills are developing, it is critical that normal walking speed be incorporated into the regimen. We have seen patients who could walk with fairly "normal" kinematics while using biofeedback, but when they were asked to walk at a normal pace (about 1 cycle per second), their control disappeared. We had neglected to train for the correct timing and speed of movement.

In summary, effective kinematic and kinetic biofeedback must start with appropriate goals. Hemiplegic patients should generally be encouraged to flex the affected knee during stance, but above-knee amputees should not. Application of lower-limb orthoses and prostheses will interact with gait, and they may require modification of treatment goals. Biofeedback therapy should always be targeted to achieve the most energy-efficient gait possible, consistent with safety and stability.

NEW CONCEPTS AND AREAS FOR FURTHER RESEARCH

Throughout this chapter, the role of biofeedback as an adjunctive modality in rehabilitation has been emphasized. Electronic monitoring devices can only be useful in informational feedback if they provide valid and timely data for patients and therapists. Movement brings measurement problems to any electrokinesiological feedback device, but without movement, neuromuscular reeducation is pointless. Biofeedback during therapeutic exercise can be a helpful tool in increasing patient awareness, but it must not be allowed to act as a proxy for therapeutic exercise. Biofeedback is merely a powerful learning aid; by itself, it cannot strengthen muscles or increase limb mobility.

The last decade has seen a rapid expansion in the capabilities and applications of computers used in conjunction with biofeedback devices. However, computers, with their enormous memories, can easily overwhelm patients and therapists with information. Although new graphics and software programs are providing a means to simplify kinesiological biofeedback, it still remains the responsibility of therapists to provide valid therapy paradigms. With the increasing three-dimensional imaging capacity of modern medicine, one concept likely to become used in biofeedback practice will be three-dimensional limb motion feedback. Already "virtual reality" environment devices are used for entertainment, and our clinical research colleagues are using these computer-assisted three-dimensional images for biofeedback to patients. How long it will be before fully three-dimensional motion images (see, e.g., Krebs, 1992) are available for therapeutic biofeedback is anyone's guess.

Much research is required before the enormous potential of biofeedback can be fully exploited. Studies of information feedback and human information processing are far from complete. Knowledge of EMG, kinematic, and kinetic parameters and their relationship to functional activities is, at this time, quite crude. For example, one of the greatest practical impediments now facing clinicians is ignorance of the muscle force–EMG relationship during nonisometric contractions. How weight bearing and timing control are reflected by kinematic and kinetic gait measurements of persons with lower-limb disability is also unclear. Worse, little information exists on the gait patterns of slow-walking normal persons; current data are primarily from young normal subjects.

Perhaps the ultimate biofeedback device is a feedback robot. Work is currently underway at the Massachusetts Institute of Technology with robot-aided rehabilitation of upper-extremity function after stroke and other neurological disorders (Krebs, Volpe, Aisen, & Hogan, 2000). The goal of such research is to increase the productivity and quality of rehabilitation for neurological disorders.

Electronic advances should continue to be exploited clinically to the advantage of disabled populations, of which biofeedback is a very promising adjunctive modality for neuromuscular reeducation.

GLOSSARY

ACETYLCHOLINE. Transmitter released by a motor neuron that diffuses across the synaptic cleft to begin a muscle action potential.

AGONIST. A muscle directly involved in contraction and opposed by the action of an antagonist muscle, which needs to relax for proper function of the agonist muscle. For example, to bend the elbow, the biceps brachii muscle, as the agonist, contracts, and the triceps muscle is the antagonist. Contrast with *antagonist*, below.

ANKLE DORSIFLEXOR. A muscle that flexes or turns the foot upward, toward the extensor (anterior) aspect of the leg. (See also *anterior tibialis*, below.)

ANTAGONIST. A muscle that opposes or resists the action of an agonist muscle or prime mover. Can impede the action of another muscle. Also, balances opposite forces, thus helping produce smooth movement. (See *agonist*, above.)

ANTERIOR TIBIALIS (TIBIALIS ANTERIOR). Muscle that arises from the tibia to and across the ankle, and dorsiflexes the foot. (See *ankle dorsiflexor*, above.)

COMMON-MODE REJECTION RATIO (CMRR). See present text; see also Peek, Chapter 4, and Neumann, Strehl, and Birbaumer, Chapter 5, this volume.

DICHOTOMOUS. Two exclusive conditions, such as on or off.

ELECTROGONIOMETER. A potentiometer, or variable-resistor rheostat. Example of use in physical therapy is training knee flexion and, for patients with above-knee amputations, to control prosthetic knee. (See text.)

ENDOPROSTHESIS, HIP OR KNEE. A prosthesis within the hip or knee. *Endo-* is a prefix designating "within."

EXTEROCEPTION. Perception obtained via exteroceptors, which are sensory nerve terminals stimulated by the immediate external environment, such as those in the skin and mucous membranes. Contrast with proprioception.

INPUT IMPEDANCE. See Peek, Chapter 4, this volume.

KNEE ARTHROTOMY. Large surgical incision into a joint—in this case, a knee.

LOCOMOTOR. Relating to locomotion (walking) and body apparatus for locomotion.

MANUAL MUSCLE TEST (MMT). Physical therapy technique to scale muscle performance.

MEGOHM. One million ohms.

MENISCECTOMY. Surgical removal of meniscus cartilage from a knee. This is the cartilage between the ends of the bones of the thigh and lower leg.

MUSCLE ACTION POTENTIAL. Change in electrical potential of stimulated nerve or muscle fibers. Responsible for EMG signal.

OHM'S LAW. Resistance or impedance is inversely related to voltage. (See Peek, Chapter 4.)

PARETIC MUSCLES. Slight or incomplete paralysis of a muscle.

QUADRICEPS MUSCLES. The four great leg extensor muscles forming the main muscle on the front of the thigh and covering the front and side of the femur: the rectus femoris, vastus intermedius, vastus lateralis, and vastus medialis. They control movement and stability of the knee.

SARCOPLASMIC RETICULUM. "Network of fine tubules, similar to endoplasmic reticulum, present in muscle tissues. . . . Composed of or containing sarcoplasm—semifluid interfibrillary substance of striated muscle cells. The cytoplasm of muscle cells" (Thomas, 1989).

SYNAPTIC CLEFT. The narrow extracellular gap of a millionth of an inch between the pre- and postsynaptic cell membranes at the synapse (the junction between nerve cells). Nerve impulses pass through this gap from one nerve to another via release of a transmitter substance by the first nerve and reception of this substance on the next one.

TRICEPS SURAE. Triceps muscle, on the back of the upper arm.

VOLUME-CONDUCTED ARTIFACT. Signals from nearby muscles inadvertently picked up by surface electrodes on other muscles (see text).

REFERENCES

Barton, L. A., & Wolf, S. L. (1992). Is EMG feedback a successful adjunct to neuromuscular rehabilitation? *Physical Therapy Practice, 2*(2), 41–49.

Basmajian, J. V. (1974). *Muscles alive* (3rd ed.). Baltimore: Williams & Wilkins.

Batavia, M., Gianutsos, J. G., Vaccaro, A., & Gold, J. T. (2001). A do-it-yourself membrane-activated auditory feedback device for weight bearing and gait training: A case report. *Archives of Physical Medicine and Rehabilitation, 82,* 541–545.

Battye, C. K., Nightingale, A., & Whillis, J. (1955). The use of myoelectric currents in the operation of prostheses. *Journal of Bone and Joint Surgery, 37B,* 506.

Benda, B. J., Riley, P. O., & Krebs, D. E. (1994). Biomechanical relationship between center of gravity and center of pressure during standing. *IEEE Transactions on Rehabilitation Engineering, 2,* 3–10.

Berger, N., & Huppert, C. R. (1952). The use of electrical and mechanical muscular forces for the control of an electrical prosthesis. *American Journal of Occupational Therapy, 6,* 110–114.

Binder, S. A. (1981). Assessing the effectiveness of positional Feedback to treat an ataxic patient: Application of a single-subject design. *Physical Therapy, 61,* 735–736.

Cataldo, M. E., Bird, B. L., & Cunningham, C. E. (1978). Experimental analysis of EMG feedback in treating cerebral palsy. *Journal of Behavioral Medicine, 1,* 311–322.

Colborne, G. R., Olney, S. J., & Griffin, M. P. (1993). Feedback of ankle joint angle and soleus electromyography in the rehabilitation of hemiplegic gait. *Archives of Physical Medicine and Rehabilitation, 74,* 1100–1106.

Craik, R. L., & Wannstedt, G. T. (1975). The limb load monitor: An augmented sensory feedback device. In *Proceedings of a conference on devices and systems for the disabled.* Philadelphia: Krusen Research Center.

De Luca, C. J. (1994). *Surface electromyography: Detection and recording.* Boston: Neuromuscular Research Center, Boston University.

Fernie, G., Holden, J., & Soto, M. (1978). Biofeedback training of knee control in the above-knee amputee. *American Journal of Physical Medicine, 57,* 161–166.

Gable, C. D., Shea, C. H., & Wright, D. L. (1991). Summary knowledge of results. *Research Quarterly for Exercise and Sport, 62,* 285–292.

Gapsis, J. J., Grabois, M., Borrell, R M., Menken, S. A., & Kelly, M. (1982). Limb load monitor: Evaluation of a sensory feedback device for controlled weight bearing. *Archives of Physical Medicine and Rehabilitation, 63,* 38–41.

Gilbert, J. A., Maxwell, G. M., George, R. T., Jr., & McElhaney, J. H. (1982). Technical note: Auditory feedback of knee angle for amputees. *Prosthetics and Orthotics International, 6,* 103–104.

Hu, M. H., & Woollacott, M. H. (1992). A training program to improve standing balance under different sensory conditions. In M. H. Woollacott & F. Horak (Eds.), *Posture and gait: Control mechanisms.* Portland, OR: University of Portland Books.

Inglis, J., Campbell, D., & Donald, M. W. (1976). Electromyographic biofeedback and neuromuscular rehabilitation. *Canadian Journal of Behavioural Science, 8,* 299–323.

Jobst, U. (1989). Posturographic-biofeedback-training (bei gleichgewichtsstorungen). *Fortschrift für Neurologie und Psychiatrie, 57,* 74–80.

Keefe, F. J., & Surwit, R. S. (1978). Electromyographic feedback: Behavioral treatment of neuromuscular disorders. *Journal of Behavioral Medicine, 1,* 13–25.

Kegel, B., & Moore, A. J. (1977). Load cell: A device to monitor weight bearing for lower extremity amputees. *Physical Therapy, 57,* 652–654.

Koheil, R., & Mandel, A. R. (1980). Joint position biofeedback facilitation of physical therapy in gait training. *American Journal of Physical Medicine, 59,* 288–297.

Krebs, D. E. (1981). Clinical electromyographic feedback following meniscectomy: A multiple regression experimental analysis. *Physical Therapy, 61,* 1017–1021.

Krebs, D. E. (1987). *Prehension assessment: Prosthetic therapy for the upper-limb child amputee.* Philadelphia: Slack.

Krebs, D. E. (1989). Isokinetic, electrophysiologic and clinical function relationships following tourniquet-aided arthrotomy. *Physical Therapy, 69,* 803–815.

Krebs, D. E. (1990). Biofeedback in therapeutic exercise. In J. V. Basmajian & S. L. Wolf (Eds.), *Therapeutic exercise* (5th ed.). Baltimore: Williams & Wilkins.

Krebs, D. E. (1992). Seize the moment: Dynamics and estimated moments of force in locomotion analysis. In *12th Annual Eugene Michels Researchers Forum.* Alexandria, VA: American Physical Therapy Association.

Krebs, D. E., Stables, W. H., Cuttita, D., Chui, C. T., & Zickel, R. E. (1982). Relationship of tourniquet time to post-operative quadriceps function [Abstract]. *Physical Therapy, 62,* 670.

Krebs, D. E., Stables, W. H., Cuttita, D., & Zickel, R. E. (1983). Knee joint angle: Its rduionship to quadriceps femoris activity in normal and postarthrotomy limbs. *Archives of Physical Medicine and Rehabilitation, 64,* 441–447.

Krebs, H. I., Volpe, B. T., Aisen, M. L., & Hogan, N. (2000). Increasing productivity and quality of care: Robot-aided neuro-rehabilitation. *Journal of Rehabilitation Research and Development, 37,* 639–652.

Lenman, J. A. E. (1959). Quantitative electromyographic changes associated with muscular weakness. *Journal of Neurology, Neurosurgery and Psychiatry, 22,* 306–310.

Lippold, O. C. J. (1952). Relation between integrated action potentials in human muscle and its isometric tension. *Journal of Physiology, 117,* 492–499.

Moore, S., & Woollacott, M. H. (1992). The use of biofeedback devices to improve postural stability. *Physical Therapy Practice, 2*(2), 1–19.

Mulder, T., & Hulstyn, W. (1984). Sensory feedback therapy and theoretical knowledge of motor control and learning. *American Journal of Physical Medicine, 63,* 226–244.

Nelson, A. J. (1976). Fusimotor influence on performance of ankle dorsiflexors in young adults. *Physiotherapy, 62,* 117–122.

Peper, E., & Robertson, J. (1976). Biofeedback use of common objects: The bathroom scale in physical therapy. *Biofeedback and Self-Regulation, 1,* 237–240.

Popat, R. A., Krebs, D. E., Mansfield, J., Russell, D., Clancy, E., Gill, K. M., & Hogan, N. (1993). Quantitative assessment of four men using above-elbow prosthetic control. *Archives of Physical Medicine and Rehabilitation, 74,* 720–729.

Schleenbaker, R. E., & Mainous, A. G. (1993). Electromyographic biofeedback for neuromuscular reeducation in the hemiplegic stroke patient: A meta-analysis. *Archives of Physical Medicine and Rehabilitation, 74,* 1301–1304.

Schmidt, R. A. (1988). *Motor control and learning: A behavioral emphasis* (2nd ed.). Champagne, IL: Human Kinetics.

Sheldon, J. H. (1963). The effect of age on the control of sway. *Gerontologia Clinicica, 5,* 129.

Sherman, R. A., & Arena, J. G. (1992). Biofeedback in the assessment and treatment of low back pain. In J. V. Basmajian & R Nyberg (Eds.), *Spinal manipulation therapies.* Baltimore: Williams & Wilkins.

Shiavi, R., Champion, S., Freeman, F., & Griffin, P. (1981). Variability of electromyographic patterns for level-surface walking through a range of self-selected speeds. *Bulletin of Prosthetic Research, 10*(35), 5–14.

Thomas, C. L. (Ed.). (1989). *Taber's cyclopedic medical dictionary.* Philadelphia: Davis.

Wannstedt, G. T., & Herman, R M. (1978). Use of augmented sensory feedback to achieve symmetrical standing. *Physical Therapy, 58,* 553–559.

Warren, C. G., & Lehmann, J. F. (1975). Training procedures and biofeedback methods to achieve controlled partial weightbearing: An assessment. *Archives of Physical Medicine and Rehabilitation, 56,* 449–455.

Winstein, C. J., Christensen, S., & Fitch, N. (1993). Effects of summary knowledge of results on the acquisition and retention of partial weight bearing during gait. *Physical Therapy Practice*, 2(4), 40–51.

Winstein, C. J., Gardner, E. R., McNeal, D. R., Barto, P. S., & Nicholson, D. E. (1989). Standing balance training: Effect on balance and locomotion in hemiparetic adults. *Archives of Physical Medicine and Rehabilitation*, 70, 755–762.

Winter, D. A. (1984). Pathologic gait diagnosis with computer-averaged electromyographic profiles. *Archives of Physical Medicine and Rehabilitation*, 65, 393–398.

Wirta, R. W., Taylor, D. R., & Finley, F. R. (1978). Pattern-recognition arm prosthesis: A historical perspective—A final report. *Bulletin of Prosthetic Research*, 10(30), 8–35.

Wolf, S. L., & Binder-MacLeod, S. A. (1982). Use of the Krusen limb load monitor to quantify temporal and loading measurements of gait. *Physical Therapy*, 62, 976–982.

Wooldridge, C. P., Leiper, C., & Ogston, D. G. (1976). Biofeedback training of knee joint position of the cerebral palsied child. *Physiotherapy Canada*, 28, 138–143.

Yang, J. F., & Winter, D. A. (1984). Electromyographic amplitude normalization methods: Improving their sensitivity as diagnostic tools in gait analysis. *Archives of Physical Medicine and Rehabilitation*, 65, 517–521.

Zachazewski, J. E., Riley, P. O., & Krebs, D. E. (1993). Biomechanical analysis of body mass transfer during stair ascent and descent in normal subjects. *Journal of Rehabilitation Research and Development*, 30, 412–422.

CHAPTER 23

Biofeedback-Assisted Musculoskeletal Therapy and Neuromuscular Reeducation

ERIC R. FOGEL

This chapter focuses on selected biofeedback techniques for specific applications in physical therapy and muscle reeducation. I discuss the rationale and limitations of specific clinical biofeedback techniques that can help patients become more aware of how to use their bodies and aid their learning.

The therapy techniques of physical rehabilitation differ in many ways from other biofeedback interventions. The differences include the patient's neurological status, structural deformities, and levels of awareness. The feedback process is "assistive," because the feedback information acts as an adjunct to the therapist's knowledge and skills in assisting the therapy.

Using biofeedback instrumentation expands the patient's natural and internal biofeedback by making the patient more aware of self-induced changes. Physical and occupational therapies always try to help patients increase their physiological self-regulation within their natural environments. External biofeedback offers unique chances for such help to be more direct and effective. The major advantages are the increased speed of the information and the therapist's more accurate observation of the physiological activity and changes. Therapists help patients change their awareness and reactions, and help them incorporate new physical activities into new routines and habits.

To work more effectively with biofeedback, all therapists from all disciplines should understand learning theories, including operant conditioning. Therapists set up goals and help patients develop new skills, feelings, routines, and functions that improve patients' lives. There is a constant need for reassessment and changing of therapy programs. Therapy is an interaction between the therapist and the patient, with the biofeedback instrument functioning as an observer and partner. There are conditions when patients need feedback time alone to practice newly developed skills and further advance these skills toward becoming habits. I do not advise leaving rehabilitation patients alone with augmented biofeedback when they are first trying to change physiological activity.

During therapy, many events often take place that are beyond therapists' understanding of patients' needs. A therapist in one discipline often lacks training and experience in other disciplines. Such a therapist could miss a deteriorating situation or one that is inconsistent with positive change. Ethical clinicians practice within the scope of their professional education, training, and licensure. Therefore, interdisciplinary referral and cooperation are essential to successful therapy.

To set up biofeedback within musculoskeletal and neuromuscular reeducation, one must follow sound therapy practices of rehabilitation programs. External biofeedback instruments cannot substitute for a good evaluation, realistic therapy, and proper consideration of the patient's physiological and environmental limitations. Although augmented biofeedback can speed up therapy, one must still work toward realistic goals. In clinical applications, one must measure a patient's rate of progress in terms of "functional improvement."

Wolf, Regenos, and Basmajian (1977) developed a measurement scale for grading patients as they make functional progress. This scale is particularly applicable to patients who have had cerebrovascular accidents (CVAs). One must not make the mistake of only assessing a patient's improvement in terms of muscle activity measured by the instruments. I discuss this further in the section of this chapter on instrumentation.

Research criteria often differ from clinical criteria. The goal of clinical therapy is patient improvement. In addition to providing information for learning, biofeedback can provide a valuable source of added documentation for "functional" clinical improvements approaching therapy goals. Statistically significant changes are insufficient justification for protocols using biofeedback.

It is important to stress that therapists must have the necessary skills to help patients become aware of that which the therapists are trying to convey. It is essential to know what the instrumentation capabilities are, and how to focus and reinforce patients' attention to information shown by the instruments. Later in this chapter, I discuss various procedures that help accomplish this in clinical applications.

Before discussing criteria for starting biofeedback, I remind therapists that their attitudes and interests in the therapy and patient can be strong positive reinforcers. A therapist's absence from the room and/or a rigid therapy regimen can often be interpreted by a patient negatively and can contribute to a lack of success.

CONSIDERATIONS IN IMPLEMENTING AND USING BIOFEEDBACK THERAPY

For criteria for when to use biofeedback, research by Wolf (1982) showed that decreased proprioceptive awareness may be one of the crucial factors in muscle reeducation. A patient compensates somewhat for the lack of position perception with muscle or positional feedback. However, the transference of skills to activities of daily living (ADLs) depends upon the patient's ability to derive other forms of "self-feedback." The patient must incorporate new skills into new movement patterns.

One clear advantage of electromyographic (EMG) biofeedback, as in the treatment of peripheral nerve injury, is its ability to help the patient to exercise an affected muscle before he or she has perceptible muscle movement. Thus, with an incomplete lesion, biofeedback allows for developing activation and functional use via feedback from the remaining intact motor units.

Basmajian's (1977) research showed that humans can control single motor units. Therapists hope to get muscle *hypertrophy* or *budding* to occur through actively exercising the remaining motor units. (Note that, as in other chapters, italics on first use of a term indicate that the term is included in the glossary at the chapter's end.) It is not clear that feedback can increase the chance of *sprouting* or *budding*. However, active exercises with strength developments and motor unit recruitment or muscle activation may increase the chances of "functional improvement." This leads to a second criterion.

One must establish whether the final goal of therapy is mostly strength or refined control. An example of a strength goal is strengthening the quadriceps to support the knee. If refined control is the goal sought, then the chances of improvement lessen if the patient's diagnosis involves loss of motor units, such as with anterior poliomyelitis. Improvements in facial expression or hand control are other typical goals involving refined control.

Proper diagnosis, appropriate and complete evaluation, and careful planning are needed for successful results. Learning may be accelerated by developing progressive exercise homework that is directly connected to actual events learned by the patient at the clinic. Studies by Wolf (1982) indicate that the retention of skills and the transference of them to daily living are much more successful if the strength is coupled with the functional activity during the therapy process.

A third factor affecting biofeedback implementation is the presence of both normal and pathological reflex activity. Historically, clinical and research reports first indicated the possibility of reducing spasticity with the use of biofeedback. I have observed that some patients improve their ability to control the secondary effects caused by spasticity and can reduce the number of reflex spasms. I believe it is a secondary effect resulting from the maintained reduction of muscle tone, which also may reduce the stress on the protective reflex system. During exercise programs, I have found it helpful to stretch the involved muscle, teach maintenance of this lengthened state, and strengthen the *antagonist* muscle to maintain the integrity of the corrected position. When working with patients who have spasticity, I believe that this process may allow for a possible resetting of the muscle tone protection system (as in ankle clonus). The clonus activity may change from stretch-induced, passive dorsiflexion at 25° plantar flexion to a delay at 5° dorsiflexion. The arc of clonus is thus brought within functional levels. I discuss the use of reflex activity positioning to facilitate activities later in this chapter.

Many patients come for therapy following traumatization of a body part (physical or psychological) and "splinting" or "bracing" muscle activity developed to protect that body segment. Such muscle activity initially may have had functional value, by preventing movement, providing security, and (in broad terms) shielding an area from further trauma. The duration and frequency of the "protective spasm" may determine the level of structural change that occurred in the muscle. A realistic and functional goal for corrective change is to bring the patient to the point of maximum pain-free use of the affected body part, rather than a goal based on an instrument's numerical readouts.

Chronically increased muscle tone distorts the sensory perception of a body part. After therapeutic correction, a therapist may often hear the patient say, "That doesn't feel right to me." The patient must then learn to become comfortable with the corrected position and incorporate it into his or her daily activities.

The process of becoming aware of one's body is often contingent on many physical and emotional factors. Teaching someone to change his or her "body image" may require an interdisciplinary approach with careful operant conditioning. Classic examples of diagnoses with distorted sensory perception are CVA, reflex sympathetic dystrophy, amputation, and severe trauma. Some clinicians may show surprise at how much more easily instrumentation-based feedback can communicate information to patients than methods without the instruments. A therapist's more complicated and uncertain verbal attempts may be very confusing to a patient with sensory distortion. The instrument can become a patient's only contact with his or her internal environment. An old but still useful article by Marinacci and Horande (1960) discusses the use of EMG feedback for muscle reeducation, the causes of loss of body use, return of muscle function, and progression of return.

In summary, I remind clinicians to be aware of each patient's presenting diagnosis and all physical and psychological factors, as well as the need to set realistic goals based on stages of graduated progression and to change the patient's therapy program periodically.

REINFORCEMENT AND PUNISHMENT

Positive reinforcement is usually more effective than negative reinforcement or punishment. However, application of aversive consequences to a competing, undesired behavior can sometimes be useful when paired with positive reinforcement to strengthen a specific, desired alternative behavior. Therapists must tailor consequences for each patient (Brudny, Grynbaum, & Korein, 1974).

TREATMENT DEVELOPMENT

It is important to use biofeedback within a conceptual approach. Awareness therapy is a concept running through all of the therapies I use, although it is not the only conceptual approach for using biofeedback. In the discussion that follows, I assume that the suggestions are only selected possible methods for managing difficult therapy situations.

When treating a patient with an upper-motor-neuron disorder, such as that resulting from a CVA, the practitioner must first assess dominant reflex patterns and functional capabilities. One directs progressive goals for learning toward EMG-assisted control over parts of neurological reflex patterns. The patient strengthens "static controlled behavior" and then progresses to actively disrupting these patterns during activity. The newly learned skills are directed toward more functional patterns. This treatment approach is founded on Brunnstrom's (1970) approach to therapy.

One may use other forms of therapy while simultaneously providing EMG biofeedback. The EMG feedback continuously informs the patient of muscle status regarding activity or inactivity. By repeatedly attending to the signal, the patient remains aware of "what is going on." Two additional approaches toward muscle reeducation are proprioceptive neuromuscular facilitation (Knott & Voss, 1969) and the use of facilitation and inhibition vibratory techniques as suggested by Hagbarth and Eklund (1969) and Hagbarth (1973). During vibratory facilitation techniques, the EMG feedback signals the patient to be attentive to changing muscle status.

One may evoke muscle reactions by using other facilitation or inhibition techniques. Rapid stretching of a muscle or reducing the stretch placed on a muscle will each cause a change in muscle tone. One then directs therapy efforts toward making the patient recognize and be able to reproduce the target response. The patient must work to maximize the control of this activity and to incorporate this activity into functional patterns.

Failure to control environmental factors during therapy sessions may lead to false or misleading feedback signals. For this reason, proper structuring of therapy sessions is critical. Important questions to ask oneself while designing the therapy session are these: (1) Is the monitor site "gravity-dependent" or supported? (2) Is a monitored muscle being stretched quickly or over a prolonged period of time? (3) Does the patient's body position facilitate or inhibit muscle influencing sensory input patterns? Case descriptions presented later in this chapter suggest some positional and environmental controls. Therapists familiar with manual muscle-testing positions (Hislop & Montgomery, 2002) can use this knowledge to isolate target muscles in an attempt to create greater specificity of signal.

Many patients have secondary factors associated with their condition. Thus it is often necessary to attend to these needs first. The therapist must create an environment where such a patient can learn new tasks without being distracted by interfering dominant patterns and pain. Thus any overriding dominant symptoms must be eliminated. Later in this chapter, I discuss a progression of techniques that I have found helpful for controlling the secondary symptoms and promoting the desired goal.

At this point I mention the importance of patients' developing responsibility for their own health care. There are various available assessment methods to determine how patients relate to their condition. The therapist must not allow patients to isolate their learning to the clinic environment. Each patient should understand the instrumentation and how it provides a means to increase physiological control elsewhere. Homework assignments and training sessions should be structured around functional activities. The more closely a learned activity resembles an ADL, the greater the chance the patient will learn it as part of his or her normal routine.

A GENERAL TREATMENT STRATEGY

Patients often are in pain or have some debilitating aspect to their posture when they first present for treatment. Many patients have various means of achieving instant relief, but these are usually of short duration. One goal of therapy is to provide a means for correction of long duration and for prevention of a return of symptoms. A corrective therapy process may be long in duration when compared to the patient's own quick relief methods. Therapists often need to provide temporary relief before trying to help a patient achieve self-regulation. Compliance can increase when the patient no longer worries about the pain.

The following are the steps I use to create a positive progression with patients:

1. Pain suppression, via the most effective method. This varies among patients.
2. Awareness therapy.
   a. *Postural.*
   b. *Functional.* The goal is for patients to prevent symptoms from occurring by becoming aware of early warning signs (subclinical) that produce symptoms.
3. Self-control and preventative measures (reduction of clinical intervention).
   a. *Postural awareness* (during functional activities).
   b. *Therapeutic exercise* (to strengthen newly learned positions and postures).
   c. *Pain reduction techniques* (self-initiated methods).
   d. *Homework* (to strengthen newly learned skills during ADLs).
4. *Progressive therapeutic exercise* (with realistic goals).
   a. *Homework* (self-regulation away from the clinic).
   b. *Reassessment* (evaluation of functional value of new skills).
   c. *Progressing of program* (attempts to maximize training results).
   d. *Review.* At a later date, the therapist determines whether learned skills have become automatic and whether beneficial learning can be achieved.

During this process, the therapist's job is reevaluating and adjusting the goals for each patient. The therapist must frequently assess functional improvement and potential structural changes. One sometimes enhances additional learning with ambulatory instruments or "home trainers." I discuss these later in the chapter.

There is also a need to quantify results and measure changes in therapy programs. Beyond statistical purposes, such quantification can help justify the existence and continued use of therapies, and thereby provide the therapist with important feedback.

INSTRUMENTATION CAPABILITIES AND MEASUREMENT

Most of the therapeutic procedures described in this chapter use EMG feedback. Feedback does not have to involve elaborate or complicated instrumentation. One can use inexpensive instrumentation and devices with effective therapeutic procedures.

Neophytes in this field may consider conventional surface-electrode-based EMG biofeedback to be the answer to all of their quantification needs. There are still limitations in the use of some equipment when one is trying to monitor activity during movement. Evaluation of surface muscles during movement depends on the specificity of signal, the selection of target muscles, the interpretation of statistical recordings, the reproducibility of results, and the development of templates for movement patterns. Biomechanical evaluation of movement patterns is not merely a measurement of surface EMG activity. When a person moves, the muscle system works in an elaborate coordination of *synergists*, antagonists, *stabilizers*, and *prime movers*, whose elaborate relationship has not been clearly established. The monumental task of mapping muscle tone changes during function and dysfunction has progressed considerably during the last several years. However, we must still identify the coordination patterns that muscles utilize to create stability or movement. It is difficult to isolate one muscle as the primary cause of pattern dysfunction and create an effective feedback loop capable of teaching a controlled behavior or activity (Sella, 1998, 2000). Multisite recordings of one system of the body may be deceptively simple when compared to self-regulation during movement of all those sites. "Functional activity" again becomes the focus for therapy.

Readers might ask, "Why use biofeedback at all?" My answer would be this: "If you obtain and maintain a usable signal and transform it to a functional task, feedback can speed the learning process and increase the amount of information that a patient can learn."

To create a learning environment for a patient, a therapist must first understand certain characteristics of both the patient and the biofeedback instrument. The patient should be evaluated for sensory awareness. The choice of primary feedback should be compatible with the patient's dominant and controllable sensory system (e.g., visual, auditory, tactile, proprioceptive).

EMG remains the leading source of feedback, but there are many other forms of feedback information. Force plate feedback for proprioceptive feedback and goniometry for angular change feedback are examples. Instrument displays are now more sophisticated and often more complicated than a few years ago.

First, the placement of electrodes should isolate the muscle's signal as much as possible. The therapeutic task is to facilitate an event. The therapist should be more careful about the consistency of electrode placement across sessions and what activity is being positively reinforced.

A suggested method of controlling the feedback sampling is offered by Basmajian (1989). The area of muscle being monitored can be reduced or increased by spreading the distance between electrodes or placing them more closely aligned.

The next step is deciding whether to use continuous feedback or to set up a threshold criterion. The type used can affect the results. When using continuous feedback, one provides a patient with a signal that reflects the entire range of muscle activity. This may be more helpful in the initial learning of a new skill. Continuous feedback gives information about the total distance of the patient from the desired behavior.

Threshold feedback restricts feedback to the presence or absence of desired physiological activity. I find threshold settings helpful to refine general responses. Whether to use continuous or threshold feedback depends on the therapy goal.

Biofeedback instruments also should contain a wide range for the audio feedback and different times for the signal to cross the computer screen. This differentiates very small changes in physiological activity and helps show precise control. The audio feedback is particularly effective for ambulatory activities and those activities where visual displays are impractical. The volume control can be used for accentuating or reducing the sound.

Use of more than one channel allows one to switch target sites without repetitious preparation. Feedback instruments also should include scales (gains), such as fractions of a microvolt. This permits measurement and monitoring within a very small range of physiological activity. It helps differentiate very small changes in physiological activity and shows precise control. Ease of operation and mobility are also important.

GENERAL CLINICAL PROCEDURES

Intake Processes

First, not every patient is suitable for biofeedback. One must be selective and identify good candidates. Evaluations include physical and psychological status. The medical diagnosis provides criteria for establishing some expectations. This does not mean that patients with the same condition will have similar results, however. One must be aware of each patient's neurological progression and clinical signs of improvement versus regression, and one must constantly rate progress. When there is no progress, reevaluation may lead to work with another body part, to focus on separate functions, to the use of other techniques, or perhaps to the use of other feedback or instruments. Being aware of the patient's interest can help one modify the program.

Evaluation includes identification of any central nervous system (CNS) disorders or upper-motor-neuron lesions. Predominant reflex patterns, tonic reflexes, *hyperreflexia*, strength, range of motion, and the patient's attention span must all be part of the assessment. Peripheral nerve injuries and lower-motor-neuron lesions require several different assessments, including severity of nerve injury (complete or incomplete), the degree of sensory loss, muscle flaccidity, and whatever mental association the patient has with the body part. The degree to which the patient has phantom pain and negative emotional associations with his or her condition should be analyzed.

Included in the physical analysis is a posture component. The therapist checks the patient's structural and functional posture during both rest and activity. One must analyze how an adverse posture developed and whether it is correctable without any further detriment to the patient. There are some basic procedures that can make these tasks easier. One should first direct efforts toward reducing antagonist muscle spasm before trying to facilitate *agonist* strength. This applies to reducing splinting activity that protects or supports a joint and its associated body part. A helpful guide to targeting a muscle is to locate the pain patterns or "trigger points" (Travell & Simons, 1983), to reduce the discomfort, and then to stretch and teach spasm reduction in the involved muscles.

It is helpful to determine the speed at which a patient can release the involved muscle. My experience agrees with that of Wolf (1982) and suggests that the release of the involved muscle must be done during activities related to the functional goal. It is therefore important to use feedback while "putting the patients through their paces" in routine activities.

Frequency of Office Sessions

The frequency of office sessions is another important consideration. A therapist should tailor the frequency of sessions to each patient's needs. Normally, I see my patients three times a week until they appear to have some control of the tasks; then I reduce the frequency to create independence from both myself as the therapist and the biofeedback instruments. Sessions often last from 45 minutes to 1 hour, but may be shorter if a patient becomes too fatigued or frustrated. When the patient achieves independence from the instruments, the therapist can reduce the office sessions to one every other week for about another 6 weeks. One may then decide to discharge the patient to a home care program and again review the patient in either 3 or 6 months. The review time depends upon the severity of the condition being treated, the learned goals, and the patient's retention. Patients receiving relaxation therapy are obviously different from patients receiving neuromuscular rehabilitation and may require less frequent sessions.

Three to five feedback sessions addressing poor kinesiological or functional behavior are often appropriate for most patients. These sessions, often interspersed among other sessions, involve focusing on relief of symptoms by changing a patient's posture when it is affecting the patient's symptoms.

Home Trainer Devices and Homework

Another consideration in planning a biofeedback program is the decision whether to use "home trainer" devices. If the therapist is confident that the patient will correctly and accurately practice the intended activities, then a home unit may be considered. One must avoid home reinforcement of incorrect muscle strength or incorrect patterns. Remember that patients often practice what they do best—and often that is what the clinician is trying to avoid. Thus, if home use of an EMG instrument is encouraging the wrong goals, then it should be avoided.

Homework assignments, however, are very appropriate. Every patient has tasks to do at home. These tasks range from corrective exercises to relaxation under stressful conditions. In my practice, I often use relaxation audiotapes given with instructions and a schedule for use.

Reassessment and Evaluation

Frequent reassessment is important, and evaluation at the end of a therapy program is helpful to rate its success and determine future goals. Reevaluation involves (1) instrumentation-based data and statistical analysis; (2) functional improvement; and (3) clinical observation of the patient's attitudes, postures, and other developed behaviors.

Although statistical analyses of physiological data have limitations, those data can provide good indications of progress when carefully obtained. However, the data must agree with functional and observed changes to constitute true measure of change in the patient.

General Instructions

There is a need to use general relaxation therapy procedures in physical therapy and rehabilitation. The presenting symptoms are the first source of information about the location of muscle tension. They are the best basis for selecting the placement site(s) of electrodes to teach general relaxation as well as control of specific muscles. The initial evaluation should involve physiological recordings tailored for each patient. They are part of the total criteria used to determine monitor sites for surface EMG. There are many techniques and protocols for teaching relaxation therapy to a patient/client. Clinicians are encouraged to use procedures with which they are most familiar. Feedback augmentation can serve as an enhancement for promoting patient awareness during the learning period. One general technique can be found in the previous edition of this book (Fogel, 1995).

Diaphragmatic breathing is a valuable skill that helps produce overall patient relaxation. It also becomes a primary consideration in reduction of dysfunctional accessory muscle breathing. Techniques for instructing an individual to breathe in a diaphragmatic and relaxed manner can be found in this text and other published sources (Fogel, 1995). I generally monitor from a scapular elevator.

A general relaxation goal is to develop maintenance of relaxation under simulated daily life conditions rapidly (within seconds or a few minutes). Although one encourages longer relaxation sessions, brief relaxation periods are more practical for integration into daily life. The patient should not only relax, but become aware of developing muscle tension that leads to symptoms.

CASE DESCRIPTIONS

The following case descriptions illustrate therapy procedures and the rationale for change of both general and specific muscle tension. I discuss the use of biofeedback and how to incorporate it into each therapy program. Many of the following procedures require specific and adequate knowledge of anatomy and physiology. I remind and caution readers to avoid such therapy programs without appropriate education and training.

Each clinician bases his or her progressive therapy goals on his or her knowledge of anatomy and dynamic motion. There is a tendency to create a "cookbook" approach to learning progressions, but each patient's program must be developed according to the patient's characteristics and needs.

Many factors influence the selection of target muscle sites. For example, if one is working with body extremities, it is necessary to establish proximal joint stability before trying to teach motion. This may require working with muscles that stabilize a joint rather than move it. Peripheral joints are dependent on the stability of the proximal joints. Furthermore, one first trains proximally and then moves to distal functions. In some cases, one may find that a muscle will appear strong but actually may lack strength through normal range of motion. Fatigued muscles may lose elasticity and compensate by fibrosing in a shortened position. The patient may appear to have a shortened muscle in spasm, whereas he or she may have actually lost the ability to use that muscle during its normal function. Recent literature on surface EMG discusses possible muscle dysfunction (Sella, 1998).

Muscles must be trained during functional tasks. Each muscle may have different functions during different tasks. A muscle can work as a prime mover, a synergist, an agonist, an antagonist, or a stabilizer. During *ballistic motion*, a muscle may serve to accelerate or decelerate a body part. One must train the muscle during *eccentric* or *concentric contraction*, dependent on its specific task. One must evaluate the target muscles within their *kinetic chain*. The feedback program should not concern itself with specific cookbook protocols. The design of a program should deal with functional muscle relationships and how to adapt them to a higher level of dynamic control. Progress through a protocol comes from the evaluator's ability to recognize patient substitutions of maladaptive behavior and chronic dysfunctional patterns.

Case 1: "Splinting" of Muscle Activity Associated with Pain

Presenting Diagnosis

Cervical paraspinal muscle spasm tension with radicular symptoms peripheral to the left fourth and fifth digits.

History and Medical Information

This 30-year-old female secretary had been in three rear-end automobile accidents over 2½ years. She had cervical-area pain and spasm, with periodic symptoms of radiculitis, after each accident. After the first two accidents, her symptoms had disappeared with conventional physical therapy treatment consisting of hydrocollator packs, ultrasound, and neck-stretching exercises. She had spasms of her neck muscles and headaches averaging two per week since the third accident, and she could not control the radicular symptoms. She felt her posture was worsening, and she had become very irritable. Her cervical spine X-rays were negative for pathology, but did show signs of paraspinal muscular spasm and decreased joint spaces. A diagnostic EMG showed no abnormalities. The neurologist thought there was partial anesthesia of the fourth and fifth digits, and also of the ulnar nerve distribution proximal to the wrist.

The patient complained of soreness in the cervical paraspinal muscles and numbness in the fourth and fifth digits of her left hand. The numbness was present for 1½ weeks, and the patient reported feeling periodic weakness in her left arm. The tension headaches involved a "band"-like feeling around her head and earaches, and had now increased to three to four times per week, despite her report that her accident had been "mild." She reported that her symptoms were more severe than before, and she was "unable to get any relief." However, she had learned to "live with" the neck discomfort. Her prior therapies had addressed her symptoms, but it became clear during the evaluation that the prior therapies had not recognized or treated her deteriorating posture and bruxism. Prior dental records showed no apparent dental problems before the first accident.

Evaluation

Tightness in the upper trapezius musculature was present, with more tightness on the left side. Soreness was present in the upper and lower trapezius, posterior cervical, scaleni, and pectoral "trigger points." Tenderness was present in the left temporomandibular joint. The joint "cracked" when the patient opened her mouth, which she could do beyond normal limits. The jaw opening deviated with an S curve to the right, and the cervical anterior compartment musculature was also sore on the left. Shoulder depression did not show peripheral signs. Evaluation of spinal range of motion showed hyperextension of the cervical spine and hypoextension of the thoracic spine. She had limitation of 50% in motions of right lateral flexion and rotation to the left. She had a 33% decrease in lateral flexion to the right, and a 25% decrease in forward flexion. At the end points in ranges of motion in all directions, the patient described soreness at the left neck "trigger points" and a shooting-type sensation into her left shoulder. Muscle testing showed strength within normal limits.

Goals of Therapy

1. To limit pain and allow for increased range of motion.
2. To increase active pain-free range of motion.
3. To provide prevention techniques for home care through use of muscle awareness training and relaxation techniques.
4. To strengthen thoracic extensors, neck flexors, and other support musculature.

Treatment

Treatment began with ice massage to the cervical paraspinal musculature, and continued with active stretching followed by ultrasound. These were all attempts to reduce muscle spasm and temporarily "release" the muscles. Transcutaneous electrical nerve stimulation (TENS) was then used to suppress the pain further.

During the initial period of pain control, other modalities reduced the myofascial pain. This allowed the patient to become free of pain so she could relax her muscles without increased pain. Additional techniques to help her become more amenable to corrective posture therapy included electric acutherapy, iontophoresis with lidocaine and dexamethasone sodium phosphate, and spinal joint mobilization (for a temporarily corrected spinal position).

Muscle control techniques started after three pain-blocking sessions in 1 week. The pain-blocking modalities continued, but now generalized relaxation techniques followed the pain-blocking sessions. Relaxation included diaphragmatic breathing to reduce the patient's "neck breathing." Further assessment of muscle tension suggested increased tightness and inability to release tension quickly in the left upper trapezius and neck accessory breathing muscles.

After the patient could significantly relax her muscle activity to a low level unassisted by the therapist, she was started on a neck awareness exercise with five sessions of EMG feedback over 2 weeks. With those exercises, she learned to release her neck muscles while in different positions (see Figure 23.1). She learned to release the involved muscles and demonstrated consistent control as shown by the EMG. She then progressed to practicing the control during functional activity exercises in six sessions, twice per week. The activity involved reciprocal upper trapezius contraction and relaxation, and then strengthening of the thoracic extension while relaxing the upper trapezius muscles (see Figure 23.2).

The patient was now asymptomatic in her left hand, and the frequency of her headaches decreased to once every 2 weeks. The location of her headaches suggested left masseter involvement. These symptoms and their frequency were at about the levels that she recalled having before the third accident. Biofeedback therapy then focused on reducing masseter muscle tension. The patient showed more difficulty releasing the left masseter than the right, suggesting an imbalance in the use of her jaw muscles (Carlsson, 1975; Rugh, 1977). Therapy then proceeded with more relaxation and instructions for equalizing right- and left-jaw functions (see Figure 23.3). Progressive resistive exercises continued at home to help thoracic extension and to decrease the patient's cervical lordosis. In addition, she practiced facial exercises designed to equalize the activity of right- and left-sided facial muscles. After sessions once a week for 3 weeks, the patient was able to control the tightness of her jaw muscles and had not experienced a headache for 3 weeks.

The therapist reviewed general and specific relaxation with EMG biofeedback 2 and 4 weeks later, and again at 6 and 12 months. Follow-up at 4 years continued to show no radicular

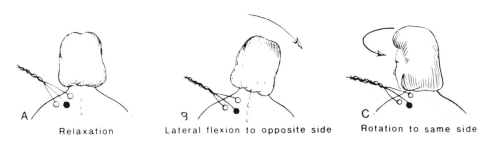

Relaxation   Lateral flexion to opposite side   Rotation to same side

FIGURE 23.1. Technique for releasing the muscles of the neck while in different positions (A–C).

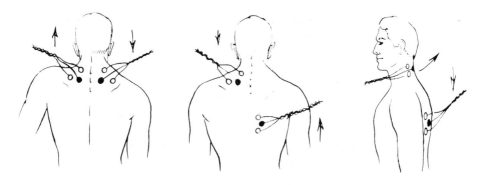

A EMG activity: Up on one side
and kept down on opposite side

B Thoracic extension while shoulders are kept down

FIGURE 23.2. (A) Reciprocal upper trapezius contraction and relaxation. (B) Strengthening of thoracic extension while relaxing the upper trapezius.

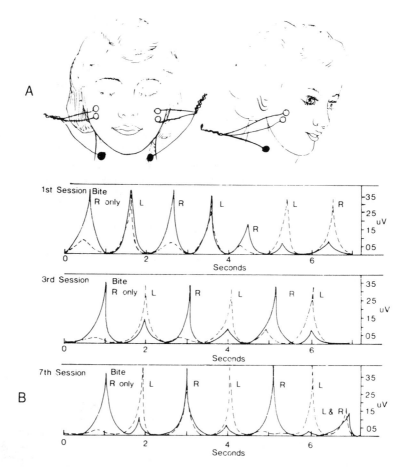

FIGURE 23.3. (A) Electrode placement for therapy to equalize right- and left-jaw functions. (B) Print-out derived from Hyperion "Bioconditioner" EMG, demonstrating the patient's progressive ability to control right- and left-bite tension.

symptoms, two or three headaches per year, 95% of full range of motion of the cervical spine, and increased thoracic range of motion. The patient continued to be aware of and attentive to her posture, and aware when she was irritating her neck. However, she reported being able to correct herself before developing symptoms.

Biofeedback therapy appeared to have helped this patient's awareness of (1) a maladaptive posture; (2) corrective positioning by use of her muscles; and (3) times when increasing muscle tension could lead to symptoms. She could prevent impending symptoms, thus requiring reduced medical care. This case illustrates the need of checking many possible factors adding to symptoms.

Case 2: Low Back Pain

Presenting Diagnosis

Low back strain/sprain with stiffness.

History and Medical Information

This 61-year-old man worked on a loading dock, lifting packages weighing up to 50 pounds. On one occasion, when bending to lift a crate off the dock, he experienced back pain immediately. One day later he felt stiffness and pain from the right lumbar 3 (L3) area to the sacroiliac and right buttock. For 3 weeks following the incident, he used home baths, showers, and hot packs, but these treatments did not decrease his symptoms. X-rays of the thoracic and lumbosacral spine were negative for pathology. He showed no neurological abnormalities.

Evaluation

The patient entered the clinic with his body held in a forward flexed position. When asked to step down on his right leg, he maintained the limb in a slight flexion at the knee. There appeared to be no lateral shift of the spinal column posture. There was a decrease in spinal range of motion as follows: a decrease of 33% in forward flexion, and a decrease of 25% in the motions of extension, extension with rotation, and lateral flexion. These motions caused pain on both right and left movement. Straight-leg raising showed tight hamstring muscles, both right and left, with the limit of elevation at 65° on the right. Muscle strength was within normal limits, and sensations appeared intact.

Goals of Therapy

1. To decrease pain.
2. To increase range of motion in the lower back.
3. To teach self-regulation for prevention of future injury.

Treatment

Therapy started with ice application, ultrasound, TENS, and spinal mobilization, all in an attempt to decrease the patient's pain and to allow for release of involved muscle groups. There was a 50% reduction in pain after six sessions spread over 2 weeks. The patient was then taught a general relaxation program. Wrist-to-wrist and diaphragmatic breathing electrode placements were used for 10 sessions (2 per week). During this period there were also three EMG feedback sessions focusing directly on reducing spasms of the patient's low back. These sessions were to create more freedom during rotation of the lower back. He was also instructed in conventional "Williams flexion exercises" with EMG electrodes on the lumbar paraspinal muscles. This electrode placement was to help call attention to relaxation in the lower back (see Figure 23.4A).

In addition, the patient learned to contract one side (hip hiking) while relaxing the opposite side. He performed this in a sitting position (see Figure 23.4B). This procedure is a generalized approach to allow increased freedom of movement for vertebral rotation. One cannot isolate specific back muscles with this electrode placement. The goal is general movement. Research at Emory Regional Rehabilitation Center (S. L. Wolf, personal communication, March 1976) suggests that spasm occurs in the deep rotator muscles lying parallel to the spinal column.

Therapy proceeded with EMG monitoring/feedback and the development of relaxation of the hamstring muscles. The patient accomplished this by passive straight-leg raising and self-controlled hamstring stretching (see Figure 23.5). The hamstring control portion lasted three sessions, two of which were provided after general relaxation therapy. General relaxation taught the patient how to relax many muscles. Functional therapy with feedback also included forward bending and maintaining a pelvic tilt position.

The patient returned to work asymptomatic. Follow-up review 1 year after the injury revealed maintenance of his asymptomatic state and full employment. Biofeedback provided an additional source of information for learning standard exercises and probably accelerated the learning process.

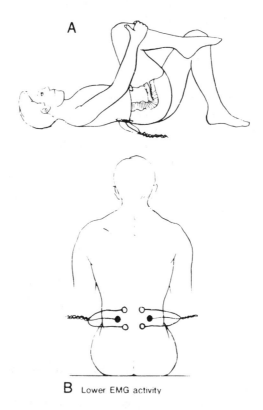

FIGURE 23.4. (A) "Williams flexion exercises." (B) Hip hiking while relaxing the opposite side in a sitting position.

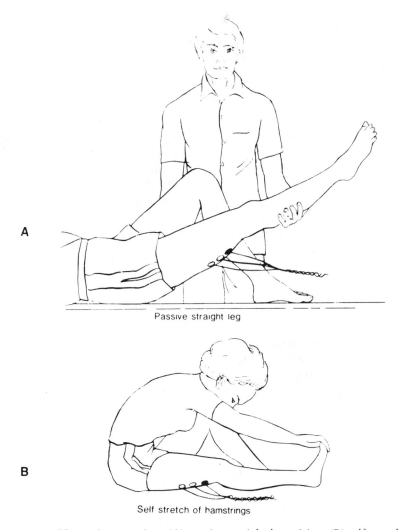

FIGURE 23.5. Hamstring exercises: (A) passive straight-leg raising; (B) self-stretching.

Case 3: Medial Meniscectomy

Presenting Diagnosis

Inability to control the left quadriceps muscle after a left-knee medial meniscectomy.

History and Medical Information

This patient was a 26-year-old woman who suffered immediate pain with twisting and popping of her left knee joint after falling down stairs. For 2 weeks she used ice applications, elevation, and immobilization to lessen the swelling and pain. The symptoms were partially controlled over the next month, but she continued to experience daily pain and began to develop a "favoring" stance; 2½ months following the accident, she began to develop locking at the knee.

An arthroscopic medial meniscectomy was performed with good healing. The left quadriceps muscle remained inactive after surgery. Despite 3 months of physical therapy to limit pain, increase range of motion, and increase strength, the patient made little to no progress. Her quadriceps muscles would not function properly, and her left knee remained sore. There was minimal muscle activity, and range of motion was 0–25° flexion without pain.

Evaluation

The patient had "trace" to "poor-minus" (15%) quadriceps activity of the left leg and was hypersensitive to touch around the knee joint. Range of motion did not improve and caused pain. The patella was fixed and nonsliding. Her skin tone was pale on the left thigh, and the left thigh was 3 inches smaller in girth than the right. Ambulation required a three-point crutch gait, and the patient exercised extreme caution before placing any weight on the left leg.

In summary, she had become extremely protective of the knee joint after experiencing pain for more than 6 months. The quadriceps functioning appeared similar to a reflex sympathetic dystrophy, but the circulation remained intact. She had disuse atrophy with decreased range of motion due to pain.

Goals of Therapy

1. To decrease knee pain.
2. To mobilize the patella.
3. To promote activity of the quadriceps.
4. To strengthen knee musculature.
5. To increase joint range of motion.
6. To improve and reeducate gait pattern.
7. To develop functional activities without feedback.

Treatment

The first step was to control pain. The next step was to desensitize the left knee with Xylocaine and iontophoresis across the kneecap, and allow the patient to experience comfort during motion. When the knee was numb, the therapist mobilized the kneecap in proximal–distal and medial–lateral directions. She held the knee fully supported in an extension position. The therapist placed EMG electrodes on the vastus medialis oblique portion of the quadriceps muscle. With EMG feedback, the patient tried to tighten the quadriceps without creating pain.

During the next session, the increased EMG activity showed that the patient could maintain longer and stronger contractions with more repetition. Pain control and mobilization continued in the third session. The next task was for the patient to try holding her knee in a straight position while support for the lower leg decreased. This slow release of muscle under tension is known as eccentric contraction (see Figure 23.6A).

During the next four sessions, the patient could maintain the increased quadriceps contraction. Therapy progressed to active terminal extension of the knee the last 15°. The patient still used ice packs prior to exercise. The EMG biofeedback came from the vastus medialis (see Figure 23.6A and 23.6C). She successfully straightened her leg, but she lacked strength. She also had protective spasm of the antagonistic muscle group, the hamstrings. In two sessions, she learned to control these spasms with self-stretching (see Figure 23.6B). The patient then began a home progressive resistive exercise program to strengthen the quadriceps.

The focus of the therapy program then switched to range of motion. The patient used EMG from the quadriceps while passively flexing the knee. Her task was to control quadriceps activity during stretch. Pain-free flexion improved over the next several sessions. She

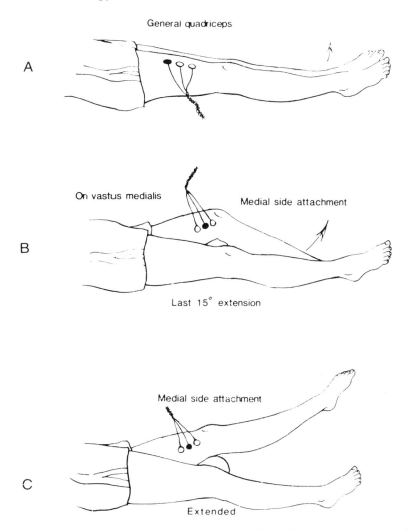

General quadriceps

A

On vastus medialis

Medial side attachment

B

Last 15° extension

Medial side attachment

C

Extended

FIGURE 23.6. (A) Eccentric contraction of the quadriceps. (B–C) Extension of the knee the last 15°, with EMG feedback from the vastus medialis.

then proceeded to practice knee strengthening, knee range of motion, and increased weight bearing (see Figure 23.7).

Gait training started when the quadriceps reached a "fair" muscle grade status (50%). While progressing from partial weight-bearing crutch gait to full weight-bearing cane gait, the patient received threshold biofeedback. Each time she extended her knee to full extension and contracted the muscle sufficiently, she received audio EMG feedback from the vastus medialis muscle (see Figure 23.8). This instruction included walking, *sidestepping*, backward walking, and pivoting. She progressed to a nonassisted gait without biofeedback in 15 sessions (see Figure 23.9). The sessions were twice a week until the last 2 sessions every 2 weeks.

At a 1½ year review, the patient maintained pain-free range of motion 0–125°. She could do three sets of 10 straight-leg raises with 22 pounds and normal-grade quadriceps activity, and terminal extension with 25 pounds. Thigh girth was equal on both legs, and her gait required no assistance with unlimited endurance.

With passive support

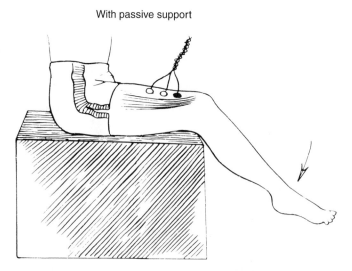

FIGURE 23.7. Relaxation of quadriceps with passive support, to aid in controlled knee flexion.

In summary, this patient learned to use her left quadriceps muscle without pain. Pain blocking was the first priority to elicit cooperation. Once the contractions were replicable, it was necessary to teach relaxation of the antagonist muscles. When she could maintain muscle integrity and support, she progressed to a gait without assistive devices. She increased her knee range of motion by actively releasing the quadriceps muscle. All activities progressed to functional patterns. Biofeedback provided her with immediate formation and reinforcement of the correct activities. Use of multiple modalities and careful progression of the therapy program were both of primary importance.

Case 4: Tendon Repair

Presenting Diagnosis

Postsurgical repair for traumatic tearing of the flexor digitorum sublimus tendons of the second, third, and fourth right-hand digits.

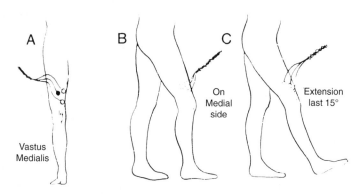

FIGURE 23.8. Extension of the knee in weight bearing, with EMG feedback from the vastus medialis.

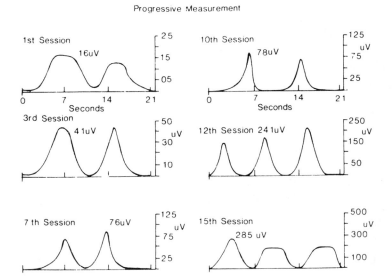

FIGURE 23.9. Printout derived from Hyperion "Bioconditioner" EMG, demonstrating the progressive strengthening of the patient's quadriceps.

History and Medical Information

The patient was a 29-year-old, right-handed man who injured his right hand when a drinking glass broke and lacerated his palm. The laceration was deep and severed the flexor digitorum sublimus tendons of the second, third, and fourth digits. Three weeks after surgical repair of the tendons, the surgical scars were healed, and therapy began. The only remaining pathology was severe limitation of finger range of motion.

Evaluation

Although the patient had active motion of his entire hand and all finger movements, there was considerable edema of the right hand. Because of edema, pain, stiffness, and muscle weakness, the patient had restriction in digital flexion. There was 75% decreased flexion at the metacarpal–phalangeal and interphalangeal joints of the right second, third, and fourth digits.

The patient showed an increase in forearm flexor and extensor muscle groups, with decreased wrist "joint play" (McMennell, 1951). He was "splinting" his forearm muscles. Passive range of motion of the joint showed limitation at endpoint because of the above-noted factors. End range of motion was "forced." Circulation and sensation were intact, except for "slight tingling" at the ends of the involved fingers. His elbow and shoulder joints were within normal limits.

In summary, prompt surgical repair maintained tendon integrity, but the forearm musculature was tight and splinting. The tightness and pain caused a decrease in range of motion. The patient was limited to gentle motion until full healing occurred.

Goals of Therapy

1. To produce full range of motion, without pain of involved fingers.
2. To provide maximum strengthening.

Treatment

Therapy began with whirlpool baths and electric acutherapy for the right hand, wrist, and forearm. The patient then received separate EMG biofeedback from the forearm extensors and flexors. First, he learned to decrease all forearm activity and allow the area to relax. Gentle passive range of motion proceeded while the patient received EMG feedback from the forearm flexor muscle group. Feedback continued during passive flexor stretching and active flexor exercise. This program continued three times per week for 3 weeks, with home exercises for range of motion without feedback.

Full exercise then started when the patient reached medical stability. The first part of the program was continued. He was instructed to increase the audio and visual EMG feedback as he began practicing stronger muscle contraction with EMG feedback from the forearm flexor muscle group. Initially, to create more muscle activity, the patient received electrical stimulation to specific muscle points. The EMG feedback came between each electrical stimulation. The patient's commands were to "hold the contraction" and keep the EMG activity as high as possible.

The patient regained 50% of the full active range of motion at the end of three sessions per week for 2 weeks. He was then seen twice per week for 4 weeks, with gradual reduction of the feedback and electrical stimulation. He regained 90% of full motion and strength after that stage. His home program was reviewed and increased to resistive exercise for the next 3 weeks. Formal treatment ended when the patient regained full strength and 95% of full range of motion. On review, 6 months later, the patient had 100% active range of motion.

In summary, this man began active exercises soon after his accident. He reduced secondary problems by limiting the swelling and decreasing splinting activity. Finally, EMG biofeedback enhanced the exercises by reinforcing his efforts.

Case 5: Peripheral Nerve Injury

Presenting Diagnosis

Left peroneal palsy.

History and Medical Information

This patient was a 32-year-old man who had fallen asleep in an "awkward position" and awakened with an inability to fully lift (dorsiflex) his left foot. He had tingling sensations in the foot and toes, and was developing progressively increased *foot slap/drop* upon heel strike during gait. Two weeks after onset of his symptoms, his muscle activity deteriorated considerably. A neurologist found no active neurological disease. X-rays were all normal, with no fractures or joint injuries evident. Circulation was intact. He was then referred for physical therapy 4 weeks after the onset of symptoms.

Evaluation

The patient presented with "trace" muscle strength of the dorsiflexors of the ankle and no pain. He walked with a foot slap. His knee and hip were normal. He had full range of motion of the ankle; his foot temperature was normal, and the skin color appeared normal. However, he remarked that he "couldn't feel what to move."

Goals of Therapy

1. To increase active muscle contraction.
2. To maintain ankle range of motion.

Treatment

Treatment began with galvanic electrical stimulation to the dorsiflexors of the left ankle. After stimulation, the patient received EMG feedback from the tibialis anterior muscle. With visual feedback, he had increased his muscle activity (see Figure 23.10). Sessions were three times a week for 2 weeks. At the end of the second week, muscle activity had increased slightly. The biofeedback helped provide awareness to aid in exercising the muscle; its use was not an attempt to change neurological growth or reinnervation.

At the end of the third week, the patient still had poor muscle strength (25%). He was then seen twice a week for 4 weeks, after which he regained 80% of his muscle strength and active joint motion. Home exercises continued throughout the therapy program. The patient refused to use an ankle dorsiflexion brace. Six months later, he had regained 100% normal muscle strength.

In summary, I assume that this man would have experienced progressive return of muscle strength without therapy. However, biofeedback and therapeutic exercise, which began immediately, helped to limit the secondary effects of paralysis and to facilitate the "feel" of proper muscle contraction. Biofeedback enhanced home exercises by helping the patient know "what to move."

Case 6: Spinal Cord Lesion

Presenting Diagnosis

Incomplete lesion of the spinal cord at C5.

History and Medical Information

This patient was a 61-year-old man who had been in excellent physical condition before suffering a spinal cord lesion. The patient had fallen and sustained an anterior dislocation lesion of the fifth cervical vertebra. At the onset, the patient was immobilized, and the cervical spine was considered stable. He received 1 year of standard physical, occupational, and recreational therapy at a spinal cord treatment center. He had more muscle control and power than expected for his condition, and could walk unassisted with a four-legged pickup walker. He had excellent muscle activity below the lesion site, but his spasticity limited his functional use of the musculature. Hyperreflexia dominated all motions, and he had little sensory awareness below the lesion. He also was experiencing loss of bowel and bladder control.

Evaluation

The primary complaint was muscle spasticity and lack of control due to hyperreflexia causing resistance to fast movements. A general measurement of patient strength showed a "fair-plus" grade (60%) in the right upper extremity and a "fair-minus" grade (40%) for the left upper extremity. The only "poor-minus" motions in the upper extremity were finger abduction and adduction and thumb opposition. The strength of the left side was basically one full muscle grade below the right side in all motions. The patient could not control flexion at his

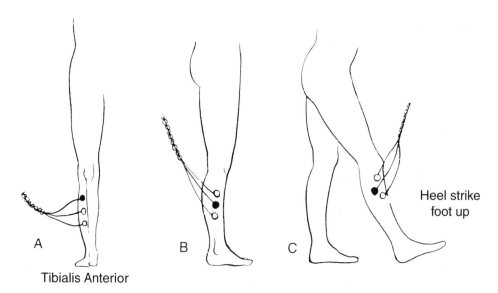

Tibialis Anterior

FIGURE 23.10. Treatment for increasing muscle activity of the ankle, with EMG feedback from the tibialis anterior muscle area.

elbow. Each time he would reach toward his mouth, he would have to overcome the resistance of his contracting triceps. Hand–finger flexor tightness restricted finger extension. He could not feel his finger positions.

In the lower extremities, the patient's hamstrings were extremely tight. The strength of the right hip extensors was graded "good," and that of the left was graded "fair-minus" (40%). Bilaterally, he had strong quadriceps. He showed weakness in his foot dorsiflexors, calf plantar flexors, and hip flexors. General muscle tone on the right was "fair-minus" (40%), and on the left "poor-minus" (15%). He could not control himself when rising from a sitting position or when sitting down into a chair. Lateral stability was poor without a walker. Both of these problems were caused by his lack of position awareness. He desired training to correct these functional deficiencies.

In summary, this man presented an example of muscle strength that was uncontrolled because of a lack of natural physiological feedback on power of his muscle contractions and joint positions. Fast, overzealous movements became restricted by an overactive stretch response. Together, these problems prevented functional movements.

Goals of Therapy

1. To decrease general muscle spasms.
2. To develop position awareness with EMG biofeedback.
3. To develop functional movements.

Treatment

Therapy started with general relaxation twice per week for 12 sessions. The first specific muscle feedback therapy used continuous EMG monitoring and feedback from the triceps and biceps muscles. I instructed the patient to relax the triceps, touch his hand to his mouth, relax the biceps, and then straighten his elbow. He learned this four-count procedure. He then learned to start his contraction more slowly and to accelerate subtly. This created less resistance to movement than quick movement did. His attempts were very successful, and the four-count cycle was increased in speed to two counts—touching the mouth and straightening the elbow.

The therapy then switched to EMG monitoring of the forearm, wrist, and finger flexor muscle groups. The patient learned to relax the flexor groups and then to extend his fingers while still relaxing the flexors. Continuous EMG feedback came from the flexor muscle group. The next step was to develop grip and release. He learned these behaviors well over 2½ months, and then he was able to feed himself independently. The strengthening and control programs progressed simultaneously, and both programs provided EMG feedback.

Therapy for the lower extremities started with facilitation feedback from the weakened dorsiflexors and plantar flexors, and relaxation of the hamstring musculature. Relaxation of the hamstrings was accomplished by progressively higher assisted straight-leg raising, performed in a supine position on a mat table. In addition, a progressive strengthening program was started for the patient's weakened muscles. The hip flexors and abdominals were specific targets. He then learned to eccentrically lower himself to a chair while receiving EMG feedback from his quadriceps. He could associate lowering into a chair with a correct amount of EMG activity fed back during the process. This process, in reverse, helped teach rising from a chair. With his head held in front of his knees, he rocked his center of gravity forward and tightened the quadriceps muscles, producing more EMG feedback. This placed him in a standing position.

I then used this procedure for developing squatting and rising from the floor. The patient also learned sidestepping and used his quadriceps as balance controllers during movement. The balance instruction taught him to maintain specific levels of EMG activity from his quadriceps during side movements. He was then transferred to a home program, with an occupational therapist and physical therapist each visiting his home one time per week. Office review sessions occurred monthly for a few months.

After 9 months of office therapy twice per week, plus the monthly review sessions, he could rise from any chair and sit down in any chair without assistance. He could rise from a floor and could crawl—both clear improvements for his functional safety. He walked unassisted with two canes, using a four-point gait. He could go up and down stairs with canes and minimal assistance. Sidestepping and lateral stability improved considerably. Upper-extremity control reached the point of unassisted feeding, and he was driving a disability-adapted car. He was also able to write with his dominant hand. Biofeedback helped him to identify the amount of muscle power needed to perform functional movements. The feedback also helped him create an awareness of the amount of muscle tension present during the various rehabilitative activities.

Case 7: CVA and Femoral Fracture

Presenting Diagnosis

Right CVA with resultant left hemiplegia. Fracture of the left femoral neck, with a femoral head prosthesis repair in the left hip. Reflex sympathetic dystrophy of the muscles distal to the fracture. Hypertension.

History and Medical Information

This patient was a 65-year-old woman who had suffered a right CVA from a ruptured aneurysm 1 year before seeing me. She had a left hemiplegia, but was able to ambulate independently with a dorsiflexion-assist leg brace and the use of a four-point cane. Her upper extremity had not responded to therapy. The left arm was spastic and carried in an elbow-flexed, internally rotated shoulder position. Nine months following the stroke, she fell and suffered a fracture of the head and neck of her left femur. A femoral head prosthesis was placed in her left femur. She lost all control of her left leg and was confined to a wheelchair. She had been walking before her fracture.

Evaluation

The patient came to me in a wheelchair and wearing a short leg brace, 1 year and 3 months after the femur fracture. She showed only trace muscle activity from the left quadriceps, as assessed by manual muscle testing. She had a predominant flexor withdrawal pattern in the lower extremity, a positive *Marie and Foix retraction sign*, and a hyperactive knee-jerk response. Joint range of motion remained full at all lower-extremity joints. When synergy patterns were used, the upper extremity showed some ability to flex at the shoulder. Her humeral head was well seated in the glenoid fossa. Upper-extremity motion was full at all joints. She appeared highly motivated for additional therapy. She wanted to increase her muscle awareness for walking and regain any possible function of her arm.

Goals of Therapy

1. To promote independent ambulation.
2. To increase function of her left arm.

Treatment

Treatment started with a program for the lower extremity. To stimulate quadriceps contraction, I tapped the patient's patellar tendon with a reflex hammer, using EMG feedback from the quadriceps muscle during this procedure. She tried to maintain the audio feedback signal and keep her leg straight during each induced contraction. After 3 weeks of twice-per-week sessions, she could initiate and maintain some muscle contraction without tapping the tendon. Muscle strength was still graded "poor-plus" (30%).

Therapy then shifted to using biofeedback with a progressive resistance exercise for the quadriceps. After two additional sessions over 6 weeks, she achieved and was maintaining a "good" muscle grade (75%). She then progressed to gait training with threshold feedback during the swing-through and heel-strike phases. She also received feedback from the tibialis anterior muscle during dorsiflexion of the foot promoted by a flexion withdrawal reflex. Training started in a 90° hip-flexed and 90° knee-flexed sitting position. As the sessions progressed, the patient performed dorsiflexion with less and less hip flexion and a straighter knee position, with biofeedback provided throughout the entire progression. These procedures were to help her perform the target skill with less and less synergy pattern facilitation. She required 20 sessions of therapy to reach a point of partially controlled dorsiflexion sufficient to clear the floor. In addition, she required review of this skill once per month. At follow-up, she still wore a short leg brace, but without a dorsiflexion assist, and remained on a progressive strengthening program.

Therapy for the upper extremity started with attempts to increase external rotation of the humerus. The target muscles for EMG monitoring were the rotator cuff muscles of the scapula. The patient retracted the humerus in the glenoid while increasing the EMG signal. The next target muscles were the rhomboids and scapular stabilizers. A flexion synergy pattern helped promote arm flexion. She then worked to strengthen external rotation retraction and shoulder girdle stability. The next arm exercise was eccentric flexion, 150° through 100° motion. She then learned to use the anterior deltoid for concentric arm flexion. (Wolf, 1982, advocates starting proximally and proceeding distally in training.)

The patient next learned to hold her arm at 90° flexion. The next progression was holding at 90° flexion while flexing and extending the elbow. A four-count progression then followed—touching her hand to her mouth, relaxing the biceps, straightening the elbow, and relaxing the triceps and arm again. The triceps and biceps each had one separate EMG monitor. The progression helped to disrupt the synergy pattern.

Feedback also proceeded from the wrist flexors and extensors. The patient first learned to relax the wrist flexors and then learned to extend her fingers while maintaining decreased flexor muscle tone (see Figure 23.11A). When she had control of the flexors, she learned to extend the thumb. This created a usable open hand. The wrist–finger training was combined with the elbow and shoulder sessions. Total upper-extremity control was then practiced in varying positions of arm flexion and abduction–adduction. She then learned grip and release with increasingly weighted objects and in varying positions. The entire process proceeded toward functional control without feedback (see Figure 23.11B).

The upper-extremity process took 4 months, at a frequency of twice per week. The goal was to teach the patient awareness and control in functional positions. To evoke initial activity, I used synergy patterns and reflex activity. The patient then progressed toward control with less reliance on therapist facilitation. In summary, this patient developed functional control of her hand and arm. She could use it in preparing meals and in other daily activities. The patient eventually became fully independent with a regular cane, and she could climb stairs and ambulate with minimal limitations. The biofeedback helped develop better control of the muscles and dominant patterns.

Case 8: Rotator Cuff Tear Caused by Motor Vehicle Accident

Presenting Diagnosis

Tear of the supraspinatus portion of the rotator cuff caused by rapid stretch during a motor vehicle accident.

History and Medical Information

This patient was a 58-year-old man who had sustained a tear of the superspinatus muscle at its transition from muscle into tendinous sheath. He had pain at the posterior portion of the left shoulder joint. Four days after the accident, he developed "severe weakness." For 2 days following the accident, he had periodic numbing along the posterior portion of the left forearm.

Evaluation

The patient presented with moderate soreness at the posterior left shoulder and considerable tenderness to palpation at the lateral portion of the superspinatus muscle. He held his left shoulder in an anterior rotated position, and the humerus was tight in the joint anteriorly and internally rotated. Posterior glide of the humerus in the glenoid showed tightness and resistance. The vertebral border of the scapula on the left was slightly winged, and the patient had a tender subscapularis "trigger point." He showed myofascial tightness over the left scapula and a "trigger point" at the infraspinatus location. Strength during external rotation of the shoulder and abduction were both reduced by 50% and painful. Shoulder range of motion was within normal limits, but showed an impingement sign at 125° forward flexion and 80° of lateral abduction.

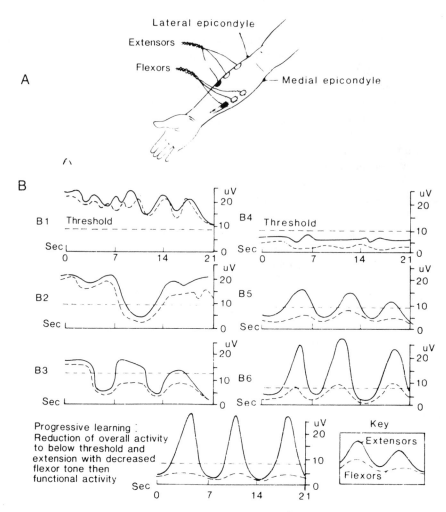

FIGURE 23.11. (A) Dual monitoring of flexor and extensor activity on two separate EMG channels. (B) Printouts derived from Hyperion "Bioconditioner" EMG, demonstrating reduction of overall activity to below threshold and extension with decreased flexor tone, and progress toward functional activity.

Goals of Therapy

1. Reduce protective spasm of the subscapularis musculature.
2. Teach patient proper use of the supraspinatus muscle (increase muscle tone).
3. Strengthen arm in all affected motions.
4. Teach home progressive resistive exercise program.

Treatment

The patient had developed a protective spasm of the subscapularis portion of the rotator cuff, and, as a result, had decreased muscle tone of the supraspinatus portion of the rotator cuff. The supraspinatus was too tender to promote increased muscle strain and needed pain-controlling therapy before muscle reeducation could begin. For three times per week in the first 2 weeks, he received various modalities consisting of electric acutherapy, ice massage, and phonophoresis with corticosteroid. Next, he received myofascial stretching of the left scapular area, followed by scapular mobilization promoting scapular glide and rotation. Posterior glide mobilization of the left humerus helped release the restricted joint. Next, muscle reeducation started with an EMG monitor on the left supraspinatus muscle. The patient pulled his arm in shoulder retraction while the therapist gave mild resistance, and the arm was in a 45° forward flexion position. (The lower scapular-to-vertebral stabilizers are excellent monitor sites for teaching scapular retraction–adduction.) When he consistently used his supraspinatus to stabilize the joint properly, exercise progressed to strengthening. He retracted the shoulder and produced EMG activity from the supraspinatus, and then performed each assigned strengthening exercise. Exercise consisted of isometric holds, isotonic movement, and isokinetic activity. During all exercises, he attended to the EMG signal.

Because of pain and tearing, the patient had lost active function of the supraspinatus muscle. He learned to use the affected muscle during all natural functioning movements. The feedback provided "muscle awareness" after the pain was controlled. Feedback also reminded the patient to stabilize his joint properly and retract his scapula during all exercise sessions. He had exercise assignments for homework. Treatment was twice a week for 6 weeks.

Case 9: Multiple Sclerosis

Presenting Diagnosis

Multiple sclerosis with complaints of knee instability and back pain.

History and Medical Information

This patient was a 54-year-old woman with a diagnosis of multiple sclerosis and lumbosacral back pain. She came to our clinic complaining of instability in both knees. She stated that she felt particularly insecure when pivoting on her legs. She felt she was "losing awareness" of her lower extremities. She had received 6 months of muscle strengthening at a major hospital's rehabilitation department.

Evaluation

The patient came to the clinic walking with a four-point pickup walker and showed considerable *hyperlordosis* of the lumbosacral spine while maintaining herself in a forward flexed position. When each leg began stance phase and weight bearing, she pulled back hard with the hamstring musculature to create a locked-knee position. She hyperextended her knees and had little to no pushoff at the end-of-stance phase, on both sides. Muscle strength in the lower extremities tested as "strong" (90–100%), but it was used only in a shortened arc of motion.

The patient had lost awareness of muscle contraction and release. She used her muscles in an all-or-none fashion. She needed feedback on when and how much to use her muscles.

Goals of Therapy

1. To increase muscle awareness for functional control of muscles during gait.
2. To teach muscle control during functional patterns.

Treatment

The patient had excellent muscle strength and a well-developed home strengthening program. Thus therapy proceeded with specific muscle pattern training. She received both EMG and force-dependent biofeedback. The first EMG monitor site was from the quadriceps muscles. First, she learned to control the feedback signal and use her muscles in a sitting, non-gravity-dependent position. She progressed to standing weight transfer, in which she was required to increase the EMG signal from each leg as she bore weight on each limb. Force feedback, dependent on body weight, came from pressure-sensitive pads placed in her shoes. With 50% of body weight transferred to the support limb, auditory feedback signaled her. She then increased the quadriceps contraction from that limb. The EMG monitor on the active quadriceps gave a threshold-dependent auditory signal showing proper levels. She progressed through various body transfers, such as sidestepping, pivoting, forward walking, and backward walking.

The next step in feedback focused on pushoff at the end-of-stance phase; EMG feedback came from both the hamstring muscles and the calf musculature. The patient first learned control of these muscle groups in a non-gravity-dependent sitting position. Then she learned to flex the knee with the hamstrings, rather than pulling back on the joint into knee extension. Exercise in a standing position started at this time. EMG feedback from the calf musculature signaled her when she was pushing with the feet. She learned to increase pushoff from midstance until the end-of-stance phase. Calf control helped to reduce knee hyperextension. Next, she learned ascending and descending stairs with increased control of the calf during both motions. Her task was to control the calf tension during eccentric release of the muscle. This occurred during lowering onto the foot and controlling heel impact while going down stairs. Then she learned to push off with the foot and calf muscles while ascending stairs. EMG feedback from the calf musculature was continuous.

The patient learned to control her movements during stair climbing and descending, pivoting, gait, and all weight transfers. Proper pushoff decreased her forward flexion position at the back and eliminated her back pain. Her greater control allowed her to perform all standing movements independently with two forearm crutches.

Treatment sessions occurred twice per week for 6 weeks, and there was one exercise review 1 month after the completion of formal therapy. Both pressure force and EMG feedback provided awareness to her, and she gained meaningful information to correct her gait. This information transferred to functional learning.

FINAL CONSIDERATIONS

There are three more general concepts important in the feedback process but not yet mentioned in this chapter. First, muscles that have been in spasm will often "overpower" the relaxed muscles; one must strengthen a weakened muscle to perform its normal function. Second, as in therapy for head control for cerebral palsy (Russell & Woolbridge, 1975), muscle or position feedback also must promote optimum joint position and the most functional posture for a particular patient. Third, one cannot train an isolated muscle without attending to its kinesiological partners.

SUMMARY

In this chapter, I have described some techniques I believe are helpful when biofeedback is used with physical therapy procedures. One must remember that feedback is simply a means for a therapist to facilitate the learning of functional awareness and control. Feedback is not the actual treatment in the present model, but rather a cluster of electronic and electromechanical instrumentation-based techniques that convey additional useful information into a common language that facilitates the use of other therapy techniques.

GLOSSARY

AGONIST. A muscle directly involved in contraction and opposed by the action of an antagonist muscle, which needs to relax for proper function of the agonist muscle. (See the glossary in Krebs & Fagerson, Chapter 22, this volume.)

ANTAGONIST. A muscle that opposes or resists the action of an agonist muscle or prime mover. (Again, see Krebs & Fagerson, Chapter 22.)

BALLISTIC MOTION. Trajectory of guided objects or projectiles.

BUDDING/GEMMATION/SPROUTING. A form of fission in which the parent cell does not divide but puts out a budlike process (daughter cell) of a small size containing its proportion of chromatin, which then separates and begins an independent existence.

CONTRACTION, CONCENTRIC. A muscle's developing enough tension to overcome resistance and move a body part.

CONTRACTION, ECCENTRIC. Resistance overcoming a muscle action and lengthening it.

FOOT SLAP/DROP. Inability to maintain a foot dorsi-flexed position or maintain eccentrically released dorsiflexion upon foot heel strike during gait.

HYPERLORDOSIS. Extreme lordosis; lordosis; a bending backwards; an anteroposterior curvature of the spine, with the convexity looking anterior.

HYPERREFLEXIA. A condition in which the deep tendon reflexes are exaggerated.

HYPERTROPHY. Overgrowth; general increase in bulk of a part or organ; not due to tumor formation.

KINETIC CHAIN. All the muscles involved in controlling and completing a functional movement. *Kinetic* relates to motion.

MARIE AND FOIX RETRACTION SIGN. Upon forcing the toes downward, the knee and hip are drawn into flexion.

PRIME MOVER. A muscle mainly responsible for directly causing an intended action or movement.

SIDESTEPPING. Lateral stepping during which no body pivoting or rotation takes place.

SPROUTING. If a portion of muscle is deprived of its innervation, nerves near the denervated portion send collaterals to those muscles. Nerve fiber ends just proximal to a lesion begin to develop buds or sprouts.

STABILIZER (FIXATOR). Accessory muscle that steadies or stabilizes a part, thus allowing more precise movements in an associated structure.

SYNERGIST MUSCLES. Muscles that act together to have a mutually helpful (cooperative) action, such as flexor muscles.

REFERENCES

Basmajian, J. V. (1977). Learned control of single motor units. In G. E. Schwartz & J. Beatty (Eds.), *Biofeedback: Therapy and research*. New York: Academic Press.

Basmajian, J. V. (Ed.). (1989). *Biofeedback: Principles and practice for clinicians* (3rd ed.) Baltimore: Williams & Wilkins.

Brudny, J., Grynbaum, B. L., & Korein, J. (1974). Spasmodic torticollis: Treatment by feedback display of EMG. *Archives of Physical Medicine and Rehabilitation, 55*, 503–408.

Brunnstrom, S. (1970). *Movement therapy in hemiplegia: A neurophysiological approach*. New York: Harper & Row.

Carlsson, S. G. (1975). Treatment of temporo-mandibular joint syndrome with biofeedback training. *Journal of the American Dental Association, 91*, 602–605.

Fogel, E. R. (1995). Biofeedback-assisted musculoskeletal therapy and neuromuscular re-education. In M. S. Schwartz & Associates, *Biofeedback: A practitioner's guide* (2nd ed.). New York: Guilford Press.

Hagbarth, K. E. (1973). The effect of muscle vibration in normal man and in patients with motor disorders. In J. E. Desmedt (Ed.), *New development in electromyography and clinical neurophysiology* (Vol. 3). Basel, Switzerland: Karger.

Hagbarth, K. E., & Eklund, G. (1969). The muscle vibrator: A useful tool in neurological therapeutic work. *Scandinavian Journal of Rehabilitation Medicine, 1,* 26–34.

Hislop, H. J., & Montgomery, J. (Eds.). (2002). *Daniels and Worthington's muscle testing: Techniques of manual examination* (7th ed.). Philadelphia: W. B. Saunders.

Knott, M., & Voss, D. (1969). *Proprioceptive neuromuscular facilitation* (2nd ed.). New York: Harper & Row.

Marinacci, A. A., & Horande, M. (1960). Electromyogram in neuromuscular reeducation. *Bulletin of the Los Angeles Neurological Society, 25,* 57–67.

McMennell, J. B. (1951). *Manual therapy* (No. 85). Springfield, IL: Thomas.

Rugh, J. (1977). *Learning differential control of balanced orofacial muscles.* Paper presented at the 8th Annual Meeting of the Biofeedback Society of America, Orlando, FL.

Russell, G., & Woolbridge, C. P. (1975). Correction of a habitual head tilt using biofeedback techniques: A case study. *Physiotherapy Canada, 27,* 181–184.

Sella, G. E. (1998). Towards an integrated approach of surface EMG utilization: Quantitative protocols of assessment and biofeedback. In *Electromyography: Applications in physical medicine* (Monograph No. 13). Woerden, The Netherlands: BFE.

Sella, G. E. (2000). *Guidelines for neuromuscular re-education: The electromyographic approach.* Martins Ferry, OH: Gen Med.

Travell, J. G., & Simons, D. G. (1983). *Myofascial pain and dysfunction: The trigger point manual.* Baltimore: Williams & Wilkins.

Wolf, S. I. (1982). *Treatment of neuromuscular problems; Treatment of musculoskeletal problems* [Two audio cassettes]. In J. Sandweiss (Ed.), *Biofeedback reviews seminars.* Los Angeles: University of California–Los Angeles.

Wolf, S. I., Regenos, E., & Basmajian, J. V. (1977). Developing strategies for biofeedback applications in neurologically handicapped patients. *Physical Therapy, 57,* 402–408.

CHAPTER 24

Psychophysiology for Performing Artists

MARCIE ZINN
MARK ZINN

We have to find some way of making the health of the performer more important than the show.
—DAVID HINKAMP, MD, MPH

EVOLUTION OF PERFORMING ARTS PSYCHOPHYSIOLOGY

Performing arts psychophysiology is the second specialty to grow out of the awareness that musicians and artists may have needs that are somewhat different from those of other patients. As a specialty, performing arts medicine was developed in the early 1980s to address the issues created by participation in a particular performing art itself (Brandfonbrener, 2000). Simply stated, it became very obvious that artists appeared to have both unique presentations of common ailments, and more specific ailments that were unique in etiology because of participation in the arts. A performing arts psychologist wrote that "psychology's role in the care of performers has lagged behind that of athletes, where special attention is given to performance enhancement, the promotion of well-being, and clinical issues in sports" (quoted in Hamilton, 1997, p. 67). Attention to such issues for performing artists is coming of age.

There are three main points of emphasis for all performing arts health care. First, performers depend heavily on the physical condition of their bodies (Harding, Brandt, & Hilberry, 1993; Hoppman & Patrone, 1989; Leijnse, 1996; Parr, 1988). The parts of the body used during performance of a musical instrument, in fact, function like an instrument; the body (the primary instrument) is just as involved in the music-making process as the chosen (secondary) instrument. Anyone can depress a piano key or pluck a violin string, but it takes a professional to turn these events into music. Performing arts medicine openly and aggressively addresses the physiology of this issue.

Second, musicians have been found to have a high prevalence and incidence of psychiatric disorders (Nagel, 1998; Ostwald, Avery, & Ostwald, 1998), including mood, anxiety, personality, somatoform, substance use, sleep, psychotic, and eating disorders (Cohen & Kupersmith, 1986; Fishbein, Middlestadt, Ottai, Straus, & Ellis, 1988; Ostwald et al., 1998). The field of applied psychophysiology and biofeedback is a profession dedicated to the research and development of clinical applications for mind–body, stress-related phenomena.

Under this paradigm, psychiatric or psychological problems will produce stress-related somatic issues.

Third, psychophysiology is frequently mentioned in various performing arts sources. Ziporyn (1984) has emphasized that psychological stress produces overall muscle tension and physical stress, which in turn predispose a performer to physical injury. Coons, Montello, and Perez (1995) found significantly depressed immune responses in musicians who used denial and avoidance coping in music performance anxiety (MPA). Craske and Rachman (1987) found that perceived skill levels in musicians were inversely related to heart rate. In addition, David Sternbach (1993) has argued that a high proportion of musicians' illnesses appear to be stress-related. And finally, Richard Lederman (1999), in his address to the Annual Symposium on Medical Problems of Musicians and Dancers, discussed the compelling evidence for the role of the autonomic nervous system in MPA and other problems—evidence that calls for the involvement of psychophysiology. More specifically, he underscored the role of an overactive sympathetic nervous system (SNS) and an underactive parasympathetic nervous system (PNS) in musicians' health problems. These issues cannot be adequately addressed by standard medical procedures.

The role of psychophysiology in performing arts appears to be twofold. Ordinarily a person who is affected by a particular disease or disorder can still function well enough in his or her profession and does not lose status as a professional. However, when an artist has any type of disease or disorder, the performance is severely compromised by the effects of the disease on the body. As a result, the artist may not be able to perform. Therefore, the presence of a disease process that is significant enough to stop participation in the art threatens the primary source of income, undermines a career, and lowers the status of the artist (Brandfonbrener, 1991; Harman, 1998; Sternbach, 1993). Two poignant examples are Gary Graffman and Leon Fleisher. Both were concert pianists whose performing careers were curtailed in the early 1980s because of disabilities involving their hands. It is common for artists to present with symptoms that impair their art, but these symptoms are not readily apparent to an observer and are often not detected by standard medical tests (Brandfonbrener, 2000). Anecdotal evidence indicates that nearly 100% of artists' problems are physiologically and psychologically "intertwined," and that nearly every patient seen in arts medicine clinics appears to have significant psychological problems exacerbating the presenting physical pathology (A. Brandfonbrener, personal communications, 1996, 1999, 2000, 2001).

PSYCHOLOGICAL AND PHYSICAL PROBLEMS OF PERFORMING ARTISTS

The largest and perhaps most famous survey concerning health issues of artists was the one conducted by Fishbein et al. (1988) at the request of the International Conference of Symphony and Opera Musicians (ICSOM). ICSOM is the union for the major orchestra and opera companies in the world. The response rate of this survey was 55%. Out of the 2212 respondents, 76% reported pain severe enough to affect their performance, and 68% reported musculoskeletal problems (with 47.4% in the neck or upper back, and 28% in the arms or shoulders). In the nonmusculoskeletal category, nearly 72% registered complaints, with MPA reported by 24%, depression by 16.6%, sleep problems by 14.2%, and acute anxiety by 13.2%.

More specifically, the existence of chronic musculoskeletal pain (Hoppman & Patrone, 1989; Roach, Martinez, & Anderson, 1994; Zaza, 1992) and tension (Brooks, 1993) is well documented in the performing arts medical literature, as are the effects of pain and tension on musicians' careers and performances (Hoppman & Patrone, 1991). Among the effects of pain and tension are severe disruptions in normal playing habits (Brandfonbrener, 1991), endurance (Roach et al., 1994), and overall control of musical output on the instrument (Ostwald & Avery, 1991). Muscle tension has also been implicated as a risk factor in repetitive strain disorder and occupation-related syndromes, such as tendonitis and peripheral nerve entrapment syndromes (Nakano, 1991).

MUSCULOSKELETAL DISORDERS OF PERFORMING ARTISTS: TREATMENT AND MANAGEMENT ISSUES

Musculoskeletal disorders are reported to be the most common occupational disorder in the arts (Bejjani et al., 1989; Bejjani, Kay, & Behnam, 1996). Psychophysiologists are well aware of the ongoing and complex subtle adjustments in muscle tension–relaxation that take place every second. Since musculoskeletal problems present such a major issue for artists and because we are aware of the problems that can arise from improper usage, it is necessary to alter assessment and history taking to include what the instrument is and what problems with the instrument there may be, including psychosocial issues. Table 24.1 (Hoppman & Patrone, 1989; Zinn Piano Program for Performing Artists; Zinn & Zinn, 2000) provides a list of history-taking items that aid in assessment of a musician.

Another ramification is the fact that musicians, once affected with musculoskeletal issues, are likely to seek therapy from nearly anyone who promises a cure, regardless of that person's training or experience. It is common to seek treatment from other musicians who have no training in any type of medical science (A. Brandfonbrener, personal communication, July 2001). Musicians wish to get better quickly, but not for the same reason as other patients. Their reason has to do with career and income; simply put, because when they can't play, they can't make money. These fast "cures" are sought in the hope that the problems really can be resolved quickly and so they do not have to leave their profession.

A third problem comes from chronic misdiagnosis. As stated before, performing arts issues are difficult if not impossible to detect with standard diagnostic procedures. Its common for physicians to advise an artist simply to "quit playing." This scenario can be incredibly frustrating and shaming for everyone involved. If a physician is not trained in performing arts issues, it is unlikely that an adequate diagnosis can be made. The doctor, feeling helpless, may implicitly "diagnose" a factitious disorder. The artist, feeling helpless, may

---

TABLE 24.1. History-Taking Items for Musicians

1. Major instrument; instrument(s) played and for how long; approximate length of practice sessions daily; recent change in instrument.

2. Practice habits: Warm-up and cool-down periods; length and frequency of sessions; length and frequency of breaks; difficulty level of pieces; movements or positions that may elicit pain or stiffness.

3. Lessons: Length of lessons; difficulty level of pieces studied; recent change in technique; change in teacher.

4. Symptoms: Onset; when playing or delayed; effect on performance; paresthesias; motor control problems.

5. Substance abuse/dependence: Alcohol, prescription medications, and nonprescription drugs. (Note that beta-blockers are often prescribed for artists.)

6. History of other types of therapy (movement therapies, physiotherapy, etc).

7. Performing history: Number of annual performances; amount of travel; opportunities for warm-up and rehearsal.

Note. Based on Hoppman and Patrone (1989) and the Zinn Piano Program for Performing Artists; Zinn and Zinn (2000).

continue in standard medical therapy, but more often will seek some alternative type of treatment.

A fourth problem is the lack of emphasis on critical thinking skills in music training. In scientific training programs, students spend a great of time learning to analyze and interpret data. Most musicians are simply not trained to think scientifically, so when they need some type of decision-making skills, they largely do not have those skills. They therefore tend to make the fundamental attribution error over and over, and fail to see the trend in their errors.

When artists present to biofeedback providers, it is likely that the artists have been rejected by physicians, have sought help from underqualified "practitioners," are faced with severe financial and career problems, and have limited ability to explore their options in an informed manner. Artists also tend to lack sufficient social support and to have high levels of chronic stress from traveling (Sternbach, 1993). Biofeedback providers will need to make a significant impact during the first visit, or the artists may not return (Wickramasekera, 1991). These clients need to see biofeedback as different from their previous experiences, and providers need to do what they can to earn their clients' trust.

USE OF SURFACE ELECTROMYOGRAPHIC FEEDBACK FOR MUSCULOSKELETAL DISORDERS IN PERFORMING ARTISTS

The error rate produced by detrimental role of sustained muscle tension (Lockwood, 1989) has been discussed in the performing arts literature since the 15th century; the damaging effects mentioned frequently in most sources are loss of control of tone and articulation, slowed movements, and pain (Gerig, 1974). Use of surface electromyographic (EMG) feedback as part of a treatment package for musicians has produced documented results for overall tension reduction in fine motor skill acquisition (French, 1980), tension relief (Levee, Cohen, & Rickles, 1976; Morasky, Reynolds, & Sowell, 1983), and muscle tension reduction in string players (Morasky, Reynolds, & Clarke, 1981) and in a woodwind player (Levee et al., 1976). (It has also been used to control MPA [LeVine & Irvine, 1984; Morasky et al., 1981], as discussed in more detail later.) In these and other studies, surface EMG (hereafter referred to simply as EMG) was superior to controls when used as the primary dependent variable. Common to these studies was the hypothesis that sustained high levels of muscle contraction inhibit smooth motor movements and contribute to fatigue in instrument playing. Richard Hoppman (1998), a performing arts medicine specialist, describes musculoskeletal pain as the most common presenting complaint of instrumentalists, and cites musculotendinous overuse as the disorder with the highest incidence rate. Overuse is discussed elsewhere as an upper-extremity disorder that has been successfully treated with EMG feedback (Spence, Sharpe, Newton-John, & Champion, 1995). What appears to be common to these early studies was the implicit expectation that overall reduction in muscle tension was the primary goal of the musicians.

Subsequent lines of evidence indicate that the problem may be a truncated tension–relaxation cycle, rather than an overall tension problem (Gerig, 1974; Montes, Bedmar, & Martin, 1993; Zinn, 1998). Between 1905 and 1921, Rudolph Breithaupt, a classical pianist and teacher, published a series of books and articles outlining the necessity of relaxation immediately after a keystroke. Professional pianists appear to relax immediately after the keystroke, making their tension–relaxation cycle more efficient and variable (Parlitz, Peschel, & Altenmuller, 1998) and extending their endurance significantly beyond that of amateurs (Penn, Chuang, & Chan, 2001).

Montes et al. (1993) addressed this issue by monitoring the abductor pollicis brevis muscle in the thumb. The underlying premise of the study was Basmajian's (1977) evidence indicating that precision in motor skill occurs as the subject learns to inhibit unnecessary muscle recruitment and muscular bracing. The subjects were taught to decrease the amount of time in their tension (keystroke)–relaxation cycle. Zinn (1998) developed a similar protocol for pianists, which involves learning to strike the piano key with enough tension to produce about 30 microvolts of EMG signal, and then to relax immediately after the keystroke (i.e., to bring the signal below 5 microvolts). Subjects were monitored in the forearm (the extensor carpi radialis and ulnaris). In a multiple-baseline-across-subjects time series design, EMG feedback to develop intrakeystroke relaxation was significantly superior to baseline (being instructed to relax to the best of their ability) among all subjects. The subjects in this study were nonmusicians (no prior musical training), aged 25–46, of both genders. Parlitz et al. (1998) measured the same phenomenon, using sensors located under the keys of a piano. They found that the more elite players had a strong keystroke followed immediately by a key duration with minimal force. A similar study of neuromuscular issues for pianists found that piano playing is primarily an experience of endurance rather than of strength (Penn et al., 2001).

Since uneconomical use of tension and force in piano playing has been shown to be a risk factor in pianists' injuries (Hoppman, 1998), it follows that biofeedback to reduce unnecessary tension is likely to be helpful in problems ranging from pain to nonoptimal performance. Other biofeedback modalities for artists are not discussed specifically in the literature; examples of using "biofeedback for general well-being," without listing what modality was used, are more common (DeLorenzo, 1990).

USE OF BIOFEEDBACK FOR ASSESSMENT AND TREATMENT OF ANXIETY AND RELATED SOMATIC SYMPTOMS

Perhaps a broader use of biofeedback for performing artists is in the assessment and treatment of anxiety and related somatic symptoms, using a number of biofeedback modalities. We (Zinn, McCain, & Zinn, 2000) found that three of the four predisposers from the High Risk Model of Threat Perception (HRMTP) (Wickramasekera, 1988) and peripheral vasoconstriction, measured 6 weeks prior to a jury exam, predicted state anxiety scores immediately after the exam ($p \leq .041$). There was also a significant ($p \leq .01$) change in hand temperature between 6 weeks prior to the jury exam and immediately following the exam. We included hand temperature as a physiological measure because of the experimental control it offers (biofeedback measurements are more resilient to experimental demand characteristics; Bordens & Abbot, 1988) and because of its reliability in measuring the stress response. Vasodilation and vasoconstriction in the periphery are exclusively sympathetically innervated and therefore provide a direct measure of ANS reactivity (Adams, Victor, & Ropper, 1997).

The somatic symptoms typical of anxiety disorders, such as cold, sweaty hands, racing heart, breathlessness, and muscle tension, are not only disruptive to normal behavior (Clark, 1996; Hope & Heimberg, 1993) but undermine musical performance (Steptoe & Fidler, 1987; Sternbach, 1993). SNS reactivity then tends to produce more anxiety, because of the increase in error rate that the SNS symptoms produce in the performance (Lederman, 1999; Lockwood, 1989).

In a sample of 51 participants (Zinn & Zinn, 2002), the hand temperature ($M = 81.37°F$) was significantly below the normal means (88.5°F) published by Blanchard (1989) (see Figure 24.1). Glenn Gould, a famous concert pianist, wore gloves with the fingertips cut out while playing the piano, because he had cold hands.

Other somatic problems experienced by musicians during performance include tremor (shaky hands, legs, etc.), heart palpitations, shortness of breath, gastrointestinal problems (nausea, vomiting, diarrhea), decreased salivation (inhibition of the PNS), and skin changes

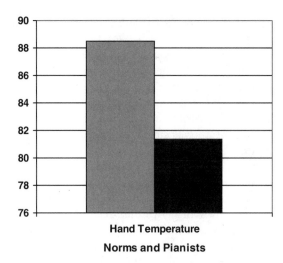

FIGURE 24.1. Hand temperature of 51 pianists compared to norms.

such as blushing and temperature regulation problems (Lederman, 1999). These problems can be modified significantly by standard biofeedback protocols that are currently in place. Since a musician has spent long hours at an instrument, it is helpful if the clinician can aid in effecting transfer of what is learned during biofeedback to the instrument. Helping the client come up with some steps to countercondition common stress reactions will likely be as helpful as anything the clinician can accomplish in the clinic. See Table 24.2 and Appendix 24.1 for some ideas.

TABLE 24.2. Some Issues in Using Biofeedback Protocols with Performing Artists

Modality	Some predominant issues	Ideas for therapy
Temperature training	Large conditioning component in practice, performance places, specific pieces of music, specific styles of playing, etc. These need to be addressed.	Home practice can include practice a desensitization procedure with gradual increases in intensity of conditioned stimuli (the instrument, music, etc.).
Muscle relaxation/control	Conditioning predominates again, but musicians have finite control already. They will have to stop at key places in their music and relax before proceeding.	During practice at home, the client can be advised to stop at every phrase ending in an important piece, and should be reminded that "old music will elicit old habits."
Deep breathing, minirelaxation, self-hypnosis	Upon questioning, it often emerges that a client rarely takes breaks, practices in dimly lit rooms with little oxygen, etc.	The client and clinician should discuss all the times that the client can stop and relax daily (during teaching, rehearsals, etc.).
Psychophysiological stress profile	A tape recording of the client's own playing is used as the stressor.	Provides major impact as to the etiology of the problem.

As noted earlier in connection with musculoskeletal disorders, history taking in relationship to the particular artist and art form is crucial. All aspects of the musician, instrument, performance places, and so forth must be known. The clinician and client should discuss how and where the client practices, how he or she sits or stands, and what about the music exacerbates the client's condition. The clinician should look for signs such as symmetry, raised shoulders, limited range of motion, and general poor posture. The client should be reminded that this is not an audition, and that he or she can relax. See Tables 24.2 and 24.3 for some treatment-planning ideas.

TABLE 24.3. **Some Issues That May Affect Treatment Planning**

Issue	What many nonmusician clients may "look like" clinically	What musicians may "look like" clinically
Appointment arrival	Varies from client to client.	Most will arrive early.
Confidentiality	An issue, but is taken for granted mostly (past experience in other medical settings). An implicit expectation.	Probably a significant issue, because their jobs may be on the line if their employers find out that they are seeking medical attention that may affect music making.
Past experience in regard to getting medical attention	Will have seen a variety of medical doctors, some alternative therapists, etc. Will expect a certain level of training in the therapist.	Will probably have seen predominantly other musicians who have no training in any type of therapy, alternative or otherwise. Will not differentiate between other musicians and qualified healers.
Motivation to participate in therapy	All ranges of motivation and premature dropout rate (common); will avoid homework and probably avoid record keeping unless clients have a profession that requires record keeping.	Highly motivated *if* they trust their clinicians. Will tend to "overdo" homework assignments and *appear* compulsive (are used to tracking their own experience).
Progress in therapy	Normal progress—what clinicians see in their clinics now. Biofeedback creates new awareness of proprioceptive cues; biofeedback will primarily serve as a learning procedure and a redirection of attention and awareness.	Rapid progress, because musicians tend to learn new musculoskeletal paradigms very quickly and efficiently. Highly developed levels of proprioceptive awareness already intact; biofeedback will primarily serve as a confirmatory procedure rather than a redirection of attention and awareness.
Payment issues	Expect insurance to pay, and therapist bills insurance.	Are used to paying "up front" and at the time of services. Private study for professionals ranges from about $80 to $200 per hour, and many musicians study privately for 20 to 30 years.

CASE EXAMPLE: PSYCHOPHYSIOLOGICAL DIAGNOSIS AND TREATMENT

The following is a case study of a classical pianist with a history of chronic muscle tension, pain in the right forearm, cold sweaty hands, and MPA. EMG biofeedback, systematic desensitization, cognitive-behavioral therapy, relaxation, self-soothing, and specific transfer of techniques were associated with a remission of symptoms and a return to a full concert and teaching schedule. The HRMTP and the Trojan Horse Procedure (Wickramasekera, 1988) were used for assessment, role induction, and stress management. The program for this client consisted of education, treatment as described above, and transfer of learning into piano practice and piano performance, including client-directed *in vivo* desensitization. This case study appears to illustrate the efficacy of this type of program for chronic pain and MPA. It also may provide insight into the nature of stress-related problems of performing artists.

This case study conceptualizes MPA as a psychophysiological disorder. It may also illustrate chronic muscle tension in music performance as a failure of adaptation—a failure of initial muscular bracing (Wickramasekera, 1988) to "adapt out" over time. Another aspect of this case is the association between increased, sustained muscle tension and anxiety disorders. This relationship has been shown to exist elsewhere, and the combination of anxiety and chronic muscle tension is more than sufficient to disrupt musical performance (Bejjani et al., 1996; Gerig, 1974; Reynolds & Clarke, 1981).

The client was a 51-year-old married female classical pianist who presented with a 37-year history of chronic muscle tension in the left trapezius region, moderate MPA, and a recent (2-year) history of dorsal forearm pain and dorsal wrist and hand pain precipitated by practicing and performance situations. Evaluations by performing arts medical specialists and other specialists (to whom she had been referred by her husband, a physician) had ruled out nerve entrapment syndromes, tendonitis, and all other physical sources of pain. The client had recently begun therapy with a board-certified psychiatrist and had been taking Tranxene, a benzodiazepine, just before performing. She reported that the Tranxene helped her anxiety symptoms, but she nonetheless found it very difficult to perform when taking it, because the sedative effects of the drug impaired her recall.

On a medical history questionnaire, the client stated that she had "physical tension caused by mental anxiety" and that she had a "continuous feeling of having to prove myself and anxiety over having to be better than others instead of just performing." The client denied a history of other physical or psychological problems, and denied substance abuse/dependence, current or past. She was not overweight and described herself as being in "excellent health." She, her husband, and their two daughters lived in the suburbs of a large city, where she taught at a prominent music school. During the initial contact, she expressed concern that others in the performing arts would find out that she was receiving treatment, which she thought would place her career at risk. She was reassured about confidentiality, and the issued was discussed at some length before treatment began.

Because of the client's problems, her performing career had virtually ended, although she was able to sustain herself teaching. Her number of yearly performances had dropped from about 25 to nearly zero. In treatment, she was instructed to play only when she was pain-free and to discontinue playing when the pain began. She was also instructed to use the benzodiazepine during rehearsal and performance, instead of performance only, to correct for state-dependent effects and allow for habituation (Klein, 1991). The psychiatrist she had been seeing was consulted, and the regimen was approved by him.

Following a performance assessment, the technique regimen she had been utilizing was hypothesized to be exacerbating her forearm pain. The exercises themselves have not been shown to be a risk factor for pain; instead, the way she conducted the exercises with sustained high levels of tension was hypothesized to be the primary factor in her pain. She was therefore instructed to discontinue that regimen until treatment began.

A J & J I-330 biofeedback unit was used to conduct the initial psychophysiological stress profile. The testing consisted of five components of 4 minutes each of physiological monitoring with four channels of physiology. The channels were peripheral skin temperature, electrodermal response (EDR), frontal EMG, and forearm EMG. Each of these components of the stress test consisted of 4 minutes (mean of 60 data points) of eyes open (EO), eyes closed (EC), stress (personally relevant stressor), and return to baseline EO and EC. Pretherapy testing demonstrated sympathetic reactivity (Rossi, 1993).

The extensor carpi radialis longus and the extensor carpi ulnaris (forearm muscles), which are central to movement of the fingers and thumb (Calais-Germain, 1993), were the specific sites monitored with the biofeedback equipment. Electrode placement was established with a standard electrode placement chart. Monitoring was done with both arms simultaneously; the signal for the right arm was in red and that for the left arm was blue, enabling the subject to discriminate between right and left. The data were collected with a standard biofeedback software program, the J & J Personal Computer Physiological Monitoring System, generating continuous visual feedback displayed to the subject on the video monitor with the computer.

Other aspects of assessment included ergonomics of the instrument; physical conditions of practice, rehearsal, and performance; and psychosocial problems, which may be present in such a case (Bejjani et al., 1996; Sataloff, Brandfonbrener, & Lederman, 1998). Initially, the client's piano practice was limited to 30–45 minutes daily. Her piano was in tune and regulated properly. Her seating height, posture, and use of her hands and arms were all within normal limits. There was no significant ulnar or radial deviation, and the wrist was not extended or flexed beyond normal limits, all of which are potential risk factors for nerve entrapment and overuse syndrome (Bejjani et al., 1996).

The HRMTP was used for psychophysiological assessment (Wickramasekera, 1988, 1998), psychophysiological role induction (Wickramasekera, 1988), and EMG stress reactivity measurement (Flor, Miltner, & Birbaumer, 1992). A personally relevant stressor, a tape recording of her own playing, was used in the stress profile, because the client stated that her forearm pain was specific to piano playing; this EMG response specificity has been demonstrated elsewhere in back pain and temporomandibular disorders (Flor et al., 1992).

Psychological testing with the HRMTP identifies psychosocial factors that are hypothesized to mediate threat perception consciously or unconsciously, regardless of the degree of physiological symptoms. These risk factors are divided into three categories: "predisposers," "triggers," and "buffers." The four predisposers are (1) high or low hypnotic ability (as measured by a standardized test of hypnotic ability); (2) cognitive catastrophizing (as measured by the Zocco [1984] catastrophizing scale); (3) high negative affect (>75%); and (4) high repression (>75%). The negative affect (trait anxiety) can be measured with the Eysenck Personality Questionnaire (Eysenck & Eysenck, 1975), and repression is measured with the Marlowe–Crowne Social Desirability Scale (Crowne & Marlowe, 1960). The predisposers are personality variables. The triggers are major life changes and accumulation of hassles or microstressors. The buffers are good social support systems, high satisfaction with that support, and good approach coping skills.

The primary goals of treatment were to reduce the client's forearm pain and left shoulder pain, treat her MPA, and increase her practice and performing stamina. The secondary goals were to establish effective transfer of these skills into her daily living, especially her practicing and performing on the piano.

The psychophysiological role induction is used to reorient the client into a psychophysiological/educational model and away from a traditional biomedical model. It provides a highly credible rationale for the client's physiological symptoms and demonstrates how cognitions alter physiology (Wickramasekera, 1988). Another function of the role induction is to turn the client into an active participant in therapy and to help him or her learn to self-monitor after therapy. The induction is therefore central to treatment. This client's profile on the HRMTP was positive for all four predisposers for somatization: absorption, suggesting high hypnotic ability (r = about .41 with hypnotic ability; Roche & McConkey, 1990), high catastrophizing, and high neuroticism + low repression score (see Table 24.4). The psychophysiological stress profile confirmed the source of the client's somatic anxiety symptoms. Her most reactive systems were hand temperature (73.1°F) and EDR (10.9 micromhos). The sources of her forearm pain were elevated EMG levels in the extensors carpi radialis longus and brevis, which are the usual sources of referred lower forearm pain (Simons, Travell, & Simons, 1999). The mean EMG level for the stress test was 4.42 microvolts; her EMG level during the stressor (an audiotape of her own playing) increased to 20.6 microvolts. Forehead tension was also high (mean = 4.41 microvolts). These results were a surprise to the client; she reported that with the exception of forearm pain and hands that "felt cold sometimes," she "felt fine." Despite the fact that the client came to treatment with considerable insight ("pain caused by mental anxiety"), she seemed most surprised to see the increased level of forearm tension when she listened to her own performance.

The client's initial forearm pain was relieved by teaching her to relax during intrakeystroke intervals and at other points of repose during a piece (during long notes, rests, etc). As a result of this intervention, the client began practicing relaxation while playing her current classical repertoire. The forearm pain ceased as a point of therapy.

The HRMTP predicts muscle spasm in people who have risk factors for stress-related somatic problems. This client reported left shoulder tension that had "existed for 38 years" (i.e., since her childhood). The position of her left shoulder was raised with regard to the right shoulder, although it felt as if the shoulders were normal to her. In other words, when she was able to lower her left shoulder to the position of the right, the client stated that the left shoulder felt significantly lower than the right. To assess this shoulder tension, which increased while she was playing, the trapezius muscles were monitored. During treatment, using the right trapezius as a control, the client was monitored for 36 sessions of EMG feedback at the piano (Figure 24.2). The initial difference between the shoulders was significant, t (1, 55) = 10.379, p = .000. The treatment continued until a nonsignificant result—(t (1, 55) = 0.539, p = .593, .800, and .809 in sessions 29, 30, and 31, respectively—was obtained for several sessions in a row. The result remained nonsignificant at follow-up.

During the course of the sessions, the client "discovered" that any type of uncertainty about the piece she was playing at the moment resulted in immediate increase in EMG. She discovered the effects of muscular bracing in response to stress (not knowing where some notes are, etc.). As a result, she was able to alter her practice habits to learn pieces more thoroughly. She was successful in altering the proprioception of her shoulders by working with herself to keep the shoulders even and remind herself that they were indeed even. Her playing became more fluent, to the degree that colleagues commented about the positive change in many aspects of her performance. Other interventions (self-hypnosis to reduce physiological reactivity just be-

TABLE 24.4. HRMTP Risk Factors at Pre- and Posttreatment

	Intake	1-yr. follow-up
Absorption	33	33
Negative affect	18	4
Catastrophizing	42	29
Repression	6	9

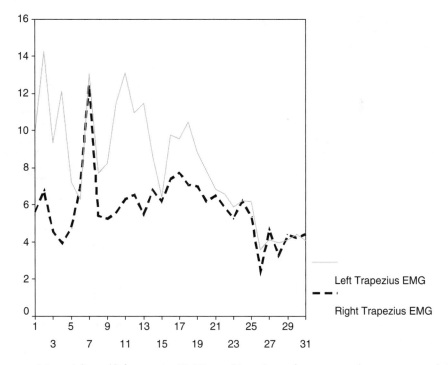

FIGURE 24.2. Mean right and left trapezius EMG over 31 sessions of neuromuscular treatment at the piano.

fore performing, keeping a mood diary, keeping a hand temperature log, etc.) were also utilized and "tested" by the patient. She was able to raise her baseline hand temperature to about 92°F, and she discontinued the Tranxene after 1 month of therapy. She learned more effective self-control and accepted more and more performance engagements as time went on, including a workshop in which she introduced some of the self-regulation skills she had learned to the workshop attendees. At a 1-year follow-up she remained symptom-free, using the skills she had learned to help her students and colleagues.

CONCLUSION

The 1999 Annual Symposium on Medical Problems of Musicians and Dancers issued a call for psychophysiology to become more involved in the study of MPA (Lederman, 1999; Sataloff, Rosen, & Levy, 1999), suggesting that neither medicine nor psychology alone is sufficient to treat MPA. Psychophysiology appears to be able to do what neither medicine nor psychiatry/psychology can do alone, and, for performing artists, appears to be necessary to keep them in their profession. From the use of a single biofeedback modality to treat overlearned muscle tension to complete psychophysiological assessment and treatment, the field of applied psychophysiology and biofeedback has a promising future in performing arts.

REFERENCES

Adams, R. D., Victor, M., & Ropper, A. H. (1997). *Principles of neurology* (6th ed.). New York: McGraw-Hill.
Basmajian, J. V. (1977). Motor learning and control: A working hypothesis. *Archives of Physical Medicine and Rehabilitation, 58*(1), 38–41.

Bejjani, F. J., Ferrara, L., Xu, N., Tomaino, C. M., Pavlidis, L., Wu, J., & Dommerholt, J. (1989). Comparison of three piano techniques as in implementation of a proposed experimental design. *Medical Problems of Performing Artists*, 4(3), 109–113.

Bejjani, F. J., Kaye, G. M., & Behnam, M. (1996). Musculoskeletal and neuromuscular conditions of instrumental musicians. *Archives of Physical and Medical Rehabilitation*, 77, 406–413.

Blanchard, E. (1989). Hand temperature norms for headache, hypertension, and irritable bowel syndrome. *Biofeedback and Self-Regulation*, 14(4), 319–331.

Bordens, K. S., & Abbot, B. B. (1988). *Research design and methods: A process approach*. Mountain View, CA: Mayfield Press.

Brandfonbrener, A. (1991). *Epidemiology of the medical problems of performing artists*. In R. Sataloff, A. Brandfonbrener, & R. Lederman (Eds.), *Textbook of performing arts medicine*. New York: Raven Press.

Brandfonbrener, A. (2000). Artists with disabilities. *Medical Problems of Performing Artists*, 15(2), 49–50.

Brooks, C. (1993). A therapist's perspective on the treatment of upper extremity nerve entrapment syndromes in musicians. *Medical Problems of Performing Artists*, 8(2), 61–69.

Calais-Germain, B. (1993). *Anatomy of movement*. Seattle, WA: Eastland Press.

Clark, D. M. (1996). Anxiety states: Panic and generalized anxiety. In K. Hawton, P. M. Salkovskis, J. Kirk, & D. M. Clark (Eds.), *Cognitive behaviour therapy for psychiatric problems*. New York: Oxford University Press.

Craske, M. G., & Rachman, S. J. (1987). Return of fear: Perceived skill and heart-rate responsivity. *British Journal of Clinical Psychology*, 26, 187–199.

Cohen, B. J., & Kupersmith, J. R. F. (1986). A study of SCL-90 scores of 87 performing artists seeking psychotherapy. *Medical Problems of Performing Artists*, 1(3), 140–142.

Coons, E. E., Montello, L. & Perez, J. (1995). Confidence and denial factors affect musicians' postperformance immune response. *International Journal of Arts Medicine*, 4(1), 4–14.

Crowne, D. P., & Marlowe, D. (1960). A new scale of social desirability independent of psychopathology. *Journal of Consulting Psychology*, 24, 349–354

DeLorenzo, L. C. (1990, March). Stage fright: The uninvited guest at performance. *Maryland Music Educator*, pp. 32–33.

Eysenck, H. J., & Eysenck, S. B. G. (1975). *Eysenck Personality Questionnaire, Form A*. San Diego, CA: Educational and Industrial Testing Service.

Fishbein, M., Middlestadt,, S. E., Ottai, V., Straus, S., & Ellis, A. (1988). Medical problems among ICSOM musicians: Overview of a national survey. *Medical Problems of Performing Artists*, 3(1), 1–14.

Flor, H., Miltner, W., & Birbaumer, N. (1992). Psychophysiological recording methods. In D. C. Turk & R. Melzack (Eds.), *Handbook of pain assessment*. New York: Guilford Press.

French, S. N. (1980). Electromyographic biofeedback for tension control during fine motor skill acquisition. *Biofeedback and Self-Regulation*, 5(2), 221–228.

Gerig, R. R. (1974). *Famous pianists and their technique*. New York: Luce.

Hamilton, L. H. (1997). The emotional costs of performing: Interventions for the young artists. *Medical Problems of Performing Artists*, 12(3), 67–71.

Harding, D. C., Brandt, K. D., & Hilberry, B. M. (1993). Finger joint force minimization in pianists using optimization techniques. *Journal of Biomechanics*, 26(12), 1403–1412.

Harman, S. E. (1998). The evolution of performing arts medicine. In R. T. Sataloff, A. G. Brandfonbrener & R. L. Lederman (Eds.), *Performing arts medicine*. (2nd ed.) San Diego, CA: Singular.

Hope, D. A., & Heimberg, R. G. (1993). Social phobia and social anxiety. In D. H. Barlow (Ed.), *Clinical handbook of psychological disorders* (2nd ed.). New York: Guilford Press.

Hoppman, R. (1998). Musculoskeletal problems in instrumental musicians. In R. T. Sataloff, A. G. Brandfonbrener, & R. J. Lederman (Eds.), *Performing arts medicine* (2nd ed.). San Diego: Singular.

Hoppman, R. A., & Patrone, N. A. (1989). A review of musculoskeletal problems in instrumental musicians. *Seminars in Arthritis and Rheumatism*, 19(2), 117–126.

Hoppman, R. A., & Patrone, N. A. (1991). Musculoskeletal problems in instrumental musicians. In R. Sataloff, A. Brandfonbrener and R. Lederman (Eds.), *Textbook of performing arts medicine*. New York: Raven Press.

Klein, S. B. (1991). *Learning: Principles and applications* (2nd ed.). New York: McGraw-Hill.

Lederman, R. (1999, June). *Medical treatment of performance anxiety: A statement in favor*. Paper presented at the Seventeenth Annual Symposium on Medical Problems of Musicians and Dancers, Aspen, CO.

Leijnse, J. N. (1996). Anatomical factors predisposing to focal dystonia in the musician's hand: Principles, theoretical examples, clinical significance. *Journal of Biomechanics*, 30(7), 659–669.

Levee, J. R., Cohen, M. J., & Rickles, W. H. (1976). Electromyographic biofeedback for relief of tension in the facial and throat muscles of a woodwind musician. *Biofeedback and Self-Regulation*, 1(1), 113–120.

LeVine, W. R., & Irvine, J. K. (1984). In vivo EMG biofeedback in violin and viola pedagogy. *Biofeedback and Self-Regulation*, 9(2), 161–167.

Lockwood, A. H. (1989). Medical problems of musicians. *New England Journal of Medicine*, 32(4), 221–227.

Montes, R., Bedmar, M., & Martin, M. S. (1993). EMG biofeedback of the abductor pollicis brevis in piano performance. *Biofeedback and Self-Regulation*, 18(2), 67–77.

Morasky, R. I., Reynolds, C., & Clarke, G. (1981). Using biofeedback to reduce left arm extensor EMG of string players during musical performance. *Biofeedback and Self-Regulation*, 6(4), 565–572.

Morasky, R. L., Reynolds, C., & Sowell, L. E. (1983). Generalization of lowered EMG levels during musical performance following biofeedback training. *Biofeedback and Self-Regulation*, 8(2), 207–216.

Nagel, J. J. (1998). Pain and injury in performing musicians: A psychodynamic approach. In R. Sataloff, A. Brandfonbrener, & R. Lederman (Eds.), *Performing arts medicine* (2nd ed.). San Diego, CA: Singular.

Nakano, K. (1991). Peripheral nerve entrapments, repetitive strain disorder, occupation-related syndromes, bursitis, and tendonitis. *Current Opinion in Rheumatology*, 3(2), 226–239.

Ostwald, P., & Avery, M. (1991). Psychiatric problems of performing artists. In R. Sataloff, A. Brandfonbrener, & R. Lederman (Eds.), *Textbook of performing arts medicine*. New York: Raven Press.

Ostwald, P., Avery, M., & Ostwald, L. (1998). Psychiatric problems of performing artists. In R. Sataloff, A. Brandfonbrener, & R. Lederman (Eds.), *Performing arts medicine* (2nd ed.). San Diego, CA: Singular.

Parlitz, D., Peschel, T., & Altenmuller, E. (1998). Assessment of dynamic finger forces in pianists: Effects of training and expertise. *Journal of Biomechanics*, 31, 1063–1087.

Parr, S. M. (1988). The effects of graduated exercise at the piano on the pianist's cardiac output, forearm blood flow, heart rate and blood pressure. *Medical Problems of Performing Artists*, 3(3), 100–104.

Penn, I. W., Chuang, T. Y., & Chan, R. C. (2001). Power spectrum analysis of first dorsal interosseous muscle in pianists. In R. J. Shephard, F. J. George, D. C. Nieman, J. S. Torg, M. L. Alexander, & W. M. Kort (Eds.), *Yearbook of sports medicine, 2001*. St. Louis, MO: Mosby.

Reynolds, C., & Clarke, G. (1981). Intensity without tension: Biofeedback. *Music Educators Journal*, 67, 52–55.

Roach, K. E., Martinez, M. A., & Anderson, N. (1994). Musculoskeletal pain in student instrumentalists: A comparison with the general students population. *Medical Problems of Performing Artists*, 9(4), 125–130.

Roche, S. M., & McConkey, K. M. (1990). Absorption: Nature, assessment and correlates. *Journal of Personality and Social Psychology*, 59, 91–101.

Rossi, E. L. (1993). *The psychobiology of mind–body healing* (rev. ed.). New York: Norton.

Sataloff, R. T., Brandfonbrener, A. G., & Lederman, R. J. (1998). *Performing arts medicine* (2nd ed.). San Diego: Singular Publishing.

Sataloff, R. T., Rosen, D. C., & Levy, S. (1999, June). *Medical treatment of performance anxiety*. Paper presented at the Seventeenth Annual Symposium on Medical Problems of Musicians and Dancers, Aspen, CO.

Simons, D. G., Travell, J. G., & Simons, L. S. (1999). *Myofacial pain and dysfunction: The trigger point manual* (2nd ed.). Baltimore: Williams & Wilkins.

Spence, S. H., Sharpe, L., Newton-John, T., & Champion, D. (1995). Effect of EMG biofeedback compared to applied relaxation training with chronic, upper extremity cumulative trauma disorders. *Pain*, 63, 199–206.

Steptoe, A., & Fidler, H. (1987). Stage fright in orchestral musicians: A study of cognitive and behavioral strategies in performance anxiety. *British Journal of Psychology*, 78, 241–249.

Sternbach, D. (1993). Addressing stress-related illness in professional musicians. *Maryland Medical Journal*, 42(3), 283–288.

Wickramasekera, I. (1988). *Behavioral medicine: Some concepts and procedures*. New York: Plenum Press.

Wickramasekera, I. (1991). Behavioral medicine: Using the High Risk Model of Threat Perception and the Trojan Horse Procedure to lead the somatizing patient out of the somatic closet. *The Clinical Supervisor*, 9(1), 59–89.

Wickramasekera, I. (1998). Secrets kept from the mind but not the body or behavior: The unsolved problems of identifying and treating somatization and psychophysiological disease. *Advances: The Journal of Mind–Body Medicine*, 14(2), 81–98.

Zaza, C. (1992). Playing-related health problems in a Canadian music school. *Medical Problems of Performing Artists*, 7(2), 48–53.

Zinn, M. L. (1998). *The use of sEMG feedback for transfer of relaxation into piano technique*. Unpublished master's thesis, Illinois Institute of Technology, Chicago.

Zinn, M. L., McCain, C., & Zinn, M. A. (2000). Musical performance anxiety and the High-Risk Model of Threat Perception. *Medical Problems of Performing Artists*, 15(2), 65–71.

Zinn, M. L., & Zinn, M. A. (2000). *Zinn piano program: Intake protocols*. Unpublished manuscript.

Zinn, M. L., & Zinn, M. A. (2002). *Hand temperature of 51 classical pianists*. Unpublished manuscript.

Ziporyn, T. (1984). Pianist's cramp to stage fright: The medical side of music making. *Journal of the American Medical Association*, 252, 985–989.

Zocco, L. (1984). *The development of a self-report inventory to assess dysfunctional cognitions in phobics*. Unpublished doctoral dissertation, Virginia Consortium for Professional Psychology.

APPENDIX 24.1. SUGGESTED PROTOCOL FOR EMG BIOFEEDBACK AT THE PIANO (WHICH CAN BE MODIFIED BY OTHER INSTRUMENTS)

This protocol (based on Zinn, 1998; Zinn et al., 2000; and Zinn & Zinn, 2002) is to be used after standard relaxation therapy has ended.

1. Client will be seated at a piano, using the approximate ergonomic conditions he or she normally utilizes for practice.

2. The electrodes will be placed on the extensor carpi radialis and ulnaris on each arm.

3. The client will first be instructed to relax completely, with his or her arms on the lap (Figure 24.3). Note that the EMG levels are very low (0.3 microvolts), reflecting the more finite muscle control typically encountered in performing arts.

4. The client will be instructed to use a normal playing position and will play a simple five-note pattern starting on C (but not middle C; the client should use the C below and the C above it, to minimize possible wrist deviation).

5. The protocol calls for the client's striking the key with a good "fortissimo" (very loud), then relaxing as much as possible immediately after the keystroke, but keeping the finger on the key (keeping the key depressed).

6. The goal is for the client to bring the relaxation EMG to as low a threshold as possible and to do so as quickly as possible. The final goal will look similar to Figure 24.4.

7. Eventually the client will be able to drop muscle tension quickly in "key" places in the piece (during rests, phrase endings, etc.) (see Figure 24.5).

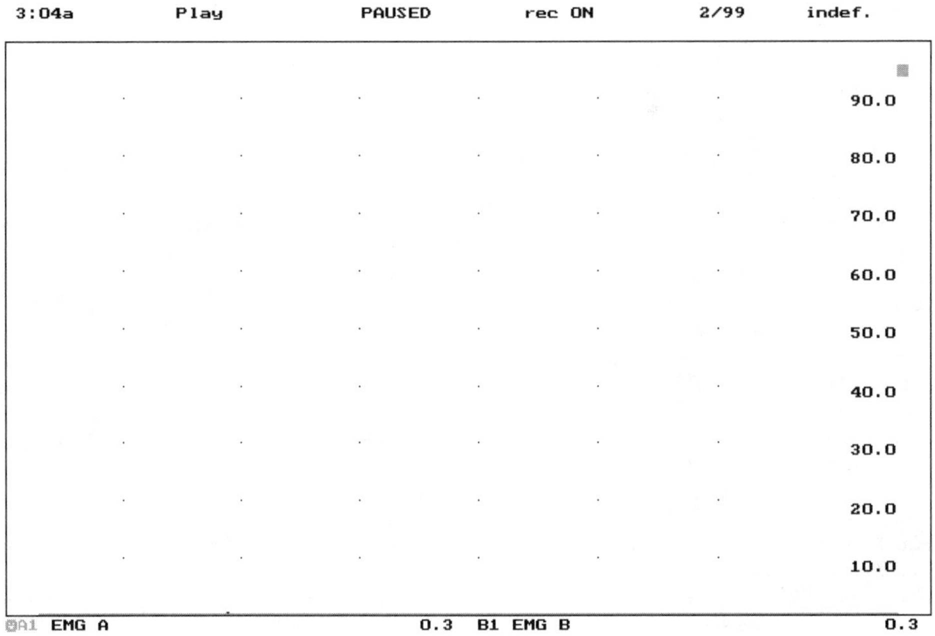

FIGURE 24.3. EMG levels of a professional pianist at the piano, with hands on lap. The pianist was instructed to "relax as much as possible." Note the small levels (0.3 microvolts).

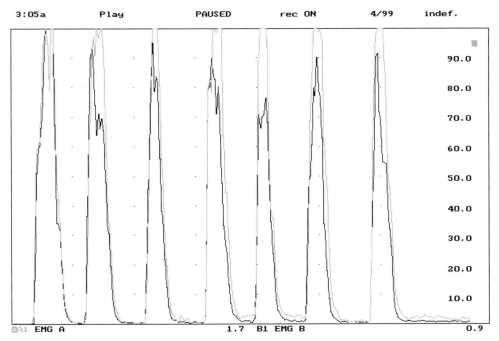

FIGURE 24.4. EMG levels of a pianist doing the "play–relax" protocol.

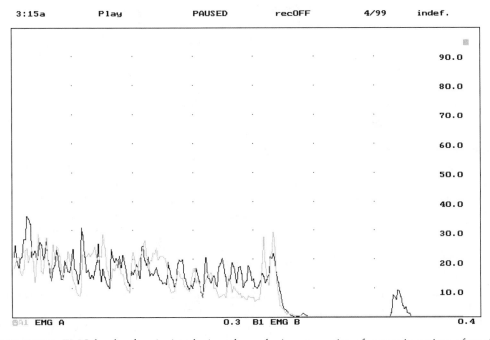

FIGURE 24.5. EMG levels of a pianist playing, then relaxing at a point of repose in a piece of music.

CHAPTER 25

Sports Psychology Applications of Biofeedback and Neurofeedback

WESLEY SIME

Psychological and physiological preparation for sport competition is the focus of intense study and highly publicized scrutiny. Physiological testing and training have evolved over the years into a sophisticated science featuring strength, conditioning, and flexibility. For each sport, there are unique training methods having direct impact upon either aerobic or anaerobic capacity (e.g., long-distance vs. sprinting events in running and swimming). There is ongoing controversy over the best methods of training to achieve an "edge" among various competitors in power sports (football, wrestling, etc.) versus graceful, aesthetically pleasing sports (gymnastics, diving, etc.). In seeking an "edge" in performance, athletes are encouraged to pursue sound nutritional and psychological approaches. The use of biofeedback, neurofeedback, and stress management in concert with sport psychology consultation can enhance healthy and safe sport performance, while also increasing an athlete's competitive advantage (Sime, 1985).

Psychological preparation of athletes for sport performance is more of an art than a science. Some coaches consider their motivational speeches and "field marshal" disciplinary strategies sufficient to inspire a psychological advantage among their athletes. However, many self-proclaimed sport "gurus" (as well as those legitimately trained and certified in the field) provide services to both individual athletes and teams, using a wide variety of methods unrelated to biofeedback. Experts come and go, but some enduring resources exist in baseball (Dorfman & Kuell, 1995; Ravizza & Hanson, 1995) and in virtually all of the Olympic sports (Thompson, Vernacchia, & Moore, 1998). The Olympic training centers in Colorado Springs and San Diego have full-time staffs of clinical psychologists, who help athletes and coaches to endure grueling training regimens and highly stressful international competition, as well as to deal with common life adjustments (leaving home, relationships, career decisions, anxiety and depression, etc.).

There is unanimous agreement among coaches, athletes, and sport psychologists that manifestations of stress and tension before and/or during competition are major threats to the success of any athlete. Logically, the prevention and treatment of stress symptoms are high priorities. However, there is very little agreement among the primary practitioners in this field regarding the use of biofeedback or neurofeedback for stress reduction or for performance enhancement. For some sports teams (e.g., football, baseball, basketball), the technology is simply overwhelming and/or too obtrusive to be used feasibly with the large number of athletes involved. On the other hand, individual athletes often seek clinical assistance from professionals who use biofeedback. This approach helps show that excess and nonfunctional psychophysiological arousal occurs in athletes under pressure, and that excess reactivity can be controlled prior to competitive performance. Sport psychologists commonly use a variety of stress-reducing and/or confidence-building techniques (e.g., relaxation, visualization, goal setting, team building, etc.) or traditional clinical approaches (cognitive-behavioral strategies, visuomotor behavior rehearsal, hypnosis, etc.) without the benefit of psychophysiological instrumentation. It is the goal of this chapter to show that biofeedback and neurofeedback can be valuable additions to this array of techniques, both with individual athletes and (under certain circumstances) with teams or groups.

Please note that I have intentionally avoided terms suggesting "treatment" or "therapy" in this context. Athletes are particularly sensitive to the implication that they need "therapy." The use of any terminology suggesting a clinical diagnosis or treatment plan can cause coaches or athletes to feel stigmatized, thus alienating them from potentially beneficial intervention. There are circumstances where serious depression and other clinical diagnoses are found among athletes and coaches, and these would warrant a more traditional clinical treatment approach. However, it is far better if the initial relationship with an athlete (or coach) is *not* predicated upon a mental health diagnosis as a premise for the work.

HISTORICAL PERSPECTIVE ON BIOFEEDBACK IN SPORT PSYCHOLOGY

The field of sport psychology emanated out of several disciplines, including physical education, the study of psychomotor behavior, coaching, and traditional clinical psychology. From 1920 to 1980, the focus was on efficient learning of physical skills; overcoming fear; going with psychological "hunches" (and overcoming "jinxes"); the effects of willpower, confidence, and sleep (or the lack of these things); motivation and pep sessions; and numerous other elementary considerations. Historically, instrumented biofeedback did not have a prominent place in any of these fields. However, research with objective measurement of outcomes and experimental manipulation of stimuli was common (Gould & Pick, 1995; Landers, 1995), and it continues to be a driving force in the field. In the early 1980s, at about the time that biofeedback was gaining a new level of credibility via certification (the Biofeedback Certification Institute of America), researchers in sports psychology began showing interest in psychophysiology (Hatfield & Landers, 1983). Along with surface electromyography (EMG), there was considerable interest in heart rate variability as measures of emotion and anxiety related to performance.

Some of the earliest practitioners in sport psychology were former coaches who had practical knowledge about mind–body interaction and sought greater wisdom from collegial interaction with exercise science and psychology colleagues. The first clinical psychologist who made advances in professional sports was Bruce Oglivie (1979), who promoted the influence of the mind upon the body in motion. His pragmatic approach was to discover dysfunctional patterns of behavior leading to competitive anxiety, while encouraging young athletes to recognize that emotional arousal was natural, but not essential to good performance. His penchant for astute observation of athletes during competition, and inquiry with them after their events provided rudimentary feedback.

The study of arousal and performance by Oglivie and others led to the application of arousal reduction and basic stress management strategies to help protect athletes from unproductive cognitive intrusions on positive imagery. These strategies included progressive relaxation, hypnosis, cognitive restructuring, visualization, mental rehearsal, self-monitoring, and stress inoculation. Other areas that were addressed included goal setting (Weinberg, 1994), imagery training (Murphy, 1994), motivation, reinforcement, self-confidence, trust, communication, cooperation, leadership, team cohesiveness, fear of failure, fear of success, control of aggressiveness, and fear of career termination (Anshel, Williams, & Williams, 2000). Those seeking to work with athletes must be aware of work in all these areas.

Emotional arousal is the primary topic in sport psychology that is commonly related to biofeedback (Gould & Udry, 1994). Some athletes rapidly become anxious and emotionally activated before and/or during performance. Worry and apprehension commonly lead to overarousal, but awareness of these reactions can be a trigger for a learned relaxation strategy. Simple heart rate elevation indicates sympathetic activation, but this can have either a positive or a negative valence. Ultimately, awareness or the quality of "felt arousal" is what differentiates supreme athletes from others whose talent is rarely consummated in high performance because they fail at anxiety reduction (Radeke & Stein, 1994).

Although arousal reduction is essential to successful performance, the more advanced use of imagery in sports incorporates awareness of arousal while seeing or feeling the virtual reality of the competitive event, as is done in visuomotor behavioral rehearsal (Suinn, 1980). This method strives to restructure a negative image of performance into a positive image. Undoubtedly, relaxation skills are an important part of facilitating imagery control, though they are not essential to a positive outcome. An advantage of biofeedback in this context is to facilitate awareness of cognitive and/or emotional intrusions upon the imagery of the athlete whose mind may waver from high-quality, positive mental imagery.

RATIONALE FOR ENHANCING PERFORMANCE FUNCTIONING WITH BIOFEEDBACK

In some highly aggressive and combative sports (football, basketball, hockey, boxing), there can be an advantage to intensifying emotional and physical reactions in the heat of competition. However, in many other sports involving finite muscle control (baseball, golf, archery, curling, diving, etc.), an athlete is at a tremendous disadvantage without total control of emotions and the attendant muscle tension. Because some athletes and coaches do not understand how emotions, physiological reactivity, and biofeedback relate to sport, it is very helpful to provide numerous, meaningful, sport-specific illustrations where athletes have "choked" under pressure. Most traditional sport psychologists have a good supply of such examples, and they are also skilled at establishing confidence, trust, and communication with both athletes and coaches.

Muscle bracing and residual tension are the classic symptoms of competitive stress. All dynamic sports (soccer, basketball, etc.) feature long periods of controlled movements ("cruising"), punctuated by moments of intense explosive efforts that require sudden elevations in intensity of muscle contraction. Controlling this range of tension to conserve energy is a difficult skill that is usually developed over time and with considerable experience. However, even veteran competitors are often vulnerable when the stakes are high and when embarrassment follows a critical loss.

Successful athletes learn to compare multidimensional components of anxiety, arousal, anticipation, and worry in good and bad performances in order to identify their unique optimal state for competition. Some need to be more relaxed, but others need to "jack up" their arousal level. Therefore, the simplistic instruction to "just relax" or "lower arousal" without consideration of these other activation components is naïve. Some common techniques to elevate arousal include getting mad at an opponent or getting charged up by the crowd's cheering. Arousal regulation is undoubtedly the most important performance enhancement technique to be considered here (Radeke & Stein, 1994). Thus more systematic assessment of athletes via applied psychophysiology and biofeedback has merit and could become more prominent.

Competitive Anxiety, Psychophysiology, and Performance

Competitive anxiety is the prevailing emotion experienced by most athletes, and sympathetic nervous system responses therein are comparable to realistic, life-threatening stress, as noted in classic studies with novice skydivers (Fenz & Epstein, 1967). Heart rate, EMG, and respiration rate are among the variables known to differentiate between the inexperienced who are fearful and the more experienced who are completely absorbed in the task. Experienced athletes routinely cope better with anxiety, because they have a greater sense of personal control over the outcome. This is manifested as greater psychophysiological self-regulation over somatic as well as cognitive components of anxiety (Hatfield & Hillman, 2001).

Some athletes perceive competitive anxiety as negative and detrimental to performance, whereas it invigorates and excites others (Page, Sime, & Nordell, 1999). In sports that require metabolic efficiency (e.g., speed and endurance events), it is clear that anxiety is associated with slower speeds and premature fatigue (Burton, 1988). Although somatic anxiety is inversely related to economy of physical performance and cognitive anxiety is directly associated with mental errors (Bird & Horn, 1990), anxiety is still a very complicated and multifaceted dimension, featuring both cognitive and somatic components as well as positive and negative interpretations during precompetitive moments (Hammermeister & Burton, 1995). Specifically, anxiety can be either facilitative or debilitative to performance, according to how the athlete appraises a particular situation (Nordell & Sime, 1993; Hale & Whitehouse, 1998). Interestingly, heart rate and state anxiety do not become unduly elevated, as long as competition is viewed as a challenge rather than a threat. Thus ancillary strategies to build confidence (such as cognitive restructuring) serve to control physiological manifestations of anxiety very well, with or without the attendant psychophysiological assessment.

In stationary, nonexertional competition (e.g., pistol/rifle shooting and archery), very subtle perceptual nuances affect the accuracy of performance dramatically, especially when somatic anxiety is significantly higher than cognitive anxiety (Gould, Petlichkoff, Simons, & Vevera, 1987). Trust, confidence, and control of somatic tension/anxiety are critical in the shooting sports, because the targets are so small and the wavering motion of the body is difficult to control completely. EMG biofeedback and meditation have been used extensively to help athletes in these sports achieve a greater sense of both cognitive (Tremayne & Barry, 2001) and physical (Solberg, Berglund, Engen, Ekeber, & Loeb, 1996) elements of "control." Others have demonstrated that empathy, use of praise, and encouragement are helpful when used adjunctively to inspire confidence and reduced anxiety necessary for optimum performance (Vealey, Armstrong, Comar, & Greenleaf, 1998).

Determining Optimal Levels of Emotion (with and without Biofeedback)

Some of the positive and productive emotions in sports include being energetic, motivated, certain, confident, purposeful, willing, resolute, and alert. Among the positive but dysfunctional emotions are being easygoing, excited, composed, relaxed, overjoyed, fearless, satisfied, exalted, and pleasant. Obviously, not all positive emotions contribute to success in sport competition. For example, after a loss in a team sport like football or basketball, coaches often are quoted in the media as saying something like, "Our players were overconfident and too relaxed for this game—that is why they lost." By contrast, there are some negative but highly functional emotions, such as being charged up, dissatisfied, attacking, vehement, intense, nervous, irritated, and provoked. Lastly, the negative and dysfunctional emotions, such as being tired, unwilling, uncertain, sluggish, depressed, lazy, distressed, sorrowful, and afraid, are almost always associated with poor performances. However, positive mood state has been shown to be a powerful component in performance, particularly where heroic efforts in strength or endurance are required (Hanin, 2000).

There are vast individual differences in the tolerable level of selected emotions, whether positive or negative, productive or dysfunctional (Vallerand & Blanchard, 2000). Addressing mood disturbances before competition is clearly relevant in influencing performance outcomes. Negative mood states, in particular, have been associated with decrements in performance efficiency, especially related to endurance sports (T. Williams, Krahenbuhl, & Morgan, 1991). Although we must not underestimate the value of simple verbal feedback regarding mood, affect, anxiety, and attitude, biofeedback can also be of tremendous use in assessing these.

Assessing Mood and Emotions in Sport Competition

One method of elucidating subtle indicators of disturbed mood is the Profile of Mood States (POMS). Prapavessis (2000) has reviewed the extensive literature on the use of the POMS in sports performance, wherein the goal is to get athletes to be cognizant of their ideal arousal level for a specific type of performance. Ironically, in a sports context, tension and anger can be either debilitative or facilitative, depending on the nature of the sport (Beedie, Terry, & Lane, 2000). For example, karate and boxing respond well to moderate amounts of tension and anger, whereas figure skating and speed skating performances break down amidst even modest levels of these two emotions. The POMS is a fairly good predictor of performance outcome from day to day (especially in short-duration events), but it is not accurate either in predicting the future level of achievement for any given athlete or in differentiating the level of accomplishment among various groups of high and low achievers. Thus the POMS is best used regularly to facilitate assessment of current mood and anxiety, in conjunction with biofeedback and other approaches.

Another concept related to regulating levels of emotion in sport is the Zone of Optimal Functioning (ZOF) theory, which translates awareness of emotional state to practical application (Hanin, 2000). The ZOF theory is a multidimensional anxiety theory; it predicts that overarousal will be associated with poor judgment and physical mistakes, whereas arousal regulation is what maintains optimal activation to be successful. Obviously, "awareness" is the critical variable in matching response to the demands at hand.

Athletes identify their idiosyncratic ZOF from past performances (in both pre- and postcompetition circumstances), such that an ideal state can be targeted and achieved by self-control with regularity (Krane, 1993). Some athletes do not perform as well as expected when they are outside their ideal zone (Annesi, 1997). On the other hand others have to give up their preferred comfort level (get beyond ideal state) to achieve personal best performance, or, in some cases, world records (Randle & Weinberg, 1997). More accurate yet unobtrusive methods of assessing this elusive emotional phenomenon are needed. Hanin (2000) relies on simple query of athletes regarding their ZOF, which is marginally reliable. Clearly this concept lends itself to further exploration with more objective psychophysiological measures, followed by carefully prescribed biofeedback applications.

Flow State: The Key to Optimal Performance

"Flow" is considered the ideal state of mind associated with achievement or optimal performance (Jackson & Csikszentmihalyi, 1999). Flow has been described as "overachieving" while "feeling terrific," "no pain," "in the zone," "total involvement," "on autopilot," "very focused," "effortless," "unbeatable," "super-alive," "floating," "composed," "tuned in," "in the groove," and "nothing else matters." The fundamentals of flow are absence of fear, awareness of objectives, clarity of goals, effortless motion, unambiguous feedback, concentration on the task, central control, loss of self-consciousness, and time warp (everything slows down).

Athletes reporting remarkable "flow state" experiences (e.g., a basketball player just couldn't miss a shot and it seemed so easy!) note retrospectively that they had total focus on performance, optimum self-awareness, and total disregard for the outcome (Jackson & Roberts, 1992). By contrast, being overly concerned with outcome was associated with worst performances. Flow appears to occur serendipitously when there is a balance between challenge and ability, so that an athlete doesn't feel threatened and keeps his or her mind on task easily. There is a feeling of control while enjoying the experience. Furthermore, the factors known to facilitate the occurrence of flow state include mental and physical preparation, confidence, clear mind, optimal motivation, and optimum arousal level (Jackson, 1995). Those seeking (but failing) to achieve "flow" usually are trying too hard, becoming overly aroused, and losing clarity of focus. Outstanding performance in a flow state is elusive and only occurs under ideal conditions of self-awareness and "letting it happen." Thus biofeedback could be one of several technological tools helpful in achieving the ideal physiological and cognitive state for allowing the "flow" experience to happen. Objectivity is needed for shaping a particular athlete's psychophysiological state—that is, doing individual profiling to create proscribed training protocols relevant to the person and to the sport.

Psychophysiological Determinants of "Running Economy"

The concept of "running economy" (RE) is relatively new to the competitive coaching world. Most coaches in endurance sports assign heavy training loads (e.g., distance traveled and speed of each set within a workout) for all athletes, and they give advice regarding technique as related to efficiency. However, efficiency for individuals of identical capacity may vary greatly (T. Williams et al., 1991). At least 50% of the variance between individuals is accounted for by RE—that is, the maximal efficiency in oxygen consumption that can be achieved at a submaximal work load. RE varies from day to day, and it can be trained up to about 30% of capacity. Thus coaches and biofeedback consultants are well advised to attend to this phenomenon.

Feedback for cardiac patients on efficiency (a clinical example of RE) is exceedingly important, because some patients are disconnected from sense of effort while walking or bicycling (Bales et al., 1990). With feedback, patients were found to be 10% more accurate in staying on target heart rate than without feedback, because of fine-tuning their "effort sense" or reconnecting awareness of effort (Noble & Robertson, 1996, pp. 157–162).

When RE was highest, distance runners in one study exhibited high levels of vigor, while tension, depression, anger, fatigue, and confusion were all low (this is known as the "iceberg profile" on the POMS). Thus an alert but relaxed state was common among the most efficient and successful athletes with high RE, who were able to extract more oxygen from each breath of air (Hatfield et al., 1992). Thus they needed less frequent inhalations for the same level of workload and were able to achieve even higher RE states with the aid of EMG biofeedback from the trapezius and forearm. Our interest, of course, is in the training effects that can be documented as a result of biofeedback intervention.

Heart rate biofeedback training plus relaxation over a 6-week period resulted in a significant increase in submaximal RE (Caird, McKenzie, & Sleivert, 1999). Both heart rate and ventilation were lowered significantly by the intervention, presumably due to a decrease in sympathetic output. It is likely that the length of training plus the regularity of the biofeedback practice sessions caused this remarkable increase in RE, while other previous studies have not showed such dramatic results. (The other studies provided EMG biofeedback together with cognitive coping, imagery, and stress inoculation, but showed less significant effects; Crews, 1992.) Even when biofeedback (provided during the exercise) was withdrawn, heart rate, ventilation, and submaximal oxygen consumption effects were still significant, demonstrating a valuable transfer of training effects. Further advances in developing user-friendly technology will make these training procedures more widespread and available to endurance athletes.

Detecting Stress, Strain, and Overload: Preventing the Risks of Overtraining

Most elite competitors in the strength and endurance sports are required to train according to "supercompensation" principles, wherein daily practices are designed to break down muscle tissue and induce intense fatigue repeatedly in order to stimulate hypertrophy in recovery. Carefully structured overtraining clearly enhances performance in the long run. Both "association" (close attention to physiological indications of effort and impending fatigue, such as respiratory and muscular strain, pain, and early signs of cramping) and "dissociation" (attending to alternative distracting variables, such as designing a "dream house" while running) are important cognitive strategies to help athletes tolerate the painful training for such endurance sports as swimming, running, and even bicycling. The irony is that the training for elite sports competition in these events may involve such intense dissociation (masking of perceptions of reality) that an athlete may occasionally lapse into debilitating changes in mood, appetite, sleep, and so on. (Kentta & Hassmen, 1998).

"Stress," "strain," "staleness," and "burnout" are common descriptors for athletes who manifest quasi-psychopathological conditions due to negative overtraining, resulting often in a "staleness syndrome" (Masters & Ogles, 1998). Depression, anger, fatigue, apathy, mental stress, irritability, indecisiveness, aggressiveness, exhaustion, and lack of concentration or energy are important warning indicators of staleness. Having an understanding of each athlete's unique stress response (in training) and knowing the realistic recovery time are critical, especially for those in preparation for championship competition (Kellmann, Altenburg, Lornes, & Steinacker, 2001). Failure to attend to these disturbances (stress responses) will result in autonomic imbalances (insufficient cortisol release) and stunted sympathetic nervous system reaction, which is caused by impairment of the pituitary–adrenal axis (Lehmann, Foster, Dickhuth, & Gastmann, 1998).

Not surprisingly, the risk of systemic illness increases too. Overtraining increases risk of infectious diseases (colds, flu) among distance swimmers and bicyclists, causing serious performance decrements (Foster, 1998; Hackney, Tearman, & Nowacki, 1990). These respiratory infections are correlated with reductions in salivary immunoglobulin A (a biochemical indicator of high stress) whenever the training loads are markedly increased (Tharp & Barnes, 1989). Other deleterious changes—neuromuscular, cardiovascular, metabolic/endocrine, and orthopedic—often occur. Common complaints include muscle soreness, chronic muscle fatigue, lethargy, apathy, appetite loss, sleep loss, mood changes, performance decline, retarded recovery after exertion, weight loss, and a physically drawn appearance. Objective diagnostic indicators include tachycardia, hypertension, amenorrhea (in women), anemia, blood glycogen depletion, low lymphocyte count, elevated body temperature, and blood cortisol. The latter accelerates fat and amino acid mobilization, which eventually causes a catabolic response in the muscle tissue, resulting in loss of body weight and muscle strength (and obviously impairing performance). Measures of elevated lactic acid following selected training sessions should forewarn coaches and athletes of impending risk.

The only effective treatments for staleness and burnout are bed rest and abstention from training, but each day of missed training compromises the chances of performing successfully in competition. Thus using applied psychophysiology wisely may make it possible to alert athletes and/or coaches to early warning signs, so that they can ward off these destructive responses. Obviously, if a biofeedback consultant observes elevated heart rate, blood pressure, and/or body temperature when an athlete is in a resting condition, it is important to inform both coach and athlete in order to help them design a more constructive training program. A simple axiom for a consultant to use when introducing biofeedback principles is "Learn to listen to your body more closely." That is, when people are hungry they eat, and when thirsty they drink. Similarly, when athletes (who are often taught to ignore their symptoms) are in pain or exhaustion, they must seek longer rest and recuperation time.

CLINICAL USE OF BIOFEEDBACK FOR INJURY PREVENTION AND REHABILITATION

Athletes in training and preparation for competition are best described as having "injuries waiting to happen" (Sime, 1998). Personal trainers and strength coaches strive to help athletes reach the upper limits of their individual tolerance when they design exercise regimens to enhance strength and endurance. Because the athletes are pressing both their physiological and psychological limits, risk of injury or emotional breakdown is great. For example, when they are lapsing into dissociative states to tolerate their training, with a "no pain, no gain" philosophy, there can be great risk of injury—especially in a sport like bicycling where a slight miscalculation might cause a life-threatening crash. However, dissociation is also a risk when it distorts accurate perception of exertion (Noble & Robertson, 1996, pp. 270–271), causing some athletes to strain muscles, sprain ankles, or even break bones (e.g., stress fractures, shin splints, etc.) because their bodies are not prepared or conditioned to handle the load.

Factors Increasing Risk of Injury

Although some injuries are unavoidable outcomes of collisions, occasional trauma, and chronic overuse (repetitive motion), there is evidence to show that many injuries are inherently associated with psychosocial factors, emotional stress, and insufficient coping skills (Andersen & Williams, 1988). Stressful life change events (e.g., marriage, divorce, financial problems, etc.), shortage of sleep, and impatience can make athletes less cautious and potentially more accident/injury-prone (J. N. Williams, Tonymon, & Andersen, 1991). Furthermore, fear, anxiety, breakdown in attentional focus, distortion in cognitive appraisal, and overall body tension result in slower reaction time. Field of vision also narrows ("tunnel vision"), increasing the risk that an athlete may trip and fall or have unnecessary collisions on the field of play (Andersen & Williams, 1999).

Others have shown that optimism, self-esteem, and a sense of hardiness are clearly associated with reduced injury rates (Ford, Eklund, & Gordon, 2000). Although the exact mechanisms of the injury–stress relationship are not clear, there is promising research suggesting that the level of residual tension in skeletal muscles surrounding the weight-bearing joints is linked to higher levels of joint and muscle trauma.

Some injuries occur because of inflexibility associated with high tension levels, which leads to more frequent joint sprains and muscle strains. EMG biofeedback has been shown to increase flexibility under normal stretching conditions (Wilson & Bird, 1981), and is even more beneficial when used on a regular basis, reinforcing retention of effects (Cummings, Wilson, & Bird, 1984). Biofeedback is particularly useful in enhancing the acute perception of effort produced in competition under high stress and tension conditions, wherein awareness usually diminishes.

Preventive and Rehabilitative Biofeedback for Injuries

Swanik, Lephart, Giraldo, DeMont, and Fu (1999) studied reactive muscle firing among females with anterior cruciate ligament (ACL) injury incurred during routine practice activities. The high incidence of ACL injuries in females is sometimes related to inadequate muscle capacity to protect the knee joint. However, the load on the ACL is a function of reactive muscle activity; the level of which is determined by kinesthetic feedback (a familiar biofeedback concept). The natural response of the body is to create muscle co-contractions in adjacent muscle groups to stabilize a joint that seems vulnerable to the load. Thus there may be excessive reactive muscle firing patterns, causing compensatory muscle activation. EMG biofeedback has been used effectively to reduce residual tension, thus allowing the ligaments of the joint to maintain functional stability. This can be done either before injury as a preventive measure, or after surgery during the rehabilitation process.

Swanik et al. (1999) obtained EMG measures of quadriceps and hamstring muscle activity during downhill walking and running to determine the peak activities during landing of each step. Downhill walking can be very traumatic on the knee joint. Greater peak activity in the quadriceps and smaller EMG activity in the hamstring areas were observed among the most vulnerable patients. Biofeedback strategies to increase the hamstring activity while reducing quadriceps activity may serve to prevent some ACL injuries. Treatment also includes strength training of the hamstring muscles to counterbalance the load.

The healing process can be enhanced with self-regulation strategies adjunctive to biofeedback (Ievleva & Orlick, 1991). Some injured athletes heal more rapidly than others, and it appears that psychosocial factors may be an important part of the healing enhancement. Positive attitude, social support, goal setting, positive self-talk, and mental imagery capability were assessed by Ievleva and Orlick in patients with knee or ankle injuries. Those athletes who had exceptionally fast recoveries also scored very high on the sum total of these psychosocial variables, while those in the slowest healing group showed very low scores. In another study, the specific effects of healing imagery on recovery from postligament surgery were remarkable (Cupal & Brewer, 2001). Significantly greater knee strength, as well as significantly less anxiety and pain for the imagery treatment group compared to placebo, appeared at 24 weeks postsurgery. Clearly, adjunctive interventions such as imagery (healing) should be used along with biofeedback to facilitate the recovery process.

Psychological Adjustment to Trauma, Injury, and Stress

The psychological trauma associated with athletic injuries, as perceived by athletic trainers, is quite dramatic (Larson, Starkey, & Zaichkowsky, 1996). In a survey of 482 athletic trainers, almost half said that every injured athlete suffers substantial psychological trauma, but only one-fourth of these trainers ever referred an athlete for counseling or to a sports psychologist for treatment. There is a need for trained clinicians in biofeedback to be resources for athletic trainers and orthopedic surgeons to provide even better rehabilitation care in facilitating positive outcome from injury. Injured athletes may exhibit anxiety, apathy, depression, hopelessness, lack of motivation, anger, aggression, withdrawal, frustration, and impatience. Furthermore, they often have a negative attitude toward injury and life; they lack self-confidence; they may lose their focus on career goals; they have poor pain tolerance; and they frequently fail to comply with rehabilitation.

Several years ago, a Division I NCAA football player with a bright future suffered a shoulder separation that kept him out of competition for 8 weeks. When complications prevented him from returning as expected, he began manifesting bizarre schizotypal symptoms. Before appropriate treatment could be introduced, this young man committed a violent crime against a helpless woman while he was in a psychotic state. His career, of course, then ended abruptly, and when treatment failed (due to withdrawal from medication), he acted out violently once again; this time, he was shot by a policeman and paralyzed from the neck down (Sime, 1997). Although this case is extreme, there are many other injured athletes who do not adjust well to the rehabilitation process, especially if progress is thwarted. Efforts to introduce therapy for prevention and treatment of injured athletes have included comprehensive programs in coping with stress (Davis, 1991). A 50% reduction in injuries in swimmers and one-third fewer injuries among football players were observed as a result of a stress management program. Adjunctive counseling therapy has been shown to be helpful with these postinjury difficulties (Anshel et al., 2000), and it should be a part of every comprehensive biofeedback program package for athletes.

IMAGERY, CONCENTRATION, METACOGNITION, AND BIOFEEDBACK

Success or failure in sport performance usually hinges on the degree to which a performer is able to maintain control of thoughts, emotions, and subtle actions that are directed toward accomplishment of specific goals. For example, the renowned golfer Jack Nicklaus once said, "I never hit a shot without first seeing it clearly in my mind." Developing control of imagery in sport is monumental. However, the ability to control images, thoughts, and emotions consistently when needed is not so easy as described by Nicklaus.

Athletes use imagery to enhance concentration on the task at hand and to block out distractions. From a coach's standpoint, imagery is an "action–language" bridge; that is, it translates verbal instruction into procedural knowledge for improving technique in performance. However, images fade quickly, especially in the face of a difficult challenge. It is not unusual to have an athlete report (after the fact) thinking about how important it is "not to think too much" just before making a critical mistake. "Metacognition" (thinking about the process of thinking) is inherently disruptive not only in sports, but in any kind of psychomotor performance. Obviously it is equally disruptive in cognitive performance (e.g., reading) as well.

Detectable Indicators of Subtle Thoughts and Positive Imagery

Historically, EMG was used to detect subtle thoughts indirectly, via elevated muscle tension of the tongue (McGuigan, 1979). As one might expect, it is very intrusive and cumbersome to attach EMG electrodes directly to the tongue. Therefore, the trend has now shifted to using simple electroencephalographic (EEG) methods for identifying the occurrence of random thoughts at the moment they appear (Sime, Allen, & Fazzano, 2001). EEG biofeedback can be useful to alert an athlete instantly when irrelevant and counterproductive thoughts appear, and to enable him or her to counteract these. For example, golfers routinely use a preshot routine (a series of thoughts, imagery, and actions repeated consistently before each shot) that is intended to consume their thought processes and prevent the intrusion of distracting thoughts or emotions (e.g., "I'll never make this shot," or "What will I do after I win this tournament?"). Mirror-like feedback of intrusive thoughts has excellent face validity in sport.

In theory, mental images are understood as products of the brain's information-processing capacity, wherein coded information stored in long-term memory becomes activated (Hecker

& Kaczor, 1988). In sports, there are several different types of imagery: (1) specific cognitive images (e.g., seeing a golf ball go in the hole), (2) general cognitive images (e.g., seeing the award ceremony that occurs after winning), and (3) motivational arousal (e.g., visualizing tremendous effort for a given event) (Martin, Moritz, & Hall, 1999). In addition, there are distinctions between "external imagery" (as a camera sees the performer) and "internal imagery" (as the performer sees the environment). The common view is that internal visual imagery is more effective than external, but not everyone agrees (Hardy & Callow, 1999). Kinesthetic and olfactory dimensions of imagery can provide an additional benefit to the advanced competitor. For instance, smelling the fresh-cut grass while seeing and then feeling a golf shot simply enriches the quality of the image of success. A common admonition in golf is "See it, feel it, then trust it as you make the shot." Obviously, it is helpful if the image is high-quality, with explicit vividness of detail (the color, feel, and even the smell of the environment).

Sports Where Imagery Has Been Prominent

Among the various sports where imagery has been systematically studied, there is considerable variation in the content and the outcomes. Figure skaters who used imagery systematically were found to be more successful than those who did not, in part because the latter group could not keep themselves from spontaneously seeing mistakes (Rodgers, Hall, & Buckolz, 1991). Gymnasts and canoeists both reported using imagery to think through rehearsals and to understand technical demands in practicing difficult moves (White & Hardy, 1998). Rock climbers demonstrated that external imagery (camera view) was best for their sport, especially when stretching to reach a distant foothold was required (Hardy & Callow, 1999). Soccer players tended to use imagery more for motivational purposes and its impact was felt more strongly in competition than in training (Salmon, Hall, & Haslam, 1994). In golf, coaches found that imagery helped in developing intrinsic motivation (Martin & Hall, 1995). That is, a group of players, assigned to use imagery before the event, spent significantly more time practicing than those who were not instructed to use it. The players using imagery also set higher goals for themselves and had more realistic expectations than those who were not given imagery instructions. Similarly, weight lifters benefited from a particular type of emotive (motivational) imagery in achieving greater strength performance (Murphy, Woolfolk, & Budney, 1988). Specifically, images of being angry or fearful enhanced strength performance, whereas the image of being relaxed was associated with decrease in strength output. Thus control of the image process is critical to the success of the competitor.

Overcoming Counterproductive/"Ironic" Intrusions: Usefulness of Biofeedback and Neurofeedback

Becoming aware of transient fluctuations in cognition and emotions requires highly disciplined monitoring of thoughts to detect subtle deviations from planned strategies (Janelle, 1999). Staying positively focused on an ideal outcome is very difficult, particularly for athletes who have "free-associating minds" that often drift to negative outcomes instead. These failures to maintain positive thoughts and emotions during performance are labeled "ironic mental processes in sport" (Janelle, 1999), because they involve tendencies to feel, act, and think in ways that are the opposite of the intended direction of the performance (self-defeating prophecies, so to speak). Whenever the cognitive load (game pressure) is either very high or very low, most athletes become more susceptible to ironic processes.

   In light of this information, it is compelling to argue that biofeedback and neurofeedback are essential in providing instantaneous feedback at the onset of ironic processes. The difficulty lies in convincing athletes and coaches that conditioning of neural processes for higher levels of focus and concentration in a resting state will transfer effectively to the competitive environment. One particular EEG biofeedback system monitors activity from 0 to 40 hertz (Hz) with an "inhibit-all" protocol displayed as a concentration line on a graph (Sime et al., 2001). Fluctuations in the line are intriguing to the user because they are directly proportional to quiet versus active mind states.

APPLIED PSYCHOPHYSIOLOGY AND BIOFEEDBACK TO ENHANCE IMAGERY

Psychophysiological measures were obtained on Olympic speed skaters at rest and during mental imagery of an intense 500-meter race (Oishi, Kasai, & Maeshima, 2000). During a 35-second period of imagery of the race, heart rate increased by 44 beats per minute and respiration rate increased to 46 cycles per minute while skin resistance decreased significantly, indicating profound intensity of imagery in this particular population of athletes. In a related study on rhythmic gymnasts shortly before competition, skin temperature dropped substantially as the level of apprehension rose before the event (Schmidt & Peper, 1992). Not surprisingly (to informed psychophysiologists), subsequent success or failure in the event was indirectly related to level of skin temperature: Those who performed better had higher skin temperature in advance.

In other research, EMG biofeedback was monitored during imagery across a variety of different sports. The effects of the imagery could be observed in the specific muscles needed for actual performance; that is, higher resting EMG was observed in leg muscles while moments of explosive jumping were being imagined in the routine (Harris & Robinson, 1986). Those who used internal imagery exhibited more EMG activity than those using external imagery, which could be an indicator of greater depth or quality of internal imagery. In a similar study, EMG biofeedback was used with gymnasts who all reported having the capability for internal imaging (Bird, 1984). Their mental rehearsal routines (in a quiet state) were associated with increases in EMG activity of 45% to 178% above resting levels. Furthermore, the configuration of the EMG profile during imagery was congruent with the actual physical demands of the gymnastic event, thus confirming that extensive absorption in the imagery process occurs during the internal imagery experience. The gymnasts actually felt small muscle contractions (during imagery) at peak moments of ballistic effort over the course of 60 seconds in the event, reflecting that it was exceptionally realistic as a high-quality imagery experience.

Temporal Indicators of Successful Imagery Performance

The quality of an imagery experience can be estimated unobtrusively simply by documenting the length of time the athlete takes to complete the experience. For example, if a gymnast's routine routinely takes 65 seconds to complete during competition, but the imagery experience (of that routine) is substantially shorter or longer than 65 seconds, the gymnast may be having a problem in imaging the difficult moves successfully. In one study, the mental imagery movement times were consistently shorter than physical routine times by only a second or two (Calmeos & Fournier, 2001). However, among those gymnasts for whom the duration of the mental rehearsal was excessively long (5–10 seconds), the extra time included perceived difficulties and possible mistakes anticipated by the gymnasts. In actual competitive situations, if the gymnasts could not perform the routine effectively "in the mind's eye" (imaging), the likelihood was significantly greater that the actual performances would be fraught with mistakes and falls. Similarly, elite speed skaters are known to be able to finish their imagery session of the race in almost exactly the same time as actual race duration (35–37 seconds).

Paradoxically, for some individuals in some sports, there may be an advantage to distorting the realistic time of the performance during imagery. Slow-motion mental rehearsal can enhance the effectiveness of practice by enriching the subject's kinesthetic involvement in the experience, and thus allowing for more accurate detection and correction of mistakes. Calmeos and Fournier (2001) found that slow-motion imagery had a very positive effect on golf putting, but was detrimental for free throw shooting in basketball among the majority of participants. On the other hand, high-speed imagery and snapshot images interspersed throughout imagery of an event such as running were found to help control for distractions. Thus a cross-country runner might visualize and feel the start of the race through the first 100 meters, then skip to the difficult hill climb, and finally envision the last quarter mile of the race anticipating a big win.

Useful Adjunctive Techniques for Imagery Enhancement

It appears obvious that imagery can be enhanced with the judicious use of both biofeedback and related adjunctive techniques. For example, imagery performed in a restricted environmental stimulation tank (REST) resulted in dart throwers' reaching higher levels of ability to focus their concentration, with concomitant improvement in accuracy (Suedfeld, Collier, & Hartnet, 1993). Although the REST procedure (lying in a tank of salt-saturated water) is obtrusive and undesirable for some, it is associated with deep levels of relaxation and may serve to facilitate greater focus and concentration, especially in conjunction with biofeedback applications.

Another important adjunctive technique is to simulate the intensity of competitive stress, anxiety, and excitement in practice sessions so that desensitization occurs (Gallego, Denot-Ledunois, Vardon, & Perruchet, 1996). For example, many consultants use tape-recorded crowd noise to challenge athletes' ability to maintain high-quality imagery under pressure. By contrast, "psyching-up" imagery has also been used effectively in preparation for a demanding muscular endurance task (Lee, 1990). Heart rate is easy to monitor and serves as a indicator of generalized arousal associated with higher-quality imagery. When visualizing the sequence of events preceding a difficult race, more successful swimmers show progressively higher heart rate than less successful performers, regardless of training or ability (Gallego et al., 1996). Being totally absorbed in the imagery experience is essential in order to achieve best outcomes upon actual performance. Absorption is a psychological concept that is measurable (Tellegen & Atkinson, 1974) and occurs concurrently with intense concentration.

RESEARCH ON TRADITIONAL PERIPHERAL BIOFEEDBACK IN SPORT PERFORMANCE

Academic sport psychologists describe biofeedback as an important tool in (1) helping an athlete learn to control activation levels, (2) helping him or her to manage emotions and mood swings, and (3) ultimately assuring physiological readiness of the body for optimum performance (Silva & Stevens, 2002). Research in sport psychology routinely includes measures of heart rate (and variability), electrodermal response (EDR), EMG, respiration (rate and respiratory sinus arrhythmia), and reaction time, in conjunction with self-report of numerous cognitive and emotional variables that may influence competitive performance (Petruzzello, Landers, & Salazar, 1991). However, as an applied technique, biofeedback is not commonly used among practicing sport psychologists. The general conclusion has been that psychophysiology may be related to performance, but that it is difficult to conduct biofeedback unobtrusively. Furthermore, some feel that the effects of biofeedback can be achieved almost as well by using adjunctive techniques (imagery, relaxation, etc.), either alone or in conjunction with professional consultation.

Although biofeedback appears to be of obvious benefit in reducing anxiety, some research suggests that anxiety is not correlated with physiological variables such as heart rate and blood pressure (Karteroliotis & Gill, 1987). On the other hand, excessive muscle tension is indirectly related to reaction time (Fontani, Maffei, Cameli & Polidori, 1999), and one of the most relevant measures for all sport performance is residual muscle tension. Thus it would be desirable to make the biofeedback of this parameter EMG available to more athletes on a regular basis for optimal performance enhancement.

In one of the earliest applications of thermal biofeedback to sports, Kappes and Chapman (1984) examined the effects of indoor versus outdoor thermal biofeedback training in improving performance in cold-weather sports. The outdoor-trained group was superior to the indoor-trained group when all groups were asked to perform outdoors. Given that football, baseball, and soccer games are traditionally played outdoors under adverse weather conditions, this approach could have considerable utility. These methods have also been used successfully in other high-risk performances involving cold, such as underwater scuba diving (Kappes, Mills, & O'Malley, 1993). Clearly hand temperature is important, as it relates to dexterity in preventing fumbles and other miscues in performance. By contrast, tolerance for heat and humidity is also a compromising variable in some sports. One study showed that exaggerated fatigue and suppressed arousal occurred during prolonged exercise in the heat (Nielsen, Hyldig, Bidstrup, Gonzalez-Alonso, & Christoffersen, 2000). Thus special efforts may be necessary to assist athletes who perform in adverse conditions of either cold or heat.

Schmidt and Peper (1992) describe unique training strategies for concentration in elite rhythmic gymnastic competition, using EDR together with heart rate biofeedback to assimilate congruence in thoughts, emotions, and stress reactions while facilitating team performance in various dance routines. A key factor was the combination of mental rehearsal with biofeedback for enhancing concentration in situations where coordination between partners was essential. The close association between vivid imagery and temperature control was an important element for these athletes' success.

Competitive golfing and rifle target shooting are two of the most intense, pressure-filled individual sports. Prapavessis, Grove, McNair, and Cable (1992) tested the effectiveness of a 6-week program for rifle shooters, designed to reduce state anxiety and enhance sport performance via thought stopping, muscle relaxation and biofeedback. A group of shooters receiving the program was contrasted with a placebo training control group. Results showed that cognitive and somatic anxiety, gun vibration, heart rate, and catecholamine levels decreased significantly in the trained group, while self-confidence and accuracy increased from baseline. A comparable study was done with elite and beginning golfers during putting performance (Boutcher & Zinsser, 1990). Both heart rate and respiratory rate decelerated significantly during 4-foot, 8-foot, and 12-foot putt performances in the trained group. Elite golfers exhibited slower heart rates than did novice golfers, suggesting an effect for experience and confidence. Past research shows that EMG is closely associated with level of competitive anxiety during performance (Caruso, Dezwaltowski, Gill, & McElroy, 1990). Furthermore, when EMG, heart rate, and respiratory rate feedback were combined, there were substantial reductions in both anxiety and frontalis muscle tension at rest and prior to competition (Blais & Vallerand, 1986).

In another series of case studies, Blumenstein, Bar-Eli, and Tenenbaum (1997) described using a comprehensive battery of psychophysiological testing and training on biofeedback apparatus to study breathing pattern, skin temperature, heart rate, GSR, and EMG (as well as EEG) in a five-step approach to mental training. Biofeedback was used in this program to help athletes regulate arousal and gain control of performance anxiety. The program represents the most comprehensive application of biofeedback available to date. The steps in the program include (1) introducing mental skills training, (2) testing and training of selected profile of biofeedback modalities, (3) extending biofeedback training together with simulated competitive stress, (4) transformation of mental training to practice, and (5) realization of the technique in competitive situations. The design of the program is elaborate, but there are, as yet, no conclusive data beyond case studies to show its effectiveness.

EEG BIOFEEDBACK AND ATTENTIONAL CONTROL IN SPORTS

"Attention" (narrowly defined in this context as subjective awareness of goals and objectives) occurs when athletes apply mental resources to informational processing, both conscious and unconscious (Simons, 1998). "Concentration" in this context is defined simply as controlling the focus of attention or giving specific direction to one's mental effort. However, there are limits to one's capacity for attention, especially with multiple tasks going on simultaneously. In general, "attention" is defined as the hypothetical process of the organism's facilitating selection of stimuli from the environment to the exclusion of other stimuli, resulting in a response to the relevant stimuli. Therein lies the biggest challenge in sport competition, that is, to be able to handle multiple tasks, while sorting and selecting the essential from the distractions and acting on the former accordingly.

Traditional sport psychologists strive to help their clients achieve greater concentration and attention to relevant details (Anshel, 1997; Sime, 2000). Knowing when and where to focus attention is difficult when lights, sun, shade, conversation, noise, and the possibility of collisions divert attention from the primary task. Traditionally, the Test of Attention and Interpersonal Style (TAIS; Nideffer, 1993) has been used to determine individual differences (self-report measures) in focus and attention to task. However, the TAIS is fraught with self-report bias and lack of objectivity (Summers, Miller, & Ford, 1991). There is a need for more direct and objective measures of attention and concentration, and the EEG is the most direct measure of the brain's attentive state. In the past, it was not thought to be a reliable measure of thought processes or cognitive states retrospectively (Brewer, Van Raalte, Linder, & Van Raalte, 1991). More recently, however, it has been suggested that the EEG can be an unobtrusive indicator of attention, providing immediate feedback of highly focused concentration and alertness (Sime et al., 2001). Two types of concentration can be distinguished on the EEG. Single-pointed concentration appears as a generalized suppression of the integrated all-band wave signal coincidental with being totally absorbed, but not action oriented. By contrast, there is an alertness/arousal state characterized by the combination of single-pointed concentration with a momentary increase in some beta frequencies. An athlete exhibits this brain wave state during periods of intense competition, especially in following a moving target visually (as in trap shooting) and anticipating necessary adjustments.

Hemispheric Shifts and Brain Wave Patterns in Athletes

The degree of attentional focus on a competitive task is related to hemispheric asymmetry, such that attending to task intensely is related to an increase in left-hemisphere alpha activity (Gannon, Landers, Kubitz, Salazar, & Petruzzello, 1992). Highly focused attention in golf coincided with similar left-hemisphere cortical activity during the last second preceding a putt, indicative of shutting down self-talk (Crews & Landers, 1993). However, with increased right-hemispheric alpha activity, there was less error in putting. Thus it appears that whereas left-hemisphere alpha increased significantly over time, it was the right-hemisphere alpha that increased momentarily and dramatically as a subject began the stroke and also made a very accurate putt.

To clarify these concepts, alpha is an idling rhythm throughout the brain, associated with shutting off unnecessary cortical activity. However, some parts of the posterior cortex are going to be turned on for almost any well-learned activity, but this cannot be observed without using specific electrode placements posteriorly. Enhancing alpha has nothing to do with increasing attention, whereas the opposite is true in the prefrontal cortex in this area. Hatfield and colleagues have examined the complex EEG activity associated with various mental states (Lawton, Hung, Saarela, & Hatfield, 1998). In essence, they conclude that an increase in left-hemispheric alpha indicates a decrease in activation (particularly in symbolic and verbal processing), thus causing a reduction in self-talk. It appears that superior performance during shooting competition (wherein the shift is toward visuospatial processing) tends to occur in the absence of thought and self-talk. Recent evidence suggests that observed EEG activity during marksmanship is due to cognitive rather that motor activity (Kerick et al., 2001). However, it appears that reduction in breathing during the shooting process may also contribute to this change in brain activity associated with increased attention. Thus both activation and inhibition of various brain areas may account for the "shifting sands" in attentional control.

Novice athletes can be successful for short periods of time, but they have to generate greater physical effort and be more volitionally determined than their more experienced competitors to hold attention levels constant. In essence, skilled and experienced competitors are very efficient in their effort (mentally and physically) such that they appear carefree in a peak performance. Novices work harder and tire earlier, eventually becoming inconsistent. To combat such fatigue, there is a psychophysiologically controlled automated feedback system using heart rate, skin conductance, and EEG (featuring beta/alpha + theta from parietal and temporal regions) to reinforce alertness and task engagement (Fremen, Mikulka, Scerbo, Prinzo, & Clouatre, 2000). This feedback procedure titrates brain wave activity at an optimal level of engagement, specifically focusing on the parietal lobes to deal with cortical attention.

Visual Attention and Eye Blink Rate: Advantages of Pre-Event "Long Gaze"

It seems clear that for many sports, but especially shooting, vision and cortical activation are important variables. In shooting, maintaining an extended gaze at the target is associated with improved performance (Janelle et al., 2000). Shooters who maintained a longer gaze in preparation for a shot also exhibited an increase in alpha and beta power in the left hemisphere and a decrease in the right, while having great success in hitting the target. This has practical implications as we examine other sports as well. Tiger Woods is described often in the news media as having a very long extended gaze, both in preparation for putts and in general as he gets more focused during tournament competition. No other golfer is so frequently observed to have such a long gaze, and obviously Tiger Woods is viewed at this writing as the best player in the world. A small coincidence, perhaps—but not likely.

However, it has been demonstrated that visual attention must be suppressed during preshot moments to achieve an automatic flow during shots on target (Loze, Collins, & Holmes, 2001). The EEG differences in the occipital lobe revealed that alpha was increased during best shots and decreased during worst shots, indicative of very low visual attention to pistol and target—almost as if the shooter did better when he or she acted indifferent and stopped trying so hard. Furthermore, when shooters rejected a shot (pulled down after aiming for 10–20 seconds), they invariably had exhibited too much beta power during the preparatory period, indicative of too much cognitive activity (Hillman, Apparies, Janelle, & Hatfield, 2000). This activation has been shown to be a limiting factor among sharpshooters when EDR, thermovascular, and cardiorespiratory measures were also taken. Good performance depended upon physiological indicators of mastery of emotional reactivity and greater concentration time. Similarly, it has been demonstrated that a particular pattern of EDR and heart rate prior to and shortly after the shot is indicative of success or failure (Tremayne & Barry, 2001). The experts showed a slow reduction in skin conductance and heart rate prior to the shot and a slow rebound increase immediately after the shot, which were not observed in less skilled shooters.

Studies on psychological momentum and confidence in target shooting and archery revealed that perceptions were often in error and performance decreased when false EEG feedback was provided (Kerick, Iso-Ahola, & Hatfield, 2000; Landers et al., 1991). When the correct EEG feedback (alpha and beta waves in left hemisphere) was provided, performance improved. As suggested in the studies described above, if right-hemisphere beta activity occurred at the time of the shot, there was too much cognitive processing going on and the performance deteriorated. Thus little or no conscious thought is congruent with successful performance. Athletes report that their "minds were blank," they operated "on feel," or they were "totally concentrated on the target" during epochs of great success in shooting. This results in momentum that builds toward greater optimism, confidence and increased focus, mind–body synchrony, and control.

Practical Applications of Neurofeedback in Sports

User-friendly technology to facilitate optimal training procedures has been developed in the last few years. Whereas the majority of EEG training is done at selected sites, using filters for specific frequencies (a complicated, delicate procedure requiring extensive training), sport psychology consultants are more interested in simple practical methods. One approach to optimizing performance is to generalize across the spectrum of 0–40Hz and improve it on a moment-to-moment basis. It is now possible to use neurofeedback with the precision necessary to actually separate levels of concentration and alertness at every moment during biofeedback and performance (Sime, 2000). It is also possible to train clients by providing feedback during their visualization of performance, thereby eliminating problems produced by movement artifacts (Sime et al., 2001).

Although some professionals have had success with athletes using high-tech clinical hardware and software in the office setting, I am inclined to take the technology to the sport environment and to employ a user-friendly application. Toward that end, I have chosen to use an EEG biofeedback system that monitors 0–40 Hz with an "inhibit-all" protocol displayed as a concentration line on a graph, as mentioned earlier (Sime et al., 2001). Fluctuations in the concentration line are directly proportional to quiet versus active mind states.

When I demonstrate the EEG feedback to an athlete, I simply record a 30-second trace of the line wavering up and down in accordance with my own random thoughts or absence thereof. Then I can review the tracing with the athlete, sharing specific examples of random thoughts that appear at various points along the line. Each trace is clearly indicative of my either having been totally absorbed (desired outcome) or distracted by noises in the hall, thoughts of urgency and exigencies, or the like. An early warning of intruding thoughts appears on the graph in the form of an sudden upward shift (spiking). Then I shift the feedback to the athlete and let him or her discover a similar pattern of fluctuating focus of attention. The sensors are relatively unobtrusive (recorded from the frontal lead placement, Fp) near the executive control center of the brain. When the athlete (e.g., a golfer) becomes totally absorbed in precise thoughts or actions, the brain wave pattern flattens out at a low level, while a second graph measuring a derivation of high beta reflects coincidental periods of alertness at critical moments before the shot. The goal is to increase the athlete's awareness of spontaneous thoughts and emotions, and to subsequently learn how to suppress these distracting cognitions at critical moments (e.g., just before a golf swing).

The ultimate benefits of neurofeedback training in the competitive sport environment include shaping the executive attention network toward greater focus of attention; intensifying alertness and arousal where needed; reducing mental fatigue by reinforcing brief, relaxing microbreaks; developing sequential-patterns absorption (concentration), followed by highly intense alertness/action; then shifting to microbreaks for recovery; and, lastly, reducing awareness of crowd noise and slippage into negative self-talk.

HEART RATE VARIABILITY AND RESPIRATORY SINUS ARRHYTHMIA TRAINING IN SPORT PSYCHOLOGY

Ideal Patterns in Athletes

The natural pattern of fluctuation in heart rate (rise and fall) in accordance with each inhalation–exhalation cycle is a healthy, functional response that can be either enhanced or disrupted by emotions and various behavioral changes. When beat-to-beat heart contractions are monitored with a finger plethysmograph sensor or an electrocardiogram (for greater accuracy), and when computer software measures are taken of the time interval between beats, the variation in heart rate can be determined second by second. In general, a smooth, sine-wave-like heart rate variability (HRV) pattern indicates more balanced autonomic nervous system functioning, or what some describe loosely as "physiological entrainment." Considerable evidence suggests that when the oscillations in heart rate are restricted and irregular in pattern (instead of flowing in sine-wave-like patterns up and down), there is a higher risk of mortality from myocardial infarction (Hymes & Nuernberger, 1991; Kleiger, Miller, Bigger, Moss, & The Multicenter Post-Infarction Research Group, 1987). A decrease in HRV amplitude and complexity in various frequency bands is a predictor of mortality among people with heart failure and myocardial infarction. It follows that HRV is also an indicator of greater autonomic nervous system balance and thus related to physical performance.

Using slow respiration together with respiratory sinus arrhythmia (RSA) biofeedback to influence individual heart rate rhythm, Vaschillo, Visochin, and Rishe (2001) demonstrated a return to physiological entrainment, as manifested by more balanced central nervous system functioning and cessation of sympathetic dominance in elite athletes under the pressure of competition. As a result, heart rate decreased (while HRV increased), blood pressure normalized, and hand temperature increased. The increase in sympathovagal balance and subsequent HRV is also associated with an important endurance factor called "airway hyperresponsiveness" that occurs in athletes. Langdeau, Turcotte, Desagne, Jobin, and Boulet (2000) found that parasympathetic tone was higher in athletes, and that this allowed for distended airways and greater airflow during heavy exercise that required maximum oxygen uptake. The ability to relax and achieve the ideal HRV state appears to be inherently critical in world-class endurance competition. Other benefits may exist related to strength and muscle contraction.

Among 30 elite wrestlers, half did 20 minutes of RSA biofeedback daily for 10 consecutive days, and the rest did no respiratory training (Vaschillo et al., 2001). The trained group showed a significant increase in reaction time, as well as speed of recovery in relaxation of the quadriceps femoris muscle, compared to no change in the control group. In a study of cross-country skiers and canoeists (Hedelin, Bjerle, & Henriksson-Larson, 2001), peak torque (strength), reaction time, oxygen consumption, and HRV at rest were measured before and after physical exercise training. Oxygen consumption was directly related to HRV among the most fit athletes, and the parasympathetic response inherent in HRV was positively associated with supraconditioning levels in all the athletes.

RSA has been used as an indicator of cardiovascular neuroregulation in other athlete populations (Strano et al., 1998). Athletes generally have a slow, deep, and regular breathing pattern at rest, leading to increased parasympathetic activity similar to that produced during RSA training. The ratio of low-frequency to high-frequency power that exists therein reflects sympathovagal balance, which is desirable in preparation for any athletic performance. Although these effects tend to occur naturally, as a part of the physical training, they are especially prominent in sports where aerobic or anaerobic conditioning includes running, jumping, and swimming (Spalding, Jeffers, Torges, & Hatfield, 2000).

Effects of Exercise and Emotions on HRV

Higher aerobic fitness levels are associated with strong vagal influences on the myocardium, resulting in modulations in cardiac reactivity during psychological stress and recovery. Thus it would be very logical to assume that simply including aerobic training in all sport training would facilitate a valuable trophotropic response with respect to controlling the effects of competitive stress. For example, archers and rifle shooters, who have absolutely no need to be aerobically fit in order to release the arrow or pull the trigger in competition, still run in preparation for competition. Their coaches routinely ask these traditionally sedentary athletes to become more physically fit anyway, in part because the exercise training induces a vagally mediated parasympathetic effect that slows heart rate and enhances the emotional control needed in competition. Spalding et al. (2000), among others, have demonstrated this effect, noting also that those with the lowest resting heart rates did exhibit greater parasympathetic effect due to the RSA training. Surprisingly, however, they could not show that higher fitness level that produced the bradycardia at rest was due exclusively to enhanced parasympathetic influence. Apparently, healthy young athletes have very robust parasympathetic nervous systems regardless of fitness level, yet are exceptionally vulnerable to emotional psychophysiological reactions to competitive stress.

The effects of emotions on HRV are well documented, but it is the potential to shift emotional states with an increase in HRV via RSA biofeedback that is most critical in sport competition and performance in many other settings (stage, theater, music, etc.). Positive emotions elicited in this manner have been associated with sympathovagal balance, whereas anger has been associated with significantly increased sympathetic activation (McCraty, Atkinson, Tiller, Rein, & Watkins, 1995). Although the health impact of this training is most dramatic in reducing hypertension and risk of fatal heart attack, other benefits to the athlete include a sense of well-being that induces confidence and thus further assures health and well-being.

CREDENTIALING AND PREPARATION TO USE BIOFEEDBACK IN SPORTS

There are two approaches to preparing for biofeedback-related work with athletes and coaches. Most clinicians and even many education specialists in biofeedback do not have a background in sport competition, or the necessary vocabulary to communicate comfortably with coaches and athletes. As such, it is hard for them to break into the sport psychology field and become successful. Thus it is wise for most biofeedback practitioners to seek collaboration with a well-trained sport psychology professional in their geographic location. A practitioner and a sport psychologist do not need to be next-door neighbors, but for best communication and cooperation, it is helpful to be within easy driving distance (even though telephone and e-mail may be the primary modes of communication). This is the easiest and most appropriate approach to take for most aspiring biofeedback therapists who want to extend their practice into performance enhancement, especially at the team level. Obviously, if an individual athlete wishes to seek assistance for relaxation or stress concerns, a therapist can function independently. However, even with the individual athletes, it is helpful to have the consultation of an informed colleague in sport psychology.

For those biofeedback providers who want to become fully trained and certified in sport psychology, there is a second approach. The Association for the Advancement of Applied Sport Psychology (AAASP) offers a certification program that serves a variety of well-trained specialists. For example, individuals who have a clinical or counseling background and who have taken a certain number of courses in sport science are eligible for AAASP certification. Many clinical or counseling psychologists have made this transition and become highly specialized in this exciting field. Most professionals in the biofeedback field will probably need additional training, workshops, or coursework in biomechanics, motor learning, and/or exercise physiology to meet the certification criteria. For more information on credentialing in this field, contact the AAASP Sport Psychology at http://www.aaasponline.org.

BIOFEEDBACK MODALITIES AND ADJUNCTIVE METHODS MOST COMMONLY USED IN SPORTS

The most common biofeedback modalities that sports psychologists utilize include heart rate (and its variability), respiration, peripheral temperature, EMG, EDR, and EEG. Unfortunately, there is not much definitive information about specific protocols and selected parameters to use with different sports. The studies described in this chapter provide the most common and apparently most relevant parameters for the particular sport training situations identified. Regarding adjunctive techniques, there is considerable evidence indicating that relaxation strategies (autogenic training, progressive relaxation, and other methods of interrupting the arousal responses) do work effectively to reduce preperformance anxiety (Gould & Udry, 1994). The quieting reflex (Stroebel, 1982) is a method that I use and recommend to athletes regularly. Guided imagery and visualization of preperformance routines (as well as performance itself) are very common among nearly all sport psychologists. There are a number who use hypnosis following the methods of Lars Eric Unestahl, who uses the term "inner mental training" to destigmatize the reference to hypnosis or self-hypnosis in this context (Unestahl, 1986). Eye movement desensitization and reprocessing (EMDR) is also a technique that has considerable value in sport settings, where bad performances with public humiliation are easily categorized as microtraumas. Among golfers, the usual preshot routine includes many repetitions of the look up to the target and back to the ball. As such, it may be that some golfers are naturally carrying out a rudimentary form of the EMDR technique. "Purist" practitioners of the method might argue differently, but it is likely that some potential clearing effect is occurring with each repetition of the look up and back down at the ball.

Software applications that serve as adjunctive methods for neurofeedback are also very important in garnering the attention of athletes, who are easily distracted. Some of these include BrainTrain, ThinkFast, and the Metronome (Cram & Charbonneau, 2002).

USING BIOFEEDBACK TO DEMONSTRATE PSYCHOPHYSIOLOGY TO COACHES AND ATHLETES

I consider the use of home trainer (or stand-alone) biofeedback equipment to be absolutely essential in field demonstrations to coaches and/or groups of athletes. Being able to show dramatic illustrations of stress reactions often serves to break down the barriers and soften the stigmas that ordinarily separate athletic performance from psychology. I find demonstrations especially helpful in the development of rapport with a larger group, after which time individual athletes may seek further information in casual conversation.

Providing illustrations of classic stress responses is an important consideration before embarking upon the use of clinical computerized biofeedback protocols in an office. With the availability of liquid crystal display projectors and laptop computers, it is becoming easier to bring the biofeedback lab to the sport setting and demonstrate methods to small or large audiences.

In large team situations, there is very little opportunity to work individually with the athletes. However, if they can see and experience vicariously the psychophysiology demonstrations, then it seems easier to engage them in individual consultation. I feel it is very important to be able to take the technology to the athletes and coaches by making group presentations. For many athletes, getting them to identify their emotional states during a period of high-stress competition can be difficult. Describing how they themselves make use of their awareness of signs and symptoms of stress to trigger ancillary efforts to defuse the symptoms (hot shower, massage, relaxation, etc.) may be an effective beginning with the athletes.

A Rich Source of Information in a Simple Handshake

In demonstrating typical stress responses under pressure of competition, one can gather a great deal of information from a simple handshake. The hands reveal peripheral temperature differences, as well as EDR (palmar sweating) information, instantaneously and unobtrusively. The emotional state of an athlete (like that of anyone else) is revealed easily by the observation of the extremes—either cold, sweaty hands or warm, dry hands. Obviously, there are numerous gradients in between (e.g., cool but dry hands or warm and damp hands). If an athlete is even close to having cold, sweaty hands, this is a clear indication that he or she is experiencing some level of stress symptoms. These symptoms are not uncommon, even among very successful performers in anticipation of a big game. Of course, it is often likely that the athlete may dissipate some of the nervous reactions soon after the start of competition. However, for a kicker who is about to step onto the field to try a 50-yard game-winning or -losing field goal late in the game, there is no time to work off the stress reactions naturally.

Many other sports involve quick, short-term performances. Divers have a 10- to 20-second time period to go from board or platform into the water; gymnasts have a 45- to 90-second window of opportunity to perform most of their routines. Interestingly, gymnasts use an extraordinary amount of powdered chalk on their hands for all events that require gripping the apparatus. Obviously, palmar sweating reactions are so predominant in competition that coaches and gymnasts consider it an automatic safety precaution to use chalk (and sometimes leather hand grips as well) to prevent slips and falls.

Consider also that skilled football and basketball players handle a slippery leather ball, flicking passes and making shots requiring great dexterity. Coaches and athletes uniformly seem unaware that greatly reduced peripheral blood flow and cold hands impair dexterity. I often use a classic example to reinforce this point with coaches and athletes.

In a Division I football game played in a Southern state, the outdoor temperature was 98° F, but on the field with the AstroTurf it was 110° F. The game was close, and the rookie running back was supposed to catch the pass from the quarterback on an option play. The crowd roared as the quarterback came under the center. The quarterback took the snap and passed the ball toward the running back, who reached for it—but, as if in slow motion, the ball floated in the air endlessly. It was obvious that the running back wanted the ball immediately in his urgency to grab it and run.

As the ball came closer, the crowd hesitated in anticipation along with the player, and then slow motion suddenly became real time and reality took over. When the ball hit the player's hands, it was as though they were as hard as rock. The ball bounced off his hands and into the arms of an opposing lineman. The young man had fumbled away a great scoring opportunity—but, more than that, he had lost a little of the trust his coaches had in him, and he knew it. It was very embarrassing and very discouraging for him.

When he came off the field, no one consoled him; everyone knew how badly he felt, so they avoided him. As he approached the sideline, I offered him reassurance in the form of the "two-hand" shake customary among players, coaches, and consultants in tough situations. I was shocked to observe that his hands were ice-cold, on a day when the field temperature was 110° F. At first I wondered how this young man could have ice-cold hands, and then I realized that the excitement, the anticipation, the anxiety, and the stress of the big game had caused him to have greatly reduced peripheral blood flow. Upon reflection, is it any surprise that he dropped the ball?

Case Study

Golf is my passion, and it is the most prominent sport where stress and mental mistakes are highlighted regularly in news media video clips. It is clearly an ideal setting for sport psychology and biofeedback, as we often see professional golfers parade their sport psychologists proudly in public, while other macho athletes in baseball and football are terribly secretive about seeking any kind of psychological assistance. Thus it was a pleasant, but not unexpected, surprise when I got a call from a friend, Rick, (a psuedonym) several years ago indicating that he wanted to subcontract biofeedback services from me for his "renowned" golf client. Initially I tried to have his client work with another highly regarded biofeedback specialist in the city where he lived (for his own convenience), but the golfer spent so little time at home that he never got around to meeting with this specialist. Thus I gladly arranged my travel schedule to meet with the client at a tournament site (in Florida) in March while the snow still covered the ground at my own residence in Nebraska.[1]

I took advantage of Rick's invitation to walk the course along with him during the tournament, observing Rick's golf client from "outside the ropes."[2] It was a remarkable learning experience to be mentored in the heat of competition. I felt like an apprentice learning "on the job" as he talked me through the steps in the process of observing critical events on the course, to be analyzed later with Rick's client. Such issues as "what factors contributed to your nervousness over that shot compared to other shots of the day?" were the topic of our conversation.

After the round of competition, Rick invited me "inside the ropes" amidst heavy security on the practice putting green to meet his client, whom I shall refer to using the pseudonym, "Shivas Irons."[3] Rick told me his client, "Shivas" would likely give us only about 10 minutes since he was an adult with ADD who had a very short attention span for academic content or intellectual conversation. However, by the end of the day, I actually had spent 6 hours with this client, instead of only 10 minutes, largely because I had brought to his attention technology and expertise that he had never seen before, and this intrigued him. Thus for my initial opportunity to work in professional golf at the highest level, I had access to one of the top players in the game all because of biofeedback technology. However, it should be noted that numerous other golfers still hesitate to engage in biofeedback consultations because they are either afraid of the technology or put off by it. It is a matter of personal preference.

At the outset of my initial consultation, I chose to begin with the EDR parameter because it is not too invasive and would likely give immediate and fairly dramatic illustration of stress, arousal, and anxiety, or so I thought. When I put the sensors on Shivas' fingers, I was a little surprised to discover that he had absolutely no moisture on the skin surface of his hand. I should have guessed that the demonstration was at risk of failure, in part because Shivas was feeling so relaxed in his own home. In addition, however, it should be noted that because golfers have calluses on the volar surface of their hands, from gripping and swinging the club 1,000 or more times a day, the eccrine glands simply do not emit as much moisture through the high resistance surface area; thus SCL and SCR are notably lower in this population (see Neumann, Strehl, & Birbaumer, Chapter 5 on Instrumentation, this volume). Thus when the EDR instrument failed to register a reading, and no sound (i.e., no biofeedback) was emitted during the baseline, I nearly panicked. Fortunately a moment later my effort to demonstrate classic stress reactions with EDR was saved by a humorous set of circumstances described in the following scene.

Shivas was sitting in his recliner, alongside a room full of exercise equipment (used for his physical exercise), seemingly "tied down" to the biofeedback equipment (to be used to "exercise" his brain). Rick suggested that maybe it was too cool in the room and asked if he should adjust the thermostat. Shivas proceeded to tell Rick how to adjust the thermostat, but the system had such a complicated array of sophisticated controls that Rick was unable to adjust it. With each subsequent attempt at instructing Rick to find the right button to no avail, Shivas became more and more frustrated because he desperately wanted to jump up and do it himself. At that moment, the EDR unit came alive and began to sing a high-pitched alerting sound indicative of the sympathetic nervous system arousal Shivas was experiencing. Rick and Shivas both stopped the chatter immediately and were astounded at the meaningfulness of this incident. They realized, without much explanation, that because Shivas was the host in his own house he felt responsible for our comfort and further that he should be able to control things. When the thermostat was beyond his direct control and when he felt inadequate in communicating the necessary action, that caused him to be remarkably stressed. From that point on, I had the rapt attention of both Rick and Shivas.

Later we moved on to the EMG demonstration. At that time, I carried with me an old J & J M-52 portable EMG that works very well for demonstrations with its light bar and raspy feedback tone. Rick was interested in seeing how muscle tension affected his client's golf putting, so we went to his indoor putting green. For this demonstration, I used a modified FpN placement (see Schwartz and Andrasik, Chapter 14 and the Appendix to Chapter 14, this volume), with one sensor over the masseter muscle and the other in the posterior cervical region (right side for a right-handed putter). It turned out to be an ideal placement for demonstrating the importance of relaxed face and neck muscles just prior to putting a ball.

I adjusted the threshold of the EMG so that Shivas could stop the raspy feedback signal completely as the tension diminished, just prior to taking the putter back to strike the ball. Golfers rely on "feel" for the delicate effort required in putting accurately, and residual tension clouds their perception of feel. Thus it is very logical for the golfer to value using biofeedback technology for enhancing the "feel" of the putt. In my opinion, consultants must emphasize this point in marketing their services.

Once again I was in a technical advisory role, working for Rick as I trudged around the green behind Shivas with his "tether" (cable) to my portable EMG unit. I needed to adjust the threshold occasionally, from one putt to the next, if the variable gain setting was not providing the appropriate feedback about the tension level in Shivas' face and neck muscles. The goal was for Shivas to become much more relaxed immediately prior to taking the club back to make the putting movement. During this period of practice and experimentation with the EMG, Rick asked several questions and made numerous comments relating the information from the biofeedback signal to other work he had done with Shivas in the past. It was a wonderful illustration of interactive consultation, featuring the benefit of instantaneous, valid feedback confirming what the expert observer (Rick) had only surmised was accurate in the past.

After we finished the biofeedback work to everyone's satisfaction, Shivas offered Rick and me refreshments and eventually grilled brisket of beef for dinner, including us with his extended family in a very intimate setting. It was a tremendous affirmation of the apparent success of these biofeedback demonstrations and of the appreciation that followed our efforts. In the ensuing weeks, Shivas had a very dramatic resurgence in his golfing performance, as Rick continued the consultation, thus extending the effects of our initial biofeedback work into his daily routine (i.e., "transfer of training"). After a lackluster start to the season, Shivas won the U.S. Open and one other major event in the last half of the season. I felt very privileged to have spent a day in the life of this legendary golfer, and I am confident that, in some cases, merely demonstrating the subtle changes in autonomic nervous system arousal via EMG or EDR may be sufficient to enhance acute awareness of behavioral control. In effect, I believe that highly gifted athletes have the innate capacity to continue discovering related subtle mind–body interactions of importance long after an experience of biofeedback.

In the past three years, I have done less biofeedback with EMG and EDR and much more with neurofeedback. In my opinion, neurofeedback has even greater potential for successful consultation with golfers because of the wide range of subtle nuances in cognition and muscular control associated with negative self-talk, self-doubt, self-recrimination, and apprehension, and at the other extreme, the anticipation of accolades if and when the shot goes in the hole. To affirm this potential, note that one year after this experience with Shivas, I consulted extensively with one of his friends at a time when he was in a slump. In my experience, once the athlete sees the connection (via direct neurofeedback in vivo, that is, during a practice effort) between random, seemingly uncontrolled subtle cognitions and the slight breakdown in swing performance associated with these negative thoughts, they then can apply other structured techniques to minimize these unnecessary and disruptive cognitions. The key factor in this consulting effort is to enhance player awareness of the principles so they can take on better intuitive observational skills related to their ideal performance state.

SUMMARY AND CONCLUSIONS

The psychological preparation of athletes for competition could be described as "taking the brain to the weight room." That is, the athletes are being mentally conditioned to withstand the rigors of fatigue, time pressure, undue expectations, and crowd pressure to give them the possibility of meeting or exceeding their performance goals. Biofeedback technology and skills training can and should be an integral part of an athlete's training regimen. Competition stress, anxiety, and residual tension are common antecedents of performance, and biofeedback is the most objective way of assessing as well as controlling these variables in the long run. Although emotions that run high can be the fuel of record-breaking performances, when they are not well controlled in precompetition, they can be deleterious. The goal of performance enhancement efforts is to channel emotions, anxiety, and stress into the "flow state" or the ZOF, as described earlier. One example of the ideal performance state is the achievement of an optimal RE (i.e., maximum speed and efficiency), also as described earlier. In some cases, dissociation can be helpful to achieve an ideal state, but in other circumstances the blocking of emotions and feelings of fatigue results in burnout from overtraining.

Biofeedback can be an essential component in the prevention of and rehabilitation from injury. For the trauma, pain, and frustration of rehabilitation, instrumented reinforcement (biofeedback) of progress can provide inspiration and consolation, whichever is needed more. In addition, I am convinced that neurofeedback may be one of the most effective ways of making an athlete truly accountable for achieving and maintaining an ideal imagery (visualization) session. Similarly, neurofeedback has potential to help in controlling intrusive negative thoughts (ironic processes). In addition to the EEG, which may hold the greatest promise for performance enhancing effects, the traditional biofeedback modalities (heart rate, respiration or HRV, EMG, EDR, and temperature) are all important elements in psychological preparation for sport. Simple observation of eye blink rate (versus long gaze at a target), hand shake (noting temperature and sweating), game-like concentration tests are all important adjuncts for the sport psychologist. Lastly, the standard adjunctive methods of relaxation, goal setting, autogenic training, hypnosis, mental rehearsal, and team building are foundations of a comprehension performance enhancement training program.

Seeking collaboration and consultation with a sport psychologist is one way for a biofeedback practitioner to get started working with athletes. It is also possible to take a program of studies in sport science and related areas, and to seek certification from the AAASP. The use of biofeedback and neurofeedback is growing rapidly in sport psychology. In the past, there have been numerous other methods by which athletes and sport psychologists (in concert) have achieved the "flow state" or the ZOF. Although there are many roads to Rome, the technologically solid path of biofeedback skills and technology appears to be a very desirable route.

NOTES

1. One big advantage to sport psychology consultation is the opportunity to travel to either warm or cold weather venues (depending on personal preferences) where skiing or golf conditions are ideal.

2. What I learned from walking the course along with Rick was that the consultant must see the sport performance in live competition, and he/she must be on site to be "invested" with the client, giving his/her time and effort to learn well in advance of trying to provide advice, counsel, or feedback to the client.

3. The name "Shivas Irons" is historically famous to all avid golfers and golf professionals who cherish the book *Golf in the Kingdom* by Michael Murphy (1997). It is a classic tale of golf mysticism, wherein "Shivas Irons" is a teaching professional in Scotland who shares his philosophy and insight during a round of golf with the unsuspecting Michael Murphy whose life was thereafter changed forever. Michael Murphy also wrote the book, *Future of the Body*, which highlights biofeedback in a different context.

REFERENCES

Andersen, M. B., & Williams, J. N. (1988). A model of stress and athletic injury: Prediction and prevention. *Journal of Sport and Exercise Psychology, 10*, 294–306.

Andersen, M. B., & Williams, J. N. (1999). Athletic injury, psychosocial factors and perceptual changes during stress. *Journal of Sports Science, 17*(9), 735–741.

Annesi, J. (1997). Three dimensional state anxiety recall: Implications for individual's zone of optimal functioning research and application. *The Sports Psychologist 11*(1), 43–52.

Anshel, M. (1997). *Sport psychology: From theory to practice*. Scottsdale, AZ: Gorsuch Scarlsbirck.

Anshel, M., Williams, L., & Williams, F. (2000). Coping style following acute stress in competitive sport. *Journal of Social Psychology, 140*(6), 751–773.

Bales, C., Metz, K., Robertson, R., Goss, F., Cosgrove, J., & McBurney, D. (1990). Perceptual regulation of prescribed exercise. *Journal of Cardiopulmonary Rehabilitation, 10*, 25–31.

Beedie, C., Terry, P., & Lane, A. (2000). The Profile of Mood States in athletic performance meta analysis. *Journal of Applied Sports Psychology, 12*, 49–68.

Bird, A. M., & Horn, N. A. (1990). Cognitive anxiety and mental errors in sport. *Journal of Sport and Exercise Psychology, 12*, 217–222.

Bird, E. I. (1984, May). *EMG quantification of mental rehearsal*. Unpublished manuscript.

Blais, M. R., & Vallerand, R. J. (1986). Multi model effects of electromyographic biofeedback: Looking at children's ability to control pre-competitive anxiety. *Journal of Sports Psychology, 8*, 283–303.

Blumenstein, B., Bar-Eli, N., & Tenenbaum, G. (1997). A five-step approach to mental training incorporating biofeedback. *The Sports Psychologist, 11*, 440–453.

Boutcher, F. H., & Zinsser, N. W. (1990). Cardiac deceleration of elite and beginning golfers during putting. *Journal of Sport and Exercise Psychology, 12*, 37–47.

Brewer, B. W., Van Raalte, J. L., Linder, D. E., & Van Raalte, N. S. (1991). Peak performance and the perils of retrospective intraspection. *Journal of Sport and Exercise Psychology, 8*, 227–238.

Burton, D. (1988). Do anxious swimmers swim slower?: Re-examining the elusive anxiety–performance relationship. *Journal of Sport and Exercise Psychology, 10*, 45–61.

Caird, S., McKenzie, A., & Sleivert, G. (1999). Biofeedback and relaxation techniques improve running economy in sub-elite long distance runners. *Medicine and Science in Sports and Exercise, 31*(5), 717–722.

Calmeos, C., & Fournier, J. (2001). Duration of physical and mental execution of gymnastics routines. *The Sports Psychologist, 16*, 142–150.

Caruso, C. M., Dezwaltowski, D. A., Gill, D. L., & McElroy, M. A. (1990). Psychological and physiological changes in competitive state anxiety during noncompetition and competitive stress and failure. *Journal of Sports and Exercise Psychology, 12*, 620.

Cram, J., & Charbonneau, J. (2002). *Effects of interactive metronome on brain function: A single subject pre-, post- study using QEEG brain maps* [Abstract]. Unpublished manuscript, Sierra Health Institute, Nevada City, CA.

Crews, D. J. (1992). Psychological state and running economy. *Medicine and Science in Sports and Exercise, 24*, 475–482.

Crews, D. J., & Landers, D. M. (1993). Electroencephalographic measures of attentional patterns prior to the golf putt. *Official Journal of the American College of Sports Medicine, 25*, 116–126.

Cummings, M., Wilson, V., & Bird, E. (1984). Flexibility development in sprinters using EMG biofeedback and relaxation training. *Biofeedback and Self-Regulation, 9*(3), 395–405.

Cupal, D. & Brewer, B. (2001). Effects of relaxation and guided imagery on knee-strength, knee reinjury anxiety and pain following anterior cruciate ligament reconstruction. *Rehabilitation Psychology, 46*(1), 28–43.

Davis, J. (1991). Sports injuries and stress management: An opportunity for research. *The Sports Psychologist, 5*, 175–182.

Dorfman, H., & Kuell, K. (1995). *The mental game of baseball: A guide to peak performance*. South Bend, IN: Diamond Communications.

Fenz, W., & Epstein, S. (1967). Gradients of physiological arousal of experienced and novice parachutists as a function of an approaching jump. *Psychosomatic Medicine, 29*, 33–51.

Fontani, G., Maffei, D., Cameli, S., & Polidori, F. (1999). Reactivity and event-related potentials during attentional tests in athletes. *European Journal of Applied Physiological and Occupational Physiology, 80*(4), 308–317.

Ford, I., Eklund, R., & Gordon, S. (2000). An examination of psychosocial variables moderating the relationship between life stress and injury time-loss among athletes of a high standard. *Journal of Sports Science, 18*(5), 301–312.

Foster, C. (1998). Monitoring training in athletes with reference to overtraining syndrome. *Medicine and Science in Sports, 30*(7), 1164–1168.

Fremen, F., Mikulka, P., Scerbo, M., Prinzo, L., & Clouatre, K. (2000). Evaluation of a psycho-physiological controlled adaptive automation system, using performance on a tracking task. *Applied Psychophysiology and Biofeedback Journal, 25*, 103–115.

Gallego, J., Denot-Ledunois, F., Vardon, G., & Perruchet, P. (1996). Ventilatory responses to imagined exercise. *Psychophysiology, 33*, 711–719.

Gannon, T., Landers, D., Kubitz, K., Salazar, W., & Petruzzello, S. (1992). An analysis of temporal Electroencephalographic pattening prior to initiation of the arm curl. *Journal of Sport and Exercise Psychology, 14*, 87–100.

Gould, D., Petlichkoff, L., Simons, J., & Vevera, M. (1987). Relationship between Competitive State Anxiety Inventory/two subscale scores and pistol sheeting performance. *Journal of Sports Psychology, 9*, 33–42.

Gould, D., & Pick, S. (1995). Sport psychology: The Griffth era, 1920–40. *The Sport Psychologist, 9*(4), 391–405.

Gould, D., & Udry, E. (1994). Psychological skills for enhancing performance: Arousal regulation strategies. *Medicine and Science in Sports and Exercise, 26*(4), 478–485.

Hackney, A. C., Tearman, S. N., III, & Nowacki, J. M. (1990). Physiological profiles of over trained and stale athletes: A review. *Applied Sports Psychology, 2*, 21–33.

Hale, B., & Whitehouse, A. (1998). The effects of imagery-manipulated appraisal on intensity and direction of competitive anxiety. *The Sport Psychologist, 12*(1), 40–51.

Hammermeister, J., & Burton, D. (1995). Anxiety and the ironman: Investigating the antecedents and consequences of endurance athlete's state anxiety. *The Sport Psychologist. 9*(1), 29–40.

Hanin, Y. L. (2000). *Emotions in sport*. Champaign, IL: Human Kinetics Press.

Hardy, L., & Callow, N. (1999). Efficacy of external and internal visual imagery perspective for the enhancement of performance on tasks in which form is important. *Journal of Sport and Exercise Psychology, 21*, 95–112.

Harris, D. V., & Robinson, W. J. (1986). The effects of skill level on ENG activity during internal and external imagery. *Journal of Sports Psychology, 8*, 105–111.

Hatfield, B. D., & Hillman, C. (2001). The psychophysiology of sport: A mechanistic understanding of the psychology of superior performance. In R. N. Singer, H. A. Hausenblas, & C. M. Janelle (Eds.), *Handbook of research in sports psychology* (2nd ed.). New York: Wiley.

Hatfield, B. D., & Landers, D. M. (1983). Psychophysiology: A new direction of sports psychology. *Journal of Sports Psychology, 5*, 243–259.

Hatfield, B. D., Spalding, T., Mahon, A., Slatter, B., Brody, E., & Vaccaro, P. (1992). The effect of psychological strategies on cardiovascular and muscular activity during treadmill running. *Medicine and Science in Sports and Exercise, 24*(2), 218–225.

Hecker, J. E., & Kaczor, L. N. (1988). Application of imagery theory to sport psychology: Some preliminary findings. *Journal of Sport and Exercise Psychology, 10*, 363–373.

Hedelin, R., Bjerle, P., & Henriksson-Larson, K. (2001). Heart rate variability in athletes: Relationship with central and peripheral performance. *Medicine and Science in Sports and Exercise, 33*(8), 1394–1398.

Hillman, C., Apparies, R., Janelle, C. M., & Hatfield, B. (2000). An electrocortical comparison of executed and rejected shots in skilled marksmen. *Biological Psychology, 52*(1), 71–83.

Hymes, A., & Nuernberger, P. (1991). Breathing patterns found in heart attack victims. *Journal of the International Association of Yoga Therapists, 2*(25), 25–27.

Ievleva, L., & Orlick, T. (1991). Mental links to enhanced healing: An exploratory study. *The Sports Psychologist, 5*, 25–40.

Jackson, S. A. (1995). Factors influencing the occurrence of slow state in elite athletes. *Journal of Applied Sports Psychology, 7*, 138–166.

Jackson, S., & Csikszentmihalyi, M. (1999). *Flow in sport: Keys to optimal experiences and performances.* Champaign, IL: Human Kinetics.

Jackson, S., & Roberts, G. (1992). Positive performance states of athletes: Toward a conceptual understanding of peak performance. *The Sport Psychologist. 6*(2), 156–171.

Janelle, C. M. (1999). Ironic mental processes in sport: Implications for sport psychologists. *The Sports Psychologist, 13*, 201–220.

Janelle, C. M., Hillman, C. H., Apparies, R., Murray, N. P., Meli, L., Fallon, E. A., & Hatfield, B. D. (2000). Expertise differences in cortical activation and gaze behavior during rifle shooting. *Journal of Sport and Exercise Psychology, 22*, 167–182.

Kappes, B. M., & Chapman, S. J. (1984). The effects of indoor versus outdoor thermal biofeedback training in cold weather sports. *Journal of Sports Psychology, 6*, 305–311.

Kappes, B. M., Mills, W., & O'Malley, J. (1993). Psychophysiological factors in the prevention and treatment of cold injuries. *Alaska Medicine, 35*(1), 131–140.

Karteroliotis, C., & Gill, D. L. (1987). Temporal changes in psychological and physiological components of state anxiety. *Journal of Sports Psychology, 9*, 261–274.

Kellmann, M., Altenburg, D., Lornes, W., & Steinacker, J. M. (2001). Assessing stress and recovery during preparation for the world championships in rowing. *The Sports Psychologist, 15*, 151–167.

Kentta, G., & Hassmen, P. (1998). Overtraining and recovery: A conceptual model. *Sports Medicine, 26*(1), 1–16.

Kerick, S. E., Iso-Ahola, S. E., & Hatfield, B. D. (2000). Psychological momentum in target shooting: Cortical, cognitive-effective, and behavioral responses. *Journal of Sport and Exercise Psychology, 22*, 1–20.

Kerick, S. E., McDowell, K., Hung, T. M., Santa Maria, D. L., Spalding, T. W., & Hatfield, B. D. (2001). The role of the left temporal region under the cognitive motor demands of shooting in skilled marksmen. *Biological Psychology, 58*, 263–277.

Kleiger, R., Miller, P., Bigger, J., Moss, A., & The Multicenter Post-Infarction Research Group. (1987). Decreased heart rate variability and its association with increased mortality after acute myocardial infarction. *American Journal of Cardiology, 59*, 256–262.

Krane, V. (1993). A practical application of the anxiety-athletic performance relationship: The zone of optimal functioning hypothesis. *The Sport Psychologist, 7*(2), 113–126.

Landers, D. (1995). Sport psychology: The formative years, 1950–80. *The Sport Psychologist. 9*(4), 406–417.

Landers, D., Petruzzello, F., Salazar, W., Crews, D., Kubitz, K., Gannon, T., & Han, M. (1991). The influence of electrocortical biofeedback on performance in pre-elite archers. *Medicine and Science in Sports and Exercise, 23*(1), 123–129.

Langdeau, J., Turcotte, H., Desagne, P., Jobin, J., & Boulet, L. (2000). Influence of sympatho-vagal balance on airway responsiveness in athletes. *European Journal of Applied Physiology, 83*(4–5), 370–375.

Larson, G., Starkey, C., & Zaichkowsky, L. (1996). Psychological aspects of athletic injuries as perceived by athletic trainers. *The Sports Psychologist, 10*, 37–47.

Lawton, D. W., Hung, T. M., Saarela, P., & Hatfield, B. D. (1998). Electroencephalography and mental states associated with elite performance. *Journal of Sport and Exercise Psychology, 20*, 35–53.

Lee, C. (1990). Psyching up for a muscular endurance task: Effects of image content on performance and mood state. *Journal of Sports and Exercise Psychology, 12,* 66–73.

Lehmann, M., Foster, C., Dickhuth, H., & Gastmann, U. (1998). Autonomic imbalance hypothesis and over-training syndrome. *Medicine and Science in Sports and Exercise, 30*(7), 1140–1145.

Loze, G., Collins, D., & Holmes, P. (2001). Pre-shot EEG alpha power reactivity during expert air-pistol shooting: A comparison of best and worst shots. *Journal of Sports Science, 19*(9), 727–733.

Martin, K. A., & Hall, C. (1995). Using mental imagery to enhance intrinsic motivation. *Journal of Sport and Expercise Psychology, 17,* 54–69.

Martin, K. A., Moritz, S. E., & Hall, C. R. (1999). Imagery used in sport: A literature review and applied model. *The Sports Psychologist, 13,* 245–268.

Masters, K. S., & Ogles, B. (1998). Associative and disassoctive strategies in exercise and running: Twenty years later, what do we know? *The Sports Psychologist, 12,* 253–270.

McCraty, R., Atkinson, M., Tiller, W., Rein, G., & Watkins, A. (1995). The effects of emotions on short-term power spectrum analysis of heart rate variability. *American Journal of Cardiology, 76*(14), 1089–1093.

McGuigan, F. J. (1979). *Psychopedological measures of covert behavior: A guide to the laboratory.* Hillsdale, NJ: Erlbaum.

Murphy, M. (1997). *Golf in the kingdom.* New York: Penquin.

Murphy, S. (1994). Imagery interventions in sport. *Medicine and Science in Sports and Exercise, 26*(4), 486–494.

Murphy, S. N., Woolfolk, R. L., & Budney, A. J. (1988). The effects of motor imagery on strength performance. *Journal of Sport and Exercise Psychology, 10,* 334–345.

Nideffer, R. (1993). Concentration and attention control training. In J. Williams (Ed.), *Applied sport psychology: Personal growth to peak performance.* Mountain View, CA: Mayfield.

Nielsen, B., Hyldig, T., Bidstrup, F., Gonzalez-Alonso, J., & Christoffersen, G. (2000). Brain activity and fatigue during prolonged exercise in the heat. *Pflugers Archives, 442*(1), 41–48.

Noble, B., & Robertson, R. (1996). *Perceived exertion.* Champaign, IL: Human Kinetics.

Nordell, K., & Sime. W. E. (1993). Competitive trait anxiety, state anxiety, and perceptions of anxiety: Interrelationships in practice and competition. *Journal of Swimming Research, 9,* 19–24.

Ogilvie, B. (1979). The sport psychologist and his professional credibility. In P. Klavora & J. Daniel (Eds.), *Coach, athlete, and the sport psychologist* (pp. 44–55). Champaign IL: Human Kinetics Press.

Oishi, K., Kasai, T., & Maeshima, T. (2000). Autonomic response specificity during motor imagery. *Journal of Physiological and Anthropological Applied Human Science, 19*(6), 255–261.

Page, S., Sime, W. E., & Nordell, K. (1999). The effects of imagery on female college swimmers' perceptions of anxiety. *The Sports Psychologist, 13*(2), 458–469.

Petruzzello, S. J., Landers, D. M., & Salazar, W. (1991). Biofeedback and sport/exercise performance: Applications and limitations. *Behavior Therapy, 22,* 379–392.

Prapavessis, H. (2000). The POMS and sports performance: A review. *Journal of Applied Sports Psychology, 12,* 34–48.

Prapavessis, H., Grove, R., McNair, P., & Cable, N. (1992). Self-regulation training, state anxiety, and sport performance: A psychological case study. *The Sport Psychologist, 6*(3), 213–229.

Radeke, T., & Stein, G. (1994). Felt arousal, thoughts/feelings, and ski performance. *Sports Psychologist, 8,* 360–375.

Randle, S., & Weinberg, R. (1997). Multidimensional anxiety and performance: An exploratory examination of the zone of optimal functioning hypothesis. *The Sports Psychologist, 11,* 160–174.

Ravizza, K., & Hanson, T. (1995). *Heads up baseball: Playing the game one pitch at a time.* Indianapolis IN: Masters Press.

Rodgers, W., Hall, C., & Buckolz, E. (1991). Effect of an imagery training programming on imagery ability, imagery use, and figure skating performance. *Journal of Applied Sports Psychology, 3,* 109–125.

Salmon, J., Hall, C., & Haslam, I. (1994). The use of imagery by soccer players. *Journal of Applied Sports Psychology, 6,* 116–133.

Schmidt, A., & Peper, E. (1992). Training strategies for concentration. In J. Williams (Ed.), *Applied sport psychology: Personal growth to peak performance.* Mountain View, CA: Mayfield.

Silva, J., & Stevens, D. (Eds.). (2002). *Psychological foundations of sport.* Boston, MA: Allyn & Bacon.

Sime, W. E. (1985). Physiological perception: The key to peak performance in athletic competition. In J. Sandweiss & S. Wolf (Eds.), *Biofeedback and Sport Science* (pp. 33–62). New York: Plenum.

Sime, W. E. (1997, October). *Psychological issues in sport involving litigation: Case study.* Paper presented at the meeting of the American Association for Applied Sport Psychology, San Diego, CA.

Sime, W. E. (1998). Injury and career termination issues. In M. A. Thompson, R. A. Vernacchia, & W. E. Moore (Eds.), *Case studies in applied sport psychology: An educational approach.* Dubuque, IA: Kendal/Hunt.

Sime, W. E. (2000, October). *The use of biofeedback and neurofeedback in applied psychophysiology to obtain objective assessment of progress in reducing stress and tension in performance and increasing attentional focus*. Paper presented at the meeting of the American Association for Applied Sport Psychology, Nashville, TN.

Sime, W. E., Allen, T., & Fazzano, C. (2001). Optimal functioning in sport psychology: Helping athletes find their zone of excellence. *Biofeedback*, 28(5), 23–25.

Simons, J. (1998). Concentration and attention in sport. In M. A. Thompson, R. A. Vernacchia, & W. E. Moore (Eds.), *Case studies in applied sport psychology: An educational approach*. Dubuque, IA: Kendal/Hunt.

Solberg, E., Berglund, K., Engen, O., Ekeber, O., & Loeb, M. (1996). The effect of meditation on shooting performance. *British Journal of Sports Medicine*, 30, 1–5.

Spalding, T., Jeffers, L., Torges, S., & Hatfield, B. (2000). Vagal and cardiac reactivity to psychological stressors in trained and untrained men. *Medicine and Science in Sports and Exercise*, 32(3), 581–591.

Strano, S., Lino, S., Calcagnini, G., DiVirgilio, V., Ciardo, R., Cerutti, S., Calcagnini, G., & Caselli, G. (1998). Respiratory sinus arrhythmia and cardiovascular neuroregulation in athletes. *Medicine and Science in Sports and Exercise*, 30(2), 215–219.

Stroebel, C. (1982). *The quieting reflex*. New York: Putnam.

Suedfeld, P., Collier, D., & Hartnet, B. (1993). Enhancing perceptual-motor accuracy through flotation REST. *The Sport Psychologist*, 7(2), 151–159.

Suinn, R. (1980). Body thinking: Psychology of Olympic champs. In R. Suinn (Ed.), *Psychology in sports: Methods and applications*. Minneapolis, MN: Burgess Press.

Summers, J. J., Miller, K., & Ford, S. (1991). Attentional style and basketball performance. *Journal of Sport and Exercise Psychology*, 8, 239–253.

Swanik, C., Lephart, S., Giraldo, J., DeMont, R., & Fu, F. (1999). Reactive muscle firing of anterior cruciate ligament-injured females during functional activities. *Journal of Athletic Training*, 34(2), 121–129.

Tellegen, A., & Atkinson, G. (1974). Openness to absorbing and self-altering experiences ("absorption"), a trait related to hypnotic susceptibility. *Journal of Abnormal Psychology*, 83, 268–277.

Tharp, G., & Barnes, M. (1989). Reduction of immunoglobin-A by training. *Medicine and Science in Sports and Exercise*, 21, S109.

Thompson, M. A., Vernacchia R. A., & Moore, W. E. (Eds.). (1998). *Case studies in applied sport psychology: An educational approach*. Dubuque, IA: Kendal/Hunt.

Tremayne, P., & Barry, R. (2001). Elite pistol shooters: Physiological patterning of best versus worst shots. *International Journal of Psychophysiology*, 44(1), 19–29.

Unestahl, L. E. (1986). The ideal performance. In L.E. Unestahl (Ed.), *Sport psychology in theory and practice*. Orebro, Sweden: Veje.

Vallerand, R., & Blanchard, C. (2000). The study of emotions in sport and exercise: Historical, definitional and conceptual perspectives. In Y. Hanin (Ed.), *Emotions in sport*. Champaign, IL: Human Kinetics Press.

Vaschillo, E. G., Visochin, U. V., & Rishe, N. (1999). *RSA biofeedback as effective relaxation method*. Unpublished correspondence from the Pyotr Lesgaft Academy of Culture (Russia) and Rutgers Medical School, New Brunswick, NJ.

Vealey, R. S., Armstrong, L., Comar, W., & Greenleaf, C. A. (1998). Influence on perceived coaching behaviors on burnout and competitive anxiety in female college athletes. *Journal of Applied Sports Psychology*, 10, 297–318.

Weinberg, R. (1994). Goal setting and performance in sport and exercise settings: A synthesis and critique. *Medicine and Science in Sports and Exercise*. 26(4), 469–477.

White, A., & Hardy, L. (1998). An in-depth analysis of the uses of imagery by high-level slalom canoeists and artistic gymnasts. *The Sports Psychologist*, 12, 387–403.

Williams, J. N., Tonymon, P., & Andersen, M. B. (1991). The effectual stressors and coping resources on anxiety and peripheral narrowing. *Journal of Applied Sports Psychology*, 3, 126–141.

Williams, T., Krahebuhl, G., & Morgan, D. (1991). Mood state and running economy in moderately trained male runners. *Medicine and Science in Sports and Exercise*, 23(6), 727–731.

Wilson, V., & Bird, E. (1981). Effects of relaxation and/or biofeedback training upon flexion in gymnasts. *Biofeedback and Self-Regulation*, 6(1), 25–34.

PART VIII

Elimination Disorders

Urinary Incontinence
Evaluation and Biofeedback Treatment

JEANNETTE TRIES
EUGENE EISMAN

At least 13 million U.S. adults living in the community, and more than 50% of all residents in nursing facilities, suffer from urinary incontinence (UI) (Agency for Health Care Policy and Research, 1996). The direct medical costs of caring for incontinent people in the community are more than $15 billion annually, plus $35.2 billion for nursing home residents. Indirect costs (which include costs for protective garments, loss of income, and/or costs for caring for an incontinent person in the home are difficult to estimate. Moreover, the embarrassment, depression and social isolation associated with UI probably, contribute to hidden costs related to the abandonment of exercise and other activities that maintain health and well-being (Nygaard, DeLancy, Amsdorf, & Murphy, 1990).

Despite its prevalence and implications, UI is underreported, and often health care providers do not treat it comprehensively (Agency for Health Care Policy and Research, 1996). This is unfortunate, given estimates that available treatments can cure or significantly improve most forms of UI. There is a consensus that in most cases, behavioral treatments, including biofeedback, should be used before invasive treatments such as surgery. This chapter reviews essential issues and procedures related to using biofeedback for UI. (As in other chapters, italics on first use of a term indicate that the term is included in the glossary at the end of the chapter.)

ANATOMY AND PHYSIOLOGY OF MICTURITION AND URINE STORAGE

Behavioral treatments for UI aim to alter complex bladder control mechanisms that coordinate smooth and striated muscle activity. This section contains a condensed summary and not a comprehensive review of the anatomical and physiological concepts that need to be understood by therapists who use behavioral treatments for UI. We refer readers to the references and texts for further study of bladder anatomy and physiology before application of biofeedback techniques for UI (Mundy, Stephenson, & Wein, 1984; Hald & Bradley, 1982; Grey, 2000; Krane & Siroky, 1991; Torrens & Morrison, 1987; Ostergard & Bent, 1991; Wein & Barrett, 1988).

The lower urinary tract includes the distal sections of the ureters and their *ureterovesical* junction at the base of the bladder. The body of the bladder is composed of smooth muscle referred to as the *detrusor muscle*, which forms the bladder wall and is highly compliant. The detrusor provides the propulsive force that expels urine through the urethra. The prostate in the male, and the smooth and striated muscle of the urethra, are also part of the lower urinary system. Finally, the pelvic floor muscles (PFMs) connect to and support the bladder neck, the vagina (in women), and the anal canal, and have a significant influence on bladder control.

A complex set of learned and reflexive control mechanisms mediates the functions of urine storage and *micturition*. Children develop voluntary control of bladder function from ages 2 to 4. More precise regulation continues for several more years. Before that time, bladder storage and micturition are reflexively organized within the brainstem and peripheral levels. With maturation and social conditioning, the detrusor reflex becomes inhibited by cortical control that is coordinated at several levels of the nervous system, extending from the frontal lobe and sensorimotor cortex to the peripheral nervous system (Hald & Bradley, 1982). This process develops bladder compliance to larger volumes, with bladder capacity doubling between the ages of 2 and 4 years (Hald & Bradley, 1982). However, the mechanism by which this process occurs is not well understood.

Thus normal bladder function depends upon the integrative functions of the frontal lobes, the sensorimotor cortex, the thalamus, the hypothalamus, the basal ganglia, the cerebellum, specific centers in the brainstem, the spinal cord, nerve roots, and the peripheral nerves. Damage at any of these levels may lead to bladder dysfunction that is characteristic of the level of the lesion (Torrens & Morrison, 1987).

The processes of storage and micturition also involve intact efferent and *afferent activity* from the sympathetic and parasympathetic branches of the autonomic nervous system. Parasympathetic nerves coming from sacral roots 2–4 innervate the detrusor muscle. Somatic nerves from sacral levels 2, 3, and 4 innervate the striated *periurethral* and *levator ani muscles*, primarily through the *pudendal nerve*. The smooth muscle of the detrusor and the proximal portion of the urethra also receive innervation from T10–L1 segments of the sympathetic nervous system.

The Process of Micturition and Storage

Afferent signals, or sensory signals from the somatic and autonomic nerves, carry information on bladder volume to the spinal cord. This sensory feedback modulates the motor, or efferent, output to the bladder and urethra. As bladder filling continues, increased sympathetic activity closes the bladder neck and suppresses detrusor contraction at the dome of the bladder and at the parasympathetic ganglia to the detrusor. Also, somatic innervation maintains static muscle tone in the striated PFMs and periurethral muscles, producing *positive urethral pressure*. Pudendal nerve activity at the striated sphincter also inhibits bladder contraction through sacral reflexes and suprasacral control loops (Wein & Barrett, 1988; Bhatia, 1991; McGuire, 1983).

Prior to urination, there is a precipitous drop in sympathetic and somatic activity at the bladder neck and urethra, which decreases *proximal urethral resistance*. Then increased parasympathetic activity stimulates detrusor contraction. The brainstem and cortical centers coordinate these peripheral processes. With learning, cerebral and cerebellar influences develop to become the predominant inhibitory control over bladder activity.

As phases of a dynamic process, storage and micturition depend upon the coordination of several neurophysiological mechanisms. Normally, as the bladder fills, the resting pressure in the bladder remains stable, and the compliant detrusor muscle accommodates to the increased volume. In a normal adult, the first urge to void occurs between 250 and 350 milliliters. However, bladder capacity can increase easily to 400–600 milliliters. As micturition begins, bladder pressure increases because the detrusor contracts as a result of uninhibited parasympathetic activity (Hald & Bradley, 1982). Thus an indicator of dysfunction is *decreased bladder compliance* to larger filling volumes. For example, one abnormal pattern occurs when one feels the first urge to void at a low volume, quickly followed by an uninhibited bladder contraction causing incontinence.

Voluntary bladder control requires the relay of signals of increasing bladder volumes to the spinal cord and then to the cortex. From the cortex, bladder activity can be inhibited through pudendal nerve efferent excitation of the striated PFMs and the sympathetically controlled smooth muscle of the proximal urethra, which increases urethral resistance. Also, pudendal afferent activity inhibits the bladder through sacral and suprasacral reflexes. The cortex inhibits the bladder contraction as well. This occurs at the brainstem and pelvic ganglia of the parasympathetic fibers to the detrusor. Because one can control the "involuntary" bladder muscle through the voluntary nervous system, there is in place a distinct mechanism for the "reeducation" of disordered bladder function via operant learning procedures.

Once there are appropriate conditions for voiding, the voluntary PFMs and muscles of the urethra relax abruptly and completely. This signals the detrusor to contract and empty without urethral resistance. During voiding, bladder pressure increases until it exceeds urethral resistance, at which point urine is expelled. As the external urethral sphincter relaxes and the detrusor develops a sustained contraction, the most proximal portion of the sphincter "funnels."

A dysfunctional voiding pattern can contribute to various bladder disorders. For example, if urethral resistance does not decrease during micturition, detrusor contractile force or intra-abdominal pressure must increase to produce a urine flow. This voiding dysfunction can lead to bladder instability, urinary retention, ureter reflux, and UI.

UI will occur when bladder pressure exceeds maximum urethral pressure. A *negative urethral pressure* can result from either of two physiological events or a combination. One is increased bladder pressure. The other is decreased urethral pressure after relaxation of smooth and/or striated urethral muscles (Hald & Bradley, 1982). Increased bladder pressure can result from uninhibited detrusor contractions or from increased intra-abdominal pressure caused by a *Valsalva maneuver* or abdominal muscle contraction. Pressure from contracted abdominal muscles or descent of the diaphragm transmits pressure to the bladder.

Hald and Bradley (1982) outlined components that interact to maintain normal bladder function. These divisions helped us understand the pathophysiology of the various forms of incontinence as we began our work in UI.

The Bladder Factor

To maintain continence during filling, *intravesical pressure* (bladder pressure) must remain low compared to *intraurethral pressure*. During the storage phase, normal bladder compliance assures a positive pressure gradient at the urethra. Low intravesical pressure during the storage phase is disrupted:

- When the bladder becomes stiff and noncompliant due to *fibrosis*.
- When the bladder wall becomes *edematous*.
- With cancerous infiltration of bladder tissue.
- With overactivity of the detrusor muscle.
- When detrusor contractility is diminished, which allows the bladder to overdistend.

When there is a sensory deficit, the bladder may become chronically overdistended because it is allowed to fill to its physiological limit. Continued *diuresis* or increased intra-abdominal pressure then increases bladder pressure to a level that exceeds urethral pressure. The result is overflow leakage.

The Bladder Neck Factor

At the base of the bladder is an area termed the *trigone*, which is formed by the two uretervesical junctions and the bladder neck. This area takes the shape of a flat plate during storage, but forms a funnel during voiding. During storage, the bladder neck maintains its plate shape by two factors. First, when it is in its normal anatomical position, the bladder neck is located just posterior to the lower third of the pubic bone (Tanagho, 1991). Second, there is sufficient sympathetic input to the smooth muscle of the proximal urethra. The integrity of the base plate during storage provides a barrier to urine loss when pressure is transmitted to the bladder and the bladder neck. Such pressure transmission occurs with activities that increase intra-abdominal pressure, such as coughing, sneezing, or lifting.

DeLancy (1988, 1989b, 1990) suggests that the levator ani muscle lateral to the bladder neck is the essential component that supports the bladder neck. The levator ani increases urethral pressure to maintain continence during times when intra-abdominal pressure is increased, such as with coughing or sneezing. When the bladder neck has sufficient support, any increase in intra-abdominal pressure is transmitted directly to the bladder neck. Pressure transmission to the bladder neck mechanically closes it. The normal transmission of intra-abdominal pressure to the bladder neck maintains continence because it increases urethral pressure, which offsets the rise in bladder pressure associated with greater intra-abdominal pressure.

In summary, the bladder neck factor that maintains continence depends on three components to remain closed. It depends on the pliancy of the urethra, which provides a sealant-like closure. It also depends on the proper anatomical placement of the bladder neck, and on sufficient support and contraction of the levator ani muscle.

The *suspension factor* contributes to normal anatomical placement of the bladder and the bladder neck behind the pubis. The *pubourethral ligaments* suspend the bladder neck. These ligaments arise from the vagina and periurethral tissue lateral to the pelvic wall and are attached to the posterior pubic rami (DeLancy, 1989a). These ligaments support the bladder neck within the abdominal high-pressure zone. This is the position where increases in intra-abdominal pressure are sent to the bladder neck to close the urethra. However, contraction and resting tone of the PFMs provide the first level of support at the bladder neck. This is the *levator factor*, discussed next.

Because the suspension factor influences the bladder neck's position and angulation (DeLancy, 1989a), any weakness in the muscle and ligamentous support can displace the bladder neck. The displacement allows the base plate to funnel during the storage phase. When funneling occurs, a rise in intra-abdominal pressure will cause a decrease rather than an increase in urethral resistance. This increases the likelihood of UI.

The Levator Factor

The levator factor refers to *slow-twitch muscle fibers*—striated muscle fibers that maintain static muscle tone and give support to the pelvic structures (Gosling, Dixon, Critchley, & Thompson, 1981; Critchley, Dixon, & Gosling, 1980; Koelbl, Strassegger, Riss, & Gruber, 1989). In contrast, *fast-twitch muscle fibers* comprise about 20–30% of the PFMs. They provide an additional, active continence mechanism during situations of elevated intra-abdominal pressure. Muscle fiber type in relationship to specific training procedures is discussed later in this chapter.

The Smooth Muscle Factor

Smooth muscle, innervated by *adrenergic sympathetic neurons*, comprises the innermost layer of the proximal urethra. Estrogen receptors are also located in the muscle and the epithelium of the urethra. Normal urethral function depends upon the integrity of this smooth muscle factor. A clinical example of how this factor can be disturbed is found in women who note an onset of stress urinary incontinence when they started taking hypertensive medications such as adrenergic antagonists (Wall & Addison, 1990; Dwyer & Teele, 1992).

The Striated Muscle Factor

The "striated muscle factor" refers to voluntary PFM fibers in the distal one-third of the urethra and periurethral area, and includes the striated levator ani complex (DeLancy, 1989b). The fibers of the urethral sphincter are predominantly slow-twitch fibers that maintain constant tone but still have the ability to contract with greater force when needed (DeLancy, 1991). It is known that muscle activity as measured by electromyography (EMG) normally increases in the distal urethra in proportion to increased bladder volumes.

The Connective Tissue Factor and Vascular and Epithelial Factor

Collagen and *elastin* within urethral tissue provide a "connective tissue factor" that assists with urethral closure. The term "vascular and epithelial factor" implies that the urethra is a contractile tube that must be soft and compliant to close off the *lumen*. The importance of this factor is obvious in some postmenopausal women. With the loss of estrogen, there often develops atrophy of the epithelium, which is associated with vaginitis and irritability of urethral tissue. This irritability contributes to bladder symptoms such as urgency and incontinence. Moreover, all of the discussed peripheral factors are interdependent with the "central nervous system factor" that coordinates their function.

TYPES OF UI

The names of different types of UI refer to the presenting symptoms associated with each type. However, the categories are not discrete. Symptoms and etiologies often overlap within the same individual. Knowledge of the anatomy and physiology of bladder control is essential in understanding the distinctions among the various types of UI.

Stress Urinary Incontinence

Stress urinary incontinence occurs when intra-abdominal pressure exceeds urethral pressure, as with coughing or sneezing, in the absence of a detrusor contraction. The striated PFMs normally support the bladder neck and exert a closing force on the urethra during conditions of heightened intra-abdominal pressure. PFM weakness or laxity can contribute to stress incontinence. Stress incontinence is more prevalent in women as a result of pelvic floor partial *denervation* injury that occurs during childbirth (Allen, Hosker, Smith, & Warrell, 1990). Stress incontinence is also seen after *prostatectomy*, due to the disruption of the urethral sphincter or its nerve supply.

Urge Incontinence

Urge incontinence is associated with a precipitous, intense, and urgent need to urinate that cannot be inhibited. Associated symptoms include urinary frequency and low-volume urination. Urge incontinence can result from detrusor *hyperreflexia*, a neurogenic condition marked by uninhibited bladder contractions. In contrast, the term *detrusor instability* (also known as *unstable bladder*) denotes a condition where uninhibited bladder contractions occur without a neurogenic etiology.

Urge incontinence can occur without demonstrable detrusor instability. This condition is termed sensory urge incontinence. The causes of both unstable bladder and *sensory urge incontinence* are not well understood. One predisposing factor for the development of unstable bladder is the pattern of voiding against urethral obstruction. This occurs when an enlarged prostate obstructs the urethra or when the urethral sphincter fails to relax during voiding. Voiding against urethral resistance can contribute to detrusor muscle irritability and can lead to bladder wall thickening, called *trabeculation*. As these changes occur, bladder compliance decreases as the threshold for bladder contraction is lowered.

Another form of incontinence that is often seen in elderly persons is *detrusor hyperactivity with impaired bladder contractility*. Patients with this condition show symptoms of stress incontinence and will have urgency and frequency. However, they may strain to empty their bladders and may have elevated postvoid residual volumes characteristic of overflow incontinence (Resnick & Yalla, 1985).

Some patients will have symptoms of both stress and urge incontinence. This condition is called *mixed incontinence*. Normally, PFM afferent activity inhibits the bladder. When the PFMs are weak, there is a decrease in PFM inhibition of the bladder; as a result, urge symptoms may develop. In addition to the effect of diminished PFM inhibition of the detrusor, stress incontinence may contribute to sensory urgency when people develop a frequent voiding habit to avoid incontinence. Over time and the possible effect of classical conditioning, bladder volumes remain at low levels. This strategy may have the effect of lowering sensory thresholds for urge to void.

Overflow Incontinence

Overflow incontinence occurs when the bladder does not empty efficiently. The bladder becomes overly distended and incontinence occurs when, as a result of ongoing diuresis, bladder pressure exceeds urethral pressure. Overflow incontinence can develop in any condition that limits bladder emptying. This includes urethral obstruction caused by *prostatic hyperplasia*, when bladder sensation is impaired, or when bladder contractility is decreased (e.g., bladder denervation resulting from diabetic neuropathy).

Reflex Incontinence

"Reflex incontinence" occurs when normal neurological control of the bladder is disrupted as a result of trauma or disease (e.g., stroke, spinal cord injury, multiple sclerosis, Parkinson's disease, or dementia). Due to disruption in neural controls, which are primarily inhibitory, incontinence occurs when the bladder fills to its physiological limit.

BIOFEEDBACK AS A TREATMENT FOR UI

The use of biofeedback as a treatment for UI started with Kegel (1948, 1951), who observed that if the PFMs were *hypotonic*, *bladder suspension surgery* for stress incontinence was less effective. To improve contraction of the *pubococcygeus* portion of the levator ani muscle, Kegel (1948) invented the pressure perineometer. From within the vagina, his perimeometer measured the contractile force of surrounding muscle and displayed the associated pressure changes on a pressure gauge. In uncontrolled clinical observations of many women, Kegel (1951) reported significant improvements in continence. Over the years, unfortunately, clinicians have taught Kegel, or PFM, exercises without the use of his biofeedback device.

RESEARCH ON BIOFEEDBACK FOR UI

Three different biofeedback methods used over the past 25 years for UI have reinforced (1) bladder inhibition; (2) PFM recruitment; or (3) stable intra-abdominal and bladder pressures during PFM recruitment.

An early study (Cardozo, Abrams, Stanton, & Feneley, 1978; Cardozo, Stanton, Hafner, & Allan, 1978) used cystometric biofeedback to reinforce bladder inhibition in 27 female subjects with detrusor instability and urge incontinence over four to eight sessions. The authors reported a 40% subjective cure, with 44% of those reporting being cured found to have objective reduction in detrusor instability when measured by a posttreatment *cystometrogram* (CMG). Another 40% of the subjects reported subjective improvement, confirmed in 14% with the objective criteria.

Unfortunately, only 4 of 11 subjects (36%) maintained the subjective improvement rate at a 5-year follow-up (Cardozo & Stanton, 1985). This early study showed that with feedback, people could learn to inhibit detrusor activity, at least during and shortly after treatment. The relapse of symptoms may have resulted from the treatment's inattention to PFM recruitment that normally inhibits the bladder. It is possible that the initial improvement observed in these patients occurred because PFM control was inadvertently reinforced, which indirectly caused bladder inhibition. However, because PFM control had not been well established with direct reinforcement, it was extinguished over time.

In contrast to detrusor biofeedback, most studies have used EMG biofeedback or pressure measures to reinforce PFM contraction (Baigis-Smith, Smith, Rose, & Newman, 1989; Burns, Marecki, Dittmar, & Bullough, 1985; Burns, Pranikoff, Nochajski, Desotelle, & Harwood, 1990; Castleden & Duffin, 1981; Fisher, 1983; Henderson & Taylor, 1987; Susset, Galea, & Read, 1990; Rose, Baigis-Smith, Smith, & Newman, 1990; Van Kampen et al., 2000). There is broad variability in the methodology used in these studies. Most protocols make little effort to isolate the effect of the biofeedback from *bladder training* strategies and home PFM exercises. These are behavioral manipulations commonly used with biofeedback. Furthermore, most studies report treatment results in terms of reduced incontinent episodes, but do not report changes in PFM function. Due to these flaws, a recent review has concluded that PFM exercises appear to be useful in the treatment of urinary incontinence, but that biofeedback has not been shown to offer any specific benefit over PFM exercises alone (Hay-Smith et al., 2001). However, the reviewers refer to the considerable limitations in available evidence, which make comparisons across studies difficult if not impossible. Various research designs and problems are discussed below.

There are limitations with biofeedback protocols that do not control for changes in intra-abdominal pressure during PFM contraction. Increases in intra-abdominal pressure and abdominal EMG can be transmitted to PFM recordings and cause measurement artifact. Moreover, co-contraction from extraneous muscle during a PFM contraction may facilitate a stronger PFM contraction through neural processes. However, the associated increase in intra-abdominal pressure compromises continence mechanisms when the PFM are weak, because with an increase in intra-abdominal pressure, bladder pressure increases as well. Because there has been no effort to research the effect of abdominal co-contraction during PFM contraction, we have a limited understanding of how different biofeedback protocols actually change the underlying physiology and function (Tries, 1990a).

For example, Burns et al. (1990) found that biofeedback did not offer benefit above PFM exercises alone. Burns et al. (1990) compared biofeedback treatment to PFM exercises without biofeedback in 135 women. One group received verbal instructions in PFM exercises. The other group received EMG biofeedback from PFM muscle contractions only. All subjects were seen in the clinic for 20 minutes per week. There was no control for abdominal co-contraction during PFM exercise. Both treatments were compared to a control group receiving no treatment. Both treatment groups demonstrated a 54–61% reduction in incontinence, compared to a 9% reduction in the control group. There was no difference between the treatment groups. Although this study showed that PFM exercises could reduce incontinence, the biofeedback protocol lacked specificity, because abdominal co-contraction was not controlled for. Under these conditions, the biofeedback offered little benefit beyond PFM exercises alone.

In contrast, a series of studies used manometric measures of rectal and external anal sphincter pressure, and CMG measures of bladder pressure, to reinforce stability in detrusor and intra-abdominal pressures at the same time that PFM contraction was reinforced (Burgio, Whitehead, & Engel, 1985; Burgio, Robinson, & Engel, 1986; Burgio, Stutzman, & Engel, 1989b; Middaugh, Whitehead, Burgio, & Engel, 1989; Burton, Pearce, Burgio, Engel, & Whitehead, 1988). This protocol simultaneously reinforced selective PFM contraction that was isolated from abdominal contraction, and demonstrated to the patient the relationship of PFM contraction on bladder inhibition. The manometric feedback protocol has been modified by some workers (Tries, 1990a) to use surface abdominal EMG as a correlate measure of intra-abdominal pressure while intravaginal and/or external anal sphincter EMG electrodes record PFM activity.

Using manometric biofeedback, Burgio et al. (1985) reported a reduction in incontinent episodes that ranged from 81.7% to 95% in 43 male and female subjects with stress incontinence, detrusor instability, and sensory urge incontinence. A mean 3.6 treatment sessions were provided over 6–12 weeks. At a 6-month follow-up, subjects reported that they had either maintained or improved their bladder function from that reported just after treatment.

In 23 women with stress and urge incontinence, Burgio et al. (1986) compared the effects of bladder and PFM exercises with manometric biofeedback. In the group who did not receive biofeedback, the therapist placed one finger in a subject's vagina and the other hand on the subject's abdomen. The therapist provided verbal feedback as to the accuracy and intensity of the PFM contractions, and cued each subject to limit abdominal co-contraction during the PFM contraction. The biofeedback group attained a reduction in incontinent episodes of 75.9%, compared to 51% in the verbal feedback group. At a 6-month follow-up, both groups showed a slight but nonsignificant relapse in symptoms. Burgio et al. (1986) concluded that the biofeedback group showed a superior result because of the immediacy and accuracy of the instrument feedback compared to the verbal feedback.

However, Burton et al. (1988) did not show that manometric biofeedback was superior to verbal feedback for PFM contraction when combined with bladder training in 23 women with urge incontinence. Both groups showed a cure rate of 30% and a reduction in incontinent episodes of 79–82%. Improvements were maintained at 1- and 6-month follow-ups. The researchers concluded that the groups responded equally to the different treatments because the subjects had primarily urge incontinence, which was felt to be modifiable with behavioral therapy and is less reliant on precise physiological changes. The authors also suggested that the superior skill and knowledge of the therapist, who treated subjects in both groups, strongly influenced their outcomes.

In an A-B design, Burgio et al. (1989) compared the effects of timed voiding to biofeedback combined with PFM exercise in 25 patients after prostatectomy, who were grouped on the basis of symptom characteristics. Subjects with stress incontinence reduced their incontinence by 28.8% with timed voiding alone and by 78.3% from the pretreatment baseline after biofeedback. Subjects with urge incontinence showed an increase in incontinence with timed voiding alone, but after receiving biofeedback showed a 80.7% reduction in urge incontinent episodes. A third group with continual urinary leakage reported no change with timed voiding and only a 17% reduction in incontinence after biofeedback treatment. Fourteen of the 25 patients were followed at 6–12 months posttreatment. Twelve (85%) subjects maintained or improved their continence from posttreatment levels. The study concluded that patients who are incontinent after prostatectomy but do not have continual leaking are good candidates for biofeedback training.

Burgio et al. (1989b) found that subjects with continual postprostatectomy leakage developed excellent control of the external anal sphincter with biofeedback and could consciously stop the flow of urine. However, they were unable to maintain control when they did not focus attention on sphincter contraction. Although the Burgio et al. (1989b) protocol reinforced selective PFM contraction without abdominal co-contraction, the protocol did not specifically reinforce the contraction of the deeper levator ani muscle, which supports the bladder neck to provide passive occlusive resistance to urine loss. It is this area that is most likely to be damaged after prostatectomy. Our own unpublished clinical observations indicate that men with continual leakage after prostatectomies can reduce urine loss by at least 50% when provided specific reinforcement for levator ani contraction via a multiple electrode probe (MEP; see below).

O'Donnell and Doyle (1991) obtained significant reductions in incontinence in 20 elderly inpatient men over age 65 receiving biofeedback, compared to a no-treatment control group of 28 men. Surface electrodes were placed at the external anal sphincter and on the abdominal muscles to reinforce selective PFM contraction. During treatment, sterile water was infused into the bladder until subjects reported a sensation of needing to void. The subjects were then reinforced to use the selective PFM contractions to inhibit bladder urgency. Treatment totaled 20 sessions over 5 weeks.

In the most important study to date, Burgio et al. (1998) compared drug therapy, an attention control, and behavioral treatment that included manometric biofeedback in a randomized placebo-controlled trial with elderly women who had urge incontinence. Subjects attended four biweekly sessions. Incontinent episodes were reduced by 80.7% in the behavioral/biofeedback group, 68% in the drug therapy group, and 39% in the attention control group. All group differences were significant. In the behavioral/biofeedback group, 73.8% of the subjects needed only a single biofeedback session to demonstrate the ability to selectively contract the PFM without increasing intra-abdominal pressure. No subject needed more than two biofeedback treatments, although all subjects attended four behavioral sessions. Subjects in the behavioral/biofeedback group practiced daily PFM exercises and were instructed in bladder inhibition strategies. Thus substantial reductions in UI were obtained in only a few biofeedback sessions when PFM contraction was contingent upon maintaining stable intra-abdominal pressure.

Several uncontrolled reports suggest that biofeedback is effective in reducing UI in neurological patients (Middaugh et al., 1989; Tries, 1990a, 1990b). These reports have aimed to improve PFM coordination in addition to simply reinforcing PFM contraction. Accordingly, subjects were reinforced to contract the PFMs immediately upon perceiving urgency. Neurological injury disrupts the normal coordination between the smooth bladder muscle and the striated sphincter during voiding, causing a condition called *detrusor–sphincter dyssynergia*. Detrusor–sphincter dyssynergia is associated with the failure of the striated sphincter to relax during voiding, often leading to incomplete bladder emptying and an elevated postvoid residual volume. Detrusor–sphincter dyssynergia can contribute to urinary tract infection and disruptions in bladder, ureters, and kidney function. To decrease detrusor–sphincter dyssynergia, Middaugh et al. (1989) and Tries (1990a, 1990b) reinforce PFM relaxation, at rest and during micturition. (See Tries & Eisman, Chapter 28, this volume, for further discussion of dyssynergia.)

In summary, the literature suggests that UI can be reduced via a treatment package that incorporates biofeedback, patient education, daily PFM exercises, and behavioral strategies that inhibit urgency. However, the mechanism for improvement has yet to be specified. Since multiple anatomical and neurological processes mediate bladder control, single-channel measurement protocols may not provide sufficient physiological information needed to optimally alter PFM and bladder function. One exception may be genuine stress incontinence. However, even for stress incontinence, Burgio et al. (1986) showed the added benefit of multi-channel biofeedback when used with Kegel exercises.

The next sections describe instrumentation and outline the essential components of a biofeedback treatment package for UI. The recommendations have evolved from personal observations of what has worked well in our clinics. Further empirical work will determine which components of treatment are most useful.

INSTRUMENTATION

To treat the various symptoms associated with incontinence, biofeedback protocols and instrumentation must be sufficiently sensitive to measure several physiological functions that contribute to bladder control. Protocols must be adequately flexible to render the physiological recordings in a meaningful form that will optimize learning for any individual patient. Accordingly, the biofeedback instrumentation should include several recording channels that measure and display changes in PFM activity and abdominal muscle activity simultaneously. In our clinics, we use computerized equipment that measures both EMG and pressure. In the past, we also used CMG biofeedback following the protocol of Burgio et al. (1985), which displays changes in bladder pressure during sterile water infusion. More recently, we have abandoned the more invasive CMG procedure except in special cases, and rely on a bladder scan to measure postvoid residual volumes and changes in bladder volumes for the treatment of urge incontinence. In place of the rectal balloon that measures intra-abdominal pressure, abdominal muscle EMG is used, which has been shown to be correlated to changes in intra-abdominal pressure (Workman, Cassisi, & Dougherty, 1992).

However, there are some disadvantages to using abdominal EMG in the place of rectal pressure. First, one may not be able to distinguish a Valsalva maneuver from an actual bladder contraction, because intra-abdominal pressure transmits directly to the bladder. A measure of rectal pressure displays a Valsalva response if present. Second, abdominal EMG measures become very attenuated on obese individuals. For this problem, one should make three adjustments: (1) using a very high-gain setting to amplify the abdominal response; (2) increasing the interelectrode distance; and (3) moving the EMG electrodes more laterally on *the external abdominal oblique muscle*, where there may be less adipose tissue, and training the patient in the *left lateral position* so that the adipose tissue is diverted to the left side of the body. However, these departures from standard placements limit the reliability of measures over sessions.

Figure 26.1 shows various types of EMG recording probes used to measure PFM intravaginally. In our clinics, we use the intravaginal probe that is seen to the far right of Figure 26.1. This probe has several advantages beyond its smaller size. Positioned above the *urogenital diaphragm*, it records EMG activity without dilating the vaginal tissue. Moreover, it can be used to record PFM activity during voiding (Eisman & Tries, 1991).

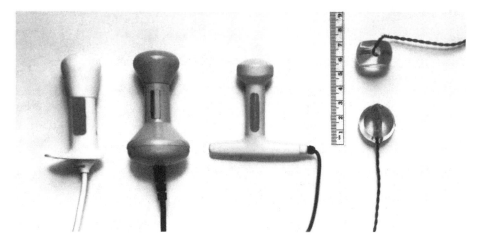

FIGURE 26.1. Various vaginal EMG probes. To the left of the ruler, three vaginal probes are shown, which dilate the vagina and protrude from the introitus. To the right of the ruler, the Eisman–Tries intravaginal probe is seen in two views to show the electrodes fixed on one end of the convex surface, with the electrode wires extending distally when the probe is placed within the vagina. The flattened surfaces of the probe conform to the cross-section of the vagina, so that when it is positioned just above the urogenital diaphragm, the flattened portions of the probe face anteriorly and posteriorly, therefore positioning the electrodes laterally.

Figure 26.2 shows various EMG probes that are used to measure EMG activity from the anal canal. In our clinic, we use the MEP. The MEP measures EMG activity at the subcutaneous or distal portion of the external anal sphincter, and also at the proximal portion of the anal canal. It therefore reflects EMG activity of the deep external anal sphincter and levator ani muscles, separately from the distal anal canal EMG (Eisman & Tries, 1993). The ability to measure EMG from two sites within the anal canal is important, because the two areas have different innervation and functions. Because the MEP is able to identify EMG specific to the levator ani, clinical observations suggest that it is valuable in treatment of stress incontinence not only in women, but also in men after prostatectomy. This observation is consistent with the anatomy. Recall that the levator ani muscle is proximal to the urogenital diaphragm and continuous from the pubis back to the *coccyx*. It functions as a support to the bladder neck, vagina, and anal canal. Therefore, in using the MEP, practitioners can differentially reinforce contraction of the deeper levator ani muscle, which normally provides tonic support to the bladder neck to maintain continence. As such, the MEP may be useful in the treatment of stress incontinence in women who cannot use or do not feel comfortable using a vaginal recording probe (e.g., women who are elderly and frail, women with vaginitis, and young girls/children).

However, in most women, we use both the MEP and a small intravaginal probe shown in Figure 26.1 to obtain simultaneous measures from three different sites within the pelvic floor. Both PFM sensors are used with a measure of abdominal EMG. Thus, in our clinics, we obtain four EMG measures during an assessment of PFM function (see Figure 26.3).

COMPONENTS OF BIOFEEDBACK FOR URINARY INCONTINENCE

Medical Assessment

Before a biofeedback evaluation and treatment begins, a medical assessment and physical examination are required to rule out neurological disorders, abdominal masses, or other

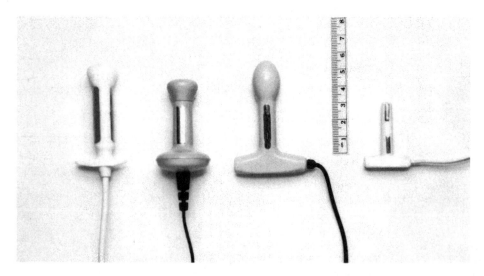

FIGURE 26.2. Various anal canal EMG probes. To the left of the ruler, three anal canal probes are shown, which have a single pair of longitudinally placed electrodes that summate EMG activity from the entire length of the anal canal. The smaller multiple electrode probe (MEP) is shown to the right of the ruler. The MEP measures surface EMG activity from two sites within the anal canal. The two bipolar electrodes adjacent to the T-handle measure subcutaneous external anal sphincter activity at the distal portion of the anal canal, while the proximal pair record activity from the deeper external anal sphincter and puborectalis muscles. The T-handle remains external to the anal verge when the probe is positioned.

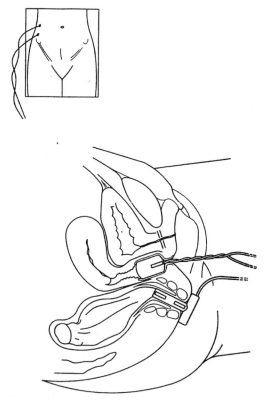

FIGURE 26.3. Schematic of the abdominal probe, Eisman–Tries intravaginal probe, and MEP placement in a sagittal view of the female pelvis.

possible causes of incontinence. A rectal exam is done to assess rectal sensation, sphincter tone, the *bulbocavernosus reflex*, the prostate gland, and the presence of fecal impaction. In women, the skin condition of the perineum is assessed, and genital atrophy, *pelvic prolapse*, and *urethral diverticula* are ruled out. In men, the perineum, the foreskin, and the glans penis are assessed for abnormalities. One also checks for lower-extremity edema. This is because the prone position may lead to fluid reabsorption in persons with increased excretion of urine (diuresis) and excessive urination at night (*nocturia*). The physical exam helps determine whether a patient needs further laboratory tests. A urinalysis is a basic test when there is urinary incontinence. One also must determine whether there are postvoid residual volumes (Agency for Health Care Policy and Research, 1996).

Verbal Interview

In the verbal interview, one gets a complete history of the onset and development of incontinence and associated symptoms. The interviewer seeks to understand the functional relationships of symptoms and obtains estimates of baseline data from which to judge the effectiveness of treatment. The following is a list of areas to cover in the interview.

1. *Situations in which urine is lost.* Is urine lost when there is an increase in intra-abdominal pressure? What are the specific activities that lead to urine loss (e.g., walking, bending, going up stairs, coughing, sneezing)? The volume of urine loss with each activity should be specified. Also, does the patient have any control of the loss of urine once it begins? Do sudden increases in intra-abdominal pressure give rise to sensations of urgency? Does the patient experience continual or intermittent leakage? Is there urine loss without awareness?

2. *Description of sensations of urgency.* What are the antecedents and consequences of urgency? For example, does the patient experience urgency in response to certain stimuli such as running water, cold weather, changing positions, coughing, or approaching the toilet? Can he or she inhibit the urgency, and if so, for how long? Does urgency occur with a full or empty bladder? To what degree is urgency associated with incontinence, and what is the volume of urine lost with each urge-incontinent episode?

3. *Nighttime voiding pattern.* How often does the patient usually void at night? What are nighttime voiding volumes? Does the patient wet the bed? Does the patient leak urine on the way to the toilet?

4. *Daytime voiding pattern.* What is the daytime voiding frequency, and what are typical voiding volumes? Do the patient's behaviors show heightened vigilance to toileting needs (e.g., does the patient void before going out of the home "just in case")?

5. *Fluid intake and urine output.* Does the patient note that drinking certain beverages (e.g., caffeinated and NutraSweet products) increases symptoms? A record of 24-hour output is useful to determine adequate hydration (see Appendix 26.1). If a patient reports output to be less than 1 liter, then input can be increased. If a patient's output is more than 2 liters, then input should be decreased.

6. *Effect of emotional arousal on symptoms.* Does the patient note an increase in symptoms when emotionally aroused?

7. *Symptoms associated with voiding dysfunction.* Does the patient report any voiding hesitancy, interrupted stream, a poor flow rate, postmicturition dribble, incomplete bladder emptying, or an inability to void with perceived bladder fullness?

8. *Reflexive control.* Can the patient quickly stop the flow of urine once it has begun? The absence of this ability does not always indicate pathology. This is because it is unphysiological to stop the flow of urine after it voluntarily starts. However, the ability to stop the urine flow in the presence of other symptoms may indicate dysfunction. For example, the ability to stop the flow without a concomitant ability to reinitiate it may be symptomatic of

nonrelaxing PFMs. Similarly, consider a patient who can readily stop and start urine flow, but who has complaints of postmicturition dribble. This suggests the presence of an uncoordinated or unstable urethral mechanism.

9. *Use of protective garments and devices.* What type of pads does the patient use, and what is the frequency of pad change? Are other supportive devices used, such as a pessary, tampons, a catheter, or a penile clamp?

10. *Bowel habits.* Does the patient have regular bowel movements without a need to strain? What is the normal stool consistency? Is there any complaint of fecal incontinence or staining?

11. *Symptom effects on lifestyle.* Has the patient restricted his or her activities as a result of bladder dysfunction? What are the direct and indirect costs to the patient (e.g., increased laundry and cost of protective padding)?

12. *Other associated symptoms.* What is the frequency of *cystitis* or bladder infection, perineal pain, and perineal skin irritation?

13. *Medical history.* A thorough medical, neurological, obstetric, and genitourinary history includes all prior treatments for bladder and bowel dysfunction.

14. *Current medications.* The practitioner must note whether there was an onset or exacerbation of bladder symptoms associated with taking certain medications. For example, women with already weakened PFMs may develop severe stress incontinence when they take an alpha-antagonist drug for hypertension (Wall & Addison, 1990; Dwyer & Teele, 1992). Conversely, any medication with anticholinergic properties may worsen urinary retention, resulting in overflow incontinence. These medications include over-the-counter agents for colds or insomnia.

15. *The symptom diary or log.* For at least 1 day before the first biofeedback session, patients record all bladder symptoms and 24-hour urine output. One can send this log (see Appendix 26.1) to the patient before the interview. The patient also maintains a log throughout treatment (see Appendix 26.2). However, the patient may not need to measure volumes after the initial evaluation, depending upon the evaluation outcome.

Accurate recording of symptoms is essential for the initial and ongoing assessment. In fact, a therapist must assertively address noncompliance to keeping the diary. If a patient is capable but unwilling to keep it, treatment may not be practical. The diary should include the following: the time of each void, the time and estimated volume of each incontinent episode, the number of pad changes, any noteworthy antecedents to and results of incontinent episodes, and associated symptoms (such as the frequency of voiding dysfunction).

Assessment with Instrumentation

Properly licensed or certified therapists whose state practice acts allows for the assessment of PFMs may conduct the physical assessment. This starts with an exam of the vagina if one uses a vaginal probe for the biofeedback. If one uses a rectal probe, then one examines the anal canal and rectum. This should be done to assure appropriate placement of the recording electrode and to assess whether the instrument measures provide a valid representation of PFM function. The following discussion outlines the EMG and manual PFM assessment that is used for bladder, bowel, and other PFM disorders.

For the vaginal exam, the patient's position is supine with the hips and knees flexed, thighs slightly abducted, and feet flat on the exam table. For the rectal exam, the patient is in the standard side-lying, left lateral position, with knees and hips flexed slightly. The left lateral position is the standard position for rectal exams because the descending colon is on the left. Also, the abdominal electrodes are superior to the table, positioned on the right abdominal muscles to decrease cardiac artifact. A pillow between the patient's knees provides a comfortable resting position that the patient can maintain over a session.

During the digital exam, the practitioner should note the resting tone of the perivaginal or anal canal muscles. With perivaginal palpation, one can assess the pubococcygeus muscle of the levator ani group. In the rectum, one feels the distal external sphincter just inside the anal canal. One palpates the *puborectalis* portion of the levator about 2.5–4.0 centimeters from the *anal verge*. One does this by gently moving the examination finger posteriorly toward the coccyx.

Then the practitioner asks the patient to contract the PFM as if trying to stop the flow of urine or passage of stool. The instruction is to hold the contraction for 10 seconds. With the therapist's other hand on the abdomen, the patient is cued to reduce abdominal activity as much as possible while contracting the PFMs. After the contraction, there is a 10-second rest period. Then the patient is asked to contract for another 10 seconds. The therapist can grade the palpated contraction on a scale of 0–5 after Laycock (1994), with grading as follows: 0, nil; 1, flicker; 2, weak; 3, moderate; 4, good; and 5, strong. The therapist records the grade together with the time in seconds that the highest grade is maintained. For example, a grade/time rating of 3/6 indicates that the patient can maintain a moderate (3) contraction for 6 seconds. One also can extend grading to include the number of repetitions of 10-second sequences and the number of fast contractions the patient can repeat (Laycock, 1994).

After the manual evaluation, the therapist positions the PFM EMG recording probe or probes. With most women seen in our clinics, we use an intravaginal probe and MEP, which are designed for use together. These probes allow for the collection of EMG from three PFM sites (the distal anal canal, the proximal anal canal, and the intravaginal site; see Figure 26.3). If these smaller probes are not used, either a vaginal or an anal probe is used to obtain a single measure of PFM function. A caution is in order: The larger probes displayed in Figures 26.1 and 26.2 are not designed for use as a pair. All PFM recordings are obtained with a bandpass filter that can maximize the muscle signal—for example, 15–80 hertz.

The therapist then places bipolar surface electrodes on the right abdominal oblique muscle, about 4 centimeters apart and 4 centimeters from the midline, with the rostral electrode placed laterally to the umbilicus and the caudal electrode placed perpendicular to the rostral electrode, just above the *anterior superior iliac spine*. The abdominal EMG channel uses a 100-200-hertz bandpass filter to minimize cardiac artifact.

To record EMG from women, an intravaginal probe is positioned first with the patient supine. Then the patient is positioned in the left lateral position with knees and hips flexed during placement of the abdominal electrodes and the MEP anal probe, as well as during the recording procedure. If one of the larger, single-channel anal probes is used, the therapist must first dilate the anal canal with a lubricated index finger as the probe is introduced into the canal with the other hand. Because of its smaller size, insertion of the MEP usually does not require prior dilation of the anal canal except when the external anal sphincter is hypertonic. After insertion, a few minutes should be allowed for the surrounding muscles to adapt before a resting baseline measure is taken. The therapist should examine the EMG baseline recording for elevated resting levels of either the abdominal muscles and/or PFMs. This indicates possible spasm or chronic muscle tension.

Next, the patient should be asked to contract the PFMs as if trying to stop the passage of gas, stool, or urine. The therapist should avoid suggesting that the patient "contract as hard as you can," because this exhortation often results in maladaptive abdominal contraction. The EMG record should be examined for PFM response latency, the signal's amplitude, the stability and endurance of the contraction, and the time it takes for the EMG signal to recover to baseline after the patient is told to relax. Also, the therapist should note the degree to which the abdominal muscles contract during PFM contraction. The patient should contract for 10 seconds several times with at least a 10- to 15-second relaxation period between each contraction. After two to three 10-second PFM contractions, the therapist should note whether the EMG shows a decrease in PFM amplitude and an associated increase in abdominal or gluteal muscle activity. Such changes indicate muscle fatigue. The baseline EMG activity should be observed between contractions, especially any increase in baseline irregularities or EMG "spiking," which could be interpreted as muscle irritability. Then the therapist should ask the patient to gently "evacuate" or "push out" the anal probe, while measuring perianal muscle relaxation and abdominal contraction.

An EMG record of a normal PFM contraction should show the following:

- Relatively low and stable baseline.
- Rapid rise to a maximum contraction.
- Stable contraction for 10 seconds.
- Short latency to return to baseline after stopping the voluntary contraction (see Figure 26.4).

Normally, the PFMs relax precipitously prior to, and during, voiding and defecation. This relaxation response can be assessed in two ways. Using the MEP, we ask a patient to perform two evacuation trials of the anal probe after the contraction trials. We ask the patient to *gently* push out the MEP as if "passing gas" for 10 seconds. After the first evacuation trial, a rest period of about 20 seconds is given, which is followed by a second evacuation trial. Measures are obtained during simulated evacuation trials to determine whether the PFMs as a group show normal muscle response flexibility, seen as relaxation below the resting baseline during the evacuation maneuver.

However, the best way to assess a voiding dysfunction is to record EMG from the PFM while the patient is voiding. Abnormal patterns of abdominal straining, detrusor–sphincter dyssynergia, voiding hesitancy, and interrupted stream can be observed during an EMG-recorded void. The therapist estimates flow rate by timing the void and then dividing volume voided by the time. (See Tries & Eisman, Chapter 28, for further discussion.)

One compares the patient's EMG with normal PFM function. Treatment then proceeds to shape the patient's responses toward a normal model. "Shaping" refers to the gradual

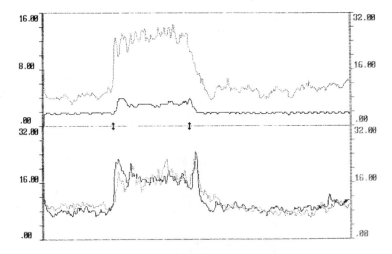

FIGURE 26.4. EMG records over 36 seconds from an asymptomatic nulliparous woman during a voluntary contraction during the time marked by the event markers. The four tracings represent EMG from (1) abdominal muscles (upper dark), (2) intravaginal muscles (upper light), (3) inner anal canal (lower dark), and (4) outer anal canal (lower light).

modification of the patient's responses through positive reinforcement of successive approximations to the ideal response.

Biofeedback Treatment Goals

After identifying functional problems and EMG abnormalities, the therapist should devise a treatment plan with specific short-term and long-term goals. The long-term goals are expected functional outcomes; the short-term goals describe the training components by which the patient will achieve the functional changes. The treatment goals listed below are typically used to document progress in quantifiable terms. However, the lists are inclusive because goals may vary for each patient, depending upon the presenting complaints.

Long-term goals may include the following:

1. Decreasing the frequency of UI episodes.
2. Decreasing urinary urgency.
3. Decreasing voiding frequency to four to eight voids during the day and one during the sleeping hours.
4. Decreasing the number and size of protective garments.
5. Decreasing voiding dysfunction and associated risk for bladder infection and instability.

Short-term goals may be as follows (some of these are discussed further in Tries & Eisman, Chapter 28):

1. Reinforcing PFM contractions toward greater stability, duration, and amplitude, to improve strength and supporting muscle tone.
2. Reinforcing selective PFM contractions without abdominal and gluteal contractions. This decreases competing responses that would increase intra-abdominal pressure, which is associated with incontinence.
3. Improving the PFM coordination by shaping phasic contractions with a short response latency and immediate recovery to baseline after voluntary contraction ceases.
4. Reducing chronically elevated PFM activity associated with pelvic pain, voiding dysfunction, or evacuation disorders.
5. Reducing strain voiding by reinforcing PFM and abdominal muscle relaxation during micturition.
6. Improving *functional bladder capacity* if abnormally small.
7. Improving the PFM coordination activity in response to urgency. When the bladder is full and the patient experiences urgency, PFM contraction that inhibits detrusor activity should be reinforced.
8. Reinforcing inhibition of the maladaptive abdominal contraction with urgency.
9. Improving discrimination of sensory cues that antedate uninhibited bladder contraction and incontinence. This should be done so that the patient learns to activate sphincter activity in a timely manner to inhibit urge and avoid incontinence.
10. Providing a home program to generalize skills learned in the clinic to the home situation.

In summary, the primary treatment goal is to optimize PFM responses that normally mediate bladder control. The patient's diary helps the therapist quantify the degree of dysfunction in terms of the number of incontinent episodes, pads used, voiding frequency, and voided volumes. The diary also documents, for third-party reimbursement, objective changes with treatment. Physiological measures document bladder capacity, endurance of stable PFM contractions, percentage of improvement in amplitude of PFM contraction over baseline, and percentage of reduction in abdominal contraction.

Training Selective PFM Contractions

If the patient complains of urinary urgency, treatment is generally focused on teaching selective PFM without abdominal contraction. With urge, the maladaptive habit of abdominal contraction increases intra-abdominal pressure and encourages urine loss rather than continence. Second, proprioceptive feedback for PFM contraction is a function of the amplitude of the contraction. Thus, when the PFMs are weak, proprioceptive feedback for contraction is diminished. If there is considerable afferent activity from substituting abdominal or gluteal muscle contraction, such activity can easily mask the weaker afferent signals from the PFMs. This "faulty feedback" in turn limits actual PFM recruitment and subsequent strengthening attempts. Moreover, afferent activity from the substituting muscles becomes associated with attempts to stop urine loss. In this way, the ineffective muscle substitution becomes conditioned to sensations of urgency, and the probability for urine loss in such situations is not changed.

Thus, to reestablish bladder control, the patient must learn to inhibit the competing and maladaptive stimulus–response patterns (urgency substitution). Furthermore, the patient must replace the faulty patterns with effective PFM contraction, which is known to suppress bladder activity via pudendal nerve afferent activity. Toward this end, one systematically shapes selective PFM recruitment, using the various features of the biofeedback protocol.

The therapist instructs the patient to contract the PFMs without contracting abdominal or gluteal muscles, displaying to the patient simultaneously the PFMs and abdominal EMG. The therapist advises the patient that the initial aim of treatment is not to produce a PFM contraction of maximum amplitude. Rather, the aim is to contract the PFMs selectively, with little co-contraction of extraneous muscles and without undue effort.

Adjusting the sensitivity settings of the feedback display permits the therapist to tailor the shaping procedure to match the patient's strength and motor control. For example, one may display abdominal EMG on a scale of 0–16 microvolts, whereas one expands the display of the PFM signal on a scale of 0–8 microvolts. This can help to reinforce submaximal contractions of the latter to help dissociate them from abdominal contractions. As skill and PFM strength improve, the therapist can display the PFM contraction using a smaller gain to reinforce contraction of greater amplitudes.

To improve PFM endurance, gradual increases in the duration of each contraction should be reinforced. As the patient improves, the contraction may be extended up to 30 seconds. The therapist should instruct the patient in diaphragmatic breathing and encourage a steady, rhythmic breathing pattern as the patient slowly begins each PFM contraction. This technique seems to establish the ability to sustain an extended PFM contraction without effort. A threshold line is useful to guide a stable contraction rather than a sawtooth display. However, caution is appropriate when one is using thresholds in the feedback display, to avoid reinforcing contractions of greater duration or amplitude at the expense of allowing abdominal/gluteal substitution (see Figure 26.5).

At each stage of treatment, the patient should practice newly acquired motor skills without feedback from the instruments to rehearse for the home exercise program. After the patient is skilled in starting and maintaining a submaximal contraction while breathing rhythmically, PFM "ramping" contractions should be included in the strengthening program. Ramping contractions are used to reinforce the normal sequence of slow-twitch to fast-twitch recruitment, to build muscle strength. However, many patients require several treatment visits to develop sufficient coordination skills to maintain the regular breathing pattern during

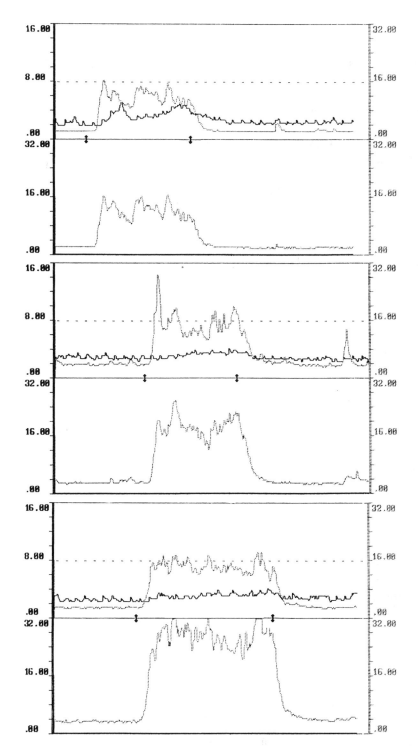

FIGURE 26.5. Abdominal and pelvic floor EMG measures using the MEP. The patient was a 62-year-old man with UI subsequent to prostatectomy. The upper dark line indicates abdominal EMG; the upper light line displays proximal anal canal measures; and the lower light line displays the distal, or outer, anal canal measures. A threshold line was set at 16 microvolts for the proximal anal canal, and the patient was reinforced to keep abdominal muscles relaxed and maintain a stable contraction. The top tracing shows a "sawtooth" recruitment pattern and the patient's tendency to use the abdominal muscles when the PFMs grew tired. The middle tracing shows greater ability to keep abdominal muscles relaxed, and the bottom tracing shows the ability to sustain a contraction for 16 seconds.

submaximal PFM contractions. Only after patients have acquired the ability to sustain the submaximal contractions while maintaining a rhythmic breathing pattern should they be advanced to perform ramping PFM contractions (see Figure 26.6).

If the patient loses urine when moving from sitting to standing, the therapist should first provide instrument feedback for PFM contraction while sitting and then continue the feedback as the patient moves to the standing position. It is often difficult for patients to recruit PFMs while standing. However, standing is the position in which patients are most often incontinent. With urge incontinence, for example, the intensity of the urge often increases as patients approach the toilet. The patients respond by rushing to the toilet, thereby contract-

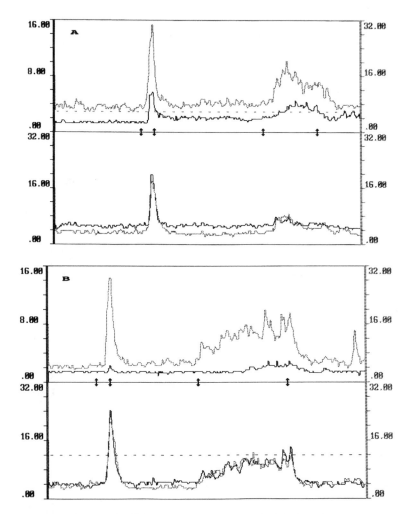

FIGURE 26.6. EMG records over 36 seconds from a 48-year-old woman with stress and urge incontinence. The four tracings represent EMG from abdominal, muscles (upper dark), paravaginal muscles (upper light), inner anal canal (lower dark), and outer anal canal (lower light). Tracing A shows early attempts to perform a quick contraction (left) followed by a sustained "ramping" contraction (right). Note inappropriate abdominal contraction, unstable vaginal recruitment, minimal anal sphincter recruitment, and muscle fatigue after only 5 seconds. In contrast, tracing B shows PFM contraction in the same patient after 4 months of training. It shows minimal abdominal substitution and the ability to systematically increase the recruitment pattern over 10 seconds with the greatest amplitude at the end of the contraction, signifying improvement in muscle endurance.

ing the abdominal muscles. Thus reinforcement for selective PFM contraction, specifically in the standing position, fosters the generalization of behavioral strategies taught to inhibit the bladder. (See "Home Program," below.)

Dyssynergia and Relaxation Training

Many patients with UI have detrusor–sphincter dyssynergia, which (as noted earlier) is characterized by a failure of the PFM and the urethral sphincter to relax precipitously before a bladder contraction and during voiding. This functional problem is not addressed with PFM strengthening. Therefore, if a voiding dysfunction is suspected, treatment must be directed toward improving PFM and urethral relaxation responses that precede urination. (See Tries & Eisman, Chapter 28.)

The Use of a Bladder Ultrasound in Place of CMG Biofeedback

A CMG is one component of the urodynamic procedures used to assess lower urinary tract function. During a CMG, the bladder is infused with either carbon dioxide or sterile water while bladder pressure is measured. The CMG evaluates the patient's sensory threshold for the first sensation of needing to void, the maximum tolerable bladder volume, bladder compliance, and the presence of bladder instability. Changes in PFM activity and abdominal muscle activity, or changes in rectal pressure, can be observed during the CMG as bladder volume is increased. CMG biofeedback allows for the direct reinforcement of bladder inhibition. However, because the CMG requires catheterization, it carries a risk of bladder infection. Over the past few years, as mentioned previously, we have limited our use of CMG biofeedback. Instead, we use an ultrasound bladder scan and oral fluid loading to indirectly assess and reinforce changes in functional bladder capacity, the patient's sensory threshold, maximum tolerable volume, and postvoid residual volumes. The postvoid residual volume gives important information about the patient's ability to empty the bladder. Interested readers will refer to texts on urodynamics for more complete descriptions of CMG diagnostic procedures and CMG biofeedback protocols (Burgio et al., 1985; O'Donnell & Doyle, 1991).

If the patient is being treated for urge incontinence, the therapist can ask the patient to fluid-load orally prior to, and at the onset of the evaluation period. During PFM biofeedback training, the therapist asks the patient to subjectively rate the sensation of bladder fullness by the following criteria (International Continence Society Committee on Standardization of Terminology, 1992): 0, no urge; 1, slight urge; 2, moderate urge ("when I would normally go the bathroom"); 3, stronger urge; and 4, overwhelming urge ("when I *must* go to the bathroom"). As soon as the patient reports a slight (1) sensation to void, the therapist checks the bladder volume using the scan and inform the patient of the volume. Then the therapist coaches the patient to remain relaxed, to breathe with the diaphragm, and to contract the PFM for several 10-second submaximal contractions. This procedure has been shown to inhibit bladder instability and urgency. To assure success when the patient is actually experiencing urgency, the patient should first practice selective PFM contractions when the bladder is empty and without a sensation of urge.

Then the patient should report his or her level of sensory urge after performing the PFM contractions. If the urge sensation diminishes, the therapist can inform the patient that bladder inhibition was successful. The patient should be instructed to use the same strategy in real-life situations during urgency. It is also useful to practice the same procedure standing so the patient feels more confident in attempting to inhibit urge while walking slowly to the toilet.

When the patient reports a sensation of urge that cannot be inhibited, or after the urge reaches a level between "moderate" and "strong," the patient should be instructed to continue the PFM contractions while the therapist removes the recording devices. The therapist then helps the patient to come to the sitting position as he or she continues to verbally reinforce submaximal PFM contraction and diaphragmatic breathing. As the patient is helped to stand, the therapist encourages the patient to remain relaxed, keeping the abdominal muscles "soft" during selective PFM contraction. Once the patient obtains a sense of control while standing, the therapist has the patient walk slowly to the toilet to void, and the voiding output as well as the postvoid residual volume is measured. Using these techniques, one often sees an increase in the patient's functional bladder capacity and a decrease in urge incontinence.

HOME PROGRAM

PFM Exercises

The home program typically includes two separate components. The first consists of PFM exercises. Typically after the first biofeedback session, therapists in our clinics give the patients written directions to perform 30 selective PFM contractions throughout the day. Patients are to divide the 30 contractions into three groups, so they perform 10 contractions lying down, 10 sitting up, and 10 while standing at different times in the day. After patients are able to selectively contract the PFMs for quick, 1- to 2-second periods, they are ready for the next step: alternating quick maximum contractions with submaximal, longer contractions that are extended over 2–3 breaths (5–10 seconds). In this way, the phasic or fast-twitch muscle fibers, as well as the slow-twitch fibers, are stimulated. Alternating the quick and sustained contractions seems to reduce fatigue. When the longer contractions are added to the program, the total number of contractions performed per day remains the same (i.e., 30 per day, divided into three exercise periods). However, an individual patient's ability to perform selective PFM contractions, as displayed during the recording procedures, determines the number and duration of the contractions assigned in the home program.

For example, consider a patient who shows PFM contractions that decay with abdominal substitution or show instability after 5 seconds. The therapist should instruct the patient to alternate 5-second contractions with the quick contractions when performing the exercises at home. Or consider the patient whose contractions show a fatigue effect shown by reduced EMG amplitudes over several trials in the office. For this patient, the therapist should recommend reducing the number of contractions performed at one time in the home program. For example, instead of having the patient practice three times a day, the same number of contractions should be spread out over more frequent practice sessions. After the patient's PFM strength improves, the home program can be modified. As the patient is able to sustain the submaximal contraction without abdominal contraction, the submaximal contraction can be increased to about 8 breaths, or 30 seconds. During the sustained contractions and during the resting period between contractions, we always have patients count breaths instead of seconds; when counting breaths, they are more likely to focus on the rhythmic breathing that we are trying to reinforce as a contingency for performing selective PFM contraction.

The patient is consistently reminded that the abdominal muscles should remain relaxed during PFM contractions. Having the patient place a hand on the lower abdomen while performing the exercises provides a gross monitor of excessive abdominal contraction. The patient should be advised to relax the PFM completely between each contraction for at least 2–3 breaths. The focus on relaxation between contraction amplifies the discriminative stimuli associated with the relaxed state in contrast to the contracted state. This is especially important for patients who have any voiding dysfunction associated with detrusor–sphincter dyssynergia. With these patients, the relaxation period between contractions should be extended to 6–10 breaths.

Once a patient shows the ability to perform the quick and submaximal contractions without using extraneous muscle co-contraction, we have the patient include "ramping" in the home program. The goal in the use of ramping contractions is to exercise the different muscle fiber types from small or slow-twitch, to large or fast-twitch, in the normal fiber recruitment sequence used as muscle demand increases. The ramping contractions start slowly but peak to a maximum effort within about 10 seconds, or 2 breaths (see Figure 26.6).

We find in our clinics that in most cases, if the patients have been appropriately trained to selectively contract the PFMs, they are able to perform the home program without the use of a home trainer. They come back to the clinic for subsequent biofeedback sessions to improve the quality of the PFM contractions at intervals that may range from 1 to 6 weeks. Thus we have not found that home trainers add to the effectiveness of treatment. On the contrary, we feel that if the home trainer does not provide feedback for abdominal muscle co-contraction, its use can deter the development of PFM contraction that is needed to improve bladder control. In the few cases where we find that PFM strength is very slow to improve (e.g., cases of severe partial denervation injury or atrophy), we are more inclined to use PFM electrical stimulation (Fall et al., 1986). We issue the patient a device that is used at home in conjunction with PFM exercises, and continue to see the patient in the clinic for biofeedback treatment and consultation.

We have learned that many practitioners tell patients to stop and start the flow of urine several times per day as a way of exercising the PFM. The presumed purpose of this exercise is to strengthen voluntary bladder control, because many patients report an inability to stop the urine flow once it begins. However, this practice is questionable, because it reinforces an abnormal response, (i.e., sphincter activity during voiding). For this reason, we *never* use this technique in our clinics. Instead, we thoughtfully alter the feedback display to shape in a stepwise fashion, approximations of the desired PFM responses until the ability to selectively contract the PFM is acquired. Our patients are uniformly instructed to relax the PFM when voiding.

Behavioral Strategies

Each patient is also given instructions in the use of bladder control strategies. The selection depends upon the symptoms reported in the bladder diary. Patients with genuine stress incontinence are told to contract the PFMs before, during, and after situations in which they are likely to lose urine (e.g., coughing, lifting, and moving from sitting to standing). This is to condition PFM activity when intra-abdominal pressure increases.

Patients with urge incontinence are instructed as follows. When a strong urge to urinate is perceived, a patient is instructed to remain quiet, relax the abdominal muscles, and breathe slowly and rhythmically. Staying relaxed, the patient contracts the PFMs three to six times to activate the detrusor–sphincter inhibitory reflex. The onset of the PFM contraction should be slow, so that the patient can maintain a rhythmic breathing pattern and avoid increasing intra-abdominal pressure. If needed, the patient may sit if this helps him or her regain control. It is important for the patient to avoid rushing, because this increases intra-abdominal pressure and urgency. After suppressing the urge, the patient decides whether voiding is still necessary and responds accordingly. If the urge returns as the patient approaches the toilet, the relax–contract cycle is repeated.

There are several bladder training protocols that encourage the gradual increase of inter-voiding intervals and *habit training* (Agency for Health Care Policy and Research, 1996; Fantl et al., 1991; Engel et al., 1990; Doughty, 2000). Habit training is a simple, timed voiding schedule without the emphasis on extending intervoiding intervals. Therapists should also read Staying Dry by Burgio, Pearce, and Lucco (1989a), which clearly outlines behavioral strategies for UI. It is for the layperson and is an excellent resource for the appropriate patient.

FREQUENCY AND DURATION OF TREATMENT SESSIONS

A practitioner often schedules the physical assessment and first biofeedback session about 1 week after the initial verbal interview. This allows one to get a baseline of bladder symptoms. The next biofeedback session is scheduled 1–2 weeks after the first session; this allows time for the patient to gain the necessary neuromotor skills required to perform selective PFM contractions for strengthening and to inhibit urgency. After that, one determines the frequency and duration of the treatment sessions by the following criteria: the severity of the problem; the motor, perceptual, and cognitive skills of the patient; and his or her ability to carry out the home program independently.

For many non-neurological patients, 6–8 sessions, scheduled over a 3- to 4-month pe-riod, are usually sufficient to attain maximum benefit from biofeedback procedures. Many patients show significant improvement in fewer sessions, and more severe cases require more frequent, direct instrument reinforcement and support from the therapist. However, atrophied muscles may require 6 months of exercise to produce optimal changes in muscle function. One may need to adjust treatment accordingly to provide support and maintain the patient's motivation. Practitioners also tailor the duration of each session for each patient. The first biofeedback session may extend from 1 to 2 hours; later treatment sessions typically last 45–60 minutes, depending upon the attention and endurance of the patient. In addition to the actual instrument feedback and reinforcement, treatment time includes other topics. The thera-pist reviews the previous week's bladder records and discusses with the patient what seems to be working and what is not working. There is continuing patient education, as well as an update and review of the home exercises and behavioral strategies.

SUMMARY AND CONCLUSION

UI is a costly and embarrassing problem that affects millions of people. Until recently, the primary treatments for UI have been surgical and pharmacological; each type is associated with known and sometimes serious risks. Because striated PFM activity mediates bladder control, one can use operant procedures with biofeedback to improve control that has been disrupted by trauma, disease, or faulty learning.

However, for biofeedback to be effective, the practitioner must have a thorough understand-ing of bladder anatomy and physiology, the behavioral principles underlying treatment, and the instrumentation. There is a clear need for more research to determine the benefit of certain bio-feedback procedures for specific symptom clusters (e.g., the conditions best suited for using CMG biofeedback or home trainers). Furthermore, biofeedback protocols must be tailored to individual patients to adjust for idiosyncratic factors such as muscle strength, coordination, endurance, and bladder characteristics. Examples of bladder characteristics are compliance, stability, and sensa-tion. These and other issues contributing to continence must be considered with each patient.

This chapter provides a primer for practitioners as they begin to prepare for using this effective biofeedback application.

GLOSSARY

ADRENERGIC SYMPATHETIC NEURONS. Neurons that carry impulses of adrenergic postganglionic fibers of the sympathetic nervous system.

AFFERENT ACTIVITY. Sensory signals from the somatic and autonomic nerves that carry information to the spinal cord.

ANAL VERGE. The external (distal) boundary of the anal canal. This is the line where the walls of the anus contact during the normal state of apposition (juxtaposition).

ANTERIOR SUPERIOR ILIAC SPINE. Blunt, bony projection on anterior portion of ilium, the large portion of the hip bone.

BLADDER SUSPENSION SURGERY. A term used to describe various types of anti-incontinence surgeries used to treat urethral hypermobility by elevating the bladder neck to its appropriate anatomic position.

BLADDER TRAINING. A behavioral strategy used primarily for urge incontinence, whereby patients systematically increase the intervoiding interval to normalize voiding frequency and increase functional bladder capacity. Patients are instructed to prolong voiding to the scheduled time using relaxation techniques, distraction, or contraction of the pelvic floor muscles (PFMs).

BULBOCAVERNOSUS REFLEX. (Also called the "bulbospongiosus reflex.") Reflex associated with the bulbospongiosus muscle, one of three bilateral superficial perineal muscles. In females, the vagina separates it from the opposite side (contralateral) muscle. It constricts (compresses) the bulbous urethra or vaginal orifice in females. Innervation of the muscle is by the pudendal nerve. The bulbospongiosus stems from the central tendon of the perineum (pelvic floor and structures of the pelvic outlet), passes around the vagina, and inserts into the dorsum of the clitoris. In men, tapping the dorsum of the penis causes the bulbocavernosus portion to retract by decompressing veins and allowing blood to flow out. The corpus spongiosum includes the urethra and ends in the glans. The dorsum of the penis is the anterior, more extensive surface of the penis continuous with the anterior abdominal wall, opposite the urethral surface, which is continuous with the scrotum. In males, it starts in the median raphe over the bulb and inserts in the root of the penis. It also compresses the urethra.

COCCYX. Three to five small, fused, rudimentary vertebrae forming the caudal extremity of vertebral column (lower back, sacrum). End of spinal column.

COLLAGEN. Fibrous insoluble protein in connective tissue, such as skin, bone, ligaments, and cartilage; it constitutes about 30% of the protein in the body.

CYSTITIS. Inflammation of the urinary bladder, usually from an infection. It is uncommon in men. Signs and symptoms include painful urination (burning or itching feeling) and increased urinary frequency or urgent need to urinate. Sometimes also present are cloudy, malodorous, bloody urine; lower abdominal pain; and slight fever. It is not serious if treated promptly, usually with antibiotics.

CYSTOMETROGRAM (CMG). A urodynamic test to assess bladder function by measuring the bladder pressure–volume relationship. One infuses either carbon dioxide or sterile water into the bladder while measuring bladder pressure and perineal muscle activity. A CMG can determine the degree of detrusor overactivity, sensation, capacity, and compliance. It always involves the insertion of a catheter into the bladder.

DECREASED BLADDER COMPLIANCE. A failure to store urine in the bladder because of a loss of bladder wall elasticity and bladder accommodation. Bladder compliance can be reduced as a result of radiation cystitis, neurological bladder disorders, or inflammatory bladder conditions such as chemical cystitis or interstitial cystitis (see *cystitis*, above).

DENERVATION. Resection or removal of a nerve to an organ or part, as can happen to a degree during childbirth (this is called "partial denervation injury").

DETRUSOR HYPERACTIVITY WITH IMPAIRED BLADDER CONTRACTILITY. A neurogenic disorder in which involuntary or uninhibited detrusor contractions coexist with bladder contractions that are inefficient in emptying the bladder without abnormal abdominal straining.

DETRUSOR INSTABILITY (UNSTABLE BLADDER). The presence of involuntary detrusor contraction in the absence of a neurological disorder.

DETRUSOR MUSCLE. *Detrusor* means "to push down"; it is a general term for any body part that pushes down. In the lower urinary system, the term refers to the smooth muscle that composes the wall of the bladder, which contracts to expel urine.

DETRUSOR–SPHINCTER DYSSYNERGIA. A discoordinated voiding pattern in which there is concurrent sphincter contraction during bladder contraction, in contrast to the normal pattern of sphincter relaxation during bladder contraction. The sphincter does not relax during voiding, and this prevents complete bladder emptying. This is normally a neurogenic condition, but the pattern can result from abnormal learning as well.

DIURESIS. Increased excretion of urine.

EDEMATOUS. Pertaining to or affected by edema (the presence of abnormally large amounts of fluid in intercellular tissue spaces of the body); usually referring to subcutaneous tissue.

ELASTIN. Yellow protein. The essential part of yellow elastic connective tissue.

EXTERNAL ABDOMINAL OBLIQUE MUSCLE. Muscle that flexes and rotates vertebral column and tenses abdominal wall, compressing abdominal viscera.

FAST-TWITCH MUSCLE FIBERS. Striated muscle fiber type with histological characteristics that provide relatively strong and phasic (quick) contractions compared to slow-twitch fibers. Some fast-twitch fibers can be conditioned to resist fatigue, but other fast-twitch fibers remain highly fatigable.

FIBROSIS. Formation of fibrous tissue, especially denoting an abnormal degenerative process.

FUNCTIONAL BLADDER CAPACITY. The maximum voided volume recorded on a voiding diary, which indicates the amount of *diuresis* that must occur before the patient feels the need to urinate.

HABIT TRAINING. A behavioral technique whereby toileting is scheduled at regular intervals that coincide with the patient's normal voiding frequency. Unlike in *bladder training* (see above), there is no effort to extend the intervoiding interval.

HYPERREFLEXIA. The presence of involuntary bladder contractions resulting from a neurological disorder.

HYPOTONIC. Diminished tone of skeletal muscles. In this chapter, diminished resistance of muscle to passive stretching.

INTRAURETHRAL PRESSURE. Pressure within the urethra, the canal conducting urine from the bladder to outside the body.

INTRAVESICAL PRESSURE. Pressure within the bladder.

LEFT LATERAL POSITION (LEFT LATERAL RECUMBENT POSITION). Position in which the person lies on the left side with right thigh and knee drawn upward. Also called an "obstetric" or "English" position (presumably based on a similarity to the manner in which women ride sidesaddle).

LEVATOR ANI MUSCLE. A large muscle that forms the pelvic floor and supports the pelvic viscera. (A *levator* is a muscle that raises a part.) It has three components, called the *pubococcygeus*, *puborectalis*, and iliococcygeus muscles. The levator ani is a heterogeneous mixture of slow- and fast-twitch muscle fibers that both supports the pelvic viscera and provides an additional occlusive force to the external urethral sphincter, especially when there is a sudden increase in intra-abdominal pressure (e.g., cough).

LEVATOR FACTOR. Slow-twitch striated muscle fibers that maintain static muscle and support the pelvic structures.

LUMEN. Cavity or channel within a tube or tubular organ.

MICTURITION. The voiding of urine.

MIXED INCONTINENCE. Stress incontinence coexisting with urge incontinence (see text).

NEGATIVE URETHRAL PRESSURE. The condition in which bladder pressure is greater than urethral pressure, at which point there is a loss of urine. To initiate micturition, a drop in urethral pressure precedes an increase in bladder pressure that is produced by a bladder contraction.

NOCTURIA. Excessive urination at night.

OVERFLOW INCONTINENCE. Overly distended bladder resulting in inefficient emptying of the bladder and incontinence. Bladder pressure overcomes urethral pressure (see text).

PELVIC PROLAPSE. Some organs of the lower abdomen sinking (prolapsing) lower. This results from stretching or slackness of the sheet of muscles and ligaments that form the pelvic floor. This sheet supports the organs of the lower abdomen, such as the bladder, uterus, and small intestines. These muscles also affect the flow of urine in the urethra as it leaves the bladder. Prolapse can result from childbirth, aging, or hereditary weakness. It is more common in elderly women and in those who have given birth to several children (e.g., uterus drooping into the vagina).

PERIURETHRAL MUSCLE. Muscle around the urethra.

PERIVAGINAL. Around the vagina.

PESSARY. An intravaginal device for supporting the uterus or rectum. It is also used for contraception.

POSITIVE URETHRAL PRESSURE. The situation in which urethral pressure is greater than bladder pressure and, as a result, storage is maintained.

PROSTATECTOMY. Surgical removal of part or all of the prostate gland.

PROSTATIC HYPERPLASIA. Abnormal multiplication or increase in the number of normal cells. Hypertrophy.

PROXIMAL URETHRAL RESISTANCE. *Proximal* means "nearer" or "closer" to any point of reference, as opposed to distal. Therefore, this term refers to resistance to urine flow that is provided at the uppermost part of the urethra.

PUBOCOCCYGEUS MUSCLE. Pertaining to the pubis and coccyx or musculus pubococcygeus. Anterior portion of the *levator ani* muscle (see above). Extends from the front of the obturator canal to the anococcygeal ligament and side of coccyx. Innervated by third and fourth sacral nerves. Helps support pelvic viscera and counters intra-abdominal pressure increases.

PUBORECTALIS MUSCLE. Pertaining to the pubis (os pubis) and rectum. The pubis is the anterior inferior part of the hip bone (os coxae) on either side. Helps support pelvic large organs and counters intra-abdominal pressure increases.

PUBOURETHRAL LIGAMENTS. The pair of fibromuscular ligaments that anchor the anterior urethra to the posterior–inferior surface of the symphysis pubis in the female. Together, the pubovesical and pubourethral ligaments provide support to the female bladder neck and anterior portion of the urethral wall.

PUDENDAL NERVE. A nerve supplying the structures of the perineum, including the genitalia, the urethral sphincter, and the external anal sphincter. The pudendum comprises the external genitalia of humans, especially females. The nerve arises from the sacral plexus by separate branches of the ventral rami of S2, S3, and S4.

SENSORY URGE INCONTINENCE. Urge incontinence without uninhibited bladder contractions (see text).

SLOW-TWITCH MUSCLE FIBERS. Striated muscle fiber type with histological characteristics that allow for the maintenance of sustained contraction over relatively long periods and contribute to the tone that closes the urethra to maintain continence.

SUSPENSION FACTOR. *Pubourethral ligaments* supporting the bladder neck.

TRABECULATION, BLADDER. *Detrusor muscle* thickening (see text).

TRIGONE. Base of the bladder.

URETEROVESICAL. Pertaining to a ureter and the bladder.

URETHRAL DIVERTICULA. Pouch or sac defect in the lining of the urethra. A *diverticulum* is a pouch or sac, either natural or from herniation, of the lining mucous membrane.

UROGENITAL DIAPHRAGM. A thin sheet of striated muscle stretching between the two sides of the pubic arch.

VALSALVA MANEUVER. Forcible exhalation effort against a closed glottis. Increases introthoracic pressure and interferes with venous return to the heart. Forced exhalation effort against occluded (pinched) nostrils and closed mouth. (See McGrady & Linden, Chapter 17, this volume.)

REFERENCES

Agency for Health Care Policy and Research. (1996, March). *Urinary Incontinence Guideline Panel. Urinary incontinence in adults: Clinical practice guidelines* (AHCPR Publication No. 96-0682. Rockville, MD: U.S. Department of Health and Human Services.

Allen, R. E., Hosker, G. L., Smith, A. R. B., & Warrell, D. W. (1990). Pelvic floor damage and childbirth: A neurophysiological study. *British Journal of Obstetrics and Gynecology, 97,* 770–779.

Baigis-Smith, J., Smith, D. A. J., Rose, M., & Newman, D. K. (1989). Managing urinary incontinence in community-residing elderly persons. *The Gerontologist, 29,* 229–233.

Bhatia, N. N. (1991). Neurophysiology of micturition. In D. R. Ostergard & A. E. Bent (Eds.), *Urogynecology and urodynamics: Theory and practice* (3rd ed.). Baltimore: Williams & Wilkins.

Burgio, K. L., Locher, J. L., Goode, P. S., Hardin, J. M., McDowell, B. J., Dombrowski, M. & Candib, D. (1998). Behavioral vs. drug treatment for urge urinary incontinence in older women: A randomized controlled trial. *Journal of the American Medical Society, 280,* 1995–2000.

Burgio, K. L., Pearce, L., & Lucco, A. J. (1989a). *Staying dry.* Baltimore: Johns Hopkins University Press.

Burgio, K. L., Robinson, J. C., & Engel, B. T. (1986). The role of biofeedback in Kegel exercise training for stress urinary incontinence. *American Journal of Obstetrics and Gynecology, 154,* 58–64,

Burgio, K. L., Stutzman, R. E., & Engel, B. T. (1989b). Behavioral training for post-prostatectomy urinary incontinence. *Journal of Urology, 141,* 303–306.

Burgio, K. L., Whitehead, W. E., & Engel, B. T. (1985). Urinary incontinence in the elderly. *Annals of Internal Medicine, 103,* 507–515.

Burns, P. A., Marecki, M. A., Dittmar, S. S., & Bullough, B. (1985). Kegel's exercises with biofeedback therapy for treatment of stress incontinence. *Nurse Practitioner, 10*(2), 28, 33–34, 46.

Burns, P. A., Pranikoff, K., Nochajski, T., Desotelle, P., & Harwood, M. K. (1990). Treatment of stress incontinence with pelvic floor exercises and biofeedback. *Journal of the American Geriatrics Society, 38,* 341–344.

Burton, J. R., Pearce, K. L., Burgio, K. L., Engel, B. T., & Whitehead, W. E. (1988). Behavioral training for urinary incontinence in elderly ambulatory patients. *Journal of the American Geriatrics Society, 36,* 693–698.

Cardozo, L. D., Abrams, P. D., Stanton, S. L., & Feneley, R. C. (1978). Idiopathic bladder instability treated by biofeedback. *British Journal of Urology, 50*(7), 521–523.

Cardozo, L. D., & Stanton, S. L. (1985). Biofeedback: A five-year follow-up. *British Journal of Urology, 56*(2), 220.

Cardozo, L. D., Stanton, S. L., Hafner, J., & Allan, V. (1978). Biofeedback in the treatment of detrusor instability. *British Journal of Urology, 50,* 250–254.

Castleden, C. M., & Duffin, H. M. (1981). Guidelines for controlling urinary incontinence without drugs or catheters. *Age and Aging, 10,* 186–192.

Critchley, H. O. D., Dixon, J. S., & Gosling, J. A. (1980). Comparative study of the periurethral and perianal parts of the human levator ani muscle. *International Journal of Urology, 35,* 226–232.

DeLancy, J. O. L. (1988). Structural aspects of the extrinsic continence mechanism. *Obstetrics and Gynecology, 72,* 296–301.

DeLancy, J. O. L. (1989a). Pubovesical ligament: A separate structure from the urethral supports ("pubo-urethral ligaments"). *Neurourology and Urodynamics, 8,* 53–61.

DeLancy, J. O. L. (1989b). Anatomy and embryology of the lower urinary tract. *Obstetrics and Gynecology Clinics of North America, 16,* 717–731.

DeLancy, J. O. L. (1990). Histology of the connection between the vagina and levator ani muscles: Implication for urinary tract function. *Journal of Reproductive Medicine, 35,* 765–771.

DeLancy, J. O. L. (1991). Anatomy of the bladder and urethra. In D. R. Ostergard & A. E. Bent (Eds.), *Urogynecology and urodynamics: Theory and practice* (3rd ed.). Baltimore: Williams & Wilkins.

Doughty, D. (Ed.). (2000). *Urinary and fecal incontinence: Nursing management* (2nd ed.). St. Louis, MO: Mosby.

Dwyer, P. L., & Teele, J. S. (1992). Prazasin: A neglected cause of stress incontinence. *Obstetrics and Gynecology, 79,* 117–121.

Eisman, E., & Tries, J. (1991). A vaginal cone for measuring EMG from the superior surface of the urogenital diaphragm. *Neurourology and Urodynamics, 10,* 409–410.

Eisman, E., & Tries, J. (1993). A new probe for measuring EMG from multiple sites in the anal canal. *Diseases of the Colon and Rectum, 36,* 946–952.

Engel, B. T., Burgio, L. D., McCormick, K. A., Hankins, A. M., Schewe, A. A., & Leahy, E. (1990). Behavioral treatment of incontinence in the long-term setting. *Journal of the American Geriatrics Society, 38,* 361–363.

Fall, M., Ahlstrom, K., Carlsson, C. A., Ek, A., Erlandson, B. E., Frandenberg, S., & Mattiasson, A. (1986). Contelle: Pelvic floor stimulator for female stress-urge incontinence. *Urology, 26,* 282–287.

Fantl, J. A., Wyman, J. F., McClish, D. K., Harkins, S. W., Elswick, R. K., Taylor, J. R., & Hadley, E. C. (1991). Efficacy of bladder training in older women with urinary incontinence. *Journal of the American Medical Association, 265,* 609–613.

Fisher, W. (1983). Physiotherapeutic aspects of urine incontinence. *Acta Obstetrica Gynecologia Scandinavica, 62,* 579–583.

Gosling, J. A., Dixon, J. S., Critchley, H. O. D., & Thompson, S. A. (1981). A comparative study of the human external sphincter and periurethral levator ani muscles. *British Journal of Urology, 53,* 35–41.

Grey, M. L. (2000). Physiology of voiding. In D. B. Doughty (Ed.), *Urinary and fecal incontinence: Nursing management* (2nd ed.). St. Louis, MO: Mosby,

Hald, T., & Bradley, W. E. (1982). *The urinary bladder: Neurology and dynamics.* Baltimore: Williams & Wilkins.

Hay-Smith, E. J., Bo, K., Berghmans, L. C., Hendricks, H. J., de Bie, R. A., & van Waalwijk, V. (2001). Pelvic floor muscle training for urinary incontinence. *Cochrane Electronic Library, 1,* CD001407.

Henderson, J. S., & Taylor, K. H. (1987). Age as a variable in an exercise program for the treatment of simple urinary stress incontinence. *Journal of Obstetric, Gynecologic, and Neonatal Nursing, 16*(4), 266–272.

International Continence Society Committee on Standardization of Terminology. (1992). Seventh report on the standardization of terminology of lower urinary tract function: Lower urinary tract rehabilitation techniques. *Scandinavian Journal of Urology and Nephrology, 26,* 99–106.

Kegel, A. H. (1948). Progressive resistance exercise in the functional restoration of the perineal muscles. *American Journal of Obstetrics and Gynecology, 56,* 238–248.

Kegel, A. H. (1951). Physiologic therapy for urinary stress incontinence. *Journal of the American Medical Society, 146,* 915–917.

Koelbl, H., Strassegger, H., Riss, P. A., & Gruber, H. (1989). Morphologic and functional aspects of pelvic floor muscles in patients with pelvic relaxation and genuine stress incontinence. *Obstetrics and Gynecology, 74,* 789–795.

Krane, R. L., & Siroky, M. B. (1991). *Clinical neuro-urology.* Boston: Little, Brown.

Laycock, J. (1994). Clinical assessment of the pelvic floor. In B. Schussler, J. Laycock, P. Norton, & S. Stanton (Eds.), *Pelvic floor re-education: Principles and practice.* London: Springer-Verlag.

McGuire, E. J. (1983). Physiology of the lower urinary tract. *American Journal of Kidney Disease, 2,* 402–408.

Middaugh, S. J., Whitehead, W. E., Burgio, K. L., & Engel, B. T. (1989). Biofeedback in treatment of urinary incontinence in stroke patients. *Biofeedback and Self-Regulation, 14,* 3–19.

Mundy, A. R., Stephenson, T. P., & Wein, A. J. (Eds.). (1984). *Urodynamics: Principles, practice, and application.* Edinburgh: Churchill Livingstone.

Nygaard, I., DeLancey, J. O. L., Amsdorf, L., & Murphy, E. (1990). Exercise and incontinence. *Obstetrics and Gynecology, 75,* 848–851.

O'Donnell, P. D., & Doyle, R. (1991). Biofeedback therapy technique for treatment of urinary incontinence. *Urology, 37*(5), 432–436.

Ostergard, D. R., & Bent, A. E. (Eds.). (1991). *Urogynecology and urodynamics: Theory and practice* (3rd ed.). Baltimore: Williams & Wilkins.

Resnick, N. M., & Yalla, S. V. (1985). Management of urinary incontinence in the elderly. *New England Journal of Medicine, 313,* 800–805.

Rose, M. A., Baigis-Smith, J., Smith, D., & Newman, D. (1990). Behavioral management of urinary incontinence in homebound older adults. *Home Healthcare Nurse, 8*(5), 10–15.

Susset, J. G., Galea, G., & Read, L. (1990). Biofeedback therapy for female incontinence due to low urethral resistance. *Journal of Urology, 143,* 1205–1208.

Tanagho, E. A. (1991). Retropubic surgical approach for correction of urinary stress incontinence. In D. R. Ostergard & A. E. Bent (Eds.), *Urogynecology and urodynamics: Theory and practice* (3rd ed.). Baltimore: Williams & Wilkins.

Torrens, M., & Morrison, J. F. B. (1987). *The physiology of the lower urinary tract.* London: Springer-Verlag.

Tries, J. (1990a). Kegel exercises enhanced by biofeedback. *Journal of Enterostomal Therapy, 17,* 67–76.

Tries, J. (1990b). The use of biofeedback in the treatment of incontinence due to head injury. *Journal of Head Trauma Rehabilitation, 5,* 91–100.

Van Kampen, M., De Weerdt, W., Van Poppel, H., De Ridder, D., Feys, H., & Baert, L. (2000). Effect of pelvic floor re-education on duration and degree of incontinence after radical prostatectomy: A randomized controlled trial. *Lancet, 355,* 98–102.

Wall, L. L., & Addison, W. A. (1990). Prazosin-induced stress incontinence. *Obstetrics and Gynecology, 75,* 558–560.

Wein, A. J., & Barrett, D. M. (1988). *Voiding function and dysfunction: A logical and practical approach.* Chicago: Year Book Medical.

Workman, D. E., Cassisi, J. E., & Dougherty, M. C. (1992). Validation of surface EMG as a measure of intravaginal and intra-abdominal activity: Implications for biofeedback-assisted Kegel exercises. *Psychophysiology, 30,* 88–93.

APPENDIX 26.1. BLADDER RECORD

Name: _____ Date: _____

(Please keep the following record for a 24-hour period—before your scheduled appointment.)

1. In the 1st column mark the time (day and night) you urinate.
2. In the 2nd column mark the volume (amount) of urine—please measure this using a plastic measuring cup or jar. Do not bring with you.
3. In the 3rd column mark the time (day and/or night) accidents occur.
4. In the 4th column describe the amount of the accident—small is a few drops—large is enough to soak through outer garments if a pad is not being worn.
5. In the 5th column describe what you were doing at the time of the accident, or what caused the accident.

URINATION RECORD		ACCIDENT RECORD		
1. Time of urination	2. Amount of urine	3. Time of accident	4. Amount large/small	5. Reason for accident

Number and type of pads used today _____.

NOTE. Do not urinate right before your scheduled appointment in the clinic—we will need you to empty your bladder as part of our evaluation.

APPENDIX 26.2. SYMPTOM LOG

Date: _9-19-94, Monday_

Time	Urinated in toilet	Small accident	Large accident	Reason for accident
6:09 AM	X			
8:47 AM	X			
10:55 AM	X		X	I think I lose urine after getting dressed.
-1:40 PM	X			
2:15 PM			X	Doing paperwork
2:45 PM		X		going down basement steps.
-4:30 PM	X		X	almost 3 hrs. since urinating in toilet.
Before 8:10 I was unable to get to toilet.		X	?	
-8:10 PM	X			
-11:10 PM	X			

Number of pads used today: _4_   Number of accidents: _4_

✴ Number of exercises: Lying _____ Sitting _____ Standing _____ Duration _____

Comments: _I should have changed my Depends more often, but I was taking care of my mother._

✴ I did all of my exercises today.

CHAPTER 27

Fecal Incontinence

JEANNETTE TRIES
EUGENE EISMAN

OVERVIEW OF THE LITERATURE

In the 1960s, a major question emerging from the fields of psychophysiology and learning theory was whether operant procedures could directly change autonomically mediated responses. Miller and DiCara (1967) researched this question using curarized animals and demonstrated that operant procedures could produce bidirectional changes in heart rate, blood pressure, and glandular activity. These findings challenged the view that smooth muscle learning was possible only through classical conditioning. However, satisfactory replication of this research has yet to occur. Thus, although numerous studies have shown that operant procedures can produce autonomic changes in noncurarized animals and humans (Bower & Hilgard, 1981), none have really employed adequate controls for skeletal muscle and central nervous system mediation.

Although specification of the mechanisms of visceral learning is of theoretical importance, it seems less so in clinical applications, because skeletal and visceral responses are inextricably linked as part of the centrally integrated response patterns (Miller, 1978). The colorectal system provides an example in which the autonomic nervous system and the somatic branch interact to maintain bowel function. This integration provides the opportunity for the use of operant procedures to alter disordered bowel function.

Reviews of the literature report that, overall, biofeedback appears to be highly effective in reducing fecal incontinence (Enck, 1993; Norton, Hosker, & Brazzelli, 2000; Heymen, Jones, Ringel, Scarlett, & Whitehead, 2001). However, comparisons among studies are difficult, owing to small sample sizes and inconsistencies with regard to methodology, selection criteria, and outcome assessment. Improvements in bowel control after biofeedback are reported to range between 64% and 70%, depending upon the methodology used. However, in light of the methodological shortcomings, these outcomes must be interpreted with caution.

The use of operant procedures to improve anorectal physiology was first reported in a single-case pediatric study (Kohlenberg, 1973). However, the seminal study of Engel, Nikoomanesh, and Schuster (1974) defined the method that was replicated by many subsequent reports. Engel et al. (1974) used a manometric three-balloon probe (described below), which simultaneously measures and allows for the reinforcement of three specific anorectal responses that maintain continence. The procedure simulated stool entering the rectum by distending a balloon placed within the rectum with air. The instructions to subjects were to attend to the sensation of rectal distension and contract the *external anal sphincter (EAS)* immediately in response, but without increasing intra-abdominal pressure. (Note that, as in other chapters, italics on first use of a term indicate that the term is included in the chapter's glossary.) The protocol used by Engel et al. (1974) addressed several essential factors that contribute to continence:

1. Awareness of sensory cues that normally signal impending loss of stool.
2. Timely EAS contraction to the perception of rectal distension.
3. Reduction of a maladaptive rise in intra-abdominal pressure that frequently accompanies EAS contraction but is counter to storage.

Thus the balloon distension procedure provided a sensory discrimination task reinforcing a response to specific cues that the patient could generalize to daily life. After one to four treatment sessions, four of the seven patients treated by Engel et al. achieved continence. Two attained significant improvement, and one patient did not complete therapy. Other uncontrolled clinical studies used similar methods and obtained comparable results (Cerulli, Nikoomanesh, and Schuster, 1979; Wald, 1981a, 1981b; Goldenberg, Hodges, Hersh, & Jinich, 1980; Riboli, Frascio, Pitto, Reboa, & Zanolla, 1988; Rao, Welcher, & Happel, 1996; Glia, Gylin, Akerlund, Lindfors, & Lindberg, 1998).

Several researchers concluded that rectal sensitivity and a short-latency EAS response to rectal distension are essential for continence. Thus improving rectal sensitivity and the EAS response time to rectal distension became primary biofeedback goals. For example, Buser and Miner (1986) reinforced immediate perception of, and EAS contraction to, rectal distension in subjects selected for having measurable delays in rectal sensation. They reported a reduction of incontinence of 92% after biofeedback.

Two studies attempted to determine which components (sensation, coordination, or strengthening procedures) of the biofeedback protocol were most effective (Latimer, Campbell, & Kasperski, 1984; Miner, Donnelly, & Read, 1990). Latimer et al. (1984) systematically introduced reinforcement for sensory discrimination, EAS strengthening, and EAS coordination in a single-case experimental design. Improvements in rectal sensation were associated with a decrease in incontinence. EAS deficits identified by manometry did not predict an individual's response to a specific biofeedback intervention. Although subjects showed greater endurance for EAS voluntary contraction and improved EAS responses to rectal distension, EAS strength as measured by maximum voluntary squeeze (VS) pressure did not change significantly.

Using a two-phase crossover design, Miner et al. (1990) compared the effects of sham sensory training, active sensory training, EAS coordination training, and EAS strength training. Improvements in rectal sensitivity were felt to contribute most to symptom reduction, because changes in EAS function were not observed. However, not all patients with improved sensation developed continence. It appears, then, that adequate sensation for rectal distension is necessary but not sufficient for continence.

It may be that EAS strength did not increase appreciably in these studies (Latimer et al., 1984; Miner et al., 1990) because reinforcement for EAS contraction was indirect, with the therapist using the feedback measures to verbally guide the patient. The degree to which a physiological variable can be shaped depends upon the accuracy and immediacy of the feedback. Verbal reinforcement cannot provide the kind of precise sensory information needed to shape approximations of the desired motor response needed to improve the quality of EAS contraction. This is especially true when trauma or disease has compromised afferent and efferent EAS activity. These protocols were also limited in improving EAS strength because little attention was given to control for increased intra-abdominal pressure during EAS contraction, which is counter to storage and limits perception of EAS contraction. Also, Miner et al. (1990) provided strength training in only three 20-minute sessions—a time that seems insufficient to strengthen weak muscles. Because the EAS strength training protocols were inadequate in these studies, it is not possible to compare the effects of strength versus sensory discrimination training.

On the other hand, some protocols have aimed to improve EAS strength. Unfortunately, measured changes in EAS strength, presumed to underlie functional improvements, have not been reported (MacLeod, 1987; Schiller, Santa Ana, Davis, & Fordtran, 1979). In a clinical series, MacLeod (1987) used an intra-anal EMG probe to treat 113 patients with incontinence from varied etiologies and reported a 63% reduction in incontinence. The procedure reinforced EAS contractions of greater amplitudes and durations up to 30 seconds. Unintentional abdominal contractions were not controlled except with verbal instruction. During the follow-up of from 6 months to 5 years, there were no reports of relapse. MacLeod (1987) concluded that EMG biofeedback is most useful for postobstetric injury, and least effective for patients with anterior resection of the rectum and those with "keyhole" anal deformities.

Recently, Heymen et al. (2000) compared the effects of rectal sensory training; EAS strength training with EMG; EAS strength training with EMG combined with rectal sensory training; EMG strength training combined with the use of a home biofeedback device; and EMG strength training combined with both sensory training and a home biofeedback device. Group sizes ranged from 8 to 10 subjects. Reductions in fecal incontinence ranged from 64% to 96% after treatment, but no difference was found between groups. This study's stated purpose was to compare the effects of different protocols. However, measures of sensation and strength, presumed to be altered by the treatments, were not included in the analysis. Given this shortcoming, the mechanism of functional improvement is not well understood.

Because of these methodological flaws, many researchers have concluded that improved continence is not necessarily associated with changes in EAS strength (Wald, 1981a; Miner et al., 1990; Latimer et al., 1984; Loening-Baucke, 1990; MacLeod, 1987; Riboli et al., 1988). However, two papers have reported increasing measures of EAS strength when subjects were given direct feedback to improve the amplitude, quality, and duration of EAS contractions that was contingent upon maintaining stable intra-abdominal pressure (Whitehead, Burgio, & Engel, 1985; Chiarioni, Scattolini, Bonfante, & Vantini, 1993). Chiarioni et al. (1993) obtained an overall 85% reduction in incontinence in 14 subjects with chronic diarrhea who had not benefited from prior medical treatment. There was an associated improvement in the ability to sustain an EAS contraction, from 19.2 seconds to 38.3 seconds. All nine patients reporting complete resolution of incontinence could sustain a 30-second EAS contraction after treatment.

Chiarioni et al.'s findings differ from those of Loening-Baucke (1990), who used a similar patient population. In the Loening-Baucke study, one group was given biofeedback plus conventional medical treatment. A second group received only conventional therapy. The reduction of incontinence was about 50% in both groups, and no difference was found between groups in EAS strength after therapy. Therefore, the author concluded that biofeedback was not effective, and attributed the low 50% improvement in both groups to the sample population (i.e., patients with diarrhea). However, the Chiarioni et al. (1993) used a similar sample. Upon examination of the methods used, it appears that these two studies obtained disparate results because they used different training procedures. Although Loening-Baucke (1990) trained coordinated EAS contraction to rectal distension, there was no attempt to reinforce EAS contraction of sufficient duration to exceed the time required for recovery of *internal anal sphincter* (IAS) inhibition following rectal distension. Nor is it possible to check the adequacy of the home training program, because data for the number of Kegel exercises per day were not reported. In contrast, Chiarioni et al. (1993) reinforced selective EAS contractions of greater amplitudes for up to 30 seconds, but without abdominal co-contraction in response to rectal distension. In addition, Chiarioni et al. (1993) assigned a vigorous home exercise program that included 20 EAS contractions lasting 30 seconds each, three times per day.

Like many biofeedback applications, those for fecal incontinence employ various adjunctive manipulations in addition to operant conditioning of targeted physiological responses. These adjunctive procedures include bowel or habit training, dietary manipulations, and the use of medications. Most reports have not controlled for the effect of these procedures. Moreover, most studies do not control for nonspecific effects associated with biofeedback therapy; these include attention from a concerned health care professional, increased awareness of the physiology that occurs when the anal canal is instrumented, and the use of a symptom diary.

At the very least, the literature indicates that sensitivity to rectal distension is essential to achieve continence, and that biofeedback therapy is effective in improving rectal sensation. However, the association between measures of EAS strength and clinical outcome has not been consistent across studies. As a result, the degree to which improved strength contributes to continence, and to sensation itself, is unknown. The disparity between obtained changes in sensation compared to sphincter strength probably correlates with the underlying physiological mechanism(s) altered by specific biofeedback procedures. On the one hand, sensation consistently improves with biofeedback. In fact, some studies report improvement with as little as one treatment session (Buser & Miner, 1986; Cerulli et al., 1979; Goldenberg et al., 1980). Because this improvement occurs rapidly, it seems to be associated with relearning of neurophysiological patterns that are essentially intact but not used because of faulty sensation.

On the other hand, it is unlikely that sensory discrimination and EAS coordination training alone will alter muscle tone or strength sufficiently to improve EAS weakness and bowel control when EAS weakness is the primary contributor to incontinence. Thus, when the muscles are weak but sensation is intact, symptom reduction depends on changing EAS strength through an extended and well-designed exercise protocol. Chiarioni et al. (1993) took this approach with patients having diarrhea and incontinence who were able to improve both EAS coordination in response to rectal distension and increase the EAS strength. Thus it is both possible and desirable to include a well-designed protocol for EAS strengthening in any biofeedback protocol for fecal incontinence.

EMG data obtained in our clinics indicate that if biofeedback is directed toward training patients to selectively contract the EAS without abdominal contraction, there may be an actual decrease in measures of EAS strength when posttreatment measures are compared to those obtained prior to the biofeedback (Tries, 2000). We hypothesize that the decrease in pelvic floor muscle (PFM) measures occurs because the pretreatment PFM measures reflect facilitation from co-contracting abdominal and gluteal muscle. When this co-contraction is decreased with biofeedback, the PFM measures also decrease to a degree. Thus the removal of the extraneous muscle co-contraction confounds comparisons of pretreatment to posttreatment measures of PFM strength. This may be why many studies have failed to show changes in EAS strength after biofeedback. This confounding effect should be considered when the effectiveness of various biofeedback protocols is being assessed.

STRUCTURE AND FUNCTION OF THE RECTUM AND ANUS

A biofeedback therapist treating fecal incontinence must have a comprehensive understanding of the structure and dynamic function of the PFMs, the rectum, and the anal canal; the pharmacological effects of the various drugs on bowel activity; the influence of diet on bowel control; and the degree to which the measurement methods characterize the pathophysiology. The following discussion should be viewed only as a brief outline, and the reader is referred to the sources cited for a more complete treatment of the anatomical and physiological factors that influence continence.

Anatomy and Physiology

The rectum is the most distal portion of the colon. It extends from the sigmoid segment to the anal canal. It is 12–15 centimeters long in adults and consists of circular and longitudinal smooth muscle layers, like the rest of the colon. When gas or feces move into the rectum, it expands to accommodate the larger mass. Sensory nerves within the rectal walls and nearby striated muscle provide a subjective sensation of fullness and cause the urge to defecate. Contraction of the large colon and rectum provides the propulsive force to move stool toward and through the anal canal.

The anal canal pierces the PFMs posteriorly. These muscles, as a group, are referred to as the *levator ani muscle*; they enclose the entire base of the bony pelvis and give off components that surround the urethra, the vagina (in women), and the anal canal. The levator ani provides the primary support for all the organs of the lower abdomen, forming the levator plate. This muscle plate positions and stabilizes the various structures of the lower abdomen and pelvis. It gives off muscle fibers that funnel down to, and interdigitate with, the fibers of the EAS that surround the anal canal. The levator ani has three parts: the puborectalis, the pubococcygeus, and the iliococcygeus muscles.

The puborectalis muscle has considerable importance in the maintenance of bowel continence. The puborectalis forms a sling that extends from the pubis back and around the junction between the rectum and the anal canal. The puborectalis is normally in a state of contraction during the storage phase and maintains an acute angle between the rectum and the anal canal. According to some authorities, this anorectal angle is the most critical factor in the maintenance of continence (Henry & Swash, 1985). For example, if trauma or birth defect compromises the puborectalis, incontinence is almost inevitable. On the other hand, a strong puborectalis can compensate even for a disordered IAS or EAS. For a more complete discussion of the PFMs, see any comprehensive anatomy text—for example, Netter (1989) or Moore (1992).

As shown in Figure 27.1, the terminal portion of the rectum narrows into the anal canal. The anal canal length is 2.5–3.0 centimeters. It has a thickening of the circular smooth muscle layer that extends down from the rectum. This thickened portion is the IAS and normally is in a state of near-maximal contraction (Henry & Swash, 1985) during the storage phase. According to the classic view, the EAS is composed of three separate bundles of striated muscle fibers. Two EAS bundles (the deep and superficial) surround the IAS at the proximal portion of the anal canal. The third, the subcutaneous, is caudal to the IAS and encircles the terminal portion of the anal canal. The EAS and PFMs always maintain slight muscle tension during the storage phase.

The IAS relaxes several times per hour, and this allows small amounts of rectal material to enter the anal canal. This material reaches the receptor-rich anoderm, which allows for the discrimination of air, liquid, or solid. When the IAS is tonically contracted, its resting pressure provides a passive barrier to the small amounts of gas or feces that might otherwise seep out. However, when the IAS relaxes to sample the rectal contents, the EAS must contract momentarily to prevent fecal seepage. When defecation is desired, the puborectalis, the EAS, and the IAS relax simultaneously and completely. This allows for the unresisted passage of stool through the anal canal.

Because rectal distension is the stimulus for IAS relaxation, the EAS must contract immediately with distension to prevent the accidental loss of stool. Contraction of the EAS is

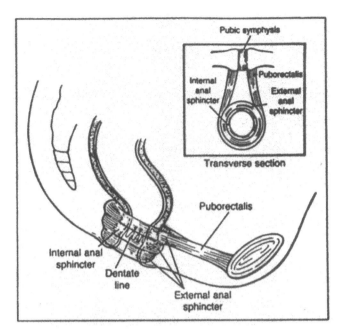

FIGURE 27.1. Anatomy of the anal canal, rectum, and distal colon, showing some of the physiological mechanisms for preserving continence. From Madoff, Williams, and Caushaj (1992, p. 1003). Copyright 1992 by Massachusetts Medical Society. All rights reserved. Reprinted by permission.

brief. However, it is of sufficient duration to allow the rectum to accommodate to the new volume of rectal contents and for the IAS to regain its contracted state. The urge to defecate ends with rectal accommodation until more material moves into the rectum, again producing distension.

The EAS contraction to rectal distension is so well learned that it occurs without conscious attention and is frequently labeled an unconditioned reflex. However, research shows that the response does not occur if a person fails to sense rectal distension even when the distension is of sufficient magnitude to produce IAS relaxation. In addition, patients can inhibit the EAS response to distension when instructed to do so, indicating that the response is in fact under learned control (Whitehead, Orr, Engel, & Schuster, 1981).

Manometry

Much of our understanding of anorectal function comes from *anorectal manometry*, which is also used for biofeedback. One type of manometry is pneumatic and uses the Schuster anorectal probe, which measures simultaneously the responses of the IAS and EAS to rectal distension by simulating feces entering the rectum (Schuster, Hookman, Hendrix, & Mendeloff, 1965).

The pneumatic manometry system has three major components: (1) the three-balloon rectal probe; (2) pressure transducers; and (3) a polygraph, chart recorder, or computer that records three or more channels. Figure 27.2 shows the rectal probe placed within the rectum and anal canal.

Briefly, the rectal probe consists of a double balloon tied around a hollow metal cylinder. The balloons are inserted into the anal canal so that the proximal balloon is positioned at the level of the IAS and the distal balloon is at the EAS. A third balloon, the rectal balloon

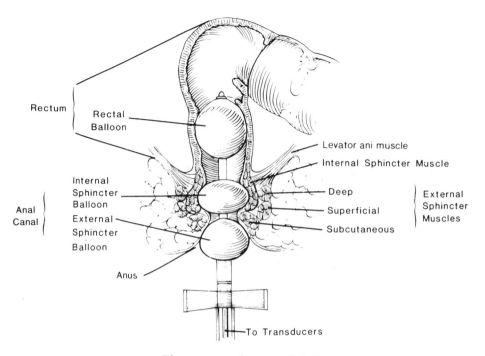

FIGURE 27.2. The rectum and anus with balloons in place.

is connected to a length of tubing that is threaded through the metal cylinder holding the IAS and EAS balloons. The rectal balloon is inserted into the patient's rectum about 10 centimeters from the anal opening. Each balloon is connected to a separate pressure transducer by polyethylene tubing. The transducers produce three measurements displayed on a polygraph or computer screen.

To record baseline pressures, one places the balloons within the anal canal and rectum, and inflates each of them which 10 cubic centimeters of air. (See the section on manometric assessment for a description of the insertion.) Typically, the EAS tracing will be fairly stable. The IAS and rectal tracings may exhibit a slow waveform associated with respiration. There is a sharp pressure rise in the rectal tracing as air enters the rectal balloon. Withdrawal of the air results in a quick return to baseline. When the volume of rectal distension is above the patient's sensory threshold (15 cubic centimeters is normal), the IAS tracing will show an initial pressure increase and then will drop to below baseline levels. The initial increase represents the puborectalis *stretch response*, and the pressure drop indicates the *IAS inhibitory reflex*. The IAS inhibitory response may occur even if the patient does not experience the subjective sensation of distension. The magnitude and duration of the IAS relaxation have a positive correlation with the magnitude of rectal distension. Relaxation of the IAS occurs even when one does not immediately withdraw the distending volume. If the distension is maintained, the relaxation may be prolonged, but after a while, the IAS will return to baseline as the rectum accommodates to the distending volume.

The EAS tracing will show a sharp increase of pressure with an acute distension of the rectal balloon. The pressure will gradually return to baseline over the next 5–10 seconds (see Figure 27.3A). Prolonged rectal distension results in an EAS response of longer duration. As is true for the IAS, the greater the rectal distension, the larger the EAS response (see Figure 27.3B).

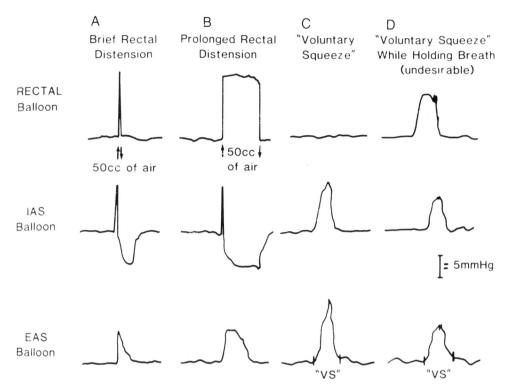

FIGURE 27.3. Sample polygraph records showing normal and sphincter function. (A) Normal EAS response (≥ 25 mm Hg) and normal IAS response (initial pressure rise followed by relaxation) to rectal distension by 50 cc of air. (B) Normal EAS and IAS responses to prolonged rectal distension. (C) Normal EAS contraction in response to verbal instructions to "squeeze" without rectal distension. IAS pressure increases, since there is no rectal distension to stimulate the relaxation reflex, and the EAS muscle may indirectly produce pressure on the IAS balloon. (D) Same responses as in C, but holding of the breath results in a weaker EAS contraction.

When a voluntary EAS contraction (vs) is produced without rectal distension, a pressure increase is seen in both the IAS and EAS tracings (see Figure 27.3C). The IAS balloon records the increase in pressure because the puborectalis and EAS surround the IAS. Without rectal distension and the associated IAS relaxation reflex, the IAS balloon provides a measure of squeeze pressure in the proximal anal canal.

Some individuals show a rise in pressure in the rectal balloon tracing during an EAS voluntary contraction (see Figure 27.3D). This response reflects an increase in intra-abdominal pressure from abdominal muscle contraction and breath holding. Although a slight increase in rectal pressure is normal with EAS contraction, a large increase is maladaptive, because pressure in the rectum pushes stool out and is the pattern of evacuation.

PATHOPHYSIOLOGY AND IMPLICATIONS FOR THERAPY

Medical and postsurgical conditions that can lead to fecal incontinence can be grouped into five general categories, based on the pathophysiology directly responsible for the incontinence (Madoff, Williams, & Caushaj, 1992). However, any individual patient may exhibit more than one of these deficits:

1. Impaired rectal sensation.
2. Inadequate contraction of the EAS.
3. Poor resting tone of the IAS.
4. Diminished rectal capacity.
4. Incomplete relaxation or paradoxical contraction with defecation.

Damage to afferent nerve fibers or to sensory areas in the brain can impair rectal sensation. Chronic dilation of the rectum that occurs with severe constipation can also reduce rectal sensation. Regardless of the etiology, failure to perceive rectal distension has deleterious effects on continence. Normally, IAS relaxation occurs frequently through the day. This intermittent IAS relaxation allows some rectal contents to contact the anoderm, which is rich in sensory receptors. This "sampling" enables the individual to determine whether the contents of the rectum are gas, liquid, or stool. The person can then plan a course of action. That is, he or she can pass gas, find a toilet, or contract the EAS to inhibit the bowel movement. If rectal sensation is impaired, however, an EAS contraction does not occur concurrently with the IAS relaxation, and there is no closure of the distal anal canal as the proximal canal expands. Fecal matter sampled in the anal canal seeps outward without increased pressure at the outer anal canal.

Manometry tests rectal sensation and the EAS response to rectal distention. Normally, the EAS automatically contracts at all levels of rectal distention that are perceptible. This contraction is called the "rectosphincteric response." The amplitude of the rectosphincteric response varies as a function of both the volume of the rectal distension and the patient's perception of the stimulus. It is therefore an index of the integrity of the sensorimotor system.

An attenuated rectosphincteric (stretch) response to distension can still result in urgency or incontinence, even with normal sensation and squeeze pressures. Diminished stretch responses are seen in a muscle with low resting tone and suggest that the sensorimotor response loops of that muscle are impaired. Sensations for rectal distension occur not only in the walls of the rectum, but also within the PFMs (Henry & Swash, 1985). Thus hypotonic PFMs reduce the rectosphincteric response to distension by limiting the proprioceptive signals typically produced by that distension. Without an adequate proprioceptive signal, the patient has little warning for the movement of stool into the rectum. As a result, he or she cannot respond with a timely EAS contraction to close the anal canal and push the fecal material back into the rectum. Patients with this problem often perceive and report the need to have a bowel movement as being "too late." Improving sphincter tone with exercise may enhance the efficiency of the stretch receptor response, thus providing such a patient with a more timely warning for loss of stool.

Impaired EAS strength or muscle tone may result from partial denervation injury to the PFMs and anal sphincter. A frequent cause for partial denervation is stretch injury during childbirth, especially where there is a prolonged second-stage labor (Allen, Hosker, Smith, & Warrell, 1990). Reduced EAS strength may also result from damage to the sphincter muscle itself, such as from anal surgery, radiation, or a vaginal–rectal tear during childbirth. In these cases, incontinence occurs because the pressure from descending stool and contracting colon overcomes a low EAS squeeze pressure.

The striated puborectalis muscle surrounds and supports the IAS smooth muscle at the inner anal canal. Because of this arrangement, both smooth and striated muscle contribute to the IAS pressure recorded with manometry.

Poor IAS resting tone is often caused by damage to the IAS during anal or rectal surgery. Examples are imperforate anus repair, ileal–anal anastomosis, or hemorrhoidectomy. Poor IAS tone also may result from chronic dilation of the sphincter with constipation. In this case, normal resting tone may be restored after the patient has been disimpacted and the rectum remains empty with regular toileting. One can palpate diminished IAS resting tone during digital examination. If the involuntary IAS has a low resting baseline, the IAS relaxation reflex will show only a small-amplitude change during manometric rectal distension. This is because the basal muscle activity is so low that there is a limited range for muscle inhibition. If, however, the IAS smooth muscle is intact but the surrounding puborectalis muscle has low supporting tone, the IAS inhibitory response will be extreme, because IAS inhibition is unopposed by any surrounding striated muscle support.

If rectal sensation and EAS contraction are adequate, individuals with poor IAS resting tone will not usually experience gross incontinence. However, they may experience seepage of liquid stool and gas in amounts too small to produce a perceived rectal distension stimulus. The EAS will then fail to contract. Alternatively, they may complain of an urgent call to produce stool where there is a limited ability to inhibit a bowel movement after perceiving the sensation. This urgency may occur because the IAS inhibition and surrounding puborectalis tone contribute significantly to the sensation for impending fecal loss. These muscles provide the first place of resistance to loss of stool or gas. When the inner anal canal has low tone, the functional length of the canal shortens. This means that the compromised anal canal has a limited area in which to elevate pressure effectively to provide resistance to fecal loss.

Rectal compliance is the ability of the rectum to adapt to a fecal mass without a sustained elevation in rectal pressure. One determines compliance by the elasticity of the rectal tissue and the degree to which the activity of the smooth muscle of the colon and rectum can be inhibited. Rectal capacity decreases when the rectal walls become noncompliant as a result of inflammation or from a reduction of the size of the rectum or colon. Noncompliance may accompany active ulcerative proctitis, scarring from rectal surgery or chronic inflammatory disease. If the rectum does not stretch and remains noncontractile to accommodate increasing amounts of stool, there is a resultant increase in rectal pressure, which may overwhelm even the strongest EAS contraction. Also, when the colon is irritable, strong colonic contractions may inhibit a weak sphincter through neural feedback loops. The spontaneous EAS contraction that normally occurs with rectal distension not only increases pressure in the anal canal, but also inhibits colonic contraction. This reduces rectal pressure until a desired evacuation time. Thus this inhibitory effect usually reduces the need for a sustained EAS contraction to maintain continence. However, when sensory or motor deficits diminish the intensity of the EAS response, there is disinhibition of the colon from this source of control. With the loss of inhibition, incontinence is more likely to occur, because rectal pressure overwhelms the anal canal squeeze pressure.

Signs of limited rectal capacity include frequent and unformed bowel movements, urgent calls to produce stool, and explosive bowel movements. One can assess rectal compliance with manometry by first distending the rectal balloon with 20 cubic centimeters of air, then maintaining the distension for 2 minutes, and increasing the distending volume by 20 cubic centimeters of arm a stepwise fashion up to 200 cubic centimeters. If the rectum is compliant, the rectal channel will show a drop in pressure following the initial pressure increase. However, there will not be a return to baseline until withdrawal of the air from the rectal balloon. If the rectum is noncompliant, rectal pressure will remain high, or there will be extreme variations in pressure that indicate rectal contraction.

"Paradoxical PFM contraction" refers to an abnormal pattern of sphincter contraction, rather than relaxation, during defecation attempts. This coordination deficit causes an outlet obstruction constipation and straining with stool. Failure to relax the sphincter during defecation should always be assessed when one is treating incontinence, because many patients become incontinent as a result of procedures done to correct the very complications that result from long-term constipation and inappropriate defecation patterns—for example, repair of *rectocele* or *prolapse*, as well as hemorrhoidectomy. Furthermore, chronic straining with stool causes PFM denervation that contributes to PFM weakness and incontinence. Therefore, patients presenting with incontinence can have both EAS weakness and a disordered defecation pattern, which prevent complete evacuation of stool with toileting. One symptom of incomplete evacuation is postdefecation seepage. (See Tries & Eisman, Chapter 28, this volume for a further discussion of paradoxical PFM contraction.)

The degree to which biofeedback will be successful often depends upon the degree to which the underlying physiology has been disrupted. When EAS strength is impaired but rectal sensation is adequate, biofeedback therapy is usually very effective if treatment is directed toward increasing EAS strength and endurance. If the sensory deficit is slight to moderate, rectal sensation often improves with therapy. Less notable outcomes are obtained in those patients who, after a bowel training program to keep the rectum empty, do not come to sense large volumes of rectal distension (e.g., 50 cubic centimeters). Individuals with inadequate IAS resting tone and an absent IAS inhibitory reflex may benefit from biofeedback therapy, but the outcomes are inconsistent. These patients may develop greater control over gross incontinence, but they may continue to have some seepage. Because biofeedback procedures do not directly influence the IAS, which is an involuntary muscle, improvement in patients with poor IAS resting tone is a function of increasing the tone and strength of the striated puborectalis muscle, which surrounds the IAS and contributes to the functional length of the anal canal. Improving puborectalis muscle strength may also improve sensitivity for rectal distension by improving the efficiency of the stretch response.

After a surgical reduction of the size of the rectum or where there is scare tissue, rectal compliance may not be significantly alterable. In this case, biofeedback may still improve continence by improving EAS strength to offset elevations in rectal pressure. If the noncompliance is physiological (e.g., rectal spasm), biofeedback may improve compliance as a result of greater rectal inhibition provided by a more effective EAS contraction.

In addition to the physiological deficits discussed above, incontinence may result from the following:

1. Decreased motivation to emit the EAS response (e.g., among senile, psychotic, or mentally retarded patients).
2. Chronic functional constipation that leads to overflow.
3. Functional diarrhea.

In these cases, habit training is the primary intervention.

TREATMENT

Treatment Providers

Biofeedback procedures for fecal incontinence involve minimal risk to the patient, but they are invasive. The therapist must be well trained to perform digital rectal examination, which is done as part of the assessment and before insertion of the rectal probes. Improper insertion of the Schuster balloon probe into a badly damaged rectum can perforate the rectal wall. Although this is unlikely, peritoneal infection can have severe consequences, including death. Also, fecal incontinence and associated bowel disorders exist concurrently with other medical disorders. Patients are often taking various medications that influence bowel function. Thus a biofeedback practitioner treating fecal incontinence must work closely with a physician.

The successful application of biofeedback for incontinence is highly dependent upon the knowledge and skill of the health care professional applying this therapy. This knowledge encompasses evaluation techniques; anatomical and physiological correlates of the types and symptoms of bowel dysfunction; instrumentation; and behavioral principles that guide the procedures.

Because most patients are embarrassed in the initial session and anxious about the procedures, a therapist must be quite sensitive to a patient's emotional needs. The rationale for the procedures should be explained in a clear and reassuring manner. The therapist should respect the patient's modesty by keeping the individual covered as much as possible. A bathroom adjoining the examination/treatment room provides privacy for patients to clean themselves and dress.

Because the causes of incontinence are often multifactorial, the more inclusive the measures and displays, the more comprehensive the treatment for the variations of symptom patterns. In our clinics, we require at least three surface electromyographic (EMG) channels for all patients with fecal incontinence, because we use the multiple electrode probe (MEP) and abdominal EMG recording sensors. In women, we also use an intravaginal probe in addition to the MEP, to obtain as complete an assessment as possible of PFM function. (See Figures 26.1, 26.2, and 26.3 in Tries & Eisman, Chapter 26, this volume). The MEP measures muscle activity at the distal EAS and also at the proximal anal canal, which reflects both deep EAS and puborectalis muscle activity. The intravaginal probe measures activity just above the urogenital diaphragm. Manometric equipment is used to test and train for rectal sensory deficits.

Whom to Treat?

It makes sense to provide biofeedback therapy to many patients with fecal incontinence even when the potential benefit is uncertain. Often there is significant functional improvement in a few sessions, especially if rectal sensitivity is disturbed and the patient responds initially to the sensory training described below. To be optimally effective, the treatment must become a problem-solving process that uses information gained from the physiological measures and the symptom diary to help patients generalize physiological changes into daily life.

The physicians who refer patients to our clinic will often use biofeedback before corrective surgery, because the treatment can improve anorectal function and therefore may improve surgical outcome. In addition to EAS strengthening, the biofeedback assessment can identify maladaptive habits such as paradoxical EAS contraction with defecation, which can be altered before surgery. Thus the beneficial effects of the surgical correction are not undone postsurgically.

Some patients, however, are not likely to benefit from biofeedback treatment. These include patients who have little or no motivation to achieve continence or who cannot follow directions—for example, patients with advanced dementia, psychosis, or severe mental retardation, as well as children under age 4. Other patients who may have limited improvement are those who, even after a bowel habit program to empty the rectum of stool, have a rectal sensory deficit of greater than 50 cubic centimeters.

BIOFEEDBACK PROCEDURES FOR BOWEL DYSFUNCTION

Functional Evaluation

After the patient's thorough medical exam, the practitioner or therapist undertakes a functional evaluation of the patient's bowel patterns and symptoms. A complete medical history of the patient should be obtained, including a detailed history of the incontinence problem (e.g., the onset of symptoms, a description of bowel patterns prior to the appearance of symptoms). The following questions should be included:

1. When was the onset of the incontinence, and what were the changes in bowel habits over the years?
2. What has been the duration of the fecal incontinence?
3. Were there any precipitating illnesses, surgery, or social/psychological issues associated with incontinence?
4. What is the frequency of bowel movements?
5. What size and consistency are the bowel movements?
6. Is it necessary to strain with a bowel movement? Is discomfort associated with the passage of stool?
7. Is there any feeling of incomplete evacuation? Is incomplete evacuation followed by incontinence?
8. What are the effects of various foods and other factors on bowel function?
9. Is there an urgent call to produce stool (i.e., the patient fears incontinence will occur if toileting is not immediate)?
10. What is the approximate time from this urge (if any) to accidental loss of stool?
11. What is the frequency of incontinent events? When the patient is incontinent, what amount and consistency of stool are produced? (The patient should be asked to distinguish stains from small amounts of stool, small amounts from large amounts, and liquid stool from solid stool.)
12. Can the patient control flatus? Can the patient pass flatus?
13. When do incontinent events occur? For example, do they occur after meals or following an incomplete evacuation? Are they nocturnal and/or diurnal?
14. What is the relationship of symptoms to diet or activity?
15. Is sensation for stool in the rectum blunted? Can the patient distinguish gas from stool?
16. What is the percentage of bowel movements controlled?
17. Are there factors that increase or decrease the likelihood of incontinence (e.g., type of activity, availability of restrooms, and anxiety)?
18. What type and number of protective pads are used?
19. What are the present medications?
20. Is assistance required to have bowel movements (i.e., laxatives, enemas, suppositories, or manual removal of stool from the rectum)?
21. Is pelvic or anal pain a problem?
22. Is there abdominal cramping? Is it associated with meals?
23. Does the patient have any bladder symptoms, such as incontinence, urgency, frequency, voiding hesitancy, or incomplete voiding?

The patient should be asked to articulate how the problem interferes with everyday life, interpersonal relationships, and self-concept. Also, the therapist should try to determine the degree to which emotional stress affects symptoms, without diminishing the effect of the physical etiology, even when that etiology is unclear. Patients must feel free to discuss the feelings of frustration and despair that are common among people with bowel disorders.

The patient should be instructed to complete a daily symptom diary. It should include bowel frequency; incontinence episodes; feelings of incomplete evacuation; stool consistency; strain or discomfort with passage of stool; use of enemas or laxatives; and other significant information related to the patient's complaints. Ideally, the patient completes the diary for about

1 week before the initial physical evaluation and during the entire treatment. The diary documents subtle changes that guide the treatment, and thus helps maintain the patient's motivation. Analyzing the diary with the patient during each office session impresses the patient with the importance of keeping the diary.

Physical Evaluation

The physical evaluation includes a digital exam and EMG of the anal canal and abdominal muscles. It may also include manometric evaluation of the anus and rectum, to assess rectal sensitivity and IAS and EAS function; this is discussed separately below.

Digital Exam

Before the manometric exam, a digital rectal exam is necessary to assess the following:

1. The EAS and IAS resting tone, felt as resistance to the finger during insertion.
2. The EAS contraction strength around the finger when the patient is instructed to squeeze.
3. The strength of the contraction of the puborectalis sling muscle when the patient is instructed to squeeze.
4. The presence of any discomfort when the puborectalis muscle is stretched posteriorly toward the coccyx. (Discomfort with this stretch may indicate excessive muscle tone, spasm, or trigger points.)
5. The size of the rectal ampulla. (Excess dilation of the rectum beyond the normal dilated state, or megarectum, suggests chronic constipation.)
6. The presence of stool in the rectum. (In a normally functioning bowel, the rectum is empty. The presence of stool suggests constipation or incomplete evacuation.)
7. The presence of strictures or scarring that may inhibit the passage of stool or limit rectal compliance.

EMG Assessment

In our clinics, we generally assess PFM function with EMG prior to the manometric assessment. The MEP (see Figure 26.2 in Chapter 26) is used for all assessments of anal canal function, because it differentiates muscle activity at the distal anal canal from the proximal portion of the anal canal. Obtaining measures from two different sites within the anal canal is useful when one is training patients to recruit muscles specifically from the weakest area. The MEP is also useful when relaxation needs to be reinforced in a specific area of the PFMs that may have become hypertonic to compensate for a weaker area. The development of such hypertonicity can contribute to a disordered defecation pattern or to *levator syndromes*, and will limit the effectiveness of the strength training if not resolved. EMG probes with a single pair of longitudinally placed electrodes summate activity across the entire length of the anal canal, and therefore cannot be used for such specific training. The smaller size of the MEP makes it more readily accepted by pediatric patients and parents. In women, the small intravaginal EMG probe (Figure 26.1) is used simultaneously with the MEP, because fecal incontinence is often associated with PFM partial denervation injury. Moreover, most women referred with fecal incontinence also have urinary incontinence. Thus we use four EMG channels to assess PFM function in women: abdominal, distal anal canal, proximal anal canal, and intravaginal EMG measures. (See Figure 26.3. See Chapter 26 for the EMG PFM assessment protocol.)

The Manometric Assessment

The manometric evaluation assesses rectal sensitivity and the functional integrity of the anal canal. These characteristics cannot be determined with EMG measures of strength. Accordingly, manometric testing is an important part of the assessment and treatment of fecal incontinence. This chapter only discusses the use of the pneumatic Schuster probe. However, a perfusion catheter system can also be used for manometry and biofeedback.

Insertion of the Schuster Probe

A condom placed over the Schuster balloon probe eases its cleaning. The condom covers the balloon with considerable slack over the balloon system, and the base of the condom just covers the T-handle. This allows advancement of the rectal balloon to about 10 centimeters above the base of the EAS balloon. It is helpful to mark the rectal tube where it should line up with the base of the cylinder. This helps assure sufficient insertion into the rectum.

The balloons should be deflated before insertion, and the three-chamber assembly should be lubricated well. First, the therapist should dilate the opening of the anal canal with a lubricated index finger. (This is a good time to conduct the full digital exam and helps the therapist visualize the anorectal angle during the balloon insertion.) With the other hand, the therapist should begin to insert the rectal balloon. With the tip of the rectal balloon, some pressure should be placed against the dilating finger. In this way, the therapist eases the rectal portion of the probe into the anal canal while it is dilated.

Once the rectal portion of the balloon is inserted, the therapist should remove the dilating finger and grasp the T-handle with the same hand, then guide the passage of the cylinder into the canal. The anorectal angle bends posteriorly. Thus the direction of the insertion pressure may change from rostral to slightly posterior as the rectal balloon passes above the puborectalis muscle. Only one-third to one-fourth of the EAS balloon is visible with a properly placed Schuster probe. Figure 27.2 shows proper placement.

With the apparatus held to prevent it from slipping, the therapist should inject 10 cubic centimeters of air into the IAS balloon. Inflation should produce a slight inward tug on the cylinder. The therapist should then place 10 cubic centimeters of air in the rectal balloon, and then inflate the EAS balloon with 10 cubic centimeters of air. Potential difficulties include the following:

1. If the rectum is full of firm stool, it may be difficult or impossible to advance the rectal balloon.

2. If the rectal balloon does not inflate or does so only with difficulty, the therapist should check for a bent tube or look to see whether the tube moved back into the cylinder.

3. If the patient has a wide anal opening, the balloon apparatus may repeatedly slip out despite proper placement and inflation. The therapist can hold the device in place by taping the crossbar of the cylinder to the patient's buttocks. However, this will probably amplify the size of the EAS responses, because contractions of the gluteal muscles exert more pressure on a taped EAS balloon.

4. When the puborectalis is in spasm, passage of the probe into the canal may be uncomfortable. If discomfort persists, it may not be possible to continue with the examination. In this event, the therapist must use an EMG probe without a retaining bulb (e.g., the MEP) initially, until the patient learns to relax the spasm.

5. Where there is considerable scar tissue or irritability of the rectal wall, there also may be discomfort. This leads to false measurements. If this occurs, the therapist should use less

than the 10-cubic-centimeter inflation bolus to set the balloons. Obviously, the alteration in the standard preparation should be noted.

The Assessment Itself

Manometric examination provides the following information:

1. The threshold of rectal sensation. This is 10–15 cubic centimeters for normal individuals.

2. The presence or absence of the IAS inhibitory reflex.

3. The integrity of the rectosphincteric response to rectal distension. The rectosphincteric response is an automatic EAS contraction that occurs when the rectum is distended. Normal persons show some EAS contraction in response to rectal distension even without instructions to squeeze. They also exhibit larger EAS responses with larger distending volumes.

4. The threshold for the IAS inhibitory reflex and the EAS response. In normal individuals, both should occur with distension of 10–15 cubic centimeters.

5. The timing of the IAS reflex and the EAS response. Both responses should occur immediately after rectal distension, although the IAS takes several seconds to reach its maximum inhibition. The normal inhibitory response lasts for 5–20 seconds after the rectal stimulus. The time depends upon the size of the stimulus. The greater the stimulus, the longer the inhibition reflex. In contrast, the EAS response reaches its maximum contraction within 1 second of the rectal stimulus.

6. The maximum VS pressure recorded from the EAS when the patient is instructed to squeeze without rectal distension. This is greater than 20 millimeters of mercury for normal subjects.

7. The degree to which there is a maladaptive increase in intra-abdominal pressure during sphincter contraction.

Examples of abnormal sphincter responses are shown in Figure 27.4. Compare these with the normal responses illustrated in Figure 27.3.

The manometric assessment is conducted as follows. The therapist/examiner should tell the patient that during the evaluation, small amounts of air will be put into the rectal balloon and immediately withdrawn. During the assessment, the patient's eyes are closed or the recording display is blocked from the patient's view. Also, the rectal balloon is inflated out of the patient's sight.

To demonstrate the procedure, the examiner should inflate the rectal balloon with a bolus of air—usually starting with 30–50 milliliters of air, and progressing up to 150 milliliters if the patient is not sensitive to the initial inflation. The examiner should instruct the patient as follows: Each time air is put into the rectal balloon, the examiner will ask, "Did you feel that?" However, there will also be times when the therapist will not inflate the rectal balloon and will still ask, "Did you feel that?" These "catch" trials control for the tendency to respond to the demand characteristics of the test rather than to the actual stimulus.

After asking the patient to close his or her eyes, the examiner administers rectal distension trials in a descending order of 50, 40, 30, 20, 15, 10, and 5 milliliters. After each distension, the air is withdrawn immediately, except for the initial 10 milliliters used to position the balloon. The examiner should wait until the pressures return to baseline before giving the next distension (about 30 seconds). The absolute sensory threshold is the lowest volume of air the patient perceives in three consecutive trials. Pressure changes in response to each distension should be examined. The sensory threshold is associated with the amplitude of rectosphincteric response

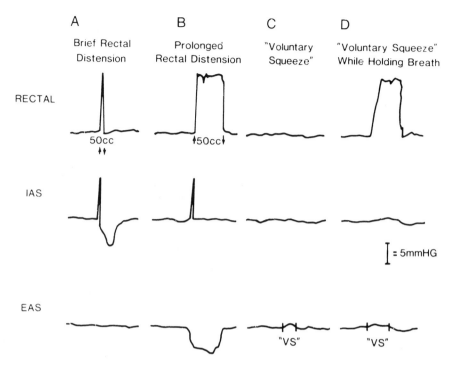

FIGURE 27.4. Sample polygraph records showing abnormal anal sphincter responses. (A) No EAS response, due to either inability to sense rectal distension or impairment of the sphincter muscle. Normal IAS relaxation response. (B) Decreased EAS pressure, due to patient's bearing down, instead of contracting the sphincter. No IAS relaxation. (Both may also occur with brief rectal distention and need not occur together.) (C) Very weak EAS contraction, due to impaired sphincter strength (may occur with or without rectal distension). (D) Very weak EAS contraction, due to either impaired sphincter strength, excessive abdominal pressure, or both.

and the amplitude and recovery of the inhibitory IAS reflex. The examiner should note and record both verbal and recorded response delays. Next, the voluntary motor response to rectal distension is observed. Here, the examiner injects an air into the rectal balloon without visual or verbal feedback to the patient. The patient is instructed to squeeze the anal sphincter when feeling this stimulus, as if trying to prevent loss of stool or flatus. The following are noted: response time, amplitude, and endurance of the EAS contraction; increases in intra-abdominal pressure; and recovery time of the IAS inhibitory response.

Next, the examiner measures the EAS maximum VS pressures over an extended contraction while the patient contracts the EAS as if trying to stop a bowel movement or the loss of flatus. As with EMG, the direction to "contract as hard as you can" should be avoided. The examiner should ask for a 10-second contraction, then have the patient rest for about 30 seconds, and repeat the contraction for one to two more trials.

In a normal manometric record, a rectal distension of 10 milliliters results in an immediate EAS contraction but IAS relaxation. The amplitude of these responses is proportionate to the volume of air inflated into the rectal balloon. The normal sensory threshold to rectal distension above an initial 10-milliliter baseline volume is in the range of 5–15 milliliters.

Guidelines to Interpret Manometric Recordings

1. The therapist should examine the tracing and compare the size, timing, and threshold of the patient's responses to normal responses.

2. If the IAS relaxation reflex is absent and the IAS resting tone is normal, it may suggest Hirschsprung's disease. However, an absent or attenuated IAS inhibitory response may result from a *nonrelaxing puborectalis muscle* that surrounds the IAS. A nonrelaxing puborectalis can mask an IAS inhibitory response because it can maintain the anal canal in a rigid, tube-like state that keeps anal pressure stable. A therapist who suspects this problem should help the patient relax and repeat the assessment. However, the nonrelaxing puborectalis muscle may be a contributor to the patient's symptoms. If this is the case, the therapist will need to address this with specific behavioral strategies.

3. The therapist should compare the rectosphincteric response to the maximum voluntary squeeze. They should be similar in amplitude. An attenuated rectosphincteric response may result from impaired sensation or low resting tone, which may decrease the stretch receptor afferent activity normally activated with distension.

4. If there is a pressure decrease in the EAS when the patient is instructed to squeeze, the patient is probably "bearing down," as is often done in defecation. Children often confuse this response with sphincter contraction.

5. If rectal pressure increases during a voluntary EAS contraction, the patient is probably increasing intra-abdominal pressure by breath holding or abdominal contraction. This maladaptive pattern is one of defecation rather than storage.

Patients with bowel dysfunction frequently show the following irregularities in their EMG and manometric records. Patients with incontinence frequently display distal and proximal anal canal EMG contraction measures that are of low amplitude and limited endurance over 10 seconds. Moreover, incontinent patients usually co-contract the abdominal and/or gluteal muscles when asked to contract the anal sphincter. When patients are asked to decrease abdominal co-contraction, a considerable decreases in EAS contraction measures are noted, indicating an inability to selectively contract the EAS. With urgency, this abdominal contraction increases intra-abdominal and rectal pressure. When the EAS is weak, an increase in intra-abdominal pressure is not offset with an adequate anal canal pressure. Thus incontinence is more likely to occur.

Patients who report having stool urgency and little warning for incontinence often show a high sensory threshold or a delayed EAS response for rectal distension. Improving rectal sensitivity is a primary biofeedback goal in this case. However, an urgent call to produce stool can also occur when rectal sensation is normal. In this case, urgency seems more a function of weak PFM efferent and afferent activity, and is associated with a attenuated or absent rectosphincteric response to distension on manometry and unstable EMG measures during sustained EAS contraction. PFM retraining often reduces bowel urgency in these patients.

Frequently, patients who report feelings of incomplete evacuation show an elevated resting EMG baseline. With the defecation maneuver, one often sees in the EAS measure either a paradoxical PFM contraction or a failure to relax. As noted earlier, the term for an inappropriate increase in muscle activity during defecation is "paradoxical PFM contraction." The term "failure to relax" is operative when muscle activity does not drop below baseline during defecation. One sees these abnormal coordination patterns in patients with outlet obstruction associated with constipation (see Chapter 28). Since many patients with fecal incontinence also have symptoms of outlet obstruction (incomplete evacuation followed by fecal seepage), paradoxical EAS activity with evacuation maneuvers should be reduced to assure optimal treatment outcome. Some patients also have difficulty appropriately raising intra-abdominal pressure with the defecation pattern. This dysfunction is seen with patients who, through maturational delays, congenital deformity, or maladaptive learning, never learned appropriate defecation patterns. Excessive EMG activity at rest also occurs in levator ani syndrome. This is a condition caused by spasm in the levator ani muscle, which produces pain and discomfort in the anal canal and pelvic floor.

BIOFEEDBACK TREATMENT GOALS

After the physiological abnormalities are identified, specific biofeedback goals for bowel dysfunction usually include shaping the following responses:

1. Selective PFM and EAS contractions of greater amplitude and duration without abdominal and/or gluteal contraction, and associated elevations in intra-abdominal pressure.
2. EAS contractions with short response latencies and with immediate recovery to baseline after voluntary contraction ceases.
3. Heightened perception to lower levels of rectal distension, paired with immediate EAS contraction and IAS inhibition.
4. PFM relaxation below resting baseline, which is concurrent with appropriate increases in intra-abdominal pressure during the defecation maneuver.
5. Reduction of elevated PFM and EAS activity, when present.

Shaping Specific Responses

Before treatment, the therapist should explain to the patient the anatomy and physiology of bowel control, stressing the interaction of PFM and colonic activity. This information should be integrated with the patient's physiological measures as they relate to the patient's bowel function.

Training Selective Sphincter Contractions

With EAS weakness or an attenuated rectosphincteric response to rectal distension, treatment should reinforce selective EAS recruitment without abdominal co-contraction or increases in intra-abdominal pressure. Such specific reinforcement is necessary, because when EAS contraction is weak, there is little proprioceptive feedback for its recruitment. Therefore, the patient may unknowingly substitute contraction of ineffective muscles for attempts at EAS contraction. The substitution limits the activation of the weak EAS, and hence it is poorly strengthened.

For guidelines to systematically shaping selective PFM recruitment, see Chapter 26. Manometry can also be used for PFM reeducation, with EAS pressure measures serving as feedback for selective PFM while intra-abdominal pressure is kept stable.

Improving Sensory Response Patterns with Rectal Distension

Manometry is used to train perception for, and the EAS response to, rectal distension. In our clinics, manometric training usually follows selective PFM contraction. To begin training, the therapist should inject a bolus of air into the rectal balloon that is of a volume that the patient perceived during the evaluation. The therapist should then immediately withdraw the air and explain the EAS and IAS responses, with the patient observing the display. The inflation is then repeated, with the patient contracting the EAS immediately following the stimulus. If abdominal pressure increases with the EAS contraction, the patient should be reminded to keep the abdominal muscles relaxed. The therapist should instruct the patient (1) to try to perceive the rectal stimulus and associate its sensation with the visual feedback and the EAS contraction, and (2) to limit any delay in the EAS response to the distension stimulus.

After the patient can immediately contract the EAS after rectal distension, the air stimulus should be given over several trials while the patient's eyes are closed. The patient should look at the display immediately after the contraction, to observe the accuracy of the response. If the patient's performance during the eyes-closed trials is equivalent to that during the biofeedback trial, the therapist should decrease the volume of rectal distension, repeating the sequence with incremental reductions down to a 5- to 10-milliliter inflation. If, in the stepwise reduction of the inflation volume, the EAS responses decay, the biofeedback trials should be repeated at the same volume.

Relaxation Therapy

With an urge to evacuate, patients often become anxious and panic—increasing the probability of incontinence, because intra-abdominal pressure increases with such anxiety. To cope, a patient should be instructed to stop activity; stand still or sit if possible; relax; and breathe in a slow, deep, rhythmic manner, using the diaphragm (see Gevirtz & Schwartz, Chapter 10, this volume). While maintaining overall body relaxation, the patient should contract the EAS selectively, to increase resistance to fecal loss and inhibit colonic activity.

In our clinic, we find that when we are measuring from three PFM sites simultaneously in women (distal anal canal, proximal anal canal and intravaginal), weakness is often noted at one recording site, but hypertonic activity is seen at the other sites. We postulate that the hypertonicity at one part of the pelvic floor is a muscle compensation response for reduced support that occurs as a result of muscle weakness at another site. We also observe that many patients with fecal incontinence show an evacuation disorder, as evidenced by paradoxical PFM contraction with evacuation maneuvers. This abnormal pattern is associated with incomplete evacuation of stool from the rectum, followed by seepage. Therefore, for biofeedback protocols to be optimally effective for those with fecal incontinence, therapy must address the hypertonicity and the associated defecation dysfunction as well as EAS weakness. We discuss these techniques in detail in Chapter 28.

Adjunctive Behavioral Procedures

Modifications in diet and bowel habits can reduce many bowel symptoms and should be implemented before biofeedback treatment begins. Research suggests that a bowel training program may contribute as much as, or more than, biofeedback therapy to the successful outcomes achieved in children with meningiomyelocele (Whitehead et al., 1982). In the initial session, the therapist should review the importance of dietary fiber and provide written guidelines regarding recommended intake and sources of dietary fiber. When stool is very loose or liquid, we often have patients increase dietary fiber by adding wheat bran to the daily diet, if a bulking agent like Metamucil is not already being used. Bran can be added to the diet slowly, starting with just 1 teaspoon a day and increasing the amount every 3 days until stool becomes a soft but formed in consistency. Bran is inexpensive, and its intake can be systematically controlled. Patients should be advised to limit foods high in fat, and the possibility of lactose intolerance should be explored. If bowel frequency with liquid stool continues, an antidiarrheal medication might be tried. Because these medicines slow colon transit time, their use is contraindicated when incontinence is associated with an impaction or incomplete evacuation.

If constipation contributes to overflow incontinence and seepage (i.e., encopresis), a bowel training program is necessary. The patient is instructed to attempt evacuation about 10–20 minutes after a meal at the same time every day, to take advantage of the *gastrocolic reflex*. The ideal time for many people to attempt evacuation is after breakfast, because the colon seems to be more active shortly after awakening. However, analysis of the symptom diary may suggest a different pattern of colonic excitability. If a bowel movement does not occur for 2 consecutive days, the patient should use an enema at the time of attempted evacuation. The patient may need stronger stimulants, such as suppositories or laxatives, to establish regular bowel patterns. However, the therapist should wean the patient from these as soon as possible. Most stool normalizers, bulk agents, and some antidiarrheal medications are nonprescription items. Nevertheless, it is a good idea to consult the patient's physician about altering their use. See Lowery, Srour, Whitehead, and Schuster (1985) and Doleys, Schwartz, and Ciminero (1981) for further information on bowel training.

The emotional and psychological benefits of exercise warrant its inclusion in a treatment program, although there is little consensus as to its effect on bowel function. For those patients who have not been on a regular exercise program and have their doctor's approval, a walking program is advantageous. It requires no specific equipment, can easily be modified to a patient's tolerance, and performance can be objectively measured by time and distance walked.

THE HOME PROGRAM

Compliance with a home program is the best predictor of success in behavioral treatment for incontinence (Millard & Oldenburg, 1983). Therefore, provision for, and compliance with, the home program are essential for the successful outcome of a biofeedback treatment.

Instruct patients to maintain a written log of the time of day for all bowel movements and incontinent episodes as an integral part of the treatment. Information such as the use of laxatives, suppositories, enemas, and sphincter exercises should also be recorded.

Daily PFM and EAS exercises are assigned to nearly all patients seen for bowel dysfunction to improve EAS coordination, strength, and endurance. (See Chapter 26.) For patients with PFM hypertonicity, practicing daily PFM exercises helps them discriminate elevated PFM activity so that when this is perceived, the patients can attempt to reduce the activity toward more normal resting levels. (See Chapter 28.)

In addition to the PFM exercises discussed in Chapter 26, patients with delayed or weak EAS responses to rectal distension should be instructed to contract the EAS when they feel any stimulus in the rectum. This conditions the automatic EAS response to rectal distension.

CLOSING REMARKS

Fecal incontinence is a troubling problem that affects many individuals and causes serious disruption in work and social activities. Furthermore, a considerable number of patients complain of both fecal and urinary incontinence. One reason this occurs is that these conditions often share the etiology of partial denervation injury at childbirth. Also, many patients complain of concurrent symptoms of disordered defecation patterns, constipation, and pelvic pain. Therefore, a clinician working in this area should be prepared to deal with the multifactorial nature of fecal incontinence and should understand, in a comprehensive way, the various functions of the pelvic floor and other factors that influence bowel function. We hope that this chapter has contributed, to some degree, to the development of such understanding.

GLOSSARY

ANAL SPHINCTERS, EXTERNAL (EAS) AND INTERNAL (IAS). The anal canal is surrounded by a voluntary or *external and sphincter (EAS)* and an involuntary or *internal anal sphincter (IAS)*. The IAS is continuous with the circular muscle layer of the colon and surrounds the superior two-thirds of the canal. The EAS blends with the puborectalis component of the *levator ani muscle* (see below) and surrounds the inferior two-thirds of the canal, external to the IAS. Nonsynchronous function of these muscles contributes to the gamut of gastrointestinal disorders, including constipation, incontinence, hemorrhoids, fistula, *prolapse*, and the like.

ANORECTAL MANOMETRY. The integrity of the anorectal muscles can be evaluated via electromyography (EMG), functionally (by how much fluid can be instilled into the rectum before leakage occurs), or manometrically (by how much pressure can be generated within the anal canal and rectum). Pressure may be measured by using a three-balloon system, commonly referred to as the "Schuster balloons," or through use of a water perfusion catheter. Changes in balloon pressure can be displayed on a computer screen and used, for example, in a biofeedback program for strengthening the EAS, to promote relaxation in the treatment of levator ani syndrome, or to improve rectal sensitivity.

GASTROCOLIC REFLEX. The increase in colonic activity that usually occurs approximately 30 minutes after a meal. Constipated patients may be advised to develop a pattern of toileting to coincide with this increased activity.

IAS INHIBITORY REFLEX. Distension of the rectum with a balloon causes relaxation (inhibition) of the IAS and contraction of the EAS. Inhibition of the IAS is an unconditioned reflex mediated by afferent impulses from stretch receptors in the walls of the rectum and, probably, in the levator plate. This reflex can occur without awareness (e.g., following spinal transection). The EAS contraction, although seemingly automatic, is a learned response that is mediated through the spinal cord and, as a consequence, disappears when the sensory component is compromised.

LEVATOR ANI MUSCLE. A large, thin sheet of muscle that forms the pelvic floor. It has three components, called the pubococcygeus, puborectalis, and iliococcygeus muscles. See the glossary in Tries and Eisman, Chapter 26, this volume, for further details.

LEVATOR SYNDROMES. A number of conditions (including proctalgia fugax, levator spasm, levator ani syndrome, and coccygodynia) characterized by different patterns of idiopathic pain in the anal and perianal regions. The pain may radiate down the legs, into the buttocks, or to the coccygeal region. These conditions are defined by exclusion because they are not referrable to any of the common disorders, such as anal fistula, abscess, hemorrhoids, or the like. There is some agreement that the underlying problem involves muscle spasm of the levator ani's component muscles. In certain cases, pelvic floor muscle (PFM) EMG values are elevated, and biofeedback directed toward normalizing function in these muscles has been successful.

NONRELAXING PUBORECTALIS MUSCLE. The contraction of the puborectalis muscle forms the acute angle between the rectum and the anal canal, and prevents the movement of material out of the rectum to maintain fecal continence. With defecation, the muscle must relax; this allows the anorectal angle to become obtuse, thereby permitting the effortless expulsion of stool. A *nonrelaxing puborectalis muscle* is one that does not relax during defecation. In many cases, this problem can be treated with biofeedback techniques.

PROLAPSE. A general term meaning "to move forward, down, or out," and subsuming several specific terms that end in "-cele" (e.g., *rectocele*, as well as "cystocele" and "enterocele"). *Rectal prolapse* is the term used to describe the condition in which the rectum moves down the anal canal. On the other hand, *rectocele* (see below) is the term used to describe the condition in which the rectum protrudes into the vagina. The severity of the condition is graded numerically; for example, a fourth-degree rectal prolapse refers to the condition in which the rectum protrudes from the anal canal.

RECTAL COMPLIANCE. When the compliant rectum is distended with a balloon or by its normal contents, there is a momentary increase in pressure; twitch diminishes rapidly as the smooth muscle relaxes to accommodate the increased volume. As the volume of material increases, the ability to accommodate it is reduced, giving rise to the feeling of urgency and the desire to defecate. However, contraction of the voluntary EAS inhibits contraction of the smooth muscle in the rectum, reducing the sense of urgency, which allows defecation to be postponed to convenient time.

RECTOCELE. The posterior wall of the vagina and the anterior wall of the rectum are in close apposition; as a result of certain poorly understood predisposing factors, the rectum may protrude into the vagina, forming a *rectocele*. The defect may be large or small, apparent only during straining, or present as a chronic condition.

STRETCH RESPONSE. A two-neuron response in which afferent activity generated by the stretching of a muscle enters the spinal cord and synapses directly with the efferent neurons to that same muscle, causing compensatory contraction or shortening of the muscle. Because only a single synapse is involved, the response occurs with a short latency.

REFERENCES

Allen, R. E., Hosker, G. L., Smith, A. R. B., & Warrell, D. W. (1990). Pelvic floor damage and childbirth: A neurophysiological study. *British Journal of Obstetrics and Gynaecology, 97,* 770–779.

Bower, G. H., & Hilgard, E. R. (1981). *Theories of learning* (5th ed.). Englewood Cliffs, NJ: Prentice-Hall.

Buser, W. D., & Miner, P. B. (1986). Delayed rectal sensation with fecal incontinence: Successful treatment using anorectal manometry. *Gastroenterology, 91,* 1186–1191.

Cerulli, M. A., Nikoomanesh, P., & Schuster, M. M. (1979). Progress in biofeedback conditioning for fecal incontinence. *Gastroenterology, 76,* 742–746.

Chiarioni, G., Scattolini, C., Bonfante, F., & Vantini, I. (1993). Liquid stool incontinence with severe urgency: anorectal function and effective biofeedback treatment. *Gut, 34,* 1576–1580.

Doleys, D., Schwartz, M. S., & Ciminero, A. (1981). Enuresis and encopresis. In E. J. Mash & L. G. Terdal (Eds.), *Behavioral assessment of childhood disorders*. New York: Guilford Press.

Enck, P. (1993). Biofeedback training in disordered defecation: A critical review. *Digestive Diseases and Sciences, 38,* 1953–1960.

Engel, B. T., Nikoomanesh, P., & Schuster, M. M. (1974). Operant conditioning of rectosphincteric responses in the treatment of fecal incontinence. *New England Journal of Medicine, 290,* 646–649.

Glia, A., Gylin, M., Akerlund, J. E., Lindfors, U., & Lindberg, G. (1998). Biofeedback training in patients with fecal incontinence. *Diseases of the Colon and Rectum, 41,* 359–364.

Goldenberg, D. A., Hodges, K., Hersh, T., & Jinich, H. (1980). Biofeedback therapy for fecal incontinence. *American Journal of Gastroenterology, 74,* 342–345.

Henry, M. M., & Swash, M. (1985). Fecal incontinence, defecation and colorectal motility. In M. M. Henry & M. Swash (Eds.), *Coloproctology and the pelvic floor: Pathophysiology and management*. London: Butterworths.

Heyman, S., Jones, K. R., Ringel, Y., Scarlett, Y., & Whitehead, W. E. (2001). Biofeedback treatment of fecal incontinence: A critical review. *Diseases of the Colon and Rectum, 44,* 728–736.

Heyman, S., Pikarsky, A. J., Weiss, E. G., Vickers, D., Norgueras, J. J., & Wexner, S. D. (2000). A prospective randomized trial comparing four biofeedback techniques for patients with faecal incontinence. *Colorectal Disease, 2,* 88–92.

Kohlenberg, J. R. (1973). Operant conditioning of human anal sphincter pressure. *Journal of Applied Behavioral Analysis, 6,* 201–208.

Latimer, P. R., Campbell, D., & Kasperski, J. (1984). A component analysis of biofeedback in the management of fecal incontinence. *Biofeedback and Self-Regulation, 9,* 311–324.

Loening-Baucke, V. (1990). Efficacy of biofeedback in improving fecal incontinence and anorectal physiologic function. *Gut, 31,* 395–402.

Lowery, S. P., Srour, J. W., Whitehead, W. E., & Schuster, M. M. (1985). Habit training as treatment of encopresis secondary to chronic constipation. *Journal of Pediatric Gastroenterology and Nutrition, 4,* 397–401.

MacLeod, J. H. (1987). Management of anal incontinence by biofeedback. *Gastroenterology, 93,* 291–294.

Madoff, R. D., Williams, J. G., & Caushaj, P. J. (1992). Fecal incontinence. *New England Journal of Medicine, 326,* 1002–1007.

Millard, R. J., & Oldenburg, B. P. (1983). The symptomatic, urodynamic and psychodynamic results of bladder re-education programs. *Journal of Urology, 130,* 715–719.

Miller, N. E. (1978). Biofeedback and visceral learning. *Annual Review of Psychology, 29,* 373–404.

Miller, N. E., & DiCara, L. V. (1967). Instrumental learning of heart rate changes in curarized rats: Shaping and specificity to discriminative stimuli. *Journal of Comparative and Physiological Psychology, 63,* 12–19.

Miner, P. B., Donnelly, T. C., & Read, N. W. (1990). Investigation of the mode of action of biofeedback in the treatment of fecal incontinence. *Digestive Diseases and Sciences, 35,* 1291–1298.

Moore, K. L. (1992). *Clinically oriented anatomy* (3rd ed.). Baltimore: Williams & Wilkins.

Netter, F. H. (1989). *Atlas of human anatomy*. Summit, NJ: CibaGeigy.

Norton, C., Hosker, G., & Brazelli, M. (2000). Biofeedback and/or sphincter exercises for the treatment of faecal incontinence in adults. *Cochrane Electronic Library, 1,* CD002111.

Rao, S. S., Welcher, K. D., & Happel, J. (1996). Can biofeedback therapy improve anorectal function in fecal incontinence? *American Journal of Gastroenterology, 91,* 2360–2366.

Riboli, F. B., Frascio, M., Pitto, G., Reboa, G., & Zanolla, R. (1988). Biofeedback conditioning for fecal incontinence. *Archives of Physical Medicine and Rehabilitation*, 69, 29–31.

Schiller, L. R., Santa Ana, C., Davis, G. R., & Fordtran, J. S. (1979). Fecal incontinence in chronic diarrhea: Report of a case with improvement after training with rectally infused saline. *Gastroenterology*, 77, 571–753.

Schuster, M. M., Hookman, P., Hendrix, T., & Mendeloff, A. (1965). Simultaneous manometric recording of internal and external anal sphincter reflexes. *Bulletin of the Johns Hopkins Hospital*, 116, 79–88.

Tries, J. (2000). *Biofeedback measures of pelvic floor muscle function in asymptomatic and incontinent women.* Unpublished doctoral dissertation. Marquette University.

Wald, A. (1981a). Biofeedback therapy of fecal incontinence. *Annals of Internal Medicine*, 95, 146–149.

Wald, A. (1981b). Use of biofeedback in treatment of fecal incontinence in patients with meningomyeloccle. *Pediatrics*, 68, 45–49.

Whitehead, W. E., Burgio, K. L., & Engel, B. T. (1985). Biofeedback treatment of fecal incontinence in geriatric patients. *Journal of the American Geriatrics Society*, 33, 320–324.

Whitehead, W. E., Orr, W. C. Engel, B. T., & Schuster, M. M. (1981). External anal sphincter response to rectal distension: Learned response or reflex. *Psychophysiology*, 19, 57–62.

Whitehead, W. E., Parker, L. H., Bosmajian, L. S., Morrell, E. D., Middaugh, S., Drescher, V. M., Cataldo, M. F., & Freeman, J. M. (1982). Behavioral treatment of fecal incontinence secondary to spina bifida [Abstract]. *Gastroenterology*, 82, 1209.

The Use of Biofeedback for Pelvic Floor Disorders Associated with a Failure to Relax

JEANNETTE TRIES
EUGENE EISMAN

To a considerable degree, the pelvic floor muscles (PFMs) mediate bowel, bladder, and sexual activity. In Chapters 26 and 27, we have discussed the role of the PFMs in preserving continence. The biofeedback techniques described in those chapters improve continence mainly by improving PFM coordination and strength. However, disruption of PFM function can lead to symptoms other than incontinence, which is narrowly defined as the unwanted loss of urine or stool. This chapter is intended to outline some biofeedback applications for PFM dysfunction other than those directed toward improving strength. However, the reader should understand that more often than not, disorders of PFM function overlap. Undoubtedly, techniques discussed in this chapter will be used with those outlined in Chapters 26 and 27, when therapists treat incontinent patients. Conversely, therapists treating disorders discussed in this chapter will also use the PFM strengthening techniques outlined in the previous chapters.

A REVIEW OF PELVIC FLOOR ANATOMY

We begin with a brief review of pelvic floor anatomy (largely in women, since the great majority of patients treated for the disorders described in this chapter are female). In the earlier chapters, we have defined the PFMs as a group of muscles that span the inferior, or underlying, surface of the bony pelvis. The PFMs include the deeper muscular body of the levator ani, which is pierced by the urethra, the anal canal, and the vagina, and gives off fibers that interdigitate with the muscular and fascial fibers surrounding each orifice and its associated organ structure (i.e., the bladder neck and distal portion of the rectum). Peripheral to the levator ani is the diamond-shaped perineum, which can be divided into two triangular parts by a line between the ischial tuberosities. The divisions of the perineum are called the urogenital diaphragm, located anteriorly, and the anal triangle, which is posterior to the ischial tuberosities. The superficial transverse perinei, the bulbocavernosus and ischiocavernosus muscles, are located within the superficial compartment of the urogenital diaphragm; they function to stabilize and compress the vaginal opening and erectile tissue. The deep perineal compartment of the urogenital diaphragm contains the deep dorsal vein and the dorsal nerves, arteries, and veins to the clitoris. The muscular components of the deeper urogenital diaphragm include the transversus vaginae muscles. The external anal sphincter (EAS) is located within the anal triangle and is peripheral to the levator ani. See Figure 28.1 and Retzky, Rogers, and Richardson (1996) for an excellent summary of female pelvic floor anatomy.

The various muscles within the pelvic floor and perineum function both synchronously and asynchronously, depending upon the activity performed. For example, it is abnormal to urinate and defecate at the same time. Therefore, with urination, the EAS remains contracted to maintain closure pressure at the anal canal, while the anterior portions of the PFMs and the urethral sphincter relax in order for the bladder neck to drop, funnel, and open. Yet, as a group, the PFMs contract in concert to offset sudden increases in intra-abdominal pressure such as coughing.

At rest, when the rectum and bladder are relatively empty, the PFMs remain slightly contracted as a result of a small amount of alpha motor neuronal activity. This activity provides resting tone to the pelvic floor, which supports the visceral structures and maintains closure pressure at the urethra and anal canal. As the volume in the rectum or bladder increases, the PFMs gradually become more active to maintain positive closure pressure at the urethra or anal canal. Increased PFM efferent activity is also associated with greater afferent activity, which inhibits smooth colorectal or bladder muscle through sacral and suprasacral reflex loops. The inhibition of the smooth bladder and colorectal muscle allows for the accommodation of urine or stool during the storage phase.

Conversely, when evacuation or urination is desired, there is a precipitous drop in PFM activity at the respective area. This relaxation allows the angle at either the vesicle neck or

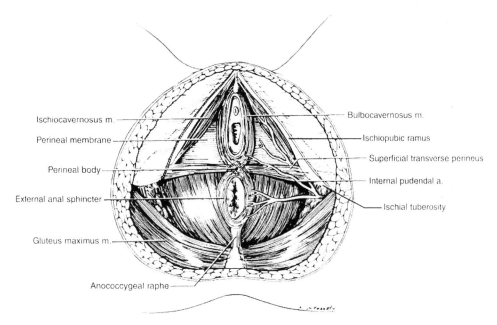

FIGURE 28.1. An inferior view of the female pelvic floor through the anal triangle. The superficial compartment of the urogenital triangle surrounds the vagina and the urethra. From Retzky, Rogers, and Richardson (1996, p. 13).

the anorectum to straighten, resulting in dilation of the urethra or anal canal. Urethra or anal canal pressure drops, reducing resistance to passage of urine or stool. PFM relaxation is associated with reduction in pudendal nerve afferent activity, which disinhibits the smooth muscle fibers of the bladder or colorectum. With the disinhibition, an efficient contraction of the bladder or colorectum can occur in order to propel stool or urine from the body. (See Chapters 26 and 27 for further discussion.) If the sequence of PFM relaxation followed by smooth muscle contraction is disturbed during voiding or evacuation, various bowel and bladder symptoms may develop. Symptoms associated with such failure to relax may include voiding hesitancy and interrupted stream, straining with evacuation or voiding, constipation, incomplete evacuation, elevated postvoid residual volumes, bladder infection, or bowel and bladder irritability. These symptoms are seen in such conditions as encopresis and enuresis, which are now thought to be associated in many cases with a failure for the PFM to relax as the underlying mechanism for abnormalities in bowel and bladder control. With the disruption in the normal interaction between the smooth muscle of the colon and bladder with the PFM, other structural deficits such as bladder trabeculation, megarectum, rectocele, and partial PFM denervation might develop.

The PFMs also participate in sexual arousal and orgasm, and may aid in the transport of sperm to the ovum (Ganong, 2001). For example, the ischiocavernosus muscles compress the crura of the clitoris to impede venous return and therefore maintain erection of the clitoris. At the end of the plateau stage of the sexual response and during orgasm, impulses from the pudendal nerve produce rhythmic contractions of the bulbocavernosus, ischiocavernosus, and EAs muscles (Masters, Johnson, & Kolodny, 1994). Many women referred to our clinic for such problems as dyspareunia, vulvodynia, and vaginismus respond well to PFM neuromuscular reeducation and biofeedback.

In summary, the pelvic floor muscles mediate the following functions:

1. Support the pelvic visceral structures.
2. Provide passive occlusive force at the urethra and anal canal at rest to maintain storage.
3. Provide dynamic occlusive force at the urethra and anal canal to maintain storage with increases in intra-abdominal pressure (e.g., a cough or sneeze).
4. Inhibit activity in the smooth muscle of the bowel and bladder, to control urgency and maintain storage.
5. Allow for the passage of stool and urine during evacuation.
6. Disinihibt colorectal and bladder activity to facilitate smooth muscle propulsive activity, which assists the evacuation of urine and stool.
7. Participate in sexual arousal and orgasm.

DISORDERS INVOLVING FAILURE TO RELAX THE PFMS

The techniques we have described in Chapters 26 and 27 improve PFM strength and coordination in response to stimuli from the bladder and rectum. The general goal of these procedures is to enhance the supportive and closure functions at the urethra and anal canal. The strengthening procedures also improve *voluntary* inhibition of bladder and bowel, resulting in increased storage capacity. This improvement comes about because increased contractile function of the PFMs results in greater afferent activity, which provides the basis for increased inhibition of the bowel and bladder.

On the other hand, an open sphincter and a propulsive force from the bladder or colorectal muscle are required for evacuation or voiding. When the PFMs fail to relax below the resting baseline during evacuation or voiding, the interaction between the striated PFMs and the smooth colorectal or bladder muscle is disrupted. For example, if the EAS and the puborectalis muscles fail to relax during defecation, the anal canal does not dilate, and resistance to the passage of stool remains. This resistance is associated with abdominal straining, which has pervasive adverse effects. Straining with stool can contribute to partial denervation injury of the PFMs, which may lead to incontinence (Swash, 1990). Straining is also associated with the development of fissures in the anal canal, rectal prolapse, rectocele, and hemorrhoids.

Physiologically, the failure of the PFMs to relax during defecation can also decrease the propulsive action of the smooth colorectal muscle, because if the PFMs remain contracted, the afferent activity from their contraction can inhibit activity in the colorectal muscle. A cycle develops, which leads to constipation or incomplete evacuation because the contractility of the colorectal muscle is diminished, and straining alone is ineffective in emptying the rectum completely. As straining with stool continues, the EAS becomes weakened, and its function is disrupted. Fecal seepage may then occur when stool remains in the distal portion of the rectum.

Children who withhold stool serve as a clinical example of how the failure to relax the PFMs disrupts smooth muscle function. A common precipitating factor for the withholding of stool in young children is an aversion to toileting acquired during an earlier, painful passage of a large, hard stool. The withholding of stool, however, is associated with increased voluntary PFM activity that inhibits peristalsis and leads to the accommodation of larger amounts of stool in the colon. Chronic accommodation of stool distends the fibers of the colorectal muscle and ultimately diminishes its propulsive ability, resulting in colonic inertia. The latter condition allows a large volume of stool to accumulate, distending the colon and rectum. The EAS is reflexively inhibited by this chronic distention, and this allows dilation of the anal canal, which allows fecal matter to seep around the bolus of stool that remains in the rectum. This disorder is called "encopresis." Reports indicate that biofeedback treatment, combined with bowel management techniques, is effective in decreasing abnormal activity of both the PFMs and the EAS, thereby reducing encopresis and constipation (Brown, Donati, Seow-Choen, & Ho, 2001; Choi et al., 2001; Dailianas et al., 2000; Emmanuel & Kamm, 2001; Mimura, Roy, Storrie, Kamm, 2000). Moreover, Emmanuel and Kamm (2001) have found that constipated patients who learn to relax the PFMs and alter the outlet obstruction also show improved colonic transit times after therapy, thereby reversing the abnormal inhibitory effect of excessive PFM activity on the smooth colorectal muscle.

The failure to relax muscles that surround the urethra and bladder neck prior to and during urination can have equally dire effects on bladder function. If the PFMs fail to relax with voiding, pressure at the urethra remains high at the onset and during voiding. In this case, bladder pressure must increase in order to propel urine through the urethra. The heightened bladder pressure results from a complex set of sacral and brainstem reflexes that increase the intensity of the detrusor contraction to overcome urethra resistance. If the reflexive increase in bladder pressure is not sufficient to overcome urethral resistance, the individual will augment bladder pressure by increasing intra-abdominal pressure, or will strain to void. Chronic straining to void is nearly always an indication for the presence of a voiding dysfunction.

Failure to relax the pelvic floor and periurethral muscles during voiding is termed "detrusor–sphincter dyssynergia." This condition occurs with neural impairment, but also develops from maladaptive learning. It is often associated with bladder irritability that develops as a result of the abnormally elevated pressure in the bladder. As the voiding dysfunction continues, the bladder wall may become thickened or trabeculated. With these changes, the threshold for the sensation of fullness and contraction is lowered, leaving the bladder irritable and unstable. Ultimately, functional bladder capacity decreases, and the patient may experience bladder urgency and frequency with and without incontinence. The term "functional bladder capacity" refers to the degree of diuresis that can occur before bladder symptoms appear, as opposed to "absolute bladder capacity," which is an objective assessment of bladder size. Other symptoms associated with dyssynergic voiding include elevated postvoid residual volumes and painful bladder spasm. In severe cases, detrusor–sphincter dyssynergia can lead to chronic bladder infection, ureter reflux, and kidney disease.

In our clinics, we see a considerable number of children referred for enuresis, with and without daytime wetting. We observe that in addition to having a small bladder capacity, these children display a voiding dysfunction characterized by a failure to relax the PFMs just before and during voiding, when measured on our biofeedback instruments. We feel that in many of these cases, the voiding dysfunction, with its associated changes in bladder physiology, is the underlying cause for the enuresis. With all referrals for enuresis, therefore, we assess for the presence of a voiding disorder and treat it specifically. Our observations are supported by several reports that demonstrate the effectiveness of behavioral treatment and biofeedback in reducing voiding dysfunction and associated incontinence in children who have failed to improve with more traditional medical treatments or with behavioral treatments such as the pad and bell (Combs, Glassberg, Gerdes, & Herowitz, 1998; De Paepe et al., 1998, 2000; Pfister et al., 1999; McKenna, Herndon, Connery, & Ferrer, 1999; Yamanishi et al., 2000).

A CASE EXAMPLE

Figure 28.2 (graphs A–C) shows a series of surface electromyographic (EMG) measures taken from an 8-year-old girl with enuresis that started when she was about age 4, during a period of considerable emotional trauma that included placement in a foster home because of parental neglect and abuse. Associated symptoms included daily passage of hard stool with straining. She had a small bladder capacity, reporting in the clinic a moderate urge to void with only 134 cubic centimeters in the bladder, as measured by ultrasound. There was a postvoid residual volume of 34 cubic centimeters. Normally, a healthy bladder should empty completely during urination. Therefore, the finding of a postvoid residual volume indicates a voiding dysfunction. EMG measures of PFM activity were obtained using a multiple electrode probe (MEP) and abdominal surface electrodes, as described in Chapter 26.

In Figure 28.2A, PFM baseline EMG measures show elevated levels at rest. A voluntary PFM contraction is associated with extraneous abdominal contraction, but in this case this may have been a function of the novel situation and the child's lack of awareness of how to contract the PFMs. When the child was asked to evacuate the MEP, paradoxical PFM activity can be seen in Figure 28.2B. Again, there is usually a novelty in performing an evacuation maneuver in the left lateral position; therefore, initial measures that indicate a paradoxical PFM contraction should be repeated after instructions and biofeedback have been given to reinforce appropriate PFM relaxation with a gentle evacuation maneuver. If after several practice trials, a patient still has difficulty producing a PFM relaxation response with evacuation of the recording probe, the paradoxical EMG activity observed may reflect actual PFM dyssynergia. In this case, the paradoxical activity persisted after initial biofeedback was given to reduce the abnormal activity.

Figure 28.2C shows EMG measures taken from the same child during voiding after she reported a moderate urge to void. To perform a voiding EMG study of any patient, we tape the MEP in place at the T-handle, using a tape that is easily removed after the recording procedures. We either use a commode chair, or place the recording equipment close to the toilet. The volume voided is measured with a urine receptacle placed on the commode

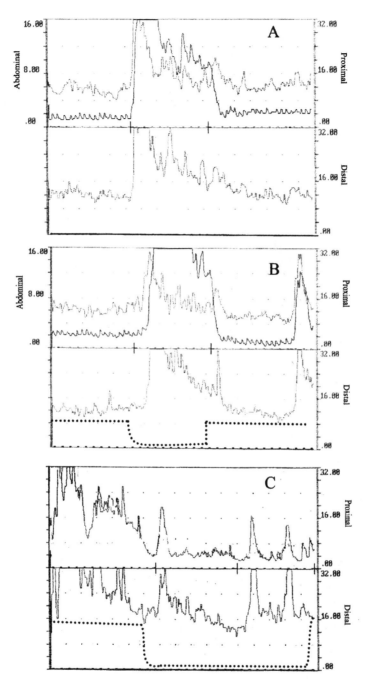

FIGURE 28.2. A series of EMG measures taken from an 8-year old girl with enuresis and voiding dysfunction. The proximal anal canal EMG, which reflects puborectalis activity, is seen in the top half of each graph (the lighter line) and is scaled on the right vertical axis. Abdominal EMG (dark line) is scaled on the left vertical axis on the top half of graphs A and B. Abdominal EMG, has been removed in graph C for simplification. The distal anal canal EMG is seen on the bottom of each graph. The dark, dotted line in graphs B and C indicate the normal expected EMG pattern for both PFM measures. Graph A shows EMG during baseline, voluntary PFM contraction (between the event markers) and recovery. Graph B shows EMG during a simulated evacuation maneuver. Graph C shows PFM EMG as measured by the MEP during a void. In graph C, the first event marker to the left indicates when the child was told to void. The middle mark indicates when the flow began, and the mark to the right indicates when the flow stopped.

chair. (Males can void directly into a urinal.) In Figure 28.C, the recordings to the left of the first event marker show the EMG while the patient was preparing to sit on a commode chair. The first event marker to the left indicates when the child was told that she could begin voiding. The middle marker indicates the moment the flow was heard by the therapist, and the last marker indicates when the child stated that she had finished voiding. The solid lines on the top and bottom halves of the graph trace the expected pattern of PFM relaxation during a void.

The voiding record shows that the child's PFMs failed to relax prior to the onset of voiding and remained contracted during the entire void. Moreover, during the void, there were spiking increases in the EMG activity. Given this record, it can be assumed that while this child voided, her urethral resistance remained high and actually increased at moments. Therefore, the voiding pressure in the bladder was elevated relative to normal voiding pressures. The chronic increase in bladder pressure gave rise to bladder irritability, with the subsequent symptom of enuresis. During the day, this child could avoid incontinence by voiding at the first sensation to void. However, while she was sleeping, her small bladder capacity and lowered threshold for contraction precluded her from responding in a timely manner to avoid incontinence.

Biofeedback/behavioral treatment is initially focused on reducing the voiding dysfunction, and then on improving functional bladder capacity. Early in the biofeedback treatment, patients are coached to identify the PFMs and then to lower the resting baseline. After learning to lower the resting baseline, they are taught, during simulated evacuation maneuvers, to relax the PFMs to a level below the resting baseline. The instruction is to "drop" the EMG activity. This "dropping" response produces an elongation of the PFMs from the resting state and is required in order for the bladder neck to elongate and form a funnel, so that voiding is not resisted at the urethra. After the PFM activity can be reduced at both rest and during evacuation maneuvers, a patient is given instrumental feedback while voiding. While voiding, the patient is reinforced for relaxing the PFMs prior to and throughout the void. (See the discussion of biofeedback relaxation techniques, below.) To increase functional bladder capacity, we use the techniques of fluid loading and the bladder scan for urge incontinence described in Chapter 26.

CONDITIONS THAT RESPOND TO PFM BIOFEEDBACK RELAXATION THERAPY

In addition to voiding dysfunction, enuresis, encopresis, and constipation, PFM therapy that includes relaxation techniques may be useful in the treatment of vulvodynia, vaginismus, and various other complaints of pelvic pain (Glazer, Rodke, Swencionis, Hertz, & Young, 1995; McKay et al., 2001). However, like biofeedback studies for incontinence, studies using biofeedback for pelvic pain lack sufficient controls to determine the precise mechanisms that underlie reported improvements. For optimal clinical outcome, biofeedback for PFM dysfunction is used with other behavioral treatments that are directed specifically toward the disorder treated. For example, for encopresis and constipation, bowel management techniques are used with the PFM biofeedback. The reader should see Doughty (2000) for an excellent overview of bowel management techniques. Treatment of pelvic pain disorders often requires assessment and attention to musculoskeletal impairments, such as postural abnormalities, that might contribute to the pelvic pain (Nitsch, 2001). Therefore, for treatment to be successful, the therapist must have a thorough knowledge of the anatomy and physiology of each disorder treated and the other adjunctive behavioral strategies.

USING BIOFEEDBACK TO TEACH PFM RELAXATION

The following sequence is generally followed when one is teaching PFM relaxation. Patients are reinforced to do the following:

1. Lower PFM resting baseline activity.
2. Selectively contract the PFMs for quick and sustained contractions.
3. Reduce the latency to relax the PFMs after voluntary contraction.
4. Elongate the PFMs with varying degrees of increased intra-abdominal pressure, as with a Valsalva maneuver.
5. Relax and elongate the PFMs prior to and during voiding.

Generally, PFM relaxation therapy takes place within the same session when the patient is taught to perform the selective PFM contractions described in Chapters 26 and 27. When a patient performs a PFM contraction, we always instruct the patient to relax the PFMs to a low baseline between each contraction trial, even when PFM relaxation is not a primary goal. When biofeedback is specifically directed toward reducing PFM hypertonus, the following procedures are useful.

An abdominal channel is generally used in PFM relaxation therapy. Patients who hold excessive tension in the pelvic floor often show elevated abdominal measures as well. Biofeedback reinforcement for abdominal relaxation, in conjunction with instruction in diaphragmatic breathing, leads to relatively quick awareness and control of excessive abdominal muscle tension. Moreover, abdominal muscle relaxation is often associated with concomitant PFM relaxation. Therefore, as patients acquire awareness and control over elevated abdominal muscle activity, they also have the means for generalizing the relaxation to the PFMs.

After a patient can control abdominal muscle activity, therapy proceeds to reinforce selective PFM contraction followed by relaxation. Figures 28.3 and 28.4 show a series of EMG recordings from a patient who was being treated for dyspareunia and outlet obstruction constipation with associated PFM dyssynergia. Figure 85.3A shows the PFM dyssynergia at the proximal and distal portions of the anal canal with a simulated evacuation maneuver. However, note the normal relaxation response in the vaginal recording, indicating that the patient's PFMs showed disparate function and dysfunction. In Figure 28.3B, the therapist set a threshold line on the EMG channel measuring activity from the distal anal canal. The patient was reinforced to (1) keep the abdominal muscles relaxed at rest with verbal cueing by the therapist and abdominal EMG biofeedback; (2) selectively contract the PFM without abdominal contraction; (3) keep the PFM activity below a visual threshold between each voluntary contraction; and (4) reduce PFM latency to return to the resting baseline immediately after voluntary contraction.

After the first PFM contraction trial (left) seen in Figure 28.3B, there was an approximate 11-second delay before the distal anal canal EMG returned to the resting baseline. An extended latency to relax after voluntary contraction is a sign of PFM hypertonus. With the second contraction trial in Figure 28.3B, the latency to return to baseline was reduced to 7 seconds. In Figure 28.3C, the latency was reduced to about 1 second, indicating improved control over distal EAS hypertonus.

Audio feedback is often used with visual feedback to shape PFM relaxation below a set threshold. A caution with the use of audio feedback is that if the threshold is set much above the actual PFM resting baseline, the audio feedback is given continuously; as a result, the audio signal loses its function as a discriminative stimulus for small reductions in PFM activity. We find that if the threshold is set at or just below the actual resting level, audio feedback

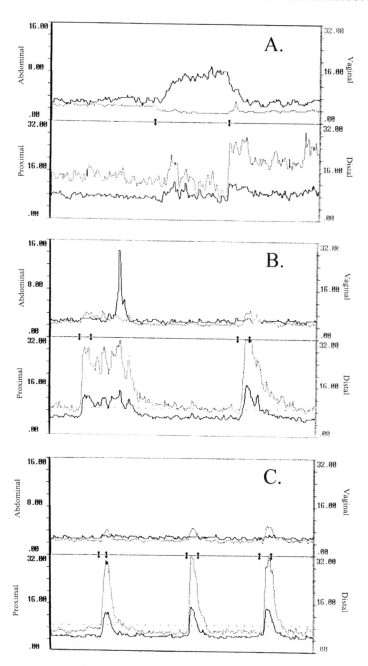

FIGURE 28.3. EMG measures from a 34-year-old multiparous woman with complaints of incomplete evacuation of stool, constipation, abdominal pain, and dyspareunia. On the top of each graph, abdominal EMG (dark) is scaled on the left vertical axis, and vaginal EMG (light) is scaled on the right. On the bottom of each graph, proximal anal canal EM (dark) is scaled on the left, while the distal anal canal EMG is scale on the right. Graph A shows elevated EMG activity at baseline and paradoxical activity, with an evacuation maneuver seen between the two event markers. Graph B shows initial training to contract the PFM (between each pai f event markers) and relax immediately after the contraction. A long latency to relax is seen in the contraction trial to the left. Graph C shows the acquisition of an improved PFM contraction and relaxation pattern.

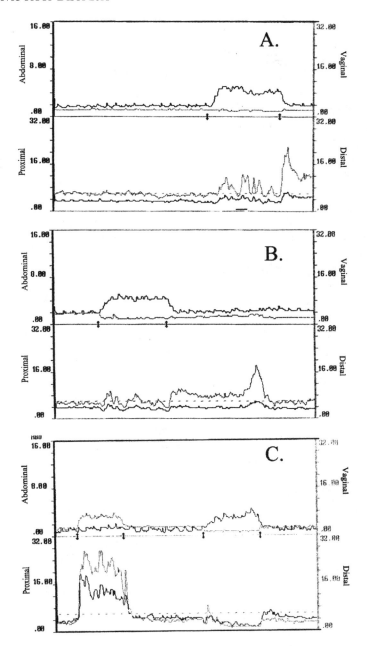

FIGURE 28.4. EMG measures from the same subject as she improved her PFM relaxation responses during simulated evacuation maneuvers. In graph A and B, note the progression in seconds below a threshold line seen in the bottom of each graph during simulated evacuation maneuvers (time between event markers). In graph C, flexibility in PFM control is seen as the patient contracted the PFM (left), then reduced EMG below the threshold during recovery, and then relaxed the PFM further, elongating the muscle fibers during a simulated evacuation maneuver.

reinforces only momentary and possibly random reductions in the PFM activity, thereby shaping a patient's PFM activity toward a lower resting baseline. When the patient learns to keep the EMG below the audio threshold about 40–50% of the time, the threshold can again be lowed by a small increment so the patient receives feedback about 10–15% of the time. As the patient learns to lower the PFM resting baseline and the threshold is reached about 50% of the time, the threshold lowered again.

After the patient has acquired some ability to lower the PFM baseline at rest, and immediately following a voluntary contraction, a PFM relaxation response that drops below the resting baseline during evacuation maneuvers is reinforced. Recall that at rest, the PFMs maintain some small level of activity to maintain closure pressure at the anal canal and urethra. However, evacuation and voiding require a flexibility of the PFMs to relax below the resting level, to a near-quiescent state, and for the muscle fibers to elongate. Therefore, for such conditions as voiding dysfunction and outlet obstruction constipation, biofeedback is used to train the motor pattern that is associated with the normal descent of the pelvic floor.

Figure 28.4A shows a feedback display after the same patient whose records are shown in Figure 28.3 had been reinforced to lower abdominal and PFM resting baseline activity, to contract the PFM, and to reduce latency to return to baseline after PFM contraction. In Figures 28.4A and 28.4B, the patient was asked to perform an evacuation maneuver and bring the distal anal canal measure below the threshold line. The patient received audio feedback when the distal EAS activity was below the threshold. In Figure 28.4A, the time below threshold was about 3 seconds within an 8-second evacuation trial. In Figure 28.4B, time below the threshold was 7 seconds within a 10-second evacuation trial. Figure 28.4C shows measures taken in the fifth and last treatment session. The patient reported that she had reduced the time needed to evacuate from 30 minutes to less than 5 minutes and could evacuate without straining. Her bowel movement frequency had increased from one bowel movement per week to every other day. Her complaints of dyspareunia were resolved. The left side of Figure 28.4C shows an improved voluntary contraction, with a short delay to return to baseline after voluntary contraction. On the right side of Figure 28.4C, an improved evacuation maneuver is seen, with a normal relaxation response seen in both the proximal and distal anal canal measures. The EMG activity drop below the resting baseline was stable for 8 seconds of a 9-second evacuation maneuver.

We find that many patients having PFM dyssynergia have difficulty learning the normal relaxation response during simulated evacuation maneuvers. We inform our patients that the learning (or relearning) of this normal pattern generally requires more practice trials than does the learning of selective PFM contraction. Visualization of the expected changes in the anatomy during biofeedback helps in the acquisition of the PFM relaxation responses, as does the adoption of "passive attention" that is used in the learning of other physiological responses (Peper, 1979).

SUMMARY

Bowel, bladder, and sexual activity require more than PFM strength, tone, and coordination. The PFMs must be able to relax to a normal resting level. Moreover, the PFMs must have sufficient flexibility to allow the muscle fibers to elongate at appropriate times for evacuation, voiding, and sexual activity. Therefore, in most biofeedback applications for disorders associated with PFM dysfunction, the assessment procedures must examine the proficiency of the pelvic floor in the performance of all its roles to include the relaxation responses that allow normal evacuation and voiding. In many cases, biofeedback techniques must then be directed toward improving not only PFM strength and coordination, but relaxation responses as well. We hope that this chapter will provide practitioners with some insight into the methods used to reinforce the necessary PFM relaxation responses.

REFERENCES

Brown, S. R., Donati, D., Seow-Choen, F., & Ho, Y. H. (2001). Biofeedback avoids surgery in patients with slow-transit constipation: Report of four cases. *Diseases of the Colon and Rectum, 44,* 737–739.

Choi, J. S., Hwang, Y. H., Salum, M. R., Weiss E. G., Pikarsky, A. J., Norgueras, J. J., & Wexner, S. D. (2001). Outcome and management of patients with large rectoanal intussusception. *American Journal of Gastroenterology, 96,* 740–744.

Combs, A. J., Glassberg, A. D., Gerdes, D., & Herowitz, M. (1998). Biofeedback therapy for children with dysfunctional voiding. *Urology, 52,* 312–315.

Dailianas, A., Skandalis, N., Rimikis, M. N., Koutsomanis, D., Kardasi, M., & Archimandritis, A. (2000). Pelvic floor study in patients with obstructive defecation: influence of biofeedback. *Journal of Clinical Gastroenterology, 30,* 115–116.

De Paepe, H., Hoebeke, P., Renson, C., Van Laecke, E., Raes, A., Van Hoecke, E., Van Daele, J., & Vande Walle, J. (1998). Pelvic-floor therapy in girls with recurrent urinary tract infections and dysfunctional voiding. *British Journal of Urology, 81,* 109–113.

De Paepe, H., Renson, C., Van Laecke, E., Raes, A., Vande Walle, J., & Hoebe, P. (2000). Pelvic-floor therapy and toilet training in young children with dysfunctional voiding and constipation. *International British Journal of Urology, 85,* 889–893.

Doughty, D. (Ed.). (2000). *Urinary and fecal incontinence: Nursing management* (2nd ed.). St. Louis, MO: Mosby.

Emmanuel, A. V., & Kamm, M. A. (2001). Response to a behavioral treatment, biofeedback, in constipated patients is associated with improved gut transit and autonomic innervation. *Gut, 49,* 214–219.

Ganong, W. (2001). *Review of medical physiology.* New York: Lange Medical Books/McGraw-Hill.

Glazer, H. I., Rodke, G., Swencionis, C., Hertz, R., & Young, A. W. (1995). Treatment of vulvar vestibulitis syndrome with electromyographic biofeedback of the pelvic floor musculature. *Journal of Reproductive Medicine, 40,* 283–290.

Masters, W. H., Johnson, V. E., & Kolodny, R. C. (1994). *Heterosexuality.* New York: HarperCollins.

McKay, E., Kaufman, R. H., Doctor, U., Berkova, Z., Glazer, H., & Redko, V. (2001). Treating vulvar vestibulitis with electromyographic biofeedback of pelvic floor musculature. *Journal of Reproductive Medicine, 46,* 337–342.

McKenna, P. H., Herndon, C. D., Connery, S., & Ferrer, F. A. (1999). Pelvic floor muscle retraining for pediataric voiding dyfunction using interactive computer games. *Journal of Urology, 162,* 1056–1062.

Mimura, T., Roy, A. J., Storrie, J. B., & Kamm, M. A. (2000). Treatment of impaired defecation associated with rectocele by behavioral retraining (biofeedback). *Diseases of the Colon and Rectum, 43,* 1267–1272.

Nitsch, W. (2001). Chronic pelvic pain in women: etiology and intervention—a review of the literature and its implication for physical therapists. *Physical Therapy: Journal of the Section on Women's Health, 25,* 7–12.

Peper, P. (1979). Problems in biofeedback: an experimental analogy—urination. In E. Peper, S. Ancoli, & M. Quinn (Eds.), *Mind/body integration: Essential readings in biofeedback.* New York: Plenum Press.

Pfister, C., Dacher, J. N., Gaucher, S., Liard-Zmuda, A., Grise, P., & Mitrofanoff, P. (1999). The usefulness of a minimal urodynamic evaluation and pelvic floor biofeedback in children with chronic voiding dysfunction. *International British Journal of Urology, 84,* 1054–1057.

Retzky, S. S., Rogers, R. M., & Richardson, A. C. (1996). Anatomy of female pelvic support. In L. T. Brubaker & T. J. Saclarides (Eds.), *The female pelvic floor: Disorders of function and support.* Philadelphia: F. A. Davis.

Swash, T. (1990). The neurogenic hypothesis of stress incontinence. *Ciba Foundation Symposium, 151,* 156–175.

Yamanishi, T., Yasuda, K., Murayama, N., Sakakibara, R., Uchiyama, T., & Ito, H. (2000). Biofeedback training for detrusor overactivity in children. *Journal of Urology, 164,* 1686–1690.

CHAPTER 29

Irritable Bowel Syndrome

MARK S. SCHWARTZ

SAMI R. ACHEM

Irritable bowel syndrome (IBS) is one of the most common disorders encountered by gastroenterologists. Yet treatments focused on gastrointestinal (GI) factors are often unsuccessful, and psychophysiological and psychosocial factors that contribute to the experience of pain and to pain behaviors are often not taken into consideration (Drossman et al., 2000b). GI tests are typically normal in IBS (Drossman et al., 2000b; Van Dulmen, Fennis, & Bleijenberg, 1996).

This chapter discusses issues and information sought or needed by practitioners and students of applied psychophysiology who evaluate and treat persons with IBS, and the rationale for including relaxation, biofeedback, and other nonmedical therapies as part of multi-component treatment for IBS.[1] (As in other chapters, italics on first use of a term indicate that the term is included in the glossary at the chapter's end.)

DEFINITIONS, SYMPTOMS, FEATURES

The diagnosis of IBS rests primarily on symptoms. There is no biological test or marker indicative of this disorder. Investigators use symptom-based criteria to define IBS. One of the most widely employed and recognized criteria sets was developed by Manning, Thompson, Heaton, and Morris (1978). They noted four common symptoms among those with IBS: (1) pain eased after bowel movement, (2) looser stools at the onset of pain, (3) more frequent bowel movements at onset of pain, and (4) abdominal distension.

More recently, a group of international experts gathered in Rome at two separate meetings to provide a contemporary definition of this disorder, taking into consideration new research information and striving to improve clarity (Thompson et al., 1999). The results of the most recent meeting have resulted in a new proposed consensus, summarized as follows:

at least 12 weeks or more, which need not to be consecutive, in the preceding 12 months of abdominal discomfort or pain that has two out of three features:

1) Relieved with defecation; and or
2) Onset associated with a change in frequency of the stool; and or
3) Onset associated with a change in form (appearance) of stool. (Thompson et al., 1999, p. 1144)

The above are in the absence of structural and metabolic abnormalities to explain the symptoms.

Clinical Evaluation

The diagnosis of IBS involves the recognition of certain symptoms consistent with this disorder (see above) and the exclusion of medical conditions that resemble IBS (see below).

Lower abdominal pain aggravated by meals and relieved by defecation, small stools, persistent or recurrent symptoms, and worsening of symptoms during periods of stress all tend to add to a positive diagnosis of IBS. In contrast, onset after age 50, nocturnal symptoms, fever, weight loss, dehydration, rectal bleeding or steatorrhea (fat in the stool), leukocytosis, an increased *erythrocyte sedimentation rate (ESR)*, anemia, and/or hypokalemia (low potassium) indicate an organic process and must be evaluated further.

A dietary history is important to review the potential exacerbating role of products containing lactose, alcohol, caffeine, or fat, or products causing gas. Psychological disorders, especially panic disorder, depression, and somatization disorder, are frequently associated with symptom reporting.

The differential diagnosis is broad. The diagnostic approach includes consideration of several disorders, based on the dominant clinical symptom. The following is a partial list of disorders that may be considered in the evaluation of IBS:

Bloating: Lactose intolerance, malabsorption of other carbohydrates (e.g., fructose, sorbitol), partial bowel obstruction, intestinal pseudo-obstruction.

Diarrhea: Lactose and carbohydrate malabsorption, *inflammatory bowel disease (IBD)*, ulcerative colitis, malabsorption disorders, parasites (giardia, amoeba), microscopic colitis, bile-induced diarrhea, laxative abuse, mastocytosis, HIV-associated diarrhea, tumors producing hormones (e.g., 5-hydroxy indol acetic acid (5-HIAA), gastrin, vasoactive intestinal polypeptide (VIP), calcitonin, glucagon, etc.; such tumors are rare).

Constipation: Medications, endocrinopathies (hypothyroidism, hypoparathyroidism), colon malignancy, diverticular disease, lack of dietary fiber, and decreased consumption of oral liquids.

Abdominal pain: Peptic ulcer disease, gallbladder disease, pancreatic neoplasm, or pancreatitis.

Depending on clinical features, one should also consider other entities, such as endometriosis, mesenteric insufficiency, Addison's disease, porphyria, heavy-metal poisoning, and angioedema.

For the majority of young patients (under 45 years of age), a basic evaluation including a careful history, physical exam, testing for occult blood in stool samples, basic laboratory tests (a *complete blood count* [CBC], ESR, serum chemistries), and perhaps a *flexible fiberoptic procto sigmoidoscopy (FlexSig)* should suffice. In some cases or in individuals over 45 years of age, endoscopy, *barium enemas*, computed tomography (CT), or *colonoscopy* with biopsies may be needed. Examples of patients who may need the latter approaches are those with atypical or alarming symptoms, family history of colon cancer or IBD, refractory symptoms, changes in symptom pattern, or late onset of symptoms (over 45 years of age).

When the initial evaluation is completed, symptomatic treatment can be started and the condition reevaluated in 4–6 weeks. This approach allows a conservative assessment over two or three points in time before additional studies are considered.

It is common for patients with IBS to complain of other upper GI symptoms, such as heartburn and belching. In addition, fibromyalgia, headaches, backache, genitourinary symptoms, and psychological dysfunction are frequently observed in these patients. However, these symptoms are not essential to diagnose IBS.

Alarming Symptoms

Patients with IBS do not have a structural or mucosal inflammatory disease. Therefore, the presence of any of the symptoms listed below should raise the possibility of an alternative diagnosis and should prompt further diagnostic investigations:

1. Fever.
2. Rectal bleeding or Hemoccult-positive stools.
3. Symptoms that awaken the patient from sleep.
4. Weight loss and or loss of appetite.
5. Anemia.
6. Abnormal findings on physical exam (patients with IBS have a normal exam, with the exception of a palpable and tender sigmoid).

Diagnostic Tests

Although there is no laboratory study that can help in the diagnosis of IBS, laboratory, radiographic, and endoscopic tests are frequently done in patients with suspected IBS—primarily to exclude other disorders resembling this condition. As noted above, laboratory studies often include a CBC and ESR; they may also include liver and pancreatic chemistries, electrolytes, and urinalysis.

Patients with diarrhea usually require stool samples to search for ova and parasites. The type of radiographic evaluation varies according to the patient's symptoms. For instance, those with abdominal pain frequently receive abdominal ultrasound and/or CT of the abdomen and pelvis. In addition, small-bowel series and upper endoscopy or colonoscopy may also be included in the evaluation of some of these patients. Again, in IBS all these studies are typically unrevealing.

Symptom Measures

A symptom diary or log consists of rating the severity of the common and major IBS symptoms. Points to consider in designing a log of IBS symptoms are compliance, practicality, symptom selection, rating system, frequency of ratings, other data (e.g., medications, dietary, stress, smoking, activity), consistency with published systems, avoidance of relying on *global ratings*, and coexisting symptoms and disorders.

The selection of symptoms should be tailored to the patient in clinical practice. In a standardized program treating many patients and collecting clinical research data, practitioners will probably include several or all of them. However, for an individual patient, one can often select fewer—those symptoms that are present and of most concern. Some of the following symptoms are not specific for IBS (e.g., soiling, nausea, gas), even for those patients with diagnosed IBS. However, including them can sometimes have clinical use.

- Abdominal pain or discomfort.
- Abdominal pain or discomfort relieved with bowel movement.
- Diarrhea (loose or watery stool).
- Loose stool or more frequent stools at onset of pain.
- Urgency.
- Soiling.
- Constipation or hard stool.

- Straining to have a bowel movement.
- Feeling of incomplete emptying.
- Bloating or feeling of abdominal distension.
- Passage of mucus.
- Bowel gas/flatulence.
- Nausea or vomiting.

A rating scale in which 0 = "not present," 1 = "mild," 2 = "moderate," 3 = "severe," and 4 = "disabling" can be used. Each term should be defined for patients. Some researchers use 0 to indicate that a symptom was "not a problem" and 4 to reflect a "debilitating problem." However, this does not appear to allow for the clear nonexistence of a symptom. Furthermore, the term "debilitating" is a complex one. Certainly IBS can be debilitating (i.e., weakening, devitalizing, or enfeebling). However, a person may feel that way with severe symptoms, yet may not report disability in functioning and working. We assume that a practitioner also wants to know whether the symptoms disabled or actually incapacitated a person. We suggest considering the terms "disabling" or "incapacitating."

Ratings for IBS symptoms could follow this 6-point rating scale: 0 = "no symptoms," 1 = "slight or not a problem," 2 = "mild intensity," 3 = "moderate intensity," 4 = "severe," and 5 = "disabling or incapacitating." Bennett Tennant, Piesse, Badcock, and Kellow (1998b) used these frequency-based ratings: 0 = "not a problem"; 1 = "once only in the 2-week period"; 2 = "occurred more than once each week"; and 3 = "occurred almost every day, or daily." Bennett et al. (1998a) also used the following severity ratings: 0 = "symptom not occurred"; 1 = "mild severity (no remedy sought, no remedy tried)"; 2 = "moderate severity (remedy sought, but daily activities were not affected)"; and 3 = "severe (interfering with daily activities)."

Medications should be included in the diary, especially those that can cause IBS symptoms and those prescribed to treat symptoms. Dietary information (e.g., ingestion of caffeine, milk products, or nondigestible carbohydrates such as cabbage and beans) and information on other factors (e.g., stress that could affect IBS symptoms) should also be considered.

Another decision is whether to get these ratings once a day in the evening or multiple times per day. Increased compliance and fewer data to review and analyze are advantages of once-a-day ratings. However, recalling in the evening symptoms that occurred 12 or more hours earlier may be less accurate than obtaining ratings periodically throughout the day. Therefore, a practitioner should consider obtaining multiple ratings each day (e.g., early morning, late morning or midday, late afternoon or early evening, and late evening), and should tailor the number and specific times to each patient.

Yet another possibility is the *Composite Primary Symptom Reduction* (CPSR) Score, developed by the State University of New York (SUNY)–Albany group. One calculates separately a Symptom Reduction Score (SRS) for two or three of the primary presenting symptoms. The Albany group used abdominal pain, diarrhea, and constipation. To get each SRS, one subtracts the average symptom rating for a follow-up period from the average rating during a baseline period. The baseline period is 2–4 weeks, and the Albany group typically used 2 weeks for the follow-up period. One then divides this by the baseline average and multiplies this by 100 to get each SRS (e.g., a Diarrhea Reduction Score, a Constipation Reduction Score, and a Pain and Tenderness Reduction Score). Then one can assess the percentage of improvement for the composite of symptoms (e.g., "much improved" = 75–100%, "improved" = 50–74%, "slightly improved" = 20–49%, "unimproved" = 0–20%, and "worse" = less than 0%) (Blanchard, Schwarz, & Neff, 1988a; Blanchard et al., 1992b). The CPSR Score is the total of the SRSs divided by the number of scores (e.g., 2 or 3). That is, one adds the SRSs and divides this sum by the number of symptoms.

One can argue whether or not this is a better way to assess improvement in clinical practice. One must have baseline and follow-up periods of equal durations, as well as the time to do the calculations (or a computer program to ease the calculations). One could analyze the differences for each symptom. Ideally, practitioners will get pretreatment baseline data and also follow-up data for at least 1 year. However, getting pretreatment baseline data is not always feasible or prudent in clinical practice. Practitioners often need to adapt their procedures from the ideal to the pragmatic.

We advocate not relying entirely on global ratings, because they sometimes markedly overestimate benefit compared to daily symptom data. For example, in one study 71% of the patients who did not improve their symptoms significantly rated themselves as quite competent in learning to overcome IBS symptoms (Blanchard et al., 1992b, p. 188). Global self-improvement ratings at 1-year follow-up showed about 70% improvement among 17 patients, compared to about 35% improvement as indicated by the CPSR Score (Schwarz, Blanchard, & Neff, 1986). This difference is substantial. However, inspection of the table (Schwarz et al., 1986, p. 195) of the CPSR Score and global ratings showed adequate consistency between these two measures for 8 of the 14 subjects.

In the first systematic study of the relations among three common outcome measures—the CPSR Score, patient global ratings, and physician global ratings—Meissner, Blanchard, and Malamood (1997) found these independent measures to be significantly related. Some consider the CPSR Score close to a gold standard as an IBS outcome measure. However, as these authors note, the CPSR Score (as used by the Albany group) assesses only three of the many IBS symptoms, and one might ask patients to select their own three most troublesome symptoms, creating a composite score tailored for each person. The problem with the latter approach is that it would create problems with comparing studies. Other limitations of the CPSR Score are that it does not assess quality of life (QOL), life interference, or medical care utilization.

The IBS-QOL Questionnaire was developed by Patrick, Drossman, Frederick, DiCesare, and Puder (1998) and further validated by Drossman et al. (2000a), who showed that it changes significantly with treatment, at least in referral-based patients with moderate and severe IBS. This questionnaire contains 34 items with 1–5 responses each. It is listed in the Appendix of the Patrick et al. (1998) paper, but to reproduce or use it one needs permission from one of the senior authors[2] and from Novartis Pharmaceuticals Corporation. Added support for the use of the IBS-QOL is that it "can accurately assess response to treatment" (Drossman et al., 2000a, p. 1005).

The main point of this discussion as a whole is to use daily ratings whenever possible. Remember that IBS is at least sometimes coexistent with other disorders (e.g., fibromyalgia syndrome, migraines, chronic fatigue, mood disorders, and anxiety disorders). These can affect the specificity of the symptoms, compliance with keeping the log, and the accuracy of the log. This potential complication suggests the need for using less ambiguous symptoms and ratings.

INCIDENCE AND PREVALENCE

There are reports that 8–17% of the general population has IBS symptoms (Whitehead, Winget, Fedoravicius, Wooley, & Blackwell, 1982; Talley, Zinsmeister, Van Dyke, & Melton, 1991; Whitehead, 1992a, 1992b). The Mayo Clinic Health Letter ("Irritable Bowel Syndrome," 1992) refers to "about one in five adult Americans" with symptoms of IBS (p. 1). Estimates indicate that 28% of patients in gastroenterologists' practices, 41% of all patients wth functional GI disorders, and 12% of primary care patient have IBS (American Gastrointestinal Association, 1997; Mitchell & Drossman, 1987).

PSYCHOLOGICAL FACTORS

Health Care Seeking

We must be careful what we assume about people with IBS, especially in medical settings. Perhaps fewer than half of people with IBS symptoms seek medical help ("Irritable Bowel Syndrome," 1992; Herschbach, Henrich, & von Rad, 1999). Moreover, in this population, the presence of and role of psychological factors in IBS symptoms do not receive similar support in all studies (Drossman et al., 1988; Whitehead, 1992a, 1992b). Most of these individuals are psychologically healthy. Some reports show that most community people with IBS believe that psychological stress stimulated their IBS symptoms. The reactions to stress and to experiencing emotional distress can exacerbate IBS, and the relationship between psychological factors and IBS has much research support. However, other reports suggest more modest relationships.

Among those persons with IBS symptoms, more and/or different psychological distress is found among those seeking health care than among the general population of persons with IBS (Blanchard & Malamood, 1996; van der Horst et al., 1997; Herschbach et al., 1999; Thompson, Heaton, Smyth, & Smyth, 2000). Persons with IBS symptoms who seek medical care may be more fearful of having serious disease; may be more depressed and/or more emotional; may view their overall health as less satisfactory; and/or may be more somatically focused, than other people with IBS symptoms (Whitehead, Bosmajian, Zonderman, Costa, & Schuster, 1988; Drossman et al., 1988; Drossman, 1994; van der Horst et al., 1997). For many patients with IBS, psychological issues may not be major aggravating factors. Nevertheless, health care professionals do encounter many other people who seek help and who often show psychological distress and a relationship of this distress to their symptoms.

Etiological Mechanisms (Physiological and Psychological)

The cause of IBS remains an enigma. Several mechanisms have been noted that lead to or aggravate IBS. These individual mechanisms are not mutually exclusive. The understanding of these mechanisms and identification of the prevailing one in a given patient may help optimize the therapeutic approach. The main disturbed mechanisms recognized in patients with IBS are altered motor function, abnormal visceral perception, infectious factors or inflammation, psychological factors, luminal factors, and a neurotransmitter imbalance.

• *Altered motor function.* Multiple studies have recognized abnormal motor function in IBS. However, the general consensus is that the basal motor parameters patients with IBS are no different from those of healthy subjects. In addition, there is a poor correlation between abdominal pain and abnormal motility, except for cramping abdominal pain in some patients with IBS (high-amplitude *peristaltic* contractions in the ileum). There is no consensus on the pattern of motility associated with diarrhea and constipation or alternating diarrhea–constipation. In severe idiopathic constipation, there is delay in colon transit.

• *Visceral hyperalgesia.* Ritchie (1973) documented that patients with IBS reported abdominal pain at lower volumes of balloon distension of the colon than did normal subjects. Similar observations have been confirmed by other investigators and extended to other functional disorders, such as noncardiac chest pain, nonulcer dyspepsia, and sphincter of Oddi dysfunction. Accordingly, it is considered that the altered sensation (abdominal pain, bloating) represents visceral hyperalgesia.

• *Infection and inflammation.* Experimental studies have shown that the excitability of a sensory neuron can be increased by applying a stimulant that induces local inflammation.

For instance, instillation of intracolonic mustard (2 milliliters, 5%) "awakens" silent or sleeping nociceptors and induces an increased response to balloon distension (Laird et al., 2000; Laird, Souslova, Wood, & Cervero, 2002). This is a concept termed "sensitization." This experimental evidence suggests that unknown irritants or neurotransmitters (see below) may contribute to the production of symptoms in IBS. There is also evidence that inflammation of the enteric mucosa or neural structures initiates or perpetuates the symptoms of IBS (Stewart, 1994; McKendrick, & Read, 1994). This information suggests that subgroups of patients with IBS may have developed their symptoms following an infectious process.

• *Psychological factors*. Psychological symptoms are common among patients with IBS, as alluded to in the previous section. Patients with IBS tend to be more preoccupied with illness than normal subjects. The most common symptoms reported include anxiety, somatization, hostility, phobia, and paranoia. Psychological factors including acute stress and overt psychiatric disease (depression, panic disorders) can alter GI function. Although it remains to be known which comes first (the psychological problem or the IBS), combined treatment of bowel symptoms and psychiatric comorbidity results in improvement in over 50% of patients with such comorbidity.

• *Luminal factors*. Luminal factors probably aggravate the underlying IBS rather than being the cause. Malabsorbed carbohydrates such as lactose, fructose, and sorbitol can imitate the clinical syndrome of IBS or precipitate it (food allergens may also play a role in a subset of patients with IBS). Thus in some patients dietary factors seem to play an important role, and exclusion diets have been found to have beneficial effects for selected patients (Goldstein, Braverman, & Stankiewicz, 2000; Ledochowski, Widner, Bair, Probst, & Fuchs, 2000; Rumessen & Gudmand-Hoyer, 1988).

• *Neurotransmitter imbalance*. Recent studies suggests that a neurotransmitters such as serotonin may play a role in the pathogenesis of IBS. Serotonin affects pain and GI motor activity. Preliminary evidence indicates that patients with IBS have increased serotonin levels in plasma and the rectosigmoid area (Bearcroft, Perrett, & Farthing, 1998). Several other neurotransmitters are being studied as potentially involved in the pathogenesis of IBS (substance P, calcitonin-gene-related peptide, nitric oxide, etc.) (Horwitz & Fisher, 2001).

Effects of Psychological Factors on Symptoms

One view with research support is that psychological factors probably are not a cause of IBS symptoms at least for most people with IBS. However, they may stimulate IBS symptoms in some people, and they may influence the decision to seek medical advice. The dissociation of IBS from being considered a psychophysiological disorder is a recent view (Whitehead, 1992a, 1992b, 1993; Thornton, McIntyre, Murray-Lyon, & Gruzelier, 1990; Blanchard 2001; Suls, Wan, & Blanchard, 1994).

Psychological symptoms are often comorbid factors with IBS and often serious enough to warrant treatment, whether or not they affect the IBS symptoms. Not making a diagnosis such as depression or anxiety disorder for people with IBS does not necessarily mean that they are not experiencing significant stress in their lives.

Even among a community sample of people with IBS, psychological stress may trigger or elicit changes in bowel functioning and, to a slightly lower degree, abdominal pain in many people with IBS (Drossman, Sandler, McKee, & Lovitz, 1982). Among those meeting bowel dysfunction criteria, about 84% reported that psychological factors affected changes in bowel functioning, and about 69% reported them affecting abdominal pain. Even among those not meeting bowel dysfunction criteria, about 68% said that stress affected changes in their bowel patterns, and 48% said it affected their abdominal pain.

The effect of stress on bowel symptoms was also found to be significant, although less so, in research from the Whitehead group. Whitehead, Crowell, Robinson, Heller, and Schuster (1992) reported on a sample of 39 recruited women who met restrictive criteria for a diagnosis of IBS. The researchers selected the women from a large group of 383 women in the community primarily recruited for reasons other than nonbowel dysfunction.

The correlation between stress and bowel symptoms was modest in both groups: A time-lagged correlation was .33 for the whole sample. Thus Whitehead et al. (1982) concluded that only "approximately 11% of the variance in bowel symptom reports is attributable to life event stress" (p. 830). This suggests that most people who report stress as the cause of their bowel symptoms could be basing this report on infrequent events. They could be misattributing the relationship because of rarely perceived associations. The investigators based this conclusion on the total of bowel symptoms for all the subjects and across all four visits for which there were data (n = 343). They correlated *Life Experiences Survey* data (Sarason, Johnson, & Siegel, 1978) for 3 months and the frequency of bowel symptoms reported during the subsequent 3 months. They repeated this over four quarterly dates for 1 year. Stress was correlated significantly with disability days and health care utilization.

The authors acknowledge the potential for insensitivity of the stress measure. There are potential problems with relying on life events reported every 3 months. For example, daily stress might produce transient changes in bowel symptoms that are missed when people are asked to report on the relationship every 3 months. However, the authors point to the consistency of their results with other data from their laboratory when they used a more sensitive method (Haderstorfer, Whitehead, & Schuster, 1989). That method was keeping a symptom log of subjective stress and bowel symptoms four times daily for 1 week.

Very carefully analyzed evidence against a relationship between daily stress and IBS symptoms was presented by Suls et al. (1994). A total of 44 patients seeking nondrug treatment for IBS completed a daily stress event diary and rating of the most bothersome daily event over 3 weeks, along with IBS symptom ratings. Analyses were of the group and idiographic within-subject correlations of stress ratings and IBS symptoms. "The idiographic correlations indicate[d] that for only a small minority of patients [did] stress reliably predict GI symptoms" (p. 109) when the daily events list and the "most bothersome event of the day" measure were used. The authors concluded that "daily sources of stress did not have strong or consistent effects on GI symptoms in most IBS patients" (p. 110). They reported that although "a small minority . . . showed a significant pattern of positive association; some subjects showed negative associations"(p. 110).

Suls et al. (1994) readily noted that "we have no doubt that a sufficiently severe stressor can be found that will induce GI symptoms" (p. 111), but they noted that "the question we posed was whether daily problems produce symptoms in most patients" (p. 111). The authors also noted the limitation of a short time series. We did not see data for the number of IBS symptoms and comparison with the usual symptoms for these patients, or comparisons with samples in other studies.

Suls et al. (1994) went on to state that

> the link between stress and GI symptomatology may not be as straightforward as originally thought, because stress is generally presumed to be sympathetically mediated. In the GI tract, however, sympathetic innervation inhibits bowel activity, whereas parasympathetic innervation stimulates propulsive activity. Additionally, sympathetic and parasympathetic influences may not be fully reciprocal and antagonistic, so that sympathetic influence is not necessarily high when parasympathetic influence is low and vice versa. . . . [These influences] may instead be uncoupled or coupled in a nonreciprocal mode (i.e., positively correlated in their effects on end organs). (p. 111)

However, another view has been expressed by Bennett et al. (1998a), who reported that

chronic stressors and extraintestinal and emotional symptomatologies were prominent features of functional dyspepsia (FD) and irritable bowel syndrome (IBS) alone. . . . particular features were . . . highly specific for particular FD and/or IBS subgroups. The chronic threat component of social stressors predicted the nature and extent of multisystem . . . symptomatology. . . . chronic stressor provoked psychological and extraintestinal disturbance is most specific for the FD-IBS group of syndromes. (p. 414)

These authors also believe (Bennett et al., 1998b) that they are the first researchers in a longitudinal study to assess "the relation of chronic and severe life stress to subsequent symptom intensity in patients with IBS (with and without concomitant FD)" (p. 259). Severe and chronic life stress had "large and consistent effects on symptom intensity over time." The severity of the chronic threat over several months accounted for "almost all the variance within individuals in symptom intensity levels" assessed three times over 16 months. Furthermore, improvement in symptom intensity was significantly reduced by the presence of sustained intense life stress over many months. These findings were for patients and "cannot be generalized to community (non patient) IBS populations or to patients with more complex medical histories" (p. 259).

In other research, a history of at least one psychopathological disorder was significantly more prevalent among women with IBS, and among women with similar symptoms but not with an IBS diagnosis, than among women without symptoms (Levy, Cain, Jarrett, & Heitkemper, 1997; Jarrett et al., 1998). Women with IBS symptoms showed a positive relationship between psychological distress and daily GI symptom distress. Relationships between daily life stress and IBS symptoms also received support from Dancey and colleagues (Dancey, Whitehouse, Painter, & Backhouse, 1995; Dancey, Taghavi, & Fox, 1998). These and other studies support the rationale for including stress management in the treatment of persons with IBS.

Trauma History

Remote trauma in childhood, such as loss of a parent, sexual abuse, or physical abuse, is more often found among some samples of patients with IBS than among healthy controls or other medical patients with nonfunctional or psychophysiological diseases (Whitehead, 1992a; Drossman et al., 1990; Lowman, Drossman, Cramer, & McKee, 1987; Walker, Katon, Roy-Byrne, Jemelka, & Russo, 1993). "Of 206 patients, 89 (44%) reported a history of sexual or physical abuse in childhood or later in life; all but 1 of the physically abused patients had been sexually abused" (Drossman et al., 1990, p. 828). Asking questions about sexual abuse in the distant past is very delicate and fraught with complexities. There is the potential for misinterpretation of questions, as well as the complex issue of inaccurate memories. (See M. S. Schwartz, Chapter 6, this volume.)

Nevertheless, many patients with IBS do report sexual abuse experiences in their childhood before age 14 (e.g., someone threatened to have sex with a patient, forced a patient to touch the sex organs of the other person, or succeeded in having sex with a patient despite the patient's reluctance (Drossman et al., 1990). Patients are very reluctant to report this; hence practitioners "must actively seek this type of information" (p. 832). These authors acknowledged the preliminary nature of their results. Even now, no one knows whether this association occurs among people with IBS who do not consult physicians. Thus the relationship to IBS remains unclear. One must consider that the selection factors that influence some people with IBS to seek help for these symptoms could include a history of abuse.

TREATMENTS

There is an extensive literature on treatment of IBS with various psychological and psychophysiological therapies; significant clinical improvements and maintenance have been reported over one or a few years (Blanchard & Malamood, 1996). That review also noted that choices among these treatments depend on preferences of practitioners, as direct comparisons were lacking. Among existing publications, there is an edge for cognitive-behavoral therapies, but multicomponent psychological/psychophysiological treatments tailored to individual patients still have an appropriate role. The latter are especially relevant, considering the psychological factors in the backgrounds and current functioning of many persons with IBS symptoms, especially among those who are seeking help. Although there are varied and inconsistent reports, there is still sufficient support for the view that excessive stress can affect and worsen bowel symptoms (Drossman et al., 1982; Bennett et al., 1998a, 1998b; Toner, Segal, Emmott, & Myran, 2000; Blanchard, 2001). Furthermore, the rationale for various psychophysiologic interventions includes the fact that medical therapies are often insufficient or disappointing.

A Multicomponent Approach: Education, Relaxation, Biofeedback, and Cognitive-Behavioral Strategies

A multicomponent psychological/psychophysiological approach, or at least some components of such an approach, are often appropriate. Biofeedback, when used for IBS, can be a valuable part of a multicomponent program (Neff & Blanchard, 1987; Schwarz et al., 1986; Blanchard et al., 1992b). The same laboratory conducted "five small-scale replications" using the same multicomponent treatment program, which included education, thermal biofeedback, relaxation, and cognitive-behavioral stress coping strategies, consistently led to clinical improvement (reduction of symptoms by at least 50%) in 40–65% of patients with IBS (Blanchard, Schwarz, Neff, & Gerardi, 1988b; p. 187).

However, in a more extensive sample of 91 patients (Blanchard et al., 1992b), there was no difference between this multicomponent package and "an ostensible attention-placebo control" group. Most of both groups improved significantly on several key symptoms. However, the authors' logical reasoning and data supported the contention that the patients in the so-called control group converted the attention placebo into an effective treatment. This study reflects the complexities of treating people with IBS and conducting well-controlled and useful clinical research.

Further complicating interpretation of the results is the chance that this application of the multicomponent approach yielded slightly less successful results than prior applications. The authors raise this possibility themselves. They wrote that, compared to prior studies from that center, this study showed "relatively poor results with the multicomponent treatment . . . [and there were] relatively high proportions of these treated patients . . . who are . . . symptomatically worse" (Blanchard et al., 1992b, p. 188). They earlier reported only about 18% being worse in follow-up among 45 patients, compared to the 29% they were now reporting. Also, the percentage of patients improving at least 50% was slightly less in this study than in their prior studies. In this study, they reported 46% of patients improving (42/91 for the three groups and 28/61 for the two groups treated with the multicomponent treatment), compared with the nearly 58% (26/45) reported in Blanchard et al. (1988b).

One can argue that the improvements in the so-called active treatment groups resulted from expectations and other factors not intended as part of the treatment. However, as Whitehead (1992a) points out, the "maintenance of treatment gains for up to 4 years . . . argues against a placebo effect explaining all the benefits of the multicomponent treatment" (p. 607). In other words, the effect lasted a long time for a placebo.

How can a person turn an attention placebo experience into an active treatment? Blanchard et al. (1992b) discussed what the patients in this group reported. For example, the subjects used

> their meditation procedures to "relax" or "to calm" themselves, despite having been told repeatedly during treatment not to relax during the pseudo-meditation training. . . . Others reported adapting the meditative procedures as a distraction technique when faced with stressful circumstances, especially to focus their attention away from GI symptoms. (p. 187)

The patients in this group also warmed their hands significantly both within and between sessions as well as or better than the multicomponent group.

Another factor to consider is that some patients make changes in their lifestyles without telling a doctor, therapist, or experimenter. For example, when people come for treatment, they often read more about their symptoms and discuss their symptoms and treatments with others. They often pay more attention to factors they already knew or suspected would affect their symptoms but had ignored before treatment. They may recall information from articles. Some such changes are too subtle even for some patients to realize themselves. For example, their expectations may change. They may notice subtle signs of anxiety, walk more slowly, breathe differently, and relax slightly more often. They may change their eating and drinking habits. The point here is that an attention placebo is often not an ineffective experience. It can be an opportunity for many patients to make therapeutic changes. Coming for therapy may become a *discriminative stimulus* that leads to healthier behaviors.

The active treatment components, the necessary components, and the sufficient components in a multicomponent treatment of IBS remain unknown. Relaxation is probably one active component (Blanchard, Greene, Scharff, & Schwarz-McMorris, 1993). However, it is imprudent for practitioners to underestimate the potential value of positive expectations. Other applied psychophysiological components are probably active as well.

Blanchard et al. (1992a) do not give their treatment enough credit. Their statement that "any diagnosable psychopathology would be a poor prognostic indicator for the kinds of treatment used in this study" (p. 649) is unnecessary and not accurate. We do not know enough about their patients' specific anxiety and depression symptoms and diagnoses to accept that statement at face value. Nevertheless, this study helps justify the value of careful interviewing for an anxiety or depression diagnosis. One can agree that such patients may need separate therapy before or with the treatment for IBS. However, the study supports the robust nature of the treatment by showing that many patients (29%) with these diagnoses can benefit from this treatment package.

We appreciate the careful expression of doubts by Blanchard et al. (1992b). We believe, however, that practitioners may rightfully embrace a recommendation for a treatment package similar to their multicomponent treatment—including education, relaxation procedures, stress coping strategies, and thermal biofeedback—for the treatment of IBS. A critic might raise the possibility that the patient education and cognitive-behavioral components are the necessary and perhaps sufficient components (Greene & Blanchard, 1994).

Possible Psychological/Psychophysiological Treatment Components

Assertiveness and Anger Management

Assertiveness and anger management therapy may be considered for selected and motivated patients. They may be impractical for or resisted by some patients; however, one should consider them for some people with moderate or severe symptoms, and/or when one expects or observes that other therapies are not enough. Assertiveness therapy, patient education, and cognitive stress management resulted in significantly more improvement among 11 treated patients than among a waiting-list group of 10 others (Lynch & Zamble, 1989). When those in the waiting-list group received treatment, they showed significant improvement. Improvements continued 5 months later. One must be cautious about generalizations from these results, however, because only 30 of the original 80 patients contacted agreed to participate. Furthermore, 9 others dropped out of the study. As Lynch and Zamble correctly acknowledge,

> it is possible that . . . persons with certain personality features, patients with illness behavior, and persons with more severe symptoms were over-represented in the sample . . . [and that the results] are generalizable only to those who (a) are referred to gastroenterologists and (b) accept a psychological treatment rationale. (p. 521)

Relaxation Therapy Alone

There is modest support for relaxation therapy alone (Voirol & Hipolito, 1987; Blanchard et al., 1993). Although these studies were done with small series of patients, there were significant improvements in multiple outcome variables, compared to symptom monitoring or conventional medical treatment. Methodological limitations preclude confident conclusions. This single treatment component might be worth considering in a stepped-care approach for some patients. Drossman and Thompson (1992) refer to relaxation procedures as "simple." Although these at times can be simple, they often are complex and require much more than sometimes implied.

Hypnosis

Hypnosis has some reported effectiveness with IBS. Galovski and Blanchard (1998) attempted to replicate hypnotherapy treatment of IBS as reported by Whorwell, Prior, and Faragher (1984) and Whorwell, Prior, and Colgan (1987). Treatment included progressive relaxation, as well as hypnosis with gut-directed imagery (e.g., "smoothly flowing rivers and waterfalls"). When subjects receiving hypnotherapy were compared with those on a symptom-monitoring waiting list, the pretreatment to 2-month follow-up replication reported significant improvement for pain, bloating, flatulence, state and trait anxiety. Of 11 subjects treated, 9 were significantly clinically improved. See Blanchard (2001) for more on hypnosis for IBS.

Cognitive Behavioral Therapies[3]

Cognitive-behavioral therapies are appropriate for many patients with IBS (Greene & Blanchard, 1994; Payne & Blanchard, 1995; Blanchard & Malamood, 1996; Van Dulmen et al., 1996; Toner et al., 1998, 2000; Blanchard, 2001). Blanchard and Malamood (1996) reviewed the prior two studies from their group in which a total of 17 of 22 patients showed clinical improvement; they concluded that cognitive therapy has yielded stronger and more consistent results, including superiority to psychological placebo, than any other psychological treatment" (p. 242). Note that their version of treatment (Blanchard, 2001) includes relaxation training, and thermal biofeedback, as well as cognitive therapy.

Van Dulmen et al. (1996) compared a multicomponent treatment focused on cognitive-behavioral therapies to a waiting-list control. There were positive changes in multiple IBS symptoms (primarily abdominal-pain-predominant symptoms), maintenance of improvements over an average of over 2 years, and improvements in stress management strategies and behaviors. The average improvement was 37%, versus worsening of 22% of those waiting for treatment. Slightly fewer than half of the treated group improved at least 50%, compared to a small percentage of control patients. When the control patients were treated, their average improvement was comparable to those originally treated.

The treatment package was provided in eight 2–hour group sessions over 3 months. The package involved patient education based on cognitive-behavioral therapies, homework assignments and discussion, progressive muscle relaxation each session, and group conversation about the education and homework. Therapeutic strategies used included reporting increased "positive cognitions" and emotions such as "worrying less," "getting angry less frequently," and "thinking that the pain will decrease" (p. 512).

There were several strengths in this study, including symptoms rated four times daily, ratings of several complaints, a good-sized patient sample of 43, and fulfillment of several of Klein's (1988) "stringent criteria necessary for a satisfactory treatment trial" (p. 512) in IBS. Limitations included the absence of strict randomization and of an attention placebo group.

Perhaps the most ambitious and extensive study and most detailed descriptions of cognitive-behavioral therapies for IBS are those by Toner et al. (1998, 2000). One should read these sources for extensive and detailed descriptions of the cognitive-behavioral approach to IBS. In these two publications, Toner and her colleagues discuss the assumptions within their model:

- An interaction among psychosocial/psychophysiological factors contributes to perpetuating IBS symptoms and distress.
- Certain cognitions by persons with IBS lead to certain behaviors, such as further medical visits, attention and hypervigilance for somatic sensations, and increased anxiety and psychophysiological arousal.

All or some of the cognitions mentioned above may lead to heightened pain sensitivity. Persons with IBS experience amplified sensations as more intense and noxious. In turn, this may lead to thoughts and worry about medical causes being missed, thus leading to more arousal and self-inspection, and expanding somatic sensations still further.

Toner and her colleagues compared cognitive-behavioral treatment with an attention placebo and with medical treatment. The latter varied and often included medications. The preliminary analyses reported (Toner et al., 1998) supported significant improvement for multiple IBS symptoms in the cognitive-behavioral group but not in the other groups.

Biofeedback-Assisted Relaxation

One can justify biofeedback-assisted relaxation to help reduce autonomic arousal and dysregulation, and to enhance patient confidence in selected abilities for physiological self-regulation. For example, thermal biofeedback is a logical and proper component of a treatment program. However, there are limits or boundaries for clinical practice, based on the available research. There is not enough evidence to argue persuasively for always needing biofeedback to achieve improvement of IBS. Nevertheless, practitioners should consider biofeedback modalities that involve the autonomic nervous system (ANS); however, they must justify them on logical grounds for specific patients, rather than use research justification. Many practitioners make use of *cognitive restructuring* separately as part of biofeedback. Biofeedback for some patients with IBS may be part of the encouraging and cognitive restructuring process, rather than needed for the degree of relaxation achieved.

Practitioners who are knowledgeable and experienced with biofeedback take issue with the statement by Drossman and Thompson (1992) that biofeedback is "relatively expensive." It need be no more expensive than any office-based relaxation therapy or psychotherapy. Practitioners do not need to charge more because they use biofeedback instruments. The proper question to ask is "Would a form of biofeedback add something useful to the treatment of a specific patient?"

Of more direct relevance to practitioners using biofeedback is the question of autonomic differences among groups with and without IBS symptoms, differences between patients and nonpatients with IBS symptoms, and changes in response to stress among patients with IBS. Studies reviewed by Payne, Blanchard, Holt, and Schwarz (1992) support the presence of ANS reactivity.

However, not all studies have supported psychophysiological differences (e.g., ANS activity and reactivity, neuroendocrine variables) between patients with IBS and controls or versus nonpatients with IBS symptoms (Payne et al., 1992; Levine, Jarrett, Cain, & Heitkemper, 1997). These studies show the difficulties of studying these questions even in well-controlled studies, as well as the presence of some inconsistencies in published results among studies. These two studies pointed out the need for multiple physiological responses, measurements under multiple conditions, and sufficient stressors and sufficient durations of stressors, and studying patients and nonpatients with IBS symptoms. Clearly, practitioners must be cautious in interpreting psychophysiological baseline data and reactivity to cognitive and other office stress stimuli.

Nevertheless, a relationship between ANS dysfunction reflected in cardiac activity and IBS was reported by Adeyemi, Desai, Towsey, and Ghista (1999). The study group of 35 patients had primarily constipation-predominant IBS, severe abdominal distension (i.e., bloating), epigastric pain, and flatulence. The ANS dysfunction involved "increased sympathetic activity at rest and impaired suppression of parasympathetic activity during . . . stress" (p. 822).

Furthermore, among patients with IBS, increased colon motor activity is a response at least to emotional stimulation (Welgan, Meshkinpour, & Ma, 2000). These authors reported:

> Anger as well as fear, pain, and anxiety increase colon motor activity in both IBS and normal subjects, although IBS patients respond to these emotions with higher motor activity, . . . while antral motor activity did not differ significantly in our groups during rest, anger decreased antral motor activity in IBS patients and increased antral motor activity in normal controls. The difference was not attributable to a difference in anger levels, . . . Rather, the difference in the antral motor response appears to be qualitative and a possible marker for irritable bowel syndrome, . . . data further suggest that increased colon motor activity in IBS patients during emotional stress is not a result of a rise in motor activity throughout the gastrointestinal tract, but a phenomenon that may be unique to the colon in this patient population. (p. 248)

Direct Biofeedback for the Colon

Colonic Motility Sounds. Attempting to modify bowel sounds or *colonic motility sounds* using an electronic stethoscope is a very direct biofeedback method and was the first type of biofeedback used for IBS (Furman, 1973). The only published attempt to replicate the original report of success with five patients by Furman (1973) reported equivocal results with a few patients (Radnitz & Blanchard, 1988, 1989). Whitehead (1992b) concluded that this method is not very successful; he stated that it produces "relatively weak treatment effects and the technique is rarely used" (p. 69).

Rectal Feedback. Another direct biofeedback technique used transducers measuring pressure from a rectal balloon to detect contractions from pressure on the balloon. Visual feedback helped 14 of 21 patients with IBS to reduce contractile activity (Bueno-Miranda, Cerulli, & Schuster, 1976). However, a replication from the same laboratory showed that muscle relaxation and systematic desensitization-type treatments were better than the rectal balloon method and more practical (Whitehead, 1985). Based on that study and those by Radnitz and Blanchard (1988, 1989), and personal communications to Whitehead (1992a) about unpublished studies, Whitehead relegated rectal pressure feedback to the archives of biofeedback techniques for IBS. Thus direct attempts to change colonic activity are not part of current practice.

Biofeedback-Assisted Treatment for Fecal Incontinence. Other types of biofeedback can be part of treating the fecal incontinence that sometimes accompanies the diarrhea-predominant form of IBS. This can help increase awareness of anal canal sensations and strengthen external anal sphincter control. (See Tries & Eisman, Chapter 27, this volume.)

Other Therapies

Some patients need couple therapy, child management and parenting instruction, help with time use management (including improved quantity and quality of sleep), and/or therapy to work through old traumas in their lives (including abuse). Time use management covers such topics as time wasting, procrastination, perfectionism, being and feeling overburdened, and prioritizing for self-care (Schwartz, 2000).

Recent research with time series analysis of sleep disturbance and IBS symptoms the next day indicates that disturbed sleep "is associated with exacerbations of IBS symptoms" the following day (Goldsmith & Levin, 1993, p. 1812). Whether this is a direct or indirect relationship is not known, nor are the mechanisms involved; however, the implication is that "therapeutic strategies designed to reduce sleep disruption seem reasonable" (Goldsmith & Levin, 1993, p. 1813).

In today's health care climate, prudent practitioners reserve the above-described approaches for those patients who clearly need them. These interventions are for patients with moderate-intensity symptoms and a few with severe symptoms who are unresponsive to other approaches.

Drossman and Thompson (1992) understandably refer to "physician-based behavioral techniques" for patients with severe or intractable symptoms. Drossman and Thompson are gastroenterologists; we assume they agree that nonphysician practitioners can effectively be part of the team working with these patients. Overall goals include reducing maladaptive illness behaviors in this small but very disabled subset of patients.

Physicians, and increasingly primary care physicians, show an ongoing "commitment to the patient's well-being rather than the treatment of the disease" (p. 1014). Treatment decisions based on presented options become more the responsibility of the patient. Situations that facilitate or reward overfocus on symptoms (e.g., "organ recital") should be avoided.

Other Treatments to Include in Multicomponent Programs

It is patently clear that one should avoid relying exclusively on any single treatment for IBS.

Patient Education and Reassurance

Treatment should always start with patient education, to clearly explain the roles of diet, stress, aerobic exercises, psychological, and psychophysiological factors. One should reassure patients that IBS is by no means life-threatening, but acknowledge the frustrating and distressing nature of the symptoms for them. Positive expectations should be discussed prudently and realistically.

Symptom Monitoring and Modification

A symptom log should be considered for patients with moderate or severe symptoms; it is perhaps unnecessary with milder symptoms. Most logs include at least the time and degrees of the symptoms. One purpose is to identify, elicit, and emphasize such factors such as milk intolerance, caffeine, and stressors. The log should include information about eating, drinking, medications, and smoking habits.

Dietary Considerations

Practitioners often encourage people with IBS to focus on dietary intake, especially when they suspect that specific foods contribute to individuals' symptoms. There are studies that support a role for dietary factors in terms of sensitivities to foods or allergies (e.g., Georges & Heitkemper, 1994; Jarrett, Heitkemper, Bond, & Georges, 1994; Dainese, Galliani, De Lazzari, Di Leo, & Naccarato, 1999; Locke, Zinsmeister, Talley, Fett, & Melton, 2000). However, persons with IBS are often "unable to identify offending foods correctly" (Dainese et al., 1999, p. 1896).

In an extensive population-based rather than patient-based survey, "IBS was significantly associated with use of analgesics . . . for reasons other than IBS" (Locke et al., 2000, p. 157). The investigators stated that the explanation is unclear. IBS was "associated with the reporting of many food allergies or sensitivities" (p. 157) among many persons in the survey. However, no specific types of food were implicated, hence supporting the view that "people with IBS have difficulties with food in general" (p. 163). These authors "suspect that the IBS causes the food sensitivity rather than vice versa [although] . . . some IBS symptoms may be true allergic reactions" (p. 163).

Thus dietary factors, possible allergic sensitivities, and intake of some chemicals (e.g., analgesics) are appropriately part of the management of IBS; yet there is no clear support for the role of alcohol, caffeine, fat, and other dietary factors, which vary widely among persons with IBS (implicating problems with a variety of foods). Evaluating possible food allergies among persons with IBS is very complex and unclear, but is still the focus of many patients.

If there is constipation, a physician or a registered dietitian may recommend gradually adding fiber to the person's diet. This process usually starts with natural sources (e.g., fruits, vegetables, whole grains, legumes) before supplements with psyllium (e.g., Metamucil or Konsyl) are tried. Poorly digested fiber and colonic metabolism often lead to gaseousness and bloating (Drossman & Thompson, 1992), but this condition usually subsides over time.

Diarrhea may result from ingesting common irritants to the digestive tract (e.g., nicotine, alcohol, caffeine, spicy foods, orange juice and other concentrated fruit juices, raw fruits, and raw vegetables ("Irritable Bowel Syndrome," 1992, pp. 2–3). However, some research does not support this consistently (Locke et al., 2000; Dainese et al., 1999). A smaller percentage of people get abdominal cramping, gas, and diarrhea from dairy products. This is especially true for those people without lactase, the intestinal enzyme needed to digest milk sugar. Some dietetic sweeteners, such as sorbitol or fructose, can cause diarrhea. Some medications irritate bowel functioning and may require dose alteration or replacement with alternate medications. Regular aerobic exercises, including walking, are also frequently recommended for those people physically able to do them.

Some people present with very restrictive diets. In such cases, one should consider rechallenging and evaluating the effects of suspected dietary substances, to avoid unnecessary exaggeration of long-term dietary restriction and possible impairment of nutrition. An elimination diet for diarrhea-dominant IBS can help identify specific sensitivities, but it is a very complex procedure with arguable value.

In a stepped-care model, the above-described treatments are sometimes not enough, especially for patients with moderate- and severe-intensity symptoms. In such cases, pharmacotherapy should be considered, as described next. The sequence and combinations depend on health care specialty, practitioner preferences and skills, patient preferences, and financial considerations. They also depend on availability of time. The order we have followed is based partly on Drossman and Thompson (1992), who also imply no specific sequence.

Pharmacotherapy Directed at Specific Symptoms

Until more information is obtained about the precise etiology of IBS, the treatment will remain largely symptomatic. For the majority of patients with mild symptoms, dietary and lifestyle changes are usually sufficient for treatment.

For patients with moderate symptoms, pharmacological treatment aimed at the gut and behavioral treatment may be effective. For patients with severe or refractory symptoms, antidepressant medications for pain control will frequently be required, along with a multidisciplinary approach (e.g., teamwork with a psychologist and gastroenterologist).

Physicians treating patients with IBS are traditionally accustomed to the use of pharmacotherapy. In this section, we review pharmacological compounds in the treatment of IBS. Although the treatment approach is frequently based on the predominant bowel symptom (pain, constipation, or diarrhea), it is very important to recognize that symptoms commonly overlap in many patients with IBS.

Reviews of the Literature. An early critique of randomized controlled trials (Klein, 1988) found no convincing evidence to support the efficacy of any medication to treat IBS. That paper highlighted the multiplicity of problems in study design in treatment trials to that date. More recent publications continue to indicate serious design problems in pharmacological trials of patients with IBS (Jailwala, Imperiale, & Kroenke, 2000; Akehurst & Kaltenthaler, 2001).

All published English-language studies included in four database sets were reviewed by Jailwala et al. (2000). The database sets were MEDLINE (1966–1999), EMBASE (1980–1999), PsycINFO (1967–1999), and the Cochrane controlled-trials registry. The following is a summary of the findings from the Jailwala et al. (2000) study.[4]

1. *Bulking agents* (Table 29.1). Thirteen trials were available for review. The efficacy of these agents was considered "not clearly established."
2. *Smooth muscle relaxants* (Table 29.1). Sixteen trials were reviewed. The information suggested that these compounds "were beneficial for abdominal pain." These findings are also consistent with a meta-analysis that reported the beneficial effects of smooth muscle relaxants (Talley et al., 1993). Of note is that four smooth muscle relaxants are currently not approved by the U.S. Food and Drug Administration for use in the United States (cimetropium, pinaverium, otilonium, and trimebutine). Another meta-analysis of 26 randomized studies of smooth muscle relaxants confirmed these conclusions and reported significant benefit from these agents when compared to placebo (Poynard, Naveau, Mory & Chaput, 1994).
3. *Prokinetic agents (domperidone and cisapride).* Six trials were available for review, and only two found these compounds efficacious. Thus "the evidence does not support the use of cisapride and is inconclusive for the use of domperidone." Cisapride has recently been withdrawn from the market by the FDA due to concerns with cardiac arrhythmias. Domperidone is not available in the United States.
4. *Antimotility agents (loperamide).* All four available studies on loperamide found it beneficial for the treatment of diarrhea.

5. *Psychotropic agents* (Table 29.1). Seven studies were examined and reported beneficial effects in general. Global improvement was reported in five trials; four of seven trials described improvement in abdominal pain and diarrhea, but not in constipation. However, Jailwala et al. (2000) concluded that the "evidence of psychotropic agents is inconclusive, more high quality trials are needed" (p. 142). Although selective serotonin reuptake inhibitors (SSRIs) are preferred over tryciclic antidepressants because of their lower adverse-effects profile, they have not been yet critically evaluated in IBS.

6. *Peppermint oil*. Three trials were available (one was a favorable study), leading Jailwala et al. (2000) to conclude that the efficacy of this agent is "not clearly established."

In another review of the literature (Akehurst & Kalenthaler, 2001), all randomized trials of pharmacological treatment for IBS during 1987–1998 were identified, with 45 studies found. Of those, only 6 met a high standard of quality (adequate description of randomization, double-blind conditions, and description of withdrawals and dropouts). Very similar conclusions to those of Jailwala et al. (2000) were noted regarding the efficacy of bulking agents, antispasmodics/anticholinergic drugs, and psychotropic compounds. In addition, the authors concluded that there remains a strong need for well-designed randomized placebo trials that also include well-defined outcome measures.

In summary, it is apparent from the critical reviews cited here and from subsequent appraisals that despite the multiplicity of pharmacological trials completed, there are serious problems with the literature on pharmacological treatment of IBS. One of the most important findings is that the median placebo response rate is 47% (range 0–84%) (Spiller, 1999). In addition, many of the previously published studies have included few patients, and the study duration is less than 3 months. Undoubtedly, future therapeutic trials must take into consideration these flaws in study design.

The Role of Serotonin Receptors. Serotonin (5-hydroxytriptamine or 5-HT) is a major neurotransmitter in the GI tract, where large amounts are synthesized in the mucosal *enterochromaffin (EC) cells* and in enteric or small intestine neurons. It also acts as a *paracrine*-signaling molecule. It can be released in response to pressure exerted on the intestinal mucosa or by other mediators. Thus mechanical or chemical stimuli can lead to release of 5-HT by EC cells. 5-HT then initiates peristaltic and secretory reflexes. Extrinsic sensory neurons activated by 5-HT initiate bowel sensations, including nausea, bloating, and pain.

TABLE 29.1. **Some Pharmacological Agents Studied in the Treatment of IBS**

Bulking agents	Smooth muscle relaxants	Psychotropic compounds
Psyllium	Cimetropium	Nortriptyline
Coarse bran	Mebeverine	Amitriptyline
Wheat bran	Dycyclomine	Desipramine
Concentrated fiber	Trimebutine	Trimipramine
Calcium polycarbophil	Rociverine	Mepiprazole
Ispaghula husk	Diltiazem	Meprobamate
	Pinaerium	
	Otilonium	
	Pirenzipine	
	Pirifinium	

Note. The data are partly from Jailwala, Imperiale, and Kroenke (2000).

During the past decade, it has been shown that 5-HT receptors in the GI tract play an important role in the modulation of visceral sensation and gut motility. This observation has led to research for pharmacological agents that may have an effect on these receptors. Several compounds that belong to the 5-HT family have been developed and studied in IBS. They are briefly reviewed here.

- *Alosetron.* A highly potent and specific 5-HT$_3$ receptor antagonist, this drug increases colonic compliance in IBS patients. During two large placebo-controlled trials, this compound was superior to placebo in improving abdominal pain, stool consistency, stool frequency, and urgency in female patients with IBS. By contrast, no consistent improvement was seen in male patients with IBS. The only adverse effect noted was constipation (Camilleri et al., 2000). This drug was launched in the United States in March 2000 for the treatment of diarrhea-predominant IBS in women. Unfortunately, more than 50 cases of ischemic colitis were reported (some leading to death) in association with this compound. This observation led to withdrawal of alosetron from the U.S. market in 2001.
- *Tegaserod.* This is a selective partial agonist highly selective for the 5-HT^4 receptor. This compound stimulates GI motility and reduces visceral afferent sensitivity (Camilleri, 2001). Three large phase III randomized, double-blind, placebo-controlled trials (involving 799 patients or more in each trial) were completed in predominantly females (85%) with constipation-predominant IBS. These studies suggest that this compound induces significant improvements in abdominal pain and in bowel movement frequency and consistency, with minimal side effects (the most common was diarrhea). This medication has just been released for use in the United States and is becoming an important treatment option for IBS (Muller-Lissner et al., 2001; Whorwell et al., 2000; Lefkowitz, Ruegg, Shi, & Baldauf, 2000).
- *Other 5-HT agents.* Several drugs belonging to the group of 5-HT^3 receptor antagonist agents—granisetron, ondansetron, tropisetron and cilansetron are still being evaluated. Further research is needed to determine whether they will have a significant role in the treatment of IBS. Prucalopride may have a beneficial effect in patients with constipation. Studies with this compound have been suspended because of concern with tumorigenic effects in animals.

K-receptor Agonists. Alternative approaches to decreasing abdominal pain have included the use of the opioid k-receptor agonists, such as fedotizine and trimebutine. Following a double-blind controlled trial for 6 weeks in patients with IBS, fedotizine was found superior to placebo in relieving abdominal pain and bloating, without significant alterations in bowel function (Dapoigny, Abitbol, & Fraitag, 1995). Despite the apparent benefits of this agent, it has not been promoted for the treatment of IBS in the United States.

Somatostatin Analogues. Somatostatin and its analogues have an antinociceptive property in both human and animal models (Farthing, 1999). A single-case report suggests that octreotide (a synthetic analogue of somatostatin) may improve symptoms of IBS (Talley, Turner, & Middleton, 1987). Large clinical trials are needed to determine whether this agent will be efficacious in the management of IBS symptoms.

Polyethylene-Glycol Electrolyte Solutions for Constipation-Predominant IBS. In recent years, a new therapy for constipation has emerged. This therapy is based on the use of a isosmotic polyethylene-glycol electrolyte (PEG) solution. Studies in adults have shown that, compared with placebo, patients receiving PEG solutions had a significant increase in weekly bowel movement frequency at 4-week follow-up (Corazziari et al., 1996).

Psychopharmacological Treatment

Some patients with severe or intractable symptoms may benefit from antidepressants or other psychopharmacological treatments (Drossman & Thompson, 1992).

CONCLUSIONS: IMPLICATIONS AND GUIDELINES FOR TREATMENT

The guidelines and implications for treatments of IBS depend partly on the nature of and severity of the symptoms, practitioner preferences and training, available treatments, patient preferences, and practical factors. Prudent practitioners tailor graduated treatments to patients. About 70% of people with IBS have mild or infrequent symptoms with no disruptions of activities (Drossman & Thompson, 1992; Drossman et al., 1994). Primary care physicians typically see these people who have no major functional impairment or psychological disturbance. The 25% of patients with moderate symptoms experience periodic disruptions in their activities, often show more psychological distress, and use health care services more often. Gastroenterologists often see these people. The estimated 5% of patients with severe or intractable IBS symptoms fear a serious underlying disease and gravitate to tertiary medical centers. They are typically not aware of the relationship between IBS and psychological symptoms that is usually present. Their IBS symptoms do not correlate with specific stimuli, such as meals, activities, or hormonal changes.

The graduated approach described by Drossman and Thompson (1992) is an excellent model with many useful recommendations. It is similar to, but not exactly the same, as a stepped-care model. In a pure stepped-care model, practitioners move through a graduated list or hierarchy of evaluation and treatment procedures. Each step depends on the results of the prior step. It is assumed that one can start patients with the first steps.

However, in clinical practice, people present with different degrees of severity, variations of symptoms, and comorbidity with other conditions, including psychological conditions. Patients also hold various beliefs about their primary diagnosis. One can start with different combinations of treatment, rather than waiting to observe the outcome of each. Prudent practice usually involves stepped care, a multicomponent approach and long-term follow-up.

As noted earlier, a medical exam is recommended for all patients with symptoms that suggest possible IBS. This often includes laboratory tests to rule out serious organic disease. Physicians usually consider either FlexSig and a barium enema, or fiberoptic colonoscopy if a patient has never been previously examined or has not been examined in recent years. These procedures help rule out organic colonic disease in patients over age 45 with symptoms that may be IBS. Physicians should particularly consider these tests if the symptoms are new, unless the contraindications and risks for colonoscopy or a barium enema dictate otherwise for the patient. After the diagnosis of IBS is made, multicomponent treatment can include various combinations of the following:

- Baseline symptom log (optional in clinical practice) and ongoing log.
- Patient education and reassurance.
- Dietary considerations.
- Pharmacotherapy directed at specific symptoms (predominant pain, diarrhea, or constipation).
- Psychological evaluation and applied psychophysiological/behavioral treatments: relaxation therapies, biofeedback-assisted relaxation, cognitive-behavioral therapies, hypnosis, time use management, other psychological therapies (e.g., couple therapy, child management and parenting instruction, and/or work on trauma/ abuse).

- Psychopharmacological treatment.
- Intensive behavioral/specific pain management treatment for severe or intractable symptoms.

GLOSSARY

BARIUM ENEMAS. Infusions of barium that allow better viewing of the lining of the rectum, colon, and the end of the small bowel (ilium). Used in the diagnosis of colon cancer, Crohn's disease, ulcerative colitis, and polyps.

COGNITIVE RESTRUCTURING. A type of cognitive-behavioral therapy in which a person learns new expectancies and new ways to view himself or herself, others, and events.

COLONIC MOTILITY SOUNDS. Sounds that can be heard with an electronic stethoscope.

COLONOSCOPY, FIBEROPTIC. The use of a fiberoptic endoscope, a flexible instrument that transmits light, to allow examination of the colon lining from the anus to the junction (cecum) of the large and small intestines.

COMPLETE BLOOD COUNT (CBC). Common and basic blood test. Indications include a screen for possible systemic diseases, including suspected hematological (e.g., anemia, leukemia) and infectious diseases.

COMPOSITE PRIMARY SYMPTOM REDUCTION (CPSR) SCORE. One calculates separately a Symptom Reduction Score (SRS) for two or three of the primary presenting symptoms, such as abdominal pain, diarrhea, and constipation. To get each SRS, one subtracts the average symptom rating for a follow-up period from the average rating during a baseline period. The baseline period is 2–4 weeks, and the follow-up period is typically 2 weeks. Then one divides this by the baseline average and multiplies by 100 to get the SRS (e.g., a Diarrhea Reduction Score). The CPSR Score is the total of the SRSs divided by the number of scores (e.g., two or three). Developed at SUNY–Albany.

DISCRIMINATIVE STIMULUS. A specific condition when reinforcement of a behavior occurs, in comparison to other conditions (stimuli). Discriminative refers to properties of the stimulus, not the person discriminating.

ENTEROCHROMAFFIN (EC) CELLS. Group of cells in the gut that secrete serotonin, substance P, and enkephalins. There are three types: antral mucosa, duodenal, and intestinal.

ERYTHROCYTE SEDIMENTATION RATE (ESR). Blood test measuring the rate at which red blood cells settle to the bottom of a container. "If the cells settle faster than normal, this can suggest an infection, anemia, inflammation, rheumatoid arthritis, rheumatic fever, or one of several types of cancer" (Larson, 1990, p. 1283).

FLEXIBLE FIBEROPTIC PROCTOSIGMOIDOSCOPY (FLEXSIG). Examination of the lower part of the colon (sigmoid) and rectum, using a flexible lighted tube. One can see nearly 50% of colorectal cancers or polyps with FlexSig. Also used in diagnosing Crohn's disease and ulcerative colitis. One can get samples of tissue through this instrument.

GLOBAL RATINGS. Patients' estimates of their symptoms without using a specific rating scale or procedure. Often refers to retrospective estimates (e.g., "I feel 50% better," "The diarrhea is 50% better"). Often not an accurate measure of symptom change.

INFLAMMATORY BOWEL DISEASE (IBD). Usually refers to Crohn's disease and ulcerative colitis. The term "colitis" applies to inflammatory disease of the colon. The term "spastic colitis" or "spastic colon" is a misnomer for IBD.

LIFE EXPERIENCES SURVEY. Sarason's (Sarason, Johnson, & Siegel, 1978) Life Experience Scale uses a 6-point scale with positive to negative ratings.

MICROSCOPIC COLITIS. A condition seen more commonly in middle-age women, characterized by persistent diarrhea and frequently confused with irritable bowel. The diagnosis is established by the typical histological findings observed on colon biopsies obtained during colonoscopy.

PARACRINE. In endocrinology, a signaling form in which the signal-releasing cell is close to the target cell, and hence local. Examples are neurotransmitters and neurohormones.

PERISTALTIC. Pertaining to involuntary movements occurring in wavelike contractions, primarily occurring in digestive tract muscles.

ULCERATIVE COLITIS. A chronic inflammatory disease in the colon anywhere in the GI tract. Signs and symptoms include bloody diarrhea, abdominal pain, urgent bowel movements with pain, fever, weight loss, joint pain, and skin lesions.

NOTES

1. Some professionals advocate cognitive-behavioral therapies and other stress management for IBS, and exclude biofeedback and sometimes relaxation therapies from treatment. This chapter assumes that many health care professionals include relaxation therapies as part of multicomponent treatment for IBS, for selected patients for whom such therapies are indicated. Another assumption is that biofeedback is justified as part of helping some persons learn relaxation skills and/or develop self-efficacy about their relaxation skills. An additional assumption is that some professionals use relaxation procedures and biofeedback to modify patients' cognitions about their ability to regulate aspects of their physiology that they thought out of their control. Many patients with IBS also have psychological and psychophysiological conditions (e.g., anxiety, headaches, fibromyalgia) for which relaxation therapies and biofeedback are part of the treatment.

2. The Appendix of the Patrick et al. (1998) article lists the addresses of Donald L. Patrick, PhD, Department of Health Services, H689, Box 357660, University of Washington, Seattle, WA 98195-7660, and Douglas A. Drossman, MD, University of North Carolina at Chapel Hill, CB#7080, Rm. 726, Burnett Womack Building, Chapel Hill, NC 27599-7080.

3. Although some studies and reports focus exclusively on cognitive-behavioral therapies, some include other therapies (including relaxation therapies), although they call the treatment "cognitive-behavioral."

4. References for this discussion are available from us; they have been omitted here because of space limitations.

RESOURCES

Useful Web sites include the following:

    http://www.romecriteria.org
    http://www.pharma.us.novartis
    http://www.med.unc.edu/medicine/fgidc

REFERENCES

Adeyemi, E. O. A., Desai, K. D., Towsey, M., & Ghista, D. (1999). Characterization of autonomic dysfunction in patients with irritable bowel syndrome by means of heart rate variability studies. *American Journal of Gastroenterology, 94,* 816–823.

Akehurst, R., & Kaltenthaler, E. (2001). Treatment of irritable bowel syndrome: A review of randomized controlled trials. Gut, *48,* 272–282.

American Gastroenterological Association Medical Position Statement: Irritable Bowel Syndrome (1997). *Gastroenterology, 112,* 2118–2119. [also, http://www.wbsaunders.com/gastro/policy/v112n6n6p2118.html]

Bearcroft, C. P., Perrett, D., & Farthing, M. J. G. (1998). Postprandial plasma 5–hydroxytryptamine in diarrhea predominant irritable bowel. *Gut, 42,* 42–46.

Bennett, E. J., Piesse, C., Palmer, K., Badcock, C.-A., Tennant, C. C., & Kellow, J. E. (1998a). Functional gastrointestinal disorders: Psychological, social, and somatic features. *Gut, 42,* 414–420.

Bennett, E. J., Tennant, C. C., Piesse, C., Badcock, C. A., & Kellow, J. E. (1998b). Level of chronic life stress predicts clinical outcome in irritable bowel syndrome. *Gut, 43,* 256–261.

Blanchard, E. B. (2001). *Irritable bowel syndrome: Psychological assessment and treatments.* Washington, DC: American Psychological Association.

Blanchard, E. B., Greene, B., Scharff, L., & Schwarz-McMorris, S. P. (1993). Relaxation training as a treatment for irritable bowel syndrome. *Biofeedback and Self-Regulation, 18*(3), 125–132.

Blanchard, E. B., & Malamood, H. S. (1996). Psychological treatment of irritable bowel syndrome. *Professional Psychology: Research and Practice, 27*(3), 241–244.

Blanchard, E. B., Scharff, L., Payne, A., Schwarz, S. P., Suls, J. M., & Malamood, H. (1992a). Prediction of outcome from cognitive-behavioural treatment of irritable bowel syndrome. *Behaviour Research and Therapy, 30*(6), 647–650.

Blanchard, E. B., & Schwarz, S. P. (1987). Adaptation of a multicomponent treatment for irritable bowel syndrome to a small-group format. *Biefeedback and Self-Regulation, 12*(1), 63–69.

Blanchard, E. B., Schwarz, S. P., & Neff, D. F. (1988a). Two-year follow up behavioral treatment of irritable bowel syndrome. *Behavior Therapy*, 19, 67–73.

Blanchard, E. B., Schwarz, S. P., Neff, D. F., & Gerardi, M. A. (1988b). Prediction of outcome from the self-regulatory treatment of irritable bowel syndrome. *Behaviour Research and Therapy*, 26(2), 187–190.

Blanchard, E. B., Schwarz, S. P., Suls, J. M., Gerardi, M. A., Scharff, L., Greene, B., Taylor, A. E., Berreman, C., & Malamood, H. S. (1992b). Two controlled evaluations of multicomponent psychological treatment of irritable bowel syndrome. *Behaviour Research and Therapy*, 30(2), 175–189.

Bueno-Miranda, F., Cerulli, M., & Schuster, M. M. (1976). Operant conditioning of colonic motility in irritable bowel syndrome (IBS) [Abstract]. *Gastroenterology*, 91, A867.

Camilleri, M. (2001). Review article: Tegaserod. *Alimentary Pharmacology and Therapeutics*, 15(3), 277–289.

Camilleri, M., Northcutt, A. R., Kong, S., Dukes, G. E., McSorley, D., & Mangel, A. W. (2000). Efficacy and safety of alosetron in women with irritable bowel syndrome: A randomized, placebo-controlled trial. *Lancet*, 355, 1035–1040.

Corazziari, E., Badiali, D., Habib, F. I., Reboa, G., Pitto, G., Mazzacca, G., Sabbatini, F., Galeazzi, R., Cilluffo, T., Vantini, I., Bardelli, E., & Baldi, F. (1996). Small volume isomotic polyethylene glycol electrolyte balanced solution (PMF-100) in treatment of chronic nonorganic constipation. *Digestive Diseases and Science*, 41(8), 1636–1642.

Dainese, R., Galliani, E. A., De Lazzari, F., Di Leo, V., & Naccarato, R. (1999). Discrepancies between reported food intolerance and sensitization test findings in irritable bowel syndrome patients. *American Journal of Gastroenterology*, 94(7), 1892–1897.

Dancey, C. P., Taghavi, M., & Fox, R. J. (1998). The relationship between daily stress and symptoms of irritable bowel: A time-series approach. *Journal of Psychosomatic Research*, 44(5), 537–545.

Dancey, C. P., Whitehouse, A., Painter, J., & Backhouse, S. (1995). The relationship between hassles, uplifts and irritable bowel syndrome: A preliminary study. *Journal of Psychosomatic Research*, 39(7), 827–832.

Dapoigny, M., Abitbol, H., & Fraitag, B. (1995). Efficacy of the peripheral kappa agonist fedotozine versus placebo in treatment of irritable bowel syndrome. *Digestive Diseases and Sciences*, 40, 2244–2248.

Drossman, D. A. (1994). Irritable bowel syndrome: The role of psychosocial factors. *Stress Medicine*, 10, 49–55.

Drossman, D. A., Leserman, J., Nachman, G., Li, Z., Gluck, H., Toomey, T. C., & Mitchell, C. M. (1990). Sexual and physical abuse in women with functional or organic gastrointestinal disorders. *Annals of Internal Medicine*, 113, 828–833.

Drossman, D. A., McKee, D. C., Sandler, R. S., Mitchell, M., Cramer, E. M., Lowman, B. C., & Burger, A. L. (1988). Psychosocial factors in the irritable bowel syndrome. *Gastroenterology*, 95, 701–708.

Drossman, D. A., Patrick, D. L., Whitehead, W. E., Toner, B. B., Diamant, N. E., Hu, Y., Jia, H., & Bangdiwala, S. I. (2000a). Further validation of the IBS-QOL: A disease-specific quality-of-life questionnaire. *American Journal of Gastroenterology*, 95(4), 999–1007.

Drossman, D. A., Richter, J. E., Talley, N. J., Thompson, W. G., Corazziari, E., & Whitehead, W. E. (1994). *The functional gastrointestinal disorders: Diagnosis, pathophysiology and treatment*. McLean, VA: Degnon & Associates.

Drossman, D. A., Sandler, R. S., McKee, D. C., & Lovitz, A. J. (1982). Bowel patterns among subjects not seeking health care. *Gastroenterology*, 83, 529–534.

Drossman, D. A., & Thompson, W. G. (1992). The irritable bowel syndrome: Review and a graduated multicomponent treatment approach. *Annals of Internal Medicine*, 116(12, pt 1), 1009–1016.

Drossman, D. A., Whitehead, W. E., Toner, B. B., Diamant, N. E., Hu, Y. J. B., Bangdiwala, S. I., & Jia, H. (2000b). What determines severity among patients with painful functional bowel disorders? *American Journal of Gastroenterology*, 95(4), 974–980.

Farthing, M. J. G. (1999). Irritable bowel syndrome: New pharmacologic approaches to treatment. *Bailliere's Clinical Gastroenterology*, 13(3), 461–471.

Furman, S. (1973). Intestinal biofeedback in functional diarrhea: A preliminary report. *Journal of Behavior Therapy and Experimental Psychiatry*, 4, 317–321.

Galovski, T. E., & Blanchard, E. B. (1998). The treatment of irritable bowel syndrome with hypnotherapy. *Applied Psychotherapy and Biofeedback*, 23(4), 219–232.

Georges, J. M., & Heitkemper, M. M. (1994). Dietary fiber and distressing gastrointestinal symptoms in midlife women. *Nursing Research*, 43(6), 357–361.

Goldsmith, G., & Levin, J. S. (1993). Effect of sleep quality on symptoms of irritable bowel syndrome. *Digestive Diseases and Sciences*, 38(10), 1809–1814.

Goldstein, R., Braverman, D., & Stankiewicz (2000). Carbohydrate malabsorption and the effect of dietary restriction on symptoms of irritable bowel syndrome and functional bowel complaints. *Israeli Medical Association Journal*, 2(8), 583–587.

Greene, B., & Blanchard, E. B. (1994). Cognitive therapy for irritable bowel syndrome. *Journal of Consulting and Clinical Psychology*, 62(3), 576–582.

Haderstorfer, B., Whitehead, W. E., & Schuster, M. M. (1989). Intestinal gas production from bacterial fermentation of undigested carbohydrate in irritable bowel syndrome. *American Journal of Gastroenterology, 84*, 375–378.

Herschbach, P., Henrich, G., & von Rad, M. (1999). Psychological factors in functional gastrointestinal disorders: Characteristics of the disorder or of the illness behavior? *Psychosomatic Medicine, 61*, 148–153.

Horwitz, B. J., & Fisher, R. S. (2001). The irritable bowel syndrome. *New England Journal of Medicine, 344*(24), 1846–1850.

Irritable bowel syndrome. (1992). *Mayo Clinic Health Letter, 10*(12), 1–2.

Jailwala, J., Imperiale, T. F., & Kroenke, K. (2000). Pharmacologic treatment of the irritable bowel syndrome: A systematic review of randomized, controlled trials. *Annals of Internal Medicine, 133*, 136–147.

Jarrett, M., Heitkemper, M. M., Bond, E. F., & Georges, J. (1994). Comparison of diet composition in women with and without functional bowel disorder. *Gastroenterology Nursing, 16*(6), 253–258.

Jarrett, M., Heitkemper, M., Cain, K. C., Tuftin, M., Walker, E. A., Bond, E. F. & Levy, R. L. (1998). The relationship between psychological distress and gastrointestinal symptoms in women with irritable bowel syndrome. *Nursing Research, 47*(3), 154–161.

Klein, K. B. (1988). Controlled treatment trials in irritable bowel syndrome: A critique. *Gastroenterology, 95*, 232–241.

Laird, J. M., Olivar, T., Roza, C., De Felipe, C., Hunt, S. P., & Cervero, F. (2000). Deficits in visceral pain and hyperalgesia of mice with a disruption of the tachykinin NK1 receptor gene. *Neuroscience, 98*(2), 345–352.

Laird, J. M., Souslova, V., Wood, J. N., & Cervero, F. (2002). Deficits in visceral pain and referred hyperalgesia in Nav1.8 (SNS/PN3)-null mice. *Journal of Neuroscience, 22*(19), 8352–8356

Larson, D. E. (1990). *Mayo Clinic family health book.* New York: Morrow.

Ledochowski, M., Widner, B., Bair, H., Probst, T., & Fuchs, D. (2000). Fructose- and sorbitol-reduced diet improves mood and gastrointestinal disturbances in fructose malabsorbers. *Scandinavian Journal of Gastroenterology, 35*(10), 1048–1052.

Lefkowitz, M. P., Ruegg, P. C., Shi, Y., & Baldauf, C. D. (2000). Validation of a global relief measure in two clinical trials of irritable bowel syndrome with tegaserod. *Gastroenterology, 118*(4, Suppl. 2, Pt.1), A145.

Levine, B. S., Jarrett, M., Cain, K. C., & Heitkemper, M. M. (1997). Psychophysiological response to a laboratory challenge in women with and without diagnosed irritable bowel syndrome. *Research in Nursing and Health, 20*, 431–441.

Levy, R. L., Cain, K. C., Jarrett, M., & Heitkemper, M. M. (1997). The relationship between daily life stress and gastrointestinal symptoms in women with irritable bowel syndrome. *Journal of Behavioral Medicine, 20*(2), 177–193.

Locke, G. R., III, Zinsmeister, A. R., Talley, N. J., Fett, S. L., & Melson, L. J. (2000). Risk factors for irritable bowel syndrome: Role of analgesics and food sensitivities. *American Journal of Gastroenterology, 95*(1), 157–165.

Lowman, B. C., Drossman, D. A., Cramer, E. M., & McKee, D. C. (1987). Recollection of childhood events in adults with irritable bowel syndrome. *Journal of Clinical Gastroenterology, 9*, 325–330.

Lynch, P. M., & Zamble, E. (1989). A controlled behavioral treatment study of irritable bowel syndrome. *Behavior Therapy, 20*, 509–523.

Manning, A. P., Thompson, W. G., Heaton, K. W., & Morris, A. F. (1978). Towards positive diagnosis of the irritable bowel. *British Medical Journal, 2*, 653–654.

McKendrick, M. W., & Read, N. W. (1994). Irritable bowel syndrome—post-salmonella infection. *Journal of Infection, 29*, 1–3.

Meissner, J. S., Blanchard, E. B., & Malamood, H. S. (1997). Comparison of treatment outcome measures for irritable bowel syndrome. *Applied Psychophysiology and Biofeedback, 22*(1), 55–62.

Mitchell, C. M., & Drossman, D. A. (1987). Survery of the AGA membership relating to patients with functional gastrointestinal disorders. *Gastroenterology, 92*, 1228–1245.

Muller-Lissner, S. A., Fumagalli, I., Bardhan, K. D., Pace, F., Pecher, E., Nault, B., & Ruegg, P. (2001). Tegaserod, a 5-HT (4) receptor partial agonist, relieves symptoms in irritable bowel syndrome patients with abdominal pain, bloating and constipation. *Alimentary Pharmacology and Therapeutics, 15*(10), 1655–1666.

Neff, D. F., & Blanchard, E. B. (1987). A multi-component treatment for irritable bowel syndrome. *Behavior Therapy, 18*, 70–83.

Patrick, D. L., Drossman, D. A., Frederick, I. O., DiCesare, J., & Puder, K. L. (1998). Quality of life in persons with irritable bowel syndrome: Development of a new measure. *Digestive Diseases and Science, 43*, 400–411.

Payne, A., & Blanchard, E. B. (1995). A controlled comparison of cognitive therapy and self-help support groups in the treatment of irritable bowel syndrome. *Journal of Consulting and Clinical Psychology, 63*, 779–786.

Payne, A., Blanchard, E. B., Holt, C. S., & Schwarz, S. (1992). Physiological reactivity to stressors in irritable bowel syndrome patients, inflammatory bowel disease patients and non-patient controls. *Behaviour Research and Therapy, 30*(3), 293–300.

Poynard, T., Naveau, S., Mory, B., & Chaput, J. C. (1994). Meta-analysis of smooth muscle relaxants in the treatment of irritable bowel syndrome. *Alimentary Pharmacology and Therapeutics, 8,* 499–510.

Radnitz, C. L., & Blanchard, E. B. (1988). Bowel sound biofeedback as a treatment for irritable bowel syndrome. *Biefeedback and Self-Regulation, 13*(2), 169–179.

Radnitz, C. L., & Blanchard, E. B. (1989). A 1- and 2-year follow-up study of bowel sound biofeedback as a treatment for irritable bowel syndrome. *Biofeedback and Self-Regulation, 14*(4), 333–338.

Ritche, J. (1973). Pain from distension of the pelvic colon by inflating a balloon in the irritable colon syndrome. *Gut, 14,* 125–132.

Rumessen, J. J., & Gudmand-Hoyer, E. (1988). Functional bowel disease: Malabsorption and abdominal distress after the ingestion of fructose, sorbitol, and fructose-sorbitol mixtures. *Gastroenterology, 95,* 694–700.

Sarason, J. G., Johnson, J. H., & Siegel, J. M. (1978). Assessing the impact of life changes: Development of the Life Experiences Survey. *Journal of Gnsulting and Clinical Psychology, 46,* 932–946.

Schwartz, M. S. (2000). Time use management. In R. L. Bratton (Ed.), *Mayo Clinic's complete guide for family physicians and residents in training.* New York: McGraw-Hill.

Schwarz, S. P., Blanchard, E. B., & Neff, D. (1986). Behavior treatment of irritable bowel syndrome: A 1-year follow-up study. *Biefeedback and Self-Regulation, 11*(3), 189–198.

Spiller, R. S. (1999). Problems and challenges in the designs of irritable bowel syndrome clinical trials: Experience from published trials. *American Journal of Medicine, 107*(5a), 91S-97S.

Stewart, G. T. (1994). Post-dysenteric colitis. *British Medical Journal, i,* 405–409.

Suls, J., Wan, C. K., & Blanchard, E. B. (1994). A multilevel data-analytic approach for evaluation of relationships between daily life stressors and symptomatology: Patients with irritable bowel syndrome. *Health Psychology, 13*(2), 103–113.

Talley, N. J., Nyren, O., Drossman, D. A., Heaton, K. W., Veldhuyzen van Zanten, S. J. O., Koch, M. M., & Ransohoff, D. F. (1993). The irritable bowel syndrome: Toward optimal design of controlled treatment trials. *Gastroenterology International, 6,* 189–211.

Talley, N. J., Turner, I., & Middleton, W. R. (1987). Somatostatin and symptomatic relief of irritable bowel syndrome. *Lancet, ii,* 1114. (Letter).

Talley, N. J., Zinsmeister, A. R., Van Dyke, C., & Melton, L. J. (1991). Epidemiology of colonic symptoms and the irritable bowel syndrome. *Gastroenterology, 101,* 927–934.

Thompson, W. G., Heaton, K. W., Smyth, G. T., & Smyth, C. (2000). Irritable bowel syndrome in general practice: Prevalence, characteristics, and referral. *Gut, 46,* 78–82.

Thompson, W. G., Longstreth, G. F., Drossman, D. A., Heaton, K. W., Irvine, E. J., & Muller-Lissner, S. A. (1999). Functional bowel disorders and functional abdominal pain. *Gut, 45*(Suppl. 2), 1143–1147.

Thornton, S., Mclntyre, P., Murray-Lyon, I., & Gruzelier, J. (1990). Psychological and psychophysiological characteristics in irritable bowel syndrome. *British Journal of Clinical Psychology, 29,* 343–345.

Toner, B. B., Segal, Z. V., Emmott, S., Ali, A., Di Gasbarro, I., & Stuckless, N. (1998). Cognitive-behavioral group therapy for patients with irritable bowel syndrome. *International Journal of Group Psychotherapy, 48*(2), 215–243.

Toner, B. B., Segal, Z. V., Emmott, S., & Myran, D. (2000). *Cognitive-behavioral treatment of irritable bowel syndrome.* New York: Guilford Press.

Van der Horst, H. E., van Dulmen, A. M., Schellevis, F. G., van Eijk, J. T. M., Fennis, J. F. M., & Bleijenberg, G. (1997). Do patients with irritable bowel syndrome in primary care really differ from outpatients with irritable bowel syndrome? *Gut, 41,* 669–674.

Van Dulmen, A. M., Fennis, J. F. M., & Bleijenberg, G. (1996). Cognitive-behavioral group therapy for irritable bowel syndrome: Effect and long-term follow-up. *Psychosomatic Medicine, 58,* 508–514.

Voirol, M. W., & Hipolito, J. (1987). Relaxation antropoanalytique dans les syndromes de l'intestin irritable: Resultats a 40 mois. *Schweizerische Medizinische Wochenschrift, 117,* 1117–1119.

Walker, E. A., Katon, W. J., Roy-Byrne, P. P., Jemelka, R. P., & Russo, J. (1993). Histories of sexual victimization in patients with irritable bowel syndrome or inflammatory bowel disease. American *Journal of Psychiatry, 150,* 1502–1506.

Welgan, P., Meshkinpour, H., & Ma, L. (2000). Role of anger in antral motor activity in irritable bowel syndrome. *Digestive Diseases and Sciences, 45*(2), 248–251.

Whitehead, W. E. (1985). Psychotherapy and biofeedback in the treatment of irritable bowel syndrome. In N. E. Read (Ed.), *Irritable bowel syndrome.* London: Grune & Stratton.

Whitehead, W. E. (1992a). Behavioral medicine approaches to gastrointestinal disorders. *Journal of Consulting and Clinical Psychology, 60*(4), 605–612.

Whitehead, W. E. (1992b). Biofeedback treatment of gastrointestinal disorders. *Biofeedback and Self-Regulation, 17*(1), 59–76.

Whitehead, W. E. (1993). Gut feelings: Stress and the GI tract. In D. Goleman & J. Gurin (Eds.), *Mind/body medicine*. New York: Consumer Reports Books.

Whitehead, W. E., Bosmajian, L., Zonderman, A. B., Costa, P. T., & Schuster, M. M. (1988). Symptoms of psychological distress associated with irritable bowel syndrome. *Gastroenterology, 95,* 709–714.

Whitehead, W. E., Crowell, M. D., Robinson, J. C., Heller, B. R., & Schuster, M. M. (1992). Effects of stressful life events on bowel symptoms: Subjects with irritable bowel syndrome compared with subjects without bowel dysfunction. *Gut, 33,* 825–830.

Whitehead, W. E., Winget, C., Fedoravicius, A. S., Wooley, S., & Blackwell, B. (1982). Learned illness behavior in patients with irritable bowel syndrome and peptic ulcer. *Digestive Diseases and Sciences, 27,* 202–208.

Whorwell, P. J., Krumholz, S., Muller-Lissner, S., Schmitt, C., Dunger-Baldauf, C., & Ruegg, P. C. (2000). Tegaserod has a favorable safety and tolerability profile in patients with constipation-predominant and alternating forms of irritable bowel syndrome [Abstract]. *Gastroenterology,* 118 (4, Suppl. 2, Pt. 2), A1204.

Whorwell, P. J., Prior, A., & Colgan, S. M. (1987). Hypnotherapy in severe irritable bowel syndrome: Further experience. *Gut, 28,* 423–425.

Whorwell, P. J., Prior, A., & Faragher, E. B. (1984). Controlled trial of hypnotherapy n the treatment of severe refractory irritable bowel syndrome. *Lancet, ii,* 1232–1234.

Pediatric Applications

C H A P T E R   3 0

Pediatric Headache

FRANK ANDRASIK
MARK S. SCHWARTZ

PREVALENCE AND PROGNOSIS

Headaches are surprisingly common in children. Even at the young age of 3, headaches are present in 3–8% of children. This increases to about 20% at age 5, 37–52% at age 7, and 57–82% from ages 7 to 15 (see Lipton, Maytal, & Winner, 2001, for a review). A U.S. study included 3158 children ages 12–17 whose families were contacted by telephone (Linet, Stewart, Celentano, Ziegler, & Sprecher, 1989). Among the many findings were that 56% of the males and 74% of the females reported a headache in the past 4 weeks; 27% of the males and 41.4% of the females reported two or more headaches; and 4.5% of the males and 9.4% of the females reported four or more headaches in the past month. The average intensity was moderate on a 1–10 scale (4.5 for males, 4.7 for females), and the mean duration was 5–6 hours. The pain and suffering children experience can have a significant impact on every aspect of their daily lives (Bandell-Hoekstra, Abu-Saadm, Passchier, & Knipschild, 2000).

Many continue to believe that pediatric headache does not need to be taken seriously, because it will be outgrown with time. Regrettably, this does not hold true for many children so affected, as revealed by the longitudinal work of the Swedish pediatrician Bo Bille and others. Nearly five decades ago (the mid 1950s), Bille began a landmark study of about 9000 Swedish schoolchildren ranging in age from 7 to 15; his first publication (Bille, 1962) told us much about headache occurrence across gender and age. Bille was able to follow a subset of these children, all of whom were diagnosed as having migraine at a very young age, for 40 years. The majority continued to be troubled by headaches at this final follow-up assessment (Bille, 1997). Subsequent work has confirmed the enduring nature of childhood headaches (e.g., Larsson, 2002; Sillanpää, 1994; Waldie, 2001), and has reinforced the importance of early intervention for ameliorating current symptoms and preventing adult symptoms. Furthermore, there are indications that childhood headaches have increased in prevalence over the past decades (Sillanpää & Anttila, 1996).

DIFFERENTIAL DIAGNOSIS AND ASSESSMENT

Diagnosis and medical evaluation for pediatric patients with headache proceeds much as it does for adult patients (Holden, Levy, Deichmann, & Gladstein, 1998; Rothner, 2001). We have pointed out the difficulties in making accurate diagnoses of adult headaches in Chapter 14 of this volume. Pediatric practitioners and researchers believe that it is even more difficult to make specific headache diagnoses for children, because many features depart from those typically seen in adults (Silberstein, 1990; Winner, Wasiewski, Gladstein, & Linder, 1997). Confounding factors may include the regular use of analgesics or ergot derivatives, which often can transform migraines and episodic tension headaches into chronic daily headaches (Gladsten & Holden, 1996). Some professionals believe that in teenagers, "masked depression" is often associated with chronic tension-type headache (Silberstein, 1990). We note that depressed teenagers are very unlikely to admit to being depressed on the more obvious self-report depression measures; thus the clinical interview may be a better assessment method for co-occurring psychological states. Silberstein (1990) looks for "evidence of sleep disturbance, loss of energy, loss of interest, and diminished ability to concentrate. The child frequently looks and behaves depressed but denies depressed affect" (p. 721). However, it may also be worth noting that all or most of the symptoms mentioned by Silberstein (1990) are also those symptoms that result from sleep deprivation—a common self-imposed behavior pattern in adolescents.

McGrath and Koster (2001) provide a number of helpful suggestions for conducting the initial interview, assessing and quantifying headaches, and tracking change over time.

TREATMENT: A STEPPED-CARE APPROACH

As for adult headache, we advocate a stepped or stratified approach to the treatment of pediatric headache, possibly beginning with identification and modification of obvious triggers and contributing factors (Andrasik, Blake, & McCarran, 1986; McGrath & Hillier, 2001). Dietary factors are commonly addressed at an early stage (Rossi, Bardare, & Brunelli, 2002; see also Block, Schwartz, & Gyllenhaal, Chapter 9, this volume). Silberstein (1990) suggests the following:

- Reassure the family that the condition is benign.
- Recommend adjustments in the child's lifestyle, including "regular bedtime, a reasonable meal schedule, and the avoidance of overload in activities" (p. 722).
- Help the family identify and eliminate headache triggers ("physical exertion, hunger, noise, traveling, light glare, certain foods, and head trauma"; p. 722).
- "In children with a disturbed home life, significant depression, or abuse, family and individual psychotherapy is indicated" (p. 722).

Prudent practitioners will also consider medications, depending in part on the frequency of the headaches, the severity and durations of the headaches, and the effectiveness of simple analgesics. Prophylactic medications are useful for some children with chronic headaches, especially those who have "severe, frequent attacks" and those "complicated by neurological symptoms" (Silberstein, 1990). See Levin (2001), Pothmann (2002), and Winner (2001) for a more complete discussion of medication approaches. The use of medications does not preclude the use of biofeedback and relaxation.

As with adults, various nonpharmacological therapies have been investigated for treating recurrent headaches in children; chief among these are relaxation, biofeedback, and cognitive-behavioral therapies. Larsson and Andrasik (2002) found over 10 investigations of varied forms of relaxation, applied in varied settings (clinics and schools) and by varied personnel (therapists, teachers, nurses, etc.). Generally positive effects have been obtained, pointing to the robustness of this approach (Hermann, Kim, & Blanchard, 1995). These treatments have typically involved the following components:

- Discrimination training, focusing on identification of tense and relaxed larger muscle groups.
- Differential relaxation.
- Cued relaxation.
- Minirelaxation, focusing on a limited number of muscles in the head, neck, or shoulder.
- Application of techniques in everyday life.

Among biofeedback modalities, thermal (autogenic) and surface electromyographic (EMG) biofeedback have been studied the most extensively for pediatric headache. Efficacy studies (Holden, Deichmann, & Levy, 1999; McGrath, Stewart, & Koster, 2001) and meta-analyses (see Figure 30.1, which illustrates data from Hermann et al., 1995) confirm their clinical utility and comparative efficacy with regard to certain medications. The use of other biofeedback modalities, such as electroencephalographic (Siniatchkin et al., 2000) and blood volume pulse biofeedback, remains in the infancy stage (Andrasik, Larsson, & Grazzi, 2002). Several investigations have revealed reasonable maintenance effects over time (Grazzi et al., 2001; see studies reviewed in Larsson & Andrasik, 2002), although at least one has been less positive (Kuhn & Allen, 1993). Unfortunately, minimal attention has been directed at identifying predictors of initial and enduring responses to treatment. A recent meta-analysis has shown that these biofeedback treatments lead to more positive clinical outcomes (but not greater levels of physiological control) when used with children than when applied with adults (Sarafino & Goehring, 2000; see Figure 30.2). These findings support the notion that children may be especially good candidates for biofeedback (Attanasio et al., 1985). Children appear to display a greater placebo response (Bussone, Grazzi, D'Amico, Leone, & Andrasik, 1998; Hermann et al., 1995), which may account in part for the enhanced overall effects.

Cognitive therapy or cognitive stress coping training has been much less investigated, but it too has promise. With one exception (Richter et al., 1986), cognitive approaches have

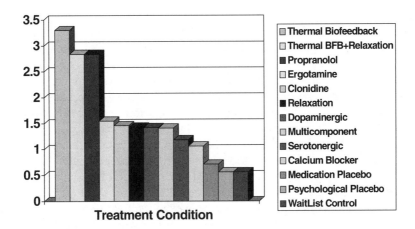

FIGURE 30.1. Within-group effect size values for behavioral and pharmacological treatments for childhood migraine. For this type of effect size, values greater than 1 reflect medium to large effects. The data are from Hermann, Kim, and Blanchard (1995).

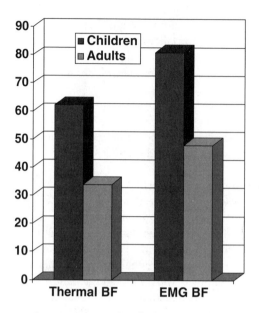

FIGURE 30.2. Mean percentage improvement in headache activity for children and adults by thermal and EMG biofeedback (BF). Values are subject-weighted means. The number of subjects and the number of studies upon which the values are based are as follows: children's thermal BF (65/6), children's EMG BF (19/4), adults' thermal BF (243/15), and adults' EMG BF (238/25). The data are from Sarafino and Goehring (2000).

been combined with other major treatment modalities, and the experimental designs employed have not made it possible to partial out the source of effects.

The "prudent limited office treatment" (PLOT) cost containment approach, which we have described in Chapter 14, has been extended to treating pediatric patients with headache. Preliminary investigations of children with migraines suggest that autogenic feedback may work equally well when delivered in the PLOT format, with either a child or a parent serving as the main treatment agent for the home instruction (Burke & Andrasik, 1989; Guarnieri & Blanchard, 1990; Allen & McKeen, 1991; Hermann, Blanchard, & Flor, 1997; see Haddock et al., 1997, for a quantitative review). This approach increases the need for family involvement and support, leading Guarnieri and Blanchard (1990) to speculate that environmental factors may be particularly important when such limited-contact treatments are employed (e.g., effects may be lessened when the home is somewhat chaotic or nonsupportive). This makes sense for a pediatric population, but requires further study. Cautious practitioners will check the home environment before deciding upon this approach in clinical practice. Data bearing on this point come from the investigation of Allen and McKeen (1991): Several of the children who were treated complied with relaxation, but their parents did not follow the guidelines for behavior management that were a part of the treatment package. These children then gradually worsened over treatment and subsequently did not do as well as the others. At a later follow-up, though, the children who initially responded had regressed, and differences were no longer apparent (Kuhn & Allen, 1993). Most recently, the effectiveness of single-session behavioral treatment has been examined (Powers et al., 2001). Although statistical significance was obtained, symptom reductions were only 10%, 25%, and 25% for headache severity, frequency, and duration, respectively, at a modest follow-up (average of 21 weeks). Thus more intensive therapeutic effort is needed.

Another approach to cost containment concerns group administration. This approach has been used regularly by Larsson and colleagues with relaxation approaches administered in school settings (see Larsson & Andrasik, 2002). Preliminary evidence supports the utility of a brief group behavioral treatment that is designed to be easily administered by a neurologist and to place minimal demands upon both provider and patient; this treatment too could thus actually be applied in various day-to-day medical practice settings. In this investigation (Andrasik et al., 2003), 34 children (from 9 to 16 years of age) with episodic tension-type headache were seen in small groups (3–5 individuals of similar ages) once per week for 8 weeks, with sessions limited to a maximum of 30 minutes. Each session followed the same format: practice of progressive muscle relaxation training with eight muscle groups (lower arms, upper arms, legs, abdomen, chest, shoulders, eyes, and forehead), and discussion of ways to apply relaxation to cope with headache and headache-related distress. A tape recording of the first session was provided to guide home practice. Patients were instructed to practice with the tape once per day during treatment and twice per week thereafter. A neurologist, who conferred with a behavioral psychologist, provided treatment. Statistically significant effects were found for several variables (except analgesic tablets), and most of these changes were clinically meaningful as well (≥50%). The improvements noted at the end of treatment held throughout the 1 year of follow-up. Although the reduction in analgesic tablet consumption was not statistically significant, it was sizable from a clinical perspective (i.e., it exceeded 50%). Although this investigation was uncontrolled, the magnitude of effects rivaled those of typical, more effort-intensive behavioral treatments and surpassed those that are typical for placebo effects (Hermann et al., 1995). Further research on this type of approach, with larger samples, appears warranted.

We must also point out that, as for adults, factors mediating treatment effects for children are not clear. Few straightforward relationships have been found between symptom changes and physiological changes during and across treatment sessions. Various psychological processes, such as self-efficacy and perceived control, have been proposed as important mediators (Allen & Shriver, 1997; Hermann & Blanchard, 2002). We discuss the complexity of this relationship more fully in Chapter 14.

CLINICAL CONSIDERATIONS AND "TIPS" FOR APPLYING BIOFEEDBACK AND RELATED TREATMENTS TO PEDIATRIC HEADACHE

From clinical experience in working with children and adolescents ranging in age from 6 to 17, Attanasio et al. (1985) have identified a number of advantages in working with younger individuals, which may help account for their enhanced treatment response (see Table 30.1). Certain difficulties are encountered as well (see Table 30.1), but these potential problems are easily addressed by tailoring language to children's comprehension levels, taking the time to ensure optimal understanding, decreasing the length of biofeedback trials, adding rest periods, and employing contingency management strategies to sustain performance when motivation lags.

Green (1983) provides a number of very helpful suggestions and verbatim scripts to use in teaching self-regulatory skills to very young children. Her recommendations for the practitioner include the following:

- Invite the family unit to the initial session, to prevent the child from being singled out as the "problem" or the "sick one."
- Introduce yourself as a "biofeedback teacher"—someone who teaches ideas and skills, who likes to be asked questions, and who in turn likes to ask questions.
- Demonstrate biofeedback with a response that is easily controlled or that produces a quick, discernible response (EMG from the forearm, electrodermal response while playing a guessing game).

TABLE 30.1. Advantages and Disadvantages of Treating Children with Biofeedback

Advantages

- Increased enthusiasm
- Quicker rate of learning
- Less skepticism about self-control procedures
- Greater confidence in special abilities
- Increased psychophysiological lability
- Few previous failure experiences with treatment
- Increased enjoyment when practicing
- Increased reliability of symptom monitoring

Disadvantages

- Briefer attention span
- Off-task behaviors during session
- Fear and apprehension about equipment
- Intolerance of minor discomfort in removing sensors
- Possible complications created by emotional and psychological problems
- Reduced ability to comprehend treatment rationale and procedures
- Possible complications of scheduling
- Lack of standardized electrode placements

Note. Based on Attanasio et al. (1985).

- Incorporate adjunctive techniques, such as belly or diaphragmatic breathing (see Gervirtz & Schwartz, Chapter 10, this volume), body scanning, the "limp rag doll" technique, and imagery.

Although fairly straightforward translations of biofeedback and related treatments developed for adult patients have met with much success in pediatric populations, it is likely that these effects could be enhanced by adding a developmental perspective to evaluation and treatment. Marcon and Labbé (1990) discuss cognition, self-regulation, psychosocial factors, and other issues that arise at various stages of development. Some of the examples reviewed concern conceptualizations of pain; differences in language, time perception, and approaches to tasks; and varied abilities to comprehend the notion of severity. Marcon and Labbé also point to the importance of considering environmental influences on headache, specifically attention from family members and teachers.

Allen and Shriver (1998) provide a concrete illustration of this last point. They randomly assigned children and adolescents (ages 7–18) with migraines to either standard thermal biofeedback or biofeedback combined with "pain behavior management" training for parents. Parents assigned to the latter condition were instructed to minimize reactions to pain behavior displays; to insist upon participation in normal, planned activities to the extent possible; and to praise and support biofeedback practice. Thermal biofeedback led to significant improvement (as expected), but the addition of parent training added a further significant increment to treatment. The combined treatment group obtained greater overall reductions in headache frequency, had a larger percentage of patients displaying clinically significant improvements (reductions greater than 50%), and revealed better adaptive functioning (i.e., pain led to less interference in daily activities). Benefits from the addition of parent behavior management training have not been uniformly demonstrated, however (Kröner-Herwig, Mohn, & Pothmann, 1998).

As noted above, a PLOT approach can work for pediatric patients, but this approach increases the need for family involvement and support. The practitioner should check the home environment before deciding upon this approach.

Finally, it is instructive to add here that some children, like some adults, "prefer the feedback and do less well without it. Other patients seem to be bothered by the feedback" (Duckro & Cantwell-Simmons, 1989, p. 432). "In either case, the information is still useful for the therapist" (p. 432).

SUMMARY AND CONCLUSIONS

Relaxation and varied biofeedback treatments for pediatric patients with headache have been repeatedly investigated and have been shown to be of clinical value. In fact, the magnitude of improvement is greater than that typically seen when these same procedures are applied with adult patients. The limited work with cognitive-based approaches is similarly supportive. A stepped-care approach is appropriate for many of these patients, although the treatment must be tailored to the individual patient.

REFERENCES

Allen, K. D., & McKeen, L. R. (1991). Home-based multicomponent treatment of pediatric migraine. *Headache*, *31*, 467–472.

Allen, K. D., & Shriver, M. D. (1997). Enhanced performance feedback to strengthen biofeedback treatment outcome with childhood migraine. *Headache*, *37*, 169–173.

Allen, K. D., & Shriver, M. D. (1998). Role of parent-mediated pain behavior management strategies in biofeedback treatment of childhood migraines. *Behavior Therapy*, *29*, 477–490.

Andrasik, F., Blake, D. D., & McCarran, M. S. (1985). A biobehavioral analysis of pediatric headache. In N. A. Krasnegor, J. D. Arasteh, & M. F. Cataldo (Eds.), *Child health behavior: A behavioral pediatrics perspective*. New York: Wiley.

Andrasik, F., Grazzi, L., Usai, S., D'Amico, D., Leone, M., & Bussone, G. (2003). Brief neurologist-administered behavioral treatment for pediatric headache with 1 year follow-up. *Neurology*, *60*, 1215–1216.

Andrasik, F., Larsson, B., & Grazzi, L. (2002). Biofeedback treatment of recurrent headaches in children and adolescents. In V. Guidetti, G. Russell, M. Sillanpää, & P. Winner (Eds.), *Headache and migraine in childhood and adolescence*. London: Martin Dunitz.

Attanasio, V., Andrasik, F., Burke, E. J., Blake, D. D., Kabela, E., & McCarran, M. S. (1985). Clinical issues in utilizing biofeedback with children. *Clinical Biofeedback and Health*, *8*, 134–141.

Bandell-Hoekstra, I., Abu-Saadm, H. H., Passchier, J., & Knipschild, P. (2000). Recurrent headache, coping, and quality of life in children: A review. *Headache*, *40*, 357–370.

Bille, B. (1962). Migraine in school children. *Acta Paediatrica Scandinavica*, *51*(Suppl. 136), 1–151.

Bille, B. (1997). A 40-year follow-up of school children with migraine. *Cephalalgia*, *17*, 488–491.

Burke, E. J., & Andrasik, F. (1989). Home- vs. clinic-based biofeedback treatment for pediatric migraine: Results of treatment through one-year follow-up. *Headache*, *29*, 434–440.

Bussone, G., Grazzi, L., D'Amico, D., Leone, M., & Andrasik, F. (1998). Biofeedback-assisted relaxation training for young adolescents with tension-type headache: A controlled study. *Cephalalgia*, *18*, 463–467.

Duckro, P. N., & Cantwell-Simmons, E. (1989). A review of studies evaluating biofeedback and relaxation training in the management of pediatric headache. *Headache*, *29*, 428–433.

Gladstein, J., & Holden, E. W. (1996). Chronic daily headache in children and adolescents: A 2-year prospective study. *Headache*, *36*, 349–351.

Grazzi, L., Andrasik, F., D'Amico, D., Leone, M., Moschiano, F., & Bussone, G. (2001). Electromyographic biofeedback-assisted relaxation training in juvenile episodic tension-type headache: Clinical outcome at three year follow-up. *Cephalalgia*, *21*, 798–803.

Green, J. A. (1983). Biofeedback therapy with children. In W. H. Rickles, J. H. Sandweiss, D. Jacobs, & R. N. Grove (Eds.), *Biofeedback and family practice medicine*. New York: Plenum Press.

Guarnieri, P., & Blanchard, E. B. (1990). Evaluation of home-based thermal biofeedback treatment of pediatric migraine headache. *Biofeedback and Self-Regulation, 15,* 179–184.

Haddock, C. K., Rowan, A. B., Andrasik, F., Wilson, P. G., Talcott, G. W., & Stein, R. J. (1997). Home-based behavioral treatments for chronic benign headache: A meta-analysis of controlled trials. *Cephalalgia, 17,* 113–118.

Hermann, C., & Blanchard, E. B. (2002). Biofeedback in the treatment of headache and other childhood pain. *Applied Psychophysiology and Biofeedback, 27,* 143–162.

Hermann, C., Blanchard, E. B., & Flor, H. (1997). Biofeedback treatment for pediatric migraine: Prediction of treatment outcome. *Journal of Consulting and Clinical Psychology, 85,* 611–616.

Hermann, C., Kim, M., & Blanchard, E. B. (1995). Behavioral and prophylactic pharmacological intervention studies of pediatric migraine: An exploratory meta-analysis. *Pain, 20,* 239–256.

Holden, E. W., Deichmann, M. M., & Levy, J. D. (1999). Empirically supported treatments in pediatric psychology: Recurrent pediatric headache. *Journal of Pediatric Psychology, 24,* 91–109.

Holden, E. W., Levy, J. D., Deichmann, M. M., & Gladstein, J. (1998). Recurrent pediatric headaches: Assessment and intervention. *Journal of Developmental and Behavioral Pediatrics, 19,* 109–116.

Kröner-Herwig, B., Mohn, U., & Pothmann, R. (1998). Comparison of biofeedback and relaxation in the treatment of pediatric headache and the influence of parent involvement on outcome. *Applied Psychophysiology and Biofeedback, 23,* 143–157.

Kuhn, B. R., & Allen, K. D. (1993). *Long-term follow-up of a home-based multicomponent treatment for pediatric migraine.* Poster presented at the 27th Annual Meeting of the Association for Advancement of Behavior Therapy, Atlanta, GA.

Larsson, B. (2002). Prognosis of recurrent headaches in childhood and adolescence. In V. Guidetti, G. Russell, M. Sillanpää, & P. Winner (Eds.), *Headache and migraine in childhood and adolescence.* London: Martin Dunitz.

Larsson, B., & Andrasik, F. (2002). Relaxation treatment of recurrent headaches in children and adolescents. In V. Guidetti, G. Russell, M. Sillanpää, & P. Winner (Eds.), *Headache and migraine in childhood and adolescence.* London: Martin Dunitz.

Levin, S. D. (2001). Drug therapies for childhood headache. In P. A. McGrath & L. M. Hillier (Eds.), *The child with headache: Diagnosis and treatment.* Seattle, WA: IASP Press.

Linet, M. S., Stewart, W. F., Celentano, D. D., Ziegler, D., & Sprecher, M. (1989). An epidemiologic study of headache among adolescents and young adults. *Journal of the American Medical Association, 261,* 2211–2216.

Lipton, R. B., Maytal, J., & Winner, P. (2001). Epidemiology and classification of headache. In P. Winner & A.D. Rothner (Eds.), *Headache in children and adolescents.* Hamilton, Ontario, Canada: BC Decker.

Marcon, R. A., & Labbé, E. E. (1990). Assessment and treatment of children's headaches from a developmental perspective. *Headache, 30,* 586–592.

McGrath, P. A., & Hillier, L. M. (2001). Recurrent headache: Triggers, causes, and contributing factors. In P. A. McGrath & L. M. Hillier (Eds.), *The child with headache: Diagnosis and treatment.* Seattle, WA: IASP Press.

McGrath, P. A., & Koster, A. L. (2001). Headache measures for children: A practical approach. In P. A. McGrath & L. M. Hillier (Eds.), *The child with headache: Diagnosis and treatment.* Seattle, WA: IASP Press.

McGrath, P. A., Stewart, D., & Koster, A. L. (2001). Nondrug therapies for childhood headache. In P. A. McGrath & L. M. Hillier (Eds.), *The child with headache: Diagnosis and treatment.* Seattle, WA: IASP Press.

Pothmann, R. (2002). Medical prophylaxis in childhood migraine. In V. Guidetti, G. Russell, M. Sillanpää, & P. Winner (Eds.), *Headache and migraine in childhood and adolescence.* London: Martin Dunitz.

Powers, S. W., Mitchell, M. J., Byars, K. C., Bentti, A. L., LeCates, S. L., & Hershey, A. D. (2001). A pilot study of one-session biofeedback training in pediatric headache. *Neurology, 56,* 133.

Richter, I. L., McGrath, P. J., Humphreys, P. J., Goodman, J. T., Firestone, P., & Keene, D. (1986). Cognitive and relaxation treatment of paediatric migraine. *Pain, 25,* 195–203.

Rossi, L., Bardare, M., & Brunelli, G. (2002). Migraine and diet. In V. Guidetti, G. Russell, M. Sillanpää, & P. Winner (Eds.), *Headache and migraine in childhood and adolescence.* London: Martin Dunitz.

Rothner, A. D. (2001). Differential diagnosis of headache in children and adolescents. In P. A. McGrath & L. M. Hillier (Eds.), *The child with headache: Diagnosis and treatment.* Seattle, WA: IASP Press.

Sarafino, E. P., & Goehring, P. (2000). Age comparisons in acquiring biofeedback control and success in reducing headache pain. *Annals of Behavioral Medicine, 22,* 10–16.

Silberstein, S. D. (1990). Twenty questions about headaches in children and adolescents. *Headache, 30,* 716–724.

Sillanpää, M. (1994). Headache in children. In J. Olesen (Ed.), *Headache classification and epidemiology.* New York: Raven Press.

Sillanpää, M., & Anttila, P. (1996). Increasing prevalence of headache in 7-year-old schoolchildren. *Headache, 36,* 466–470.

Siniatchkin, M., Hierundar, A., Kropp, P., Kuhnert, R., Gerber, W. D., & Stephani, U. (2000). Self-regulation of slow cortical potentials in children with migraine: An exploratory study. *Applied Psychophysiology and Biofeedback, 25,* 13–32.

Waldie, K. (2001). Childhood headache, stress in adolescence, and primary headache in young adulthood: A longitudinal cohort study. *Headache, 41,* 1–10.

Winner, P. (2001). Triptans in childhood and adolescence. *Seminars in Pediatric Neurology, 8,* 22–26.

Winner, P., Wasiewski, W., Gladstein, J., & Linder, S. (1997). Multicenter prospective evaluation of proposed pediatric migraine revisions to the IHS criteria. *Headache, 37,* 545–548.

CHAPTER 31

Pediatric Applications Other Than Headache

TIMOTHY P. CULBERT
GERARD A. BANEZ

Health care service and delivery paradigms for children continue to evolve, and as they do, there is clear recognition of the complex interplay of mind and body evident in virtually all manifestations of disease, illness, health and wellness. The mainstream pediatric literature continues to see an increase in the publication of papers on mind–body techniques, and this increase parallels the increasing recognition of psychophysiological problems in pediatric care (Starfield & Borkowf, 1969; Sharp & Pantell, 1992; Sugarman, 1996). The field of biofeedback as applied to pediatric populations is poised to make a major contribution in both the assessment and treatment of many common childhood biobehavioral (or psychophysiological) disorders, because it provides concrete evidence for mind–body links and offers a means to address both somatic and emotional/behavioral components of these complex problems (Culbert, Kajander, & Reaney, 1996; Smith, 1991; Barowsky, 1990).

Scientific research, ongoing studies, and clinical experience suggest that biofeedback and related self-regulation techniques are effective and will play increasingly prominent roles in well-child care, school settings, performance enhancement of all kinds, and the care of children with chronic illness and disability (Sussman & Culbert, 1999). This chapter briefly reviews the relationship of biofeedback to other relevant areas of pediatric care; describes features of biofeedback as applied to children and adolescents that differentiate it from adult approaches; and reviews biofeedback applications for specific childhood disorders. (Note: Biofeedback for pediatric headache, electroencephalographic [EEG] biofeedback for attention-deficit/hyperactivity disorder [ADHD], and heart rate variability [HRV] training are reviewed in other chapters of this book.)

WHY BIOFEEDBACK, WHY NOW?

As is the case in adult medicine, pediatric health professionals continue to see an increasing percentage of patients presenting with psychophysiological disorders and psychosocially mediated morbidity. Studies suggest that as many as 25% of children and adolescents experience these multidimensional problems (Brugman, Reijneveld, Verlhulst, & Verloove-

Vanhorick, 2001). As we identify more young patients with mind–body difficulties, it is important to develop and offer therapies that explicitly acknowledge this linkage and that proceed to assist children with both components. Biofeedback provides an ideal strategy with which first to educate pediatric patients about this mind–body link, and then to help them develop appropriate self-regulatory skills (Culbert, Kajander, & Reaney, 1996; Andrasik & Attansio, 1985). One can imagine the relevance of this strategy on a spectrum that includes health/ wellness promotion and peak performance training on one end, and the remediation of specific psychophysiological dysfunction on the other.

Biofeedback is culturally syntonic with today's computer-savvy youth, and therefore provides an immediate "connection" and point of multimedia interest that can help in engaging pediatric patients in ways that traditional talk therapies may not (Culbert, Reaney, & Kohen, 1994). In our experience, this engagement in the process of understanding mind–body connections and the cultivation of lowered states of arousal often enhances positive rapport with children or adolescents and allows them to "open up" in ways that standard therapeutic approaches may not (Culbert, 1999).

For the therapist, biofeedback lends precision to the process of behavioral therapy, particularly when "relaxation" is a goal. Relaxation is often subjectively defined as feeling "loose," "good," or "comfortable." Biofeedback allows a therapist to define it more clearly as a state of lowered sympathetic nervous system (SNS) arousal and/or a more desirable balance in parasympathetic nervous system–SNS activity. In addition, biofeedback can allow a therapist to observe physiological reaction patterns in a patient when discussing certain key topics or themes. This is helpful in then demonstrating to a client the mind–body connection in concrete, immediate terms. For children, this aspect of treatment is powerful—being able to actually show them how "a change in your thinking has caused a change in your body's reactions"! Particularly in pediatric patients with somatoform disorders and stress-related symptoms, this invaluable information and the insight provided allow them to move forward more quickly in the therapeutic process.

SELF-REGULATION SKILLS TRAINING

It is useful to think of biofeedback within a class of skills that involve self-regulation:

> Biofeedback
> Relaxation/mental imagery (self-hypnosis)
> Cognitive-behavioral therapy
> Diaphragmatic breathing
> Meditation
> Autogenics
> Progressive muscle relaxation
> Mind–body education

These skills all empower patients to focus their minds in ways that positively influence their bodies (Sussman & Culbert, 1999). In children's language, this means teaching them to "be the boss of your body!" Self-regulation techniques can also be described as strategies that help people to discover and cultivate their innate healing abilities. Examples of such techniques include the voluntary modulation of specific physiological functions, the directed use of mental imagery and therapeutic suggestion, self-monitoring, enhancing somatic awareness, and control of positive and negative self-talk tendencies. These strategies are commonly blended together in clinical practice.

Training of self-regulatory ability, when considered within a developmental context, is consistent with children's natural drives for mastery and autonomy (Dixon & Stein, 2000). Through the use of these self-initiated and self-guided strategies, individuals participate actively in the control and remediation of impairing symptoms. With the acquisition of self-regulation skills, children and adolescents are encouraged to take "ownership" of their personal challenges, and then to utilize their own talents and abilities in facilitating their own progress toward the attainment of the desired level of health and wellness.

BIOFEEDBACK IN THE CONTEXT OF COMPLEMENTARY AND ALTERNATIVE MEDICINE

Another reason biofeedback is becoming an attractive strategy in pediatric health care is that it offers a nonpharmacological alternative for certain childhood disorders (e.g., headaches). The movement toward more participatory, natural, self-directed therapies is an essential factor in the growth of the area of complementary and alternative medicine (CAM) (Gaudet, 1998). The National Center for Complementary and Alternative Medicine (NCCAM) of the National Institutes of Health describes five domains of CAM, with biofeedback falling within the domain designated as "mind–body therapies" (NCCAM, 1999). CAM use is growing in pediatrics as it is in the adult population, with the use of mind–body therapies (including biofeedback) leading the way (Kemper, 2000). A recent survey of pediatricians (Sikand & Laken, 1998) revealed that more than 50% of those surveyed reported that they would be willing to refer a pediatric patient for a CAM therapy. The CAM therapy these pediatricians identified as being the most likely for referral was biofeedback! Epidemiological studies identify the use of CAM by children and adolescents as ranging from 11% of patients in pediatric primary care, to 42% of patients in pediatric hematology/oncology, and to 73% in one group of homeless youth (Spigelblatt, Laine-Ammara, Pless, & Guyver, 1994; Kemper & Wornham, 2001; Breuner, Barry, & Kemper, 1998).

PHYSIOLOGICAL CONTROL IN CHILDREN

Research over the past 30 years demonstrates that children and adolescents are capable of voluntarily modulating physiological processes, including peripheral temperature, muscle activity, breathing, brain electrical activity, and certain aspects of immune function such as salivary immunoglobulin A (Labbe, Delaney, Olson, & Hickman, 1993; Olness, 1997; Hewson-Bower & Drummond, 1996; Olness, Culbert, & Uden, 1989; Delaney, Olson, & Labbe, 1992). In fact, studies suggest that children are generally better than adults in many self-regulatory skills. Children make excellent biofeedback subjects (Attansio et al., 1985), for reasons that include the following:

Children are more enthusiastic.
Children are less skeptical about self-control procedures.
Children have confidence in their special abilities.
Children have more psychophysiological lability.

Because children are developmentally prone to using fantasy, it is important to understand the role that mental imagery can naturally play in biofeedback and relaxation therapy. The links between certain thoughts or types of mental imagery and specific physiological response patterns are well documented. For example, mental rehearsal of an activity such as an athletic routine or playing a musical instrument can result in autonomic nervous system (ANS) responses that are similar to the activity itself—often with increased SNS activity, including increased heart rate (Lee & Olness, 1996; Wang & Morgan, 1992). Children can be taught to cultivate certain kinds of mental-imagery as a way of achieving a desirable level of control in a certain physiological parameter. For example, utilizing imagery about warm thoughts and relaxing, pleasant sensations can facilitate peripheral temperature change. Clinical experience suggests images of relaxing experiences will more typically facilitate a lowered state of SNS arousal, as evidenced by lower heart rate, increased peripheral temperature, or decreased electrical skin conductance.

In addition to mental imagery, certain emotional states are capable of eliciting strong physiological response patterns (Cacioppo, Klein, Berntson, & Hatfield, 1993). Directed cultivation of such emotions as love, warmth, and feelings of safety and support may help in eliciting desirable patterns of physiological response, such as improved HRV, decreased electrodermal activity (EDA), or increased peripheral temperature (Institute for HeartMath®, 1997).

To date, no true "standards" have been established for "normal" baseline measurements of ANS functions in children and adolescents, such as peripheral temperature, EDA, or surface electromyographic (EMG) activity. Boyce, Chesney, and Kaiser (1990) assessed the physiological concomitants of stress and anxiety in preschool children, and noted a wide range of individual responses across a variety of autonomic and immunological measures. The lack of normative data on physiological baseline data in children is a limiting factor in research in this area.

It is also clear that like adults, certain children may demonstrate significant lability across a number of physiological measures, while others may be "hot responders" in only one modality. In our own experience, it is not necessarily true that children need to achieve absolute thresholds in terms of a given physiological response to achieve symptom resolution. For example, adult protocols commonly call for a peripheral temperature above 95°F or an EMG level below 3 microvolts. Many pediatric patients show improvement in target symptoms with a physiological response that is trending in the right direction consistently.

DEVELOPMENTAL CONSIDERATIONS

In work with children and adolescents, each encounter must be crafted in a way that attends to the specific developmental stage, sensory preferences, attention span, personal interests, and learning style of the patient at hand (Reaney & Kohen, 1998). This requires not only appropriate knowledge of developmental stages and capabilities, but also flexibility on the part of the therapist. The length, frequency, and content of biofeedback training sessions may need to be adjusted to fit the unique needs of each patient, with younger children often needing shorter, more frequent sessions. Single sessions can be broken up by changing feedback modalities, games, or audio settings. Young children can easily utilize mental imagery to enhance the relaxation process as they imagine "being in a favorite place." They may also tolerate and in fact benefit from more directive approaches. For older children, it is often useful to appeal to their desire for mastery and give more detailed explanations of therapy goals.

TREATMENT PLANNING

Our clinical experience suggests that, as a general guideline, most pediatric patients can achieve positive outcomes with 8–10 sessions lasting 30–45 minutes each, scheduled 1–2 weeks apart.

All children should be asked to participate in daily self-monitoring as part of their treatment plan. Rewards are appropriate early in the treatment process as way to reinforce cooperation and practice. Daily practice at home and/or school is essential for success.

The "discern–control–generalize" model offers a useful paradigm within which to consider therapy and session planning with pediatric clients. In the "discern" phase, clients are taught about mind–body links and assisted in discriminating differences in states of relaxation and tension. In the "control" phase, children are coached to master specific skills (e.g., diaphragmatic breathing, decreased trapezius muscle tone) and to achieve consistent trends or goals for a specific physiological function over a defined period of time. The final and most important stage is the "generalize" phase, when patients learn to apply their self-regulation skills in the real-life situation at the desired time. Helping children to transfer the skills learned in the office includes identification of environmental cues and situational triggers that remind them when to use these abilities. Parents and teachers may get involved at this step and assist in cueing the children when desirable. Mental imagery is commonly utilized as a practice strategy at this stage, to offer the chance for "imaginal" or *in vitro* rehearsal of a real-life situation where the individual wishes to apply a new skill.

THERAPEUTIC COMMUNICATION AND THE BIOFEEDBACK–HYPNOSIS INTERFACE

Careful attention to the content and structure of language is a key ingredient in therapeutic communication with children and adolescents (Reaney & Kohen, 1998). Daniel Kohen, Karen Olness, and others in the field of pediatric hypnosis and hypnotherapy have contributed to a large volume of literature on this essential aspect of all pediatric clinical encounters (Olness & Kohen, 1996). They point out that children frequently and spontaneously move in and out of altered states of awareness, within which they experience heightened suggestibility. Careful attention to the way in which language is used with children in these "alternative states" is essential. Markers of these "hypnotic" states include focused attention, absorption, and curiosity. Many children who are receiving biofeedback therapy clearly (and actually quite commonly) move into an altered state as they become relaxed. In this state, attention is narrowly focused, they are more aware of internal events and sensations, and they are ready to facilitate change more readily (physiological and perceptual shifts).

While in such a state of consciousness, children are more receptive to therapeutic suggestion. Therefore, language used during these encounters must be carefully tailored to do the following:

Convey positive expectancy.
Be permissive (as opposed to directive).
Maximize the fit with the child's interest and personality.
Respect and reflect developmental ability.
Evoke a sense of wonder/curiosity.
Include appropriate suggestions to enhance functioning and/or control of symptoms.

With biofeedback, game formats (some of which are described below) lend themselves nicely to therapeutic metaphors involving notions of self-control relevant to a given child and his or her presenting problem. In working with pediatric populations, it is not enough for clinicians to be technically competent; they must also be able to approach each child in a developmentally sensitive manner, to establish rapport, and to utilize words and language strategically.

HARDWARE AND SOFTWARE CHOICES

Children in today's society are accustomed to viewing high-quality video graphics in TV, video games, and movies. Biofeedback training using game formats is appealing for many youngsters and serves as an engaging treatment "hook." Video games are designed to be "intrinsically motivating," and we can learn from this experience and design the same features into successful pediatric biofeedback treatment strategies (Malone, 1991). The three essential elements identified are those of fantasy, curiosity, and challenge. Selecting and varying audio and video screens with pediatric patients can be essential in holding attention and "connecting" with young patients. Some examples of software we have found useful follow.

The BioIntegrator 4.0 (available from Bio Research Institute, 331 East Cotati Avenue, Cotati, CA 94928) contains a very useful "Puzzle" function, which allows children to create a complete jigsaw puzzle picture as they control a physiological function and move toward a preset threshold in a desired fashion. The speed with which pieces appear, the pattern in which they appear, and the associated audio feedback component can all be manipulated to increase reinforcement value and hold interest. A number of pictures are available, including animals, airplanes, and artwork. The "Mandala" displays in this same system include colorful geometric patterns that "animate" or move at threshold, and also contain games involving achieving point totals and colorful dots. (See Figure 31.1.)

Heartmath, Inc. (Heartmath, 14700 West Park Avenue, Boulder Creek, CA 95006) produces an HRV hardware–software package called the Freeze-Framer® as part of its "emotional management enhancement" product line, which is appealing to children and adoles-

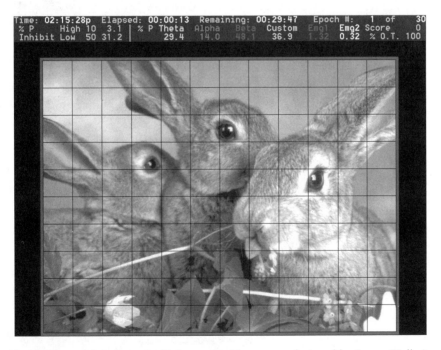

FIGURE 31.1. This graphic is from the BioIntegrator Plus system designed by Steven Wall. A modality is selected and a desired range of control is set by the therapist. The patient then chooses a favorite picture, which will gradually appear as jigsaw puzzle pieces "clicking in" to place as they successfully control the chosen physiologic function. An audio feedback reward can also be provided. Copyright 2003 by Steve Wall, Bio Research Institute. Reprinted with permission.

cents. Three games included in this package make it fun for patients to gain control of their emotional state and cultivate a lowered state of arousal. Child-friendly formats include a black-and-white picture that turns to color with improved HRV, a balloon that lifts off and flies over a beautiful landscape, and a rainbow that builds and completes with a pot of gold at the end. (See Figure 31.2.)

Me2, Inc. (Me2 Limited, 7609 Mountain Park, Concord, OH, 44060) produces a CD-ROM-based game called The Mind/Body Game, which plugs into a desktop or laptop personal computer. This game utilizes skin conductance level to teach children how changes in thinking can create a change in physiological response pattern. The child chooses one of three animated animals and the animal's expression changes from a frown to a smile as the child becomes more relaxed.

Although it is an an older system, the J & J I-330 (available from J & J Enterprises, 22797 Holgar Court NE, Poulsbo, WA 98370) includes game interfaces that are simple yet effective in engaging young patients. These include the stoplight game, river rafting, the egg catching game and kaleidoscope.

Thought Technology's Biograph software (together with Procomp Hardware; both available from Thought Technology, 2180 Belgrade Avenue, Montreal, QC H4A 2L8 Canada) offers several child-friendly game animations/graphics, including a morphing "smiley face" and a moving sunset; it also has a relay feature available that can trigger an external device as a reward. Moving animation screens on the Biograph X disc with appealing musical instrument digital interface audio song options include a cartoon dog, a spaceship landing sequence, a bowling game, and a flower that opens and closes at a preset threshold. (See Figure 31.3.)

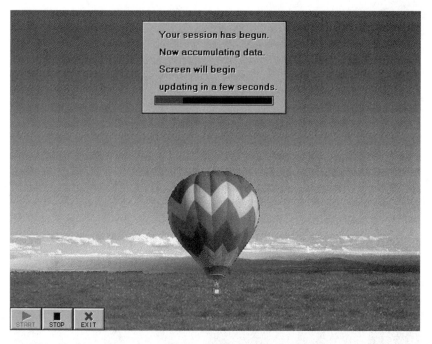

FIGURE 31.2. This graphic is from a game sequence provided as part of the "Freeze-Framer" software from HeartMath, LLC. The patient is coached through diaphragmatic breathing and positive emotional imagery exercises to achieve a desired "entrained" level of heart rate variability to cause the balloon to fly over some beautiful landscapes. Graphic provided by Quantum Intech, Inc. with permission. Copyright 2001 by Intech, Inc.

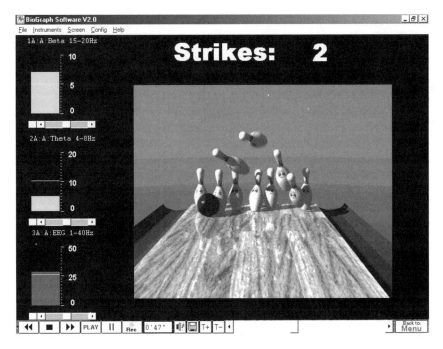

FIGURE 31.3. This graphic is from the Biograph software (Animation X software CD) developed by Thought Technology, Ltd. for their ProComp hardware line. The software can be programmed so that the patient is rewarded by bowling a strike and enjoying preselected audio reinforcement when they achieve a desired threshold for the specified modality. With children we use EDA, EMG, and peripheral temperature as typical modalities with this game. Graphic reprinted with permission of Thought Technology, Ltd.

We have also found that home training devices—such as hand-held EMG trainers (U-control, available from Thought Technology Ltd.), temperature bands (Dermatherms from Sharn, Inc., 4801 George Road, Tampa, FL 33634), temperature dots (biodots), and EDA units (available from Thoughtstream, Mindplace Marketing, Seattle, WA www.mindplace.com), are very helpful in promoting home practice. Customized calendars and stickers offer an engaging way for kids to track progress. In addition, we have created a clinical handout series, symptom-monitoring sheets, and other worksheets describing practice strategies for our pediatric patients as well.

CLINICAL APPLICATIONS OF BIOFEEDBACK WITH CHILDREN

There are many applications for biofeedback in childhood disorders, both as a primary treatment modality and as an adjunctive approach (see Table 31.1). Literature supports the fact that with regard to biofeedback, children often perform better than adults (Andrasik & Attansio, 1985). There is also evidence for age-related performance differences across different groups of children, which reflect cognitive, learning, motivational, and related developmental phenomena (Suter & Loughry-Machado, 1981; Sussman & Culbert, 1999). The following sections provide a review of recognized areas of biofeedback intervention with children and adolescents.

TABLE 31.1. Biofeedback and Self-Regulation Skills: Review of Evidence for Pediatric Applications

Disorder	BF treatment	Modalities
Pain		
Headache	Primary or adjunctive	EMG, TMP
Other chronic pain	Adjunctive	PNG, EMG, TMP
Acute pain and needle phobia	Adjunctive	EDA, PNG
Anxiety/stress-related disorders	Adjunctive	PNG, EDA, HRV
Sleep disorders	Primary or adjunctive	EMG, PNG
Enuresis	Primary	EMG, manometric, alarm
Encopresis	Primary or adjunctive	EMG, manometric
ANS dysregulation		
Raynaud's	Adjunctive	TMP, EDA
Reflex sympathetic dystrophy/complex regional pain syndrome	Adjunctive	TMP, EDA
Hypertension	Adjunctive	EDA, PNG, HRV, BP
Irritable bowel syndrome	Adjunctive	EDA, PNG, TMP, HRV
Hyperhidrosis	Adjunctive	EDA, HRV
Neuromuscular rehabilitation	Primary or adjunctive	EMG
Attention-deficit/hyperactivity disorder	Adjunctive	EEG, EMG
Learning disorders	Adjunctive	EEG, EMG
Seizure disorders	Adjunctive	EEG
Repetitive behaviors		
Tics/Tourette's disorder	Adjunctive	EEG, EMG, EDA
Habit disorders	Adjunctive	EMG, PNG
Impulse control problems	Adjunctive	EDA, HRV, PNG
Chronic illness		
Asthma	Adjunctive	EMG, PNG, HRV
Hematology/Oncology	Adjunctive	TMP, PNG
Peak performance training	Adjunctive	EMG, EEG, HRV

Note. TMP, peripheral temperature; EMG, electromyography; PNG, pneumography; EEG, electroencephalography; EDA, electrodermal activity; HRV, heart rate variability; BP, blood pressure.

Disorders of Elimination (Encopresis and Enuresis)

Biofeedback is increasingly used in the treatment of encopresis and enuresis, either as the primary treatment modality or as an adjunctive therapy. Biofeedback for these disorders can be used to assess the physiological mechanisms felt to underlie or be associated with a child's soiling or wetting accidents (e.g., EMG monitoring of a weak external anal sphincter), and treatment effects are specific to the type of biofeedback used. A fair amount of research on biofeedback for these disorders exists, and clinical implications are emerging. (See Tries & Eisman, Chapters 26 and 27, this volume, for more complete discussions.)

Encopresis

Biofeedback treatment of encopresis typically involves some combination of the following: training in discriminating the sensation of rectal distension, strengthening of the external anal sphincter via EMG training, training in the synchronization of internal and external anal sphincter responses, and (for those with pelvic floor dyssynergia or paradoxical contraction) training in the coordination of abdominal and pelvic floor musculature for elimination. The type of biofeedback used is a function of the physiological mechanisms hypothesized to underlie the child's soiling. For example, if a child's soiling is felt to be associated with poor sensation of the urge to produce stool, training aimed at improving rectal sensation is indicated. When soiling is associated with poor control due to a weak external anal sphincter, sphincter strengthening via EMG biofeedback may be appropriate.

The majority of existing research appears to focus on biofeedback treatment of encopresis associated with pelvic floor dyssynergia or paradoxical contraction. "Pelvic floor dyssynergia" refers to the abnormal closure of the anal canal during straining for defecation. Children with dyssynergia squeeze their buttocks and hips during attempts to defecate and are unable to relax their external anal sphincter. These abnormal defecation dynamics are thought to develop in response to past painful bowel movements. To control the amount of stool being passed and protect against pain, the child squeezes the anal canal during defecation. Assessment of pelvic floor dyssynergia uses surface EMG electrodes to monitor abdominal muscles and an anal sensor (or surface EMG electrodes just outside the anal opening) to evaluate the child's ability to maintain external anal sphincter relaxation while contracting abdominal muscle. If there is dyssynergia between the two muscle regions, biofeedback is used to teach appropriate responses.

Numerous uncontrolled studies suggest that this type of biofeedback is an effective adjunctive treatment for encopresis (see Loening-Baucke, 1996, for an excellent review of this literature). The findings from controlled studies, however, have not been as positive (Brooks et al., 2000). Though some controlled investigations have found that biofeedback is beneficial (e.g., Loening-Baucke, 1990; Wald, Chandra, Gabel, & Chiponis, 1987), other studies have reported that the addition of biofeedback to standard medical management does not increase effectiveness of treatment (e.g., Cox, Sutphen, Borowitz, Kovatchev, & Ling, 1998; Cox, Sutphen, Ling, Quillian, & Borowitz, 1996; Nolan, Catto-Smith, Coffey, & Wells, 1998; Van der Plas et al., 1996), even for those children who positively evidence pelvic floor dyssynergia. In one study that suggested the benefits of biofeedback treatment (Loening-Baucke, 1990), no statistically significant differences in comparison to the control group were found at long-term follow-up (Loening-Baucke, 1995). The results of controlled studies have been described by some investigators (e.g., Loening-Baucke, 1996, as disappointing. Others, such as McGrath, Mellon, and Murphy (2000), point out methodological problems (e.g., subject selection, varying types/methods of treatment) that complicate the process of evaluating the efficacy of this treatment. At present, existing data do not support the use of biofeedback as the sole treatment for encopresis. In clinical practice, we encourage consideration of brief biofeedback treatment, typically no more than two to four sessions, for children who have pelvic floor dyssynergia and are not showing a positive response to standard medical management. To be most helpful, such treatment needs to be provided within the context of a comprehensive biobehavioral treatment of encopresis, including bowel cleanout, a regular sitting schedule, medications, and dietary restrictions/recommendations.

Enuresis

A variety of biofeedback approaches can play important roles in the comprehensive management of dysfunctional voiding in children (Schulman, Quinn, Plachter, & Kodman-Jones, 1999). Though not always categorized as a biofeedback technique, the urine or enuresis alarm has been presented in previous editions of this text (Schwartz & Associates, 1987, 1995) as a biofeedback device for children with nocturnal enuresis. The modern urine alarm consists of a small, transistorized unit that is worn on the body and is activated with urination during sleep. A typical urine alarm protocol (Houts, 1990; Schmitt, 1990) requires that the child wear and turn on the alarm every night during the treatment period. When the alarm rings, the child is to wake, stop the flow of urine, go to the bathroom, and finish voiding. He or she is to then put wet sheets and clothes in the laundry, put a clean sheet on the bed, and reattach the alarm. Use of the urine alarm continues until the child achieves 14 consecutive dry nights. At that point, a simple overlearning procedure can be implemented to prevent relapses and build more confidence (Houts, 1990). The urine alarm is not intended to serve as a punishment; rather, it sets up a "dilemma" for the child, requiring that he or she be rudely awakened while rested and comfortable. It is thought that by awakening quickly to the alarm, the child eventually learns by conditioning or approximation to awaken to the internal stimulus of a full bladder (Schmitt, 1997).

A growing body of literature, including numerous controlled studies, has documented the efficacy of the urine alarm as a treatment for nocturnal enuresis. In their systematic literature review, Mellon and McGrath (2000) identify the urine alarm as a necessary and, for many children, sufficient component in the treatment of enuresis. Utilizing rigorous criteria to evaluate the empirical support for various enuresis treatments, they conclude that the urine alarm is an effective treatment that meets criteria for the highest level of support. When compared to desmopressin acetate (DDAVP) and imipramine, the two drugs commonly used in treatment of enuresis, the alarm fares the best in terms of cure and relapse rates, risks, and cost (Schmitt, 1997). Although these drugs may be helpful for short-term use, they do not produce a permanent cure. The cures associated with the urine alarm endure and hold up over time.

The clinical challenges in successfully implementing urine alarm treatment are the time and effort required, for both child and parent(s). In our practice, we have found that clear, accurate instructions and appropriate expectations (e.g., that treatment may require 12 weeks or even more) are essential. Evaluating and eliciting child and parental motivation and commitment are critical to outcome. The important message is that the urine alarm can be very effective but also labor-intensive. For some children who have not responded to other treatments, compliance with the urine alarm can be enhanced through the combined use of the alarm and DDAVP. After the child is dry for 3 weeks, the dosage of the drug is decreased gradually. The combination of DDAVP and the alarm is reportedly most helpful for children with severe wetting and those with behavioral and familial problems (Bradbury & Meadow, 1995).

More conventional biofeedback techniques are increasingly used in the treatment of children who have dysfunctional voiding and diurnal enuresis. For example, when detrusor–sphincter dyssynergia is associated with diurnal incontinence, EMG and urodynamic biofeedback are used to teach coordination of detrusor contraction and sphincter relaxation (Yamanishi et al., 2000). Biofeedback therapy for adult urinary incontinence is common, and emerging evidence suggests its promise for children who have daytime wetting (e.g., Combs, Glassberg, Gerdes, & Horowitz, 1998; Porena, Costantini, Rociola, & Mearini, 2000; Kjolseth, Monster-Knudsen, & Madsen, 1993).

In our practice, we recently used EMG biofeedback as an adjunctive therapy in the treatment of a 16-year-old female who developed increased urinary urge and frequency after a urinary tract infection. Though her history was negative for wetting accidents, she was reporting urge and voiding every 15–20 minutes. Daily functioning was significantly impaired, with many days of school missed and a significant decrease in peer activities. EMG biofeedback was used to demonstrate normal urethral sphincter strength and teach pelvic floor strengthening exercises. It was incorporated into a comprehensive treatment, including voiding schedule, strengthening exercises, relaxation breathing, and coping self-statements. After six sessions, she reported less frequent urge and was voiding every 90–120 minutes. Day-to-day activity was normalized soon thereafter. Despite the fact that the biofeedback component was explicitly conceptualized as an adjunctive technique, she reported at the conclusion of treatment that the biofeedback was the most helpful treatment technique. According to her report, evidence of adequate sphincter strength via EMG increased her perceptions of control and greatly enhanced her confidence in the ability to maintain bladder control.

Acute, Chronic, and Recurrent Pain

Chronic and recurrent pain in children and adolescents is a significant problem with a high prevalence worldwide (McGrath & Finley, 1999). As is the case with adults, research on pediatric pain has expanded dramatically, and new approaches to pain have crossed disciplinary boundaries.

As described by Andrasik and Schwartz (Chapter 30, this volume), biofeedback has arguably become the treatment of choice for pediatric headache. In addition, clinical experience suggests that biofeedback and self-regulation techniques such as relaxation/mental imagery and diaphragmatic breathing are also very helpful in working with a variety of pediatric pain issues. These include chronic pain (e.g., pain associated with juvenile rheumatoid arthritis, cancer, sickle cell disease, and burns, as well as recurrent abdominal pain [RAP] and fibromyalgia), needle phobia, and acute procedural pain, although the literature is somewhat limited (Knudson-Cooper, 1981; Lavigne, Ross, & Berry, 1992; Varni, Walco, & Katz, 1989; Kuttner, 1989; Shapiro, 1995).

There is unanimous support in the literature for psychological approaches to pain when dealing with children (McGrath, 1990). Strategies include educating a child about the pain when it is procedure-related; maximizing a sense of participation, choice, and control with the child; and using such techniques as breathing, relaxation, positive self-talk, distraction, and imagery. Although the mechanisms of therapeutic change are not entirely known, these techniques are quite effective. The "neuromatrix" and "gate" theories of pain suggest the ability of the central nervous system (CNS) to down-regulate pain conduction via descending pathways (Melzack, 1999). Melzack's neuromatrix paradigm describes a complex interplay of CNS and peripheral nervous system components with learned, conditioned, and inherited pain reaction patterns.

The anxiety that accompanies pain is often as important to address as the pain itself (Kuttner, 1989). Biofeedback can be creatively incorporated into treatment strategies for children with needle phobia/procedural pain and anxiety, as the following case illustrates.

Abbi, a 12-year-old, was referred for self-regulation training for control of severe needle phobia. She needed immunizations within a few weeks to go on a family overseas trip. The referring pediatrician had been unsuccessful in gaining Abbi's cooperation for these vaccinations. She uncontrollably screamed and cried, and her parents and the professional staff were at a loss as to how best to help her.

Abbi only recalled one other experience a few years back, when she had venipuncture, that required more than one attempt to get the sample. She recalled feeling "out of control" as people held her down. Since that time, she had had a strong fear of needles. She expressed her desire to help herself.

During the first session, Abbi was introduced to basic EMG biofeedback and breathing therapy, emphasizing control and mastery themes. Abbi enjoyed this and did well. During the next session, she was introduced to EDA, as an easy way for her to track her own nervous system's anxiety responses to needles. Over that and the two subsequent sessions, Abbi focussed on controlling her SNS response with graduated exposure to elements of the vaccination experience. She learned to control her breathing, heart rate, and SNS activity as reflected in maintenance of low EDA readings. She particularly liked the biofeedback screen called Kaleidoscope (mentioned earlier), in which she erased a complex design of colorful lines and shapes as she decreased her EDA to the desired threshold level (below 5 micromhos).

A vaccination visit plan was then discussed and role-played using actual equipment, but stopping short of giving the injection. Abbi practiced by playing the nurse and giving a play vaccination, maintaining good control, and noticing how proud she felt. The following week in the biofeedback room, with her EDA sensor attached and running, Abbi demonstrated her self-regulation skills by keeping her EDA at desired levels, staying in control, and receiving her vaccination with minimal distress. She was quite proud of her accomplishment.

Needle phobia is a common problem in a variety of settings for children of all ages. Many children report afterwards that the anticipatory anxiety and emotional distress are often worse than the actual "shot" itself. As Abbi's case illustrates, direct desensitization with the monitoring of a relevant physiological modality such as EDA (or breathing or heart rate) offers an excellent opportunity to extinguish fear and reinforce the desired behavioral change. The engaging nature of visual feedback and the ability to set concrete "goals" are helpful for many young children in reinforcing their sense of control. Finally, the use of these techniques can heighten curiosity and thereby enhance the focus on something other than the injection pain. Even if simply used for distraction, biofeedback-based approaches can provide great benefit for children during procedural pain. Also, by reinforcing an enhanced sense of control in young patients, biofeedback training serves as a great metaphor for mastering pain (e.g., "If you can control this physiological function, you can also control the pain").

Studies suggest that up to 34% of the world's children suffer from RAP (Faull & Nicol, 1986). In a recent study, Humphreys and Gevirtz (2000) evaluated the efficacy of four treatment protocols, three of which included biofeedback, in the treatment of RAP. The study involved 64 children (mean age 9.75 years) with diagnosed RAP, who were randomly assigned to one of four groups:

1. Fiber-only comparison group
2. Fiber and biofeedback-assisted cultivation of lowered arousal.
3. Fiber, biofeedback, and cognitive-behavioral intervention.
4. Fiber, biofeedback, cognitive-behavioral intervention, and parent support.

The biofeedback component involved thermal biofeedback. All three treatment groups (groups 2–4) demonstrated significant within-session increases in peripheral temperature. Subjects reported significantly reduced abdominal pain. The authors concluded that increased dietary fiber coupled with biofeedback-assisted cultivation of lowered arousal was effective and efficient as a treatment for RAP.

Studies suggest that thermal feedback is a helpful component in pain control for individuals with arthritic joint pain related to bleeding disorders such as hemophilia (Varni, 1981; Varni & Gilbert, 1982). Temperature feedback may also play a supportive role for children with sickle cell disease (Hall, Chiarucci, & Berman, 1992).

Repetitive Behavioral Patterns (Habit Disorders, Impulse Control Problems, and Tics)

Patients with tics, Tourette's disorder, thumbsucking, nailbiting, bruxism, rumination, and picking behaviors may derive substantial benefits from behavioral therapies (Blum, 1999; Peterson, Campise, & Azrin, 1994) and self-regulation therapy which includes biofeedback (Leung & Robson, 1991; Kohen, 1991; Culbert et al.,1994). Repetitive behaviors often share a characteristic quality of being somewhat automatic, almost involuntary, and (for many children) stress- or anxiety-related. Some problems, like tic behaviors, are largely involuntary but can be voluntarily suppressed for varying lengths of time. Others, like thumbsucking, are really more under volitional control, and when brought to conscious awareness can be fully eliminated.

A conceptual model that is useful identifies several of the common elements seen in repetitive behavior patterns and their associated treatment strategies:

Repetitive behavior component	Treatment strategy
Automaticity of behavior	Pattern interruption practice
Anxiety/stress	Relaxation therapy
Deficient self-control	Ego strengthening/reinforcement
Poor somatic awareness	Self-awareness therapy

Biofeedback can help with each of these elements in a habitual or recurrent behavioral pattern.

Thumbsucking provides a good example. To bring the thumbsucking behavior into focus and awareness, we have patients identify their "high-risk" times of day, when they would tend to exhibit this behavior the most. We then have them focus their practice efforts during those times. We have them self-monitor and rate themselves on a visual analogue scale as to how much thumbsucking they are doing at a given time each day. With better awareness of their pattern, they can then begin to interrupt or change it, so it is not so "automatic." We can assign a competing behavior that is more adaptive (e.g., squeezing a "koosh" ball") to be done each time they feel the urge to perform the target habit, as another way of interrupting the usual cycle.

Biofeedback can be a helpful self-awareness teaching tool (Bakal, 1999). For example, in patients with thumbsucking, we have utilized forearm EMG biofeedback as way to increase self-awareness and, at the same time, to interrupt the automatic nature of the behavior. EMG sensors are placed on the forearm of the same side of the thumb that a child prefers to suck. An EMG threshhold value is then set so that when the child's arm is resting comfortably in his or her lap in a relaxed manner, the child is rewarded with engaging audio and visual feedback (spinning shape, more points, a green light). When the subject brings the hand up to his or her mouth to suck the thumb, the threshold event is triggered so that the enjoyable feedback (audio and visual) he or she was receiving freezes (and in one software program it can actually be set to give them a red light). With several repetitions, the child becomes much more aware of the arm and thumb coming up to the mouth and the muscles that this movement involves. The child can then learn to practice being more aware of this by closing his or her eyes and visualizing a traffic light image. When the child is moving the arm and thumb up, he or she can see a red light, which is the cue to stop. When the child is keeping the thumb out of the mouth and resting the arm comfortably, he or she can visualize a green light, which is the reinforcing cue to continue with that behavior. The child can then incorporate this sequence into a mental imagery (self-hypnosis) exercise to be practiced several times a day in the appropriate setting. In addition, for children in whom anxiety and stress "drive" or maintain a habitual behavior, treatment to lower SNS arousal (any biofeedback modality) can also be useful. These biofeedback-based approaches are blended with the appropriate operant elements in an overall plan.

One of us (Culbert) has found that relaxation therapy for children with mild to moderate tics and Tourette's disorder is often very helpful in reducing tic frequency and severity and in facilitating a sense of control for these children (Kohen & Botts, 1987). Surface EMG work in and around the area of motor involvement is useful, as is more general biofeedback for lowered arousal. It is well described for children with tics/Tourette's disorder that tic behaviors (vocal or motor) are more likely to occur with increased frequency and severity in the context of emotional arousal, whether this is associated with stress, excitement, or rage (Michultka, Blanchard, & Rosenblum, 1989). Therefore, emotional self-regulation therapy via biofeedback is useful for enhancing emotional and somatic awareness and in cultivating control of lowered states of arousal. O'Connor, Gareau, and Borgeat (1995) describe the successful use of EMG training in nine patients with tics to improve discrimination of levels of muscle contraction and to modify muscular control. Although these were adults (aged 23–49 years) with tics, the findings are applicable to pediatric patients as well.

A few studies have suggested a possible role for biofeedback in the treatment of pediatric rumination syndrome. "Rumination" is defined as the repeated regurgitation of food, with weight loss or failure to gain expected weight, developing after a period of normal functioning. The partially digested food is brought back into the mouth and then ejected from the mouth or reswallowed (American Psychiatric Association, 1994). In individuals with mental retardation, the prevalence of rumination is 6–10% (Fredericks, Carr, & Williams, 1998). Khan, Hyman, Cocjin, and DiLorenzo (2000) describe a multimodality approach for both nutritional and behavioral rehabilitation of 12 pediatric patients with rumination disorder (age range 9–19). None of the children in this case series were developmentally delayed. A combination of cognitive-behavioral therapy with relaxation and biofeedback was used in 7 of the 12 patients, with good benefit. Unfortunately, the authors do not give any methodological detail in terms of the specific type of biofeedback that was provided.

EMG biofeedback with a masseter placement can be useful in treating bruxism in children and adolescents (Feehan & Marsh, 1989; Schneider & Peterson, 1982). (See Glaros & Lausten, Chapter 15, this volume.)

Studies suggest that biofeedback, arousal management, and relaxation can be effective components of therapeutic programming for children, adolescents, and adults with anger management problems (Snyder, Kymissis, & Kessler, 1999; Corder, Whiteside, & Haizlip, 1986). Our clinical experience also suggests that biofeedback can be a useful adjunct in behavioral therapy approaches for children and adolescents with anger management and impulse control problems. Many times these maladaptive behaviors occur in response to predictable situational or interpersonal triggers, and result in somewhat stereotypical (negative) emotional arousal patterns and associated behavior.

Biofeedback can help children to understand and get better at discerning states of emotional arousal early, and then allow them the time and strategy to deescalate and make an appropriate behavioral choice. This fits well into the traditional five-step cognitive-behavioral problem-solving framework (Kendall & Braswell, 1986):

1. Stop! (Take a deep breath.)
2. Identify the problem. (Ask yourself, "Why am I feeling this way?")
3. Generate a few response options. (What can I do about it?)
4. Choose the best option and do it!
5. Evaluate what happened. (How did it go?)

Biofeedback-based relaxation therapy can help greatly with the steps in this process by helping children to identify and then control excessive emotional arousal early in the process. Instead of acting out this emotional state impulsively, they can learn to go through this problem-solving process in a more directed manner. Preliminary experience with a number of adolescents presented with anger management challenges indicates this to be a useful clinical approach (Culbert & Bonfilio, 1998).

Anxiety and Stress-Related Problems

Anxiety, fear, and stress evoke the familiar "fight or flight" repertoire of psychophysiological responses in people at all developmental life stages. Modern research has established that anxiety disorders are among the most common of all childhood psychiatric disorders, yet scientific study of effective treatments remains quite limited (Bernstein & Borchardt, 1991). Anxiety and stress-related problems include panic attacks, somatoform disorders, separation anxiety, specific phobias, school avoidance, posttraumatic stress disorder, and generalized anxiety disorder. This group of relatively common childhood conditions represents a domain for which biofeedback, relaxation, and self-hypnosis are very promising (Gagnon, Hudnall, & Andrasik, 1992; Gil, Perry, & King, 1988; Hobbie, 1989; Kendall, 1994; Kendall, Howard, & Epps, 1988; Young, Montano, & Goldberg, 1991).

A study by Kendall (1994) demonstrated that a cognitive-behavioral treatment program that included relaxation therapy was effective for children diagnosed with anxiety disorders. Although in this study the relaxation technique was not taught with biofeedback, it supports relaxation as a useful element. A systematic review of cognitive-behavioral approaches for the anxious child reveals that many of these successful approaches include a relaxation and/or breath control component (Kendall et al., 1988).

Psychologist David Mars (1998) reports on individuals with panic attacks (including children) who have been treated very effectively with breath control therapies, including capnography (the measurement and feedback of end-tidal CO_2 values). Physiologically, people with anxiety, particularly panic attacks, often hyperventilate (overbreathe), driving their CO_2 values down; this in turns upsets the acid–base balance of the body. In response, the body decreases cerebral blood flow, which can then contribute to cognitive distortions that perpetuate the panic cycle and that interfere with self-control and recovery. When these patients learn to breathe properly, to a normal level of exhaled CO_2 (38–42 torr), they restore proper physiological balance and then are able to think more coherently, which enhances the ability to utilize behavioral strategies in recovery.

Clinical experience suggests that EDA, HRV, peripheral temperature, and diaphragmatic breathing (pneumography or capnography) are all quite helpful for young patients with anxiety/stress symptoms. Using home and school training devices such as temperature-sensitive dots or bands is also helpful as a way of helping children self-monitor and self-cue in settings where they are experiencing SNS overarousal.

Children and adolescents may experience stress in many forms: physical, medical, cognitive, emotional, psychosocial, and cultural. Biofeedback and relaxation therapies can help pediatric patients cope with a variety of stressful conditions and situations. Our experience suggests that stress management approaches incorporating biofeedback as a component of group therapy with children and adolescents are also very helpful and engaging. Techniques such as progressive muscle relaxation, self-hypnosis, and autogenics can also be very useful when integrated with biofeedback strategies in this population (Smith & Womack, 1987).

The "quieting reflex" (QR) concept was discovered in 1974 by Charles Stroebel as an outgrowth of work on stress management work. It has been adapted for use with children

(Stroebel & Stroebel, 1984) and called the "Kiddie QR." This program is divided into brief, sequential exercises including the use of child-oriented images and metaphors. The QR teaches children to pause and discriminate body arousal states. This can be nicely integrated with biofeedback monitoring to teach self-control and the achievement of an adaptive homeostatic physiological state.

Sleep Disorders

Disorders of initiating and maintaining sleep are fairly common in childhood and adolescence; in fact, surveys indicate that 25% of children and adolescents experience some sort of sleep disturbance (Mindell, 1993). Many times, childhood sleep disturbance includes a behavioral component or is secondarily related to a psychological disturbance (such as anxiety or depression). In addition, the sleep system is exquisitely sensitive to stress. Stress, anxiety, and excessive psychophysiological arousal can all inhibit normal sleep patterns. For these reasons, biofeedback and related strategies are often very useful for pediatric sleep disorders.

A successful strategy for children or adolescents with sleep onset difficulty as described by Barowsky, Moskowitz, and Zweig (1990) involves teaching these patients to reduce psychophysiological arousal through bifrontal EMG and thermal biofeedback. As they become more relaxed and less aroused from a CNS standpoint, they transition into sleep more easily, thus decreasing sleep latency. Diaphragmatic breathing, EDA, and bitrapezius EMG work are also useful. A study that included adolescent patients with insomnia demonstrated that those receiving both frontal EMG biofeedback and progressive muscle relaxation showed improvements in sleep onset time, relative to controls (Freedman & Papsdorf, 1976).

For children with insomnia, night terrors, and nightmares, the coupling of relaxation therapy with positive, comforting mental imagery at bedtime can provide an effective approach (Kohen, Mahowald, & Rosen, 1992; King, Cranstoun, & Josephs, 1989; Anderson, 1979).

ANS Dysfunction

Clinical experience as well as the knowledge of the etiological role of ANS imbalance suggests that children with disorders of ANS dysfunction, including Raynaud's disease/phenomenon, reflex sympathetic dystrophy (now called complex regional pain syndrome), hyperhidrosis, essential hypertension, and irritable bowel syndrome, may benefit from biofeedback targeted at SNS overactivity, albeit the pediatric-specific literature is limited (Athreya, 1994; Barowsky, Zweig, & Moskowitz, 1987; Ewart, Harris, & Iwata, 1987; Freedman, Ianni, & Wenig, 1983; Lightman, Pochaczevsky, & Ilowite, 1987; Olssen & Berde, 1993, Olness, 1990; Silber & Majd, 1988; Wilder et al., 1992). EDA, peripheral temperature, HRV training, and breath control work have been particularly useful in these populations in the authors' clinical experience. In patients with Raynaud's disease/phenomenon, learning to warm the fingers and toes in the face of a cold stressor in the office provides a useful generalization strategy.

Neuromuscular Rehabilitation

The benefits of biofeedback in rehabilitation are reviewed in a previous chapter, however a few comments on pediatric applications are warranted. Child psychologists, physiatrists and physical therapists are documenting the many benefits of EMG work in pediatric rehabilitation. Children with spina bifida, cerebral palsy, traumatic brain injury, burns, and complications related to CNS tumors may all benefit from biofeedback (primarily EMG) (Allen, Bernstein, & Chait, 1991; Brucker & Buleava, 1996; Brundy, Grynbaum, & Korein, 1974; Finley, Niman, Standley, & Wansley, 1977; Cataldo, Bird, & Cunningham, 1978; Toner,

Cook, & Elder, 1998; Bertoti & Gross, 1988; Nash, Neilson, & O'Dwyer, 1989; Colburne, Wright, & Naumann, 1994; Murdoch, Pitt, Theodoros, & Ward, 1999). Therapeutic applications of biofeedback in this area include

Proprioceptive awareness development
Muscle reeducation
Strength and endurance training
Muscle tone down-training
Gait analysis and retraining
Bowel and bladder control training
Correction of drooling
Head control and postural training
Enhancement of speech
Treatment of torticollis

Pediatric psychologist Jeff Bolek, PhD (1998), who practices at the Cleveland Clinic Children's Hospital for Rehabilitation in Ohio, appropriately points out that with EMG biofeedback in this setting, the type of reinforcer used with each pediatric patient is vitally important. Asking patients what they prefer for a reward is a start. One adolescent whom he worked with was happy to have a particular song played. Some brain-injured children prefer tactile stimulation, such as vibrating rubber tubes placed around the shoulders. The olfactory sense is not processed by the thalamus, and therefore scents may be a desirable reward. Battery-operated toys that are connected to the biofeedback equipment, and that "turn on" (via a biofax relay box) when a desired threshold is attained, are also favorites in his clinical work. The design of reinforcement intervals and the scheduling of training sessions (blocked versus intermittent) are crucial to success as well (Bolek, 1998).

Chronic Illness

Behavioral treatment procedures, including biofeedback, are finding wide application as adjunctive treatments in the management of children with chronic debilitating medical conditions (Masek, Fentress, & Spirito, 1981; McQuaid & Nassau, 1999). Pediatric subspecialty care has evolved to a point where many patients with significant childhood chronic illness can be medically stabilized and have significantly improved longevity compared to 30 years ago. However, being stable from a medical standpoint does not ensure that these children are functioning without impairment. Chronic illness can have many biobehavioral, academic, and social sequelae that we are beginning to see more clearly. Biofeedback and self-regulation are ideal strategies to assist pediatric populations with chronic illness in optimizing function and performance across all domains of daily activity. Psychological and behavioral treatments in the context of chronic illness have particular relevance in four domains: pain management, treatment compliance (adherence), health locus of control issues, and stress management.

Asthma

In 1982, Creer, Renne, and Chai suggested that the investigation and treatment of asthma requires a collaboration between medicine and psychology because the "physical and psychological factors are inextricably interwoven." It is generally well accepted that behavioral interventions as adjunctive treatments for asthma are essential for many patients. In some children, asthma episodes may be emotionally triggered. Effective biofeedback-based interventions have included bifrontal EMG, airway feedback, pneumography, capnography, and HRV (Kotses & Glaus, 1981; Kotses et al., 1991; Lehrer, Sargunaraj, & Hochron, 1992).

Cystic Fibrosis

Spirito, Russo, and Masek (1984) describe the need for behavioral interventions and stress management in children with cystic fibrosis. They describe the successful application of biofeedback, relaxation, and behavioral counseling in a group of patients aged 13–23. Delk, Gevirtz, Hicks, Carden, and Rucker (1994) examined the effects of respiratory muscle feedback on lung function in a group of subjects aged 10–41 years. A significant treatment effect was observed for the biofeedback group relative to controls, with improvement in several pulmonary function measurements.

Insulin-Dependent Diabetes Mellitus

It has been suggested that patients with insulin-dependent diabetes mellitus (IDDM) may be particularly susceptible to stress-induced hyperglycemia and to stress effects on metabolic control. Therefore, stress management training has been proposed as one option for enhancing glycemic control in these individuals. Rose, Firestone, Heick, and Faught (1983) used a multiple-baseline design in a study of five adolescents with poorly controlled IDDM. Improved diabetic control occurred when behavioral treatment was introduced. A study of biofeedback-assisted stress management included a 17-year-old individual with IDDM who experienced benefit from a protocol that included frontal EMG (Rosenbaum, 1983).

Alcoholism

Brief biofeedback-assisted autogenic therapy ($n = 12$) led to enhanced sense of internal locus of control after the training procedure, relative to a control condition ($n = 13$), for adolescents with alcoholism. The treatment protocol included four weekly sessions of finger temperature monitoring during a taped autogenic relaxation exercise (Sharp, Huford, Allison, Sparks, & Cameron, 1997).

Hematology/Oncology

Studies in a variety of childhood cancers and hematological disorders (e.g., sickle cell disease) support the role of self-regulation therapy for children. Specifically, a number of studies support the use of relaxation, mental imagery (self-hypnosis), distraction, relaxation, and cognitive-behavioral strategies for the procedural pain and anticipatory nausea issues that are commonly encountered (Kuttner, Bowman, & Teasdale, 1988; Labaw, Holton, Tewell, & Eccles, 1975; LeBaron & Hilgard, 1984; Kaufman, Tarnowski, & Olson, 1989; Zeltzer, Dolgin, LeBaron, & LeBaron, 1991). Video games are also helpful as a cognitive distraction in reducing chemotherapy-related distress (Kolko & Rickard-Figueroa, 1985; Redd & Andrykowski, 1982). In our experience, biofeedback protocols for children can be set up like a video game experience (Culbert et al., 1994). Therefore, biofeedback can be a very helpful adjunctive technique for this population. A study in adults with chemotherapy-related side effects of cancer treatment indicated that temperature and EMG biofeedback reduced some physiological indicators of arousal after treatment, but that relaxation alone reduced nausea and anxiety during chemotherapy (Burish & Jenkins, 1992).

Taken together, this literature supports the benefits of lowered arousal, directed therapeutic imagery, breath control, and distraction. There was no study specific to the use of biofeedback for this purpose in children, but the fact that relaxation is generally supported as helpful suggests that biofeedback can be appropriately employed for this purpose. Our clinical experience with many oncology patients supports this notion as well. Training in controlled diaphragmatic breathing as measured by pneumography, coupled with positive mental imagery, has been very useful for these patients. Research into immune system function suggests that children can voluntarily learn to modulate certain aspects of immune function with self-directed relaxation/mental imagery techniques (Olness et al., 1989; Hewson-Bower & Drummond, 1996; Noll, 1988; Surman, Gottlieb, & Hackett, 1972).

Learning Disorders and School Performance

Although it is beyond the scope of this chapter to cover this topic in detail, it is important to point out that biofeedback with children is moving beyond clinical health care settings and into the schools. Over 20 years ago, Joe Kamiya (1979) wrote: "The potential role of biofeedback in education is unique. Whereas other modes of education are basically addressed to the individual's development of interaction skills and coping abilities with the external environment, biofeedback is a way to help the individual cope with the internal environment" (p. 24). Interest in biofeedback as a means to enhance learning and classroom performance seemed to peak in the 1970s, with a number of innovative programs in Colorado, Minnesota, South Dakota, and Indiana (Reaney, Sugarman, & Olness, 1998). More recently, Daniel Hamiel (personal communication, March 2000) reports great success with a biofeedback-based stress management program for all ages in schools in Israel. According to Hamiel, teachers in the United States are also finding emotional management training that includes HRV biofeedback very helpful in settings for emotionally/behaviorally challenged youth. Neurofeedback, as described elsewhere in this book, is helping children with a variety of learning and attentional problems. Peripheral biofeedback modalities such as EDA and EMG continue to have utility in school settings for children with ADHD, learning difficulties such as poor handwriting, and performance anxiety.

Biofeedback has great promise as an intervention strategy for children in a variety of educational settings, and is an ideal tool for enhancing physical, attentional, emotional, and social regulation skills. Studies indicate that children with learning disorders (LDs) and children with a variety of cognitive deficits can be successfully coached in relaxation, biofeedback, and self-regulation. For example, a group of children with LDs were able to demonstrate twice the peripheral temperature control ability than children without LDs, after five biofeedback sessions that included a consistent reinforcer (Hunter, Russell, Russell, & Zimmerman, 1976). In one early study, Guralnick and Mott (1976) described breath control therapy with an 11-year-old male diagnosed with perceptual–motor disabilities in an LD program. This boy demonstrated a chaotic, shallow breathing pattern, marked by his inability to control the volume of inhalation–exhalation. This led to problems with speech production patterns. Eight 30-minute sessions of strain-gauge-based biofeedback resulted in markedly improved voluntary breath control.

Mangina and Beuzeron-Mangina (1992) describe a psychophysiological assessment method that differentiates children with LDs from children without LDs, based on bilateral EDA differences. They go on to define the relationship between "optimal physiological activation" states during certain types of cognitive stimulation and Mangina's method of optimizing these states.

Several authors have described the use of EMG biofeedback in the treatment of writing problems with school-aged children. Studies have utilized bifrontal EMG (Hughes, Jackson, Dubois, & Erwin, 1979) and forearm EMG (Carter & Russell, 1980; Cobb & Evans, 1981). In these studies, the main goal was to reduce muscle tension to a level that allowed for easier, more fluid writing. This may suggest that in general, that as children become more relaxed, they can experience performance improvements—perhaps in part because of reduced muscular and ANS "interference" (Andrasik & Attansio, 1985)

Other academic, attentional, and emotional control and enhancement procedures that primarily utilize EEG biofeedback are very promising and are reviewed elsewhere in this text (see Lubar, Chapter 18, and Monastra, Chapter 19, this volume). It should be pointed that although most of the recent literature on biofeedback interventions for children with ADHD has focused on neurofeedback procedures, EMG biofeedback and other basic relaxation procedures may still be of some value for many children in this population (Braud, 1978; Braud, Lupin, & Braud, 1975; Lee, 1991).

A new CNS biofeedback application that appears promising is called "hemoencephalography" (HEG). (Note: We wish to acknowledge information provided by William Mize, MD [personal communication, March 2001] for this section.) As measured by functional magnetic resonance imaging (fMRI) studies, cortical circulation is closely coupled to neuronal activation (Posner & Raichle, 1998). HEG, a red/infrared-light-energy-sensing system, allows for imaging (Villringer & Chance, 1997) and neurobiofeedback directly on cortical circulation. This system directly engages discrete cellular assemblies in one volume of targeted tissue. This contrasts with traditional neurofeedback, which modifies the amplitude or phase relationships of selected waveforms in the EEG at a given location, using an operant conditioning paradigm (Nash, 2000). These waveforms have multiple determinants, both proximal and distal to the site of therapy (Nunez, 1995). HEG exists in two forms: an active light-emitting system (the more common technology), which interacts directly with vascular systems and the neuronal cells they support; and a passive technology (PIR HEG), which senses infrared energy, a metabolic output from a targeted brain volume.

The more common active system consists of a double-output light source tuned to hemoglobin light absorption phenomena linked to the oxygenation level of red blood cells (Jobsis, 1977; Benaron, Kurth, Steven, Delivoria-Papadopoulos, & Chance, 1995). A photo sensor detects the light energy reflected back from the brain tissue and produces a signal based on the ratio of the energy measured in different wavelengths. Thus, as oxygenated capillary beds are recruited by a subject performing HEG biofeedback, the signal increases. This form of HEG exercises cortical and adjacent subcortical tissue volumes of ≤ 1 cm^3 directly below the device. Its purpose is to stimulate brain function and related supporting circulation through activating the tissue immediately below the apparatus. The passive system does not emit light, but senses a band of infrared light energy (wavelength 7–14 microns). This more diffuse system is designed to be unaffected by ambient light and receives energy output from cortical and subcortical tissue in a spherical volume no less than 32 millimeters in diameter (golf ball size) directly under the sensing element.

Active HEG biofeedback has been studied in a mixed population of patients (Toomin et al., 2001): 16 adults with a diverse array of brain disorders affecting attention and cognition, and 11 children with attention and/or learning problems. HEG biofeedback was applied frontally for 10 minutes each to F_{p1}, F_{p2}, and F_{pz} (total therapy time per session, 30 minutes) for 10 sessions approximately 1 week apart. Using the patients as their own controls, scores on the Test of Variables of Attention (TOVA; a standardized computer measure of attention) rose from a baseline group mean of 87.4 (standard mean for normal subjects is 100) to 98.4 after treatment. These patients showed a comparable rise in general cognitive function (13.8%; $p < .001$, $df = 15$) as measured by the computerized Microcog system. This treatment effect as measured by the TOVA is similar in magnitude to that achieved by traditional neurobiofeedback in 20–40 sessions. HEG is felt by Toomin and colleagues to be more efficient because it is more direct in its application to neural anatomy than EEG wave training. Before-and-after single-photon emission computed tomography (SPECT) images (see Figures 31.4A and 31.4B) of patients treated with HEG biofeedback (30 sessions of 30 minutes each) show significant increases in circulatory patterns at

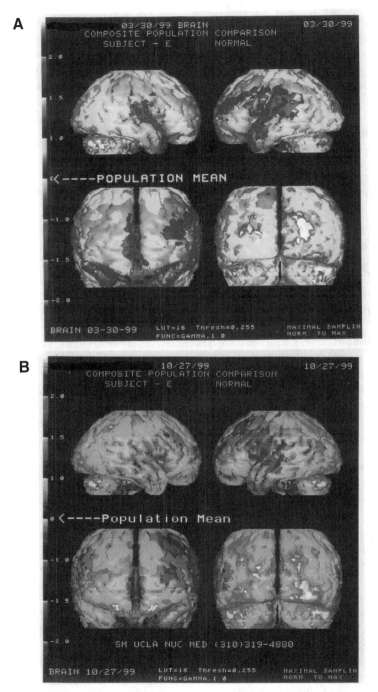

FIGURE 31.4. (A) SPECT images of a patient before HEG therapy. (B) SPECT images of the same patient after HEG therapy.

rest, over broad cortical areas; that is, the increases appear not to be confined to the areas treated directly. This suggests that activation of the prefrontal cortex through autoregulation may recruit broader neural areas through cortical relationships. It is unknown whether these distant effects are due to therapeutic "coupling," which has been observed in pilot studies between comparable loci in either hemisphere, or whether it is due to homeostasis following changes induced by HEG therapy. Neurotherapy, by modifying EEG variables, is thought to challenge the brain toward improved self-regulation of arousal, attention, and affect. In this regard, HEG is like other forms of neurotherapy that have more than local effects. HEG is a new and promising addition to the growing neurofeedback armamentarium.

CONCLUSIONS/LOOKING AHEAD

It has become evident that pediatric health care professionals and educational professionals urgently need training in a new array of skills that can be helpful in confronting the new psychophysiological and psychosocial morbidities challenging today's youth and families. The effects of stress and psychosocial dysfunction may well continue to play out in adulthood. Studies now indicate that over half of all visits to primary care physicians are related to psychosocial problems that present as common physical complaints. How better to reduce or prevent the occurrence of somatic and psychophysiological disorders in adults than to teach self-regulation at all ages? Biofeedback and related self-regulatory skills could possibly become core competencies in pediatric training as a way of addressing these problems. Wickramasekera, Davies, and Davies (1996) state that "Clinical, educational and research projects are needed in nonpsychiatric primary care settings" (p. 222), and go on to propose that psychophysiology laboratories should be established in primary care residency programs.

The psychophysiological disorders that represent a growing component of the "new morbidity" in pediatrics are not going to go away. Because of this, it is fair to say that the future of biofeedback and applied psychophysiology in pediatric medical, educational, psychological, and community-based settings is limitless. There is a pressing need to train more child health care and educational professionals in biofeedback and self-regulation skills. It is exciting to imagine the possibilities. What if . . .

> . . . every child and adolescent received "stress inoculation" as part of standard well-child care or as part of the health education curriculum at all levels of schooling?
>
> . . . every child diagnosed with asthma, diabetes, cancer, or other chronic or life-threatening illnesses received intensive training in self-regulation skills via biofeedback-based protocols, at the time of diagnosis?
>
> . . . every pediatric inpatient learned about nonpharmacological, self-regulatory strategies, including biofeedback, to control procedural and postoperative pain and anxiety?
>
> . . . every child with headaches or RAP received thermal or HRV biofeedback as part of the first-line approach to their treatment?
>
> . . . every school had biofeedback equipment readily available, so that kids with anger management, attentional, or performance anxiety issues could learn about ways to self-regulate these functions through biofeedback right in their classroom environment?
>
> . . . all kids had access to optimal performance "coaching" for musical, athletic, public speaking, and other performance activities?

Pediatrics as a field has begun to move in the right direction with the publication of *Bright Futures: Guidelines for Health Supervision of Infants, Children, and Adolescents* (Green,

1994)—a set of recommendations and materials reflecting the consensus opinion of more than 100 multidisciplinary experts, and emphasizing a biopsychosocial approach to well-child care and anticipatory guidance. The ubiquitous effects of stress on youth in modern society are also acknowledged. Goals espoused in these guidelines include a mandate to transform the process of health supervision to include giving each young person ways to "cope with stressful life experiences, have high self-esteem, acquire a sense of self-efficacy, and the belief the he/she can succeed in life" (Green, 1994, p. xiii). The benefits of collaboration between pediatric primary health care providers and mental health professionals in helping children with stress management and related adaptive and coping strategies are also reviewed. Therapeutic approaches contained within the fields of applied psychophysiology and biofeedback can play a key role in these efforts as ideal, child-friendly strategies.

Research on the use of biofeedback and self-regulation skills with young people has grown substantially in the past 25 years, and study results are exceedingly positive in almost all areas examined. Furthermore, children and adolescents find biofeedback very desirable, engaging, and nonthreatening as a treatment strategy. This makes it an ideal therapeutic vehicle for addressing the biobehavioral, psychosocial, and academic challenges being confronted by today's youth.

REFERENCES

Allen, K. D., Bernstein, B., & Chait, D. H. (1991). EMG biofeedback treatment of pediatric hyperfunctional dysphonia. *Journal of Behavior Therapy and Experimental Psychiatry, 22*, 97–101.

American Psychiatric Association. (1994). *Diagnostic and statistical manual of mental disorders* (4th ed.). Washington, DC: Author.

Anderson, D. (1979). Treatment of insomnia in a 13-year old boy by relaxation training and reduction of parental attention. *Journal of Behavior Therapy and Experimental Psychiatry, 10*, 263–265.

Andrasik, V., & Attansio, V. (1985). Biofeedback in pediatrics: Current status and appraisal. In M. Wolraich & D. Routh (Eds.), *Advances in developmental and behavioral pediatrics*. Greenwich, CT: JAI Press.

Athreya, B. (1994). Vasospastic disorders in children. *Seminars in Pediatric Surgery, 3*, 70–78.

Attansio, V., Andrasik, F., Burke, E., Blake, D., Kabela, E., & McCarran, M. (1985). Clinical issues in utilizing biofeedback with children. *Clinical Biofeedback and Health, 8*, 134–141.

Bakal, D. (1999). *Minding the body: Clinical uses of somatic awareness*. New York: Guilford Press.

Barowsky, E. I. (1990). The use of biofeedback in the treatment of disorders of childhood. *Annals of the New York Academy of Sciences, 602*, 221–233.

Barowsky, E. I., Moskowitz, J., & Zweig, J. B. (1990). Biofeedback for disorders of initiating and maintaining sleep. *Annals of the New York Academy of Sciences, 602*, 97–103.

Barowsky, E. I., Zweig, J. B., & Moskowitz, J. (1987). Thermal biofeedback in the treatment of symptoms associated with reflex sympathetic dystrophy. *Journal of Child Neurology, 2*, 229–232.

Benaron, D. A., Kurth, C. D., Steven, J. M., Delivoria-Papadopoulos, M., & Chance, B. (1995). Transcranial optical path length by near infra-red phase-shift spectroscopy. *Journal of Clinical Monitoring, 11*, 109–117.

Bernstein, G., & Borchardt, C. (1991). Anxiety disorders of childhood and adolescence: A critical review. *Journal of the American Academy of Child and Adolescent Psychiatry, 30*, 519–532.

Bertoti, D., & Gross, A. (1988). Evaluation of biofeedback seat insert for improving active sitting posture in children with cerebral palsy. *Physical Therapy, 68*, 1109–1113.

Blum, N. (1999). Repetitive behaviors. In M. D. Levine, W. B. Carey, & A. C. Crocker (Eds.), *Developmental–behavioral pediatrics* (3rd. ed.). Philadelphia: Saunders.

Bolek, J. (1998). Surface EMG applications of pediatric biofeedback in rehabilitation settings. *Biofeedback, 26*, 21–23.

Boyce, T., Chesney, M., & Kaiser, P. (1990). Development of a protocol for measuring cardiovascular response to stress in preschool children. *Journal of Developmental and Behavioral Pediatrics, 11*, 214–217.

Bradbury, M. G., & Meadow, S. R. (1995). Combined treatment with enuresis alarm and desmopressin for nocturnal enuresis. *Acta Paediatrica, 84*, 1014–1018.

Braud, L. (1978). The effects of frontal EMG biofeedback and progressive relaxation upon hyperactivity and its behavioral concomitants. *Biofeedback and Self-Regulation, 3*, 69–89.

Braud, L., Lupin, M., & Braud, W. (1975). The use of electromyographic biofeedback in the control of hyperactivity. *Journal of Learning Disabilities, 8*, 21–26.

Breuner, C., Barry, P. J., & Kemper, K. (1998). Alternative medicine use by homeless youth. *Archives of Pediatrics and Adolescent Medicine, 152,* 1071–1075.

Brooks, R., Copen, R., Cox, D., Morris, J., Borowitz, S., & Sutphen, J. (2000). Review of the treatment literature for encopresis, functional constipation and stool-toileting refusal. *Annals of Behavioral Medicine, 22,* 26–27.

Brucker, S., & Buleava, V. (1996). Biofeedback effect on EMG response in patients with spinal cord injury. *Archives of Physical Medicine and Rehabilitation, 77,* 133–137.

Brugman, E., Reijneveld, S., Verhulst, F., & Verloove-Vanhorick, P. (2001). Identification and management of psychosocial problems by preventative child health care. *Archives of Pediatrics and Adolescent Medicine, 155,* 462–469.

Brundy, J., Grynbaum, B., & Korein, J. (1974). Spasmodic torticollis: Treatment by feedback display of the EMG. *Archives of Physical Medicine and Rehabilitation, 55,* 403–408.

Burish, T. G., & Jenkins, R. A. (1992). Effectiveness of biofeedback and relaxation training in reducing the side effects of cancer chemotherapy. *Health Psychology, 11,* 17–23.

Cacioppo, J., Klein, D., Berntson, G., & Hatfield, E. (1993). The psychophysiology of emotion. In M. Lewis & J. Haviland (Eds.), *Handbook of emotions.* New York: Guilford Press.

Carter, J., & Russell, H. (1980). Biofeedback and academic attainment of LD children. *Academic Therapy, 15,* 483–486.

Cataldo, M., Bird, B., & Cunningham, C. (1978). Experimental analysis of EMG feedback in treating cerebral palsy. *Journal of Behavioral Medicine, 1,* 311–321.

Cobb, D., & Evans, J. (1981). The use of biofeedback techniques with school aged children exhibiting behavioral and/or learning problems. *Journal of Abnormal Child Psychology, 9,* 251–281.

Colburne, R. G., Wright, V. F., & Naumann, S. (1994). Feedback of triceps surae EMG in gait of children with cerebral palsy: A controlled study. *Archives of Physical Medicine and Rehabilitation, 75,* 40–45.

Combs, A. J., Glassberg, A. D., Gerdes, D., & Horowitz, M. (1998). Biofeedback therapy for children with dysfunctional voiding. *Urology, 52,* 312–315.

Corder, B., Whiteside, R., & Haizlip, T. (1986). Biofeedback, cognitive training and relaxation techniques as multimodal adjunct therapy for hospitalized adolescents: A pilot study. *Adolescence, 21,* 339–346.

Cox, D. J., Sutphen, J., Borowitz, S., Kovatchev, B., & Ling, W. (1998). Contribution of behavior therapy and biofeedback to laxative therapy in the treatment of pediatric encopresis. *Annals of Behavioral Medicine, 20,* 70–76.

Cox, D. J., Sutphen, J., Ling, W., Quillian, W., & Borowitz, S. (1996). Additive benefits of laxative, toilet training, and biofeedback therapies in the treatment of pediatric encopresis. *Journal of Pediatric Psychology, 21,* 659–670.

Creer, T., Renne, C., & Chai, H. (1982). The application of behavioral techniques to childhood asthma. In D. Russo & J. Varni (Eds.), *Behavioral pediatrics: Research and practice.* New York: Plenum Press.

Culbert, T. (1999). Biofeedback with children and adolescents. In C. Schaefer (Ed.), *Innovative pyschotherapy techniques in child and adolescent therapy* (2nd ed.). New York: Wiley.

Culbert, T., & Bonfilio, S. (1998). Integrating biofeedback and cognitive-behavioral therapy for children with anger management problems. *Biofeedback, 26,* 27–29.

Culbert, T., Kajander, R., & Reaney, J. (1996). Biofeedback with children and adolescents: Clinical observations and patient perspectives. *Journal of Developmental and Behavioral Pediatrics, 17,* 342–350.

Culbert, T., Reaney, J., & Kohen, D. (1994). Cyberphysiologic strategies for children: The clinical hypnosis/biofeedback interface. *International Journal of Clinical and Experimental Hypnosis, 42,* 97–117.

Delaney, D. C., Olson, K., & Labbe, E. E. (1992). Skin temperature biofeedback: Evaluation of non-clinical children's responses. *Journal of Behavior Therapy and Experimental Psychiatry, 23,* 37–42.

Delk, K., Gevirtz, R., Hicks, D. A., Carden, F., & Rucker, R. (1994). The effects of biofeedback assisted breathing retraining on lung functions in patients with cystic fibrosis. *Chest, 105,* 23–27.

Dixon, S., & Stein, M. (2000). *Encounters with children* (3rd ed.) St. Louis, MO: Mosby/Year Book.

Ewart, C. K., Harris, W. L., & Iwata, M. M. (1987). Feasibility and effectiveness of school based relaxation in lowering blood pressure. *Health Psychology, 6,* 399–416.

Faull, C., & Nicol, A. (1986). Abdominal pain in 6 year olds: An epidemiologic study in a new town. *Journal of Child Psychology and Psychiatry, 27,* 251–260.

Feehan, M., & Marsh, N. (1989). The reduction of bruxism using contingent EMG audible biofeedback: A case study. *Journal of Behavior Therapy and Experimental Psychiatry, 20,* 179–183.

Finley, W., Niman, C., Standley, J., & Wansley, R. (1977). Electrophysiologic behavior modification of frontal EMG in cerebral-palsied children. *Biofeedback and Self-Regulation, 2,* 59–78.

Fredericks, D., Carr, J., & Williams, W. (1998). Overview of treatment of rumination disorder for adults in a residential setting. *Journal of Behavior Therapy and Experimental Psychiatry, 29,* 31–40.

Freedman, R., Ianni, P., & Wenig, P. (1983). Behavioral treatment of Raynaud's disease. *Journal of Consulting and Clinical Psychology, 51,* 539–549.

Freedman, R., & Papsdorf, J. (1976). Biofeedback and progressive relaxation treatment of sleep–onset insomnia: A controlled, all-night investigation. *Biofeedback and Self-Regulation*, 1, 253–271.

Gagnon, D., Hudnall, L., & Andrasik, F. (1992). Biofeedback and related procedures in coping with stress. In A. La Greca, L. Siegel, J. L. Wallander, & C. E. Walker (Eds.), *Stress and coping in child health*. New York: Guilford Press.

Gaudet, T. (1998). Integrative medicine: The evolution of a new approach to medicine and medical education. *Integrative Medicine*, 1, 67–73.

Gil, K. M., Perry, G., & King, L. R. (1988). The use of biofeedback in a behavioral program designed to teach an anxious child self-catheterization. *Biofeedback and Self-Regulation*, 13, 347–355.

Green, M. (Ed.) (1994). *Bright futures: Guidelines for health supervision of infants, children, and adolescents*. Arlington, VA: National Center for Education in Maternal and Child Health.

Guralnick, M., & Mott, D. (1976). Biofeedback training with a learning disabled child. *Perceptual and Motor Skills*, 42, 27–30.

Hall, H., Chiarucci, D., & Berman, B. (1992). Self-regulation and assessment approaches for vaso-occlusive pain management for pediatric sickle cell anemia patients. *International Journal of Psychosomatics*, 39, 28–33.

Hewson-Bower, B., & Drummond, P. (1996). Secretory immunoglobulin A increases during relaxation in children with and without recurrent upper respiratory tract infections. *Journal of Developmental and Behavioral Pediatrics*, 17, 311–316.

Hobbie, C. (1989). Relaxation techniques for children and young people. *Journal of Pediatric Health Care*, 3, 83–87.

Houts, A. C. (1990). *Parent guide to enuresis treatment* (5th ed.). Memphis, TN: Author.

Hughes, H., Jackson, K., DuBois, E., & Erwin, R. (1979). Treatment of handwriting problems utilizing EMG biofeedback training. *Perceptual and Motor Skills*, 48, 603–606.

Humphreys, P., & Gevirtz, R. (2000). Treatment of recurrent abdominal pain: Components analysis of four treatment protocols. *Journal of Pedeatric Gastroenterology and Nutrition*, 31, 47–51.

Hunter, S., Russell, H., Russell, E., & Zimmerman, R. (1976). Control of fingertip temperature increases via biofeedback in learning-disabled and normal children. *Perceptual and Motor Skills*, 43, 743–755.

Institute for HeartMath®. (1997). *HeartMath® research overview*. Boulder Creek, CA: Author.

Jobsis, F. F. (1977). Non-invasive infra-red monitoring of cerebral O_2 sufficiency, blood volume, HbO_2–Hb shifts and blood flow. *Acta Neurologia Scandinavica*, 64(Suppl. 452).

Kamiya, J. (1979, May). Applications of biofeedback in developmental education. *Newsletter of the American Psychological Association*, pp. 24–25.

Kaufman, K., Tarnowksi, K., & Olson, R. (1989). Self-regulation treatment to reduce the aversiveness of cancer chemotherapy. *Journal of Adolescent Health Care*, 10, 323–327.

Kemper, K. (2000). Holistic pediatrics = good medicine. *Pediatrics*, 105, 214–218.

Kemper, K., & Wornham, W. (2001). Consultations for holistic pediatric services for inpatients and outpatient oncology patients at a children's hospital. *Archives of Pediatrics and Adolescent Medicine*, 155, 449–453.

Kendall, P. (1994). Treating anxiety disorders in children: Results of a randomized clinical trial. *Journal of Consulting and Clinical Psychology*, 62, 100–110.

Kendall, P., & Braswell, L. (1986). Medical applications of cognitive-behavioral interventions with children. *Journal of Developmental and Behavioral Pediatrics*, 7, 257–264.

Kendall, P., Howard, B., & Epps, J. (1988). The anxious child: Cognitive-behavioral treatment strategies. *Behavior Modification*, 12, 281–310.

Khan, S., Hyman, P., Cocjin, J., & DiLorenzo, C. (2000). Rumination syndrome in adolescents. *Journal of Pediatrics*, 136, 528–531.

King, N., Cranstoun, F., & Josephs, A. (1989). Emotive imagery and children's nighttime fears: A multiple baseline design evaluation. *Journal of Behavior Therapy and Experimental Psychiatry*, 20, 125–135.

Kjolseth, D., Monster-Knudsen, L., & Madsen, B. (1993). Urodynamic biofeedback training for children with bladder–sphincter dyscoordination during voiding. *Neurology and Urodynamics*, 12, 211–221.

Knudson-Cooper, M. S. (1981). Relaxation and biofeedback training in the treatment of severely burned children. *Journal of Burn Care and Rehabilitation*, 2, 102–110.

Kohen, D. P. (1991). Applications of relaxation and mental imagery (self-hypnosis) for habit problems. *Pediatric Annals*, 20, 136–144.

Kohen, D. P., & Botts, P. (1987). Relaxation-imagery (self-hypnosis) in Tourette's syndrome: Experience with four children. *American Journal of Clinical Hypnosis*, 29, 227–237.

Kohen, D. P., Mahowald, M.W., & Rosen, G. M. (1992). Sleep terror disorder in children: The role of self-hypnosis in management. *American Journal of Clinical Hypnosis*, 34, 233–234.

Kolko, D., & Rickard-Figueroa, J. (1985). Effects of video games on the adverse corollaries of chemotherapy in pediatric oncology patients: A single case analysis. *Journal of Consulting and Clinical Psychology*, 53, 223–228.

Kotses, H., & Glaus, K. (1981). Applications of biofeedback to the treatment of asthma: A critical review. *Biofeedback and Self-Regulation*, 6, 575–593.

Kotses, H., Harver, A., Segreto, J., Glaus, K., Creer, T., & Young, G. (1991). Long-term effects of biofeedback induced facial relaxation on measures of asthma severity in children. *Biofeedback and Self-Regulation*, 16, 1–21.

Kuttner, L. (1989). Management of young children's acute pain and anxiety during invasive medical procedures. *Pediatrician*, 1639–1644.

Kuttner, L., Bowman, M., & Teasdale, M. (1988). Psychological treatment of distress, pain, and anxiety for young children with cancer. *Journal of Developmental and Behavioral Pediatrics*, 9, 374–381.

Labaw, W., Holton, C., Tewell, K., & Eccles, D. (1975). The use of self-hypnosis by children with cancer. *American Journal of Clinical Hypnosis*, 17, 233–238.

Labbe, E., Delaney, D., Olson, K., & Hickman, H. (1993). Skin-temperature biofeedback training: Cognitive and developmental factors in a non-clinical child population. *Perceptual and Motor Skills*, 76, 955–962.

Lavigne, J. V., Ross, C. D., & Berry, S. L. (1992). Evaluation of a psychological treatment package for treating pain in juvenile rheumatoid arthritis. *Arthritis Care and Research*, 5, 101–110.

LeBaron, S., & Hilgard, J. R. (1984). *Hypnotherapy for pain in children with cancer.* Los Altos, CA: Kauffman.

Lee, L., & Olness, K. (1996). Effects of self-induced mental imagery on autonomic reactivity in children. *Journal of Developmental and Behavioral Pediatrics*, 17, 323–327.

Lee, S. W. (1991). Biofeedback as a treatment for childhood hyperactivity: A critical review of the literature. *Psychological Reports*, 68, 163–192.

Lehrer, P., Sargunaraj, D., & Hochron, S. (1992). Psychological approaches to the treatment of asthma. *Journal of Consulting and Clinical Psychology*, 60, 639–643.

Leung, A., & Robson, W. (1991). Bruxism: How to stop tooth grinding and clenching. *Postgraduate Medicine*, 89, 167–171.

Lightman, H. I., Pochaczevsky, R., & Ilowite, N. T. (1987). Thermography in childhood reflex sympathetic dystrophy. *Journal of Pediatrics*, 11, 551–555.

Loening-Baucke, V. A. (1990). Modulation of abnormal defecation dynamics by biofeedback treatment in chronically constipated children with encopresis. *Journal of Pediatrics*, 116, 214–222.

Loening-Baucke, V. A. (1995). Biofeedback treatment for chronic constipation and encopresis in childhood: Long-term outcome. *Pediatrics*, 96, 105–110.

Loening-Baucke, V. A. (1996). Biofeedback training in children with functional constipation: A critical review. *Digestive Diseases and Sciences*, 41, 65–71.

Malone, T. (1991, December). What makes computer games fun? *BYTE*, pp. 258–277.

Mangina, C., & Beuzeron-Mangina, H. (1992). Psychophysiological treatment for learning disabilities: Controlled research and evidence. *International Journal of Psychophysiology*, 12, 243–250.

Mars, D. (1998). Biofeedback assisted psychotherapy using multimodal biofeedback including capnography. *Biofeedback*, 26, 4–7.

Masek, B., Fentress, D., & Spirito, A. (1981). Behavioral treatment of symptoms of childhood illness. *Clinical Psychology Review*, 4, 561–571.

McGrath, P. (1990). *Pain in children: Nature, assessment and treatment.* New York: Guilford Press.

McGrath, P., & Finley, G. A. (1999). *Chronic and recurrent pain in children and adolescents.* Seattle, WA: IASP Press.

McGrath, M. L., Mellon, M. W., & Murphy, L. (2000). Empirically supported treatments in pediatric psychology: Constipation and encopresis. *Journal of Pediatric Psychology*, 25, 225–254.

McQuaid, E., & Nassau, J. (1999). Empirically supported treatments of disease-related symptoms in pediatric psychology: Asthma, diabetes, and cancer. *Journal of Pediatric Psychology*, 24, 305–328.

Mellon, M., & McGrath, M. (2000). Empirically supported treatments in pediatric psychology: Nocturnal enuresis. *Journal of Pediatric Psychology*, 25, 193–214.

Melzack, R. (1999). From the gate to the neuromatrix. *Pain*, 6 , S121–S126.

Michultka, D., Blanchard, E., & Rosenblum, E. (1989). Stress management and Gilles de la Tourette's syndrome. *Biofeedback and Self-Regulation*, 14, 115–123.

Mindell, J. (1993). Sleep disorders in children. *Health Psychology*, 12, 151–162.

Murdoch, B., Pitt, G., Theodoros, D., & Ward, E. (1999). Real-time continuous visual biofeedback in the treatment of speech breathing disorders following childhood traumatic brain injury: Report of one case. *Pediatric Rehabilitation*, 3, 5–20.

Nash, J. K. (2000). Treatment of attention deficit hyperactivity disorder with neurotherapy. *Clinical Electroencephalography*, 31, 30–37.

Nash, J., Neilson, P., & O'Dwyer, N. (1989). Reducing spasticity to control muscle contracture of children with cerebral palsy. *Developmental Medicine and Child Neurology*, 31, 471–480.

National Center for Complementary and Alternative Medicine. (NCCAM). (1999). National Institutes of Health, Bethesda, Maryland 20892. www.nccam.nih.gov.

Nolan, T., Catto-Smith, T., Coffey, C., & Wells, J. (1998). Randomised controlled trial of biofeedback training in persistent encopresis with anismus. *Archives of Disease in Childhood, 79,* 131–135.

Noll, R. (1988). Hypnotherapy of a child with warts. *Journal of Developmental and Behavioral Pediatrics, 8,* 357–358.

Nunez, P. (1995). *Neocortical dynamics and human EEG rhythms.* New York, NY: Oxford University Press.

O'Connor, K., Gareau, D., & Borgeat, F. (1995). Muscle control in chronic tic disorders. *Biofeedback and Self-Regulation, 20,* 111–122.

Olness, K. (1990). Reflex sympathetic dystrophy: Treatment of children with cyberphysiologic strategies. *Swedish Journal of Hypnosis, Psychotherapy, and Psychosomatic Medicine, 17,* 15–18.

Olness, K. (1997). Clinical applications of biofeedback with hypnosis. *Hypnosis, 24,* 70–73.

Olness, K., Culbert, T., & Uden, D. (1989). Self-regulation of salivary immunoglobulin A by children. *Pediatrics, 83,* 66–71.

Olness, K., & Kohen, D. (1996). *Hypnosis and hypnotherapy with children* (3rd ed.). New York: Guilford Press.

Olssen, G., & Berde, C. (1993). Neuorpathic pain in children and adolescents. In N. Schechter, C. Berde, & M. Yaster (Eds.), *Pain in infants, children and adolescents.* Baltimore: Williams & Wilkins.

Peterson, A., Campise, R., & Azrin, N. (1994). Behavioral and pharmacological treatments for tic and habit disorders: A review. *Journal of Developmental and Behavioral Pediatrics, 15,* 430–441.

Porena, M., Costantini, E., Rociola, W., & Mearini, E. (2000). Biofeedback successfully cures detrusor-sphincter dyssynergia in pediatric patients. *Journal of Urology, 163,* 1927–1931.

Posner, M. I., & Raichle, M. (1998). The neuroimaging of human brain function. *Proceedings of the National Academy of Sciences USA Online, 95*(3).

Reaney, J., & Kohen, D. (1998). Reaching the child: Developmental considerations and therapeutic communication in pediatric biofeedback. *Biofeedback, 26,* 33–35.

Reaney, J., Sugarman, L., & Olness, K. (1998). Taking biofeedback to where the kids are. *Biofeedback, 26,* 30–32.

Redd, W., & Andrykowski, M. (1982). Behavioral intervention in cancer treatment: Controlling aversion reactions to chemotherapy. *Journal of Consulting and Clinical Psychology, 55,* 391–395.

Rose, M., Firestone, P., Heick, H., & Faught, A. (1983). The effects of anxiety management training on the control of juvenile diabetes mellitus. *Journal of Behavioral Medicine, 6,* 381–395.

Rosenbaum, L. (1983). Biofeedback assisted stress management training for insulin-treated diabetes mellitus. *Biofeedback and Self-Regulation, 8,* 519–532.

Schmitt, B. D. (1990). Nocturnal enuresis: Finding the treatment that fits the child. *Contemporary Pediatrics, 7,* 70–97.

Schmitt, B. D. (1997). Nocturnal enuresis. *Pediatrics in Review, 18,* 183–191.

Schneider, P., & Peterson, J. (1982). Oral habits, considerations in management. *Pediatric Clinics of North America, 29,* 523–546.

Schulman, S., Quinn, C., Platcher, N., & Codman-Jones, C. (1999). Comprehensive management of dysfunctional voiding. *Pediatrics, 103,* e31.

Schwartz, M. S., & Associates. (1987). *Biofeedback: A practitioner's guide.* New York: Guilford Press.

Schwartz, M. S., & Associates. (1995). *Biofeedback: A practitioner's guide* (2nd ed.). New York: Guilford Press.

Shapiro, B. (1995). Treatment of chronic pain in children and adolescents. *Pediatric Annals, 24,* 148–157.

Sharp, C., Huford, D., Allison, J., Sparks, R., & Cameron, B. (1997). Facilitation of internal locus of control in adolescent alcoholics through brief biofeedback-assisted autogenic relaxation training procedure. *Journal of Substance Abuse Treatment, 14,* 55–60.

Sharp, L., & Pantell, R. (1992). Psychosocial problems during child health supervision visits: Eliciting, then what? *Pediatrics, 89,* 619–623.

Sikand, A., & Laken, M. (1998). Pediatricians' experience with complementary/alternative medicine. *Archives of Pediatrics and Adolescent Medicine, 152,* 1059–1064.

Silber, T., & Majd, M. (1988). Reflex sympathetic dystrophy in children and adolescents. *American Journal of Diseases of Children, 142,* 1325–1330.

Smith, M. (1991). Biofeedback. *Pediatric Annals, 20,* 128–134.

Smith, M., & Womack, W. (1987). Stress management techniques in childhood and adolescence. *Clinical Pediatrics, 26,* 581–585.

Snyder, K., Kymissis, P., & Kessler, K. (1999). Anger management for adolescents: Efficacy of brief group therapy. *Journal of the American Academy of Child and Adolescent Psychiatry, 38,* 1409–1416.

Spigelblatt, L., Laine-Ammara, G., Pless, I., & Guyver, A. (1994). The use of alternative medicine by children. *Pediatrics, 94,* 811–814.

Spirito, A., Russo, D., & Masek, B. (1984). Behavioral interventions and stress management training for hospitalized adolescents and young adults with cystic fibrosis. *General Hospital Psychiatry, 6,* 211–218.

Starfield, B., & Borkowf, F. (1969). Physicians' recognition of complaints made by parents about their children's health. *Pediatrics, 42,* 168–172.

Stroebel, C., & Stroebel, E. (1984). The quieting reflex: A psychophysiological approach for helping children deal with healthy and unhealthy stress. In J. Humphrey (Ed.), *Stress in childhood*. New York: AMC Press.

Sugarman, L. (1996). Hypnosis in primary care pediatric practice: Developing skills for the new morbidity. *Journal of Developmental and Behavioral Pediatrics*, 17, 300–306.

Surman, O., Gottlieb, S., & Hackett, T. (1972). Hypnotic treatment of a child with warts. *American Journal of Clinical Hypnosis*, 15, 12–14.

Sussman, D., & Culbert, T. (1999). Pediatric self-regulation. In M. Levine, W. Carey, & A. Crocker (Eds.), *Developmental–behavioral pediatrics* (3rd ed.). Philadelphia: Saunders.

Suter, S., & Loughry-Machado, G. (1981). Skin temperature biofeedback in children and adults. *Journal of Experimental Child Psychology*, 32, 77–87.

Toner, L., Cook, K., & Elder, G. (1998). Improved ankle function in children with cerebral palsy after computer-assisted motor learning. *Developmental Medicine and Child Neurology*, 40, 829–835.

Toomin, H., Remond, A., Toomin, M., Marsh, R., Kozlowski, G., Kimble, M., & Mize, W. (2001). *Intentional increase of cerebral blood oxygenation: A brain exercise therapy*. Manuscript submitted for publication.

Van der Plas, R. N., Benninga, M. A., Buller, H. A., Bossuyt, P. M., Akkermans, L. M., Redekop, W. K., & Taminiau, J. A. (1996). Biofeedback training in treatment of childhood constipation: A randomized controlled study. *Lancet*, 348, 776–780.

Varni, J. (1981). Self-regulation techniques in the management of chronic arthritic pain in hemophilia. *Behavior Therapy*, 12, 185–187.

Varni, J., & Gilbert, A. (1980). Self-regulation of chronic arthritic pain and long-term analgesic dependence in a hemophiliac. *Rheumatology and Rehabilitation*, 61, 375–379.

Varni, J., Walco, G., & Katz, E. (1989). Assessment and management of chronic and recurrent pain in children with chronic diseases. *Pediatrician*, 16, 56–63.

Villringer, A., & Chance, B. (1997). Non-invasive optical spectroscopy and imaging of human brain function. *Trends in Neuroscience*, 20, 435–442.

Wald, A. (1981). Use of biofeedback in the treatment of fecal incontinence in patients with meningomyelocele. *Pediatrics*, 68, 45–49.

Wald, A., Chandra, R., Gabel, S., & Chiponis, D. (1987). Evaluation of biofeedback in childhood encopresis. *Journal of Pediatric Gastroenterology and Nutrition*, 6, 554–558.

Wang, Y., & Morgan, W. P. (1992). The effect of imagery perspectives on the psychophysiological responses to imagined exercise. *Behavioral Brain Research*, 52, 167–174.

Wickramasekera, I., Davies, T., & Davies, S. (1996). Applied psychophysiology: A bridge between the biomedical model and the biopsychosocial model in family medicine. *Professional Psychology: Research and Practice*, 27, 221–223.

Wilder, R., Berde, C., Wolohan, M., Vieyra, M., Masek, B., & Mitchell, L. (1992). Reflex sympathetic dystrophy in children. *Journal of Bone and Joint Surgery*, 74, 910–919.

Yamanishi, T., Yassuda, K., Murayama, N., Sakakibara, R., Uchiyama, T., & Ito, H. (2000). Biofeedback training for detrusor overactivity in children. *Journal of Urology*, 164, 1686–1690.

Young, M. H., Montano, R. J., & Goldberg, R. L. (1991). Self-hypnosis, sensory cueing, and response prevention: Decreasing anxiety and improving written output of a pre-adolescent with learning disabilities. *American Journal of Clinical Hypnosis*, 34, 129–136.

Zeltzer, L., Dolgin, M., LeBaron, S., & LeBaron, C. (1991). A randomized controlled study of behavioral intervention for chemotherapy distress in children with cancer. *Pediatrics*, 88, 34–42.

PART X

Other Applications

CHAPTER 32

Diabetes Mellitus

ANGELE McGRADY
BARBARA BAILEY

This chapter first describes the characteristics of diabetes mellitus and discusses the traditional management of the disease. It then explores the impact of psychological variables and lifestyle factors on the control of diabetes. The chapter mainly addresses general clinical procedures for treatment with biofeedback and relaxation combined with traditional medical therapy. We discuss recommendations for types of and number of treatment sessions, home practice, and communication with a patient's physician. Next, we summarize important considerations in using biofeedback for persons with diabetes, and we discuss possible contraindications to treatment. A brief summary of research studies is given at the end of the chapter. (As in other chapters, italics on first use of a term indicate that the term is included in the glossary at the end of the chapter.)

More empirical research is necessary to establish and advance a psychophysiological approach to diabetes. However, the overall results are encouraging, and practitioners using relaxation and biofeedback can welcome referrals of patients with diabetes. Treatment of patients with diabetes involves particular risks and requires specialized knowledge. Thus practitioners using relaxation and biofeedback must have this knowledge and work as part of a treatment team.

DEFINITIONS AND TYPES OF DIABETES MELLITUS

Definition

Diabetes mellitus is a chronic disorder of metabolism affecting about 16 million people, or 6–7% of the United States population (Diabetes Research Working Group, 1999). High blood glucose (sugar), known as *hyperglycemia*, characterizes diabetes. Hyperglycemia results from either relative or absolute insulin deficiency. Glucose is one of the products that results from the breakdown (metabolism) of ingested food, principally carbohydrates. Glucose is the body's main fuel source and typically the brain's only energy source. Blood glucose levels are recorded as milligrams per deciliter or as millimoles per liter (abbreviated mg/dl and mmol/l, respectively, with specific numbers).

The glucose level in the blood normally rises after a meal. This increase prompts the pancreas, an organ that lies behind the stomach, to secrete the regulatory hormone called insulin. By combining with cell surface receptors, insulin allows glucose to enter cells and increases storage of fatty acids, amino acids, and glucose. The counterregulatory hormone, glucagon, is also released by the pancreas. Glucagon mobilizes glucose, fatty acids, and amino acids from storage sites into the blood when needed. Other counterregulatory hormones—namely, epinephrine, growth hormone, and cortisol—are also important to maintain normal blood glucose between meals (Goodman, 1994). The capillary blood glucose level in people without diabetes is less than 110 mg/dl preprandially (fasting) and less than 140 mg/dl 2 hours postprandially (Lebovitz, 1998). In people with diabetes, either the pancreas is not able to produce enough insulin, the cells are unable to use insulin efficiently, or both. In either case, hyperglycemia ensues because the cells are not able to use glucose for energy, and the liver continues to release glucose from glycogen stores or make more glucose from precursors (gluconeogenesis).

Physicians base the diagnosis of diabetes on fasting blood glucose levels and on the 2-hour postprandial (postload) values. The fasting plasma glucose threshold for diabetes is 126 mg/dl (7.0 mmol/l) on two separate occasions, while 110–125 mg/dl fasting glucose now comprises a new category termed "impaired glucose metabolism" (Shaw, Zimmet, McCarty, & de Courten, 2000). An important laboratory test commonly performed on the blood of people with diabetes is that of glycosylated hemoglobin (*hemoglobin A1c*). This test, used to assess glycemic control, reflects the average blood glucose level for the preceding 2–3 months. The normal range depends to some extent on the laboratory method. In our laboratory, the normal range is 4.0–6.0%. The recommended hemoglobin A1c goal is less than 7%, with action suggested if it is greater than 8% (Lebovitz, 1998). *Fructosamine*, another laboratory test done on the blood plasma, represents the average blood glucose for the preceding 2–3 weeks. Although hemoglobin A1c is the gold standard in diabetes management, fructosamine more accurately reflects recent interventions to control blood glucose. In our laboratory, the ranges are 200–272 mmol/l for normal individuals, and up to 381 mmol/l for persons with controlled diabetes (Armbruster, 1987; Springer, 1989). However, many authorities do not commonly use the test for fructosamine because it is less reliable. Physicians order these tests because they are useful for assessing glycemic control and treatment efficacy for a longer period than the daily capillary measurements (American Diabetes Association [ADA], 2001).

Types of Diabetes

There are two main types of diabetes mellitus: Type 1 and Type 2. Type 1 diabetes was previously written as Type I and referred to as "insulin-dependent" or "juvenile-onset" diabetes. Type 2 was formerly known as Type II, "non-insulin-dependent," or "adult-onset diabetes." Changes in terminology were adopted in 1997 when new recommendations were made about the diagnosis and classification of the disease (Lebovitz, 1998). Thus we use the new terminology throughout this chapter. In Type 1 diabetes, the pancreas makes minimal or no insulin, so the person needs to administer injections of insulin daily to keep the blood glucose level under control. People usually develop this type of diabetes before age 30, and the signs and symptoms of the disease may appear abruptly. The classic symptoms are *polydipsia* (excessive thirst), *polyphagia* (excessive hunger), and *polyuria* (excessive urination). The person may also report weight loss, blurred vision, increased fatigue, and delayed wound healing. About 5–10% of the population with diabetes has Type 1.

Most people with diabetes (90–95%) have Type 2, in which the pancreas produces reduced, normal, or even above-normal amounts of insulin, but blood glucose levels remain higher than normal. *Insulin resistance* plays a key role in this type of diabetes. People with Type 2 diabetes usually develop it after age 40, and symptoms of hyperglycemia appear gradually. They are often obese and have a family history of the disorder. African Americans, Hispanics, and Native Americans are at higher risk for diabetes than people of European descent. Type 2 diabetes may be accompanied by essential hypertension and hyperlipidemia (excess lipids) (American Diabetes Association [ADA], 2000).

TRADITIONAL MANAGEMENT OF DIABETES MELLITUS

There is no cure yet for either type of diabetes. However, one can manage the disease with a combination of diet, physical activity, and/or pharmacological therapies. Management requires lifelong daily attention. Self-management is a "set of skilled behaviors engaged to manage one's own illness" (Goodall & Halford, 1991, p. 1). Educating patients to carry out the prescribed regimen is the cornerstone of treatment (Lebovitz, 1998). The "Standards of Medical Care for Patients with Diabetes Mellitus" (ADA, 2000) indicate that education for self-management is a necessary component of the overall management plan, and the individual's role in self-care needs to be addressed at the initial and ongoing visits. A team of health care professionals can best provide individualized, comprehensive instruction. In addition, patients can use the resources provided by the ADA and the American Association of Diabetes Educators to initiate and maintain a healthy lifestyle. Consult the "Resources" section at the end of the chapter for further information.

EDUCATION

People with diabetes can learn from diabetes educators specific behaviors to keep their blood glucose level within an acceptable range. Adhering to a treatment regimen requires that people with diabetes acquire certain knowledge and skills to attain glycemic control. Primarily, they need to take an oral agent and/or administer insulin to lower their blood glucose level. Learning how to use a blood glucose meter to check the blood glucose level and interpret results is vital in both Type 1 and Type 2 diabetes mellitus. Specific dietary principles must be understood, and previous patterns of eating must be modified. Practitioners and diabetes educators encourage regular physical activity to assist in lowering the blood glucose level and to achieve and maintain desired weight. Stress management is also an important component of total diabetes management.

In summary, unhealthy lifestyle (particularly poor eating habits) and inactivity set the stage for the development of Type 2 diabetes. In order to compensate for the effects of both Type 1 and Type 2 diabetes, each person faces the challenges of adjustments from prior living habits. The integration of new skills and activities into an established daily routine may be difficult and stressful. Practitioners and diabetes educators also direct education toward management of the acute and chronic complications of the disease.

PHARMACOLOGICAL THERAPY

Insulin

The types of insulin differ in their onset of action, peak, and duration. The type of insulin used determines the time for an insulin dose to begin to lower the blood glucose, the time to reach its peak effect, and the duration of the effect (see Table 32.1). One cannot take insulin orally because it is destroyed by the stomach's digestive juices. Thus one injects insulin into the subcutaneous fat tissue with a needle and syringe. Suitable injection sites include the ab-

TABLE 32.1. Types and Action of Insulin

Types	Examples	Onset	Peak	Duration
Rapid-acting	Lispro	0.25–0.5 hr.	0.5–1½ hr.	4–6 hr.
Short-acting	Regular	0.5–1 hr.	2–3 hr.	6–8 hr.
Intermediate-acting	NPH	2–4 hr.	6–10 hr.	14–18 hr.
	Lente	3–4 hr.	6–12 hr.	16–20 hr.
Long-acting	Ultralente	6–10 hr.	10–16 hr.	20–24 hr.
Premixed combinations				
70/30 (70% NPH, 30% Regular)		0.5–1 hr.	Dual	14–18 hr.
50/50 (50% NPH, 50% Regular)		0.5–1 hr.	Dual	14–18 hr.
75/25 (75% NPL, 25% Lispro)		0.25–0.5 hr.	Dual	14–18 hr.

Note. The data are from Lebovitz (1998, p. 187).

domen (which is the preferred site), upper arms, anterior thighs, and buttocks. The absorption rate is quickest from the abdomen, next from the arms, and slowest from the thighs and buttocks. It is recommended that injections be properly rotated within a site according to a site rotation plan because random rotation of injections between sites leads to greater glucose fluctuation. Physicians prescribe the type(s) and frequency of insulin injections. They base this on the patient's weight, the degree of glycemic control desired, the patient's response to insulin, and the patient's projected level of physical activity. Alternatives to the traditional insulin injections with a syringe are (1) continuous subcutaneous insulin infusion (insulin pump), (2) insulin pens, and (3) jet injectors.

Oral Glucose-Lowering Agents

Oral glucose-lowering agents are tablets prescribed for people with Type 2 diabetes. These agents are not insulin. Thus they are not effective or appropriate for individuals who have Type 1 diabetes and should not be used during *diabetic ketoacidosis* (DKA; see subsequent discussion), sepsis, surgery, pregnancy, or other stress during which control fluctuates. There are five classes of oral agents that can be used as monotherapy, with other oral agents or in combination with insulin: (1) sulfonylureas (which stimulate the pancreas to secrete more insulin), (2) meglitinides (which stimulate the pancreas to secrete more insulin), (3) biguanides (which keep the liver from producing too much glucose), (4) alpha-glucosidase inhibitors (which slow the breakdown of carbohydrate in the intestine), and (5) thiazolidinediones (which make muscle cells more sensitive to insulin). (See Table 32.2.) More specific information about each agent—pharmacodynamics, dosage, administration, contradictions, and adverse reactions—should be obtained from the product literature of the manufacturer.

Self-Monitoring of Blood Glucose

Methods for self-monitoring of blood glucose (SMBG) have markedly improved over the last two decades as a result of advances in technology and the relative ease of performing the procedure (ADA, 1994). People with diabetes typically monitor their blood glucose with a home blood glucose meter by applying a small amount of blood obtained from a fingertip or alternate site (e.g., arm or leg) to a test strip. The blood glucose meter gives a precise number

TABLE 32.2. **Types and Actions of Oral Medications**

Class	Generic name	Brand name	Comments
Sulfonylureas	First generation:		Second-generation agents are more effective at lower doses and have fewer side effects. Hypoglycemia may be a problem if meals are skipped or with renal dysfunction. Should not be used by patients with significant liver or renal impairment
	Tolbutamide	Orinase	
	Acetohexamide	Dymelor	
	Tolazamide	Tolinase	
	Chlorpropamide	Diabinese	
	Second generation:		
	Glyburide	DiaBeta Micronase Glynase Prestabs	
	Gilipizide	Glucotrol Glucotrol XL (extended release)	
	Glimepiride	Amaryl	
Meglitinides	Repaglinide Nateglinide	Prandin Starlix	A dose needs to be taken with each meal and large snacks. May cause low blood sugar if a meal is skipped.
Biguanides	Metformin	Glucophage	Initial side effects: Nausea, diarrhea, decreased appetite, gastrointestinal distress. Should be taken with a meal. Not recommended for patients with renal or liver dysfunction, heart failure, age over 80, or history of excessive alcohol use. Needs to be stopped before surgery, acute myocardial infarction and cerebrovascular accident tests using intravenous contrast dye, severe dehydration.
Alpha-glucosidase inhibitors	Miglitol	Precose Glyset	Side effects: diarrhea, gas, bloating. Need to start at a low dose and increase slowly. Should not be used by patients with cirrhosis, inflammatory bowel or intestinal disease, chronic ulceration, or partial bowel obstruction.
Thiazolidinediones	Rosiglitazone Pioglitazone	Avandia Actos	Must check liver function tests before starting treatment and repeat every other month for the first year, then periodically. Maximum effects may take up to 12 weeks.
Combination oral agents	Glyburide + Metformin	Glucovance	Action, side effects, and contra-indications are the same as those of each single drug.

Note. The data are from Bristol-Myers Squibb (2000) and Lebovitz (1998).

showing the actual blood glucose level. The frequency of SMBG needs to be individualized and is influenced by various factors, such as willingness of the person to do self-testing, insurance coverage for durable medical equipment and test strips, the intensity of the prescribed regimen, and the perceived use and benefits of test results.

Health care professionals must competently offer patients the necessary education and training to perform SMBG. For example, an improperly done blood test that does not follow the manufacturer's directions may produce an inaccurate result. Blood glucose meters need to be calibrated correctly, checked for quality control regularly (using the control solution provided by the manufacturer), and stored properly. In addition, the person with diabetes should be evaluated on how well he or she performs a blood test and the accuracy of his or her log book. Encouragement for daily monitoring should be offered.

The results of SMBG provide valuable information about the person's management of the disease and effectiveness of the prescribed treatment regimen. Most meters in current use have the capability to download data to a personal computer and then to analyze stored data. Computer software programs are available from meter manufacturers for specific meters (Streja, 2000). Charts, graphs, and statistical information that are generated from the data are useful in identifying patterns of glycemic control and assisting health care providers in prescribing or altering pharmacological therapy, diet, and activity. The U.S. Food and Drug Administration has recently approved a noninvasive monitoring device, for adults, as a prescription product. It measures blood glucose collected through the skin, instead of in the blood. Educational programs on the product for physicians and diabetes educators are available.

COMPLICATIONS OF DIABETES

Both acute and chronic complications can occur in persons with Type 1 and Type 2 diabetes mellitus. The acute complications discussed below are *hypoglycemia*, DKA, and hyperglycemic hyperosmolar nonketotic syndrome (HHNS). The chronic complications discussed later may appear after an individual has had diabetes for years and can seriously affect many organ systems of the body. Both types of complications are discussed briefly, since the management of diabetic complications, excluding hypoglycemia, remains within the purview of the patient's physician.

Acute Complications

Hypoglycemia

Hypoglycemia refers to a low blood glucose level (below 70 mg/dl), precipitated by such variables as too high a dose of insulin or oral glucose lowering agent, a delayed or skipped snack/meal, insufficient carbohydrate intake, more physical activity than usual, or a combination of these (Funnell, 1998). The initial warning signs and symptoms (adrenal stage) are those associated with increased sympathetic nervous system activity: sweating, hunger, tachycardia, anxiety, weakness, occasional nausea and vomiting, increased blood pressure, cold hands, and hyperalertness. The cerebral stage of hypoglycemia occurs when there is a severe lack of glucose supplied to the brain, termed *neuroglycopenia*. Symptoms consist of confusion and inability to concentrate. Hypoglycemia can progress to the point of unresponsiveness, seizures, and coma (Havlin & Cryer, 1988).

Persons with diabetes need to check their blood glucose level when they experience mild signs and symptoms of hypoglycemia. If monitoring equipment is unavailable or if it is impractical to do SMBG, they must assume that the symptoms are the result of hypoglycemia and provide immediate self-treatment.

Treatment of hypoglycemia consists of eating or drinking something containing carbohydrate to raise the blood glucose level quickly. The person should ingest 10–15 grams of a quick-acting carbohydrate (Funnell, 1998). Examples of foods that can provide this amount of carbohydrate are 4 ounces of fruit juice, 4 ounces of regular (not sugar-free) soft drink, 8 ounces of low-fat milk, 1 tablespoon of honey, 6–8 Life Savers, or 3 glucose tablets. After self-treatment, it may take 10–15 minutes before the person feels better. Some people are frightened by hypoglycemia and overtreat themselves, causing a rebound hyperglycemia. SMBG is recommended after treatment, to verify that the blood glucose level has increased and returned to normal. If the next scheduled snack or meal is more than 30 minutes away, the person should eat a starch and protein (e.g., cheese and crackers) to prevent the blood glucose level from going down again. For episodes of severe hypoglycemia where the person is unresponsive and unable to swallow, someone should give the person an injection of glucagon to raise the blood glucose level. If glucagon is not available, emergency medical assistance should be enlisted immediately.

Some individuals who have diabetes (usually Type 1) for many years may develop *hypoglycemia unawareness*. That is, they lose the capacity to recognize early warning signs and symptoms of low blood sugar. This happens because of an absent or diminished counterregulatory hormone (epinephrine) response. As a result, these people may experience episodes of severe hypoglycemia that require a glucagon injection by another person and/or emergency medical assistance. Patients who experience hypoglycemia unawareness should be encouraged to monitor their blood glucose levels regularly. They should treat themselves with glucose promptly if their blood glucose level is <70 mg/dl or if they recognize signs and symptoms of hypoglycemia. Family members should also be educated about hypoglycemia and trained to observe signs and symptoms of low glucose. A glucagon emergency kit is available by prescription and should be kept for home use.

Diabetic Ketoacidosis

DKA results from a profound insulin deficiency and is a more common complication of Type 1 than of Type 2 diabetes. Key features of DKA usually include a blood glucose level greater than 250 mg/dl, a positive test for *ketones*, dehydration, and electrolyte imbalance. Precipitating factors that can lead to DKA are acute illness, infection, or inadequate insulin dose (Funnell, 1998).

Hyperglycemic Hyperosmolar Nonketotic Syndrome

HHNS occurs from a relative lack of insulin and is more common in persons with Type 2 diabetes, especially elderly individuals. HHNS is also characterized by high (>800 mg/dl) blood glucose levels, severe dehydration, and neurological deficits. Unlike DKA, there is usually an absence of acidosis (Funnell, 1998). Both DKA and HHNS are serious conditions that require urgent intervention by a physician.

Chronic Complications

Persons with either Type 1 or Type 2 diabetes mellitus are at risk for developing chronic *microvascular complications* and *neuropathy* (see below). These serious health problems can develop in individuals after they have had diabetes for years. However, it remains unclear why some people with diabetes develop them, whereas others do not. Nonetheless, recent research emphasizes the importance of good glycemic control and use of pharmacological therapy to prevent or delay the occurrence of complications.

The Diabetes Control and Complications Trial (DCCT) was a large-scale trial of more than 1400 patients with Type 1 diabetes mellitus. The purpose of the study was to determine the effect of intensive therapy of diabetes on the incidence of long-term complications. Half of the patients continued their usual care, and the other half received intensive treatment (three to four injections per day and multiple monitoring of blood glucose). Results were striking. The intensive therapy group decreased average blood glucose and glycosylated hemoglobin. Long-term complications of the eye, kidney, and nervous system were reduced by more than one-half (DCCT Research Group, 1993).

The United Kingdom Prospective Diabetes Study (UKPDS) was the largest and longest study of glycemic control and chronic complications; it looked at over 5000 people with new-onset Type 2 diabetes. This randomized clinical study compared the effects of intensive therapy (involving the use of several oral and antidiabetic agents and insulin) with the effects of conventional treatment on the development of chronic complications of the disease. Upon completion of this 10-year study, the intensive therapy group attained a hemoglobin A1c level of 7.0%, whereas the control group's value was 7.9%. Analysis of the data revealed that intensive treatment resulted in a significant reduction in complications of the disease (UKPDS Group, 1998a, 1998b).

Microvascular Complications

Microvascular complications involve the small blood vessels in the eye (retinopathy) and kidney (nephropathy). Damage occurs to the small blood vessels in the retina, causing leakage or bleeding in the eye. Damage to and hemorrhage of the fragile blood vessels of the eye (e.g., microaneurysms, as in *background diabetic retinopathy*) may result in loss of vision if not treated. Patients should schedule at least an annual visual examination with an ophthalmologist.

Approximately 30% of persons with Type 1 diabetes who have diabetic nephropathy will progress to end-stage renal disease. Damaged glomeruli (filtering units of the kidneys) can no longer adequately filter waste products, resulting in increased accumulation of these waste products in the blood. Strong predictors of diabetic nephropathy are chronic poor glycemic control and the duration of the disease. If the kidneys fail, individuals will require hemodialysis or peritoneal dialysis to remove waste products of metabolism. Kidney transplantation is an alternative to dialysis in some persons (Lebovitz, 1998).

Macrovascular Complications

Macrovascular complications refer to damage to larger blood vessels of the body. There are three major types of macrovascular disease: coronary artery disease, cerebro artery disease (cerebrovascular), and peripheral vascular disease. Therefore, myocardial infarctions, cerebrovascular accidents, and lower-extremity amputations occur two to three times more frequently among people with diabetes than in the general population (Funnell, 1998).

Diabetic Neuropathy

There are two major categories of neuropathy, or problems with nerve function due to diabetes (Funnell, 1998).

1. Diffuse polyneuropathy involves multiple nerves and is chronic and progressive in nature, with increased morbidity and mortality. Treatment focuses on attaining better glyce-

mic control, pain management, and prevention of further dysfunction and injury (e.g., foot ulcers or amputation).

   a. Sensory polyneuropathy is the most common type and affects almost 75% of patients. Symptoms are progressive and increase with severity and duration of diabetes. An example is distal symmetrical sensorimotor polyneuropathy (e.g., numbness, tingling, and loss of sensation of the hands and lower extremities).

   b. Autonomic neuropathy involves involuntary control of bodily function. Examples include the following:

   • Neurogenic bladder.
   • Sexual dysfunction (e.g., impotence, decreased vaginal lubrication).
   • Gastroparesis (abnormal emptying of stomach contents).
   • Fecal incontinence and nocturnal diarrhea.
   • Orthostatic hypotension.
   • Painless heart attack.
   • Hypoglycemia unawareness.
   • Anhidrosis (lack of sweating).
   • Abnormal pupillary dysfunction.

   2. Focal neuropathy involves individual nerves of the body and occurs less often. Symptoms are acute and self-limited. Episodes are unpredictable, not specific to diabetes, and not associated with duration of the disease. Examples include (a) mononeuropathy or multiplex neuropathy, (b) plexopathy (e.g., femoral neuropathy), (c) radiculopathy (e.g., intercostal neuropathy), and (d) cranial neuropathy (e.g., diabetic ophthalmoplegial neuropathy).

THE ROLE OF PSYCHOLOGIGAL STRESS IN DIABETES

The Effects of Stress on Metabolism

Several models describe the impact of stress on metabolism as it relates to the etiology and maintenance of diabetes (Glasgow et al., 1999; Peyrot, McMurry, & Kruger, 1999; Surwit & Feinglos, 1988). Emotional distress or events perceived as challenging by the individual activate several physiological pathways. Stimulation of the sympathetic nervous system releases glucagon from the pancreas and decreases secretion of insulin. Decreased parasympathetic (vagal) nerve activity also results in less insulin. These autonomic imbalances result in lower blood levels of insulin, decreased entry of glucose to cells, and hyperglycemia. In addition, sympathetic stimulation causes the release of catecholamines (epinephrine and norepinephrine) from the adrenal medulla. These hormones also have an anti-insulin effect contributing to the hyperglycemia.

   The other pathway activated during stress is via the anterior pituitary gland. This gland causes the adrenal cortex to release cortisol, and the pituitary to release growth hormone. It also causes the thyroid gland to release thyroxine, although this has more to do with long-term regulation than with acute variations in glucose. These hormones stimulate biochemical processes (glycogenolysis and gluconeogenesis) in the liver, resulting in increased blood glucose. Lack of insulin makes glucose unusable. The tissues' inability to use glucose increases hepatic and adipose tissue *lipolysis* (metabolism of fat for energy). Increased blood levels of fatty acids and ketones in the urine may result in hyperlipidemia and DKA.

   Thus these models propose that stress increases blood glucose through sympathetic and adrenal medullary pathways. Imbalance in the function of the hypothalamic–pituitary–adrenal axis heightens the probability of accumulation of fat in the viscera, which increases insulin resistance (Björntorp & Rosmond, 1999). A single stressor, however, can actually decrease blood glucose in some persons under laboratory conditions. Individuals react to stress with either hypo- or hyperglycemia (Gonder-Frederick, Carter, Cox, & Clarke, 1990). Nonetheless, chronic severe stress may have a continuing disruptive effect on blood glucose, elevating average blood glucose levels, and increasing variability. Whether stress is associated with the onset of Type 1 or Type 2 diabetes remains unclear. Since stress-induced overeating results in obesity, which is a major predictor of Type 2 diabetes, poor dietary habits are indirectly correlated with onset of diabetes.

The Effects of Stress on the Person with Diabetes

Psychological factors can have an impact on the individual's ability to adjust to diabetes, whether the disease starts in adolescence or adulthood (Cox & Gonder-Frederick, 1991). Receiving the diagnosis itself may be a traumatic event. Initially there may be a sense of relief, because before the diagnosis the person was feeling very sick, weak, and tired without knowing why. However, most individuals go through a grief process after being told the diagnosis. Components of this process consist of anxiety, fear, denial, anger, bargaining, depression, and finally acceptance. Immediately after diagnosis, many patients feel overwhelmed by the amount of information they must absorb and what they need to do to implement and maintain glycemic control. Sometimes many educational sessions are necessary before a person feels competent to manage his or her disease. Nonetheless, knowledge gained does not mean that the person has accepted the disease, will adhere to the treatment regimen, or will achieve glycemic control. Living with diabetes and adjusting to changes in management produces distress (Rubin & Peyrot, 2001). Worsening of the disease or development of complications present further challenges to control and acceptance.

Acute and chronic stress may affect management of diabetes in several ways. Acute and severe distress distract some patients from attending to their usual self-care regimen. For example, they may miss an insulin dose, overeat, skip a meal, and/or decrease the frequency of blood glucose monitoring. During periods with frequent daily stress, some people with diabetes sacrifice their usual self-care activities, and instead concentrate on managing the stress. This can lead to poor glycemic control. Forgetting or deliberately omitting insulin is a common cause of ketoacidosis requiring hospitalization (Wilkinson, 1987). A person's perception of stress and its effects can strongly influence the neural and endocrine impact on blood glucose. Individuals competent in stress management may show only minor, short-lasting blood glucose instability under stressful conditions.

The number of stressful life events has been correlated with Type 2 diabetes. Persons of low socioeconomic status are at higher risk for diabetes, partially due to the increased stress of a noisy environment, financial challenges, and crowded living conditions (Wamala, Wolk, & Orth-Gomer, 1997). Persons exposed to frequent or long-lasting stress may develop an attitude of hopelessness if they are unable to cope with the demands made upon them (Mooy, de Vries, Grootenhuis, Bouter, & Heine, 2000). In fact, depressive symptoms have a major impact on the daily life of persons with diabetes, and clinical depression has a worse course in persons with diabetes (Gavard, Lustman, & Clouse, 1993). Glycohemoglobin values were higher in those individuals (with either Type 1 or Type 2 diabetes) who had active mood or anxiety disorders (Lustman, Griffith, & Clouse, 1988). A recent meta-analysis points to a doubling of the odds of clinical depression (depression requiring treatment) in patients with diabetes (Anderson, Freedland, Clouse, & Lustman, 2001).

In summary, the behavioral model focuses on lifestyle and adherence to regimen, while the psychophysiological model emphasizes neuroendocrine pathways. Stress can trigger unhealthy changes in behavior, as well as decrease the effectiveness of hypoglycemic agents (Peyrot et al., 1999).

TEAM APPROACH IN USING BIOFEEDBACK-ASSISTED RELAXATION WITH DIABETIC PATIENTS

Members of the Team

The team approach is optimal for working with patients with diabetes. Assessing the psychological and physiological effects of stress, stress management, and biofeedback on blood glucose control is necessary. In addition to a physician with special expertise in diabetes, the team consists of at least a certified biofeedback practitioner, a certified diabetes educator, and the patient. The team works together in evaluating the effects of treatment on the physiological and psychological aspects of glycemic control. The quality of the relationship between the team and the patient is critical for successful management. Good communication and trust between the patient and the provider have been shown to be associated with better adherence and lower glycosylated hemoglobin levels (Ciechanowski, Katon, Russo, & Walker, 2001).

The Biofeedback Practitioner

A "biofeedback practitioner" is a general term that includes any of various professionals with differing qualifications and competencies in addition to biofeedback. For the present discussion, we assume that this is a properly qualified and credentialed professional. Whoever is in this role must be state-licensed to conduct the specified parts of the evaluation and treatment. If not, then the team also needs another properly credentialed professional, such as a psychologist. In some medical settings, a registered dietitian is a useful part of the team. Most biofeedback practitioners do not have expertise in diabetes education and management. Thus, when these practitioners treat patients with diabetes, they need to know the basic pathophysiology of diabetes and the fundamentals of medical diabetes management. In summary, the team should involve a physician, a biofeedback therapist, a diabetes educator, dietitian, a psychologist or other mental health care provider, and the patient.

Role of the Mental Health Practitioner Who Uses Biofeedback

The psychologist practitioner carries out an initial interview with the diabetic patient to determine stress-related physical and emotional symptoms. One assesses the patient's perception of the effects of stress on his or her blood glucose and his or her perceived capabilities and management strategies (see M. S. Schwartz, Chapter 6, this volume). Psychological testing may also be used to assess the person's levels of depression, anxiety, and anger. The diagnostic evaluation also establishes the presence of emotional conditions and any comorbid illnesses.

This practitioner also conducts a psychophysiological assessment. Practitioners differ on the specifics of this assessment, but often monitor multiple modalities. These often include muscle tension, skin conductance, blood flow in the hands (via skin temperature), heart rate, and breathing during the resting baseline, and during and after various standard office stressors (see Arena & Schwartz, Chapter 7, this volume). Our clinic measures forehead muscle tension with surface electromyography (EMG), heart rate, blood pressure, and finger temperature while patients sit quietly with their eyes closed, then under mental stress conditions, and finally while the patients attempt to relax without instructions.

The practitioner provides biofeedback, relaxation therapies, and stress management. Relaxation and biofeedback can help patients feel more in control of their physiology, their psychological state, and their illness. Furthermore, decreased plasma levels of stress hormones and sympathetic activity mediate lowered arousal (Benson, Beary, & Carol, 1974) and diminished hyperglycemia.

The mental health practitioner can also treat the comorbid emotional illnesses with psychotherapy. In particular, cognitive-behavioral therapy has been effective in improving mood and in facilitating self-management of blood glucose in persons with diabetes (Lustman, Freedland, Griffith, & Clouse, 1998). Patients whose mood or anxiety disorders are not responsive to psychotherapy should be referred to their physician for medication management. Serotonin reuptake inhibitors have a positive effect on mood as well as a beneficial effect on blood glucose (Goodnick, Henry, & Buki, 1995).

Role of the Diabetes Educator

The diabetes educator, as well as the physician, can interpret blood glucose values because he or she understands the effects of hypoglycemic medications, diet, and exercise on blood glucose. In addition, the educator should consider collaborative goal setting with the patient to emphasize the importance of patient self-care (Anderson et al., 1995). In a study of Type 1 diabetes, structured diabetes education was associated with feelings of greater independence, better self care and improved blood glucose over the short and the long term (Howorka et al., 2000). The educator also obtains information about the person's diabetes care regimen, using the following outline.

History

1. Year of diagnosis and symptoms that led to the diagnosis.
2. Family history of diabetes.
3. Other medical problems.
4. Use of prescription and nonprescription medications, nutritional supplements, and herbal products.
5. Self-concept/self-image relative to diabetes.
6. Previous diabetes education.

Medical Treatment Regimen for Diabetes, Knowledge, and Management

1. Medications
    a. Insulin: Type(s), source; frequency of injections; prescribed doses; injection site(s); problems with preparing or giving injections; knowledge of onset, peak, and duration of action.
    b. Oral glucose-lowering agents: Types, dosage, and knowledge of effects.
2. Diet: Usual caloric intake; restrictions; mealtimes; types and amounts of food; meal-planning skills; compliance problems.
3. Activity/exercise: Types, frequency, duration; impediments to activity.
4. SMBG: Type of blood glucose meter; frequency and time(s) of testing; record keeping; and any monitoring problems.
5. Weight, height. Calculate the body mass index.

Acute/Chronic Complications of Diabetes, Knowledge, and Management

1. Hypoglycemia: Frequency of episodes; signs and symptoms; usual causes.
    a. Treatment(s): Use of a glucagon emergency kit; availability of a quick-acting carbohydrate source.
    b. Precautions: Wearing a Medic-Alert or similar bracelet or necklace; carrying a wallet card.

2. Ketoacidosis and HHNS: Number of episodes since diagnosis; cause(s) for episode(s); knowledge of testing of urine for ketones when ill.

Education and Instruction

With the information above, one identifies the patient's knowledge, current self-management, self-care deficits and problems, and capabilities to make appropriate decisions and manage his or her disease. This information provides the basis for instructing the patient about diabetes care and addressing problems with daily management during later sessions.

USING BIOFEEDBACK AND RELAXATION WITH PATIENTS WITH DIABETES MELLITUS

Choice of Patients

Type of Diabetes

See the research summary at the end of the chapter for details of controlled studies of the use of biofeedback-assisted relaxation with persons with Type 2 and Type 1 diabetes.

Time since Diagnosis and When to Start Biofeedback

Starting at the time of diagnosis, patients with diabetes need to adjust their lifestyle and behavior significantly. They must incorporate diabetes management behaviors into their daily routine. Psychosocial adjustment to both Type 1 and Type 2 diabetes is often problematic. Therefore, counseling and supportive psychotherapy can be useful during the early weeks and months after diagnosis. However, beginning a rigorous biofeedback-assisted relaxation program may not be appropriate soon after diagnosis. Adding the clinic appointments for biofeedback and home practice requirements necessary to learn relaxation techniques might overload the resources of the patient. Furthermore, it would be difficult to attribute improvement in glycemic control to the biofeedback and relaxation, because the patient would be starting multiple new behaviors concurrently.

Another reason for deferring biofeedback during the first year after diagnosis is the so-called diabetic *honeymoon period*. This phenomenon is the partial or complete remission of the signs and symptoms of diabetes soon after the onset of Type 1 diabetes, when the pancreas temporarily produces insulin. The blood glucose level may stabilize at close to normal, and the need for exogenous insulin may decrease significantly or completely. This period may last 1, several, or (rarely) 12 months (Beaser, 1995). One could mistakenly attribute a decreased need for exogenous insulin to the biofeedback and stress management treatment instead of to temporary pancreatic insulin production. When the honeymoon period ends and the patient's beta cells are no longer capable of producing insulin, the patient could misattribute the renewed need for exogenous insulin as a total failure of the self-regulation process.

Within a stepped-care model, one might consider starting more conservative relaxation therapy within 12 months after diagnosis for selected patients. For example, one could start with relaxation instructions and printed patient education about relaxation. The material should include information to avoid misattributions about blood glucose changes during the honeymoon period. Treatment could then proceed to office-based biofeedback-assisted relaxation after 1 year.

Acknowledged Impact of Stress

Patients must at least partially accept the idea that stress can have a negative impact on glycemic control. Increased average blood glucose, a wider range of values, an increase in fasting blood glucose, higher insulin requirement, and sometimes more frequent hypoglycemia are common stress effects reported by patients. If a patient is unaware of or rejects the correlation between stress and blood glucose, then perhaps stress is less of a factor than diet or inactivity in affecting that person's blood glucose. However, the person may not understand the effects of stress on physiological function in general and on blood glucose in particular. In this case, the patient should be educated about stress and its relationship to blood glucose. This can improve awareness of the effects of daily hassles and increases the chance for psychophysiological therapy in normalizing blood glucose levels.

Cooperation with the Patient's Physician

The physician must approve the referral for biofeedback and should agree to be available for consultation as needed. The biofeedback practitioners should document the patient's glucose data before, during, and after a biofeedback-assisted relaxation treatment program. These data should be shared with the patient's physician during and after treatment. The physician should also disclose pertinent data about the patient's other medical problems, particularly those related to diabetes (such as hypertension and hyperlipidemia), and the current therapy of those disorders.

The physician should give the patient guidelines to adjust daily insulin dosages depending on his or her blood glucose values. The patient can adjust the dosages when the blood glucose level exceeds an acceptable level and the patient cannot explain the hyperglycemia by diet, exercise, or insulin. One can use algorithms to make insulin adjustments. For example, some individuals use a "split-and-mixed" insulin regimen, such as using intermediate-acting and short-acting insulin twice a day. Physicians may instruct them to increase one type of insulin by a predetermined number of units to compensate for unexplained hyperglycemia. For circumstances such as illness that immediately increase the body's insulin requirement, physicians may prescribe supplementary doses of short-acting regular insulin to prevent progressive loss of glycemic control (Skyler, Skyler, Seigler, & O'Sullivan, 1981).

Reduction of insulin doses or oral hypoglycemic agents may become necessary as a patient progresses with biofeedback therapy. Equally important, patients with severe and unresolved glycemic control problems should be instructed to contact their physicians for guidance and possible changes in their medical treatment regimen.

Adherence to the Prescribed Medical Regimen

Patients who consistently do not comply with recommendations for diet, prescribed glucose-lowering medication, and/or blood glucose monitoring are not good candidates. They probably will not comply with relaxation practice assignments. Furthermore, improved adherence to the medical regimen may result in better glucose control, but it will confound interpretation of the effects of biofeedback treatment on blood glucose.

Physical Setting

An office for treating diabetic patients needs to maintain sources of quick-acting carbohydrates. Examples are fruit juice, glucose tablets, and regular (not sugar-free) soft drinks. A meter to test for blood glucose, including test strips and lancets, should be available. The equipment to download and calculate average values is helpful but not necessary. A diabetes manual such as *Therapy for Diabetes Mellitus and Related Disorders* (Lebovitz, 1998) is useful.

Evaluation of Outcome

The primary treatment outcome measure is blood glucose. We use six indicators of blood glucose to evaluate end-of-treatment outcome, but other medical clinics may use other indexes and criteria. Our values are calculated from about 50 measurements made before and the same number after completion of therapy. The indicators we use are these:

1. Average blood glucose level.
2. Percentage of the values above 200 mg/dl.
3. Percentage of morning (fasting) values between 80 and 120 mg/dl.
4. Number of hypoglycemic episodes (or values equal to or below 50 mg/dl). This value is primarily applicable to Type 1 diabetes.
5. Average predinner blood glucose (applicable primarily to Type 2 diabetes).
6. Hemoglobin A1c (indicates average blood glucose during the past 2–3 months).

A secondary outcome variable is dosage of glucose-lowering medication. We compare the number of tablets of oral glucose-lowering medication or number of units of rapid, intermediate and long-acting insulin used before and after therapy.

GENERAL CLINICAL PROCEDURES

Goals

The goals of biofeedback-assisted relaxation are to do the following:

1. Increase the person's ability to perceive and effectively manage stress.
2. Decrease the stress-mediated neural and endocrine systems' effects on blood glucose and insulin utilization.
3. Reduce average blood glucose, increase the percentage of fasting blood glucose values at target range, and (over the long term) decrease glycosylated hemoglobin.
4. Reduce dosage of hypoglycemic medication if blood glucose levels are well controlled at entry.

Baseline: Blood Glucose Monitoring

Practitioners must have sufficient data about glycemic control before starting biofeedback for patients with Type 1 or Type 2 diabetes. We suggest at least 2 weeks (fasting and evening measurements) of blood glucose data. A practitioner should try to assess the accuracy of a patient's blood glucose values reported during the initial interview and reassess after treatment. Patients can make gross errors in self-reports of blood glucose values (Mazze, Shamoon, Pasmantier, Lucido, & Murphy, 1984). In these cases, the therapist can recommend a meter with a memory. Some meters permit downloading the data to a computer that prints blood glucose results with the date and time of each test. One can compare these data to the patient's log book results. Occasionally, an individual feels under great pressure to produce "good data" for the practitioner. One must review such a patient's blood glucose data carefully and with sensitivity and consideration of his or her efforts in maintaining good glycemic control. Regular blood glucose monitoring must continue during treatment.

Patients should be requested to bring their meter and blood glucose log book to all treatment sessions. The practitioner should review blood glucose values with them, discuss trends in glycemic control, and address problems with glycemic control such as hypoglycemia. A positive attitude toward good self-management should be encouraged. If necessary, the practitioner should contact the physician to adjust the medical treatment regimen.

It also may be helpful for patients to record daily stressful events and the time of occurrence of situations that the patient finds difficult. This helps identify work and family stressors to be discussed later in the stress management or psychotherapy intervention. As mentioned earlier, physiological assessment and psychological testing occur during baseline and at the end of treatment.

One must check body weight, particularly for patients with Type 2 diabetes and for persons who are overweight, when treatment starts. Weight loss and accompanying decreases in blood glucose level may require adjustment of the medication dose. Furthermore, when significant weight loss occurs during treatment, one cannot attribute decreases in blood glucose solely to relaxation or biofeedback therapies. We recommend weekly weighing for Type 2 patients, and pretreatment and end-of-treatment weighing for patients with Type 1 diabetes.

Relaxation Therapy

Relaxation therapies involve slow diaphragmatic breathing (see Gevirtz & Schwartz, Chapter 10, this volume), meditation, autogenic phrases, and/or progressive muscle relaxation. One also may use "positive imagery" with other relaxation therapies (Davis, Eshelman, & McKay, 1995). The person's blood glucose level should be measured before and after at least the first relaxation session. In our program, most sessions include instruction and practice of autogenic phrases. About one-fourth of the sessions involve progressive relaxation.

Biofeedback

Office sessions should not be scheduled at times of low blood glucose or within an hour after strenuous exercise. A practitioner should not proceed with a relaxation or biofeedback session if a patient is experiencing hypoglycemic symptoms, because biofeedback may lower glucose levels even more. The practitioner should wait until symptoms have resolved and it has been confirmed (by measurement) that the blood glucose levels have increased to normal levels.

We offer therapy encompassing 12 sessions. Each 1-hour session consists of counseling for 15 minutes, a 5-minute EMG and thermal baseline, 15 minutes of biofeedback, 5 minutes of debriefing, and 15–20 minutes of reviewing blood glucose logs. The relaxation therapies can be coupled with EMG or thermal biofeedback. One may use one or multiple sites for EMG. Selection depends on the results of the pretreatment psychophysiolgocial profile or known tension areas for individual patients.

Thermal biofeedback can be used with most patients, since loss of thermal sensation in the hands is uncommon and occurs late in the progression of peripheral neuropathy. A single-case study (Bailey, Good, & McGrady, 1990) reported that a patient with Type 1 diabetes learned to increase finger temperature despite sensory deficits. The patient had little sensation of changes in hand temperature, yet she could warm her hands. There is encouraging evidence that thermal biofeedback is useful in maintaining circulation to the hands and feet (Rice & Schindler, 1992).

Home Practice of Relaxation

We recommend starting with once- or twice-daily practice of relaxation for 15–20 minutes. The biofeedback practitioner, the diabetes educator, and the patient determine the optimal time(s) for practice. This is important so that relaxation practice does not coincide with times of peak insulin action and thus increase the risk for hypoglycemia. Patients with Type 1 diabetes should avoid relaxation practice after 9 P.M. to prevent potential exacerbation of nighttime hypoglycemia (Bendtson, Gade, Thomsen, Rosenfalck, & Wildschiodtz, 1992). Patients with Type 2 diabetes are at significantly lower risk for nighttime hypoglycemia and therefore can safely use relaxation techniques at bedtime.

At about the midpoint of treatment, we recommend starting minirelaxation periods many times per day for 30–60 seconds each. The diabetic person may use these periods in various ways, such as deep breathing when monitoring his or her blood glucose. Between the application of the blood on the test strip in the glucometer and the display of the result, there is usually a brief waiting period. The suggestion to use this time for a minirelaxation is usually very well accepted by patients. Patients with Type 1 diabetes can also use minirelaxation after 9 P.M.

Review of Blood Glucose and Insulin Data

In our setting, patients with Type 1 diabetes spend 15–20 minutes each session with a diabetes educator, to review their blood glucose documentation and to identify trends of hypoglycemia or hyperglycemia. The educator discusses possible reasons for the identified trend(s) and suggests strategies to avoid recurrences. He or she also notes the relaxation practice times and scrutinizes relaxation's effects on the next blood glucose value. Patients with Type 2 diabetes need less intense scrutiny, but are checked by a nurse or diabetes educator at monthly intervals.

Long-Term Follow-Up

There are no long-term follow-up studies with diabetic populations treated with biofeedback or relaxation. However, we suggest periodic follow-up sessions as is common practice when treating other chronic disorders. The practitioner and the patient determine the timing of the follow-up office sessions. At follow-up, glycemic control, self-care, and continued use of relaxation techniques are evaluated.

FINDING PATIENTS WITH DIABETES APPROPRIATE FOR BIOFEEDBACK

Many practitioners and researchers work in large hospitals or medical clinics that treat many patients with diabetes mellitus. Professionals in other settings can locate patients who may benefit from biofeedback-assisted relaxation treatments through various sources. Local hospitals may have diabetes care centers. Patient support groups are common. The local office of the ADA may print a monthly newsletter and may hold regular meetings for people with Type 1 or Type 2 diabetes mellitus. For information about basic and clinical research in diabetes, several professional journals are good sources of information. Examples are *Diabetes Care, The Diabetes Educator, and Practical Diabetology*. Subscriptions to *Diabetes Self-Management* and *The Diabetes Forecast* are useful for patients.

POSSIBLE CONTRAINDICATIONS TO TREATMENT

The following concerns have been brought to our attention and require comment.

1. *Patients can misinterpret hypoglycemia as anxiety. This can happen.* Many of the symptoms associated with hypoglycemia are also characteristic of an anxiety reaction. These

include sweating, cold hands, hyperalertness, and tachycardia. Indeed, the symptoms of hypoglycemia and the symptoms of the stress response are both caused by excess sympathetic, adrenal medullary, and adrenal cortical activity. In fact, epinephrine, cortisol, and glucagon are critical to compensate for hypoglycemia (Ganong, 1997). If a person is experiencing hypoglycemia but interprets it as anxiety, his or her blood glucose may continue to decrease to dangerous levels while the patient attempts to "relax away" the symptoms. Therefore, patients should be instructed in the appropriate response to the symptoms of hypoglycemia. First, they should test blood glucose to check for low blood sugar. Then they should treat appropriately with a quick-acting source of carbohydrate, followed by retesting. Relaxation will *not* stop the symptoms of hypoglycemia.

It may be possible to use biofeedback to help patients differentiate the stress response from hypoglycemia. For example, increased facial muscle tension, commonly experienced during a stress response, is not a common sign of hypoglycemia. Learning to discriminate facial muscle tension using EMG biofeedback may help some patients to distinguish the two states. This suggestion is anecdotal and is not documented in research studies; it thus requires testing. The only accurate way of identifying hypoglycemia is testing the blood.

2. *People with diabetes use hyperventilation to counteract acidosis; therefore, they should be taught deep breathing. This is not true.* Acidosis stimulates hyperventilation. In persons with and without diabetes, the respiratory system attempts to compensate for shifts in blood acidity (see Gevirtz & Schwartz, Chapter 10, this volume; Fried, 1993; Timmons & Ley, 1994). People with diabetes may automatically hyperventilate in their attempt to re-regulate blood acidity through respiratory compensation. However, instructions or training to breathe slowly and deeply with the diaphragm do not and cannot override the strong signals from the brain's respiratory center. If a patient is acidotic, attempts at voluntary control of breathing are overridden quickly. Patients should also test their urine for ketones, to distinguish DKA from hyperventilation secondary to anxiety.

What are the implications for using slow, deep diaphragmatic breathing with patients with diabetes? One should question the patient about any history of ketoacidosis and assess hyperventilation (see Gevirtz & Schwartz, Chapter 10). One should also observe and measure breathing during the initial interviews and when the patient practices breathing therapy procedures. SMBG must continue throughout treatment, and the data must be used to monitor any changes in average blood glucose levels.

3. *People who are diabetic and depressed may experience a worsening of their diabetes if they participate in biofeedback assisted relaxation programs. This is not true.* Diabetic patients with clinical depression will probably not benefit from biofeedback-assisted relaxation programs, but it is unlikely that their diabetes will worsen as a result of psychophysiological therapy. Clinical depression needs to be treated with antidepressant medication or psychotherapy before patients begin biofeedback assisted relaxation to improve motivation for treatment. In addition, the selective serotonin reuptake inhibitors seem to have an independent blood-glucose-lowering effect (Goodnick et al., 1995).

4. *Deep relaxation has a tendency to lower blood glucose to hypoglycemic levels. This is very unlikely.* Very early reports (e.g., Fowler, Budzynski, & Vandenbergh, 1976) expressed concerns about the effects of biofeedback on blood glucose in patients with Type 1 diabetes, because of possible hypoglycemia. However, at the time of that case study, SMBG was uncommon and meters were expensive and difficult to use. That case study patient did not monitor blood glucose daily. We suggest that the risks of using biofeedback-assisted relaxation in Type 1 and Type 2 diabetes are low if SMBG is in place and if a trained professional is available to interpret those glucose records. The practitioner should be aware of the possibility of hypoglycemia if patients are not maintaining proper nutrition, or are exercising excessively and not eating additional food to compensate for the synergistic effect of exercise and insulin. Pa-

tients with either type of diabetes who are not monitoring and recording blood glucose and medication data are not good candidates for biofeedback or relaxation treatment.

RESEARCH SUMMARY

The following is a brief summary of research (excluding single-case studies) that has considered the effects of biofeedback or relaxation for patients with Type 1 or Type 2 diabetes. A detailed description and a critique of the studies are beyond the scope of this chapter.

Rosenbaum (1983) treated four patients with Type 1 and two with Type 2 diabetes with biofeedback, relaxation, and family therapy. She presented the results in a case-study-type format and followed the patients for up to 4 years. Five of the six patients showed improvement in at least one of three outcome measures: average plasma glucose, insulin dosage, and/or range of blood glucose. There were no complications related to biofeedback treatment.

Surwit and Feinglos (1983) used biofeedback and relaxation in a hospital setting to treat six patients with Type 2 diabetes, and compared these to another six patients without such treatment. The treated patients had five daily sessions of progressive relaxation and EMG biofeedback, and they significantly improved their glucose tolerance. There were no changes in insulin sensitivity or glucose-stimulated insulin secretory activity.

Seven patients with Type 1 diabetes were treated with biofeedback-assisted relaxation (EMG and thermal). Four of the seven achieved a decrease in units of insulin required to maintain control of blood glucose (Guthrie, Moeller, & Guthrie, 1983).

Five diabetic patients who monitored blood glucose daily and whose diabetes was well controlled on insulin participated in a study by Landis et al. (1985). Treatment consisted of 15 weekly 1-hour sessions of biofeedback-assisted relaxation and three subsequent monthly sessions. Therapists used EMG, thermal, and skin conductance feedback. Average glucose levels and insulin remained stable during treatment. However, in four of the five patients, the median and the range of values for blood glucose decreased.

One study focused on 20 patients with poorly controlled Type 1 diabetes (Feinglos, Hastedt, & Surwit, 1987). The study used glycohemoglobin to assess outcome. Ten patients received EMG biofeedback-assisted progressive muscle relaxation, and 10 patients received no treatment. Treatment consisted of 1 week of in-hospital training followed by 6 weeks of practicing relaxation at home. There was no improvement in glycohemoglobin or total insulin dose reported in the trained group compared with the untrained group.

We (McGrady, Bailey, & Good, 1991) randomly assigned 18 patients with Type 1 diabetes to a treatment or a no-treatment group. Patients in the former group received 10 sessions of relaxation therapy (8 of autogenic relaxation and 2 of progressive relaxation). EMG and thermal biofeedback were used to facilitate learning the relaxation response. The experimental and control groups differed significantly on three criteria of improvement: the average level of blood glucose, the percentage of blood glucose values above 200 mg/dl, and the percentage of fasting blood glucose values at target. There were no significant changes in the insulin dosages in either group. A second controlled study of 16 patients confirmed the positive effects of biofeedback-assisted relaxation on blood glucose (McGrady, Graham, & Bailey, 1996). However, a third study utilizing the same experimental design failed to replicate the significant advantage for the group receiving biofeedback and relaxation (McGrady & Horner, 1999). Patients without depressive symptoms were able to lower blood glucose as in the previous studies, but those with symptoms of depression, high anxiety, and frequent daily hassles did not lower blood glucose, possibly due to poorer compliance.

No increment in outcome was reported when EMG biofeedback and progressive relaxation were added to intensive medical therapy in a group of patients with Type 2 diabetes.

However, persons with higher emotional lability and sympathetic neural activity were the best responders (Lane, McCaskill, Ross, Feinglos, & Surwit, 1993). Jablon, Naliboff, Gilmore, and Rosenthal (1997) also failed to show improvements in glucose, despite reductions in muscle tension and anxiety in patients with Type 2 diabetes. A recent study (Surwit et al., 2002) found that group-based stress management led to improved glycohemoglobin values over a 1-year period. This is the first large scale study that demonstrated lower hemoglobin A1c after stress management in Type 2 diabetes. Preliminary data collected in our laboratory from 10 patients with Type 2 diabetes and some concurrent depressive symptoms revealed significant decreases in blood glucose and glycohemoglobin. Treatment consisted of EMG and thermal biofeedback, relaxation therapy, home practice, and problem solving. We emphasized increasing patients' sense of control over their physiological responses to stress, which include elevated blood glucose. An antidepressant was prescribed for patients with clinical depression before initiation of biofeedback-assisted relaxation. These findings suggest that depressive symptoms must be addressed before biofeedback-assisted relaxation begins (McGinnis & McGrady, 2002).

CONCLUSION

Research using biofeedback, relaxation, and stress management as adjunctive treatments for persons with diabetes mellitus is encouraging. The theoretical framework underlying stress-induced increases in blood glucose and stress-reduction-mediated decreases supports continued trials of biofeedback. However, treatment of these patients using behavioral therapies is often complicated by comorbid psychiatric disorders. Further controlled trials of biofeedback in diabetic patients, in which mood and anxiety disorders are identified and concurrently treated, should help clarify the efficacy controversy. Recent advances in knowledge of the immune aspects of diabetes may further the understanding of psychoneuroimmunological factors in the regulation of blood glucose. Rapid improvements in technology allow diabetic patients and their health care providers to anticipate fewer invasive procedures, better glycemic control, and a more normal life.

Learning relaxation techniques with biofeedback may be a valuable adjunct to usual medical care of this chronic illness. Certainly, the adjunctive techniques cannot substitute for diet, activity, hypoglycemic medication, or blood glucose monitoring. However, patients with diabetes can achieve better self-care by learning psychophysiological self-regulation, including various types of stress management. Patients frequently report a greater sense of control as a result of biofeedback, which in turn facilitates a sense of empowerment. Because self-care is indeed the cornerstone of glycemic control, the self-regulatory therapies such as relaxation with biofeedback are logical components of overall management of diabetes. More research is necessary to determine ideal selection of patients and the most efficacious relaxation and biofeedback procedures.

GLOSSARY

BACKGROUND DIABETIC RETINOPATHY. Microaneurysms in the retina.

DIABETIC KETOACIDOSIS (DKA). An acute complication of diabetes caused by a deficiency of insulin and resulting in hyperglycemia, ketosis, acidosis, dehydration, and electrolyte imbalance.

FRUCTOSAMINE. A laboratory serum test that measures the amount of glycated protein and indicates the level of glycemic control for the preceding 2–3 weeks.

HEMOGLOBIN A1c. A laboratory blood test measuring the percentage or fraction of hemoglobin that has glucose attached. The test is used to evaluate glycemic control for the preceding 2–3 months.

HONEYMOON PERIOD. Phenomenon that may occur shortly after the onset of Type 1 diabetes, in which there is partial or complete remission of signs and symptoms of the disease. It may last up to 12 months.

HYPERGLYCEMIA. Increased blood glucose.

HYPOGLYCEMIA. An acute complication of diabetes in which the blood glucose level is low (<70 mg/dl). This can result from an imbalance of activity, food intake, and/or hypoglycemic medication.

HYPOGLYCEMIA UNAWARENESS. Lack of recognition of the early warning signs and symptoms of low blood sugar. This may result from an absent and/or diminished counterregulatory hormone response. The person may experience episodes of severe hypoglycemia requiring the use of glucagon and/or emergency medical treatment.

INSULIN RESISTANCE. A condition in which glucose is unable to enter cells because there are fewer insulin receptors on the cell surface. Combination between insulin and these receptors is necessary for glucose entry.

KETONES. Chemicals formed during the metabolism of fat. Normal blood and urine concentration is low. Excessive ketones may accompany insulin deficiency in Type 1 diabetes.

LIPOLYSIS. Metabolism of fat for energy.

MACROVASCULAR COMPLICATIONS. Damage to larger blood vessels of the body involving the coronary arteries, cerebral arteries, and peripheral blood vessels.

MICROVASCULAR COMPLICATIONS. Changes in the small blood vessels in the eyes (retinopathy) and kidneys (nephropathy), which may lead to blindness and kidney failure, respectively.

NEUROGLYCOPENIA. Deficiency of any or all glucose in the brain.

NEUROPATHY. Damage to nerve cells of the body that results from diabetes.

POLYDIPSIA. Excessive thirst.

POLYPHAGIA. Excessive hunger.

POLYURIA. Excessive urination.

ACKNOWLEDGMENTS

We thank endocrinologist Thomas P. Fox, MD, of Mayo Clinic Jacksonville for his review of drafts of this chapter. His comments and suggestions were very helpful. This does not imply his endorsement of the content of this chapter.

RESOURCES

The following Web sites are useful:

American Diabetes Association (ADA): http://www.diabetes.org
National Institute of Diabetes and Digestive and Kidney Diseases (NIDDK): http://www.niddk.nih.gov
Joslin Diabetes Center: http://www.joslin.harvard.edu

The American Association of Diabetes Educators can be contacted at 1-800-TEAM-UP-4 to obtain a list of educators in each state. In addition, the ADA can provide a list of education programs (e.g., inpatient, outpatient, physician offices, clinics) that have met the National Standards for Diabetes Self-Management Education Programs. This information can be obtained from the ADA Web site (see above) or through one of its publications, *The Diabetes Forecast.*

REFERENCES

American Diabetes Association (ADA). (1994). Consensus statement: Self-monitoring of blood glucose. *Diabetes Care, 17*, 81–86.
American Diabetes Association (ADA). (2000). Standards of medical care for patients with diabetes mellitus. *Diabetes Care, 23*(Suppl. 1), S32–S42.
American Diabetes Association (ADA). (2001). Tests of glycemia in diabetes. *Diabetes Care, 24*(Suppl. 1), S80–S82.

Anderson, R. J., Freedland, K. E., Clouse, R. E., & Lustman, P. J. (2001). The prevalence of comorbid depression in adults with diabetes. *Diabetes Care, 24,* 1069–1078.

Anderson, R. M., Funnell, M. M., Butler, P. M., Arnold, M. S., Fitzgerald, J. T.. & Feste, C. C. (1995). Patient empowerment. *Diabetes Care, 18,* 943–949.

Armbruster, D. A. (1987). Fructosamine: Structure, analysis and clinical usefulness. *Clinical Chemistry, 33,* 2153–2163.

Bailey, B. K., Good, M. P., & McGrady, A. V. (1990). Clinical observations on behavioral treatment of a patient with insulin-dependent diabetes mellitus. *Biofeedback and Self-Regulation, 15,* 7–13.

Beaser, R. S. (1995). *The Joslin guide to diabetes.* New York: Simon & Schuster.

Bendtson, I., Gade, J., Thomsen, C. E., Rosenfalck, A., & Wildschiodtz, G. (1992). Sleep disturbances in IDDM patients with nocturnal hypoglycemia. *Sleep, 15,* 74–81.

Benson, H., Beary, J. F., & Carol, M. P. (1974). The relaxation response. *Psychiatry, 37,* 37–46.

Björntorp, P., & Rosmond, R. (1999). Visceral obesity and diabetes. *Drugs, 58*(Suppl. 1), 13–18.

Bristol/Myers Squibb. (2000). *Learn about better ways to lower your blood sugar: Questions and answers about Glucovance.* Princton, NJ: Author.

Ciechanowski, P. S., Katon, W. J., Russo, J. E., & Walker, E. A. (2001). The patient–provider relationship: Attachment theory and adherence to treatment in diabetes. *American Journal of Psychiatry, 158,* 29–35.

Cox, D. J., & Gonder-Frederick, L. A. (1991). The role of stress in diabetes mellitus. In P. M. McCabe, N. Schneiderman, T. M. Field, & J. S. Skyler (Eds.), *Stress, coping and disease.* Hillsdale, NJ: Erlbaum.

Davis, M., Eshelman, E. R., &McKay, M. (1995). *The relaxation and stress reduction workbook.* Oakland, CA: New Harbinger.

Diabetes Control and Complications Trial (DCCT) Research Group. (1993). The effect of intensive treatment of diabetes on the development and progression of long-term complications in insulin-dependent diabetes mellitus. *New England Journal of Medicine, 329,* 977–986.

Diabetes Research Working Group. (1999). *Conquering diabetes: A strategic plan for the 21st century* (NIH Publication No. 99-4398). Washington, DC: National Institutes of Health.

Feinglos, M. N., Hastedt, P., & Surwit, R. S. (1987). Effects of relaxation therapy on patients with Type I diabetes mellitus. *Diabetes Care, 10,* 72–75.

Fowler, J. E., Budzynski, T. H., & Vandenbergh, R L. (1976). The effects of an EMG biofeedback relaxation program on the control of diabetes. *Biofeedback and Self-Regulation, 1,* 105–112.

Fried, R. (1993). Respiration in stress and stress control. In P. Lehrer & R. L. Woolfolk (Eds.), *Principles and practice of stress management* (2nd ed., pp. 301–331). NewYork: Guilford Press.

Funnell, M. (Ed.). (1998). *A core curriculum for diabetes education* (3rd ed.). Chicago: American Association of Diabetes Educators.

Ganong, W. F. (1997). *Review of medical physiology* (18th ed.). Greenwich, CT: Lange Medical.

Gavard, J. A., Lustman, P. J., & Clouse, R. E. (1993). Prevalence of depression in adults with diabetes. *Diabetes Care, 16,* 1167–1178.

Glasgow, R. E., Fisher, E. B., Anderson, B. J., LaGreca, A., Marrero, D., Johnson, S. B., Rubin, R. R, & Cox, D. J. (1999). Behavioral science in diabetes. *Diabetes Care, 22,* 832–843.

Gonder-Frederick, L. A., Carter, W. R., Cox, D. J., & Clarke, W. L. (1990). Environmental stress and blood glucose change in insulin-dependent diabetes mellitus. *Health Psychology, 9,* 503–515.

Goodall, T., & Halford, N. K. (1991). Self management of diabetes mellitus: A critical review. *Health Psychology, 10,* 1–8.

Goodman, M. A. (1994). *Basic medical endocrinology* (2nd ed.). New York: Raven Press.

Goodnick, P. J., Henry, J. H., & Buki, V. M. (1995). Treatment of depression in patients with diabetes mellitus. *Journal of Clinical Psychiatry, 56,* 128–136.

Guthrie, D., Moeller, T., & Guthrie, R. (1983). Biofeedback and its application to the stabilization and control of diabetes mellitus. *American Journal of Clinical Biofeedback, 6,* 82–87.

Havlin, C. E., & Cryer, P. E. (1988). Hypoglycemia: The limiting factor in the management of insulin-dependent diabetes mellitus. *Diabetes Educator, 14,* 407–411.

Howorka, K., Pumpria, J., Wagner-Nosiska, D., Grillmayr, H., Schlusche, C., & Schabmann, A. (2000). Empowering diabetes out-patients with structured education: Short-term and long-term effects of functional insulin treatment on perceived control over diabetes. *Journal of Psychosomatic Research, 48,* 37–44.

Jablon, S. L., Naliboff, B. D., Gilmore, S. L., & Rosenthal, M. J. (1997). Effects of relaxation training on glucose tolerance and diabetic control in Type II diabetes. *Applied Psychophysiology and Biofeedback, 22,* 155–169.

Landis, B., Jovanovic, L., Landis, E., Peterson, C. M., Groshen, S., Johnson, K., & Miller, N. E. (1985). Effects of stress reduction on daily glucose range in previously stabilized insulin-dependent diabetic patients. *Diabetes Care, 8,* 624–626.

Lane, J. D., McCaskill, C. C., Ross, S. L., Feinglos, M. N., & Surwit, R. S. (1993). Relaxation training for NIDDM. *Diabetes Care, 16,* 1087–1094.

Lebovitz, H. E. (Ed.). (1998). *Therapy for diabetes mellitus and related disorders* (3rd ed.). Alexandria, VA: American Diabetes Association.

Lustman, P. J., Freedland, K. E., Griffith, L. S., & Clouse, R. E. (1998). Predicting response to cognitive behavior therapy of depression in Type 2 diabetes. *General Hospital Psychiatry, 20*, 302–306.

Lustman, P. J., Griffith, L. S., & Clouse, R. E. (1988). Depression in adults with diabetes. *Diabetes Care, 11*, 605–612.

Mazze, R. S., Shamoon, H., Pasmantier, R., Lucido, D., & Murphy, J. (1984). Reliability of blood glucose monitoring by patients with diabetes mellitus. *American Journal of Medicine, 77*, 211–217.

McGinnis, R., & McGrady, A. (2002). *Role of mood in outcome of biofeedback assisted relaxation in type 2 diabetes mellitus.* Unpublished observations.

McGrady, A. V., Bailey, B. K., & Good, M. P. (1991). Controlled study of biofeedback-assisted relaxation in Type I diabetes. *Diabetes Care, 14*, 360–365.

McGrady, A. V., Graham, G., & Bailey, B. (1996). Biofeedback assisted relaxation in insulin dependent diabetes: A replication and extension study. *Annals of Behavioral Medicine, 22*(3), 155–169.

McGrady, A. V., & Horner, J. (1999). Role of mood in outcome of biofeedback assisted relaxation therapy in insulin dependent diabetes mellitus. *Applied Psychophysiology and Biofeedback, 24*, 79–88.

Mooy, J. M., de Vries, H., Grootenhuis, P. A., Bouter, L. M., & Heine, R. J. (2000). Major stressful life events in relation to prevalence of undetected type 2 diabetes. *Diabetes Care, 23*, 197–201.

Peyrot, M., McMurray, J. F., & Kruger, D. F. (1999). A biopsychosocial model of glycemic control in diabetes: Stress, coping and regimen adherence. *Journal of Health and Social Behavior, 40*, 141–158.

Rice, B. I., & Schindler, J. V. (1992). Effect of thermal biofeedback-assisted relaxation training on blood circulation in the lower extremities of a population with diabetes. *Diabetes Care, 15*, 853–858.

Rosenbaum, L. (1983). Biofeedback-assisted stress management for insulin-treated diabetes mellitus. *Biofeedback and Self-Regulation, 8*, 519–532.

Rubin, R. R., & Peyrot, M. (2001). Psychological issues and treatments for people with diabetes. *Journal of Clinical Psychology, 57*, 457–478.

Shaw, J. E., Zimmet, P. C., McCarty, D., & de Courten, M. (2000). Type 2 diabetes worldwide according to the new classification and criteria. *Diabetes Care, 23*, B5–B10.

Skyler, J. S., Skyler, D. L., Seigler, D. E., & O'Sullivan, M. J. (1981). Algorithms for adjustment to insulin dosages by patients who monitor blood glucose. *Diabetes Care, 4*, 311–318.

Springer, R. (1989, January–February). Glycated protein tests. *Diabetes Self-Management*, pp. 44–46.

Streja, D. (2000). Blood glucose meters with storage capability: Computer-assisted analysis of data. *Practical Diabetology, 19*(3), 7–18.

Surwit, R. S., & Feinglos, M. N. (1983). The effects of relaxation on glucose tolerance in noninsulin dependent diabetes mellitus. *Diabetes Care, 6*, 176–179.

Surwit, R. S., & Feinglos, M. N. (1988). Stress and autonomic nervous system in Type II diabetes. *Diabetes Care, 11*, 83–85.

Surwit, R. S., van Tilburg, M. A., Zucker, N., McCaskill, C. C., Parekh, P., Feinglos, M. N., Edwards, C. L., Williams, P., & Lane, J. D. (2002). Stress management improves long-term glycemic control in Type 2 diabetes. *Diabetes Care, 25*, 30–34.

Timmons, B. H., & Ley, R. (Eds.). (1994). *Behavioral and psychological approaches to breathing disorders.* New York: Plenum Press.

United Kingdom Prospective Diabetes Study (UKPDS) Group. (1998a). Intensive blood glucose control with sulfonylureas or insulin compared with conventional treatment and risks: Complications in patients with Type 2 diabetes (UKPDS 33). *Lancet, 352*, 837–853.

United Kingdom Prospective Diabetes Study (UKPDS) Group. (1998b). Effect of intensive blood glucose control with metformin on complications in overweight patients with Type 2 diabetes (UKPDS 34). *Lancet, 352*, 854–865.

Wamala, S. P., Wolk, A., & Orth-Gomer, K. (1997). Determinants of obesity in relation to socioeconomic status among middle-aged Swedish women. *Preventive Medicine, 26*, 734–744.

Wilkinson, G. (1987). The influence of psychiatric, psychological and social factors on the control of insulin-dependent diabetes mellitus. *Journal of Psychosomatic Research, 31*, 277–286.

Tinnitus

Nothing Is as Loud as a Sound You Are Trying Not to Hear

HERTA FLOR
MARK S. SCHWARTZ

SCOPE OF THE PROBLEM

"Tinnitus" is derived from the Latin word *tinnire*, which means "to ring," and refers to the perception of an auditory stimulus without an external source of sound (Hazell & Jastreboff, 1990). Tinnitus is commonly classified as "objective" or "subjective." Objective tinnitus refers to sounds that are produced in or close to the auditory system and are in principle audible to an external listener. They may be related to vascular disorders, *otoacoustic emissions*, or tensor tympany syndrome. (As in other chapters, italics on first use of a term in text indicate that the term is included in the glossary at the chapter's end.) It is often possible to identify the underlying cause and thus cure the problem. Subjective tinnitus is only audible to the patient and may be related to hearing loss, noise exposure, or *Menière's disease*. The objective–subjective distinction has been criticized, because tinnitus is always a subjective experience and always has a physiological correlate, even if the sounds the patient hears are not directly audible or measurable by an outside observer. In addition, vascular tinnitus can often only be heard by the person with tinnitus.

In only a small proportion of tinnitus cases can an internal source of the sound be identified (see below). In most cases, the perception of tinnitus cannot be explained by an abnormality in the auditory pathways. Tinnitus affects about 35–45% of the population at some point in their lives; however, only about 1–2% experience major interference and seek medical attention (Kirsch, Blanchard, & Parnes, 1989; Nadol, 1993; Parving, Hein, Suaducani, Ostri, & Gyntelberg, 1993; Schleuning, 1991). There are about 1.7–3.4 million persons with severe tinnitus in the United States, and more than 800,000 are seriously disabled by it. Although it affects people of any age, most persons with tinnitus are age 40 or older. There is no gender difference. When the tinnitus becomes chronic, it usually lasts forever. Tinnitus can be described as constant or intermittent; it can affect both ears or be unilateral; it can be similar to a pure tone or can be "noisiform" and take on many characteristics, such as "whistling, ringing, roaring, humming, buzzing, static, whooshing, chirping, like running water, among others, or combinations of these noises" (Ince, Greene, Alba, & Zaretsky, 1987, p. 175). Tinnitus is often associated with "hyperacusis," which is an "exceptionally acute sense of hearing . . . used to denote a painful sensitiveness to sounds" (*Dorland's Illustrated*

Medical Dictionary, 1988, p. 790). To date there are no studies that can explain why some persons learn to live with tinnitus without major problems, and why others suffer so much that they become disabled, sleepless, and depressed.

PATHOPHYSIOLOGY AND PSYCHOLOGICAL CONCEPTS OF TINNITUS

Medical Variables

Tinnitus must be viewed as a multifactorial problem whose cause is in most cases unknown. The most common reasons for the onset of tinnitus are *otological*. Factors that initiate the experience of tinnitus are chronic exposure to noise, acute noise trauma of the ear, or sudden hearing loss. More than two-thirds of patients with tinnitus complain of hearing loss. In rare cases, tinnitus may be related to damage to the eighth nerve, due to a tumor that can be detected by computerized tomography or magnetic resonance imaging (cf. Weissman & Hirsch, 2000). Vascular causes include abnormal communications between the arterial and venous systems (Levine & Snow, 1987) and congenital vascular abnormalities. Tinnitus may also be the consequence of traumatic brain injury, degenerative brain disease, an ischemic insult, or multiple sclerosis. In addition, a long list of medications can induce tinnitus, ranging from salicylates to Emla cream (the American Tinnitus Association provides such a list on its Web site; see the "Resources" list at the end of the chapter). Therefore, an intensive medical workup by an otolaryngologist (and, if indicated, additional specialists) must always precede any psychological intervention.

Neurophysiological Considerations

In most cases, no clear physiological cause of the tinnitus can be detected. A large number of theoretical models on the pathophysiology of tinnitus have been proposed. For example, the neurophysiological model of Jastreboff (1990; see also Jastreboff & Jastreboff, 2000) assumes that abnormalities both in cochlear function and in the processing of the tinnitus-related signal lead to the chronic condition of tinnitus. He postulates four components that determine the tinnitus experience: (1) the generation of tinnitus-related neuronal activity in the periphery, which initiates the problem but has little to do with its perpetuation; (2) the detection of this signal in subcortical centers; (3) the perception and evaluation of the signal in cortical areas; both of which may be exaggerated and lead to (4) the consequence of a sustained activation of the limbic system and autonomic nervous system (ANS) that create the emotional distress related to tinnitus (see Figure 33.1). Although widely cited and employed as a basis of what Jastreboff calls "tinnitus retraining therapy," the model is very vague with respect to the mechanisms that lead to the initiation and maintenance of the tinnitus, and it is not specific enough to lead to circumscribed empirical research (cf. Kröner-Herwig et al., 2000).

Other models have postulated disorders in specific portions of the auditory pathway (such as alterations in afferent or afferent discharge, cross-talk between adjacent nerve fibers, central nervous system [CNS] hypersensitivity, edge effects, and dysfunctions in transmitter and cellular mechanisms), or have drawn parallels between mechanisms of neural plasticity that contribute to chronic pain and tinnitus (for overviews, see Kaltenbach, 2000; Moller, 2000). Animal models of induced tinnitus as well as imaging studies have suggested that the auditory cortex and limbic structures may primarily be altered by the experience of tinnitus, and that it is very unlikely that tinnitus is generated in the auditory pathway (Wallhäuser-Franke, Braun, & Langner, 1996; Mühlnickel, Elbert, Taub, & Flor, 1998).

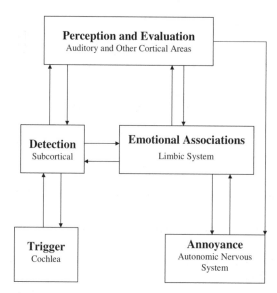

FIGURE 33.1. A block diagram of the development of tinnitus. Adapted from Jastreboff, Gray, and Gold (1996). Copyright 1996 by the *American Journal of Otology*. Adapted by permission.

Cerebral Correlates of Tinnitus

Several studies have recently attempted to examine the cerebral correlates of the experience of tinnitus by analyzing patients with tinnitus in periods with no or less tinnitus versus current or high tinnitus. Other studies have exposed patients with tinnitus and healthy controls to varying sounds and have examined how these were processed. For example, Mühlnickel et al. (1998) used magnetoencephalographic recordings to study the representation of pure tones in the tonotopic map of patients with tinnitus and healthy controls. They found that the representation of the tinnitus sound had shifted from the straight line that usually characterizes the relationship of tone frequency and location of tone representation in primary auditory cortex. In the patients with tinnitus, the representation of the tinnitus frequency had moved into an area adjacent to the normal tonotopic representation, and this shift was highly positively correlated with the severity of the tinnitus as assessed by the Multidimensional Tinnitus Inventory (see below and Figure 33.2). Mühlnickel et al. concluded that tinnitus might have some similarity to the phenomenon of phantom limb pain, which they had previously found to be associated with a comparable type of cortical change. In patients with upper-extremity amputations, the cortical representation of the lip adjacent to the amputated hand or arm had shifted into the cortical hand area, and the magnitude of this shift was found to be highly correlated with phantom limb pain (Flor et al., 1995). Mühlnickel et al. suggested that this change in auditory cortical representation, called *cortical reorganization* or *cortical plasticity*, might be the neural correlate of the perception of tinnitus.

Similar conclusions were reached by Lockwood et al. (1998, 1999), who located patients who possessed the unusual ability to exert substantial voluntary control over the loudness of their tinnitus by performing an orofacial movement (jaw clenching). Their positron emission tomography study showed that tinnitus activated the auditory cortex as well as limbic areas, and that the patients also responded with widespread cortical activation to pure tone stimulation. This is an intriguing finding, that appears to lend support also to the notion that orofacial muscle activity may be a factor contributing to tinnitus, although only few patients with tinnitus exhibit this phenomenon. (Among 1000 respondents to the most recent American Tinnitus Association survey, only 0.2% appeared to show the phenomenon; G. Reich,

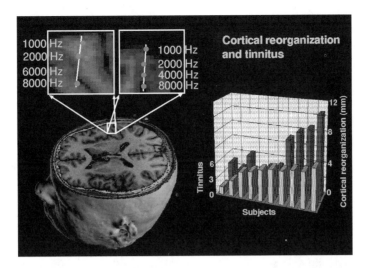

FIGURE 33.2. On the left side, the tonotopic map of a patient with tinnitus is presented, compared to the tonotopic map of a healthy control. Note that the tinnitus frequency deviates from this map. On the right, the association between tinnitus severity and deviation from the tonotopic map is depicted: The larger the deviation, the more intense the tinnitus. Based on Mühlnickel, Elbert, Taub, and Flor (1998).

personal communication to Lockwood et al., 1998, p. 117.) However, we need to know more about the survey questions to know more about the unusualness of this orofacial tinnitus induction. Parallel studies in patients with phantom limb pain have shown that most patients are not aware that this type of phenomenon (elicitation of phantom sensation by stimulation or movement) exists at all. Lockwood et al. (1998, 1999) speculate that there may be aberrant neural connections with auditory portions of the brain. Furthermore, they speculate from their data that the neural systems mediating tinnitus may be linked to systems controlling emotions via the hippocampus—a portion of the limbic system that is the gateway to centers mediating emotional control, as well as an important component of memory systems. Like the severity of phantom limb pain, the severity and the psychological impact of tinnitus may depend on the nature and extent of plastic change in the central auditory system. Several other imaging studies have likewise found abnormal activation in the auditory cortex and the limbic system in patients with tinnitus and in healthy controls exposed to aversive noise (e.g., Andersson et al., 2000; Mirz, Gjedde, Sodkilde-Jorgensen, & Pedersen, 2000). Taken together, these studies suggest that the auditory cortex and limbic areas are always involved in the processing of tinnitus sounds. It remains to be determined to what extent the limbic activation is a cause or a consequence of the problem. Additional active areas such as frontal or parietal activations may depend on the specific sample or task used.

Psychophysiological Models

Some experts believe that stress, physical tension in cephalic and neck muscles, and cognitive factors either are among the causes of tinnitus or can accentuate its severity and associated distress for some patients (e.g., Schleuning, 1991; Rubinstein, 1993; Jakes, Hallam, McKenna, & Hinchcliffe, 1992). This is part of the rationale for using relaxation therapies, biofeedback, and cognitive-behavioral stress management. Rubinstein (1993) provides an extensive review of the proposed relationship between *craniomandibular disorders* (*CMDs*) and tinnitus. He studied patients being evaluated for CMDs, others being evaluated for tinnitus, and epidemiological samples. He concluded that there is an association between CMD signs/symptoms and tinnitus. He based this partly on the common association of tinnitus in patients with headaches, fatigue/tenderness in jaw muscles, pain on palpation of masticatory muscles, and impaired mandibular mobility compared to epidemiological samples. Many people with tinnitus report that mandibular movements and bruxism, jaw tenderness/fatigue, and/or pressure on the temporomandibular joint (TMJ) influence and correlate with fluctuations in tinnitus, vertigo, and hyperacusis. Rubinstein's (1993) review and studies support both *stomatognathic* and biofeedback treatments for reducing or eliminating tinnitus in selected patients.

Psychological Models

Psychological models of tinnitus emphasize that *habituation* to tinnitus fails to occur in some patients, and that this lack of habituation is accompanied by high arousal levels and the acquisition of emotional significance by the tinnitus sound (Hallam, Rachman, & Hinchcliffe, 1987). Andersson (2001) emphasizes that the changing nature of the tinnitus sound prevents habituation from occurring. The cognitive disruption resulting from this lack of habituation leads to conditioned emotional reactions to the tinnitus. It is also assumed that the focusing of attention on tinnitus leads to dysfunctionl appraisal and evaluation, followed by dysfunctional coping and operant factors (avoidance behaviors) that again increase annoyance related to the tinnitus, as well as discomfort and suffering (cf. Kröner-Herwig et al., 2000). The cognitive model of tinnitus complaints assumes that the attention given to the tinnitus noises is a major contributing factor creating the disturbing effects. If a person views these as threatening or implying future loss, then the result is more likely to be emotional distress. Furthermore, attending to the tinnitus interferes with other adaptive activities. This leads to views of the noises as being more intrusive and affecting concentration and sleep. It may be that long-term insomnia predating the tinnitus may increase the risk of disturbed sleep after tinnitus starts (Hallam, Jakes, & Hinchcliffe, 1988).

ASSESSMENT OF TINNITUS

Table 33.1 presents the essential components of a multiaxial tinnitus assessment, modeled after the Multiaxial Assessment of Pain (cf. Turk & Rudy, 1988).

Audiological and Psychophysical Examination

A good audiological examination is needed. This should include the assessment of the frequency and intensity of the tinnitus, the minimal masking level, "residual inhibition" (see below), and the assessment of hearing loss. Since the loudness as well as the frequency of tinnitus is often very variable, measures that characterize tinnitus should be obtained. First, consider giving patients a tape that contains a collection of typical tinnitus sounds prepared by the American Tinnitus Association. The patients rate on a visual analogue scale how similar this type of sound is to their own tinnitus. This gives an estimate of the qualitative aspects of the tinnitus sounds. The patients then have to match both the frequency and the loudness of their tinnitus to sounds that are presented to them. Finally, *audiological masker* is used to test at what level of masking sound a patient no longer perceives his or her tinnitus (minimal masking level), and also to test whether "residual inhibition" is present (i.e., whether the use of a sound in the tinnitus frequency leads to a temporary reduction of the tinnitus sound).

Tinnitus Characteristics and Psychosocial Variables

Table 33.2 summarizes the items to be covered in a structured tinnitus interview, as presented by Andersson (2001). This basic information includes duration of tinnitus; possible causes

TABLE 33.1. **Multiaxial Assessment of Tinnitus**

- Audiological assessment and psychophysical testing
  - Pitch
  - Loudness
  - Maskability
  - Residual inhibition
  - Quality
- Verbal/subjective level
  - Tinnitus interview
  - Multidimensional Tinnitus Inventory (MTI) or other tinnitus questionnaire
  - Tinnitus diary
  - Tinnitus-related catastrophizing
  - Anxiety
  - Stress
  - Depression
- Behavioral level
  - Avoidance of noise
  - Other tinnitus-related avoidance behaviors
- Psychophysiological assessment
  - Stress-related muscle tension
  - Autonomic responding
  - Deviations from the tonotopic map
  - Cortical responses to sound
- Determination of patient profiles and differential indication for treatment

Note. Based on Turk and Rudy (1988).

(e.g., acoustic trauma, infection, head trauma, and hearing loss); location (right, left, or bilateral); severity; type (e.g., single or multiple sounds, continuous or intermittent sound, or pulsating); quality of sounds; past and present treatments; medications; and the temporal nature of the tinnitus. The interview also covers the effects of tinnitus on patients' lives and methods the patients use to manage it. Other sample interviews have been published by Andersson, Lyttkens, and Larsen (1999) and Hiller, Goebel, and Schindelmann (1999).

For a measure of tinnitus disturbance, a rating system that separates activity from rest and sleep conditions (Podoshin, Ben-David, Fradis, Gerstel, & Felner, 1991) is useful. Table 33.3 presents both this rating system and a slight elaboration of it. Podoshin et al. used a 0–4 scale; however, the proposed 0–5 scale makes it more comparable to the scales and rating forms often used by practitioners treating headaches and other pain symptoms. Some wording changes have also been made. Both rating scales are presented here for interest and consideration.

The Tinnitus Effects Questionnaire (TEQ; Hallam et al., 1988; Jakes et al., 1992) exists in a 52-item version and a 33-item revised version. The four scores derived from the revised version of the scale are as follows: Emotional Distress, Auditory Perceptual Difficulties, Insomnia, and Irrational Beliefs. The last claims to measure absolutist, all-or-none thinking, as well as catastrophic beliefs about tinnitus. Based on studies by Hallam et al. (1988) and Jakes et al. (1992), sensory and perceptual problems only partially overlap with the emotional distress people report. A good discussion of item development and factor analyses is the Hallam et al. (1988) article.[1] A factor analysis of a German translation of the TEQ showed five factors (Hiller & Goebel, 1992).[2]

TABLE 33.2. Items to Be Covered in a Structured Tinnitus Interview

- Background data (age, etc.)
- Hearing loss and use of hearing aids
- Tinnitus localization
- Events associated with the onset of tinnitus
- Tinnitus grading:
    - I. Only audible in silent environments
    - II. Audible only in ordinary acoustic environments, but masked by loud environmental sounds; it can disturb going to sleep, but not sleep in general
    - III. Audible in all acoustic environments; disturbs going to sleep; can disturb sleep in general; and is a dominating problem that affects quality of life
- Variation in tinnitus loudness
- Attention directed toward tinnitus on an ordinary day
- Most problematic situations associated with tinnitus
- Time of the day most problematic
- Possibility of doing something to lessen the problems with tinnitus
- Possibility of changing the loudness of the tinnitus
- Situations when the tinnitus is less problematic
- Avoidance of situations and activities because of tinnitus
- Psychological consequences of tinnitus
- Sleep problems (hours of sleep per night, sleep onset latency, awakenings during the night, time awake in the morning)
- Influence of background sounds or noises on tinnitus
- Masking of tinnitus by background sounds
- Noise sensitivity, including hyperacusis
- Influence of stress and fatigue
- Influence of weather
- Medication and their effects on tinnitus
- Use of caffeine and its effects on tinnitus
- Alcohol use and its effects on tinnitus
- Tobacco use effects on tinnitus
- Role of relatives/significant other when coping with tinnitus
- Major or minor changes in tinnitus characteristics since onset
- Tolerance of tinnitus in relation to onset (e.g., much better or much worse)
- Earlier or ongoing treatments for tinnitus and hearing loss (including counseling)
- Perceived cause of tinnitus
- Problems with headache
- Dizziness or unsteadiness
- Muscular tension (in face, jaw, shoulder)
- Earlier or ongoing psychiatric consultations/treatments
- Attitude toward tinnitus
- Attitude toward referral to a psychologist
- Presentation of a cognitive-behavioral model of tinnitus annoyance, and checking for acceptance of the model and the approach to treatment

Note. Adapted from Andersson (2001). Copyright 2001 by Thieme Medical Publishers. Adapted by permission.

TABLE 33.3. Two Tinnitus Rating Systems

During activity

    0 = No tinnitus

    1 = Mild tinnitus without disturbance

    2 = Moderate, which disturbs but does not affect activity

    3 = Severe, which affects activity

    4 = Very severe, which renders activity impossible

During rest

    0 = No tinnitus

    1 = Mild tinnitus without disturbance

    2 = Moderate, which disturbs but does not affect sleep

    3 = Severe, which affects sleep

    4 = Very severe, which causes severe insomnia and spontaneous arousals

During activity

    0 = No sound even when thought about

    1 = Slight; barely can hear the sound; ignored or forgotten about often

    2 = Mild; aware all the time, but no interference with any activity

    3 = Moderate; disturbing; some interference with activities

    4 = Severe; much interference with activities

    5 = Very severe; incapacitating; makes specific activities impossible

During rest and at bedtime

    0 = No tinnitus, even when thought about during rest or trying to sleep

    1 = Slight; barely aware; ignored at times; can rest and sleep well

    2 = Mild; aware all the time, but no interference with rest or sleep

    3 = Moderate; disturbing; some interference with sleep

    4 = Severe; much interference with sleep

    5 = Very severe; interference with rest; causes severe insomnia and spontaneous awakenings from sleep

Note. Based on Podoshin, Ben-David, Fradis, Gerstel, and Felner (1991).

Interference with Daily Activities (IWDA; Jakes, Hallam, Rachman, & Hinchcliffe, 1986) is a 23-item checklist also called the Tinnitus Activity Schedule. It purports to measure the number of activities affected by tinnitus. Sample activities are reading newspapers, watching television, relaxing during the day, and dealing calmly with problems. Patients rate each activity on a scale from O to 2: 0 = "not at all," 1 = "a little," and 2 = "a lot." Another measure to consider is the Iowa Tinnitus Handicap Questionnaire (Kuk, Tyler, Russell, & Jordon, 1990).

Based on the West Haven–Yale Multidimensional Pain Inventory (Kerns, Turk, & Rudy, 1985), the Multidimensional Tinnitus Inventory (MTI) was designed to assess psychosocial aspects of tinnitus. The questionnaire consists of three parts, with section 1 including 28 items that assess Tinnitus Severity, Interference Related to Tinnitus, Affective Distress, Life Control, and Social Support. Section 2 consists of 14 items and assesses responses of significant others to the problem, which can be characterized as either solicitous or punishing/ignoring. Section 3 consists of 11 items asking about daily activities. The scale has good reliability and validity, and is reproduced in Figure 33.3 (see Mühlnickel et al., 1998; Flor, Hoffmann, Struve, & Diesch, 2002).

FIGURE 33.3. Multidimensional Tinnitus Inventory (MTI).

Name: _____ Date: _____

Instructions: An important part of our evaluation includes examination of tinnitus from **your** perspective. You know your tinnitus better than anyone, so the information you give is very helpful in planning a treatment program for you.

Please read each question carefully and then do your best to answer each one. **Do not skip any questions**. If there is a question that you think does not apply to you, please **circle the number** of that question. After you have completed the questionnaire, check your responses to make sure that you have answered each question. Please use the last page to add any additional information or comments that you think would be of help to us in better understanding your tinnitus problem.

A. Some of the questions in this questionnaire refer to your "significant other." A significant other is *a person with whom you feel closest*. This includes *anyone* that you relate to on a regular or infrequent basis. It is very important that you identify someone as your "significant other." Please indicate below who your significant other is (check one):

Spouse	Partner/companion	Housemate/roommate
Friend	Neighbor	Parent/child/other relative
Other (please describe): _____		

B. Do you currently live with this person?   Yes   No

When you answer questions in the following pages about "your significant other," always respond in reference to the specific person you just indicated.

Section 1

This part asks questions to help us learn more about your tinnitus and how it affects your life. Under each question is a scale to mark your answer. Read each question carefully, and then **circle a number** on the scale under that question to indicate how the specific question applies to you. An example may help you to better understand how you should answer these questions.

Example

How nervous are you when you ride in a car when the traffic is heavy?

0	1	2	3	4	5	6
Not at all nervous						Extremely nervous

If you are *not at all* nervous when riding in a car in heavy traffic, you would want to **circle** the number 0. If you are *very nervous* when riding in a car in heavy traffic, you would then **circle** the number 6. Lower numbers would be used for less nervousness, and higher numbers for more nervousness.

Please answer the following questions:

1. Rate the level of your tinnitus at the *present moment*.

0	1	2	3	4	5	6
No tinnitus						Very intense tinnitus

2. In general, how much does your tinnitus interfere with your day-to-day activities?

0	1	2	3	4	5	6
No interference						Extreme interference

3. Since the time your tinnitus began, how much has your tinnitus changed your ability to work?
(_____ Check here if you are not working for reasons other than your tinnitus.)

0	1	2	3	4	5	6
No change						Extreme change

4. How much has your tinnitus changed the amount of satisfaction or enjoyment you get from taking part in social and recreational activities?

0	1	2	3	4	5	6
No change						Extreme change

5. How supportive or helpful is your spouse or significant other (*this refers to the person you indicated above*) to you in relation to your tinnitus?

0	1	2	3	4	5	6
Not at all supportive						Extremely supportive

6. Rate your overall mood during the *past week*.

0	1	2	3	4	5	6
Extremely low						Extremely high

7. How much has your tinnitus interfered with your ability to get enough sleep?

0	1	2	3	4	5	6
No interference						Extreme interference

8. On the average, how severe has your tinnitus been during the *last week*?

0	1	2	3	4	5	6
Not at all severe						Extremely severe

9. How able are you to predict when your tinnitus will start, get better, or get worse?

0	1	2	3	4	5	6
Not at all able to predict						Very able to predict

10. How much has your tinnitus changed your ability to take part in recreational and other social activities?

0	1	2	3	4	5	6
No change						Extreme change

11. How much do you limit your activities in order to keep your tinnitus from getting worse?

0	1	2	3	4	5	6
Not at all						Very much

12. How much has your tinnitus changed the amount of satisfaction or enjoyment you get from family-related activities?

0	1	2	3	4	5	6
No change						Extreme change

13. How worried is your spouse (significant other) about you because of your tinnitus?

0	1	2	3	4	5	6
Not at all worried						Extremely worried

14. During the *past week,* how much control do you feel you have had over your life?

0	1	2	3	4	5	6
No control						Extreme control

15. On an average day, how much does your tinnitus vary (increase or decrease)?

0	1	2	3	4	5	6
Remains the same						Changes a lot

16. How much suffering do you experience because of your tinnitus?

0	1	2	3	4	5	6
No suffering						Extreme suffering

17. How often are you able to do something that helps to reduce your tinnitus?

0	1	2	3	4	5	6
Never						Very often

18. How much has your tinnitus changed your relationship with your spouse, family, or significant other?

0	1	2	3	4	5	6
No change						Extreme change

19. How much has your tinnitus changed the amount of satisfaction or enjoyment you get from work?
(_____ Check here if you are not presently working.)

0	1	2	3	4	5	6
No change						Extreme change

20. How attentive is your spouse (significant other) to you because of your tinnitus?

0	1	2	3	4	5	6
Not at all attentive						Extremely attentive

21. During the *past week*, how well do you feel you've been able to deal with your problems?

0	1	2	3	4	5	6
Not at all						Extremely well

22. How much control do you feel you have over your tinnitus?

0	1	2	3	4	5	6
No control at all						A great deal of control

23. How much has your tinnitus changed your ability to do household chores?

0	1	2	3	4	5	6
No change						Extreme change

24. During the *past week*, how successful were you in coping with stressful situations in your life?

0	1	2	3	4	5	6
Not at all successful						Extremely successful

25. How much has your tinnitus interfered with your ability to plan activities?

0	1	2	3	4	5	6
No change						Extreme change

(cont.)

FIGURE 33.3. (cont.)

26. During the *past week,* how irritable have you been?

0	1	2	3	4	5	6
Not at all irritable						Extremely irritable

27. How much has your tinnitus changed your friendships with people other than your family?

0	1	2	3	4	5	6
No change						Extreme change

28. During the *past week,* how tense or anxious have you been?

0	1	2	3	4	5	6
Not at all tense or anxious						Extremely tense and anxious

Section 2

In this section, we are interested in knowing how your spouse (or significant other) responds to you when he or she knows you have tinnitus. On the scale listed below each question, **circle a number** to indicate how often your spouse (or significant other) responds to you in that particular way when you have tinnitus.

Please answer all of the 14 questions.

1. Ignores me.

0	1	2	3	4	5	6
Never						Very often

2. Asks me what he or she can do to help.

0	1	2	3	4	5	6
Never						Very often

3. Tries to distract me.

0	1	2	3	4	5	6
Never						Very often

4. Gets irritated with me.

0	1	2	3	4	5	6
Never						Very often

5. Takes over my jobs or duties.

0	1	2	3	4	5	6
Never						Very often

6. Talks to me about something else to take my mind off the tinnitus.

0	1	2	3	4	5	6
Never						Very often

7. Gets frustrated with me.

0	1	2	3	4	5	6
Never						Very often

8. Tries to get me to rest.

0	1	2	3	4	5	6
Never						Very often

9. Tries to involve me in some activity.

0	1	2	3	4	5	6
Never						Very often

10. Gets angry with me.

0	1	2	3	4	5	6
Never						Very often

11. Gets me medication.

0	1	2	3	4	5	6
Never						Very often

12. Encourages me to work on a hobby.

0	1	2	3	4	5	6
Never						Very often

13. Gets me something to eat or drink.

0	1	2	3	4	5	6
Never						Very often

14. Turns on the TV to take my mind off my tinnitus.

0	1	2	3	4	5	6
Never						Very often

Section 3

Listed below are 11 daily activities. Please indicate *how often* you do each of these by circling a number on the scale listed below each activity. Please complete all 11 questions.

1. Reading.

0	1	2	3	4	5	6
Never						Very often

2. Work on a hobby.

0	1	2	3	4	5	6
Never						Very often

3. Go out to eat.

0	1	2	3	4	5	6
Never						Very often

4. Watch TV.

0	1	2	3	4	5	6
Never						Very often

5. Listen to the radio/music.

0	1	2	3	4	5	6
Never						Very often

6. Relax quietly.

0	1	2	3	4	5	6
Never						Very often

7. Go to a movie or theater.

0	1	2	3	4	5	6
Never						Very often

8. Visit friends.

0	1	2	3	4	5	6
Never						Very often

10. Take a trip.

0	1	2	3	4	5	6
Never						Very often

11. Go to a concert.

0	1	2	3	4	5	6
Never						Very often

Scoring key for the MTI:

Section I:
Tinnitus Severity: 1 + 8 + 15 + 16
Interference Related to Tinnitus: 2 + 3 + 4 + 7 + 10 + 11 + 12 + 18 + 19 + 23 + 25 + 27
Affective Distress: 6 + 26 + 28
Life Control: 9 + 14 + 17 + 21 + 22 + 24
Social Support: 5 + 13 + 20
Divide sum by the number of items completed per scale; values range from 0 to 6.

Section II:
Solicitous responses: 2 + 3 + 5 + 6 + 8 + 9 + 11 + 12 + 13 + 14
Punishing/ignoring responses: 1 + 4 + 7 + 10

Section III:
Activities in the house: 1 + 2 + 4 + 5 + 6
Activities out of the house: 3 + 7 + 8 + 9 + 10 + 11
Total activities: Total sum

A tinnitus diary is an important instrument for both assessment and treatment of patients with tinnitus. A typical tinnitus diary contains information about the loudness of the tinnitus, the annoyance related to tinnitus, the interference of tinnitus with daily activities, the patients' mood, daily stressors, effects of tinnitus on sleep, and the use of tinnitus treatments (including their efficacy) (see Figure 33.4). It gives information about the fluctuation of tinnitus, about variables that are associated with it, and about the relationship of tinnitus severity and annoyance. During treatment, it may provide important feedback about the patients' adherence to treatment, and it helps to document treatment-related changes.

Additional questionnaires that may be useful are measures of depression and anxiety, as well as the magnitude of somatic symptoms. In addition, catastrophizing related to the experience of tinnitus is routinely assessed, in order to determine to what extent maladaptive cognitive evaluations exist (see Figure 33.5).

Behavioral Assessment

The extent to which patients with tinnitus avoid situations of noise or other situations related to their tinnitus should be assessed. This information can be taken from the interview, the MTI, and the tinnitus diary. It is often useful to include patients' significant others in this assessment, because they often have noticed avoidance behavior better than the patients have. It is also important to determine to what extent there is positive reinforcement for tinnitus. These avoidance behaviors, as well as positive responses to tinnitus, must be addressed in treatment.

Psychophysiological Assessment

Biofeedback practitioners should consider using both psychological and physical stress induction methods to determine to what extent elevated levels of muscle tension might contribute to the experience of tinnitus. Ask patients to imagine stressful situations, as well as situations when their tinnitus was especially severe, while assessing tension from several head-related muscle groups (such as the temporalis, masseter, sternocleidomastoid, frontalis, trapezius, and splenius capitis). Physical tests may include clenching the teeth, listening to loud noise, relaxing in silence, or others, depending on the factors that aggravate tinnitus as determined from the interview. Try to always include heart rate or skin conductance as indicators of general ANS arousal, and also to control for the effectiveness of stress induction procedures. Electroencephalographic or magnetoencephalographic recordings or functional magnetic resonance imaging can be used to test for cortical and other cerebral responses that may be deviant in patients with tinnitus.

Identification of Subgroups and Patient–Treatment Matching

The MTI and related information can be used to classify patients into subgroups that might differentially profit from various types of tinnitus treatments. One group—termed "highly physiologically reactive"—is characterized by elevated muscle tension levels and heightened stress reactivity. For those patients, surface electromyographic (EMG) biofeedback combined with stress management training is the most appropriate intervention. A second group of patients is depressed and shows a lack of coping skills, as well as excessive attention to the tinnitus sounds. For these patients, a cognitive-behavioral approach may be best suited. Patients with hyperacusis and phonophobia (a severe fear of exposure to sound), and those who are being reinforced for tinnitus and show severe avoidance behaviors, may need exposure

FIGURE 33.4. Tinnitus diary.

Code No.: _____ Date: _____ Day: Mo Tu We Thu Fr Sa Su

1. How *severe* was your tinnitus today?

Morning (6–12)	0	1	2	3	4	5	6	7	8	9	10
Afternoon (12–6)	0	1	2	3	4	5	6	7	8	9	10
Evening (6–12)	0	1	2	3	4	5	6	7	8	9	10
Night (12–6)	0	1	2	3	4	5	6	7	8	9	10

Not at all   Very severe

2. How much has your tinnitus *bothered* you today?

Morning (6–12)	0	1	2	3	4	5	6	7	8	9	10
Afternoon (12–6)	0	1	2	3	4	5	6	7	8	9	10
Evening (6–12)	0	1	2	3	4	5	6	7	8	9	10
Night (12–6)	0	1	2	3	4	5	6	7	8	9	10

Not at all   Very severe

3. Did you have trouble *sleeping* because of the tinnitus?
   0   1   2   3   4   5   6   7   8   9   10
   Not at all   Very much

4. How would you describe your *mood* today?
   0   1   2   3   4   5   6   7   8   9   10
   Very bad   Very good

5. How *stressed* did you feel today?
   0   1   2   3   4   5   6   7   8   9   10
   Not at all   Very much

6. Did you take any *medications* today?

Medication	Amount	Time
_____	_____	_____
_____	_____	_____

7. Did anything special occur today (e.g., illness, stress)? If yes, what?
_____
_____

8. Did you notice anything that made the tinnitus better or worse? If yes, what happened?
_____
_____

9. Protocol of exercises:

Begin _____ End _____	Bothered by tinnitus before:	0	1	2	3	4	5	6	7	8	9	10
Begin _____ End _____	Bothered by tinnitus after:	0	1	2	3	4	5	6	7	8	9	10
Begin _____ End _____	Bothered by tinnitus before:	0	1	2	3	4	5	6	7	8	9	10
Begin _____ End _____	Bothered by tinnitus after:	0	1	2	3	4	5	6	7	8	9	10
Begin _____ End _____	Bothered by tinnitus before:	0	1	2	3	4	5	6	7	8	9	10
Begin _____ End _____	Bothered by tinnitus after:	0	1	2	3	4	5	6	7	8	9	10

Not at all   Very much

training; that is, they need to learn to tolerate increasing levels of sound and habituate slowly to noise and tinnitus. Rather than combining all those treatment strategies, we suggest that the therapist pinpoint the core problems of the patient and then use the treatment that is best suited for the specific problem. We suspect that the low success rates found for some biofeedback and behavioral procedures in some studies may be related to the fact that the researchers did not select the patients carefully enough for treatment and may have targeted problems that were not relevant for parts of their samples.

FIGURE 33.5. Tinnitus-related self-statements.

Name: _____   Date:_____

Most of the time we have an internal conversation with ourselves. We ask ourselves, for example, to do certain things; we blame ourselves if we make a mistake; and we reward ourselves for our accomplishments. When we have tinnitus, we also say certain things to ourselves that are different from what we say when we are feeling good. Below we have listed typical thoughts of people with tinnitus. Please read each of the statements, and then mark how often you have this thought when your tinnitus is severe. Please circle the appropriate number on the scale, ranging from 0 = "almost never" to 5 = "almost always."

	Almost never					Almost always
1. If I stay calm and relax, things will be better.	0	1	2	3	4	5
2. I cannot stand this tinnitus any longer.	0	1	2	3	4	5
3. I can do something about my tinnitus.	0	1	2	3	4	5
4. No matter what I do, my tinnitus doesn't change anyway.	0	1	2	3	4	5
5. I need to relax.	0	1	2	3	4	5
6. I'll manage.	0	1	2	3	4	5
7. I need to avoid noise.	0	1	2	3	4	5
8. I will soon be better again.	0	1	2	3	4	5
9. This will never end.	0	1	2	3	4	5
10. I am a hopeless case.	0	1	2	3	4	5
11. There are worse things than my tinnitus.	0	1	2	3	4	5
12. I can cope with it.	0	1	2	3	4	5
13. When will it get worse again?	0	1	2	3	4	5
14. This tinnitus is driving me crazy.	0	1	2	3	4	5
15. I can't go on any more.	0	1	2	3	4	5

Scoring key:
Catastrophizing: 2 + 4 + 7 + 9 + 10 + 13 + 14 + 15
Coping: 1 + 3 + 5 + 6 + 8 + 11 + 12
Divide by the number of items completed; range, 0–5.

TREATMENTS

Several qualitative and quantitative reviews on the efficacy of psychological interventions for tinnitus have been published in recent years (Kirsch et al., 1989; Andersson, Melin, Hägnebo, Scott, & Lindberg, 1995; Wilson & Henry, 1993; Andersson & Lyttkens, 1999). They all agree that psychological interventions are to date the most effective treatments for tinnitus. The interventions that have so far been tested in controlled studies include EMG biofeedback, relaxation, hypnosis, support/counseling, therapeutic noise, and cognitive-behavioral treatments. Also discussed here are *matching-to-sample feedback*, Jastreboff's tinnitus retraining therapy, and techniques aimed at altering cortical plasticity.

EMG Biofeedback

Publications about biofeedback treatments for tinnitus include both case reports and controlled group outcome studies (e.g., Grossan, 1976; House, Miller, & House, 1977; Borton, Moore, & Clark, 1981; Elfner, May, Moore, & Mendelson, 1981; Duckro, Pollard, Bray, &

Scheiter, 1984; Walsh & Gerley, 1985; Haralambous et al., 1987; Kirsch, Blanchard, & Parnes, 1987). Conclusions are promising but mixed. Several studies and case reports suggest that relaxation and EMG biofeedback can at least reduce the subjective disturbance and annoyance resulting from tinnitus. Some reports suggest that these treatments may reduce the severity or loudness of the tinnitus, although this is much less clear. The methodological flaws in some of the studies are serious. These include lack of control groups, lack of baseline data, and reliance on anecdotal reports. Another serious flaw is using only global measures that probably markedly overestimate improvement. Other studies used insufficient biofeedback, and some studies lack documentation of physiological changes in the biofeedback modalities. Controlled studies typically do not show significant changes in objective measures of tinnitus intensity. Objective audiological support is typically lacking.

Increasing physiological self-regulation of striated head muscles and ANS arousal may provide patients with a better sense of control. It can also help them focus their attention away from the tinnitus. However, we do not know whether relaxation and biofeedback have any direct effect on the physiological mechanisms of tinnitus. Paradoxically, audiological evaluations sometimes show increases in the audio intensity needed to mask the sound even with decreased subjective ratings of severity. For example, Kirsch et al. (1987) reported that three of six subjects were initially in the 35- to 95-decibel range and showed an increase 1 month after treatment. The other three subjects showed either very little or considerable reduction in masking intensity.

CMDs or *temporomandibular disorders* (*TMDs*) are probably a common cause of, or factor contributing to, subjective tinnitus (Schleuning, 1991; Rubinstein, 1993). See Glaros and Lausten (Chapter 15, this volume) for a discussion of the rationale for relaxation and biofeedback therapies for TMDs. One can logically extrapolate this rationale to treating selected patients with tinnitus for whom TMDs appear to be at least a contributing factor.

For instance, a female patient age 40 had daily tinnitus for 5 months. She had had sensorineural hearing loss in one ear since childhood, and wore a hearing aid. The place she worked for many years had undergone a major transition a few months before her symptoms began. She did not tolerate changes well. She also had a history of teeth clenching and grinding since childhood, as well as a major lateral malocclusion. She had used an athletic mouthguard nightly for years to prevent occlusal wear, but had also avoided dentists for years. Her TMJ areas and the sides of her face were more tense since the tinnitus started.

Treatment involved a dental consultation and proper mouthguard for sleep, an EMG biofeedback assessment, and biofeedback-assisted relaxation. It was not clear whether the increased stress emitted increased bruxing that brought about the tinnitus. Increased stress may have led to bruxing and tinnitus independently. Treatment focused initially on reducing the TMD symptoms. When last seen a few weeks after the first visit, she reported no tinnitus symptoms for 3 weeks.

Otolaryngologists and other physicians who see patients with tinnitus often seek help in managing some of these patients from practitioners who use applied psychophysiological treatments. The focus in the remainder of this section is on biobehavioral management and treatments for subjective tinnitus.

Patients often rate noticeable improvement in their ability to manage the stress of tinnitus after biofeedback/relaxation treatment, and they often report much satisfaction with treatment. This may result from a sense of well-being and better management of associated symptoms. An illustration is a comment from a patient with chronic and disabling subjective tinnitus whom one of us (M. S. Schwartz) treated. He reported dramatic and positive changes in his sleep and life after two office visits and a multicomponent behavioral treatment including passive relaxation. He said, "The sound is still the same, but it does not bother me the way it did. I now start sleep fast and feel much better during the day."

Research and clinical speculations suggest other ways in which biofeedback and related procedures might help subjective tinnitus. These include distractor effects, habituation, cognitive changes, sleep improvement, and/or lowered physiological tension and arousal. (These are not listed here in any order of preference. The "Speculations . . ." section of this chapter contains a discussion of these.)

Other factors that may accentuate tinnitus severity include depression and anxiety. Some antidepressant medications help these depressed patients with tinnitus (Schleuning, 1991; Dobie, Sakai, Sullivan, Katon, & Russo, 1993).

It can be concluded from the published research that a positive relationship exists between applied psychophysiological therapies and improvements in the subjective well-being of many patients with tinnitus. Applied psychophysiological therapies include not only relaxation and biofeedback, but cognitive-behavioral therapies. The review by Kirsch et al. (1989) speculates about differences among the results of various studies and the methodological shortcomings of many of them. This includes the lack of sufficient information in many studies. Nevertheless, Kirsch et al. conclude that "improvements can occur on self-reported annoyance, intrusiveness, and coping ability" (p. 63). This review reported about the same state and trait anxiety levels for patients with tinnitus as for general medical/surgical patients. This argues against the idea that these patients are more anxious than other patients.

A study by Podoshin et al. (1991) not only supported the use of biofeedback for tinnitus, but claimed it produced better results than a medicine used to treat tinnitus and vertigo. The biofeedback involved 30-minute sessions with bifrontal EMG and visual and auditory feedback. Advantages of the study included comparisons with other active treatments (medication and acupuncture) and multiple control conditions (placebo biofeedback and placebo medication). All the nonbiofeedback groups did more poorly than the biofeedback group of 10 patients (6 male patients, 4 female patients; mean age 56, range 47–66 years). Unfortunately, no information was provided about the biofeedback instruments and procedures, and no EMG data were presented.

Evaluation of tinnitus with an audiological procedure for matching the frequency and intensity of the tinnitus with tones showed no change in pitch (presumably in any group, but this was not clear) (Podoshin et al., 1991). Subjective ratings were the indicators of improvement, which was most significant while resting. The ratings dropped from an average of 2.7 (moderate to severe) to 1.6 (mild to moderate). For the most part, ratings were slightly higher during rest, as expected. This study showed that EMG biofeedback can be better than some other treatments. However, it fell short in the use of biofeedback procedures. Also, the study did not provide the types of data practitioners need and expect to see in published studies using biofeedback.

There are no significant correlations between audiological measures of tinnitus intensity and self-reported ratings of disturbance (Kirsch et al., 1987). An important methodological note is that tinnitus intensity can vary. Thus ratings provide an index over days and weeks, whereas masking measures reflect only one specific moment. Other studies also show little, if any, correlations between audiological measures of intensity and self-reported ratings of disturbance. In the Kirsch et al. (1987) study, there were substantial drops in frontal EMG from a 5-minute baseline to the last 5 minutes of most of the six relaxation and two EMG feedback sessions. These drops were much more than during session one. The researchers limited the EMG feedback to the frontal area, which is not "the best measure of overall muscle relaxation," as Kirsch et al. (1987, p. 303) would have us believe. There also were not enough data to justify their statement that subjects showed "successful learning of the relaxation techniques, as indicated by the EMG data" (p. 310). In addition, there was no specification of whether or not the therapist was with the subjects during the sessions. Kirsch et al. (1987) reported a 40-minute session.

In general, most studies of biofeedback treatment for tinnitus to date have failed to include stress management components into their training and often have only attended to resting baseline levels, which have been shown to be less characteristic of a disorder than stress reactivity levels (cf. Flor & Turk, 1989). In addition, most studies have not selected patients in whom a relationship of tinnitus and elevated tension levels of stress reactivity levels could be documented.

Relaxation, Hypnosis, Support/Counseling, and Therapeutic Noise

Several studies have examined the effect of such procedures as relaxation, self-hypnosis, and support/counseling. In the meta-analysis by Andersson and Lyttkens (1999), only two hypnosis studies were included, both with positive effect size. Education/information/support alone showed mixed results in the meta-analysis, but some effect in a study by Attias et al. (1993)—who demonstrated, however, the highest effects for a self-hypnosis treatment, whereas tinnitus masking alone had no effect. The data on relaxation training alone are mixed. Several studies did not report any effects (e.g., Ireland, Wilson, Tonkin, & Platt-Hepworth, 1985; Dineen, Doyle, & Bench, 1997; Dineen, Doyle, Bench, & Perry, 1999), and the meta-analysis by Andersson and Lyttkens (1999) shows partially negative or very low effect sizes combined with high effect sizes for the Ireland et al. (1985) study. A study by Davies, McKenna, and Hallam (1995) found applied relaxation training to be as effective as a cognitive-behavioral treatment. Support or counseling seemed to have only little effect, as the Andersson and Lyttkens (1999) meta-analysis suggests. The use of broad-band white noise as suggested by Jastreboff was tested in the study by Dineen et al. (1997, 1999) and was not found to produce any specific effect on tinnitus, except for better coping in those with low coping ability. In most studies, tinnitus-related annoyance and other affective variables were altered, rather than tinnitus loudness.

Cognitive-Behavioral Treatment

Cognitive-behavioral therapies can help patients change their thoughts about their symptoms and can help reduce the anxiety and physical tension that often accompany the symptoms. In the meta-analysis by Andersson and Lyttkens (1999), the cognitive-behavioral treatments showed the highest effect sizes; however, only two biofeedback studies were included in this review. Kirsch et al. (1989) also encouraged more investigation of cognitive techniques. Jakes et al. (1992) reported on a controlled group outcome study of cognitive techniques. The value of cognitive therapy received support from this well-controlled group design with 84 subjects. They started with 2 weeks of baseline. They then compared 30 subjects receiving 5 weeks of group cognitive therapy (GCT), subjects in three other treatment groups, and a waiting-list control group. The other treatment groups received a masker therapy, a placebo masker, or a combination of GCT and a masker. Follow-up assessment was at 3 months. Measures included the TEQ and IWDA. "Only patients receiving GCT (with or without a masker) were significantly improved over baseline on a tinnitus distress questionnaire" (p. 67), although this "emerged only at the 3-month follow-up assessment" (p. 78). Other studies have confirmed that cognitive-behavioral treatments mainly influence the amount of annoyance related to tinnitus, but not tinnitus loudness (e.g., Davies et al., 1995; Henry & Wilson, 1996).

Part of the value of the Jakes et al. (1992) study is its support for the potential use of cognitive therapy in the treatment package for subjective tinnitus. However, one cannot conclude that it is better than biofeedback or combinations of comprehensive cognitive-behavioral, biofeedback, and relaxation treatments.

The research and clinical insights of Podoshin et al. (1991) add other valuable information. For example, they point out potential compliance problems with daily logs of symptoms. They note the potential for countertherapeutic effects when therapists try to monitor some people closely. The "Implications . . ." section below contains ideas gleaned partly from their report.

Matching-to-Sample Feedback

The interesting technique of matching-to-sample feedback is worth noting as innovative and as an example of direct rather than indirect feedback. First reported by Ince and colleagues with 2 cases, they also provided a single-group design with 30 patients (Ince et al., 1987). In the Ince et al. (1987) procedure, researchers matched audiometrically produced sounds to each subject's perception of the tinnitus sound and fed back that sound. They determined thresholds for the specific tinnitus sound of each person. They used white noise, narrow-band noise, pure tone sound, or a combination of sounds. Based on each person's description, the experimenter selected a decibel level, a frequency level, and a stimulus. Each subject guided the adjustment process to help make the stimulus sound as close as possible to the tinnitus sound. The experimenter then slightly reduced the loudness of the stimulus. The goal was to reduce the tinnitus matched to the new loudness level. At the end of each 60 seconds, each subject reported whether the tinnitus reduction matched the external stimulus. If so, there was another reduction of 5 decibels of the external stimulus after a 30-second rest period. This process continued for up to 15 trials or until the tinnitus stopped.

Everyone had 12 or fewer sessions, and the investigators encouraged practice many times a day with the self-regulation method. The authors noted that those who practiced the required task as instructed "tended to improve more rapidly than those who did not" (p. 180). However, "exactly how often the participants did practice and precisely how they practiced between sessions are not known" (p. 180).

The Kirsch et al. (1989) review reported that "nearly all subjects demonstrated a marked reduction in tinnitus loudness, with 84 percent reducing the tinnitus by 10–62 [decibels] and several eliminating the tinnitus completely" (p. 61). The review acknowledged their impressive results, but cautioned readers that global self-reports alone were the basis for assuming generalization outside the office session, and there were no long-term follow-up data. Moreover, fatigue or habituation of the auditory system could have accounted for the changes observed in the office.

Tinnitus Retraining Therapy

Tinnitus retraining therapy has been propagated by Jastreboff (e.g., Jastreboff & Jastreboff, 2000) and consists of extensive counseling combined with the use of *audiological sound generators*, with the goal of decreasing both cortical and ANS activity associated with the tinnitus problem. According to Jastreboff and Jastreboff, this treatment needs to span at least 18 months to be successful. Although this intervention has received much attention over the past few years, neither its content nor its efficacy has been clearly documented. No manual for the treatment is available, and it is probably also not needed, simply because the treatment consists only of some general counseling and the use of sound generators. The patients are counseled not to avoid noise and sounds, but rather to avoid silence, in order to heighten the level of stimulation related to nontinnitus sounds. They are also told that the tinnitus should not be masked by a sound generator, but that it should remain audible, and that the sound generator should merely provide enrichment of environmental sounds. Patients with hearing loss are fitted with hearing aids—not necessarily to improve hearing, but to increase the level of input to the ear and the higher brain centers. The Jastreboffs place their patients in five categories ranging from 0 to 4 and suggest somewhat different combinations of their procedures, depending on the presence or absence of hearing loss, hyperacusis, life impact, and the presence of sound-induced exacerbation. As Kröner-Herwig and her collaborators (2000) justly point out, there is surprisingly little evidence for the efficacy of this treatment, despite the claims of Jastreboff and his colleagues that it is highly effective.

Treatment Directed toward the Alteration of Cortical Plasticity

Based on the Mühlnickel et al. (1998) study showing plastic alterations in auditory cortex, and reports in the animal literature that sensory discrimination training can alter the tonotopic map in auditory cortex (Recanzone, Schreiner, & Merzenich, 1993), Flor, Hoffmann, Struve, and Diesch (in press) have devised several procedures designed to directly alter the brain activity of patients with tinnitus. "Auditory training therapy" determines the tinnitus frequency and then presents pairs of tones close to the tinnitus frequency to a patient, who has to discriminate these tones and receives feedback on the accuracy of the discrimination. The tones are successively moved closer together to make the tasks more and more difficult. The therapy is modeled after the work of Recanzone et al. (1993), who found an expansion of frequencies that were presented in animal experiments. Similar changes in the representation of sounds were also reported in healthy humans by Mennig, Roberts, and Pantev (2000). In an initial study with thirteen patients, Flor et al. (in press) found significant changes in tinnitus severity and annoyance in the treatment group.

A second type of intervention to alter the representation of sound in the brain was first described by Pantev, Wollbrink, Roberts, Engelien, and Lütkenhöner (1999) in healthy humans. These authors showed that the use of a notch filter when a piece of music was played to subjects over an extended period of time led to a decrease of the space this notched-out frequency occupied in primary somatosensory cortex. Flor and colleagues have used this principle to notch out the tinnitus frequency and have combined these techniques with the discrimination procedures described above. It is, however, still too early to determine whether these additional techniques have an additive effect.

IMPLICATIONS, GUIDELINES, AND LIMITS

Intake and Assessment of Tinnitus

- Include pre- and posttreatment audiological assessments.
- Consider including patients who suffer from severe tinnitus. Expect that extreme distress and suicidal thoughts will characterize some patients.
- Ask questions about sleep problems predating the tinnitus.
- Consider daily self-report records about how bothersome the tinnitus is during activities, rest, and sleep.
- Expect improvement to be in the form of less disturbance during rest and sleep than during activities.
- Expect improvement from the moderate-to-severe range to the mild-to-moderate range.
- Consider periodic sample weeks for getting symptom logs.
- Consider using the IWDA, the TEQ, and/or the MTI.
- Some patients will improve at or about five sessions. However, review progress at about five sessions, and consider more sessions if the data justify it.
- Plan on office follow-up rather than relying on phone follow-up.

Interventions

- Consider multiple stress management therapies, such as multiple relaxation therapies, biofeedback-assisted muscle and ANS relaxation, and cognitive-behavioral therapies.
- Consider using bifrontal EMG feedback at least for some patients, but also consider using the frontalis–posterior neck EMG placement to assess temporalis and occipitalis tension better.
- Consider passive relaxation rather than tense–release procedures, especially for the cephalic and neck muscles.
- Include visual rather than audio feedback, which might confound the results. If audio feedback must be used, then consider sounds that the patient selects as pleasant and useful, rather than limiting the sounds to a predetermined type. (Some of the published reports used clicks.)
- Include cognitive-behavioral therapy focused at least on the beliefs assessed by the TEQ, other measures, and interviews.
- Consider graduated exposure procedures. For example, use relaxation with biofeedback and cognitive procedures while the patient gradually moves in 1- to 5-decibel steps from a state in which an audiologist ideally masks the tinnitus to the least-masked state.
- If there is serious depression, treat it. Include cognitive therapy and address topics in addition to the tinnitus.
- Consider group treatment; however, realize that many patients need individual treatment.
- Assume that some patients are unwilling to accept the idea of learning how to adapt to the tinnitus. They remain focused on finding physical causes and total cures.
- Assume that many patients do accept the rationale and premises of the behavioral explanations and therapies.
- Consider investing time in patient education.
- Assume that the positive effects of treatment may "sink in" after cessation of formal treatment, especially if the treatment is only a few sessions.
- Consider using behavioral and cognitive-behavioral techniques, such as distraction techniques (like those used in cognitive pain management), modification of underlying assumptions, and problem-solving techniques.
- Consider treatments such as medications and/or audiological maskers/sound generators.
- Consider gradual exposure to sound for patients with hyperacusis and for those who avoid sound and noisy environments due to their tinnitus.
- Consider the use of hearing aids in patients with hearing loss.

SPECULATIONS ON HOW BIOFEEDBACK WORKS FOR TINNITUS

One way in which biofeedback and relaxation may work for tinnitus is that they have "distraction" effects. These treatments help people focus on other body areas, on the feedback stimuli, on breathing, and on other cognitive activities. Patients may become more adept at distraction as they reduce the tension, arousal, and cognitions associated with focusing on the tinnitus. This may be especially applicable during rest and when efforts to sleep.

Another possibility is that "habituation" effects occur after repeated exposure to the tinnitus during relaxation and biofeedback sessions in the office and at home. This alone would not explain improvements in patients with long-term, chronic tinnitus. However, there could be some habituation when a gradual exposure procedure is combined with physiological and cognitive changes.

Cognitive changes include positive expectations and decreased thoughts of helplessness or other anxious cognitions. Successfully challenging and refuting thoughts of the tinnitus as a catastrophe and a disabling condition could be very helpful here, as these methods are with some other symptoms. Biofeedback probably functions in both feedforward and feedback ways to guide, reinforce, and convince people of their psychophysiological self-regulation and dexterity. It could similarly affect some patients with tinnitus.

Improved sleep may play an important role. For a variety of reasons, many of these patients seem to achieve improved sleep. This factor could affect a variety of daytime symptoms, including the ability to adjust to the primary symptoms. People with psychophysiological sleep-onset insomnia often benefit from relaxation and cognitive strategies at bedtime. At least for some people, this result is probably the result of changed cognitions at bedtime.

We know of no research that has studied sleep efficiency, sleep architecture, and related sleep parameters among patients with tinnitus receiving the behavioral interventions discussed here. However, it is a logical speculation that decreased time to sleep onset and reduction of other symptoms associated with sleep deprivation may help. They certainly may result in an increased sense of general well-being, neurocognitive efficiency, and confidence in managing otherwise more distressing symptoms.

The speculations above do not exclude the potential role of reduced physiological muscle tension and sympathetic nervous system arousal, although there is not enough direct evidence for accepting the specific role of these factors. For selected patients with evidence of TMDs, such as teeth clenching and grinding, this explanation may play an important role.

Other factors are also of potential relevance. During a focused intervention, some patients may make other changes without telling a practitioner or research investigator (e.g., decreasing or stopping caffeine usage, stopping or changing medication, or getting their ears cleaned out by an otolaryngologist). They may also change some stressful parts of their lives without telling a practitioner. They may get a bedside sound masker, or audiotapes of pleasant sounds, or music that helps them adapt and sleep better. Practitioners should not assume that patients will report all these changes; they should ask tactfully.

In conclusion, relaxation therapies, EMG biofeedback, and cognitive-behavioral therapy can help in the management of subjective tinnitus for some people.

GLOSSARY

AUDIOLOGICAL MASKERS OR SOUND GENERATORS. One type of treatment for tinnitus. A small instrument is worn in the ear and produces more acceptable noise than the noise in the ear. Some favor a sound that can mask the tinnitus (in this case, the instrument is called a *masker*). Others insist that a low-level white noise that does not mask the tinnitus sound is better (in this case, the instrument is called a *sound generator*).

CORTICAL REORGANIZATION (CORTICAL PLASTICITY). A change in the functional architecture of the sensorimotor areas of the cortex related to injury or stimulation and learning.

CRANIOMANDIBULAR DISORDERS (CMDs). Pertaining to the head and mandible. Sometimes used interchangeably with *temporomandibular disorders* (see below).

HABITUATION. Adaptation or adjustment to novel conditions or stimuli, such as an office, instrumentation, psychophysiological recordings, or auditory or visual stimuli.

MATCHING-TO-SAMPLE FEEDBACK. An experimental procedure for treating tinnitus, which involves matching audiometric produced sounds to each person's perception of a tinnitus sound, and feeding back that sound. Developed by L. P. Ince and colleagues (1987).

MENIÈRE'S DISEASE. A disorder in which an increased fluid level in the labyrinth of the inner ear leads to disturbances in the production and resorption of fluid in the endolymph.

OTOACOUSTIC EMISSIONS. Ear sounds originating in the ear that can be objectively determined.

OTOLOGICAL. Pertaining to otology, the branch of medicine dealing with medical/surgical treatments of the ear.

STOMATOGNATHIC. Denoting the mouth and jaws together.

TEMPOROMANDIBULAR DISORDERS (TMDs). Pertaining to disorders involving the temporal and mandibular areas of the head. (See also Glaros & Lausten, Chapter 15, this volume.)

ACKNOWLEDGMENT

We thank Dagmar Hoffmann for help with figures and tables and with the editing of the references.

NOTES

1. The questionnaires are not yet published or available in the United States. Until there is a publisher of the English version, readers should consider writing to R. S. Hallam, PhD, for copies. His address is Psychology Department, University of East London, Romford Road, London E15 4LZ, United Kingdom. (See also Resources)
2. Scales of the Hiller and Goebel (1992) analysis:

1. Cognitive and Emotional Distress (8 core items, 12 associated items) (27.2% of variance).
2. Intrusiveness (5 core items, 3 associated items) (6.7% of variance).
3. Auditory and perceptual difficulties (5 core items, 2 associated items) (5.4% of variance).
4. Sleep disturbances (4 core items) (4.9% of variance).
5. Somatic Complaints (3 core items) (3.4% of variance).

The core and associated items constituting each scale are as follows:

1. Core items = 3, 13, 17, 21, 27, 43, 44, 47; associated = 1, 5, 8, 11, 16, 18–20, 28, 37, 39, 41.
2. Core items = 7, 10, 15, 35, 48; associated = 5, 20, 34.
3. Core items = 9, 14, 26, 33, 38; associated = 2, 50.
4. Core items = 4, 12, 31, 36.
5. Core items = 22, 25, 51.

RESOURCES

Relevant Web sites include the following:

http://www.tinnitus-pjj.com (Jastrebroff's Web site, with information on tinnitus retraining therapy).
http://www.tinnitus.org (Hazell's home page, with information about tinnitus retraining therapy, guidelines, and examples for patients).
http://www.tinnitus-audiology.com (Oregon Tinnitus and Hyperacusis Treatment Center, with sound samples, a discussion group for sufferers, examples of tinnitus types and diagnoses, treatments, and medications).
http://neuro.bio.tu-darmstadt.de/langner/tinnitus-html/english/tinnitus.htm (Langner's Web site, with facts about tinnitus, sound examples, self-help information).
http://www.ata.org (American Tinnitus Association, with information about tinnitus, program of the association, large bibliography).
http://www.ohsu.edu/ohrc/tinnitusclinic/index.htm (Oregon Health Sciences University Tinnitus Clinic, with broad information on tinnitus, treatments, things to avoid).
http://www.barajas.vanaga.es/tinnitus/tq.htm

The following books are useful as bibliotherapy for patients:

Habets, B. (1998). *The tinnitus handbook.* New York: United Research.
Henry, J. L., & Wilson, P. H. (2001). *Tinnitus: A self-management guide for the ringing in your ears.* Boston: Allyn & Bacon.
Kellerhals, B., & Zogg, R. (1999). *Tinnitus rehabilitation by retraining: A workbook for sufferers, their doctors and other health care professionals.* Farmington, CT: Karger.

Sheppard, L., & Hawkridge, A. (1997). *Tinnitus: Learning to live with it.* New York: Ashgrove Press.
Vernon, J. A. (1997). *Tinnitus: Treatment and relief.* Boston: Allyn & Bacon.
Vernon, J. A., & Sanders, B. T. (2001). *Tinnitus: Questions and answers.* Boston: Allyn & Bacon.

REFERENCES

*Literature especially recommended for practitioners.

*Andersson, G. (2001). The role of psychology in managing tinnitus: A cognitive behavioral approach. *Seminars in Hearing, 22,* 65–76.
*Andersson, G., & Lyttkens, L. (1999). A meta-analytic review of psychological treatments for tinnitus. *British Journal of Audiology, 33,* 201–210.
Andersson, G., Lyttkens, L., Hirvelä, C., Fumark, T., Tillfors, M., & Fredrikson, M. (2000). Regional cerebral blood flow during tinnitus: A PET case study with lidocaine and auditory stimulation. *Acta Otolaryngologica, 120,* 967–972.
*Andersson, G., Lyttkens, L., & Larsen, H. C. (1999). Distinguishing levels of tinnitus distress. *Clinical Otolaryngology, 24,* 404–410.
Andersson, G., Melin, L., Hägnebo, C., Scott, B., & Lindberg, P. (1995). A review of psychological treatment approaches for patients suffering from tinnitus. *Annals of Behavioral Medicine, 17,* 357–366.
Attias, J., Shemesh, Z., Sohmer, H., Gold, S., Shoham, C., & Faraggi, D. (1993). Comparison between self-hypnosis, masking and attentiveness for alleviation of chronic tinnitus. *Audiology, 32,* 205–212.
Borton, T. E., Moore, W. H., Jr., & Clark, S. R (1981). Electromyographic feedback treatment for tinnitus aurium. *Journal of Speech and Hearing Disorders, 46,* 39–45.
Davies, S., McKenna, I., & Hallam, R. S. (1995). Relaxation and cognitive therapy: Controlled trial in chronic tinnitus. *Psychological Health, 10,* 129–143.
Dineen, R., Doyle, J., & Bench, J. (1997). Managing tinnitus: A comparison of different approaches to tinnitus management training. *British Journal of Audiology, 31,* 331–344.
Dineen, R., Doyle, J., Bench, J., & Perry, A. (1999). The influence of training on tinnitus perception: An evaluation 12 months after tinnitus management training. *British Journal of Audiology, 33,* 29–51.
Dobie, R. A., Sakai, C. S. Sullivan, M. D., Katon, W. J., & Russo, J. (1993). Antidepressant treatment of tinnitus patients: Report of a randomized clinical trial and clinical prediction of benefit. *American Journal of Otology, 14,* 18–23.
Dorland's illustrated medical dictionary (27th ed.). (1988). Philadelphia: Saunders.
Duckro, P. N., Pollard, C. A., Bray, H. D., & Scheiter, L. (1984). Comprehensive behavioral management of complex tinnitus: A case illustration. *Biofeedback and Self-Regulation, 9,* 459–469.
Elfner, L. F., May, J. G., Moore, J. D., & Mendelson, J. M. (1981). Effects of EMG and thermal training on tinnitus: A case study. *Biofeedback and Self-Regulation, 6,* 517–521.
Flor, H., Elbert, T., Knecht, S., Wienbruch, C., Pantev, C., Birbaumer, N., Larbig, W., & Taub, E. (1995). Phantom-limb pain as a perceptual correlate of cortical reorganization following arm amputation. *Nature, 375,* 482–484.
Flor, H., Hoffmann, D., Struve, M., & Diesch, E. (2002). *The Multidimensional Tinnitus Inventory.* Manuscript submitted for publication.
Flor, H., Hoffmann, D., Struve, M., & Diesch, E. (in press). Effects of an auditory discrimination training on tinnitus. *Applied Psychophysiology and Biofeedback.*
Flor, H., & Turk, D. C. (1989). Psychophysiology of chronic pain: Do chronic pain patients exhibit symptom-specific psychophysiological responses? *Psychological Bulletin, 105,* 215–259.
Grossan, M. (1976). Treatment of subjective tinnitus with biofeedback. *Ear, Nose, and Throat, 55,* 314–318.
Hallam, R. S., Jakes, S. C., & Hinchcliffe, R. (1988). Cognitive variables in tinnitus annoyance. *British Journal of Clinical Psychology, 27,* 213–222.
*Hallam, R. S., Rachman, S., & Hinchcliffe, R. (1987). Psychological aspects of tinnitus. In S. Rachman (Ed.), *Contributions to medical psychology.* Oxford: Pergamon Press.
Haralambous, G., Wilson, P. H., Platt-Hepworth, S., Tonkin, J. P., Rae Hensley, V., & Kavanagh, D. (1987). EMG biofeedback in the treatment of tinnitus: An experimental evaluation. *Behaviour Research and Therapy, 25,* 49–55.
Hazell, J. W., & Jastreboff, P. J. (1990). Tinnitus: I. Auditory mechanisms: A model for tinnitus and impairment. *Journal of Otolaryngology, 19,* 1–5.
Henry, J. L., & Wilson, P. H. (1996). The psychological management of tinnitus: Comparison of a combined cognitive educational programm, education alone and a waiting-list control. *International Tinnitus Journal, 2,* 9–20.
Hiller, W., & Goebel, G. (1992). A psychometric study of complaints in chronic tinnitus. *Journal of Psychosomatic Research, 36,* 337–348.

Hiller, W., Goebel, G., & Schindelmann, U. (1999). Developing a structured interview to assess audiological, aetiological and psychological variables of tinnitus. In J. Hazell (Ed.), *Proceedings of the Sixth International Tinnitus Seminar*. Cambridge, England: Tinnitus and Hyperacusis Centre.

House, J. W., Miller, L., & House, P. R. (1977). Severe tinnitus: Treatment with biofeedback training. *Transactions of the American Academy of Ophthalmology and Otolaryngology, 84*, 697–703.

*Ince, L. P., Greene, R. Y., Alba, A., & Zaretsky, H. H. (1987). A matching-to-sample feedback technique for training self-control of tinnitus. *Health Psychology, 6*, 173–182.

Ireland, C. E., Wilson, P. H., Tonkin, J. P., & Platt-Hepworth, S. (1985). An evaluation of relaxation training in the treatment of tinnitus. *Behaviour Research and Therapy, 23*, 423–430.

Jakes, S. C., Hallam, R. S., McKenna, L., & Hinchcliffe, R. (1992). Group cognitive therapy for medical patients: An application to tinnitus. *Cognitive Therapy and Research, 16*, 67–82.

Jakes, S. C., Hallam, R. S., Rachman, S., & Hinchcliffe, R. (1986). The effects or reassurance, relaxation training and distraction on chronic tinnitus sufferers. *Behaviour Research and Therapy, 26*, 497–508.

Jastreboff, P. J. (1990). Phantom auditory perception (tinnitus): Mechanisms of generation and perception. *Neuroscience Research, 8*, 221–254.

Jastreboff, P. J., Gray, W. C., & Gold, S. L. (1996). Neurophysiological approach to tinnitus patients. *American Journal of Otology, 17*, 236–240.

*Jastreboff, P. J., & Jastreboff, M. M. (2000). Tinnitus retraining therapy (TRT) as a method for treatment of tinnitus and hyperacusis patients. *Journal of the American Academy of Audiology, 11*, 162–177.

*Kaltenbach, J. A. (2000). Neurophysiologic mechanisms of tinnitus. *Journal of the American Academy of Audiology, 11*, 125–137.

Kerns, R. D., Turk, D. C., & Rudy, T. E. (1985). The West Haven–Yale Multidimensional Pain Inventory. *Pain, 23*, 345–356.

*Kirsch, C. A., Blanchard, E. B., & Parnes, S. M. (1987). A multiple-baseline evaluation of the treatment of subjective tinnitus with relaxation training and biofeedback. *Biofeedloack and Self-Regulation, 12*, 295–311.

*Kirsch, C. A., Blanchard, E. B., & Parnes, S. M. (1989). A review of the efficacy of behavioral techniques in the treatment of subjective tinnitus. *Annals of Behavioral Medicine, 11*, 58–65.

*Kröner-Herwig, B., Biesinger, E., Gerhards, F., Goebel, G., Greimel, K. V., & Hiller, W. (2000). Retraining therapy for chronic tinnitus: A critical analysis of its status. *Scandinavian Audiology, 29*, 67–78.

Kuk, F. K., Tyler, R S., Russell, D., & Jordan, H. (1990). The psychometric properties of a tinnitus handicap questionnaire. *Ear and Hearing, 11*, 434–445.

Levine, S. B., & Snow, J. B., Jr. (1987). Pulsatile tinnitus. *Laryngoscope, 97*, 401–406.

Lockwood, A. H., Salvi, R. J., Burkard, R. F., Galantowicz, P. J., Coad, M. L., & Wack, D. S. (1999). Neuroanatomy of tinnitus. *Scandinavian Audiology Supplement, 51*, 47–52.

Lockwood, A. H., Salvi, R. J., Coad, M. L., Towsley, M. L., Wack, D. S., & Murphy, B. W. (1998). The functional neuroanatomy of tinnitus: Evidence for limbic system links and neural plasticity. *Neurology, 50*, 114–120.

Mennig, H., Roberts, L. E., & Pantev, C. (2000). Plastic changes in the auditory cortex induced by intensive frequency discrimination training. *Neuroreport, 11*, 817–822.

Mirz, F., Gjedde, A., Sodkilde-Jorgensen, H., & Pedersen, C. B. (2000). Functional brain imaging of tinnitus-like perception induced by aversive auditory stimuli. *Neuroreport, 11*, 633–637.

Moller, A. R. (2000). Similarities between severe tinnitus and chronic pain. *Journal of the American Academy of Audiology, 11*, 115–124.

Mühlnickel. W., Elbert, T., Taub, E., & Flor, H. (1998). Reorganization of auditory cortex in tinnitus. *Proceedings of the National Academy of Sciences USA, 95*, 10340–10343.

Nadol, J. B., Jr. (1993). Hearing loss. *New England Journal of Medicine, 329*, 1092–1102.

Pantev, C., Wollbrink, A. Roberts, L. E., Engelien, A., & Lütkenhöner, B. (1999). Short-term plasticity of the human auditory cortex. *Brain Research, 842*, 192–199.

Parving, A., Hein, H.O., Suadicani, B., Ostri, B., & Gyntelberg, F. (1993). Epidemiology of hearing disorders. *Scandinavian Audiology, 22*, 101–107.

*Podoshin, L., Ben-David, Y., Fradis, M., Gerstel, R., & Felner, H. (1991). Idiopathic subjective tinnitus treated by biofeedback, acupuncture and drug therapy. *Ear, Nose and Throat Journal, 70*, 284–289.

Recanzone, G. H., Schreiner, C. E., & Merzenich, M. M. (1993). Plasticity in the frequency representation of primary auditory cortex following discrimination training in adult owl monkeys. *Journal of Neuroscience, 13*, 87–103.

Rubinstein, G. (1993). Tinnitus and craniomandibular disorders: Is there a link? *Swedish Dental Journal Supplement, 95*, 1–45.

*Schleuning, A. J., II. (1991). Management of the patient with tinnitus. *Medical Clinics of North America, 75*, 1225–1237.

Turk, D. C., & Rudy, T. E. (1988). Toward an empirically-derived taxonomy of chronic pain patients: Integration of psychological assessment data. *Journal of Consulting and Clinical Psychology, 56*, 233–238.

Wallhäuser-Franke, E., Braun, S., & Langner, G. (1996). Salycylate alters 2-DG uptake in the auditory system: A model for tinnitus? *Neuroreport, 8,* 1585–1588.

Walsh, W. M., & Gerley, P. P. (1985). Thermal biofeedback and the treatment of tinnitus. *Laryngoscope, 95,* 987–989.

Weissman, J. L., & Hirsch, B. E. (2000). Imaging tinnitus. *Radiology, 216,* 342–349.

Wilson, P. H., Haralambous, G., Ireland, C., Platt-Hapworth, S., & Tonkin, J. (1987). Psychological management of tinnitus: Effects of relaxation training and biofeedback. In H. Feldmann (Ed.), *Proceedings III International Tinnitus Seminar.* Karlsruhe, Germany: Harsch.

Wilson, P. H., & Henry, J. L. (1993). Psychological approaches in the management of tinnitus. *Australian Journal of Otolaryngology, 1,* 296–302.

Fibromyalgia Syndrome

MARK S. SCHWARTZ
JEFFREY M. THOMPSON

Relaxation therapies with surface electromyographic (EMG) biofeedback are part of acceptable treatment protocols for fibromyalgia syndrome (FMS) and related diagnoses. Patient education literature from the American College of Rheumatology (ACR), the American Fibromyalgia Syndrome Association, and journal articles support these treatments for FMS and related conditions (McCain, 1990; Thompson, 1990, 2000; see also the "Resources" section at the end of the chapter). These treatments are most effective as components of a multidisciplinary treatment program.

These patients are very commonly seen by practitioners (particularly mental health professionals) who use biofeedback for reasons in addition to muscle pain (e.g., history of emotional trauma, psychological problems, irritable bowel syndrome [IBS], anxiety disorders, migraine headaches, depression). Thus it is important to have an understanding of the multiple facets of this disorder. (As in other chapters, italics on first use of a term indicate that the term is included in the glossary at the chapter's end.)

TERMS AND DEFINITIONS

The most widely used term and the term now accepted by the ACR is "fibromyalgia syndrome" (FS or FMS; abbreviated in this chapter as FMS) (Wolfe et al., 1990). However, the disorder is often referred to only as "fibromyalgia." Specific criteria for diagnosis are found in many references, including those by Thompson (2000), Wolfe et al. (1990), and Okifugi and Turk (1999); they include widespread pain of greater than 3 months' duration and 11 of 18 "tender points." The history of the terms is discussed by Thompson (1990, 2000). There is abundant literature discussing other related diagnoses and terms, and how they are different from, overlap, and blend into FMS (Thompson, 1990, 2000; Wolfe et al., 1990).

Gradual onset of symptoms is typical among persons diagnosed with FMS. However, substantial subsets of these patients report physical or emotional traumas that immediately precede or seem to precipitate the FMS onset. The nature of the relationship is unclear. Physical traumas include motor vehicle accidents, surgery, work-related injuries, and viral illness (Aaron et al., 1997).

The terms *tension myalgia* and *myofascial pain syndrome* (MPS) typically refer to more localized muscle pain without systemic symptoms. The distinctions blur, however, when one observes (1) that patients can start with local or regional pain that later becomes widespread; and (2) that multiple sites can occur among patients with MPS, with systemic symptoms emerging later (Thompson, 1990, 1996). This concept of a continuum of pain, in which FMS represents only one end of the spectrum of muscle pain and not a distinct disease entity, is gaining more widespread acceptance (Wolfe, 1997; Bennett, 1999).

Tension myalgia is a term that covers the spectrum of muscle pain, from localized to whole-body. It is no longer used professionally, because of the widespread use and acceptance of the terms FMS and MPS. It is still useful in patient education, because it is descriptive and avoids the "baggage" of the term FMS (e.g., the premature elevation of FMS to the status of disease by the lay public and the medicolegal system). Myalgia is what the patients feel—pain in the muscles and their attachments. Tension is what is seen clinically in most patients—the increased muscle tension due to motor dysfunction, overuse, deconditioning, and/or postural stress (which is often made worse by psychological stressors). This overactivation, inability to relax, and incoordination are among the targets for the use of surface EMG (hereafter referred to simply as EMG) biofeedback.

PREVALENCE AND EPIDEMIOLOGY

It is difficult to estimate the prevalence of a condition for which there are still disagreements about terminology and definitions. However, estimates for the United States, England, and Scandinavia suggest that from about 1% to 11% of the population is affected (Croft, Rigby, Boswell, Schollum, & Silman, 1993; Schochat, Croft, & Raspe, 1994). These estimates include from 3 to 6 million Americans (Baumstark & Buckelew, 1992; Donaldson, Sella, & Mueller, 1998a). In rheumatology offices, the prevalence estimate ranges from 15% to 20%. Thus, whatever definition and criteria are used, this is a common set of symptoms.

HEALTH CARE SEEKING: PSYCHOLOGICAL FACTORS

Related to prevalence, as well as etiology and treatment, are the factors that lead persons with FMS symptoms to seek medical care. Medical care seeking among patients with FMS is associated with a history of diagnosable psychological problems and more psychological distress (Aaron et al., 1996). There is also support for the view that emotional trauma is a major factor predicting medical care seeking among these patients (Aaron et al., 1997): Reported trauma is more common among patients with FMS than among nonpatients with FMS, but emotional trauma was the only significant predictor of seeking health care. A history of physical abuse or sexual/physical abuse was not predictive in this study. This implies that people with FMS who seek medical care for FMS and/or for other pain symptoms are different from persons with FMS who do not seek such help. At least with women, an emotional trauma history appears to contribute to psychological and psychophysiological changes that have a major impact on seeking health care.

ETIOLOGIES / MECHANISMS

The confusion surrounding the definition of muscle pain syndromes is mirrored in the search for an etiology. Most of the early explanations addressed local muscle pain and focused on abnormalities of the muscle. Specific histological changes have eluded investigators. The current theory for MPS and trigger points involves abnormalities of the motor end plate (the area where nerves connect to muscles) (Simons & Travell, 1999). Most recent theories regarding FMS and widespread muscle pain focus on changes in the central nervous system (CNS) with sensitization of pain mechanisms (Bennett, 1999). The central mechanism theories invoke abnormalities in one or more of the following: the neuroendocrine system (the *hypothalamic–pituitary–adrenal* axis (Crofford, 1996; Crofford Engleberg, & Demitrack, 1996) and *hypothalamic–pituitary–thyroid axis*[1] (Abud-Mendoza et al., 1997), neurotransmitters (e.g., serotonin, calcitonin-gene-related peptide, others), *substance P* (Russell, 1998; Russell et al., 1994; Weigent, Bradley, Blalock, & Alcaron, 1998), and/or growth hormone (Thompson, 2000; Okifuji & Turk, 1999; Bennett, 1999; Fransen & Russell, 1996).

Part of the problem is that FMS is not a homogeneous disorder. There are many likely pathways to the final result of chronic widespread pain and dysfunction. Early, when the pain is more localized and the patient has few systemic or psychological symptoms, the major problem may well be a disordered motor system. As the pain becomes chronic and widespread, and interferes with function, the complexities of a chronic pain syndrome (with all the biopsychosocial problems implied by that term) arise. In any given patient, a different set of factors may be playing the major role in that patient's pain syndrome.

A preliminary but integrated and dynamic process model (Okifuji & Turk, 1999) captures the diversity and complexity of FMS. This model integrates premorbid factors, precipitating factors, and stress responses. The importance of these factors varies from person to person. A major implication of this model is that one treatment will not be effective for all or most persons with FMS. Tailoring and matching treatments to patients will improve efficacy.

SYMPTOMS AND MEASURES: GUIDELINES AND IMPLICATIONS

Pain

Tender Points and the Tender Point Index

Tender points and widespread pain are among the cardinal FMS symptoms. There are nine bilateral pairs of sites. For details and anatomical figures, see Starz, Sinclair, Okifuji, and Turk (1997), Okifuji, Turk, Sinclair, Starz, and Marcus (1997), Thompson (1990), Wolfe et al. (1990), and Okifuji and Turk (1999). These areas are suboccipital, low cervical/*sternomastoid*, mid-upper *trapezius*, origin of *supraspinatus* above medial scapula, near junction of second rib to sternum, outer side of elbow, upper outer gluteal, side of upper thigh, and inner knee above kneecap.

There have been attempts to quantify tender points to provide a measure of disease activity, especially for use in outcome studies. With the Tender Point Index (TPI), one palpates with about 4 kilograms of pressure the 18 specified body sites and a few control sites not expected to be tender. Early versions of the TPI (Wolfe et al., 1990; Russell, Fletcher, Michalek, McBroom, & Hester, 1991) used a 5-point scale from 0 to 4. This has been further standardized with detailed procedures and a 0–10 interval scale, the Manual Tender Point Survey (MTPS; see Starz et al., 1997, and Okifuji et al., 1997, for the detailed manual). The advantage of the interval scale in the MTPS (rather than the ordinal 0–5 scale in the TPI) is that it allows for the use of parametric statistics. Unfortunately for clinical practice, the detailed procedures take 5–7 minutes to complete, and there is a very poor relationship between the various tender point counts and other measures of patient well-being besides the level of distress (Wolfe, 1997).

Widespread Pain

Widespread pain present for 3 months or longer is a useful criterion in terms of sensitivity and specificity, but describes 11% of the general population (Croft et al., 1993). According to the original ACR system (Wolfe et al., 1990), pain is widespread when the following are all present. Pain is in the left and right side of the body, and pain appears above and below the waist. The patient also must report *axial skeletal pain*: pain in areas of the cervical spine, anterior chest, thoracic spine, or low back. Shoulder pain on either side and buttock pain on either side fulfill the side criteria. Low back pain fulfills the lower segment criteria. An example of widespread pain is "right shoulder, left buttock, and thoracic spine" (Wolfe et al., 1990, p. 163). See MacFarlane, Croft, Schollum, and Silman (1996) for a proposed refinement of the definition.

Measures of Pain

Dolorimetry. A *dolorimeter* measures the sensations from pressure to pain at tender soft tissue sites (Wolfe et al., 1990; Russell, 1990). It consists of a pressure algometer with a spring-loaded gauge capped with a flat circular rubber or cork stopper. Based on using this at the specified body sites, one calculates a Dolorimeter Pain Index (DPI). Objectivity, reliability, and standardization are all better with the DPI than with at least the original TPI scoring system. Advantages include indicating exact pressure applied. However, tender point pain tolerance varies greatly, depending on the surface size of the dolorimeter and on the pressure and rate (Okifuji et al., 1997). It is used in some research with FMS and has potential value for medicolegal cases, but it is not necessary and not recommended in routine clinical practice. Wolfe et al. (1990) and others have concluded that digital palpation of tender points is more discriminatory than dolorimetry is. A practitioner should consider getting the same measures at regular intervals to assess response to therapy systematically. Because pain thresholds can vary throughout the day and from day to day for a given individual (Gudni Thorsteinsson, MD, personal communication, June 1994), one should also consider multiple measures at different times of the day and over multiple days before, during, and after treatment.

Self-Report Pain Intensity and Pain Affect Rating Scales. A *visual analogue scale (VAS)* is a good method for measuring pain intensity in patients with FMS. It is often a 10-centimeter line with the ends labeled as extremes of pain, such as from "no pain" to "pain as bad as it could be" (Jensen & Karoly, 1992). Patients are asked to mark the line at the point that best indicates their pain intensity. The distance from no pain to their mark is the intensity score, usually measured in millimeters. Careful explanations and patient practice reduce errors for patients, such as some elderly persons and others.

Alternative versions of this method, known as "graphic rating scales," may be easier for some patients to understand (Jensen & Karoly, 1992). These scales use numbers from 0 up to 10, or adjectives such as "mild," "moderate," and "severe." Jensen and Karoly also recommend not using the VAS as the primary or only pain intensity measure. They describe and illustrate other self-report scales and procedures.

There are several measures of pain affect worth considering for patients with FMS. Examples are verbal rating scales and a VAS (Jensen & Karoly, 1992). A VAS for pain affect will have endpoints labeled something like "not bad at all" and "the most unpleasant feeling possible for me." Jensen and Karoly (1992, p. 143) state that "by far the most widely used measure of pain affect is the Affective subscale of the McGill Pain Questionnaire (MPQ)." The MPQ, originally developed by Melzack (1975), is presented and discussed in detail by

Melzack and Katz (1992). For other pain measures, see Turk and Melzack (1992). However, it is yet unknown whether measures of pain affect will add anything meaningful to assessing patients with FMS.

Sleep Disturbance

Poor sleep is an almost universal finding among patients with FMS. They typically awaken with fatigue, and they often have trouble starting and maintaining sleep. Moldofsky (1990) and his group investigated an anomalous electroencepalographic (EEG) phenomenon during non-rapid-eye-movement (NREM) sleep, *alpha–delta sleep* (also known as "alpha EEG NREM sleep anomaly"), and referred to FMS as a "nonrestorative sleep syndrome." However, the meaning of this sleep anomaly is unclear: Perlis et al. (1997) were "unable to confirm that there was a relationship between alpha sleep and the myalgia syndrome of fibromyalgia," although noting that "the association of myalgia symptoms with alpha sleep may be evident only with more objective measures of pain" (p. 278). Further lack of support for this relationship was noted by Shaver et al. (1997), who did not find the alpha intrusions during NREM sleep among a small group of women with FMS, although the study did support "more early night transitional sleep (stage 1) . . . , more sleep stage changes . . . and higher sleep fragmentation index" (p. 247) in this group. The relationship between poor sleep and significantly more pain has received support from Affleck, Urrows, Tennen, Higgins, and Abeles (1996), who studied 50 women with FMS; they noted that "the within-person association favored the hypothesis that sleep difficulties precede, rather than follow, increased pain during the day" (p. 367), although there was support for a bidirectional relation between the sequence of sleep and attention to pain. Thus disturbed sleep (including lighter and less consolidated sleep in the first part of the night) is associated with FMS, but the relationship between alpha EEG NREM sleep and FMS is unreliably observed across studies, and hence is unclear.

Other Symptoms

The list of other symptoms often reported by persons with FMS is extensive and described in many references. Readers are directed to various references (Jacobsen, Petersen, & Danneskjold-Samsoe, 1993; see also the "Resources" section). Fatigue is common and relates to the sleep disturbance. Other symptoms include (but are not limited to) stiffness, headaches, face pain, insomnia, irritable bowel, genitourinary problems, paresthesias, ambient temperature and other environmental sensitivities, noncardiac chest symptoms, breathing symptoms, neurocognitive deficits, depression, and anxiety. A useful measure that attempts to cover the major components of FMS, including pain and function, is the Fibromyalgia Impact Questionnaire (Burckhardt, Clark, & Bennett, 1991).

PSYCHOLOGICAL FACTORS, PROBLEMS, AND DIAGNOSES

Substantial numbers of patients with FMS have and/or had significant psychological problems. Nonpatients with FMS, however, have a much lower rate of psychological problems and may not differ in this regard from the general population (Daily, Bishop, Russell, & Fletcher, 1990; Yunus, Ahles, Aldag, & Masi, 1991; Turk & Flor, 1989; Aaron et al., 1996; Alexander et al., 1998). Thus medical care seeking appears associated with a history of diagnosable psychological problems.

This does not mean that psychological/psychiatric problems have an etiological role in FMS. Research on that topic does not reliably support the psychogenic model. However, there is much support for the presence of psychological problems in the histories of many persons with FMS (Çeliker, Borman, Öktem, Gökçe-Kutsal, & Başgöze, 1997; Keel, 1998; Aaron et al., 1996; Kurtze, Gundersen, & Svebak, 1998). Stress, reactions to stress, anxiety, and depression can have an impact on FMS symptoms and their severity, as well as on treatment (e.g., Russell et al., 1991). As noted earlier, emotional trauma is a major factor predicting medical care seeking among patients with FMS (Aaron et al., 1996).

Physical and Emotional Trauma

Reported trauma is more common among patients with FMS than among nonpatients with FMS. Emotional trauma is defined in this context as death or severe health problem in the family, marital stress, surgery, and others. Aaron et al. (1996) found that patients with a trauma history sought help from more physicians and had more visits than patients without a trauma history. Emotional trauma was also associated with more disability than was either physical trauma or no trauma. Emotional trauma was associated with more fatigue severity than physical trauma. Higher rates of disability compensation were found among patients with physical trauma history. However, there were no significant differences between the physical and emotional trauma groups with respect to pain intensity or tender points. Thus emotional trauma predicts medical care seeking (perhaps due to more fatigue and functional disability), and physical trauma predicts compensation for disability.

Stress

The greater daily stress experienced by patients with FMS includes a broad spectrum of items beyond illness, income, or education (Daily et al., 1990). Daily and colleagues noted that their results did not clarify "whether stress precedes or follows changes in disease activity and impact" (p. 1384). They also pointed out that patients with FMS may be hypersensitive and thus may overreport daily stress. Daily et al.'s patients reported more pain, including more pelvic and stomach pain, more use of pain medications, and more fatigue. They also reported more use of outpatient medical services for non-FMS problems and more functional disability, and were described as showing more hypervigilance, lower pain thresholds, and lower tolerance for a variety of stimuli. These results were supported by McDermid, Rollman, and McCain (1996), but not all studies have supported the hypervigilance.

Self-Efficacy

One should consider evaluation of patients' self-efficacy with regard to FMS and pain management. Buckelew et al. (1996) reported that pretreatment self-efficacy was associated with better physical activity in patients with FMS, and changes in self-efficacy were associated with other physical indications of better outcome.

Neurocognitive Issues

Grace, Nielson, Hopkins, and Berg (1999) reviewed and improved on prior studies of neurocognitive issues in FMS. They concluded that subsets of patients with FMS show substantial impairments on measures of immediate and delayed memory and of sustained attention/concentration. The perceived problems are often greater than the objective deficits, yet objective deficits do exist. The memory impairments probably reflect attentional factors that affect memory, rather than a primary memory problem. A major implication of these findings is for treatments that require patients to learn a lot of new information and develop new skills. The authors suggest providing frequent repetitions, furnishing supplementary written materials, and helping patients with ways to compensate for problems in memory and sustained attention.

In summary, practitioners should consider a tailored evaluation at least for depression, anxiety, neurocognitive functioning (e.g., immediate memory, basic and sustained attention/concentration), self-efficacy, daily stress, emotional traumas, sexual and physical abuse, anger, symptom impact, and attitudes about illness/pain.

COMORBID DISORDERS

FMS overlaps with multiple disorders. One group of investigators coined the term "affective spectrum disorder" to signal the potential linkage with conditions that respond at least somewhat to antidepressant medications (Hudson & Pope, 1989, 1990; Hudson, Goldenberg, Pope, Keck, & Schlesinger, 1992). Another and more recent conceptualization linking multiple disorders is by Yunus (1996), who developed the concept of "dysregulation spectrum syndrome" (DSS) reflecting the overlap of systemic and regional disorders. Yunus notes nine conditions besides FMS in his DSS family: chronic fatigue syndrome, IBS, tension and migraine headaches, temporomandibular joint syndrome, MPS, primary dysmenorrhea, periodic limb movement disorder, and "restless legs" syndrome. According to this view, these so-called DSS conditions are thought to share several characteristics (Yunus, 1996) and are thought to respond to centrally acting therapies. The high comorbidity begs for explanation and has important implications for clinical practice aside from questions of etiology. For example, the coexistence of other symptoms and disorders for which there is published support for the use of relaxation therapies and biofeedback (e.g., headaches, anxiety, IBS) helps justify using them for many patients with FMS.

TREATMENTS[2]

Methodological Considerations and Adherence/Compliance

First, one must consider that there are large differences between patients with FMS treated in research settings and those treated in clinical practice (Okifuji & Turk, 1999). It is also difficult for patients to adhere to treatments that are more demanding in terms of time, effort, and/or complexity (e.g., exercise, relaxation therapies, cognitive-behavioral approaches). In one multidisciplinary treatment program (Turk, Okifuji, Sinclair, & Starz, 1998), there was a meaningful change in pain after treatment for about 40% of the patients. Turk et al. also demonstrated that responses to treatment varied across subgroups of patients. The patients who showed the most improvement from the treatment were coping poorly, perceiving disability, and showing emotional distress with high levels of pain. This group responded better than those for whom the distress and disability were associated with interpersonal problems (who showed no improvement), and also better than a third group whose members were already coping better before treatment (Okifuji & Turk, 1999).

Another important factor relevant here is compliance/adherence to treatment (e.g., Vlaeyen et al., 1996). Turk and Gatchel (1999, p. 490), referring to Kerns, Rosenberg, Jamison, Caudill, and Haythornthwaite (1997), remind us that "not all patients are equally ready for treatment." They also remind us that at least for some persons with chronic pain, psychological interventions can be effective, but adherence by patients with chronic pain is very low. This can and probably does result in some treatments' being viewed as ineffective "when [they] may in fact have been very effective for those who adhered to the prescriptive behaviors" (p. 490).

Thus, to improve treatment efficacy, practitioners should consider the following:

- Working toward matching treatments to subgroups of patients with FMS.
- Helping to overcome impediments for patients accepting and applying therapy recommendations.
- Doing whatever can be done to help patients overcome obstacles to adherence.
- Examining studies for subgroups of factors facilitating or impeding adherence.

Relaxation Therapies, EMG Biofeedback, and Closely Related Applied Psychophysiological Therapies

The National Fibromyalgia Partnership (see the "Resources" section) includes varied relaxation therapies and biofeedback in its list of treatment and management approaches. There is sufficient support for including relaxation therapies without or with EMG biofeedback as part of treatment programs for FMS (Buckelew et al., 1998; Sarnoch, Adler, & Scholtz, 1997; Keel, Bodoky, Gerhard, & Müller, 1998; Ferraccioli et al., 1987; Martin et al., 1996; Gunther, Mur, Kinigadner, & Miller, 1994; Kaplan, Goldenberg, & Galvin-Nadeau, 1993). However, few of these studies allow examination of the independent effects of relaxation therapies and/or EMG biofeedback. Thus there is no firm support for the role of relaxation therapies and/or EMG biofeedback when used alone.

Older Studies

Ferraccioli et al. (1987) used single-channel frontal EMG with audio feedback and with eyes closed, a very modest form of EMG biofeedback. They included an unspecified version of *progressive muscle relaxation*. It appears that there were 21 treatment sessions after the first baseline session. The study reported significant improvements at the end of treatment and at 6-month follow-up. The authors used the number of tender points, pain intensity rated on a VAS, and morning stiffness as criteria. The authors deserve recognition for their early contribution, as well as for treating only patients resistant to prior medical treatment with *nonsteroidal anti-inflammatory drugs (NSAIDs)*.

The same investigators reported a later trial of biofeedback with 10 of 24 female patients with FMS who were studied for other purposes (Ferraccioli et al., 1990). The focus of the study was neuroendocrinological. They compared patients with FMS and those with other chronic pain conditions (e.g., rheumatoid arthritis, low back pain) and found that 15 of the 24 women (62%) with FMS had one or more abnormal hormone levels when "the strictest criteria" (p. 871) were used. They speculate that patients without these hormone imbalances can benefit from relaxation and EMG biofeedback, compared to those with such imbalances. In the three pain conditions studied, the authors found support for the hypothesis that "chronic pain and stress are important determinants of neuroendocrinologic abnormalities especially at the hypothalamic–pituitary–thyroid axis" (p. 872).

There was no specific information about the biofeedback and relaxation. It is indeed unfortunate that the specific role of biofeedback, and relaxation for that matter, was left so unclear. Nevertheless, several of the patients participating did get better compared to their prior treatments and compared to a group receiving false EMG biofeedback. Psychopathological factors, such as depression, resulted in poor outcome.

The relationship among the abnormal hormone levels, FMS, and response to biofeedback and relaxation remains unclear. Nevertheless, the neuroendocrinological results have potential implications for practitioners treating FMS with relaxation and biofeedback. Of the 10 patients, there were 7 without neuroendocrinological abnormalities, and 6 of these showed benefit of 50% or more improvement in tender points, MPQ scores, and VAS scores with 15 biofeedback sessions and practice. None of the 3 patients with the defined abnormalities showed benefit from this treatment.

Later Studies

Sarnoch et al. (1997) was not a treatment study, yet was supportive of EMG biofeedback in the treatment of FMS. This study of 18 patients with FMS focused on discrimination of levels of muscle activity in the right trapezius and then relaxation. The biofeedback was limited to audio only, with eyes closed, and only from the trapezius, and the relaxation was limited to at least 15 minutes daily of trapezius relaxation. Nevertheless, Sarnoch et al. reported improved muscular sensitivity with a few sessions, as well as slightly reduced muscle activity, and these findings were statistically associated with a reduction of pain reports. They described their results as consistent with findings from other studies focusing on dysfunctional muscular sensitivity and activity. Examples include an inability to relax between muscle contractions while performing dynamic movements (p. 1043, referring to Elert, Rantapää-Dahlqvist, Henrikson-Larsen, & Gerdle, 1989) and a slower muscular relaxation rate following voluntary hand grip exercises (p. 1043, referring to the work of Backman, Bengtsson, Bengtsson, Lennmarken, & Henriksson, 1988). The paper also refers to consistency with work by Flor, Schugens, and Birbaumer (1992).

Keel et al. (1998) studied the combination of self-help therapies with cognitive relaxation, and exercises for a subset of patients with FMS. The treatment group of 14, mostly females, involved 15 weekly group sessions lasting about 2 hours each, with 20- to 30-minute segments of information, self-control, gymnastics, autogenic relaxation, and discussion. The control group of 13 patients had 15 sessions of 45–60 minutes focused on autogenic relaxation.

The use of autogenic therapy is understandable, considering where the study was conducted (in the German-speaking part of Switzerland); however, it is not akin to the progressive relaxation techniques, as the authors contend. Practice instructions were only for daily use (and thus were insufficient, at least logically), and there was no evidence for adherence. Furthermore, because no biofeedback or psychophysiological measures were used, we have no way of knowing whether or not there was any psychophysiological progress and for whom. Some critics would also point to the group format as a limitation for learning and monitoring the effectiveness of relaxation therapy. Physical exercises included stretching and aerobic exercises, but here too, no adherence measures and no measures of muscle strength or endurance were mentioned. The Okifuji and Turk (1999) view that "one size does not fit all" is supported, in that a minority of persons improved modestly. We have insufficient information about the role of any of the treatment elements.

One of the most ambitious studies we found on this topic was that by Buckelew et al. (1998). The study was designed to assess treatment efficacy of biofeedback/relaxation, exercises, and a combination, using several outcome measures, with long-term follow-up. The study compared 29 patients receiving biofeedback/relaxation, 30 receiving exercises, 30 receiving the combination, and 30 in an attention control group. The patients were recruited subjects from a large number of patients' medical charts, and essentially all were females.

There was modest but significant improvement on pain and psychological distress in within-group analyses, with all the treatment groups showing improvements on some measures, including the TPI and self-efficacy, at posttreatment. Only the combination group maintained this improvement at 3 months, however. The attention control group worsened at every point. On the TPI, the control group's worsening contrasted with the treatment groups' improving, thus leading to speculation that intervention may prevent increased tenderness—a conclusion that needs further study and, if valid, would be worthwhile.

Therapy took place once a week for 1.5–3 hours for 6 weeks. The relaxation and biofeedback consisted of cognitive and muscle relaxation, and EMG for one site (one trapezius). Patients were asked to practice at least two additional times per week. No specifics were given for relaxation or for biofeedback. Therapists were described as "trainers," had bachelor's and master's degrees, and had 1–5 years' experience.

Exercise involved active range-of-motion work; specific strengthening; low- to moderate-intensity aerobic walking; work on posture and body mechanics; and use of heat, cold, and massage. There were validity checks for the measures. Most improvements were significant; here again, however, only a subset of patients using a variety of procedures got better.

The Bottom Line

The ambitiousness and efforts of Buckelew and her colleagues, and Keel and her colleagues, are commendable. It is very frustrating that the results were so modest. Based on the review above, these and the other studies do not allow an understanding of the specific role of biofeedback and related applied psychophysiological approaches in the treatment of FMS.

Relaxation therapies and biofeedback still seem logical to include, and there is modest support for their use, but there is still very little research. If these therapies do help significantly, the changes are modest and occur for a minority of patients.

Unfortunately, the existing studies with relaxation and biofeedback do not report much about what they did, provided whatever they did for short times, focused on one muscle, did not provide much daily relaxation, did not provide much information about adherence to recommended procedures, and/or did not provide stress management (e.g., time use management) to facilitate adherence. The complexity of FMS, as Okifuji and Turk (1999) describe, suggests more extensive therapies, as well as tailoring of therapies to individuals.

To properly evaluate relaxation procedures, patients need to use more extensive relaxation daily, rather than once a day or two to three times a week. Adherence to those recommendations may continue to be a problem.

If we assume that a history of abuse or of other emotional and physical traumas has a significant psychobiological impact on the development and maintenance of FMS symptoms, illness behaviors, health care seeking, and medication use, then treatment should include a focus on this for some patients. However, some problems with this approach are that it would have to be added to the other approaches, would be expensive to institute, and would be problematic financially when reimbursement for those services is very low and limited. Furthermore, many of these patients do not want to pursue such treatment, and potential risks are encountered when those doors are opened.

Other Treatments

Parts of this section are based on the work of Thompson (2000), Okifuji and Turk (1999), and the National Fibromyalgia Partnership (see the "Resources" section). Many practitioners treat FMS with a multifaceted, multidisciplinary approach. Seldom is an isolated treatment successful, since FMS affects multiple aspects of a patient's well-being. Treatment strategies that address the muscle dysfunction/deconditioning, sleep disturbance, and psychological issues (including patient self-efficacy) seem to have the best chance of success. Some treatment approaches that can complement relaxation therapies and biofeedback are presented below.

Patient Education

Patient education is the most important initial step in treatment, and includes correcting myths and misattributions about FMS. Morrow's (1999) brief article on biofeedback can be given to patients.

Work on Body Mechanics

Work on body mechanics includes checking and correcting posture, body mechanics during lifting and other activities, and anatomical factors (e.g., a short leg).

Medications

The only medications that have been shown to be effective for FMS are those related to improving sleep quality and those used to treat concomitant disorders (e.g., depression, anxiety). They all seem to work in some way with the serotonin system. Medications used include the following:

- *Amitriptyline* (Elavil), trazodone (Desyrel), or cyclobenzaprine (Flexeril) at bedtime in very low doses, to improve sleep and perhaps reduce pain.
- Selective serotonin reuptake inhibitors (SSRIs) for depression. Some physicians use SSRIs in combination with trazodone (or other medications) to improve sleep, even in patients who are not clinically depressed (Goldenberg, Mayskiy, Mossey, Ruthazer, & Schmic, 1996).
- New NSAIDs (e.g., Celebrex and Vioxx), to inhibit the prostaglandin cyclooxygenase enzyme, which causes inflammation and pain. Since there is no inflammation in FMS, the only use for these medications is as mild analgesics. Less expensive alternatives would be more appropriate (e.g., ibuprofen, acetaminophen).
- Other analgesics (e.g., tramadol [Ultram]), unless patients are sensitive to codeine preparations or unless other contraindications exist.
- Benzodiazepines (e.g., diazepam [Valium], alprazolam [Xanax], lorazepam [Ativan], clonazepam [Klonopin]), sometimes used for anxiety and muscle spasms. Risks include dependency and side effects. Not useful for treating FMS itself.
- Sleep medications (e.g., zolpidem tartrate [Ambien], sonata), sometimes for short intervals. Over-the-counter sleep aids are to be avoided.

Exercise

Low-impact cardiovascular aerobic exercises—such as fast walking, warm-water walking/exercises, bicycling, cross-country skiing, or use of a treadmill or other machines—are appropriate for selected patients if they can tolerate them. Goals include preventing muscle atrophy, promoting circulation of blood to muscles and connective tissues, building strength, and increasing endurance. The key is to start very slowly and proceed gradually. Because patients with FMS have a reduced tolerance for muscular exertion, the exercise should not be painful. The results of a 14-week program with submaximal aerobic exercise (45 minutes three times a week) followed over 4 years provided support for the use of this type of program, but efficacy depended largely on adherence to the regimen (Wigers, Stiles, & Vogel, 1996).

Other support for exercise treatment for FMS was reported by Martin et al. (1996). They focused on muscle strengthening, endurance, and flexibility with a 1-hour program (20-minute submaximal fast walk, 20-minute flexibility work, and 20-minute muscle strengthening). The patients did this three times a week for 6 weeks. In this short time, these patients did a little better; three differences were statistically significant, compared to results for those receiving relaxation training alone.[3] There were significant drops in tender point counts, decreased pain sensitivity in the tender point areas, and improved aerobic fitness. A major purpose of that study was to show that patients with FMS could participate in this type of program without adverse effects.

Even healthy persons have difficulty adhering to physical fitness programs. An attempt to make fitness exercises more appealing involved low-impact aerobic dance, but this study did not show significant improvements in FMS symptoms (Nørregaard, Lykkegaard, Mehlgen, & Danneskiold-Samsøe, 1997, cited in Okifuji & Turk, 1999).

Physical Therapies

For selected patients, physical therapies may include posture work, massage, stretching, Pilates, physical conditioning, and other therapies (e.g., heat, high galvanic stimulation, *spray and stretch*) focused on myofascia and *trigger points*.

Occupational Therapies

Examples of occupational therapies used for FMS include ergonomics and pacing of activities.

Sleep Hygiene

Sleep hygiene and related behavioral methods to improve sleep are prudent and common.

Cognitive-Behavioral Therapy/Stress Management

For selected patients, stress management and cognitive-behavioral therapy may be justifiable. They can help patients manage daily stress, other sources of stress, and adjustment to symptoms. Effective time use management may include reducing overload, reducing disorganization, managing procrastination and perfectionism, and other aspects. Bradley (1989) described procedures, experimental research designs, and methodology features for studies of behavioral programs. It should be noted that "cognitive-behavioral" intervention is often not strictly cognitive-behavioral; it is often multicomponent treatment and includes multiple types of relaxation therapies. Strictly cognitive-behavioral therapy focuses on negative/maladaptive thinking (e.g., hopelessness), self-statements, and cognitive distractions. However, some research does not support the additive value of cognitive therapies (Vlaeyen et al., 1996), at least within comprehensive and time-consuming treatment programs for patients with limited education and with moderate to severe disability.

Other Approaches

Other approaches (e.g., nutrition, acupuncture) are mentioned here only for the sake of completeness.

If all of the approaches described above are insufficient, some practitioners consider injections along with spray and stretch techniques, but these are most effective for the more localized muscle pain syndromes

EEG Biofeedback/Neurofeedback

EEG biofeedback/neurofeedback/EEG-driven stimulation (EDS) are intriguing and promising additions to the array of interventions for FMS (Donaldson, 1998, 1999; Donaldson, Nelson, & Schulz, 1998b; Mueller, Donaldson, Nelson, & Layman, 2001). Interested readers should read at least these articles for the details. The rationale for these approaches is discussed in the publications by Stuart Donaldson and his colleagues. As noted earlier, FMS involves decreased concentration, decreased immediate memory, and problems with multitasking (Grace et al., 1999). These are sometimes referred to as "fibro-fog." This has been assumed by some to be associated with the waking EEG. EDS is one type of EEG neurotherapy intervention.

> The EDS neurotherapy system . . . may be understood . . . as an interactive EEG entrainment device. . . . [It] monitors the patient's EEG in the 0–30 Hz frequency band from a single monopolar electrode . . . to set the rate of the frequency-modulated light stimulation that is fed back to the patient to entrain the EEG. (Mueller et al., 2001, p. 935)

A preliminary study (Mueller et al., 2001) involved a series of 30 patients who had EDS treatments until their EEG showed stability and a more normal pattern with reduced delta and theta. There were also patient reports of "increased cognitive clarity, improved sleep, increased mental and physical energy, reduced affective disturbances, and increased awareness of localized as opposed to generalized pain" (p. 939). The patients had an average total of 37 (SD = 15–16) EDS sessions (range from 16 to 80). They also had an average of 2 EMG treatments, 5–6 physical therapy sessions, and 7 massage therapy sessions. There was a decrease in patients' use of prescription and nonprescription drugs. The authors discussed the reasons why they thought that the EDS added to the positive treatment results, although they acknowledge that multimodal intervention is needed for patients with FMS: "It would appear that EDS may have contributed a specific and necessary ingredient that was the prime initator of therapeutic efficacy . . . this is only a tentative conclusion" (p. 948).

Thus it appears that EEG biofeedback/EDS may be considered as treatment options by some practitioners for at least some patients. Well-controlled research studies will be very welcome. Shorter interventions will also be welcome (and probably necessary, if this approach is ever to become available and practical to most patients).

IMPLICATIONS, GUIDELINES, AND LIMITS

One must tailor treatment to the individual patient, and it is helpful to treat patients with FMS in close collaboration with physicians in proper specialties.

For many patients, muscle relaxation with at least EMG biofeedback to enhance general relaxation and to treat specific body areas may be appropriate. Multiple muscle sites and simultaneous EMG channels can be used with patients in multiple postures or positions, during multiple stressor conditions, and in responses to and with recovery after various body movements.

As just noted, EEG biofeedback/EDS as described by Donaldson (1998, 1999) and Mueller et al. (2001) may be options considered by some practitioners for at least some patients; again, however, the presence of supportive controlled research data would be very welcome.

Finally, one should consider using these treatments within a stepped-care model. That is, one could use these therapies after stopping unsuccessful treatments or after reaching a plateau in progress from other treatments. Treatment depends on the individual patient and preferences of the practitioner and patient. A baseline is ideal but often not practical in clinical practice. Practitioners will tailor the sequence and content.

- Baseline.
- Patient education and reassurance.
- Normalization of sleep and treatment of depression if present; medications may be necessary.
- Physical therapies, with a focus on a home program of stretching and aerobic fitness.
- Relaxation and EMG biofeedback.
- EEG biofeedback/EDS (tentative).
- Psychological assessment.
- Stress management and cognitive-behavioral therapies.
- Other treatments as needed.

CONCLUSION

Multiple types of relaxation therapies and biofeedback are parts of multicomponent and multidisciplinary treatments for many patients with FMS.

The treatment algorithm proposed by Thompson (1996, 2000) provides a useful model for planning treatment. Practitioners often combine treatments, and this is often proper.

Psychological and psychophysiological factors often play a large role in the disorder known as FMS. These factors undoubtedly influence whatever CNS processes are involved in the pathophysiology of FMS. Applied psychophysiological interventions (e.g., relaxation therapies, EMG biofeedback, EEG biofeedback/EDS, cognitive-behavioral therapies, other behavioral and stress management therapies) can have an impact on patients' attitudes and beliefs about symptoms and functioning, as well as on physiology and pain.

We look forward to research studies and clinical treatment details regarding the theories, treatment approaches, and implications of Donaldson and colleagues' EEG-based approach. We also look forward to further guidelines and instructions for tailoring treatments and matching treatment to patients. Finally, we look forward to pharmacological and other biological advances offering substantial improvements in the biological systems that need repairing and regulating.

GLOSSARY

ALPHA–DELTA SLEEP. Anomalous sleep phenomenon, originally described by Hauri and Hawkins (1973), wherein alpha electroencephalographic (EEG) activity (7.5–11 hertz) occurs in non-rapid-eye-movement (NREM) sleep. The occurrence of alpha during delta or slow-wave (stages III and IV) sleep is characteristic and gives this finding its name (Fredrickson & Krueger, 1994); the alpha is thought to interfere with restorative nature of the delta sleep stage. The "alpha waves are not regularly accompanied by EMG, respiratory, or other physiological evidence of arousal" (Fredrickson & Krueger, 1994, p. 530). This anomaly is found in many (but not all) persons with FMS, and in people with other medical conditions. It is also known as "alpha EEG NREM sleep anomaly" (Moldofsky, 1990). Patients with FMS often complain of light and interrupted sleep, feeling unrefreshed and tired upon awakening, daytime fatigue, stiffness, and muscle aching, but not usually excess daytime sleepiness. Thus FMS is sometimes referred to as a "nonrestorative sleep syndrome." One must differentiate the presence of increased alpha waves during sleep from causes such as from the use of sedative/hypnotics or stimulants that also can produce alpha and background fast activity.

AMITRIPTYLINE. A tricyclic antidepressant drug. Trade names, Elavil and Endep. Proposed mechanisms include increased synaptic norepinephrine or serotonin (5-HT), inhibited 5-HT and norepinephrine reuptake, effects on 5-HT_2 receptors, and decreased beta-receptor density.

AXIAL SKELETAL PAIN. Pain in areas of the cervical spine, anterior chest, thoracic spine, or low back.

DOLORIMETER. An instrument to measure the severity of tenderness at the soft tissue sites. It consists of a pressure algometer with a spring-loaded gauge capped with a flat circular rubber or cork stopper about 1.5 centimeters in diameter. One advances the instrument at increments of about 1 kilogram per second and asks the patient to say when it feels painful.

HYPOTHALAMIC–PITUITARY–THYROID AXIS. A term reflecting the interrelationship among the hypothalamus, pituitary, and thyroid glands.

MYOFASCIAL PAIN SYNDROME (MPS). Common term for muscle strain resulting in tissue damage. Focus is often on trigger points and a palpable band of tight muscle versus multiple tender points in FS. (See text.)

NONSTEROIDAL ANTI-INFLAMMATORY DRUGS (NSAIDs). Aspirin and other salicylates, indomethacin (Indocin), ibuprofen (Advil, Motrin-IBS, Nuprin), naproxen, and fenoprofen (Nalfon) are examples.

PROGRESSIVE MUSCLE RELAXATION. A very common type of muscle and general relaxation developed by Dr. Edmund Jacobson. Starts with tensing and releasing of specific muscle groups and progresses to tensing larger groups, discriminating between tension in selected areas and relaxation in others, and eventually to releasing muscle tension without tensing. The tensing–releasing portion is sometimes mistakenly used alone.

SPRAY AND STRETCH (STRETCH AND SPRAY). The use of ethyl chloride to relieve musculoskeletal pain and allow stretching of the muscles. It inactivates myofascial trigger points more quickly than local injections or other methods. Although the spray occurs first, the stretch is the necessary component, and the spray merely eases the stretch.

STERNOMASTOID (STERNOCLEIDOMASTOID). Muscles connecting the sternum (breastbone) and the clavicle (collarbone) to the mastoid process of the temporal bone at the nuchal line of the occipital bone (back of the lower part of the ear). These muscles rotate and extend the head, and flex the vertebral column.

SUBSTANCE P. Neurotransmitter that signals the brain to register pain. Patients with fibromyalgia have elevated substance P (Weigent et al., 1998) compared to controls.

SUPRASPINATUS. A deep muscle in the upper back and shoulder area under the trapezius. It abducts (draws away) the arm.

TENSION MYALGIA. Common term used to describe many muscle pain disorders. Implies that muscle tension is caused by spasm, poor posture, overuse, and other factors.

TRAPEZIUS. Large triangular muscle of the neck, shoulders, and midback regions. Supports the shoulders and postural control of the shoulder girdle, even when a person is standing at rest. Participates with the levator scapulae to raise the shoulders. Participates with other muscles for other movements such as abducting the arm. Has three sets of fibers—upper, middle, and lower. Each set can function separately with other muscles with similar function, or the three sets can work together to rotate the scapula.

TRIGGER POINTS. One or more hyperirritable spots within the belly of a muscle. So named because, when stimulated, it tends to cause referred pain in distinct distributions. Defined by Travell and Simons (1983) as follows: (1) tender area within a muscle belly; (2) pressure on it causes pain and/or tingling in specific distribution; (3) the muscle shortens, resulting in reduced range of motion, and stretching or contracting the muscle causes pain; (4) muscle feels taut at and around the trigger point; (5) stimulating the TrP (by snapping it or needling it) often causes muscle contraction; (6) injection of a local anesthetic into the trigger point eliminates the local and referred pain.

VISUAL ANALOGUE SCALE (VAS). A straight line, usually 10 centimeters long, with ends labeled as the extremes of pain intensity (e.g., "no pain" to "pain as bad as it could be") or pain affect (e.g., "not bad at all" to "the most unpleasant feeling possible for me"). Alternative versions may have specific points along the line labeled with intensity-denoting adjectives or numbers; these versions are called "graphic rating scales." The distance from the "no pain" (or "not bad at all") end to the mark made by the patient is the pain intensity (or pain affect) score.

NOTES

1. Both terms, hypothalamic–pituitary–adrenal axis and hypothalamic–pituitary–thyroid axis are discussed in the literature on fibromyalgia.

2. The order of treatments in this section does not necessarily represent the order of clinical preference or research support. Putting psychophysiological treatments first reflects the focus of this chapter.

3. This was reported by Okifuji and Turk (1999) as "similar to those findings from the aerobic training alone" (p. 240), but the other group did not receive aerobic training. The differences were statistically significant, although the clinical significance was unclear and one of the three differences was partly due to "difficult to explain" worsening of the relaxation on one measure of aerobic fitness.

RESOURCES

Useful Web sites include the following:

http://www.afsafund.org (The American Fibromyalgia Syndrome Association; information about FMS, and a list and detailed descriptions of research funded by this group).

http://www.fmpartnership.org (The National Fibromyalgia Partnership; this site contains a list and description of federally funded research, a monograph on FMS, and publications of this organization).

REFERENCES

Aaron, L. A., Bradley, L. A., Alarcón, G. S., Alexander, R. W., Triana-Alexander, M., Martin, M. Y., & Alberts, K. R. (1996). Psychiatric diagnoses in patients with fibromyalgia are related to health care-seeking behavior rather than to illness. *Arthritis and Rheumatism, 39*(3), 436–445.

Aaron, L. A., Bradley, L. A., Alarcón, G. S., Triana-Alexander, M., Alexander, R. W., Martin, M. Y., & Alberts, K. R. (1997). Perceived physical and emotional trauma as precipitating events in fibromyalgia. *Arthritis and Rheumatism, 40*(3), 453–460.

Abud-Mendoza, C., Magana-Aquino, M., Medina, R., Grimaldo, J. I., Rodriquez-Rivera, G., & Gonsalez-Amaro, R. (1997). Hypothalamus–hypophysis–thyroid axis dysfunction in patients with refractory fibromyalgia. *Arthritis and Rheumatism* (Abstract Suppl.), *40*(9), p. S189.

Affleck, G., Urrows, S., Tennen, H., Higgins, P., & Abeles, M. (1996). Sequential daily relations of sleep, pain intensity, and attention to pain among women with fibromyalgia. *Pain, 68,* 363–368.

Alexander, R. W., Bradley, L. A., Alarcón, G. S., Triana-Alexander, M., Aaron, L. A., Alberts, K. R., Martin, M. Y., & Stewart, K. E. (1998). Sexual and physical abuse in woman with fibromyalgia: Association with outpatient health care utilization and pain medication usage. *Arthritis Care and Research, 11*(2), 102–115.

Backman E., Bengtsson, A., Bengtsson, M., Lennmarken, C., & Henriksson, K. G. (1988). Skeletal muscle function in primary fibromyalgia: Effect of regional sympathetic blockade with guanethidine. *Acta Neurologica Scandinavica, 77*(3), 187–191.

Baumstark, K. E., & Buckelew, S. P. (1992). Fibromyalgia: Clinical signs, research findings, treatment implications, and future directions. *Annals of Behavioral Medicine, 14*(4), 282–291.

Bennett, R. M. (1999). Emerging concepts in the neurobiology of chronic pain: Evidence of abnormal sensory processing in fibromyalgia. *Mayo Clinic Proceedings, 74,* 385–398.

Bradley, L. A. (1989). Cognitive-behavioral therapy for primary fibromyalgia. *Journal of Rheumatology, 16* (Suppl. 19), 131–136.

Buckelew, S. P., Conway, R., Parker, J., Deuser, W. E., Read, J., Witty, T. E., Hewett, J. E., Minor, M., Johnson, J. C., Van Male, L., McIntosh, M. J., & Kay, D. R. (1998). Biofeedback/relaxation training and exercise interventions for fibromyalgia: A prospective trial. *Arthritis Care and Research, 11*(3), 196–209.

Buckelew, S. P., Huyser, B., Hewett, J. E., Parker, J. C., Johnson, J. C., Conway, R., & Kay, D. R. (1996). Self-efficacy predicting outcome among fibromyalgia subjects. *Arthritis Care and Research, 9*(2), 97–104.

Burckhardt, C. S., Clark, S. R., & Bennett, R. M. (1991). The Fibromyalgia Impact Questionnaire (FIQ): Development and validation. *Journal of Rheumatology, 18,* 728–733.

Çeliker, R., Borman, P., Öktem, F., Gökçe-Kutsal, Y., & Başgöze, O. (1997). Psychological disturbance in fibromyalgia: Relation to pain severity. *Clinical Rheumatology, 16*(2), 179–184.

Crofford, L. J. (1996). The hypothalamic–pituitary–adrenal stress axis in the fibromyalgia syndrome. *Journal of Musculoskeletal Pain, 4*(1/2), 181–200.

Crofford, L. J., Engleberg, N. C., & Demitrack, M. A. (1996). Neurohormonal perturbations in fibromyalgia. *Baillieres Clinical Rheumatology, 10*(2), 365–378.

Croft, P., Rigby, A. S., Boswell, R., Schollum, J., & Silman, A. (1993). The prevalence of chronic widespread pain in the general population. *Journal of Rheumatology, 20,* 710–713.

Daily, P. A., Bishop, G. D., Russell, I. J., & Fletcher, E. M. (1990). Psychological stress and the fibrositis/fibromyalgia syndrome. *Journal of Rheumatology, 17*(10), 1380–1385.

Donaldson, C. C. S. (1998). EEG-driven stimulation: Hitting the "reset button" in fibromyalgia patients. *Fibromyalgia Frontiers*, 6(4), 1–3, 12–13.

Donaldson, C. C. S. (1999). The pain of fibromyalgia: A message for the practitioner. *Biofeedback*, 27(3), 11–12.

Donaldson, C. C. S., Nelson, D. V., & Schulz, R. (1998b). Disinhibition in the gamma motoneuron circuitry: A neglected mechanism for understanding myofascial pain syndromes? *Applied Psychophysiology and Biofeedback*, 23(1), 43–57.

Donaldson, S., Sella, G. E., & Mueller, H. H. (1998a). Fibromyalgia: A retrospective study of 252 consecutive referrals. *Canadian Journal of Clinical Medicine*, 5(6), 116–127.

Elert, J. E., Rantapää-Dahlqvist, S. B., Henrikson-Larsen, K., & Gerdle, B. (1989). Increased EMG activity during short pauses in patients with primary fibromyalgia. *Scandinavian Journal of Rheumatology*, 18, 321–323.

Ferraccioli, G., Cavalieri, F., Salaffi, F., Fontana, S., Scita, F., Nolli, M., & Maestri, D. (1990). Neuroendocrinologic findings in primary fibromyalgia (soft tissue chronic pain syndrome) and in after chronic rheumatic conditions rheumatoid arthritis, low back pain). *Journal of Rheumatology*, 17(70), 869–873.

Ferraccioli, G., Ghirelli, L., Scita, F., Nolli, M., Moozzani, M., Pontana, S., Scorsonelli, M., Tridenti, A., & DeRisio, C. (1987). EMG-biofeedback training in fibromyalgia syndrome. *Journal of Rheumatology*, 14, 820–825.

Flor, H., Schugens, M. M., & Birbaumer, N. (1992). Discrimination of muscle tension in chronic pain patients and healthy controls. *Biofeedback and Self-Regulation*, 17(3), 165–177.

Fransen, J., & Russell, I. J. (1996). *The fibromyalgia help book: Practical guide to living better with fibromyalgia.* St. Paul, MN: Smith House Press.

Fredrickson, P. A., & Krueger, B. R. (1994). Insomnia associated with specific polysomnographic findings. In M. H. Kryger, T. Roth, & W. G. Dement (Eds.), *Principles and practice of sleep medicine* (2nd ed.). Philadelphia: W. B. Saunders.

Goldenberg, D., Mayskiy, M., Mossey, C., Ruthazer, R., & Schmic, C. (1996). A randomized double blind crossover trial of fluoxetine and amitriptyline in the treatment of fibromyalgia. *Arthritis and Rheumatism*, 39, 1852–1859.

Grace, G. M., Nielson, W. R., Hopkins, M., & Berg, M. A. (1999). Concentration and memory deficits in patients with fibromyalgia syndrome. *Journal of Clinical and Experimental Neuropsychology*, 21(4), 477–487.

Gunther, V., Mur, E., Kinigadner, U., & Miller, C. (1994). Fibromyalgia: The effect of relaxation and hydrogalvanic bath therapy on the subjective pain experience. *Clinical Rheumatology*, 13, 573–578.

Hauri, P., & Hawkins, D. R. (1973). Alpha–delta sleep. *Electroencephalography and Clinical Neurophysiology*, 34, 233–237.

Hudson, J. I., Goldenberg, D. L., Pope, H. G., Jr., Keck, P. E., Jr., & Schlesinger, L. (L992). Comorbidity of fibromyalgia with medical and psychiatric disorders. *American Journal of Medicine*, 92, 363–367.

Hudson, J. I., & Pope, H. G. Jr. (1989). Fibromyalgia and psychopathology: Is fibromyalgia a form of "affective spectrum disorder"? *Journal of Rheumatology*, 16(Suppl. 19), 15–22.

Hudson, J. I., & Pope, H. G. Jr. (1990). Affective spectrum disorder: Does antidepressant response identify a family of disorders with a common pathophysiology? *American Journal of Psychiaty*, 147, 552–564.

Jacobsen, S., Petersen, I. S., & Danneskjold-Samsoe, B. (1993). Clinical features of patients with chronic muscle pain B with special reference to fibromyalgia. *Scandinavian Journal of Rheumatology*, 22, 69–76.

Jensen, M. P., & Karoly, P. (1992). Self-report scales and procedures for assessing pain in adults. In D. C. Turk & R. Melzack (Eds.), *Handbook of pain assessment.* New York: Guilford Press.

Kaplan, K. H., Goldenberg, D. L., & Galvin-Nadeau, M. (1993). The impact of a meditation-based stress reduction program on fibromyalgia. *General Hospital Psychiatry*, 15(5), 284–289.

Keel, P. J. (1998). Psychological and psychiatric aspects of fibromyalgia syndrome (FMS). *Zeitschrift für Rheumatologie*, 57(2), 97–100.

Keel, P. J., Bodoky, C., Gerhard, U., & Müller, W. (1998). Comparison of integrated group therapy and group relaxation training for fibromyalgia. *The Clinical Journal of Pain*, 14, 232–238.

Kerns, R. D., Rosenberg, R., Jamison, R., Caudill, M. A., & Haythornthwaite, J. (1997). Readiness to adopt a self-management approach to chronic pain: The Pain Stages of Change Questionnaire (PSOCQ). *Pain*, 72, 227–234.

Kurtze, N., Gundersen, K. T., & Svebak, S. (1998). The role of anxiety and depression in fatigue and pattens of pain among subgroups of fibromyalgia patients. *British Journal of Medical Psychology*, 71, 185–194.

MacFarlane, G. J., Croft, P. R., Schollum, J., & Silman, A. J. (1996). Widespread pain: Is an improved classification possible? *Journal of Rheumatology*, 23, 1628–1632.

Martin, L., Nutting, A., Macintosh, B. R., Edworthy, S. M., Butterwick, D., & Cook, J. (1996). An exercise program in the treatment of fibromyalgia. *Journal of Rheumatology*, 23, 1050–1053.

McCain, G. A. (1990). Management of the fibromyalgia syndrome. In J. R. Fricton & E. A. Awad (Eds.), *Advances in pain research and therapy: Vol. 17. Myofascial pain and fibromyalgia.* New York: Raven Press.

McDermid, A. J., Rollman, G. B., & McCain, G. A. (1996). Generalized hypervigilance in fibromyalgia: Evidence of perceptual amplification. *Pain*, 66, 133–144.

Melzack, R. (1975). The McGill Pain Questionnaire: Major properties and scoring methods. *Pain, 1*, 277–299.

Melzack, R., & Katz, J. (1992). The McGill Pain Questionnaire: Appraisal and current status. In D. C. Turk & R. Melzack (Eds.), *Handbook of pain assessment*. New York: Guilford Press.

Moldofsky, H. (1990). The contribution of sleep–wake physiology to fibromyalgia. In J. R Fricton & E. A. Awad (Eds.), *Advances in pain research and therapy: Vol. 17. Myofascial pain and fibromyalgia*. New York: Raven Press.

Morrow, S. (1999). Biofeedback: Teaching better muscle awareness. *Fibromyalgia: Wellness letter, 2*(2), 1–2.

Mueller, H. H., Donaldson, C. C. S., Nelson, D. V., & Layman, M. (2001). Treatment of fibromyalgia incorporating EEG-driven stimulation: A clinical outcomes study. *Journal of Clinical Psychology, 57*(7), 933–952.

Okifuji, A., & Turk, D. C. (1999). Fibromyalgia: Search for mechanisms and effective treatments. In R. J. Gatchel & D. C. Turk (Eds.), *Psychological factors in pain: Critical perspectives*. New York: Guilford Press.

Okifuji, A., Turk, D. C., Sinclair, D., Starz, T. W., & Marcus, D. A. (1997). A standardized manual tender point survey: I. Development and determination of a threshold point for the identification of positive tender points in fibromyalgia syndrome. *Journal of Rheumatology, 24*, 377–383.

Perlis, M. L., Giles, D. E., Bootzin, R. R., Dikman, Z. V., Fleming, G. M., Drummond, S. P. A., & Rose, M. W. (1997). Alpha sleep and information preocessing, perception of sleep, pain, and arousability in fibromyalgia. *International Journal of Neuroscience, 89*, 265–280.

Russell, I. J. (1990). Treatment of patients with fibromyalgia syndrome: Considerations of the whys and wherefores. In J. R. Fricton & E. A. Awad (Eds.), *Advances in pain research and therapy: Vol. 17. Myofascial pain and fibromyalgia*. New York: Raven Press.

Russell, I. J. (1998). Cerebrospinal fluid (CSF) substance P (SP) in fibromyalgia (FMS): Changes in CSP SP over time, parallel changes in clinical activity, *Arthritis and Rheumatism* (Abstract Suppl.), *41*(9), S256.

Russell, I. J., Fletcher, E. M., Michalek, J. E., McBroom, P. C., & Hester, G. G. (1991). Treatment of primary fibrositis/fibromyalgia syndrome with ibuprofen and alprazolam: A double-blind, placebo-controlled study. *Arthritis and Rheumatism, 34*(5), 552–560.

Russell, I. J., Orr, M. D., Littman, B., Vipraio, G. A., Alboukrek, D., Michalek, J. E., Lopez, Y., & MacKippip, F. (1994). Elevated cerebrospinal fluid levels of substance P in patients with the fibromyalgia syndrome. *Arthritis and Rheumatism, 37*(11), 1593–1601.

Sarnoch, H., Adler, F., & Scholtz, O. B. (1997). Relevance of muscular sensitivity, muscular activity, and cognitive variables for pain reduction associated with EMG biofeedback in fibromyalgia. *Perceptual and Motor Skills, 84*, 1043–1050.

Schochat, T., Croft, P., & Raspe, H. (1994). The epidemiology of fibromyalgia. *British Journal of Rheumatology, 33*, 783–786.

Shaver, J. L. F., Lentz, M., Landis, C. A., Heitkemper, M. M., Buchwald, D. S., & Woods, N. F. (1997). Sleep, psychological distress, and stress arousal in women with fibromyalgia. *Research in Nursing and Health, 20*, 247–257.

Simons, D. G., & Travell, J. G. (1999). *Myofascial pain and dysfunction: The trigger point manual* (2nd ed., Vol. 1). Baltimore: Williams & Wilkins.

Starz, T. W., Sinclair, J. D., Okifuji, A., & Turk, D. C. (1997). Putting the finger on fibromyalgia: The Manual Tender Point Survey. *Journal of Musculoskeletal Medicine, 14*, 61–67.

Thompson, J. M. (1990). Tension myalgia as a diagnosis at the Mayo Clinic and its relationship to fibrositis, fibromyalgia, and myofascial pain syndrome. *Mayo Clinic Proceedings, 65*, 1237–1248.

Thompson, J. M. (1996). The diagnosis and treatment of muscle pain syndromes. In R. L. Braddom (Ed.), *Physical medicine and rehabilitation*. Philadelphia: Saunders.

Thompson, J. M. (2000). The diagnosis and treatment of muscle pain syndromes. In R. L. Braddom (Ed.), *Physical medicine and rehabilitation* (2nd ed.). Philadelphia: Saunders.

Travell, J. G., & Simons, D. G. (1983). *Myofascial pain and dysfunction: The trigger point manual*. Baltimore: Williams & Wilkins.

Turk, D. C., & Flor, H. (1989). Primary fibromyalgia is greater than tender points: Toward a multi-axial taxonomy. *Journal of Rheumatology, 16*(Suppl. 19), 80–86.

Turk, D. C., & Gatchel, R. J. (1999). Psychosocial factors and pain: Revolution and evolution. In R. J. Gatchel & D. C. Turk (Eds). *Psychological factors in pain: Critical perspectives*. New York: Guilford Press.

Turk, D. C., & Melzack, R. (Eds.). (1992). *Handbook of pain assessment*. New York: Guilford Press.

Turk, D. C., Okifuji, A., Sinclair, J. D., & Starz, T. W. (1998). Interdisciplininary treatment for fibromyalgia syndrome: Clinical and statistical significance. *Arthritis Care and Research, 11*, 186–195.

Vlaeyen, J. W., Teeken-Gruben, N. J., Goossens, M. E., Rutten-van Mölken, M. P., Pelt, R. A., van Eek, H., & Heuts, P. H. (1996). Cognitive-educational treatment of fibromyalgia: A randomized clinical trial. I. Clinical effects. *Journal of Rheumatology, 23*, 1237–1245.

Weigent, D. A., Bradley, L. A., Blalock, J. E., & Alarcon, G. S. (1998). Current concepts in the pathophysiology of abnormal pain perception in fibromyalgia. *American Journal of Medical Science, 315*(6), 405–412.

Wigers, S. H., Stiles, T. C., & Vogel, P. A. (1996). Effects of aerobic exercise versus stress management treatment in fibromyalgia. *Scandinavian Journal of Rheumatology, 25,* 77–86.

Wolfe, F. (1997). The relation between tender points and fibromyalgia symptom variables: Evidence that fibromyalgia is not a discrete entity in the clinic. *Annals of Rheumatological Diseases, 56,* 268–271.

Wolfe, F., Smythe, H. A., Yunus, M. B., Bennett, R. M., Bombardier, C., Goldenberg, D. L., Tugwell, P., Campbell, S. M., Abeles, M., Clark, P., Gam, A. G., Farber, S. J., Fiechtner, J. J., Franklin, C. M., Gasstter, R. A., Hamaty, D., Lessard, J., Lichtbroun, A. S., Masi, A. T., McCain, G. A., Reynolds, W. J., Tomano, T. J., Russell, I. J., & Sheon, R. P. (1990). The American College of Rheumatology 1990 criteria for the classification of fibromyalgia: Report of the multi-center criteria committee. *Arthritis and Rheumatism, 33*(2), 160–172.

Yunus, M. B. (1996). Dysfunctional spectrum syndrome: A unified concept for many common maladies. *Fibromyalgia Frontiers, 4*(4), 1–3, 8.

Yunus, M. B., Ahles, T. A., Aldag, J. C., & Masi, A. T. (1991). Relationship of clinical features with psychological status in primary fibromyalgia. *Arthritis and Rheumatism, 34*(1), 15–21.

Treating Special Populations

MARK S. SCHWARTZ
FRANK ANDRASIK

TREATING PEOPLE WITH DEVELOPMENTAL DISABILITES

Little is known about the clinical utility of biofeedback and related procedures for people with developmental disabilities, although the work of Calamari, Geist, and Shahbazian (1987) points out the potential of surface electromyographic (EMG) biofeedback. The research to date (Lindsay, Baty, Michie, & Richardson, 1989) has mainly focused on a special relaxation approach developed by Shilling and Poppen (1983), termed *behavioral relaxation training* (BRT). This approach is illustrated in the following case. (Note that, as in other chapters, italics on first use of a term indicate that the term is included in the chapter's glossary.)

A Case Report

Michultka, Poppen, and Blanchard (1988) applied BRT to treat the migraine and frequent tension-type headache symptoms of a 29-year-old male patient with severe functional retardation. At age 7, he was diagnosed with autism, which was attributed to anoxia at birth. Administration of the Stanford–Binet Intelligence Scale at age 26 revealed an IQ below 30. He used one- and two-word phrases and *echolalia* to express himself and was inconsistent in responding to requests. However, he revealed some gross and fine motor skills, and he could complete some basic self-care skills. He was also able to verbalize headache presence by stating, "I have a headache."

BRT consisted of modeling, prompting, feedback, and positive reinforcement for sequentially shaping and reducing tension in 10 muscle groupings. The therapist began by demonstrating how to relax the hands, applying the BRT procedures as appropriate, and continuing with the next posture (attempts to have the client demonstrate both tension and relaxation proved to be too difficult). Relaxed postures were required to be maintained for increasingly longer intervals in order for verbal reinforcement to be delivered (beginning with 5 seconds and continuing to 60 seconds). A relaxed posture was considered to be acquired when it could be maintained for two 60-second intervals. A small amount of iced tea was used to reinforce compliance, in addition to the verbal reinforcement. Nineteen sessions were used in all (10 for acquisition training, 9 for proficiency training).

The Behavioral Relaxation Scale (BRS) was administered during the final 10 minutes of each session in order to assess relaxation progress. With the BRS, the client was shown to demonstrate a high level of skill proficiency (90%), which was maintained over a 3-month follow-up period. More importantly, BRT led to marked improvement: Both headache complaints and medication consumption (staff-verified) decreased by approximately 50%.

Implications and Limits

Michultka et al. (1988) reveal the potential of BRT for teaching relaxation to individuals with moderate to severe developmental disabilities, and for treating headaches in this population. The use and adaptation of BRT procedures for anxiety in people with severe developmental disabilities have support (Lindsay et al., 1989). A major advantage of these procedures is that they do not require the conceptual awareness that is needed (but is difficult to achieve by people with severe retardation) for other forms of relaxation. As Lindsay et al. (1989) describe the sequence,

> The instructor demonstrates the unrelaxed and relaxed states in each area and then helps the person to copy the relaxed behaviors . . . in a comfortable chair. [The person is] . . . asked first to watch the unrelaxed behaviour and then to watch and imitate the relaxed behaviour . . . with manual guidance if necessary. (pp. 133–134)

There is potential cost-effectiveness in using this treatment for this population, because it minimizes professional time and reduces the time and expense for management. Furthermore, there is less need for medical attention and tests, and there exists a potential for at least partial home care rather than only residential care.

The limits of the Michultka et al. (1988) report include possible staff bias in reporting complaints of headache and medication use. There were also problems with compliance and the length of treatment because of the patient's behavioral problems. No physiological data could be collected because of the subject's motor behavior. Finally, the *A-B design* did not allow clear evidence of a treatment effect for the headache symptoms.

Lindsay and his colleagues (Lindsay, 1988; Lindsay et al., 1989) also warn that this "powerful psychological technique" may be abused for people with mental retardation if it is used solely to keep them quiet and manageable, rather than "as a beginning to a treatment program whereby [such a] person is introduced to more adaptive and stimulating opportunities" (Lindsay et al., 1989, p. 139).

TREATING OLDER/ELDERLY PEOPLE

The frontier for applications of biofeedback and related procedures with older or elderly[1] persons involves improving selection and refining treatment procedures. Motivated, creative developers and settlers will follow the trailblazers in this area.

It was once commonly assumed that biofeedback therapies were for young and middle-aged people. It was assumed further that people beyond middle age probably could not learn psychophysiological self-regulation, because it was too complicated and subtle. Researchers and clinical practitioners eager to show success focused on younger patients. Changes have occurred only gradually in reports about biofeedback for older and elderly people (Andrasik, 1991).

Mannarino (1991) has reminded us that by the year 2020, nearly 29% of us are projected to be aged 65 or older, and 4.1% to be aged 80 or older. The latter group will be over 12 million strong. The belief in inevitable decline in physical, mental, and sexual functioning with age was previously accepted as fact. However, according to a former director of the National Institute on Aging, we now know that this "inevitable decline" is a myth (Williams,

1991). Most older and many elderly persons continue to function very well. Data from 1983–1984,[2] based on household interviews of civilians, indicated that in each of two age groups 75 years and over (75–84 years, and 85 years and over), 35% reported being in excellent or very good health (Mannarino, 1991, p. 392). Williams (1991) praised Warner Schaie (1983, 1989) as providing "the best longitudinal data on a population followed from age 50 through the 80s" (p. 340); he described Schaie's data as showing "no consistent decline in mental function until the middle 80s" (p. 340). Williams (1991) also cited evidence that although there is considerable variability, stability holds for other organ systems as well.

There is much research support showing that older/elderly adults have a substantial reserve capacity and are capable of increasing their performance on tests of fluid intelligence as a consequence of guided instruction in problem-solving strategies by an "expert" tutor (Baltes, Sowarka, & Kliegl, 1989). These investigators at the prestigious Max-Planck-Institute for Human Development and Education in Berlin subsequently showed that similar training benefits could occur without a special tutor (in a sample with an average educational level of 10.7 years). These individuals' reported subjective health was better than average; they could learn to solve a variety of tasks and novel problems; and they could do this with or without guided help.

There are many disorders for which applied psychophysiology and biofeedback can be used as interventions for older/elderly persons. These include headaches, neuromuscular rehabilitation, chronic pain, hypertension, chronic constipation, urinary and fecal incontinence, irritable bowel syndrome, *dysphagia*, balance and equilibrium, and diabetes. Because of space limitations, we can only describe a few of these here.

Chronic Headaches

Abrahamson (1987) reviewed the data of Blanchard, Andrasik, Evans, and Hillhouse (1985), who had reported difficulty treating older/elderly patients with very chronic headaches. She reported that she had successfully treated patients aged 60–76 years with a variety of symptoms, and she reflected on her own therapy procedures. The group at the State University of New York–Albany was already examining its own data with a larger sample (Kabela, Blanchard, Appelbaum, & Nicholson, 1989). They focused on an uncontrolled series of 16 patients with headache aged 60–77, of whom 10 achieved the success criterion of 50% or greater improvement. These patients accomplished this despite the fact that 5 of them had reported headaches for 40–60 years; others reported headaches for 10–25 years.

Arena, Hightower, and Chang (1988) published the first prospective study of muscle relaxation treatment of older/elderly patients with tension headaches. They reported that 70% of their sample significantly improved with eight sessions over 6 weeks. They also published the first prospective study of surface EMG (hereafter referred to simply as EMG) biofeedback in the treatment of an older population with tension headaches (Arena, Hannah, Bruno, & Meador, 1991). Here the focus was on a sample of eight patients, with an average age of 65 (range 62–71), who had had at least 30 years of headaches. Their procedures (see Schwartz & Andrasik, Chapter 14, this volume) were adapted to meet the needs of older patients. On a standard headache index, four patients were shown to improve 53–89%, and three others improved 35–45%. It should be noted that three of the four successfully treated patients were among their oldest patients, including the very oldest.

Chronic Pain

Middaugh and her colleagues at the Medical University of South Carolina have made important and useful inroads into the frontier of biofeedback applications to older patients, especially those with chronic musculoskeletal back pain and other chronic pain conditions (Middaugh, Levin, Kee, Barchiesi, & Roberts, 1988; Middaugh, Woods, Kee, Harden, & Peters, 1991; Middaugh, Kee, & Peters, 1992; Middaugh & Pawlick, 2002). They initially compared the results of 59 older patients with 58 younger patients treated in a multidisciplinary chronic pain rehabilitation program. The average age of the older patients was 63, compared with age 37 for the younger. Middaugh et al.'s program involved both inpatients and outpatients, with a variety of pain types. Most of the patients had musculoskeletal back pain (73% of the older and 83% of the younger). The biofeedback and relaxation involved 8–12 sessions of muscle relaxation, breathing, and EMG biofeedback.

The EMG biofeedback typically focused on the upper trapezius muscles for patients with cervical pain and on the lumbar paraspinous muscles for patients with low back pain. With EMG biofeedback, patients practiced muscle relaxation during various activities, such as sitting, standing, walking, and performing daily activities (e.g., writing and simulated driving). Psychophysiological goals included reaching hand temperatures of 93.5°F or higher and respiration rates of 12 breaths per minute or lower. Goals for EMG included reaching 25 microvolts (peak-to-peak[3]) or less during baselines while sitting or standing, and recovery within 15 seconds.

Before therapy, only two of the eight older patients with chronic cervical pain could relax the upper trapezius muscles during a sitting baseline. They could not recover to a criterion level of relaxation rapidly after three shoulder shrugs and releases. After therapy, six of the eight older patients met both criteria. Among the six younger patients with chronic cervical pain, only one patient met both criteria (Middaugh et al., 1991). The older patients also met the criteria for hand temperature and respiration rate; in these respects, there were no differences between the groups. For the present discussion, the important point is that "biofeedback/ relaxation . . . did not pose special problems for older chronic pain patients . . . compared to younger patients with similar diagnoses and duration of pain who were receiving treatment in the same multidisciplinary treatment program" (Middaugh et al., 1991, p. 376).

The larger sample reported by Middaugh et al. (1992) lent further support for these conclusions. Both groups showed reduced ratings of maximum pain. The 17 older patients, aged 55–78, reduced their use of health care services by 93% and reduced their use of pain-related medications 64% (Middaugh et al., 1988). Middaugh and Pawlick (2002) recently replicated these positive findings with a larger clinical sample. In fact, in this latest trial, greater reductions in pain occurred for the older patients.

Older/elderly people can and do make targeted psychophysiological changes, and they often can do as well as (or better than) younger patients on changing pain ratings. In contrast to statements by some authors (e.g., Kaplan & Kepes, 1989) who speculate that biofeedback may be "less suitable" for patients over age 70, biofeedback and relaxation procedures are as proper with them as they are with younger patients.

Constipation

The highly successful use of EMG biofeedback for constipation resulting from *paradoxical puborectalis contraction* has been demonstrated primarily with older/elderly patients. The report by Heyman and Wexner (1993) gives the average age of their 39 patients as 62.6; the oldest patient was 84! See more discussion of this application in Tries and Eisman, Chapter 28 of this volume. For the present discussion, the conclusion is that practitioners must not exclude older and elderly patients from this treatment.

Incontinence

Other examples of successful applications of biofeedback for older/elderly patients include applications for fecal incontinence (Whitehead, Burgio, & Engel, 1985) and urinary incontinence (McDowell, Burgio, Dombrowski, Locher, & Rodriguez, 1992; Middaugh, Whitehead, Burgio, & Engel, 1989).

The average age of the 18 patients with fecal incontinence selected for treatment by Whitehead et al. (1985) was 73; the range was 65–92 years! These patients significantly increased sphincter strength with biofeedback. There was more than a 75% decrease of incontinence for 10 of the patients (77%). At 6 months, 60% of the patients maintained their improvement, and 42% did so at 1 year (Whitehead et al., 1985). The criteria for these percentages were being continent or soiling less than once per month. Of those patients who were unsuccessful, two had severe dementia, and one revealed "gross loss of sensation for rectal distension" (p. 323). Five patients maintained continence at 1 year. We may also note that three patients had debilitating and progressive illnesses, which probably resulted in the relapses.

Significantly, a 92-year-old male patient initially did very well reducing the incontinence from 3.5 to 0.7 incidents per week. The next oldest patients, aged 81 and 78, did very well after treatment and at both follow-up assessments. The purpose here is mainly to show the value of this therapy for elderly patients. Urinary incontinence after strokes in four older patients was the focus of the Middaugh et al. (1989) series. The strokes had occurred 8 months, 2, 4, and 10 years earlier among these patients; their ages ranged from 61 to 69 years. All "achieved and maintained continence" (p. 3).

The 27 women and 2 men with urinary incontinence in the McDowell et al. (1992) series had an average age of nearly 75, with a range of 56–90 years. Most (n = 21) had a mixed type of urinary incontinence, and 7 had only the urge type. Many of the patients selected and doing well had several other significant health problems, including depression, stroke, diabetes, and parkinsonism. The 29 selected patients were among 70 initially referred and evaluated. The others were "ineligible based on their mental status, urologic findings, or more urgent medical problems" (p. 374). One cannot assess the specific need for biofeedback in this multicomponent treatment study. However, that is not the point of including it here. The point is that the selected patients could participate adequately with the biofeedback procedures and showed excellent results. The average weekly number of accidents dropped from 16.9 to 2.5. Individual patients reduced their accidents an average of 81.6%, and 10 of the 29 patients became continent.

Conclusion

Using biofeedback and other applied psychophysiological therapies with older/elderly people is no longer a frontier position. It has progressed into a major development in the heartland. One clearly sees that being over age 65 is no longer a criterion for excluding patients from or denying them such treatments.

TREATING PEOPLE DIAGNOSED WITH SCHIZOPHRENIA

People diagnosed with schizophrenia have a variety of symptoms for which tension reduction treatments might help. However, people so affected obviously also have a variety of behaviors and other characteristics, including psychomotor deficits and medication effects, that interfere with relaxation therapies and biofeedback-assisted procedures. Goals typically do not target the underlying problem—that is, whatever is causing the constellation of behaviors called schizophrenia. Goals more appropriately include changing such behaviors as excess muscle tension.

For early work applying biofeedback to this population, one looks to only five studies found by Pharr and Coursey in their 1989 review (Acosta, Yamamoto, & Wilcox, 1978; Nigl & Jackson, 1979; Weiner, 1979; Keating, 1981; Wentworth-Rohr, 1981). Employing relaxation and biofeedback with such patients is obviously extremely challenging, and few professionals have ventured into this area. The first four reports included 14 inpatients and 12 outpatients; the Wentworth-Rohr study included 45 inpatients. A subsequent single-case report (Stein & Nikolic, 1989) showed that a patient diagnosed with *undifferentiated schizophrenia* could accept and participate in relaxation therapies and biofeedback. The patient experienced a clinically significant reduction of anxiety, according to self-report measures. The authors described interesting modifications of treatment procedures, such as role reversals. More recent research has again substantiated the value of various self-regulatory treatments for this population (Rickard, Collier, McCoy, Crist, & Weinberger, 1993; Starkey, Deleone, & Flannery, 1995). Furthermore, few negative side effects have been reported (Rickard, McCoy, Collier, & Weinberger, 1989).

The paper by Pharr and Coursey (1989) supported the use of EMG feedback for lowering muscle tension. Using the right forearm extensor muscles and a frontal placement, they compared EMG feedback from a meter and an audio tone for patients who received seven sessions. They noted that some people diagnosed with schizophrenia could tolerate EMG biofeedback for periods up to 40 minutes, with a typical session being divided into four 10-minute phases (baseline, forearm feedback, frontal feedback, and postsession monitoring). Even when taking medications such as *chlorpromazine*, *lithium*, and antiparkinsonian agents, these patients significantly reduced their muscle tension levels. Baseline EMG values (defined as the "integrated absolute levels, microvolts per minute, of muscle tension over 1-minute periods of both sites combined," p. 234) were very high throughout: 36 and 30 microvolts in sessions 1 and 2, and approximately 22 microvolts by sessions 6 and 7. The postsession EMG level showed no decrease at the end of session 1. However, there were large decreases in subsequent sessions: Activity decreased to 20 microvolts in sessions 4–6, and further to 15 microvolts in session 7. The variances remained sizable. One comparison group received progressive relaxation via an audiotape, while another served as a control group and merely listened to audiotaped information on adjustment taken from two psychology texts. Neither of these two comparison groups showed improvement.

The value of this study lies in its uniqueness at the time. It provided a controlled investigation of biofeedback for patients diagnosed with schizophrenia. It showed that many of these patients would participate in such treatment and could reduce muscle tension. There were also some positive global behavior changes in social behavior, based on the Nurses' Observation Scale for Inpatient Evaluation. These are encouraging, although they need replication and extension.

It is useful to have models within which to plan and develop interventions. A paper by Spaulding, Storms, Goodrich, and Sullivan (1986) reviews and offers a useful guide and perspective for including relaxation therapies and biofeedback in multimodal treatments of patients with schizophrenia. They focus on the vulnerability–stress model of schizophrenia in which persons with schizophrenia are assumed to have lower thresholds for disorganization that contribute to vulnerability. Stress increases arousal, which brings many competing responses to the same strength, leading to intrusion of inappropriate responses. Interventions that reduce arousal and lower the strengths of competing responses should reduce psychological deficits. These authors concluded:

> Arousal-reducing, attentional, and cognitive interventions are appropriate for . . . schizophrenic disorders. . . . Remediation . . . may facilitate the effectiveness of neuroleptic medications, social skills training, and family therapy. (p. 560)

Spaulding et al. (1986) also proposed that patients with schizophrenia can be taught to manage their own arousal during prodromal and postacute phases. They further asserted that relaxation techniques are very useful and "a popular modality in service programs for severely disordered psychiatric patients" (p. 565). Referring partly to work by Ford, Stroebel, Strong, and Szarek (1982), they added that "biofeedback may prove to be a useful adjunct to . . . arousal-reduction techniques in schizophrenics" (p. 565).

Treatment Considerations

The work of the late I. Wentworth-Rohr (1988) provides helpful clinical guidelines for using biofeedback with these patients. His experience and clinical wisdom suggested that practitioners should pay meticulous attention to patients' questions and apprehensions, and should devote extra time to making sure that patients have a clear and concrete understanding of the source of the signal. He used EMG, temperature, and electrodermal biofeedback, with a variety of relaxation techniques. He emphasized the need for working with only cooperative patients who were not experiencing overtly psychotic episodes.

Wentworth-Rohr carefully explained relaxation techniques "as taking one's attention and mind and placing them where one wants to." He discouraged free association and any techniques or statements that suggested "letting the mind go blank or empty. . . ." He reminded patients "to maintain their attention (passively) on their body regions, rather than to allow their minds or attention to drift off." He encouraged "recollection of an experience of self-adequacy and a sense of tranquility." If the frontal EMG fell to less than 2 microvolts (with the bandpass set at 100–200 hertz), and respiration became obviously slow and shallow, he lessened the relaxation depth by instructing patients to recall specific scenes or images. He apparently was trying to avoid having patients fall asleep or slip into "ego regression."

In his 1988 report, Wentworth-Rohr noted there were an average of three presenting complaints for those patients for whom biofeedback and behavior therapy were appropriate, with the number of complaints ranging from one to five. The average duration was about the same for each complaint. The average number of treatment sessions was 11–12, and the range was 1–32. There were 9 or more sessions for 29 of the 45 patients. It is not clear how many of these sessions were exclusively or mostly for biofeedback, and that is a major limitation. However, Wentworth-Rohr and his colleagues used biofeedback with nearly all the patients in the series, and the case examples focused on biofeedback. Relaxation and biofeedback were core parts of the treatment.

Wentworth-Rohr (1988) reported significant and lasting improvements in 29 of 46 symptoms, with improvement requiring nine or more sessions. Follow-up time averaged 14 months and ranged from 6 to 46 months. Of the original 45 patients, 31 could be followed. Of these, 22 had received 9 or more sessions. Of these, the six who had 9–11 sessions improved on more problems (14/18; $p < .018$) than those with more sessions or fewer sessions. Of the 16 with 12–32 sessions, most improved (29/46 problems; $p < .077$). This compares with poor improvement for those with eight or fewer sessions (5/22). Wentworth-Rohr and colleagues did not control for psychotropic medications, which is significant, because 35 of the 45 patients were using such medications.

Other guidelines for working with these patients derive from Liberman, Nuechterlein, and Wallace (1982, as reported by Spaulding et al., 1986). These are provided below, following several recommendations by Wentworth-Rohr (1988).

Implications

Many patients diagnosed with schizophrenia can participate in treatments involving relaxation and biofeedback modalities. Wentworth-Rohr (1988) recommends that clinicians do the following:

- Select cooperative patients who are not overtly psychotic.
- Consider patients in the prodromal, postacute, and chronic stages.
- Consider special treatment procedures for this population.
- Expect physiological changes to occur in the desired direction, even with patients taking a variety of very potent psychotropic medications.
- Do not expect new symptoms to develop. A small percentage (9% or 4/45, in Wentworth-Rohr's [1988] sample) of patients may show worsening of symptoms, but this is unlikely to be due to treatment.
- Use uncluttered visual displays. For example, display one or two channels rather than more. Keep other information off the screens if possible.
- Repeat steps often before moving to new tasks.
- Recognize that muscle tension is often much higher in these patients than in most other patients.
- Consider role reversals when teaching relaxation and using biofeedback. For example, allow a patient to teach you a procedure with and without the biofeedback.
- Expect that significant reduction of psychophysiological tension may start within the first sessions, but that successful reduction of symptoms and maintenance are likely to require nine or more sessions with most of these patients.

Liberman et al. (1982) add these guidelines:

- Eliminate all clutter and other distracting stimuli in the treatment room.
- Divide the tasks into simple steps. Use shortened versions of relaxation procedures.
- Use graphic charts with clear and simple information to show patients their progress.
- Use praise for proper and correct responding, and mild criticism contingent on improper and incorrect responses.

The use of biofeedback and related treatments with this population should encourage practitioners to work with these and other severely impaired patients. A diagnosis of schizophrenia and the presence of psychotropic medications should not deter practitioners. The combination of medication with biofeedback treatments may be needed for these patients. It is not yet possible to separate the effects of the nonpharmacological treatments. We address one final topic: There is growing evidence that patients with schizophrenia can learn to regulate cortical activity (Gruzelier, 2000; Schneider et al., 1992). With further work and development, such approaches may prove to be particularly helpful for targeting the attentional, motivational, and arousal dysregulations that characterize patients with severe psychiatric disturbances.

TREATING PEOPLE WITH PHANTOM LIMB PAIN

"Phantom limb pain" is pain experienced in a body part that no longer exists because of traumatic or surgical amputation. The missing body part is usually a foot, lower leg, hand, or arm. Most people with phantom limb pain also experience stump pain; "pure" phantom pain is less common. Nerves in the residual limb probably seldom, if ever, become normal. These nerves have limited protection. Poorly fitted prostheses and painful sores create volleys of signals to the brain. According to Sherman, Arena, Sherman, and Ernst (1989), these and other stump problems probably stimulate the brain centers that were formerly reactive to the removed portion of the limb. *Receptor interneurons*, formerly associated with the amputated portion of the limb, may detect signals produced by intact nerves from the residual limb. They reach the *sensory and motor homunculus* along tracks formerly associated with the amputated portion of the limb; thus the brain interprets them as starting from the phantom part. Irritation of the stump increases phantom pain, and resolving the stump problem should help reduce this pain. Increased muscle tension in the residual limb precedes sensations of cramping phantom pain (Sherman et al., 1989; Sherman, Greffin, Evans, & Grana, 1992). These careful researchers cautiously state that "this evidence can not prove that cramping phantom pain is actually caused by increased muscle tension, but it certainly increases the likelihood that it is the underlying cause" (Sherman et al., 1992, p. 73). It is less clear but "highly likely that changes in muscle tension are also related to onset of . . . shocking–shooting phantom pain" (p. 73). A detailed discussion of this mechanism may be found in Sherman et al. (1989).

Definitions, Incidence, and Features

"Burning" and "cramping," alone or together, are two very common descriptions of phantom limb pain, as is "tingling." Other less common descriptions are "shooting," "shocking," "stabbing," "throbbing," and "twisting" pain. The focus on and distinction between burning and cramping are important, because Sherman et al. (1989) suggest that skin temperature biofeedback is more effective for burning pain and that EMG biofeedback is more effective for cramping pain. Among military veterans with amputations, 80% report significant phantom pain. For the vast majority of individuals with amputations, none of the standard treatments provides significant and lasting benefit (Sherman & Sherman, 1985; Sherman et al., 1989). Most patients in the series reported by Sherman and colleagues had unilateral amputations above or below the knee. There were also patients with bilateral, at-shoulder, at-hip, toe, above-elbow, and below-elbow amputations in this series. Some had had the amputations within the past 1–2 years; however, most of the amputations had occurred many years before the subjects entered Sherman et al.'s studies. The reasons for the amputations included war injuries, vehicular accidents, vascular problems, and diabetes.

Comparison of cortical somatotropic maps and phantom limb phenomena for four patients with traumatic amputations and phantom pain, five with congenital absence of an upper limb, and five healthy control subjects showed significant shifts in cortical representation among the group with traumatic amputations, but none among the group with congenital limb absence or the control subjects. This is consistent with the rarity of phantom limb phenomena among individuals with congenital missing limbs (Flor et al., 1998). The estimated base rate for nonpainful phantom limb phenomena is between 7% and 18% for adults with congenital limb absence. Even among the three individuals with congenital missing limbs in the Flor et al. (1998) study who sustained stump trauma, none of them developed phantom phenomena; this finding is contrary to other reports that intense input results in late-developing phantom limbs in such patients. Other research concludes that the "development of phantom limbs and phantom pain [is] closely tied to experience rather than to genetic determination" (Montoya et al., 1998, p. 1101).

Biofeedback Treatment

EMG biofeedback from the major muscles of the residual limb is the preferred modality for cramping phantom pain. Skin temperature biofeedback to help increase peripheral blood flow is the modality that Sherman's group uses for burning pain. Relaxation procedures are an important part of both treatments. There is good support for the use of biofeedback for phantom limb pain (Sherman, 1989, 1997; Sherman et al., 1989; Belleggia & Birbaumer, 2001).

A case study of much importance was recently reported by Belleggia and Birbaumer (2001), who successfully treated a 69-year-old man with phantom pain in the right arm

3 years after an amputation at the right wrist after an accident. The pain was rated 7 of a possible 10 before amputation, with pressure feelings from the fingers to elbow, and then burning and shooting phantom pain 1 month after the amputation. He also felt flexed fingers, a fist, and cold at that time, and rated the phantom pain as 8 of 10. There was no stump pain and no prosthesis.

Intervention involved two phases of six sessions each. The first focused on increasing awareness of sensations and muscle tension in the stump via increasing and decreasing tension. The second phase focused on increasing stump temperature to decrease the burning phantom pain. In the two phases, after baselines, there were first increases and then decreases in EMG at the stump, and then increases in temperature, with each change involving alternating feedback and no feedback (each for 6 minutes).

Skin temperatures decreased during baseline for the stump but not the intact arm. During biofeedback-assisted treatment, skin temperature in the stump increased by about 2°C (from 30.4°) to about 32°), and EMG decreased. "Telescoping" (retraction of the phantom limb into the stump) occurred during treatment, with the phantom fingers moving to the stump and without the patient's perceiving the arm. The phantom fingers remained open and relaxed instead of in a fist, and the pain rating decreased to 3 of 10. At 3 and 12 months, the pain rating was 0. At 12 months there was more telescoping, with only some fingers vaguely felt on the stump. The telescoping was consistent with a negative correlation between phantom limb pain and telescoping, although this is not always observed (Flor, Birbaumer, & Sherman, 2000).

Clinical Response and Outcome

The contributions of Sherman and colleagues to understanding and treating phantom pain with biofeedback date back nearly three decades (Sherman, 1976; McKechnie, 1975; Sherman, Gall, & Gormly, 1979). The original series of 16 cases was followed for 1–5 years, and 88% of these patients maintained their pain reduction (Sherman et al., 1989). Sherman and colleagues' treatment consists of EMG and/or thermal biofeedback and at least muscle relaxation. They expressed cautious optimism about their report of thermal biofeedback for 30 patients, whose pain was presumably related to peripheral vasoconstriction (Sherman et al., 1989). Their rationale for relaxation and thermal biofeedback is straightforward: Decreased blood flow to the residual limb results in phantom pain, usually involving burning and sometimes throbbing and tingling sensations. Sherman et al. (1989) state that "several lines of logic and evidence increase the likelihood that changes in blood flow in the peripheral limb are the cause of the change in phantom pain" (p. 270).

Other Treatments

Muscle relaxation procedures are used for both types of phantom limb pain. The rationale is to decrease muscle tension and help increase blood flow by decreasing vasoconstriction. Sherman et al. (1989) note that when the pain is due to vasoconstriction, "any method that increases blood flow to the residual limb should attenuate the pain" (p. 272). Medications for achieving increased blood flow are important for patients with extensive peripheral vascular disease, who have severe problems with peripheral blood flow (Sherman & Barja, 1989).

Another very important, exciting, and efficacious rehabilitation approach, developed in a line of research originated and continued by Edward Taub and many associates, is called "constraint-induced movement therapy." A functional prosthesis (of the Sauerbruch type) permits carrying out a wide variety of activities, effectively thereby enhancing substantial use of the remaining part of the limb. The Sauerbruch prosthesis connects an arm muscle to a prosthetic hand that allows contraction and relaxation of the muscle to control the prosthetic hand. This permits massed practice many hours per day over consecutive days. The rationale for this approach with patients who have phantom limb pain is that, as with patients recovering from stroke, this excites the part of the cerebral cortex that innervates the muscles in the residual limb and leads rapidly to normalizing the relevant parts of the sensory and motor homunculus. Weiss, Mittner, Adler, Brükner, and Taub (1999), in a preliminary yet very encouraging study, compared a group of patients with amputations who were using the Sauerbruch prosthesis to a control group using a cosmetic prosthesis of little functional value. As predicted, five of the seven subjects with the Sauerbruch prosthesis who had previously had phantom limb pain reported disappearance of the pain. One went from unbearable pain (10 on a 0–10 scale) to no pain. In contrast, none of the subjects using the cosmetic prosthesis reported disappearance of their pain, and several reported increased pain. "The presumed mechanism [is] an increase in use-dependent (afferent-increase) cortical reorganization that reverses the cortical reorganization of the afferent-decrease type . . . highly correlated with phantom limb pain" (Weiss et al., 1999, p. 134).

Psychological Factors and Measures

As with other types of chronic pain, psychological factors such as stress and fatigue can worsen phantom limb pain. However, based on a comprehensive reexamination of the literature and their own experience, Sherman et al. (1989) do not believe that psychological variables *cause* the pain. The self-report measures used to assess chronic pain and psychological problems in this population should thus be the same as for other conditions in which psychological factors can worsen or exacerbate pain.

Cortical Reorganization, Neural Plasticity, and Some Implications

Phantom limb pain is related to cortical reorganization; hence it reveals "plasticity," or the ability of the brain to change its topography or physical characteristics as a result of events that affect the body—in this case, loss of a limb and biofeedback-assisted intervention (Birbaumer et al., 1997; Knecht et al., 1995, 1998; Flor et al., 1995; Montoya et al., 1997, 1998; Ramachandran & Rogers-Ramachandran, 2000). This is an extremely important, exciting, and very promising area of research, with substantial heuristic value and clinical implications.

Implications and Limits

The following are recommendations for practitioners in this area:

- Assess the phantom limb pain and factors that might worsen and relieve it.
- For cramping pain, use EMG biofeedback from the residual limb.
- For burning pain, use skin temperature biofeedback from the stump area.
- Use muscle relaxation procedures and other relaxation procedures that can reduce muscle tension and increase blood flow.
- Consider medications for peripheral vasodilation for selected patients.

There appear to be multiple ways, including biofeedback, relaxation, and constraint-induced movement therapy, to reduce and stop phantom limb pain. Research on phantom limb pain has resulted in considerable research support for the presence of cortical plasticity or reorganization, which is associated with changes in pain and related sensations.

SUMMARY

This chapter has highlighted the use, potential, and support for biofeedback and other forms of applied psychophysiological interventions for four special populations: people with severe developmental disabilities, older/elderly persons, patients diagnosed with schizophrenia, and patients with phantom limb pain.

GLOSSARY

A-B DESIGN. A single-case experimental design in which an intervention or treatment (B) follows a baseline (A).

BEHAVIORAL RELAXATION TRAINING (BRT). A set of special relaxation procedures developed by Poppen and colleagues (Schilling & Poppen, 1983). It includes modeling, prompting, verbal feedback, and positive reinforcement of relaxed and unrelaxed overt behaviors and postures in 10 areas of the body. The goal is to teach relaxed postures associated with reduced muscle tension, but it avoids focusing on internal states and sensations of relaxation that people with severe mental retardation and others with severe disabilities may find very difficult to grasp. BRT is often used with the Behavioral Relaxation Scale (BRS; Poppen & Maurer, 1982) to help document the relaxation behaviors.

CHLORPROMAZINE. A phenothiazine derivative used as a major tranquilizer.

DYSPHAGIA (APHAGIA). Difficulty swallowing.

ECHOLALIA. Stereotyped repeating of the words or phrases of another person.

HOMUNCULUS, SENSORY AND MOTOR. *Homunculus* literally means "a little man." The sensory and motor homunculus is the proportional representation of various parts of the body in the sensory and motor areas of the cerebral cortex. The representation is proportional to the amount of cortical area associated with sensory and motor innervation density of the body parts, rather than to the size of the body parts themselves. For example, the lips and fingers have a relatively large representation in the sensory area. In the motor area, the fingers, hand, and lips have a relatively large representation.

LITHIUM. Lithium salts (lithium carbonate), commonly used to treat bipolar disorder by attentuating mood swings, especially the manic phase.

PARADOXICAL PUBORECTALIS CONTRACTION. Dyscoordination of the external anal sphincter and puborectalis muscles. Tightening of these muscles during attempts to defecate. Causes functional outlet obstruction, also known as "dyschezia" or difficult or painful evacuation of feces. Other terms for this condition are "anismus" and "pelvic floor outlet obstruction syndrome" (see Tries & Eisman, Chapter 28, this volume).

RECEPTOR INTERNEURONS. Interneurons are between the primary afferent (sensory) neuron and the final motor neuron. Also, neurons whose process is entirely within a specific area and that synapse with neurons extending into that area. Synapse is the junction between nerve cells.

SCHIZOPHRENIA, UNDIFFERENTIATED. Presence of symptoms that meet the general criteria for schizophrenia but not those for any of its subtypes.

NOTES

1. There are no agreed-upon age criteria for separating young adulthood, middle age, and "elderly" status. If 40–55 is considered middle age (as it is by some), then being elderly starts at 56. Mark S. Schwartz was 53 when the second edition of this book was published. He noted then that his preference was to define "elderly" as beginning at age 65. He added that when he got near age 65, he might adjust that age slightly. He currently proposes ages 20–29 as young adulthood, 30–39 as high young adulthood, 40–54 as middle age, 55–64 as upper middle age, 65–74 as older age, and 75+ as elderly status. (Note that Schwartz is age 61 at this writing! People aged 75+ are very different from people aged 55–64, and the two groups should not be lumped together.

2. Data from the National Health Interview Survey (Division of Health Interview Statistics, National Center for Health Statistics).

3. Peak-to-peak microvolts are about three times higher than root mean square and integral average microvolts (see Peek, Chapter 4, this volume).

REFERENCES

Treating People with Developmental Disabilities

Calamari, J. E., Geist, G. O., & Shahbazian, M. J. (1987). Evaluation of multiple component relaxation training with developmentally disabled persons. *Research in Developmental Disabilities, 8,* 55–70.

Lindsay, W. R. (1988). *The assessment and treatment of anxiety and phobia in people with a mental handicap.* Workshop presented for the British Institute of Mental Handicap.

Lindsay, W. R., Baty, F. J., Michie, A. M., & Richardson, I. (1989). A comparison of anxiety treatments with adults who have moderate and severe mental retardation. *Research in Developmental Disabilities, 10*(2), 129–140.

Michultka, D. M., Poppen, R. L., & Blanchard, E. B. (1988). Relaxation training as a treatment for chronic headaches in an individual having severe developmental disabilities. *Biofeedback and Self-Regulation, 13*(3), 257–266.

Poppen, R., & Maurer, J. P. (1982). Electromyographic analysis of relaxed postures. *Biofeedback and Self-Regulation, 7,* 491–498.

Shilling, D., & Poppen, R. (1983). Behavioral relaxation training and assessment. *Journal of Behavior Therapy and Experimental Psychiatry, 14,* 99–107.

Treating Older People

Abrahamson, C. F. (1987). Response to the challenge: Effective treatment of the elderly through thermal biofeedback combined with progressive relaxation. *Biofeedback and Self-Regulation, 12*(2), 121–125.

Andrasik, F. (1991). Aging and self-regulation: An introduction and overview. *Biofeedback and Self-Regulation, 16*(4), 333–336.

Arena, J. G., Hannah, S. L., Bruno, G. M., & Meador, K. J. (1991). Electromyographic biofeedback training for tension headache in the elderly: A prospective study. *Biofeedback and Self-Regulation, 16*(4), 397–390.

Arena, J. G., Hightower, N. E., & Chang, G. C. (1988). Relaxation therapy for tension headaches in the elderly: A prospective study. *Psychology and Aging, 3,* 96–98.

Baltes, P. B., Sowarka, D., & Kliegl, R. (1989). Cognitive training research on fluid intelligence in old age: What can older adults achieve by themselves? *Psychology and Aging, 4*(2), 217–221.

Blanchard, E. B., Andrasik, F., Evans, D. D., & Hillhouse, J. (1985). Biofeedback and relaxation treatments for headache in the elderly: A caution and a challenge. *Biofeedback and Self-Regulation, 10*(1), 69–73.

Heyman, S., & Wexner, S. (1993, March). EMG biofeedback retraining for paradoxical puborectalis contractions in patients with chronic constipation. In *Proceedings of the 24th Annual Meeting of the Association for Applied Psychophysiology and Biofeedback*, Los Angeles. Wheat Ridge, CO: Association for Applied Psychophysiology and Biofeedback.

Kabela, E., Blanchard, E. B., Appelbaum, K. A., & Nicholson, N. (1989). Self-regulatory treatment of headache in the elderly. *Biofeedback and Self-Regulation, 14*(3), 219–228.

Kaplan, R., & Kepes, E. (1989, October). *Pain problems over 70 and under 40 years.* Paper presented at the Eighth Annual Meeting of the American Pain Society, Phoenix, AZ.

Mannarino, M. (1991). The present and future roles of biofeedback in successful aging. *Biofeedback and Self-Regulation, 16*(4), 391–397.

McDowell, J., Burgio, K. L., Dombrowski, M., Locher, J. L., & Rodriguez, R. (1992). An interdisciplinary approach to the assessment and behavioral treatment of urinary incontinence in geriatric outpatients. *Journal of the American Geriatrics Society, 40*(4), 370–374.

Middaugh, S. J., Kee, W. G., & Peters, J. R. (1992, March). Physiological response of older and younger pain patients to biofeedback-assisted relaxation training. In *Proceedings of the 23rd Annual Meeting of the Association for Applied Psychophysiology and Biofeedback, Colorado Springs.* Wheat Ridge, CO: Association for Applied Psychophysiology and Biofeedback.

Middaugh, S. J., Levin, R B., Kee, W. G., Barchiesi, F. D., & Roberts, J. M. (1988). Chronic pain: Its treatment in geriatric and younger patients. *Archives of Physical Medicine and Rehabilitation, 69,* 1021–1026.

Middaugh, S. J., & Pawlick, K. (2002). Biofeedback and behavioral treatment of persistent pain in the older adult: A review and a study. *Applied Psychophysiology and Biofeedback, 27,* 185–202.

Middaugh, S. J., Whitehead, W. E., Burgio, K. L., & Engel, B. T. (1989). Biofeedback in treatment of urinary incontinence in stroke patients. *Biofeedback and Self-Regulation, 14,* 3–19.

Middaugh, S. J., Woods, E., Kee, W. G., Harden, R. N., & Peters, J. R. (1991). Biofeedback-assisted relaxation for the aging chronic pain patient. *Biofeedback and Self-Regulation, 16*(4), 361–376.

Schaie, K. W. (1983). The Seattle longitudinal study: A 21-year exploration of psychometric intelligence in adulthood. In K. W. Schaie (Ed.), *Longitudinal studies of adult psychological development*. New York: Guilford Press.

Schaie, K. W. (1989). Perceptual speed in adulthood: Cross-sectional and longitudinal studies. *Psychology and Aging, 4*, 443–453.

Whitehead, W. E., Burgio, K. L., & Engel, B. T. (1985). Biofeedback treatment of fecal incontinence in geriatric patients. *Journal of the American Geriatrics Society, 33*(5), 320–324.

Williams, T. F. (1991). Health care trends for older people. *Biofeedback and Self-Regulation, 16*(4), 337–347.

Treating People Diagnosed with Schizophrenia

Acosta, F., Yamanoto, J., & Wilcox, S. (1978). Application of electromyographic feedback to the relaxation of schizophrenic, neurotic and tension headache patients. *Journal of Consulting and Clinical Psychology, 46*, 383–384.

Ford, M., Stroebel, C., Strong, P., & Szarek, B. (1982). Quieting response training: Treatment of psychophysiological disorders in psychiatric inpatients. *Biofeedback and Self-Regulation, 7*, 331–339.

Gruzelier, J. (2000). Self regulation of electrocortical activity in schizophrenia and schizotypy: A review. *Clinical Electroencephalography, 31*, 23–29.

Keating, C. (1981). *Exploration of a combined program of electromyographic biofeedback and progressive relaxation as a treatment approach with schizophrenics*. Unpublished doctoral dissertation, Michigan State University.

Liberman, R. P., Nuechterlein, K., & Wallace, C. (1982). Social skills training and the nature of schizophrenia. In J. Curran & P. Monti (Eds.), *Social skills training*. New York: Guilford Press.

Nigl, A., & Jackson, B. (1979). Electromyographic biofeedback as an adjunct to standard psychiatric treatment. *Journal of Clinical Psychology, 44*, 433–436.

Pharr, O. M., & Coursey, R. D. (1989). The use and utility of EMG biofeedback with chronic schizophrenic patients. *Biofeedback and Self-Regulation, 14*(3), 229–245.

Rickard, H. C., Collier, J. B., McCoy, A. D., Crist, D. A., & Weinberger, M. B. (1993). Relaxation training for psychiatric inpatients. *Psychological Reports, 72*, 1267–1274.

Rickard, H. C., McCoy, A. D., Collier, J. B., & Weinberger, M. B. (1989). Relaxation training side effects reported by seriously disturbed inpatients. *Journal of Clinical Psychology, 45*, 446–450.

Schneider, F., Rockstroh, B., Heimann, H., Lutzenberger, W., Mattes, R., Elbert, T., Birbaumer, N., & Bartels, M. (1992). Self-regulation of slow cortical potentials in psychiatric patients: Schizophrenia. *Biofeedback and Self-Regulation, 17*, 277–292.

Spaulding, W. D., Storms, L., Goodrich, V., & Sullivan, M. (1986). Applications of experimental psychopathology in psychiatric rehabilitation. *Schizophrenia Bulletin, 12*(4), 560–577.

Starkey, D., Deleone, H., & Flannery R. B. (1995). Stress management for psychiatric patients in a state hospital setting. *American Journal of Orthopsychiatry, 65*, 446–450.

Stein, F., & Nikolic, S. (1989). Teaching stress management techniques to a schizophrenic patient. *American Journal of Occupational Therapy, 43*(3), 162–169.

Weiner, H. (1979). On altering muscle tension with chronic schizophrenia. *Psychological Reports, 44*, 527–534.

Wentworth-Rohr, I. (1988). *Symptom reduction through clinical biofeedback*. New York: Human Sciences Press.

Treating People with Phantom Limb Pain

Belleggia, G., & Birbaumer, N. (2001). Treatment of phantom limb pain with combined EMG and thermal biofeedback: A case report. *Applied Psychophysiology and Biofeedback, 26*(2), 141–146.

Birbaumer, N., Lutzenberger, W., Montoya, P., Larbig, W., Unertl, K., Töpfner, S., Grodd, W., Taub, E., & Flor, H. (1997). Effects of regional anesthesia on phantom limb pain are mirrored in changes in cortical reorganization. *Journal of Neuroscience, 15*, 5503–5508.

Flor, H., Birbaumer, N., & Sherman, R. A. (2000). Phantom limb pain. In *Pain. VIII, (3,5)* 1–4. Clinical updates, International Association for the Study of Pain.

Flor, H., Elbert, T., Knecht, S., Wienbruch, C., Pantev, C., Birbaumer, N., Larbig, W., & Taub, E. (1995). Phantom limb pain as perceptual correlate of cortical reorganization following arm amputation. *Nature, 375*, 482–484.

Flor, H., Elbert, T., Muhlnickel, W., Pantev, C., Wienbruch, C., & Taub, E. (1998). Cortical reorganization and phantom phenomena in congenital and traumatic upper-extremity amputees. *Experimental Brain Research*, *119*, 205–212.

Knecht, S., Henningsen, H., Elbert, T., Flor, H., Höhling, C., Pantev, C., Birbaumer, N., & Taub, E. (1995). Cortical reorganization in human amputees and mislocalization of painful stimuli to the phantom limb. *Neuroscience Letters, 201*, 262–264.

Knecht, S., Henningsen, H., Höhling, C., Elbert, T., Flor, H., Pantev, C., & Taub, E. (1998). Plasticity of plasticity?: Changes in the pattern of perceptual correlates of reorganization after amputation. *Brain, 121*, 717–724.

McKechnie, R. J. (1975). Relief from phantom limb pain by relaxation exercises. *Journal of Behavior Therapy and Experimental Psychiatry, 6*, 262–263.

Montoya, P., Larbig, W., Grulke, N., Flor, H., Taub, E., & Birbaumer, N. (1997). The relationship of phantom limb pain to other phantom limb phenomena in upper extremity amputees. *Pain, 72*, 87–93.

Montoya, P., Ritter, K., Huse, E., Larbig, W., Braun, C., Töpfner, S., Lutzenberger, W., Grodd, W., Flor, H., & Birbaumer, N. (1998). The cortical somatotopic map and phantom phenomena in subjects with congenital limb atrophy and traumatic amputees with phantom limb pain. *European Journal of Neuroscience, 10*, 1095–1102.

Ramachandran, V. S., & Rogers-Ramachandran, D. (2000). Phantom limbs and neural plasticity. *Archives of Neurology, 57*, 317–320.

Sherman, R. A. (1976). Case reports of treatment of phantom limb pain with a combination of electro-myographic biofeedback and verbal relaxation techniques. *Biofeedback and Self-Regulation, 1*, 353.

Sherman, R. A. (1980). Special review: Published treatments of phantom limb pain. *American Journal of Physical Medicine, 59*(5), 232–244.

Sherman, R. A. (1989). Stump and phantom limb pain. In R. K. Portenoy (Ed.), *Neurologic clinics: Pain.* Philadelphia: Saunders.

Sherman, R. A., Arena, J. G., Sherman, C. J., & Ernst, J. L. (1989). The mystery of phantom pain: Growing evidence for psychophysiological mechanisms. *Biofeedback and Self-Regulation, 14*(4), 267–280.

Sherman, R. A., & Associates. (1997). *Phantom pain.* New York: Plenum Press.

Sherman, R. A., & Barja, R. J. (1989). Treatment of post-amputation and phantom limb pain. In K. Foley & R. Payne (Eds.), *Current therapy of pain.* Grand Junction, CO: Decker.

Sherman, R. A., Gall, N., & Gormly, J. (1979). Treatment of phantom limb pain with muscular relaxation training to disrupt the pain–anxiety–tension cycle. *Pain, 22*(6), 47–55.

Sherman, R. A., Greffin, V. D., Evans, C., & Grana, A. (1992, March). Temporal relationships between change in phantom pain intensity and change in surface electromyogram of the residual limb. In *Proceedings of the 23rd Annual Meeting of the Association for Applied Psychophysiology and Biofeedback, Colorado Springs.* Wheat Ridge, CO: Association for Applied Psychophysiology and Biofeedback.

Sherman, R. A., & Sherman, C. J. (1985). A comparison of phantom sensations among amputees whose amputations were of civilian and military origins. *Pain, 28*, 285–295.

Weiss, T., Miltner, W. H. R., Adler, T., Brückner, L., & Taub, E. (1999). Decrease in phantom limb pain associated with prosthesis-induced increased use of an amputation stump in humans. *Neuroscience Letters, 272*, 131–134.

PART XI

Professional Issues

CHAPTER 36

The Application of Ethics
and Law in Daily Practice[1]

SEBASTIAN STRIEFEL

Have you ever reflected on your personal and professional values as they apply to what you do in biofeedback and applied psychophysiology? Do you know the *Practice Guidelines and Standards for Providers of Biofeedback and Applied Psychophysiological Services* (Striefel, Butler, Coxe, McKee, & Sherman, 1999) and *The Ethical Principles of Applied Psychophysiology and Biofeedback* (Association for Applied Psychophysiology and Biofeedback [AAPB], 1995)? Do you know how to resolve an ethical dilemma? Do you know how to manage and minimize risk in your professional activities? If not, read on.

The intent of this chapter is to provide basic, up-to-date ethical and legal information that affects professional practice today, some decision-making information, a review of some core ethical principles, application examples, references for further reading, and (I hope) the development of an appreciation of ongoing education as a key for maximizing ethical behavior while simultaneously minimizing provider risk. Zuckerman (2003) lists four steps for ethical self-protection: being realistic, learning the rules (e.g., laws and ethical principles), developing an ethical sensitivity (awareness), and tightening up the procedures that you use (e.g., informed consent). So keep these four steps in mind as you read this chapter. Remaining current about ethical and legal issues is essential to professional survival. Fortunately, the overall risk of litigation or ethical complaints is small for the conscientious practitioner who continually strives to be competent (Zuckerman, 2003).

DEFINITIONS

Some commonly used terms and concepts are defined in this section, and some definitions are interspersed throughout the chapter.

Values, Ethics, Ethical Principles, and Law

Professionals often try to resolve ethical situations by relying on their own personal values; however, this can be problematic, because not everyone's values are acceptable to others (Kitchener, 2000; Zuckerman, 2003). "Values," as used here, are a provider's moral likes, desires, and priorities (Kitchener, 2000; Striefel, 1997, 1998, 2003). "Ethics" simply means doing what is morally right—in other words, engaging in those behaviors that are morally correct and that are in the best interests of those served (Striefel, 1995, 2003, in press). Core or foundational "ethical principles" consist of common, moral norms that exist across time and that provide the foundation for the ethical codes developed by various health care professions (Kitchener, 2000; Striefel, 2003). An "ethical code," or what is more commonly referred to as the ethical principles of an association or profession, specifies the rules of conduct agreed upon by a professional group such as the AAPB (AAPB, 1995; Striefel, 1995, 2003, in press). Laws, on the other hand, are the minimal standards of conduct that a society will accept, as specified in legal statutes. So values, laws, foundational ethical principles, and ethical codes of conduct interact to guide professional behavior, and none of them alone provide specific solutions for how to behave in all specific situations encountered by providers (Striefel, 2003). Each provides general guidance and is subject to interpretation. Moreover, what is expected can change, based on any change in the circumstances involved.

Ethical Dilemmas

Practical difficulties faced by professionals on a daily basis center around how to deal with the ethical dilemmas that arise. An "ethical dilemma" is any controversy that involves conflicting moral principles or responsibilities in which one must choose between two rights (Corey, Corey, & Callanan, 2000; Striefel, 1986, 1995, 1999a, in press). Unfortunately, many providers do not recognize ethical dilemmas when they encounter them. As such, most ethical violations occur inadvertently, because providers are not aware of how their behavior or lack of behavior may have an adverse impact on their clients (Corey et al., 2000; Lakin, 1991). An example of an ethical dilemma is the situation in which one is the only neurofeedback provider in a geographical area and a client seeks help for a problem one is not competent to treat. Does one try to provide treatment, or let the client suffer because one is not competent in that area of practice? The dilemma is related to choosing between doing what is best for that client and operating only in areas in which one is competent. There are many potential solutions to such a dilemma, including obtaining careful informed consent, obtaining appropriate training, and seeking consultation or supervision. One must first recognize that a dilemma exists before one can deal with it appropriately (Striefel, 1995; Zuckerman, 2003). Some ethical dilemmas are inherent in the process of providing service to clients, in conducting research, and in supervising or training others. It is the practitioner's responsibility to understand the characteristics and sources of ethical dilemmas, because it is always the therapist who is the accountable party in a treatment relationship (Lakin, 1991). The good news is that almost all malpractice lawsuits arise from foreseeable problems that could have been avoided if practitioners learned to recognize and anticipate them by being proactive rather than reactive (Bennett, Bryant, VandenBos, & Greenwood, 1990; Zuckerman, 2003).

Levels of Ethical Functioning

There are two levels of ethical functioning: mandatory or lower-level functioning, and aspirational or higher-level functioning (Corey et al., 2000; Striefel, 1989a, 1995, 2003). In mandatory ethics, one does what is required by law and by the ethical principles of the group(s) to which one belongs. Doing so provides reasonably good protection against any professional or legal action that might be taken against one as a service provider. At the aspirational level of functioning, one goes beyond the minimal by striving to do what is in the best interests of the client, even though additional time and effort may be required. It includes thinking about what impacts the practitioner's actions will have on the client, and can include such activities as reading or seeking consultation. For example, suppose a practitioner is providing electroencephalographic (EEG) biofeedback (neurofeedback) services to a child with a diagnosis of attention-deficit/hyperactivity disorder (ADHD) and to the child's family. In the course of treatment, the practitioner learns that the child is being physically abused by the parent who brought the child in for treatment. Laws in all 50 states mandate that practitioners report any suspected abuse or neglect of a child to the appropriate social service agency or law enforcement agency. Mandatory ethics would dictate that a report be filed within the timeline specified in the law (often 24 hours). Aspirational ethics would encourage the practitioner to think about how best to make the report so as to keep the child and family in treatment. Additional actions could include considering how to get the family to make the report; consulting with a colleague and attorney about options to consider; and interacting with personnel from the agency to whom the report is made on how they might proceed, so that the client and family will stay in treatment. A report must still be filed within the timeline specified in the law, so it is best for practitioners who work with children to plan ahead for how they will deal with potential abuse or neglect when the situation arises. Planning ahead and being proactive constitute another example of an aspirational level of ethical functioning.

Client outcomes and the acceptance of biofeedback depend in part on the ethical activities of practitioners. As such, it is desirable for biofeedback practitioners and other professionals to strive for an aspirational level of functioning (Striefel, 1989a, 1995, 2003). When a professional group does not adhere to a reasonable level of ethical functioning, society often restricts professional practice by passing laws to ensure a certain level of functioning (Corey et al., 2000; Roswell, 1989). In addition, unethical behavior promotes higher costs for professional liability insurance (Zuckerman, 2003).

ACQUIRING APPROPRIATE ETHICAL BEHAVIOR

Required Adherence

Biofeedback practitioners should adhere to AAPB's ethical principles and practice guidelines and standards (AAPB, 1995; Striefel et al., 1999)[2] and to those of the other professional groups to which they belong (e.g., those of the American Psychological Association [APA] for psychologists). Ethics committees and the courts are increasingly holding practitioners accountable for adhering to nationally available ethical principles and practice guidelines and standards, even when practitioners are not members of a specific association (Striefel, in press, Striefel et al., 1999; Zuckerman, 2003). Remaining current requires ongoing education and effort. In fact, many states now require practitioners to obtain a specific number of continuing education hours on ethics in order to renew their licenses to practice (Striefel, 2003). Ongoing education is needed for several reasons. First, behaving ethically is much more complex today than in the past, and the situations encountered by practitioners are changing rapidly because of new laws, legal precedents, changing standards of care, and ethical code changes. Second, managed care has raised numerous ethical issues not addressed by existing ethical codes; for example, managed care companies often approve far fewer sessions than are needed to treat a client's problem (Haley et al., 1998). Finally, Internet access has raised consumer awareness and access to information about what to expect ethically and legally from practitioners (Nickelson, 2000).

How does one learn appropriate ethical behavior when each situation requires a different solution, especially since most ethical principles/codes are vague and provide only general guidance? Several behaviors are required in order for a provider to behave ethically. The keys to appropriate ethical practice are self-analysis (including awareness of personal moral values); knowledge of foundational ethical principles; ongoing education and a good professional library; written policies and procedures; and an ethical decision-making process that involves the use of supervision and consultation, as well as good documentation (Striefel, 1995). Each of these items is clarified in the sections that follow.

Self-Analysis: What Do You Believe?

It is important for every practitioner to spend some time in a self-analysis to determine what he or she believes. One way to do this is to write a self-disclosure statement that lists areas in which one is competent to practice (Striefel, 1992c, Striefel et al., 1999). Another way to do a self-analysis is to read current materials on ethical principles and moral values, and then to write out what one believes and how that corresponds with expected professional behavior. Based on a national interdisciplinary survey, Jensen and Bergin (1988) reported some universally agreed-upon values on which mental health therapists base their treatment activities. These included self-determination; development of effective strategies for coping with stress; development of the ability to give and receive affection; increasing one's sensitivity to the feelings of others; practicing self-control; having a sense of purpose for living; being honest, open, and genuine; finding satisfaction in one's work; developing a sense of identity and self-worth; being skilled in interpersonal relationships; having an appreciation for self-awareness and motivation for personal growth; and practicing good habits of physical health. How do these values compare to your own?

Foundational Ethical Principles

Some broad foundational principles on which ethical codes and principles of conduct are based follow (Striefel, 2003).

1. "Nonmaleficence" means that a practitioner or researcher should do no harm. Some practical examples include not entering into problematic multiple-role relationships with clients (e.g., no sexual contact with clients or former clients), not behaving paternalistically toward clients, and not violating confidentiality unless it is in a client's best interests or for the protection of others (Striefel, 2000, 2003).

2. "Beneficence" means that a practitioner or researcher should maximize the possible benefits of a proposed intervention (Kitchener, 2000). The central focus of health care practitioners is that of *doing good* by contributing to the health and well-being of those served (Striefel, 2000b, 2003).

3. "Respect for people's autonomy" has two related meanings. First, it means that individuals should be treated as autonomous agents capable of self-determination (Striefel, 2003). Second, it means that those with diminished capacity for autonomy should be protected (Kitchener, 2000; Striefel, 2003). Autonomy is the primary basis for informed consent and confidentiality.

4. "Fidelity" means being honest and trustworthy. It is the core ethical principle that provides guidance in terms of developing and maintaining a meaningful relationship between a practitioner and a client or a researcher and a subject (Striefel, 2000b, 2003). Confidentiality and informed consent are partially based on the principle of fidelity.

5. "Justice" means that everyone should be treated fairly (Striefel, 2003). It is the basis for not discriminating against anyone on the basis of age, gender, sexual preference, ethnicity, race, national origin, disability, language, or socioeconomic status (Kitchener, 2000).

Each provider should decide what these foundational principles and those of the AAPB mean in daily practice through reading, thought, and discussion with others.

Education and Professional Library

To maximize the probability of helping clients and to minimize the risk of injury, practitioners should participate in ongoing education by reading ethical articles and books, attending an ethics workshop at least once every 3 years, and discussing ethical issues and solutions with peers and supervisors. Most universities offer courses in ethics, and the AAPB regularly offers workshops and presentations on ethics at its meetings and workshops.

A good professional library is essential (Striefel, 1995) and should include materials such as the following:

- *The Ethical Principles of Applied Psychophysiology and Biofeedback* (AAPB, 1995), and the ethical code of one's professional discipline.
- The *Practice Guidelines and Standards for Providers of Biofeedback and Applied Psychophysiological Services* (Striefel et al., 1999), and the practice guidelines for one's discipline.
- A book on risk management, such as *Professional Liability and Risk Management* (Bennett et al., 1990).
- Relevant state laws (e.g., licensing, reporting of child abuse and neglect, records retention, commitment, billings and collections, and mental health; Striefel, 2000a, in press).
- Medicaid, Medicare, and other third-party payer regulations.
- Some good books on ethics and on law, such as *Issues and Ethics in the Helping Professions* (Corey et al., 2000); *Psychology and the Legal System* (Wrightsman, Nietzel, & Fortune, 1998); *Psychologists' Desk Reference* (Koocher, Norcross, & Hill, 1998); and *The Paper Office* (Zuckerman, 2003).

Written Policies and Procedures

Risk management is an essential component of professional practice today (Striefel, 1993b, 1995, 1999b, 2002, in press). "Risk management" can be defined as having in place well-developed written policies and procedures that are adhered to by all staff members (Striefel, 1992b; 1995); that minimize the probability of litigation or the filing of ethical complaints (Bennett et al., 1990); that encourage proactive quality control; that minimize the probability of injury or dissatisfaction by those served; that maximize the probability of professional behavior by all staff members; and that minimize staff stress (Striefel, 1992b).

Elsewhere (Striefel, 1995, 2002), I have emphasized the advantages of written policies and procedures for guiding professional practice, including the following: (1) The process of writing the policies and procedures requires a practitioner to think about what he or she is and is not doing, and about what could or should be done; (2) they provide a mechanism for increasing the probability that all people in an agency will know what is expected of them, and that they will engage in certain key activities in the same way; (3) they can be reviewed both internally and by external consultants to assure that they meet legal, ethical, and at least the minimal standards of care; and (4) when adhered to, they can help reduce the risk of malpractice litigation and the need to deal with ethical complaints. The policies and procedures should cover all aspects of practice—including, but not limited to, fees, billing and collection procedures; confidentiality; informed consent; contacting the therapist during work and personal time; termination and referral; coverage in the provider's absence; and records. (See Striefel, 1993b, 1999b, and 2002, for more specifics.)

The written policies and procedures should also include copies of all forms to be used in the biofeedback practice. Zuckerman's (2003) excellent book *The Paper Office*, Third Edition includes a variety of forms and procedures that can readily be adapted to a biofeedback practice. *The Paper Office* also includes copies of many forms on a CD-ROM. The various ethical principles to be adhered to by providers should be included in the agency's policies and procedures manual, and it is recommended that all staff members be required to sign a statement that they agree, as a condition of employment, to adhere to the ethical principles of the AAPB and those of their professional discipline (Striefel, 1995; Zuckerman, 2003). Such a policy, if enforced, would provide grounds for educating staffers, terminating unethical staffers, and emphasizing the importance of ethical behavior.

Ethical Decision Making

There are two equally important and interrelated components for ethical decision making. The first is called "ethical competence," which means knowing what to do. The second is a commitment to actually doing what one knows is right. Many practitioners are able to determine what they should do ethically, but they fail to follow through in actually doing it. For example, would you be willing to report a good friend and colleague if you became aware that he or she had committed a serious ethical violation? If not, what factors would keep you from doing so? What could you do to motivate yourself to actually report the violation? Consultation in such situations is often an important component.

All biofeedback providers need to have some model available for making ethical decisions (Koocher & Keith-Spiegel, 1998; Striefel, 1995, 1999a, 2003). It is during the decision-making process that knowledge, competence, and commitment to doing what is right are fine-tuned for guiding appropriate ethical behavior (Koocher & Keith-Spiegel, 1998). The process is the same as that used by practitioners providing other types of services, such as psychotherapy, counseling, or physical therapy. One can begin the decision-making process by answering five questions. First, "Would another reasonable practitioner in the same situation make the same decision and behave in the same way?" Second, "What do my values suggest that I should do in resolving the dilemma I have encountered?" Third, "What do ethical theories, foundational ethical principles, relevant ethical codes, practice guidelines and standards, and laws suggest or mandate as solutions?" Fourth, "Whom can I consult with or seek supervision from to identify appropriate alternatives for resolving the dilemma encountered?" Fifth, "What do those affected by the decision want to have happen, or what is in their best interest?" The answers to each of these questions can be helpful in ethical decision making, especially if applied systematically within the context of a systematic decision-making model, such as the one that follows.

Practitioners should use an ethical decision-making model repeatedly, so that it becomes an automatic habit for use when an ethical dilemma is encountered. Ethical decision making can take a few minutes or can take days or weeks, depending on how complex the issues are, the time available for making the decision, and the degree of preplanning that a practitioner has engaged in for resolving ethical dilemmas (e.g., plan for dealing with a suicidal client).

The major steps in one ethical decision-making model include the following:

1. Review the objective information available, to determine what other information is needed for resolving the situation.

2. Analyze the situation to determine whether the dilemma is an ethical one. Reviewing the foundational ethical principles provided previously can be helpful at this step. List the competing ethical positions, if possible.

3. Review the ethical principles of AAPB and of your primary discipline, along with relevant practice guidelines and standards to identify the possible options for resolving the

dilemma. List the options and the probable consequences (risks and benefits) that each option might have on each stakeholder (e.g., the client, the client's family, and you).

4. Seek appropriate consultation as needed, to ensure that personal skill deficits and biases do not cloud the decision that needs to be made, and that all possible options and consequences have been considered.

5. Review the questions listed before, and make the decision based on what you believe is the ethically correct thing to do.

6. Carry out your plan by actually doing what you believe is ethically correct. Use your consultant for support as needed to motivate you to carry out the plan. Carefully document your rationale, the decision-making process, consultation, and actions taken.

7. Evaluate the decision made, the action taken, the outcomes achieved, and take corrective action, if needed. See Striefel (1995, 1999b) for more details and flowcharts on this process, or see Koocher and Keith-Spiegel (1998) for a related discussion.

Additional questions one can ask oneself in making ethical decisions include the following (Patterson & Wilkins, 1991; MacKay & O'Neill, 1992; Striefel, 1997):

- "What are my duties and responsibilities in this situation?"
- "To whom am I responsible?"
- "How do I ethically carry out my duties and responsibilities to those I serve?"
- "Is there some potential harm to the client, and if so, is it real or hypothetical?"
- "How do I make sure that I do no harm in this situation?"
- "How do I do the most good and act fairly to all stakeholders in this situation?"

A good ethical decision-making process is essential for resolving ethical dilemmas, planning for situations that are likely to occur, preventing potential injury to clients, protecting the best interests of clients, and preventing emotional distress and risk for the practitioner.

ETHICAL APPLICATIONS

A number of principles and values are useful in guiding professional practice activities. Many of these principles are part of the AAPB's ethical principles and practice guidelines and standards (AAPB, 1995; Striefel et al., 1999). Application of these principles and values includes such concepts as respect, responsibility, competence, privacy, confidentiality, and privileged communication.

Respect

In its simplest form, "respect" can be defined as protecting client autonomy; doing no harm; and striving to maximize client benefits by doing good, being honest and trustworthy, and treating everyone fairly. Practically, respect is doing what is in the client's best interests by knowing one's professional responsibilities, remaining competent via continuing education, restricting professional activities to areas in which one is competent, and knowing and abiding by professional boundaries. See Striefel (1995) for a more detailed list of examples for showing respect for clients. This whole chapter discusses ways to show respect.

The failure to show respect for those served can result in many problems for a service provider. For example, clients who are unhappy with the way they are being interacted with are more likely to initiate action against a provider (Bennett et al., 1990). Zuckerman (2003) has pointed out that "Lawsuits represent about the last stage of breakdown in human relationships" (p. 76). The filing of an ethical complaint by a client is also an indicator of relationship problems. As such, it is strongly recommended that practitioners attend carefully to the special relationship that they have with clients, and that they address a client's complaints quickly and to the client's satisfaction. The relevant question here is this: "Do I as a service provider show respect for those I serve and for their rights?"

Responsibility

Biofeedback practitioners, like any other direct service providers, always have a responsibility ("response-ability") for what they do and do not do (Striefel, in press; Striefel et al., 1999). In addition, they have a shared legal and ethical responsibility for what those whom they supervise or employ do or fail to do. The AAPB's practice guidelines and standards provide a detailed discussion of practitioners' responsibilities (Striefel et al., 1999). See also Striefel (in press) for more information. Ethically, practitioners should strive to adhere to the highest standards of their profession. Behaving responsibly means accepting responsibility for one's own behavior and the consequences of that behavior; ensuring that biofeedback is used appropriately; and striving to educate the public concerning responsible use of biofeedback in treatment, research, and training. This statement sounds fairly straightforward, but its actual implementation in daily practice is more complex. In practice, responsible behavior means doing all those things previously discussed in terms of showing respect for clients. As such, they are not repeated here.

A professional cannot blame a client for his or her own lack of responsible behavior (Corey et al., 2000; Striefel, 1995). Those who try to blame the system or others for their own failure to accept responsibility may well be feeling powerless, and this can be detrimental to clients (Corey et al., 2000). Feelings of powerlessness may well be a sign of "burnout," of operating beyond one's level of competence, or of being in a "rut" of repeatedly doing what is comfortable. It is also an indicator that the practitioner may need to seek professional help (e.g., psychotherapy), additional training, or consultation or supervision to behave responsibly again. It may even be an indicator that it is time for the practitioner to stop seeing clients.

Responsible practice is based on informed, sound, and responsible judgment. The skills needed for a responsible practice are developed by reading, attending classes and workshops, obtaining frequent supervision and/or consultation, conducting self-evaluations, undergoing peer reviews, and knowing one's own areas of competence (Striefel, 1995, in press). One must know and abide by all relevant laws, ethical principles, and practice guidelines and standards.

Competence

The AAPB's practice guidelines and standards define "competence" to mean that "the provider has the knowledge to understand a particular client's problems and to formulate an appropriate treatment plan, has the skills needed to apply that knowledge effectively, and the judgement to use such knowledge and skills appropriately" (Striefel et al., 1999, p. 3.1). The guidelines further specify that providers will "strive to provide services only in areas in which they are competent as based on education, training and/or experience, unless appropriately supervised by a supervisor competent in the relevant skill areas" (p. 3.1). A truly competent provider recognizes his or her limitations and deficits, as well as his or her skills and strengths (Koocher & Keith-Siegel, 1998).

There are two levels of competence necessary for providing high-quality professional services (Koocher & Keith-Siegel, 1998). The first is "intellectual competence," which refers to acquisition of the knowledge needed to assess, conceptualize, plan, and conduct appropriate treatment for a specific client with specific problem(s) (Koocher & Keith-Siegel, 1998). For example, being successful in doing surface electromyographic (EMG) biofeedback with clients does not necessarily translate into doing competent neurofeedback treatment without additional knowledge and skill training. The second level of competence is "emotional competence," which refers to the provider's ability to emotionally identify and cope with the clinical material that emerges in treating clients, without letting personal biases or values negatively affect clients (Koocher & Keith-Siegel, 1998). It includes being able to deal appropriately with transference (in which a client projects unresolved issues with others onto the therapist) and countertransference (in which a therapist projects unresolved issues with others onto the client), while simultaneously caring for oneself.

Some ways for determining one's level of competence include peer review, self-awareness, evaluations of one's impact on clients, and taking exams such as those required for state licensing or Biofeedback Certification Institute of America (BCIA) certification (Striefel, in press; Striefel et al., 1999). One of the most important and meaningful methods for determining one's competence is through evaluation of one's impact on clients. If one consistently obtains positive outcomes with specific groups of clients, one is probably competent in that area. If one consistently obtains negative outcomes with a particular type of client, one needs to search further to determine whether the negative outcomes are due to some area of incompetence (e.g., using the wrong type of treatment for the client's problem) or to other factors (e.g., lack of client follow-through). Discussions with the client and with other biofeedback service providers can be useful in determining areas of competence, so that proactive activities can not only help protect the client, but prevent the filing of an ethical complaint or lawsuit against the provider (Koocher & Keith-Siegel, 1998). In addition to practicing only in those areas in which one is competent, an ethical practitioner must obtain training in new areas, and obtain appropriate supervision and/or consultation in applying these new areas to clients (Striefel, in press). Remaining competent requires ongoing training both to maintain and to expand one's areas of practice. It is unethical to exaggerate one's qualifications or skills, and engaging in such behaviors can lead to problems with clients and ethics committees, as well as possible malpractice litigation (Striefel, 1995; Striefel et al., 1999).

It is also important to be alert to signs of fatigue, burnout, and personal/emotional problems in oneself. When such conditions exist, one is more likely to make mistakes and to behave incompetently. When signs of fatigue occur, one needs to take corrective action by taking a vacation, seeking personal counseling, cutting back on work hours, or engaging in other activities that will alleviate the problem.

Privacy, Confidentiality, and Privileged Communication

"Privacy" refers to an individual's right to choose if, when, under what circumstances, and to what extent to share his or her beliefs, behavior, or opinions with others (Corey et al., 2000). The right to a certain level of privacy is guaranteed by the U.S. Constitution. A client even has a right to choose whether or not to allow his or her physiology to be recorded or seen by the provider. Informed consent (discussed later) is essential before invading this area of a client's privacy.

Two other terms have their foundation in the concept of privacy; they are confidentiality and privileged communication. "Confidentiality" can be defined as the ethical or moral responsibility of a professional to protect a client from the unauthorized disclosure of information obtained in a treatment relationship (Corey et al., 2000; Striefel, 1995, in press). "Privileged communication," a legal right defined in legal statutes, protects clients from having their confidential information revealed in a legal proceeding without their permission

(Striefel, 1995, in press). There are practical, but often complex, exceptions to implementation of both confidentiality and privileged communication.

Confidentiality

Clients should be informed of the limits of confidentiality at the onset of treatment within the informed consent process, preferably with written documentation (Striefel, 1995, Striefel et al., 1999). Some common limits of confidentiality that clients should be aware of include the following: (1) Certain laws require breaking confidentiality (e.g., all professionals must report suspected and/or actual child abuse, and some states have a "duty to warn or protect" law which requires certain professionals to break confidentiality if a client or someone else is in danger of being injured or killed); (2) if a client uses a third-party payer, certain information will be revealed; (3) if a client initiates legal action against a provider, the provider has a right to use confidential client information to the extent necessary to defend him- or herself; (4) if services are being provided under court order, confidential information will be shared; (5) if a provider will use collection agencies or a small-claims court to collect unpaid bills, financial information will be shared; (6) when a client uses his or her mental status in a legal proceeding and the practitioner has information about the client's mental status, such information will be shared; and (7) parents have a right to access information about their minor children, and adults have a right to access or release information about themselves to others (Striefel, 1995, in press; Zuckerman, 2003). If the service provider will discuss the client with a supervisor or consultant, the client should be so informed. If clients are aware of the limits of confidentiality at the onset of services, they can hypothetically (if not practically) decide whether they want to enter treatment under these conditions, and if so, how much information to reveal. It is unethical to videotape or audiotape a client without the client's permission.

Some practical components of privacy and confidentiality include assuring that (1) one's professional space has a sound barrier, so that private information from a treatment session cannot be overheard in the hall or waiting room; (2) a client's last name isn't called out in a waiting room; (3) the receptionist doesn't use client names on the telephone where others can overhear the conversation; (4) the receptionist doesn't give verbal telephone messages where others can hear them if names are used; (5) a therapist has access to only the files of his or her clients; (6) each therapist has a separate appointment book; (7) all staff members agree to keep client information private; and (8) client records are kept in locked files not accessible to those who "have no need to know" (e.g., janitors and office mates) (Striefel, 1995, 1999b). Many of the components suggested do not exist in common practice; nonetheless, failure to have them in place is technically a violation of a client's right to privacy, and providers should strive to eliminate technical violations. For example, Zuckerman (2003) suggests that instead of calling out a client's last name in the waiting room, the provider should approach the client, make eye contact, and say, "Won't you please come in?"

Privileged Communication

The client owns the "privilege" in privileged communication. Therefore, the provider cannot generally release information without the client's consent in any legal proceeding (Striefel, 1995, in press). All states have privileged communication statutes for attorneys, psychologists, and physicians. Most states also have privileged communication laws that cover other professionals, such as licensed professional counselors and social workers. It is up to individual providers to find out whether or not their services are covered by such a law. Usually the privileged communication statute is included within the specific discipline's licensing law.

When covered by law, privileged communication exists (1) if the communication originates in the belief that it will not be disclosed; (2) if the communication is made by a client or one who wishes to become one; and (3) if no casual third parties were present (Striefel, 1995). The loss of privileged communication may exist or occur (1) if a relationship is not covered by law (e.g., I know of no state that provides privileged communication for unlicensed providers); (2) if the client initiates legal action against the therapist; (3) if the client files a workers' compensation lawsuit; (4) if a casual third party is present; (5) if treatment is court-ordered; and often (6) if there is a risk of suicide or injury to others (Corey et al., 2000; Striefel, 1995, in press). Other exceptions may exist, depending on specific laws in each state.

Two good premises for you as a practitioner to operate under are these: (1) When in doubt, don't give it out—call your attorney instead (Stromberg et al., 1988); and (2) if no compelling reason exists, don't give it out without consulting with your client, even if the client initially requested that you release the information (e.g., the benefits to the client should outweigh the risks, and when that is not so, the client and his or her attorney should be aware of your concerns) (Striefel, 1989c, 1995).

Whenever a practitioner violates a client's confidentiality or reveals privileged information, it is critical to document the situation, steps taken, consultation sought, rationale used to justify it, outcome, and anything else that seems relevant (e.g., a court order by a judge). If the client or his or her attorney give permission for information to be released, a release of information form should be signed. Zuckerman (1997) suggests that the client sign three copies of the release, one for the client, one for the provider's file, and one for the person or agency receiving the information.

If a practitioner receives a subpoena for records, the practitioner should probably take several steps (Striefel, 1995; Zuckerman, 2003)—including, but not limited to, these:

1. Not giving out the records without taking time to determine what action to take legally and ethically.
2. Not removing or changing anything in the client's file (doing so could result in a contempt-of-court charge).
3. Contacting one's attorney to verify that the subpoena is legal and not just a look-alike, to clarify whether or not the records are covered by privileged communication statutes, and to seek appropriate guidance.
4. Contacting the client and/or his or her attorney to determine the desirability of compliance.
5. If there are items in the file that do not seem relevant to the case, asking for a private session with the judge, to determine whether some information can be withheld (Corey et al., 2000).

A subpoena must be responded to, but not necessarily complied with (Zuckerman, 2003). A court order, however, must be complied with, or one must appeal the decision to a higher court or risk judge imposed penalties. When a judge deems that the "common good" of society is more important that the right of the individual, he or she may issue a court order that supersedes a state's privileged communication law. Appeals are sometimes successful in maintaining confidentiality. The U.S. Supreme Court ruled in *Jaffee v. Redmond* that psychotherapists may refuse to divulge in federal court what their patients have shared with them in confidence, because such privacy is needed for establishing and maintaining the level of trust necessary for treatment to be successful (Wrightsman et al., 1998). How that decision will be applied in local or state courts, or how it might be applied to biofeedback services, is unknown at this time. New court cases and decisions can occur at any time, as such, an attorney can be useful in clarifying how case law may apply to a specific situation.

PRACTICE AREAS WITH ETHICAL IMPLICATIONS

A number of practice areas have ethical implications. Several of the major ones are discussed in the sections that follow.

Informed Consent

"Informed consent" is the process of obtaining a client's permission to engage in various treatment and related activities (Striefel, 1990a, 1995, in press). Respect for a client's right to autonomy means that he or she is entitled to the information needed to make reasonable choices (Striefel, 2003). Truthful informed consent can help establish trust and a meaningful relationship with clients by making them a meaningful part of the decision-making process. Informed consent is mandated in the AAPB's practice guidelines and standards (Striefel et al., 1999). The following components are required for informed consent to be legal and ethical (Striefel, 1990c, 1995). First, it requires that a client be given all of the information that a reasonable person would want/need in order to make a decision about how to proceed. The information should include the risks and benefits of the proposed activities (e.g., assessment or treatment) and those of the major available alternatives, including taking no action at all (Striefel, 1995, in press). Second, practitioners should carefully consider the quality of information and the manner in which it is presented, in an effort to optimize clients' ability to understand the information (Koocher & Keith-Spiegel, 1998). Asking clients questions is one way to determine if they understand the information (Striefel, in press). Third, it requires that a client give consent voluntarily, without any form of coercion. Distortion or withholding information can be considered a subtle form of coercion. The fourth requirement is that the client have the capacity to make the necessary decision(s) (Striefel, in press). Determining a client's capacity can be a simple or complex process, depending on the situation. Generally, it is assumed that an adult client has the appropriate capacity unless there is evidence to the contrary. A couple of additional terms are useful here. An "autonomous" person is one who can make free choices from the available options and is capable of knowing the difference between right and wrong. An autonomous person is assumed to be competent and is accountable for his or her behavior. There are also individuals with "diminished capacities" for autonomy. This group includes individuals who may or may not be competent to give informed consent. Some of the classes of people who fall in this category are children, individuals with certain disabilities (e.g., mental retardation and some mental illnesses), and people who are not fluent in the language of the service provider (Striefel, 1995). When one is working with an individual of diminished capacity, it is essential to get informed consent from the appropriate parent, guardian, or advocate, in addition to that of the client (Striefel, 1995). Getting actual consent, in other words, the client or advocate giving verbal or written consent is the fifth component.

A sixth consideration is to document the informed consent process. Written documentation is important if later concerns arise, if a procedure is new or is considered by many professionals to be experimental, or if unusual circumstances exist (Striefel et al., 1999). Know the laws of your state; for example, Colorado and Washington law require written informed consent by various health care professionals. Documentation can be completed by simply writing in a client's file the information provided to the client and his or her response. It is a good idea to have the client sign and date the note. If the informed consent is related to some aspect of practice that is common to many or all clients (e.g., the limits of confidentiality), then it is probably worthwhile to develop a specific form for that aspect of informed consent, including a signature block. Some areas in which informed consent should be obtained include the limits of confidentiality; fees, billings, and collection procedures; client rights; assessments; treatment approaches; touching the client (e.g., to attach electrodes); type of clothing to wear; release of confidential information; and experimental procedures (Striefel, 1990c, 1995, in press).

Informed consent is not a one-time process, nor is it a "rubber stamp" process (Striefel, 1990c, 1995). Informed consent, even if written, is useful only if the consent meets all of the requirements previously specified, and thus empowers the client as a decision maker. It is good practice to include some questions to clients as a means of determining whether or not the clients understood the information that was presented to them. For example, after presenting the needed information, one could ask, "In your own words, tell me what the risks and benefits are for obtaining biofeedback treatment for your headaches," or "What other types of treatment are available for treating your headaches, and why is biofeedback the treatment of choice for you?" Ethical complaints have been filed against AAPB members for behaviors such as (1) not obtaining informed consent before touching a client, and (2) failing to inform clients that some newer interventions for specific problems (e.g., neurofeedback for ADHD) are considered by many practitioners to be experimental. In fact, some years ago several state licensing boards required some neurofeedback providers to change their informed consent procedures and advertisements, so that clients are informed that neurofeedback is considered by some or many providers to be an experimental intervention (Striefel, 1999b, 2002). Elsewhere (Striefel, 1999b, 2002), I have provided samples of informed consent forms, a flowchart of the process, and sample statements concerning the experimental nature of an intervention. The AAPB's practice guidelines and standards specify that practitioners should address the issue of experimental interventions whenever it may apply (Striefel et al., 1999). The informed consent process allows clients to decide what they want to do in reference to what is proposed by their service provider (e.g., a client could choose to terminate treatment rather than pay a higher fee).

The informed consent process is philosophically in agreement with what biofeedback is all about. In essence, biofeedback is designed to teach clients to take control of their own physiology and other aspects of their lives—that is, to be empowered (Koocher & Keith-Spiegel, 1998; Striefel, 1995). Obtaining informed consent is one way to model for clients that they are in fact in charge of the decisions they make. Paternalistic behavior (i.e., making decisions about and for clients that they should make for themselves) in a sense tells them that the provider sees them as incapable of making decisions. Unnecessary paternalism by a service provider is unethical (Striefel, 1990c, 1995). Clients and research subjects should be informed that they can refuse to participate in any procedure, and that they can withdraw or request changes without any penalty (Striefel, 1995). Zuckerman (2003) provides one of the most useful and comprehensive discussions about informed consent, and his book includes a variety of forms and procedures for documenting informed consent. Providers can readily adapt some of his sample forms for use in their own practice activities.

Multiple-Role Relationships and Other Boundary Issues

Multiple-role relationships (often called dual relationships) occur whenever a practitioner interacts with the client in more than one role (e.g., as therapist and teacher or as therapist and supervisor) (Bennett et al., 1990; Striefel, 2000c, in press). There are many possible multiple-role relationships that biofeedback practitioners are likely to encounter, and not all of them can be avoided—nor are all of them problematic, if a practitioner is cognizant of the boundary issues involved and knows how to deal with them in an ethically appropriate manner (Striefel, 2000c, 2002, in press). Meeting client needs is the priority that should guide the practitioner's behavior when encountering and dealing with multiple-role issues. It is best to avoid potentially problematic multiple-role relationships. Some common multiple-role relationships and a couple of other boundary issues follow (Corey et al., 2000; Koocher & Keith-Spiegel, 1998; Striefel, 2000b, 2000c).

- Entering into a business relationship with a client can be problematic, because it potentially pits client needs against the financial interests of the practitioner.
- Bartering with a client over a service or product is also potentially problematic, because of the possibility that either party can be exploited or dissatisfied if either party perceives an inequity in the exchange.
- Providing treatment services to a family member or friend is potentially problematic, because of the emotional entanglements and conflicts of interest that are possible.
- Providing treatment services to an employee is potentially problematic for the same reasons as for providing treatment to family members.
- Socializing and/or becoming friends with clients or students during or after treatment or an education program is potentially problematic, because of the power differential that makes exploitation possible.
- Accepting acquaintances as clients can be problematic if equal power does not exist.
- Accepting referrals from clients or those with whom the clients have close relationships can be problematic, both because maintaining confidentiality (remembering who said what) is difficult, and because there are potential conflicts of interest between the needs of the two clients.
- Encountering clients in real-world situations where role conflicts are very likely can be problematic. For instance, in rural communities and small ethnic neighborhoods, practitioners are likely to have many chance and existing encounters with clients.
- Accepting gifts or asking clients for favors opens a practitioner up to charges of exploitation, depending on the size of the gift or favor or the frequency of gifts.
- Conducting treatment outside a professional setting should only occur when it is in the best interests of the client, and caution should be taken to not cross other boundaries (e.g., getting sexually involved with the client).

Warning Signs and Ways to Deal with Them

To deal with multiple-role relationships and other boundary issues, practitioners should learn to recognize when such a relationship or issue has arisen, and they should know how to deal with the dilemma posed. When such a dilemma cannot be avoided via referral, a practitioner should be careful to obtain full informed consent from a client. Consent should include discussing the risks and benefits associated with both roles and with other boundary issues. The nonpractitioner role may have to be put on hold temporarily or permanently (e.g., social interaction may have to cease); consultation or supervision may be essential to maintaining the best interests of the client; the practitioner's loyalties and priorities should be clarified for the client; a plan for how to proceed needs to be developed that includes how problems that may arise will be resolved; the practitioner's family needs to know that there will be times when certain social interactions will not be allowed, and that there will be no discussion when those situations arise; and the practitioner needs to learn to recognize warning signs that potential problems are arising (Striefel, 2000b, 2000c). Koocher and Keith-Spiegel (1998) and I (Striefel, 2000b, 2000c) discuss at least 15 warning signs and how to deal with them. These include occasions when a practitioner does the following (Koocher & Keith-Spiegel, 1998; Striefel, 2000b, 2000c):

1. Actively seeks opportunities to be with a client outside the treatment setting.
2. Views clients as people who are central to his or her life.

3. Excitedly anticipates a specific client's sessions.
4. Expects a client to do favors for him or her (e.g., giving the practitioner inside trading tips).
5. Wishes that a client was his or her friend, lover, or business partner instead of being a client.
6. Views a client as being in a position to advance the practitioner's position.
7. Discloses extensive details about his or her own life, and expects nurturance from the client in return.
8. Feels entitled to most of the credit if a client improves, rather than giving the client credit.
9. Notices that the interaction between the client and practitioner is becoming less and less relevant to the client's treatment goals.
10. Tries to influence aspects of a client's life that have nothing to do with treatment goals (e.g., the client's hobbies or religion).
11. Believes that he or she is the only person who can help this specific client.
12. Relies on the client's praise and presence for enhancing his or her self-esteem.
13. Allows a client to take advantage of him or her without confrontation (e.g., regularly not paying his or her bill).
14. Does not do what he or she knows is needed therapeutically, because he or she fears that the client will terminate treatment.
15. Resists terminating a client's treatment, even though the need to terminate is clear.

For most of these "warning sign" areas there are probably circumstances that would justify crossing a boundary because (1) the situation is in the best interests of the client and the risk of injury is nonexistent or low, or (2) the situation is totally unavoidable. For example, clients who are bedridden are much more receptive to in-home treatment of mental-health-related problems than they are of going to an office for treatment. When proper precautions are taken, successful treatment can be provided to clients who might otherwise not seek or participate in treatment.

Referral, consultation/supervision, informed consent, continuing education, restricting one's practice activities to certain kinds of clients, and individual psychotherapy for the practitioner are all potential solutions for dealing with the warning signs. It is best to remember the following "rules of thumb": (1) Be only a client's therapist (one role); (2) provide treatment only in your office, unless not doing so is part of the client's treatment program (e.g., *in vivo* desensitization in a natural environment) (Striefel, 1993a); and (3) provide only treatment in your office (i.e., do not socialize with clients there). Kitchener (2000) provides a table that summarizes responses to a survey of 18 multiple-role relationships, and that indicates how ethical or unethical practitioners consider each relationship (e.g., accepting gifts worth less than $10 vs. gifts worth over $50). The list overlaps with some issues identified elsewhere (Percival & Striefel, 1994). Both lists can be helpful in comparing one's own beliefs concerning various ethical issues with those of other practitioners.

Sexual Multiple-Role Relationships

Sexual relationships with clients, former clients, students, supervisees, or employees are unethical. Practitioners should not engage in such behavior, and should report other professionals who do to the appropriate licensing board and ethics committee (Corey et al., 2000; AAPB, 1995; Striefel, 1995; Striefel et al., 1999). Violation of this boundary is not accepted by any health care profession, and the consequences can be severe. It is a clear case of exploitation, and no excuse is acceptable to the courts or to ethics committees (Corey et al., 2000; Striefel,

1995). Clients suffer when practitioners exploit them by entering into sexual relationships with them (Bouhoutsos, Holroyd, Lerman, Forer, & Greenberg, 1983). In addition, in some states, it is a felony to have sexual contact with a current or former client (Corey et al., 2000; Striefel, 1989b, 1995). The provider, not the client, is always held accountable for deviations from acceptable standards of care and for the consequences that occur (Striefel, 1989b, Striefel et al., 1999). It is a sign of incompetence not to be aware of the current ethical expectations of one's profession, and it is unethical not to abide by those expectations.

Treatment

Practitioners generally have the following three functions when accepting clients for treatment: a healing function, an educational function, and a technological function in which various treatment techniques are applied to modify client behavior (Koocher & Keith-Spiegel, 1998). There are numerous guidelines on factors to consider in carrying out each of these three functions ethically. A few are mentioned here. The Association for the Advancement of Behavior Therapy (1977) has published a checklist of items to consider in developing ethical treatment plans. The checklist seems relevant to those providing biofeedback and related services, and covers such items as ethical goals, treatment options, client rights, appropriateness or referrals, and practitioner competence. The APA (1993b) has published guidelines for providing services to ethnically, linguistically, and culturally diverse populations that help clarify the educational function when one is working with clients different from oneself on any of these dimensions (Striefel, 1993c). Corey et al. (2000) have discussed the feminist perspective as it applies to the treatment of both women and men. Their primary focus is on recognizing women's individual rights, common responsibilities for both women and men as partners and as parents, questioning traditional values and roles for women, and the importance of supporting women in their pursuit of rewarding roles outside of the home and family. Each of the guidelines previously mentioned can be helpful in guiding practitioners' behavior in providing ethically appropriate treatment.

Supervision

"Supervision is the process of conveying knowledge and skills from one person to another by having one person (the supervisor) oversee the activities of another person (the supervisee)" (Striefel et al., 1999, p. 4.1). A supervisor has an ethical obligation to (1) assess the skill level of each supervisee regularly, and to give ongoing feedback to the supervisee; (2) assist the supervisee in acquiring the needed skills; (3) assure that the supervisee works with clients only in areas in which the supervisee is reasonably competent, unless the supervisor is physically present; (4) provide the level of supervision needed by the specific client and supervisee; (5) assure that supervisees behave ethically; and (6) supervise only in areas in which the supervisor is competent (Corey et al., 2000; Striefel, 1990b, 1995, in press; Striefel et al., 1999). In addition, a supervisor should strive to meet each client at least once, to assure that the supervisee has conceptualized the problem and treatment needs correctly (Striefel, 1995). Supervision should be carefully documented.

Being competent as a supervisor requires more than being assigned to a supervisory role. Competent supervision requires training, reading, ongoing monitoring, and feedback. It is unethical to take on the role of supervision if one is not competent to do so (Striefel et al., 1999). A competent professional knows what to do, how to do it, when to do it, and when to seek consultation first (Striefel, 1995; Striefel et al., 1999).

Supervisors have shared legal and ethical responsibility for the behavior of those they supervise (Striefel, 1990b, in press) and clients have a right to know the training status of a trainee and who the trainee's supervisor is. An ethical supervisor knows that it is fraud to sign insurance forms as the service provider when he or she was actually the supervisor, and will not agree to a false diagnosis just to collect from the insurance company. Some insurance companies have decided that one can sign insurance forms as a supervisor only if one was in the building where a client was seen, at the time a client was seen (i.e., available at a moment's notice).

Supervisors should manage the rights and responsibilities of supervisees carefully (Corey et al., 2000). This includes, but is not limited to, going through an informed consent process with supervisees concerning the following: approaches that will be used in supervision, how supervisees will be evaluated, supervisees' rights, limits of confidentiality for supervisees, access to records kept by supervisors about supervisees, grievance procedures, and any other expectations of supervisees (e.g., the expectation that biofeedback supervisees will adhere to the AAPB's ethical principles and practice guidelines and standards (Striefel, in press). Supervision should be an active process in which supervisees get at least 1 hour of supervision per week and such additional supervision as needed to meet the needs both of the clients served and of the supervisee. Supervisors should avoid entering into problematic multiple-role relationships with supervisees, should establish the goals (skills) to be acquired by supervisees, and should develop a plan for helping each supervisee to achieve these goals/skills. The process of supervision is very similar to that of working with a client (i.e., assessment, establishment of goals, development and implementation of an intervention plan, evaluation of outcomes, and documentation).

Availability

Once a practitioner accepts a person as a client, he or she has an ethical and legal obligation to be available when needed or to make arrangements with another competent provider to be available. This availability includes accessibility or backup services during out-of-office hours and in emergency situations. When clients are in pain (physical or psychological) and cannot reach their service provider, they often become unhappy, and some initiate action against the provider on the basis of abandonment (Striefel, 1995). Charges of abandonment can occur when a practitioner is not available and does not have backup coverage available when a client emergency occurs, when the practitioner leaves a client alone in a biofeedback session without informed consent, or when the professional does not pick up messages in a timely manner (Striefel, 1992a). A practitioner has an ethical obligation to prepare clients for the practitioner's absence for vacations, emergencies, or other absences, and needs to have a backup system in place (Striefel, 1992a). A practitioner's procedure for being contacted during out-of-office hours and for accessing emergency backup should be part of the informed consent process with clients. Clients should be given copies of appropriate telephone numbers and procedures (Striefel, 1992a).

Referrals and Termination

There are two types of referral processes. In the first, a practitioner receives a referral from another practitioner; in the second, a practitioner refers a client elsewhere. There are potential ethical issues related to each of these referral processes.

Incoming Referrals

There are a number of justifiable reasons for not accepting a person as a client: (1) The person's problem is outside the practitioner's areas of competence; (2) the practitioner's waiting list is long, and the person needs critical services now; (3) accepting the person as a client would create a problematic multiple-role relationship or conflict of interest; (4) the person cannot afford the fee charged (most providers do some pro bono services); and (5) the practitioner cannot form a good working relationship with the potential client (Striefel, 1995; Zuckerman, 2003). It is important not to refuse services to a person purely because of his or her age, gender, race, or the like—that is, not to discriminate against any class of people (which is an injustice). It is also unethical to accept every client referred on the basis that one is competent to deal with all people and all problems, unless one *is* universally competent (which is doubtful) (Striefel, 1995; Zuckerman, 2003). Exceeding one's areas of competence can readily increase a practitioner's stress level and can result in problems for clients.

In order to decide which referrals to accept as clients, a provider needs to know his or her areas of competence and limitations, may need to have available a supervisor/consultant for new areas, and definitely needs to have a systematic process available for collecting certain critical information that will be needed to decide whether the referral is appropriate (Bennett et al., 1990; Zuckerman, 2003; Striefel, in press). A process also needs to be in place for getting relevant records from other providers (with the potential client's signed release of records), for sharing critical information with the potential client (e.g., fees, collection procedures, and parking), and for interacting with the client's physician about medically related matters.

Outgoing Referrals and/or Termination

Ethically, it is essential to refer clients elsewhere and/or to terminate services in the following situations: The client needs a service that the practitioner cannot provide, even if supervision was available; the practitioner has become emotionally involved and is unable to be effective (Zuckerman, 2003, recommends that referral occur after three unsuccessful sessions); the practitioner has personal problems that interfere with his or her being able to meet the client's needs; the client is not making progress with the services provided, even after several different approaches have been tried, including the use of consultation; the client has achieved the goals of treatment; or the practitioner is moving or will no longer be able to provide services (Striefel, 1995, in press). It is not ethical to keep a client in treatment after the treatment goals have been achieved just because the practitioner needs the income.

When a practitioner is referring a client elsewhere, it is common practice to make this referral to a specific provider because he or she is known by the practitioner. Such referrals place the practitioner at risk of having acted negligently, if the new provider turns out to be incompetent for treating the client's problem or causes harm (Striefel, 1995; Zuckerman, 2003). It is a better practice to give a client the names of at least three competent providers whenever possible and let the client choose. It is also helpful to be aware of the areas of competence of other practitioners in the community, so that appropriate, low-risk referrals can be made.

Once the client has made a choice, it is useful to have him or her sign a release of information so that, when contacted by the new provider, the practitioner can share information with this provider in a timely manner. It is also useful when terminating or referring a client to review his or her file and write a summary of the services provided (Bennett et al., 1990). The practitioner should record in the file the reason for termination or referral and the details of the process used, information shared, and anything else that is important. It is unethical to hold a client's records "in bondage" just because the client did not pay his or her bill (APA, 2002).

Abandonment occurs (which is unethical) if a practitioner (1) fails to help a client who still needs services access appropriate services, or at least to help him or her identify appropriate sources for such services, before terminating; (2) terminates a client in crisis; (3) fails to recommend to a client who still needs services before terminating him or her that the client get service elsewhere; (4) has no emergency or backup coverage; or (5) fails to do a follow-up with a client who does not show up for scheduled sessions or who terminates against the practitioner's recommendation (Bennett et al., 1990; Striefel, in press; Zuckerman, 2003). Also, if a provider's policy is to terminate clients if they fail to pay their bills in a timely manner, they should be informed of that policy during the initial informed consent process.

Ethical Record Keeping

Client files and business records should be thorough and accurate (Bennett et al., 1990; Striefel, 1995, in press; Zuckerman, 2003). It is unethical not to have sufficient documentation for meeting client needs (Striefel, 1995; Zuckerman, 2003). A client's records should make clear what was done, when, why, how, by whom, and where. Client records fulfill many different purposes for different stakeholders, including serving as a means for the following: reviewing client progress; motivating the client; communicating with other service providers (with client permission); protecting the provider if a client, or someone else on the client's behalf, initiates litigation or files an ethical complaint against the provider; and testifying in court in reference to a client (e.g., workers' compensation litigation) (Striefel, 1995, in press).

It is essential to maintain a file on each client separately, to protect access to those records (locked files), and to release records only with client permission or as required by law or ethical constraints (Bennett et al., 1990). Failure to maintain adequate records is a basis for a negligence lawsuit, and inadequate records are often grounds for third-party payers (e.g., Medicare) to file fraud charges (Foxhall, 2000). The federal government is spending more than $700 million per year on combating health care fraud, and many practitioners have been found guilty of fraud because they maintained inadequate records—for example, they did not document medical necessity for services that they provided (Foxhall, 2000). Providers should know their state laws in reference to records retention, billing and bill collection, records review, and record ownership (Striefel, 1995, in press; Zuckerman, 2003). A provider should make arrangements with a colleague to maintain client records in case the provider dies or becomes disabled, so that other providers who might serve the client can access the information with client permission (Striefel, 1995). It is recommended that the complete records be retained for 3 years (this time period depends on state law) after the last contact with a client, and that a summary should be maintained for an additional 12 years (Bennett et al., 1990, APA, 1993a; Striefel, in press). The records of minors should be retained for at least 5 years after they reach the age of majority (Zuckerman, 2003). Because of the number of years after treatment in which clients are allowed to file lawsuits, it is probably best to keep a good summary forever. Computer scanners and disks make this a very viable option.

Zuckerman (2003), Bennett et al. (1990), and Striefel (in press) provide listings of the information that should be contained on an ethical and legal release-of-records form. In fact, Zuckerman (2003) provides several samples of forms to use for different release purposes. Records in a provider's files that were obtained through a release-of-records form belong to the original agency; thus it is often illegal to forward such records to other providers (Striefel, 1995; Zuckerman, 2003). Providers should not falsify anything in a client's file, nor should any insurance claims be falsified. Doing so is unethical and illegal (Bennett et al., 1990; Striefel, 1995; Striefel et al., 1999). In fact, providers should take care not to submit claims for services that do not meet the third-party payor's requirements. A practitioner in Utah was indicted on 66 counts of fraud for submitting claims to Medicare—not because the information provided was not accurate (because it was), but because he used unlicensed practitioners to provide services, which violated Medicare regulations in Utah ("Fraud," 1993). Medicare regulations vary from state to state. Foxhall (2000) provided several examples in which practitioners operating "in good faith" were found guilty of fraud because they failed to follow Medicare's rules, including keeping inadequate records and failing to demonstrate medical necessity. The APA (1993a) has published some very nice record-keeping guidelines. It also publishes monthly practice pointers at its Web site (go to http://www.apa.org/practice/pointer .html).

SUMMARY

It is important for you as a service provider to take ethics and their applications seriously. Know the emergency resources available in your community; engage in ongoing education; form a network of consultants and use them regularly; know and abide by all relevant state and federal laws, policies, and regulations, ethical principles, and practice guidelines and standards; find a competent attorney who specializes in areas related to your practice activities; know your areas of competence and limitations; be sensitive to the professional relationships you develop, especially those with clients and supervisees; document carefully; assure continuity of care for each client; get full informed consent (preferably in writing); maintain confidentiality; be open in your communication with clients and address their concerns; take seriously all threats of suicide or harm to others; do not accept all referrals, and refer to other practitioners when this is appropriate to a client's needs; think and act preventively and conservatively; do not promise cures; make accurate diagnoses; take care of your own needs and health, to avoid burnout or exploitation of clients; respect individual differences; terminate services properly; and limit your scope of practice to areas in which you are able to maintain your competence (Koocher & Keith-Spiegel, 1998; Kitchener, 2000; Striefel, 1995, 1999b, 2002; Zuckerman, 2003). Finally, develop written policies and procedures for guiding your professional behaviors in all of the aforementioned areas, as a means for behaving proactively and for aspiring to the highest level of ethical functioning.

NOTES

1. This chapter is a major revision of the chapter published in the 1995 edition of this book (Striefel, 1995).
2. Both of these documents can be obtained from the AAPB at 10200 W. 44th Ave, Suite 304, Wheat Ridge, CO 80033-2840.

REFERENCES

American Psychological Association (APA). (1993a). Record keeping guidelines. *American Psychologist*, 48(9), 984–986.
American Psychological Association (APA). (1993b). Guidelines for providers of psychological services to ethnic, linguistic, and culturally diverse populations. *American Psychologist*, 48(1), 45–48.
American Psychological Association (APA). (2002). *Ethical principles of psychologists and code of conduct.* Washington, DC: Author.
Association for Advancement of Behavior Therapy. (1977). *Checklist for the ethicality of proposed treatments.* New York: Author.
Association for Applied Psychophysiology and Biofeedback (AAPB). (1995). *The ethical principles of applied psychophysiology and biofeedback.* Wheat Ridge, CO: Author.
Bennett, B. E., Bryant, B. K., VandenBos, G. R., & Greenwood, A. (1990). *Professional liability and risk management.* Washington, DC: American Psychological Association.
Bouhoutsos, J., Holroyd, J., Lerman, H., Forer, B. R., & Greenberg, M. (1983). Sexual intimacies between psychotherapists and patients. *Professional Psychology: Research and Practice*, 14(2), 185–196.
Corey, G., Corey, M. S., & Callanan, P. (2000). *Issues and ethics in the helping professions* (5th ed.). Pacific Grove, CA: Brooks/Cole.

Foxhall, K. (2000). How would your practice records look to the FBI? *APA Monitor on Psychology, 3*(1), 1–6.

Fraud (1993, August 15). *The Herald Journal* [Logan, UT], p. 1.

Haley, W. E., McDaniel, S. H., Bray, J. H., Frank, R. G., Heldring, M., Johnson, S. B., Lu, E. G., Reed, G. M., & Wiggins, J. G. (1998). Psychological practice in primary care settings: Practice tips for clinicians. *Professional Psychology: Research and Practice, 29*(3), 237–244.

Jensen, J. P., & Bergin, A. E. (1988). Mental health values of professional therapists: A national interdisciplinary survey. *Professional Psychology: Research and Practice, 19*(3), 290–297.

Kitchener, K. S. (2000). *Foundations of ethical practice, research, and teaching in psychology.* Mahwah, NJ: Erlbaum.

Koocher, G. P., & Keith-Spiegel, P. (1998). *Ethics in psychology: Professional standards and cases.* New York: Oxford University Press.

Koocher, G. P., Norcross, J. C., & Hill, S. S., III. (1998). *Psychologists' desk reference.* Washington, DC: American Psychological Association.

Lakin, M. (1991). *Coping with ethical dilemmas in psychotherapy.* New York: Pergamon Press.

MacKay, E., & O'Neill, P. (1992). What creates the dilemma in ethical dilemmas?: Examples from psychological practice. *Ethics and Behavior, 2*(4), 227–244.

Nickelson, D. (2000). *Telecommunication trends and professional practice: Opportunities and challenges* (Practitioner Focus). Washington, DC: American Psychological Association.

Patterson, P., & Wilkins, L. (1991). *Media ethics: Issues and cases.* Dubuque, IA: Brown.

Percival, G., & Striefel, S. (1994). Ethical beliefs and practices of AAPB members. *Biofeedback and Self-Regulation, 19*(1), 67–93.

Roswell, V. A. (1989). Professional liability: Issues for behavior therapists in the 1980s and 1990s. *Biofeedback, 17*(2), 22–35.

Striefel, S. (1986, Summer). Ethical conduct in treating the sexually attractive client. *Utah Psychological Association Newsletter,* pp. 2–3.

Striefel, S. (1989a). A perspective on ethics. *Biofeedback, 17*(1), 21–22.

Striefel, S. (1989b). Avoiding sexual misconduct. *Biofeedback, 17*(2), 35–38.

Striefel, S. (1989c). Confidentiality vs. privileged communications. *Biofeedback, 17*(3), 43–46.

Striefel, S. (1990a). The informed consent process. *Biofeedback, 18*(1), 51–55.

Striefel, S. (1990b). The ethics of supervision. *Biofeedback, 18*(3), 36–37.

Striefel, S. (1990c). Responsibility and competence. *Biofeedback, 18*(4), 39–40.

Striefel, S. (1992a). Absences and interruptions of biofeedback therapy. *Biofeedback, 20*(1), 34–36.

Striefel, S. (1992b). Ethics and risk management: An introduction. *Biofeedback, 20*(2), 44–45.

Striefel, S. (1992c). Ethics and risk management: Managing risks. *Biofeedback, 20*(3), 33–34.

Striefel, S. (1993a, March). *Ethics and risk management in professional practice.* Workshop conducted at the Annual Meeting of the Association for Applied Psychophysiology and Biofeedback, Los Angeles.

Striefel, S. (1993b). Ethics and risk management: Written policies and procedures. *Biofeedback, 21*(1), 42–43.

Striefel, S. (1993c). Ethical issues in the biofeedback treatment of people different from yourself: Part 1. An overview. *Biofeedback, 21*(3), 6–7.

Striefel, S. (1995). Professional ethical behavior for providers of biofeedback. In M. S. Schwartz & Associates, *Biofeedback: A practitioner's guide* (2nd ed.). New York: Guilford Press.

Striefel, S. (1997). Duties and values: Part I. *Biofeedback, 25*(4), 3A–4A.

Striefel, S. (1998). Duties and values: Part II. *Biofeedback, 26*(2), 21A–22A.

Striefel, S. (1999a). Making the right ethical choice is not always easy. *Biofeedback, 24*(2), 4–5.

Striefel, S. (1999b). Ethical, legal and professional pitfalls associated with neurofeedback services. In J. Evans & A. Abarbanel (Eds.), *Introduction to quantitative EEG and neurofeedback.* San Diego, CA: Academic Press.

Striefel, S. (2000a). The role of aspirational ethics and licensing laws in the practice of neurofeedback. *Journal of Neurofeedback, 4*(1), 43–55.

Striefel, S. (2000b). Some core ethical principles and their application. *Biofeedback, 28*(4), 4–5, 11.

Striefel, S. (2000c). Professional boundary issues in neurofeedback and other biofeedback. *Biofeedback, 28*(3), 5, 6, and 12.

Striefel, S. (2002). Ethics and risk management. In R. Kall, J. Kamiya, & G. Schwartz (Eds.), *Applied neurophysiology and brain biofeedback.* Trevose, PA: Futurehealth.

Striefel, S. (2003). Professional ethics and practice standards in mind–body medicine. In D. Moss, A. McGrady, T. C. Davis, and I. Wickramasekera (Eds.), *Handbook of mind–body medicine for primary care.* Thousand Oaks, CA: Sage.

Striefel, S. (in press). Professional conduct. In D. Montgomery & A. Crider (Eds.), *AAPB's Professional Education Series: Introduction to general biofeedback.* Wheat Ridge, CO: Association for Applied Psychophysiology and Biofeedback.

Striefel, S., Butler, F., Coxe, J. A., McKee, M. G., & Sherman, R. A. (1999). *Practice guidelines and standards for providers of biofeedback and applied psychophysiological services.* Wheat Ridge, CO: Association for Applied Psychophysiology and Biofeedback.

Stromberg, C. D., Haggarty, D. J., Leibenluft, R. F., McMillan, M. H., Mishkin, B., Rubin, B. L., & Trilling, H. R. (1988). *The psychologist's legal handbook.* Washington, DC: Council for the National Register of Health Service Providers in Psychology.

Wrightsman, L. S., Nietzel, M. T., & Fortune, W. H. (1998). *Psychology and the legal system.* Pacific Grove, CA: Brooks/Cole.

Zuckerman, E. L. (1997). *The paper office* (2nd ed.). New York: Guilford Press.

Zuckerman, E. L. (2003). *The paper office* (3rd ed.). New York: Guilford Press.

CHAPTER 37

Other Professional Topics and Issues[1]

SEBASTIAN STRIEFEL
ROBERT WHITEHOUSE
MARK S. SCHWARTZ

DEFINITIONS AND JOB TITLES/RESPONSIBILITIES

Definitions of Biofeedback and Applied Psychophysiology

Definitions of the terms "biofeedback" and "applied psychophysiology" affect job titles and descriptions. Some professionals view the term "biofeedback" narrowly as meaning only specific instrumentation-based procedures. Other professionals view it as a shorthand term referring to a wide array of evaluative and therapeutic procedures associated within the broader rubric of "applied psychophysiology"[2] (Olson, 1995a; M. S. Schwartz, 1999; Striefel, 1999). Terms such as "augmented proprioception" and "external psychophysiological feedback" are technically more accurate, but are too cumbersome for routine professional use.

This is not the place to engage in professional polemics on this topic. (See N. M. Schwartz & Schwartz, Chapter 3, this volume, for a full discussion of the definitions issue.) See also *Applied Psychophysiology and Biofeedback* (1999), Volume 24, Number 1, for a broad discussion by M. S. Schwartz et al. of the definition of "applied psychophysiology." However, the term "biofeedback" has taken on much more meaning than the narrow conceptualization. Referring professionals, including physicians, often infer and expect more from the services associated with a broader conceptualization. National certification in biofeedback recognizes biofeedback broadly defined, and the written certification exam covers much more than instrumentation. All of this also has implications for the issue of whether biofeedback is a separate profession, which we discuss at the end of this chapter.

Implications of Various Job Titles

Individuals who are educated within a recognized health care discipline, and are state-sanctioned to practice independently, will probably retain their respective licensed titles when providing biofeedback services. Such titles are generally recognized and respected by other professionals, and imply a scope of practice that extends beyond biofeedback. Professionals from traditional health care disciplines not licensed in some or all states for independent practice (e.g., nursing and physical therapy) who use biofeedback will probably also retain their respective licensed titles. The more common titles of professionals who use biofeedback include "psychologist," "nurse," "licensed professional counselor," "psychiatrist," "physical therapist," "occupational therapist," "clinical social worker," "licensed mental health counselor," and "marriage and family counselor." Among the more common titles in usage, for those who do not have a degree or license in a recognized health care discipline, are "biofeedback therapist," "biofeedback practitioner," "biofeedback technician," "biofeedback assistant," and "certified biofeedback therapist" (sometimes abbreviated as CBT; BCIAC may be used if a therapist is certified by the Biofeedback Certification Institute of America [BCIA]).

Assistants, technicians, students, and trainees are always supervised, as implied in their titles. Some "therapists" and "practitioners" are also supervised in some settings. The degree of independence and responsibilities accorded such individuals depends on several factors, including the setting, the discipline, the laws and regulations in force, the employer, and the supervising professionals. Most persons providing biofeedback services under supervision are providing far more than only technical services.

A proper job title should accurately reflect a person's duties and status. It also helps other professionals understand the title and what to expect, and can help gain respect for a professional with that title. In addition, it facilitates the person's mobility across employment situations and state lines. Standardization of titles and functions is important for those who prefer to use "biofeedback" in their titles, or who need to do so because they have no standardized discipline or licensed title.

The BCIA establishes criteria for education, training, and supervised experience for persons qualifying for certification, regardless of their title. Considerations in developing a job description[3] include the BCIA Blueprint Knowledge Statements, or role delineations for biofeedback practitioners. The BCIA established these as necessary in 1980 (M. S. Schwartz, 1981) and updates them periodically. The BCIA statements or modifications of them could be used to formulate a job description for those providing biofeedback services.

Functions and Responsibilities of Supervised Paraprofessionals

The functions and responsibilities of a supervised biofeedback therapist depend upon such factors as education, training, experience, type of setting, client needs, state regulations, attitudes and experience of the supervising professional, relationship between the supervisor and the supervisee, malpractice insurance guidelines, and third-party reimbursement. These factors must be considered in selecting a model for the delivery of services (discussed later) and in selecting personnel to deliver the services.

The responsibilities of a supervised, qualified biofeedback therapist include at least assisting in assessment and evaluation, making decisions about patient selection, conducting physiological baselines and psychophysiological stress assessments, providing the therapy rationale and description of therapy, setting therapeutic goals, selecting body sites for feedback, conducting some or all of the biofeedback and other physiological self-regulatory therapy sessions, and keeping physiological and symptom data records. Other responsibilities of these therapists include evaluation of patient progress, teaching generalization of self-regulatory skills, conducting follow-up evaluation, helping select instrumentation and modalities, and maintaining instrumentation and supplies.

Qualified Therapists

Who are the qualified professionals who offer biofeedback therapies? How can the public and others correctly identify them? The diversity of professional degrees, licenses, titles, and

educational credentials in the field causes confusion. The answer to the question of who qualifies as a biofeedback therapist depends largely on competence and law. The practice guidelines and standards of the Association for Applied Psychophysiology and Biofeedback (AAPB)
(Striefel Butter, Coxe, McKee, & Sherman, 1999) endorse as a minimal standard for practice
for all providers of applied psychophysiological and biofeedback services, that they strive for
BCIA certification in biofeedback or the equivalent as documented by education, training,
and experience. BCIA general certification for biofeedback or specialty certification in neurofeedback is an indicator of a minimal level of competence to practice. Continuing education
is needed to remain competent, and providers are cautioned to restrict their practice areas to
those in which they are, in fact, competent and/or appropriately supervised. Through national
certification examinations and meeting the criteria specified by the BCIA, professionals can
attest to their basic levels of competence in biofeedback.

Providers are expected to practice in accordance with the laws of the state in which they
practice. This includes licensing or certification by the state, if required by law, for those who
wish to practice independently. State licensure indicates that one has at least entry-level competence to provide the services germane to the discipline in which one is licensed. The AAPB's
practice guidelines and standards specify that a biofeedback therapist should provide services
only in those areas in which he or she has competence based on education, training, and experience, unless appropriately supervised (Striefel et al., 1999). A competent biofeedback
therapist needs to know what to do (and what not to do), when and whether to do it, why,
and how to do it (Striefel, 1995; Striefel et al., 1999). Certification is different from a license
provided by a state. State laws may require that unlicensed professionals, even those certified
by a national certification agency like the BCIA, must still work under the supervision of
appropriately licensed professionals (Striefel, 1995; Striefel et al., 1999).

Assessment and Supervision

The AAPB's practice guidelines and standards (Striefel et al., 1999) clarify the expectations
for provider and supervisor competence, and provide guidance on what to strive for and what
is mandatory.

Failure to comply with state law can have severe penalties. Supervision of professionals
who are not state-approved for independent practice is particularly important, because many
professionals provide biofeedback services for medical, psychological, and dental disorders
that require specified knowledge, training, experience, and state credentials. Professionals,
licensed or unlicensed for independent practice, who do not possess the competence necessary to meet clients' needs should refer these clients elsewhere, to avoid doing them a disser-
vice by providing services that are below the expected standard of care or that might even
harm the clients. Some biofeedback therapists are not members of professional organizations
that compel following ethical and professional standards of conduct and practice. Courts are
increasingly holding such professionals to existing national ethical principles and practice
guidelines and standards (e.g., those of the AAPB), even if an individual is not a member of
a specific organization (Striefel, 1995; Zuckerman, 2003). (See Striefel, Chapter 36, this volume, for more information on these topics).

Supervisor Functions

There are supervisors who know little about biofeedback and associated therapies and do
not get involved in those aspects of therapy, and thus are not engaging in biofeedback supervision. If one is designated as someone else's supervisor, and does not provide competent
supervision, one is behaving unethically and is at risk legally. In contrast, there are supervi-

sory practitioners who are simultaneously providing the same services with other patients and working in tandem with the therapists in the treatment of some or all patients.

There are problems when a supervisor relies on a biofeedback therapist for full knowledge and experience with evaluative and therapy procedures. This is especially true if the supervisor seldom sees the patients. If the supervisor has limited experience with the procedures, he or she can provide only limited supervision. This leaves therapists who should be "supervised" on their own. An ethical and prudent supervisor who is not competent to provide supervision for biofeedback and/or related applied psychophysiological services will engage in one or more of the following activities: (1) hiring a practitioner who is competent in the necessary supervisory, biofeedback, and related skills to provide supervision of those activities for the particular organization; (2) obtaining additional training and supervision to become competent to supervise biofeedback services; and/or (3) ceasing to accept clients for biofeedback services if competent and ethical supervision is not available. Supervisors share ethical and legal responsibility for what those whom they supervise, or should ethically supervise, do or fail to do (Striefel, 1995; Zuckerman, 2003). If the supervisee is negligent, the supervisor's license, reputation, and income are at risk if a lawsuit or ethics complaint is filed. As such, it is in everyone's best interest for the supervisor not to agree to provide supervision in areas in which he or she is not competent.

Several factors influence the need for involvement of the supervising professional, including the therapist's qualifications and skills, the patients' disorders, and the complexity of the cases. Supervising professionals see the advantages of being familiar and experienced with the responsibilities of the therapists. They know that they should be able to conduct the same therapy when needed, or should arrange for a supervisor who can. (See Striefel, Chapter 36, this volume, or Striefel, 1995, for more discussion of supervision and supervisors.)

MODELS OF PRACTICE[4]

Another practical consideration related to delivering biofeedback services concerns the variety of service delivery models.

The One-Practitioner Model

The one-practitioner model is the most common model for delivering biofeedback services. In this model, one professional provides all the evaluative and therapy services. The professional either treats one patient at a time or works with a small group of patients. The one-practitioner model allows for individualization of evaluation and intervention. The group variant of this model allows providers to treat more patients and may be less expensive; however, it provides less attention to meeting the individualized needs of each patient and may not be reimbursable (see the section on coding, billing, and reimbursement later in this chapter).

Another variant of the one-practitioner model is the overlapping model. In this model, one professional uses a staggered and overlapping schedule to treat multiple patients concurrently in separate offices. The practitioner goes from room to room and patient to patient several times during each treatment session, performing different functions during each visit, such as reviewing homework and hookup, leaving client to practice alone, planning homework, and terminating the session with the client. See Olson (1995b) for more details. This model requires careful planning and disciplined scheduling. It thus limits flexibility and makes it difficult to give extra time to patients. There are many limitations to this model (Olson, 1995b). The most critical limitation concerns whether each client's needs are being met in an effective and efficient manner. Services that fall below the expected standard of care are unethical and could become problematic if a client becomes dissatisfied and decides to take action against the provider (Striefel, 1995; Zuckerman, 2003).

The Collaborative Model

In collaborative service models, one or more independently licensed professionals and a biofeedback provider deliver the services. There are five variants of this model.

The Staggered-Schedule Model

In the first variant, a biofeedback therapist provides services in the staggered or simultaneous-patients schedule of the overlapping model, described above. However, there are two providers (e.g., a licensed provider and a nonlicensed assistant), who rotate rooms and patients. Either professional may provide some or all services, depending partly on the qualifications of each, the patient, and the needs of the patient. The analogues for this model are the services provided by dentists with their dental assistants and hygienists.

The Control-Room Model: Overlapping and Group Treatment

In some settings, there is a central control room located next to two or more treatment rooms. This arrangement allows both common and tailored audiovisual feedback from and to each separate room. The instrumentation controls are in the control room. This design allows for one or two professionals to conduct evaluative and therapy sessions simultaneously in two or more rooms.

The Evaluation–Therapy Model

A third variation of the collaborative model involves delegation of specific services to different providers. For example, a licensed, supervising professional conducts the intake, periodic, and final sessions, and may provide other needed services (e.g., psychotherapy), while a biofeedback therapist conducts all or most of the biofeedback therapy sessions. The first professional obtains a history and decides whether to start therapy, provides a rationale for therapy, and selects the therapy and the procedures.

In a variation of the evaluation–therapy model, a properly trained and credentialed therapist provides the intake and initial psychophysiological assessment. The therapist discusses the case with the supervisor before proceeding with therapy. The supervising professional may also see the patient in the first session, periodically during therapy, and at the end of therapy. This allows the supervising professional to remain in close contact with the patient. It supports the therapist's role and recommendations, encourages compliance with the regimen, and allows better evaluation of progress. Therapist competence, and the relationship, communication, and trust between the professionals, are of obvious importance. The major advantages are the flexibility and lowered costs allowed by this model.

The Parallel-Treatment Model

Some independently licensed health care professionals, including physicians, dentists, and psychologists, are neither interested in conducting biofeedback therapy nor qualified to do so. Yet they may recognize the value and efficacy of biofeedback and other physiological self-regulatory therapies. Such professionals may employ a properly qualified biofeedback therapist who provides the intake, psychophysiological assessment, therapy, and follow-up, while the independently licensed professional provides his or her own specialty services. The employed bio-feedback therapist should be licensed or should receive competent supervision from someone qualified to provide biofeedback services; otherwise, the licensed professional is at unnecessary risk if something goes wrong. As suggested earlier, professionals should not hire someone to provide services they are not competent to supervise unless competent supervision is available.

This model allows for both types of intervention simultaneously or sequentially. For, example, a patient may receive psychotherapy from one mental health professional and receive relaxation and biofeedback therapies from another professional. Another example is the neurologist, internist, or dentist who requests an evaluation for relaxation and biofeedback therapies by a qualified biofeedback therapist.

Using any of the collaborative models described above, professionals can provide a wider array of biofeedback and other needed professional services than the one-practitioner model allows (e.g., a client may need biofeedback, psychotherapy, and several different medical services). More flexibility in scheduling patients and better meeting the individualized needs of clients can be other advantages, and there is less risk of professionals' developing "burnout" because of the sharing of responsibilities and support. The presence of two or more professionals can also provide a greater array of skills and experience. There is still the potential for burnout of the biofeedback therapist, and professionals must recognize and help prevent that from occurring. Some ways to prevent or lessen burnout include (1) involving the biofeedback therapist in the evaluative and decision-making process, (2) varying job responsibilities, (3) maintaining high-quality interprofessional communications, (4) providing support and positive reinforcements, and (5) providing for ongoing education and time away from the job.

The Telehealth Model

The "telehealth" model is the newest variant of the collaborative model; it generally relies on telephone line connections, computerized biofeedback equipment, and videoconferencing equipment (Striefel, 2000a). In this model, a technician is available on site to attach electrodes, turn on equipment (e.g., biofeedback and videoconferencing equipment), and provide any other support services needed on site. A competent professional in another location actually conducts the assessments, plans the intervention, and conducts treatment via two-way, telephone-based audio and video equipment. It could also be done via the Internet. The professional and the client can see and hear each other in real time, even though they may be hundreds or thousands of miles apart. This model is used to provide services in areas where competent biofeedback therapists are not available, but the services are needed (e.g., rural areas). The U.S. military uses telehealth approaches to providing biofeedback services successfully worldwide. Federal prisons also use this approach to provide a variety of health care services when professionals competent for providing specific services are not available on site; doing so eliminates the risks of transporting dangerous prisoners outside of a prison (Striefel, 2000a). Many ethical, legal, and practical issues related to using this model still need to be identified and addressed (Striefel, 2000a, 2000b).

Summary

At present, no empirical data exist to demonstrate that one model of practice is superior to another. There are advantages and disadvantages associated with each model. Many professionals, however, would agree from their own experiences that variants of the collaborative models have a higher probability of better meeting the often complex needs of their clients, especially if services are individualized to meet individual client needs. The primary considerations for selection of the model are (1) patient welfare; (2) professional qualifications, skills, and experience; (3) practical considerations; (4) cost-effectiveness; and (5) reimbursability. The criteria of efficacy and efficiency are as germane to biofeedback services as they are to other health-related services. The qualifications of all professionals involved in an evaluation and therapy program are very important, regardless of the delivery model.

Biofeedback Clinic Designs

Three types of professional arrangements are prevalent:

1. A biofeedback therapist works under the supervision of a professional who is state-credentialed for independent practice. In this case, the licensed professional also has appropriate education, credentials, and proficiency in biofeedback. Such a supervisor is engaging in ethical behavior by being competent in areas in which he or she provides supervision (Striefel et al., 1999). This arrangement has clear advantages. A prudent supervisor will train his or her supervisees, and may even require that his or her staff show at least basic knowledge and practical skills through the BCIA certification procedures.

2. A biofeedback therapist works under the direction of a licensed professional who does not have proficiency in biofeedback. If the licensed professional also serves as the supervisor, he or she is behaving unethically by supervising in areas in which he or she is not competent (Striefel et al., 1999). In addition, the supervisor is at risk financially, legally, and ethically if problems arise that results in a claim of malpractice or injury because of what the supervisee did or did not do (Striefel, 1995; Striefel et al., 1999; Zuckerman, 2003). This arrangement is not for inexperienced providers, because they will have to be competent in all areas of service or be at unnecessary risk because their supervisor is not competent in biofeedback. One of us (Striefel) has received numerous complaints from providers hired to provide biofeedback, services by a supervisor who is not competent to provide biofeedback, or from others who are concerned about such arrangements because the supervisees are coming to them for guidance on how to provide services. Once again, it is best not to enter into such an arrangement unless one is competent to provide biofeedback services independently and/or other arrangements have been made for receiving supervision and consultation if and when needed.

3. A biofeedback therapist works independently within a hospital, clinic, or educational institution. The therapist may or may not have a license as a health care provider and may receive little or no direct professional supervision. He or she must, however, be in compliance with state licensing laws. In such situations, it can be extremely useful to become a member of a peer consultation group or appropriate Internet chat line group, to have available other practitioners with whom to interact when questions or issues about biofeedback services arise.

The development of a particular clinic design depends upon the requirements of the professional setting, the budget, and the availability of skilled and otherwise qualified biofeedback providers. Practitioners may provide high-quality biofeedback therapy within any of the above-mentioned arrangements; however, each design has inherent advantages and disadvantages for the staff members involved and for the services provided.

THERAPIST PRESENCE OR ABSENCE

During what phases of physiological monitoring and feedback therapy should biofeedback therapists be present? This is a delicate, complex, and controversial question that has no one answer. Many variations exist in current practice for therapists providing biofeedback and other applied psychophysiological interventions. The variations range from therapists' always being present to therapists' seldom being present.

Several important issues must be considered in deciding when it is appropriate for the therapist to be present versus absent. Keep in mind also that the biofeedback billing codes are defined as "face-to-face." If a therapist is going to be absent from the room, the absence must be in the best interests of the client. Weiner (1998) points out that the interests, needs, and welfare of the patient must always come first. As such, therapist absences should be a planned part of a client's treatment program, and continuity of care should be ensured. It is the responsibility of the therapist to help each client achieve his or her treatment goals.

The Operant Paradigm

Well-structured biofeedback encompasses the use of operant conditioning principles. In the operant paradigm, specific and associated behaviors, including physiology, emotions, and cognitions, can be changed via the immediate consequences produced by a behavior. Consequences can increase the future likelihood of a behavior (e.g., physiological change), if the client finds the consequences desirable and reinforcing; they can decrease the future likelihood of the behavior change, if the client judges the consequence to be undesirable or punishing; and, of course, the consequences can be neutral and have no impact on the future likelihood of the behavior. The feedback that a client receives about his or her physiology during biofeedback can have any of these potential impacts. It is part of the therapist's role to help the client understand how each type of feedback is associated with his or her physiology, and to structure the feedback so that learning takes place efficiently. The learning process is faster and easier with a highly motivated and intelligent client than it is with an unmotivated client who does not want to be in treatment in the first place—for instance, a child diagnosed with attention-deficit/hyperactivity disorder (ADHD) who enjoys the reactions of others to his or her acting-out behavior.

The published literature on human learning makes clear that trial-and-error learning can be slow and inefficient, in comparison to learning in which the consequences are structured so that a person gets clear and meaningful feedback both when he or she is engaging in the correct behavior (i.e., producing the desired physiological changes) and also when he or she is not producing the desired behavior (i.e., when physiology is not changing or is going in the opposite direction from what is desired). Biofeedback equipment available today allows the therapist to give clients two different types of feedback—one following successful physiological changes, and the other following unsuccessful physiological changes. In addition, the feedback can even change in relation to the magnitude or speed of the changes produced.

Meaningful Feedback

Lights, sounds, and other types of equipment-produced feedback are not always meaningful or sufficient in and of themselves for producing the desired physiological changes, especially early in the treatment process. If they were, there would be no need for biofeedback therapists. In operant terminology, when the consequences are not sufficient for producing the desired changes in physiology, one would say either that the feedback received from the machine is by itself not functionally reinforcing enough to produce or support behavior change, or that the learning task has not been structured well enough for the person to learn the desired task. In both situations, the practitioner needs to be involved in restructuring the learning task so that the client is successful. Shellenberger and Green (1986) reported that to make biofeedback training more successful, there must be clear goals, rewards for approximating these goals, and clear instructions on how to achieve self-regulation. Can a therapist do these things if he or she is absent? What can be done to make feedback functional and reinforcing for the client, so that the client can produce the desired physiological changes? The answer is in the relationship that is established between the client and therapist.

The Therapist–Client Relationship

A key component of all successful treatment approaches, including biofeedback and other applied psychophysiological interventions, is the relationship that exists between the client and the therapist. Good relationships take time to develop, and are based in part on the number and quality of interactions that occur. With most clients, a therapist has to be present in order for a meaningful relationship to form. (This can include being present via a telehealth hookup.) If a client perceives that the therapist is interested in the client, his or her problems, and their resolution, a good relationship is likely to develop, and positive treatment outcomes are likely to occur. When a practitioner listens carefully, reflects back to the client what the client has presented as his or her concerns, makes eye contact, involves the client in treatment-related decision making (e.g., during the informed consent process), and engages in all of those other behaviors that result in the client's perceiving the therapist as trustworthy, then the therapist gains credibility. As a result, the therapist's comments become a form of feedback and reinforcement that can enhance not only the relationship, but also the learning and physiological changes that occur. If the therapist is judged by the client to be a positive influence (reinforcing), his or her comments and instructions can become antecedents for appropriate behavior and learning, and previously ineffective biofeedback can become reinforcing by being paired with the therapist. The placebo factor is influenced by the confidence and enthusiasm shown by the therapist for the intervention he or she is using, and can have a powerful effect on client outcomes (Wickramasekera, 1999). Pavlovian and operant conditioning may well be the most powerful and reliable methods for instilling expectations in humans (Wickramasekera, 1999). So the practitioner needs to be present often enough to influence the client's expectation that he or she can modify not only his or her physiology, but also the symptoms that brought the client in for treatment in the first place. Even spontaneous recovery from life-threatening diseases (e.g., cancer) can be enhanced by increasing a client's hope for recovery through what the therapist tells the client (O'Regan & Hirsberg, 1993).

If the therapist is not present to interact with the client as needed, client progress can be hindered, dissatisfaction can occur, and the client may well drop out of treatment. Most lawsuits and ethical complaints are filed when clients are dissatisfied with the interactions or lack of interactions that they are having with their therapists (Zuckerman, 2003). Practitioners should not underestimate the power of their presence, or of their verbal approval and support. So the feedback that a client receives from the biofeedback equipment can become more meaningful and can be enhanced in effectiveness when the therapist is present to help the client (1) identify new strategies for modifying physiology; (2) identify the feedback associated with both successful and unsuccessful physiological changes; and (3) identify those internal cues and external observable behaviors that are associated with success or failure (e.g., a tingling sensation in the fingers that is associated with finger temperature increases). A competent therapist is a coach who is present often enough to guide behavior so that the client successfully learns to modify his or her behavior in the desired direction. The fewer the number of errors made in learning the self-regulation skills, the faster learning will occur.

Generalization and Maintenance of Behavior Change

For the physiological changes produced to be meaningful, the client must be able to produce the changes in his or her everyday activities. The literature on treatment and the operant paradigm discusses these changes in terms of generalization and maintenance of behavior.

One component of a client's treatment plan in programming for generalization and maintenance of behavior is to plan for therapist absence. Therapist absences must be structured to occur at times, and at a frequency and duration, that will allow the client and therapist to determine whether the client has sufficiently mastered the self-regulation and other skills taught to be able to demonstrate those skills in the therapist's absence. The timing, frequency, and duration of absences will depend on the specific client; his or her age and level of motivation; the degree of learning that has occurred; and other factors relevant to the specific client.

Advantages of Therapist Presence and Absence

The advantages of therapist presence include the following:

1. The therapist can observe patients for sources of artifacts. Examples are swallowing, eyes opening or closing, shifts in hand positions, other movements, and breathing changes. Windows into therapy rooms or remote video cameras can accomplish this, but are luxuries not usually available.
2. The therapist can make treatment suggestions during and between segments of sessions (e.g., strategies to try that have been useful for other patients).
3. The therapist's presence provides more "real-life" situations for generalization to occasions when other people are present.
4. The therapist can be more flexible in altering treatment protocols or equipment settings when needed or desired.
5. The therapist can be supportive in an effort to reduce a patient's frustration during long feedback segments (longer than 20 minutes). The therapist can also stop such segments or switch to different feedback signals or modalities.
6. The therapist's presence demonstrates interest in the patient, which can be a powerful motivator.
7. The therapist can record data from the instruments in short trials, such as those of 15, 30, or 60 seconds, when automated data acquisition systems are unavailable.
8. The therapist can provide the attention that some patients expect and need.
9. The therapist can take opportunities to employ other therapy procedures during biofeedback to facilitate relaxation or neuromuscular rehabilitation.
10. The therapist's presence may sometimes permit the use of less complex and less expensive instrumentation.

The advantages of planned therapist absence include these:

1. It allows the patient to practice newly acquired physiological self-regulation skills in a safe and familiar setting, to see whether he or she can produce the desired changes with the therapist absent.
2. It can help prepare the patient for producing physiological changes in his or her own daily environment.
3. It may help reduce the cost of treatment if the therapist charges less for times during which he or she is absent.
4. It may well help the patient gain confidence in his or her self-relgulatory abilities.

Leaving Patients Alone: A Prudent Viewpoint

We offer a prudent position on leaving patients alone. The presence of a skilled and qualified therapist is a necessary part of biofeedback therapies. As noted above, there are times when it is acceptable to leave patients alone—for example, to allow patients to explore and further develop physiological self-regulation. However, such phases should occur less often than those with direct observation or with a therapist present.

We believe that it is inappropriate and unethical to provide therapy sessions with patients alone, unless such sessions are a planned part of a patient's treatment to which he or she has given informed consent, after fully understanding the implications of therapist absence. In addition, we believe that direct and nearly continuous observation of clients during treatment is needed in order for treatment to be successful, especially during the early sessions. Interacting with clients during treatment is one part of successful treatment.

We suspect that the practice of leaving patients alone for many sessions is a major concern to third-party payers, who view clinics where this occurs as "biofeedback factories" or will simply not pay for anything other than "face-to-face" treatment. Moreover, when treatment is unsuccessful, such experiences of being left alone create a negative impression of biofeedback in the minds of patients. They often drop out of treatment, do not seek biofeedback again, and tell their primary care physicians that biofeedback does not work. The motivation of some practitioners who leave their patients alone during many office sessions is unclear; however, financial factors probably motivate some such practitioners.

Suggestions for When Patients Are Left Alone

If a practitioner decides to leave patients alone, it must be as a planned part of treatment and full informed consent must have been obtained, as noted above. Thereafter, we suggest consideration of the following:

- The instruments used should allow recording and storage of all the trials of physiological data. Brief trials should be employed, to improve assessment of changes and variance among the trials. Recording many trials also allows observing outlying trials that suggest possible artifacts, such as patients' movements.
- Therapists should provide careful instructions beforehand. Patients should be told what produces artifacts, and therefore what to try to avoid or remember to note later. If there is direct observation from an observation room and an intercom, then one can substitute different statements (e.g., "I will be next door and can see and hear you. If you need me, just ask").
- Patients should be left alone only for short periods, such as 5–20 minutes.
- Ideally, there will be some type of observation.
- There should be a way for selected patients to signal therapists in case they are uncomfortable. Practitioner judgment dictates the need for a signaling system.
- Therapists should ask patients beforehand what their thoughts and feelings are about being alone. Prudent therapists know to give patients a realistic chance to express themselves. They are able to create an atmosphere in which patients are comfortable expressing themselves about any concerns. They will avoid asking a patient, "Do you want to be left alone for a while?" or "Is my presence bothering you?" Good therapists will say something like the following:

> "Sometimes patients find it distracting or a little interfering to have someone else always in the room. How would you feel about being alone for a few minutes? How much time do you think you would be comfortable being alone to explore self-regulation? Are you comfortable with being alone for 10 minutes?"

- Conscientious therapists often adjust the fees of such sessions to reflect the different costs associated with the therapists' absence. If a patient is left alone for about 15 minutes or longer, some professionals consider it excessive and inappropriate to charge the same rate as when they are present. The same rate can be justified if a therapist is observing from another room.

Suggestions for When Therapists Are Present

When a therapist is present in the room with a patient, it may be useful for the therapist to remember not to position him- or herself between the patient and the door, unless this is unavoidable. Some patients feel safer if they believe that they can leave if they want to, especially patients with a history of sexual abuse. A therapist's physical proximity to a patient should not invade the patient's sense of personal space, unless the patient understands and accepts why the therapist is so close. An observant therapist discusses these factors with a patient: distance, purpose, the patient's comfort, and where the therapist will be located so the therapist can observe and interact with the patient without being intrusive or making him or her uncomfortable. Therapists should ask patients about their thoughts and feelings about the therapists' presence. As noted above, they try to create an atmosphere in which patients feel comfortable expressing themselves.

Research

There is still very limited research about whether therapists should be or need to be present during biofeedback sessions (Borgeat, Elie, & Castonguay, 1991; Borgeat, Hade, Larouche, & Bedwani., 1980; Borgeat, Hade, Larouche, & Gauthier, 1984; Bregman & McAllister, 1983; Dumouchel, 1985). See M. S. Schwartz and Gemberling (1995) for a summary and review of that research.

There are studies that do not favor therapist presence during biofeedback sessions, although there are substantial limits in methodology and completeness in these studies. These investigators correctly note the need for much more research. Other studies suggest that the presence of therapists may be better under some conditions. For example, some research supports the clinical lore concerning the importance of individual therapist variables. As such, prudent professionals will think carefully about the relevant factors before deciding what to do. Until sufficient research and further guidelines exist, biofeedback practitioners will probably not leave most patients alone without direct observation most of the time.

WRITTEN PROFESSIONAL COMMUNICATIONS

Communications about biofeedback involve unique information. Prudent practitioners take extra care writing reports, session notes, and letters so as to maximize the benefit to clients. As Ochs (1990) notes, "A record is a trail of the problem(s), assessments, considerations, intentions, and outcomes of a particular patient's treatment process" (p. 24).

Purposes Served by Written Communications

The failure of a practitioner to keep proper records and protect patients' confidentiality is now a basis for a malpractice claim (Zuckerman, 2003). Written communications are made and copies are kept for many purposes, including (1) to help coordinate and improve the services received by clients from different practitioners; (2) to document the services provided to clients to meet legal obligations and third-party payer requirements; (3) to help practitioners defend themselves, should legal action or an ethical complaint be filed against them (inadequate documentation is one of the most common grounds for fraud charges being filed against practitioners by Medicare, as noted by Foxhall, 2000a); and (4) to comply with a profession's ethical expectations (e.g., to ensure that another provider could take over the client's treatment if a practitioner were no longer available) (Zuckerman, 2003).

General Suggestions for the Presentation of Information

Professionals, health insurance companies, and referral sources are often unfamiliar with biofeedback terminology, rationale, and procedures. Practitioners also differ in their communication methods, style, and terminology used; they often record and emphasize different information. This all affects the clarity and value of their communications.

Clear writing helps practitioners to remember what they did and to communicate that information to others. Many other people read what practitioners write, including some persons who are less or not at all familiar with biofeedback terminology and procedures—or, indeed, even with what biofeedback means. There are multiple proper ways to write professional notes and letters. See M. S. Schwartz (1995) for examples of overly brief and overly detailed notes, and discussion.

Prudent practitioners avoid misinterpreting data. They describe sessions in enough detail and clarity that others reading the description know what took place and what interpretations are being considered. Describing sessions this way may also promote questioning patients about what they were thinking about during specified phases. As well, it informs other professionals that the practitioner is being careful with interpretations.

Some readers may be thinking that it is impractical to record detailed notes. The degree of detail needed in routine clinical practice is changing rapidly, because inadequate records are now seen as evidence of substandard care, regardless of how good the actual service provided was (Weiner & Wettstein, 1993). If something is not written down, the courts and external review bodies assume that it did not occur (Foxhall, 2000a; Striefel, 1995; Zuckerman, 2003). If a third-party payer is billed for a service that was not carefully documented in accordance with the regulations of that payer (e.g., Medicare requires the record to document "medical necessity"), the provider is subject to charges of fraud—and the penalties for this can be severe, both financially and legally (Foxhall, 2000a). Do you know what constitutes "reasonable and necessary services" as defined by Medicare in your state? If you serve Medicare patients, it is essential to know how these terms are defined. The rules vary from state to state and across third-party payers. So detailed reports are better than those with very limited or no detail. The degree of detail depends on the situation and the professional. Thoughtful inclusion of details and interpretations can be educational and enhance credibility.

Inclusion of Evaluation and Treatment Information
in Reports and Peer Reviews

The interview, evaluation, psychophysiological assessment, and treatment processes are complex and involve many topics. Much information is needed in reports and notes. Furthermore, the information differs according to each client's history and each disorder being assessed and treated. Practitioners using biofeedback ask for referrals and ask third-party payers to pay for these services. Reviewers make judgments about many aspects of clinical services. It is educational to place ourselves as biofeedback practitioners in the position of others less familiar with biofeedback by imagining ourselves as those people who have questions and doubts about the value of our procedures. They are often seeking information and reassurance that the procedures used were proper and cost-effective. Were the reports and notes clear in terms of the symptoms, diagnoses, details of service and level of care provided, and progress notes (American Psychological Association [APA], 1993a)? If these items are not completely documented, or the wrong codes were used, this may be considered to be evidence that the billed services were not reasonable and medically necessary (APA, 1993a).

Referral sources, reviewers, and third-party payers care about content and clarity. Naive, incomplete, illegible, unclear, poorly worded, or careless reports, session notes, and letters detract from a professional's credibility and can raise questions about substandard care or even fraud. A self-righteous or defensive attitude on the part of practitioners preparing reports and session notes is unwise, unprofessional, and self-defeating. For example, if a service such as assessment takes longer than usual, the documentation must make clear why additional time was reasonable and necessary.

The APA has available several publications that can be useful concerning documentation. They include *Practice Pointer: The Basics of Medicare Audits* (APA, 1993b), "Record Keeping Guidelines" (APA, 1993c), and *State Medicaid Reimbursement Standards for Psychologists* (APA, 1995). (See also M. S. Schwartz, Chapter 6, and Arena & Schwartz, Chapter 7, this volume, for discussions of the intake process and baselines, respectively. See other chapters for discussions of specific disorders and information needed in reports.

Poorly worded and insufficient information in reports could reduce the chances of reimbursement and referrals. Has the essential information been included, and how well and how clearly did the practitioner present it? Ochs (1990) presents typical questions asked by review agencies. We offer a slightly modified wording of his questions without changing the substance: "Does the available documentation support this treatment for the specific symptom(s) and effects? Is the treatment proper and reasonable? Is the documentation about the biofeedback proper? Does the available documentation show a need for more treatment?"

Borrowing from Ochs (1990) again, we glean from his remarks that reviewers expect explicit statements and data about the symptoms and condition of a patient before, during, and after treatment. They look for a rationale for estimating the phases of treatment and the length of treatment, as well as for consistency of the measurement systems or symptoms and psychophysiology. For atypical or unusual treatment approaches, they need clear statements about the rationale and methods for assessing changes. Reviewers also want information about transfer of training to daily activities, and the strengths and limitations of patients. They prefer evaluations for treatment for preexisting and comorbid conditions that could interfere with treatment compliance and obtaining the desired results, and they expect that practitioners understand and accept factors that could change the treatment plan. Overall, reviewers look for active participation by practitioners in treatment.

Session Record Keeping

Biofeedback and other treatment records require detailed and precise descriptions of the sessions. Practitioners should record any events and conditions that could affect a patient's physiological functioning and data interpretation. At a minimum, the documentation should include (1) identifying data; (2) symptoms and presenting problem; (3) history of problem; (4) dates of service and length of sessions; (5) fees; (6) types of services; (7) all assessments and the rationale for using them; (8) the treatment plan; (9) any consultations obtained (including supervision); (10) summary reports and/or testing reports and supporting data; (11) release-of-records information obtained; (12) complete progress notes; (13) physiological data summaries; and (14) rationale for anything unusual in terms of assessment, length or frequency of sessions, or anything else that would document why specific services were reasonable and necessary (APA, 1993b, 1993c). In addition, notes should be signed and include the proper Current Procedural Terminology (CPT) codes for the type and duration of the session.

The discussion that follows provides a rationale and guidelines for recording selected items, especially those unique to biofeedback. Most information can be useful, is easy to record, and can help communications. Therapeutic decisions, comparisons, and communications become more difficult without some of this information.

General Information

- *Time of day* is useful if the patient's symptoms or ability to regulate psychophysiology may vary with the time of day. Biorhythms vary across the day. For example, electroencephalographic (EEG) assessments and training sessions should be conducted at the same time of day for any individual client, because of rhythmic EEG changes that occur across the 24-hour day.
- *Patient waiting time* before the physiological recordings started is sometimes useful to record, especially if the session was preceded by physical activity, caffeine or nicotine intake, or stressful events.

Non-Instrument-Related Conditions

- *Temperature (indoor/outdoor)* should be noted when indoor temperatures vary significantly or are very different from outdoor temperatures, especially if the patient just came into the office.
- *Lighting* can affect relaxation procedures, patient cognitions and comfort, and EEG or surface electromyographic (EMG) instrumentation artifact. Fluorescent lighting can sometimes affect some physiological data, such as surface EMG (hereafter referred to simply as EMG).
- *Noise* within the office or outside may affect psychophysiological reactivity.
- *Type of chair* should be noted, because sitting in a recliner or high-backed chair is not similar to most real-life conditions, and therapists often monitor and provide feedback for patients in different chairs.
- *Body position* (e.g., sitting up with head resting back and supported, sitting up with head not supported, fully reclining, and standing) is obviously also important.
- *Activity* notations are useful for therapists who vary patients' activities during monitoring and feedback (e.g., resting quietly, reading aloud, reading silently, writing, conversation, listening to someone else talk, tensing fists, typing, playing an instrument, and talking on the phone).

Instrumentation and Physiological Data

- *Electrode/sensor/thermistor sites* need to be recorded precisely enough so that other practitioners can identify the exact sites from which the data were recorded, so that they can duplicate sensor placement if needed. For example, the International 10–20 System is used for standardized electrode placement in EEG assessments or neurofeedback training.
- *Temperature measurement sites* vary, so note which hand, digit, side, and phalange are used. Different sites result in different temperatures. It is more accurate to use the term "digit" rather than "finger," and the terms "volar" and "dorsal" for the palm side and back side of the fingers, respectively.
- *EMG notations* ideally are accurate and clear. However, in routine clinical use, such specificity is often less practical and not always necessary. For routine clinical notes, such terms as "standard bifrontal," "bilateral masseters," and "bilateral posterior [or cervical] neck"

may be acceptable, through they are subject to some misinterpretation. When precision is important, the distance from standard anatomical locations and the exact spacing of the electrodes should be specified. One example of the latter is in neuromuscular recruitment. Anatomical drawings are helpful when one does not need more precision.

 • *Instrument checks and settings* should be recorded to assure that the instruments are working correctly and that the same settings can be used with this client in future sessions.

• *Battery status and battery check information* is important when one is using battery-operated instruments. The batteries should be checked before each session, unless they were just charged. This is especially useful in an office with multiple therapists using the same instruments.

• *Electrode–skin resistance or impedance* is important and depends on the type of instrumentation, recording site, chance of high resistance, and the purpose of the session. It is best to develop the habit of assuring that the impedance is in compliance with that specified by the manufacturer for the specific instrumentation being used, to ensure consistency and accuracy. One typically need not include this specific information in communications to others unless one believes that it is important in interpreting the data. It is still good practice to record the impedance level in the session notes, to ensure that this issue is attended to for every treatment session.

• *Bandpass specification* (e.g., 100–200 hertz, 20–1000 hertz for EMG) is important.

• *Response integration time (RIT)* in some stand-alone instruments is fixed, whereas other equipment permits adjustments. Computer software usually permits several choices, with very obvious differences in the visually displayed and audio signals. If the RIT is adjustable, one should check it and consider noting it, unless it is always the same. Notation is important if different therapists use the same instrument. The clinical significance of variations in RIT is unclear. However, one expects significant differences between responses to feedback with very short RITs of about 1 second or less, and responses to feedback with RITs of about 3 seconds or longer.

• *Trial durations, intertrial rest periods, and breaks* are important and should be documented. The therapist should note breaks between series of trials and the activities during breaks, such as discussions and their topics. Activities may affect physiological data and hence the starting point for the next sequence of trials. Computers automatically record the trial and intertrial durations, but not the breaks. Notation for a typical session helps those reading reports to understand the sessions and comparisons between sessions.

• *Scale/gain* affects the size or degree of changes in physiology that the instrument feeds back to the patient (similar to the magnification of a microscope). For example, displaying the EMG signal on a range of 1–11 microvolts and 72–82°F provides less information than a range of 1–5 microvolts and 77–82°F does. A patient's ability to regulate his or her physiological activity and interpretation of the data depend partly on the feedback scale. For example, the gain affects the feedback signal. Higher gains magnify or amplify physiological signals, and then changes appear larger and clearer. However, if the gain is too high, then tiny fluctuations can be annoying for some patients. Therapists can adjust the gain to fit the patient, task, and stage of progress. In stand-alone instruments, one can specify this (such as × 0.1, × 0.3, × 1, × 3, or × 10). This information should be recorded.

• *Feedback type notations* (e.g., graphic displays used, audio range, and threshold information) help the therapist remember what was used and how the patient reacted.

• *Physiological data artifacts* should be documented, including patient movements as swallowing, coughing, sneezing, yawning, and talking. Some therapists reset the recordings to stop such trials or drop them from analyses. Sometimes, however, the reduction of movement artifacts across sessions can be considered a therapy goal and a sign of the patient's increased ability to sit quietly (e.g., a patient with ADHD).

The Use of Standard Abbreviations and Symbols

The use of standard abbreviations and symbols helps professionals write notes and reports faster and in much less space. The trend is toward dictated and typed notes as practitioners adopt computer-based electronic medical records. However, some practitioners should be familiar with them when working in settings where others use them. See Table 28.2 in M. S. Schwartz (1995, p. 723) for a list of common abbreviations and symbols. A more complete listing is in *The Charles Press Handbook of Current Medical Abbreviations* (1997). See M. S. Schwartz (1995, pp. 724–725) for an example of a report of a completed patient evaluation and treatment with extensive use of abbreviations.

BIOFEEDBACK QUALITY CONTROL: EVALUATING THE THERAPIES

Society and consumers demand much from products and services. Accountability is an ever-increasing part of professional practice. Practitioners of biofeedback can protect their professional futures by understanding their legal rights, responsibilities, and limitations. This can be accomplished, at least partially, by maintaining rigorous scientific and clinical standards in research and clinical practice activities. Practitioner qualifications, treatment rationale and efficacy, billing and coding, and the duration of the effects of interventions are all subject to legal and public scrutiny. Therapists should be prudent and take appropriate proactive steps to prevent problems.

Evaluating Treatment Efficacy over Time

The purposes served by collecting data on treatment efficacy over time include the following:

- Assisting in the diagnostic process and in determination of appropriate treatment.
- Assisting in the determination of when modifications in the treatment process are needed and when termination or referral is appropriate.
- Assisting the therapist in determining when consultation or supervision is needed and in improving his or her skills for treating clients with similar problems in the future; follow-up data are particularly useful for skill improvement.
- Assisting in the process of appropriately documenting for third-party payers and others (including the client), that the treatment was reasonable and necessary, as well as what kind of progress (if any) occurred. Follow-up data is often used by third-party payers in deciding to whom they will refer patients (Stout, 1995).
- Contributing to the data base that can be used by other providers for determining what kind of treatments are appropriate for different kinds of client problems.

Research Studies

Good treatment has a rationale that is based on both published research and clinical experience. Well-designed research studies are used to establish the efficacy and effectiveness of specific clinical interventions. Follow-up data are needed to verify the durability of such interventions. Recognizing the need for routine and well-controlled follow-up studies, Miller (1974) made a recommendation that when a journal accepts a clinical outcome study, the investigator must agree to collect follow-up data for later publication. Some peer-reviewed journals typically require some follow-up, often at least 6 months and sometimes longer. Other journals require no follow-up data collection. Requiring long-term follow-up of 2–5 years is an ideal goal, but one that is seldom achieved. Miller (1983) reemphasized the importance of accountable data collection and follow-up information, such as (1) change in satisfaction level with current life; (2) days lost from work since the end of biofeedback treatment, due to the original presenting problem treated via biofeedback; (3) other treatments received for the same problem after biofeedback treatment ended; and (4) changes in medications since the end of biofeedback therapy.

Most biofeedback providers do not conduct routine follow-up because of the pressures of managed care, which today take more time and effort than in the past, leaving little energy or time for client follow-up. Interestingly, Bakal (1999) reported that patients with headache who had multiple sessions of relaxation training and biofeedback treatment often had little understanding of how to manage their symptoms without medications after treatment ended. In fact, many of the patients did not use the self-regulation skills that they had been taught, and relied on medications instead. Follow-up by the biofeedback provider would have allowed him or her to become aware of this issue and to modify the treatment program, to assure that the self-regulation skills being taught were in fact learned well enough to be applied in daily life activities.

Measurement Methods

This is not the place to debate the topic of measurement methods. The purpose here is to note that, no matter what the treatment parameters are or what level of tailoring occurs, progress needs to be measured. The patient's symptoms and disorder, as well as the provider's discipline and training, affect the choice of measurement methods used to identify changes during and after treatment.

> Since it is unlikely that any one technique will be found 100% effective for all individuals, it behooves the responsible clinician to develop a research-oriented, problem-solving approach to therapy. This requires that the therapist continually monitor his or her own skills in selecting and administering interventions and evaluate their consequences for specific types of patients. (G. E. Schwartz, 1983, p. 380.

Client progress and outcome data are essential for achieving this purpose.

G. E. Schwartz (1983) also emphasized that in addition to adequate formal training and continuing education, therapists must develop more systematic decision-making skills, and must develop both single-subject and group-oriented research approaches to evaluating treatment progress. Systematic procedures can be incorporated into any practice whereby particular interventions, singularly or in combination, can be continually assessed via feedback provided by the patient. Measurement methods used before, during, and after therapy include face-to-face interviews, telephone interviews, written questionnaires, personality assessments, symptom logs or diaries, and (of course), physiological data.

M. S. Schwartz and Fehmi (1982) offered several criteria for measuring progress, including changes in any of the following: frequency, intensity (or severity), and duration of daily symptoms and symptoms occurring during stress and higher-risk situations; medications; hospital visits; and thoughts about self-efficacy in regard to self-regulation. Changes in life, activities, environment, and family relationships are also general criteria (e.g., returning to work and maintaining normal hours at work). Practitioners should think logically about this issue in reference to each client's symptoms, diagnosis, and treatment goals (including physiological), and should consider how to determine whether the goals have been met. Writing treatment goals in observable and measurable terms is helpful in guiding the selection of progress and outcome measurement methods to use (Zuckerman, 2003). Answering questions such as the following can be helpful in determining which methods to use:

1. "What aspects of the client's physiology do I and the client hope to change via bio-feedback and other treatments, such as relaxation training? How will I measure all, or at least the most important, aspects of each?"

2. "What symptoms and aspects of each symptom do I and the client plan to change via treatment? How will I measure each of these?"

3. "What are the measurable behaviors associated with this client's diagnosis, and how do I go about measuring them?"

4. "What do the published literature and my past clinical experience tell me are impor-tant for measuring progress and outcomes for this client?"

5. "Do I expect medication use to change? How will I collaborate with this client's phy-sician on this issue and how will we track medication changes?"

6. "How will I measure the client's satisfaction with treatment progress and outcomes?"

Osgood, Suci, and Tannenbaum (1957) offered suggestions and examples for social sci-entists seeking to understand, define, and measure the elusive variable called "meaning." They stated that such an index should "be evaluated against the usual criteria for measuring in-struments" (p. 11) and should possess the following: (1) objectivity, (2) reliability, (3) valid-ity, (4) sensitivity, (5) comparability, and (6) utility. Osgood and his colleagues concluded that a 7-point bipolar scale is the most effective method for measuring subjective judgments. They based this conclusion on extensive investigations and statistical analyses with various scales. An example of their commonly used scale is presented below:

Extremely Relaxed __ __ __ __ __ __ __ *Extremely Tense*

There are numerous reliable and valid objective measures now available for many be-havioral and symptom dimensions. For examples and descriptions of many measures of the assessment of pain, see Turk and Melzack (1992). The important point is that practitioners be encouraged to measure progress.

Outcome measures are another way of documenting efficacy and can be collected by individual providers or group of providers, or by diagnosis, or both—as demonstrated by Keatley (1998) and her colleagues. Keatley and 10 other biofeedback providers looked at pre–post biofeedback measures, behavioral indices, length of treatment, types of biofeedback treat-ment, cost, quality of life, and patient satisfaction for their patients with six different pain diagnoses (low back pain, temporomandibular disorders [TMDs], cervical pain, cumalitive trauma [CT], and tension and migraine headaches). Their database not only gave them aver-age costs and protocol successes per diagnosis, but also became a powerful rationale for get-ting later patients' insurance denials reversed on appeal.

Meta-analysis is yet another way of reviewing treatment successes and failures. Here the available literature on an application is reviewed to determine the treatment effect sizes. For example, Crider and Glaros (1999) conducted a meta-analysis of EMG biofeedback treat-ment for TMDs, and were able to conclude that 69% of patients who received such treat-ment became symptom-free or were significantly improved at posttreatment follow-up. They then speculated as to why pre- to posttreatment changes in EMG activity were not necessar-ily correlated with the degree of clinical improvement. They posited alternative hypotheses about why the successes occurred, despite the lack of correlation with EMG levels. Increased proprioceptive awareness and heightened self-efficacy as a result of the biofeedback training may have been largely responsible. Such a meta-analysis may further help justify use of bio-feedback, even when a mechanism of control is not easily identifiable.

Similarly, when a precise protocol is known to have the best effects, it is important to use both the protocol and the criteria specific to that protocol. John D. Perry's (2001) critical analysis of research on what works and what does not was important in influencing the Health Care Financing Administration's 2000 decision to require all regional Medicare agencies to reimburse for biofeedback of urinary incontinence.

THE ISSUE OF REIMBURSEMENT FOR BIOFEEDBACK SERVICES

Can and should third parties reimburse for services provided by someone other than an independently licensed professional? This is a very important question and has major implications for the field of applied psychophysiology and biofeedback. The simple answer is that each payer makes its own rules, but compliance with those rules can be complex. The definition of "direct provider" is also crucial, because third-party systems often reimburse only independently licensed professionals who are *directly* providing services. The answer is further complicated because the biofeedback treatment codes have been defined or interpreted by the American Medical Association's (AMA's) CPT coding to be "face-to-face."

The term "direct" has different connotations for different professionals. It is not restricted to mean "face-to-face." *The American Heritage Dictionary for DOS* (1992) defines the word, as a verb, "to manage," "to take charge of with authority," "to aim, guide, or address (something or someone) toward a goal." These definitions do not necessarily mean "without the help of others." For example, surgeons provide "direct" services and do so with considerable help of supervised operating room personnel; supervised professionals conduct some of these services without a surgeon's presence. Similarly, physical and occupational therapists in medical settings provide a variety of clinical services without a physician's presence, yet physicians generally direct and supervise these services. Conscientious supervisors can supervise others providing therapies using clinical biofeedback, while still maintaining a "direct" relationship with the patient and the services. These other professionals should have proper education, training, and credentials as biofeedback therapists.

Medicaid regulations vary across states in terms of whether on not licensed providers can be directly reimbursed, whether a physician referral is needed, whether services can be covered if "bundled" into an array of services provided at a clinic or hospital, and whether requirements beyond licensure are required (e.g., some states require listing in the National Register of Health Service Providers) (APA, 1995). Only 11 states allowed for reimbursement of services provided by an unlicensed provider in 1995 (APA, 1995). Providers are encouraged to check with their state Medicaid office if they have questions about who Medicaid reimburses. Providers must also learn what is expected or required by the different third-party payers that they bill or that cover the services of their clients.

There are providers of biofeedback with demonstrated competence who do not have a license for independent practice. These providers must comply with the legal and ethical requirements that govern both their practice activities and those of their discipline, along with the requirements of third-party payers. These issues have been discussed in more detail earlier in this chapter and by Striefel in Chapter 36.

Third-party payers should reimburse practitioners who maintain high standards of competence, who practice prudently within a stepped-care framework, and who meet the third-party payers' requirements. Practitioners do best with the help of supervised professional assistants, including qualified and competent biofeedback therapists—when, of course, these services are reimbursable when provided by such personnel. Practitioners using prudent criteria for selecting patients for therapy may actually contain and lower overall costs to third-party payers, because successfully treated patients often use fewer health care services in the future. For example, primary care clinics that provide treatment for psychological problems have shown a 27% reduction in hospital admissions and bed use days (APA, 2000). Similar reductions in costs could well be expected for clients treated through biofeedback. With supervised therapists, practitioners often can treat more patients successfully in the same time period. The fees of supervised professionals are often less than for independently licensed and directly reimbursable professionals.

The definitions of "supervision" and guidelines for it are integral to the issue of direct services acceptable to affected parties. Note that the AAPB's practice guidelines and standards (Striefel et al., 1999) state that "a reasonable minimal level of supervision might be that which is often required in state licensing laws, i.e., at least one hour of face-to-face or other appropriate supervision for each 40-hours of services provided by the supervisee. More supervision should be provided as appropriate or necessary, based on client need [or] legal requirements" (p. 4.4). Definitions and guidelines need to reflect the many factors and circumstances in clinical settings. The APA's *General Guidelines for Providers of Psychological Services* (APA, 1987) dropped the prior limit of three "psychological assistants." However, it maintains the same concerns and attempts to discourage misuse by providing that professional psychologists be "sufficiently available to ensure adequate evaluation or assessment, intervention planning, direction, and emergency consultation" (p. 11). This dissuades supervisors from employing and trying to supervise large numbers of unlicensed people. Some state licensing laws (e.g., the psychology licensing laws of Utah and Texas) have specific requirements concerning who can be supervised, or how many supervisees there can be for one supervisor of a specific discipline.

The issue of reimbursement relates to the issue of determining who is a qualified clinical provider of biofeedback therapies. As explained earlier, BCIA certification and state licensing are two criteria for determining competence to provide services. The biofeedback credential continues to increase in credibility and recognition. For example, a preferred provider organization (PPO) in Florida reportedly uses the BCIA credential as a criterion for reimbursing biofeedback services (T. Dietvorst, personal communication, 1993), and four states now require BCIA certification or equivalent for workers' compensation biofeedback providers. This will probably become a trend as biofeedback providers educate insurance companies on their standards and the need to reimburse those demonstrating proficiency, rather than those (licensed or not) who have taken a weekend workshop or less and bill for these professional services.

Practitioners typically want to know whether their state has a utilization review law, and if so, what its provisions are. In 1993, 27 states had such laws (APA, 1993a). Some of these laws require third-party payers to disclose their utilization review criteria; others do not (APA, 1993a).

CODING, BILLING, AND REIMBURSEMENT

Coding, billing, and reimbursement are complex processes and depend on the following: the provider and which of the 21 disciplines providing biofeedback the provider belongs to; the service; the payer; charges; appropriate codes; who is billing; the governmental and regulatory guidelines governing the provider and service; and the criteria for fraud.

Coding

Practitioners need to know the commonly used diagnostic codes, including those in the *Diagnostic and Statistical Manual of Mental Disorders*, fourth edition (DSM-IV) and the *International Classification of Diseases*, 10th revision (ICD-10), as well as the latest CPT codes published by the AMA (2002), Whitehouse (1997, 1998) has provided extensive coverage and discussion of these codes. At this writing, a new CPT manual has been published (AMA, 2002). It is titled *Current Procedural Terminology: CPT 2003* and includes procedural codes (including evaluation codes) that reflect psychosocial services to patients with physical health diagnoses (AMA, 2002; Foxhall, 2000b). The codes cover cognitive, behavioral, social, and psychophysiological procedures designed to ameliorate physical health problems (Foxhall, 2000b). The code numbers are 96150–96155. However, it is doubtful if there will ever be appropriately detailed biofeedback evaluation codes (e.g., for a psychophysiological stress profile, muscle scans, dynamic muscle evaluations, EEG assessments, etc.) for general use. There is a code for EMG muscle scanning for use by physical therapists only (97750).

Prior to 1997 there was a series of CPT biofeedback codes, 90900–90915. Starting in 1997, these codes were collapsed in the CPT book into two codes, 90901 and 90911, under the category "Biofeedback." These were accompanied by two new codes 90875 and 90876 under the category "Psychiatric Therapeutic Procedures." For 1998 these code descriptions were modified and still remain (AMA, 1998, 2002) as follows:

Biofeedback
    90901 Biofeedback training by any modality
    90911 Biofeedback training, *perineal muscles,* anorectal, *or urethral sphincter,* including EMG and/or manometry (AMA, 2002, p. 340)

Psychiatric Therapeutic Procedures
Other Psychiatric Services or Procedures
    90875 Individual psychophysiological therapy incorporating biofeedback training by any modality (face-to-face with the patient), with psychotherapy (e.g., insight-oriented, behavior-modifying or supportive psychotherapy); approximately 20–30 minutes
    90876 approximately 45–50 minutes (AMA, 2002, p. 339)

The creation of these two different categories of codes has led to much confusion for providers as well as insurance companies. For example, Medicare will not reimburse for 90875 or 90876, but will reimburse for 90911 for specific incontinence diagnoses, and for 90901 for only a few muscle-related diagnoses, while defining 90901 as only

for muscle re-education of specific muscle groups or for treating pathological muscle abnormalities of spasticity, incapacitating muscle spasm, or weakness [and there is proof that] more conventional treatments (heat, cold, massage, exercise, support) have not been successful. This therapy is not covered for treatment of ordinary muscle tension states or for psychosomatic conditions. (Whitehouse, 1997, p. 9)

Some other coding guidebooks and insurance companies have assumed that such restrictions should apply for them as well. In fact, this is the narrowest definition and is not widely used elsewhere.

The confusion about which codes to use takes many forms. For example, the AMA CPT Coding Clearinghouse's response to questions one of us posed (Whitehouse, 1997) about deciding which code to use was that the type of work done is what determines which code to use on a given day, and that 90901 could be thought of as physical *training* without the *therapeutics* (i.e., psychotherapy, talking of issues, resistance, fears, pains, etc.). As for *who* can bill for these CPT codes, the AMA reminds us that although they were set up for physicians, the use of these codes is by determination of the third party payer (Whitehouse, 1997).

Codes do change, as do their uses. This often goes unnoticed by many providers, or they code according to whatever they think should be the determining factor, or they have been advised by someone else to code "creatively." However, it is the provider who is ultimately responsible for which codes are used and whether they are properly, ethically, and legally used. This necessitates keeping abreast of the codes by checking with billing/coding experts, each year's new CPT manual, any professional organizations to which the provider belongs, and to coding briefs in the professional literature (especially the briefs one might be inclined to ignore). Because biofeedback (and/or applied psychophysiology) is not recognized as an independent profession, our avenue for recommending code changes is first through the AAPB (currently the Insurance and Legislative Committee), which can then carry recommendations to our AMA-recognized representative—the APA's committee on coding, which has representation on the AMA CPT coding committees.

So how do providers decide what code to use if a third party is to pay? Besides the discussion above, the following paragraphs contain considerations we consider important. More detail is also provided by Whitehouse (1998).

Billing

There are two bottom lines for billing: (1) It is the decision of the third party whom it will reimburse, how much, for what diagnoses, and for how long; and (2) a provider must stay within the scope of practice and other statutory regulations affecting anyone providing biofeedback. This leaves the provider with several dilemmas:

1. Who checks with the third party? Many say it is the patient's responsibility, but the AAPB's practice guidelines and standards (Striefel et al., 1999) state that *providers* must obtain preauthorization and "obtain from the client or the client's insurance company the information needed to determine covered services, co-pay requirements, covered service settings, deductibles, procedure and diagnostic codes for which third-party reimbursement is available or specifically excluded, the third-party's reimbursement and provider requirements, and any other information needed to accurately and legally file an insurance claim" (p. 8.3).

2. What if biofeedback is not a covered benefit or if a practitioner is not an approved provider (e.g., not licensed or not in the managed care network, if that is required)?

3. Who is to pay initially (the client or the third party)?

4. Who gets the bill (i.e. who is billed)?

5. How are copayments handled?

6. What if there is no third party? What payment arrangements should be made with the client?

7. Should a provider reduce charges if the client cannot pay the usual fees?

8. What should be done about discrepancies between what is billed and what a third party reimburses? Does a provider write off the balance (as must be done if the provider has a contract with the insurer to accept its plan for what it pays and what the copayment is), or bill the client for the balance if possible and if the provider and client have so agreed, or adjust the fee for service, or appeal the insurance decision?

9. What if regulations governing who can provide biofeedback exclude a provider at this time?

Since there is no consistency among insurance companies on answers to these questions, here are some considerations for billing, based on our experience:

1. The AMA CPT advice is to choose the most appropriate code for the service rendered at any given time. However, it is the third party's decision as to whether it will pay, so the third party's advice should be obtained and documented.

2. Some companies consider 90876 (and 90875) as reimbursable only for licensed physicians or psychologists. Others include licensed social workers, nurses, and licensed professional counselors. Often these companies consider 90901, as for anyone else.

3. Some companies consider 90901 as the only code to use for any biofeedback service, including intake. Some of these require licensure in the above or registry in physical or occupational therapy. Some companies (e.g., some major medical and at least four workers' compensation companies) require certification (especially BCIA) in biofeedback; however, most do not at this time. Medicare sometimes reimburses for 90901 and for 90911, depending on the diagnosis and provider, but may limit the number of sessions to two to four. Certification is not known to be a requirement here, as specific licensure is.

4. Some companies (e.g., some state workers' compensation companies) make up their own codes. Some even require use of much older codes.

5. For some major medical insurers, 90901 is used only for certain medical or dental diagnoses, while 90876 is used for certain psychological diagnoses, and 90911 only for specific types of incontinence. Most of these require licensure for the provider.

6. Some companies say that licensed or BCIA-certified providers can use either 90901 or 90876, but that unlicensed and/or uncertified providers have to use 90901. Some are starting to define 90901 as a code for technicians to use.

7. Some companies allow for biofeedback, but may have another company that manages a network of providers with no biofeedback provider in it (i.e., although the insurance company would pay for needed biofeedback services. There is no provider in its network who has the competence needed to provide this service).

8. Some companies do not reimburse for biofeedback codes, but will consider biofeedback permissible (or in some cases recommend it) if included within a psychotherapy session, as long as the primary emphasis is on psychotherapy and the diagnosis is a psychiatric one that the provider is licensed to treat.[5]

9. Physicians and larger facilities (hospitals, rehabilitation centers, etc.) can employ and usually bill for services such as biofeedback by their employees. By Medicare standards, psychologists can no longer do the same. However, as with much else, reimbursement for this is at the discretion of the third party, so it is incumbent on a provider to find out what the third party's procedure is.

10. In some states, there are governmental or regulatory restrictions on who can provide biofeedback services. The APA (2002) has an online manual entitled *Medicare Handbook: A Guide for Psychologists* that should prove helpful for providers.

11. Most personal injury protection (PIP) insurance companies reimburse for biofeedback. Many reimburse without regard for who the provider is. Many reimburse at a set fee or set rate.

In short, providers need to know how their services will be covered if they want third-party payment. Once providers know what is covered, whether they are covered providers, what the reimbursement rate is, what the session limits are, and what codes to use, they can get informed consent from their clients or patients, and proceed with treatment. Our adivce continues as follows:

12. Providers who have a billing service should be sure that the service has at least this information and is not encouraging "creative" billing, the use of multiple CPT codes, or billing for charges that are for more than the usual (e.g., hourly) rate (as these are often investigated as fraudulent). Providers also should not assume that they should always bill the same code, as each company may have different requirements or recommendations.

13. It is best to ask the insurance company all of the questions posed above (see also below for the way we often ask these).

14. At this time there are no assessment/evaluation codes for biofeedback, so providers should also find out how to bill for intake sessions.

15. If providers' initial time involves extensive record review, or a special report is requested or necessary, they should find out if and how they can most properly bill for those services. Likewise, if providers want their clients to have home training tapes, books, or portable biofeedback instruments, they need to know whether a third party will pay for those or not, and whether to use 99070 or 99071 for the special coding of those or for any supplies that might be billed.

16. Some companies view billing 1 unit of time for 90901 to be 1 hour, while others see it as 1 minute, and others see it as 15 minutes. Providers should be sure to specify amount of time and cite modifier 22 if the time is more than what the company might expect.

17. A supervisor or supervisee of biofeedback services must abide by all laws, rules, and regulations of third-party payers, and must be sure that the role of each person is clearly understood in billing and in signing for billing (Striefel et al., 1999). The legal supervisor (for the services, not just for meeting certification requirements) is probably legally responsible for what and how billing is done. Perhaps the most common mistake here is to assume that the supervisor can bill for the supervisee. In many cases, the actual provider of the face-to-face services must be listed on the bill along with the supervisor. Checking the state regulations, and consulting the third party, are advisable.

18. Fraud, as defined in the new Social Security Act (Sections 1909 and 1128A), is a felony and includes "knowingly and willfully" charging in excess of state-established reimbursement rates (e.g., for Medicaid), offering or accepting kickbacks, and such practices as regularly discounting copayments and accepting only insurance-paid fees. (Witnessing the peer review processes and some of the fraud investigations across the country makes us very cautious. What seems to come up most often is billing for exorbitant amounts using multiple codes, creative coding, or excessive numbers of sessions, in cases where it appears there is routinely an attempt to find ways to get the very most money, much beyond the usual fees for service.) Since many companies are adopting the new fraud bill as a standard, more cases are being investigated and are coming to our attention. Some providers are being asked to give back what was considered double billing, for many years of service.

In other words, with billing and coding, it is best for providers not to assume that they know what to bill. Rather, they need to check out what is possible and right, or else should be prepared to make things right (even years later).

Here is a set of questions for third-party carriers, as modified from Whitehouse (1998), which should help obtain the answers needed for proper billing and coding:

1. Is biofeedback a covered benefit under this particular insurance policy?

2. If so, under what code(s)? 90901, 90911 (for incontinence only), 95957 (sometimes used for certain EEG analyses), or other (some workers' compensation use other codes; some companies use the old codes, 90900–90915)?

3. If not, is 90876 a covered code? If so, who can use it?

4. For what diagnoses is biofeedback a covered benefit? (Or: Is biofeedback a covered benefit for this diagnosis?)

5. For what diagnoses is biofeedback excluded (e.g., some companies will not cover temporomandibular joint pain, but will cover TMDs or myofascial pain?

6. Is the biofeedback for this diagnosis covered under medical, dental, mental health, or other benefits?

7. What are the biofeedback provider requirements, if any? Special licensure, special certification (BCIA or other), PPO or health maintenance organization (HMO) network, other?

8. What is the reimbursement (dollar amount or rate), and how much time is that for (e.g., minutes, blocks of 15 minutes, 60 minutes)?

9. How many sessions are allowed? (Or: What are the limits on sessions or dollar amounts?) If 90876 is allowed, can it be billed on the same day as someone also billing for 90806 Psychotherapy, since many companies allow only one psychological service charge per day?

10. Is there a deductible to be met? Is there a copay?

11. Is preauthorization required? If so, how does one get it?

12. How should one code the initial evaluation (or the biofeedback part of it)—90901, 90801, 95999, 95957, 90899, 97770, 97799, 95812, 97010, 97003, or other?

13. What is the appeal process (if reimbursement or services are denied)?

Reimbursement

Although directly related to coding and billing, reimbursement has its own concerns. One of those has to do with deciding what to charge. Most of us have a usual charge for our services. This may be based on minutes, blocks of time (e.g., 15-minute increments), regular services (e.g., 45- to 50-minute session, with the remaining time out of an hour reserved for notes, phone calls, scheduling, staffing, or other client-related business), or special services (e.g., conducting or interpreting a specialized evaluation, writing an extensive report, extensive staffing, or testifying). If the time spent with or for a client exceeds the usual time or charge, it may be possible to charge for that service or time. However, this should be done with the client's informed consent, along with information about whether the third party will pay (and, if not, with a clear understanding over what the bill is and who pays, and at what rate, full or partial).

Professionals are expected to do some pro bono or reduced-rate services. It is best to bill for such services and then to discount the amount to be written off. However, it is fraud to give everyone the same discounted rate without regard for each person's circumstances, especially if billing the insurance for the full amount. An unlicensed provider working for someone else should make his or her own determination whether to provide a service for free or for reduced charge, unless the employer is paying the provider for hours worked.

Reimbursement rates from a third party are usually set by what are called "relative values scales" and then multiplied by a conversion factor to determine the fee schedule for what that party will pay an approved or authorized provider. Reimbursement rates currently vary from about $44 to $150 for a 50- to 60-minute biofeedback session, depending on the third party and provider. Sometimes these scales are adjusted up or down by what is typically charged for a service in a state, in a part of a state, or across the country. For example, in one recent year the average charges (30th–80th percentile) across the country for general biofeedback were $82–$122, while they were $185–$230 for 90911 for incontinence, and $139–$180 for psychotherapy.

Reimbursement for EEG services or other specialty types of biofeedback may be billable under 90901 or different codes and with differing reimbursement rates, depending on the diagnosis, the type of service, and the third party. Providers should check also for what is common practice in their area of specialty, and then check with the third party.

Also to be determined at the outset of treatment is whether a client is to pay at the time of service and be reimbursed by the insurance company (the model frequently used with major medical coverage), or whether the client will pay a copay and have the insurance pay the provider the rest of the fee or what the company considers, "usual and customary" for the type of service. Workers' compensation and PIP plans usually pay the provider. Many require "timely" submission of bills, such as within 30 days of the date of service. Many also now require treatment plans and notes submitted along with the bill before they will pay. This may present an ethical dilemma over what is confidential and should not be released without client consent.

What to do about "balances due" should have informed consent, particularly if it has to be sent to collections. Sometimes balances due can be adjusted to accommodate a client's situation or the likelihood of getting reimbursed, particularly if the insurance does not or will not reimburse.

If insurance coverage is denied for a biofeedback service that a provider believes can be justified as a viable and common practice, the provider has the right to appeal the denial. Quite often the appeal will be honored if the provider furnishes information supporting the use of biofeedback for that diagnosis.

Models of Practice and Reimbursement

Most biofeedback practitioners are licensed in another field and engaged in some form of independent practice. They may bill directly for their services. They may have contractual agreements with managed care organizations through HMOs or PPOs that determine what actual fee or percentage of their fee will be reimbursed if approved. Unfortunately, many companies will not guarantee payment, but review bills after the service is provided and then determine what will be reimbursed.

Numerous biofeedback practitioners have chosen not to participate in HMOs or PPOs. Instead, they have elected to provide services on a "cash pay" basis, often at a reduced fee to encourage greater motivation and more clients. Feedback from many of these practitioners shows this to be a viable alternative.

Many biofeedback providers choose to work for a large organization, such as a hospital, a university, a research facility, or the U.S. government or military. Often there is a salary or hourly wage for patients/clients seen. Income tax laws determine whether such providers qualify as independent contractors. Usually they also have to have other places of business at which they provide services. As a contractor, one usually works for either an hourly wage, or a percentage of what is billed or what reimbursement is received.

One fairly new model is for biofeedback providers to go to various physicians, chiropractors, dentists, or other facilities and offer either to provide services there for a percentage of what is received if the other practitioners/facilities bill, or to take care of the billing themselves (or through their own billing service).

Another common model is for a biofeedback provider to become an employee of a physician, who then can bill for the provider's services (often under the physician's name, as a physician extender). Physicians have the greatest latitude in how to bill for biofeedback services.

As discussed elsewhere in this chapter (see especially below), another option that is being explored is whether biofeedback can be a licensable profession or whether certification can be required for practice in a given state.

We have now described some of the common models of how to work in the field of biofeedback and be reimbursed for it. If the field of biofeedback and applied psychophysiology continues to expand, with suffcient additional providers and options for practice, we can approach the goal of having biofeedback/applied psychophysiology in or associated with most primary care practices. Another goal, advanced in 2001 by the Colorado Association for Applied Psychophysiology and Biofeedback and the AAPB, is for biofeedback to be available in many more colleges/universities, either in the curriculum or as special services. This will provide more opportunities for employment, as well as for preventive and educational services.

IS BIOFEEDBACK A SEPARATE PROFESSION?

The answer to the question "Is biofeedback a separate profession?" seems at present to be a clear "no." Whether biofeedback can become a profession remains to be seen. The creation of a reputable and meaningful profession called "biofeedback" will take considerable resources in the form of time and effort. There are many potential obstacles that need to be overcome. Are the resources available for such an undertaking?

The Controversy

Discussions concerning this controversial issue have been going on for several years. Some argue that biofeedback is provided by members of a wide variety of health care professions, depending on the education and credentials required by the states in which they practice (Walters, 1999). Generally, the supporters of this position are individuals who can already practice independently because they have the necessary education and credentials. Others argue that sufficient knowledge and enough unique techniques exist to warrant defining biofeedback as a profession (Walters, 1999). Generally, those arguing that biofeedback should be a profession are individuals who are not currently licensed to practice independently in their states (although some of these individuals are currently practicing independently because laws in the states in which they practice have not, to date, restricted the practice to members of specific licensed disciplines). The supporters of this second position are concerned that their opportunity to practice independently may disappear in the future, as more states modify their licensing laws to include restrictions on who can practice biofeedback independently. For example, Utah and Texas have passed laws within the last several years that restrict the independent practice of biofeedback to individuals who are licensed in specific health care disciplines or are exempted in the law (e.g., members of the clergy).

In 1999, the AAPB board passed a motion and created a committee to explore the issue of what it might take for biofeedback to become a profession (Walters, 1999). This was the second time that the issue of biofeedback as a profession was studied by the AAPB. Glaros (1998) first studied this issue and concluded that biofeedback did not meet the criteria for being deemed a profession. Kall (1999) and Patterson in Kall (1999) have been working with legislators in New Jersey to draft a bill that would create a title licensing act for biofeedback practitioners. What the training curriculum, academic degrees, and supervision requirements should be have yet to be worked out.

A license by itself does not create a profession; for example, one gets a license to drive a car, but this does not make car driving a profession (Bayles, 1988). A license that does not meet the criteria common to reputable health care professions could in fact, create a professional backlash if it is seen by other licensed professionals as an attempt to license individuals who are not qualified for independent practice. A backlash could hurt the reputation of biofeedback and could make it even more difficult to have biofeedback accepted by the predominant referral sources (i.e., physicians), and to achieve acceptance and reimbursement by third-party payers. Seeking legal recognition of certification for biofeedback practitioners might meet with less resistance from other professionals than from these two groups.

Evidence against Biofeedback as a Profession

As pointed out by Glaros (1998), the characteristics that make up a profession are complex and multidimensional. Glaros (1998) stated that the published literature characterizes a profession as having the following seven characteristics: a systematic theory, professional authority, professional autonomy, community sanctions, a code of ethics, a professional culture, and a career concept. He discussed each characteristic and concluded that only the evidence for an ethics code strongly supported considering biofeedback as a profession. The other six characteristics each had some support, but not enough to permit the conclusion that biofeedback or applied psychophysiology met the criteria for a profession. Each of these six characteristics needed the support of a much stronger training component than existed at that time (or than still currently exists).

Bayles (1988) stated that no widely accepted definition for the term "profession" exists, so one must determine whether or not an occupation has the necessary features to be deemed a profession. He listed three such features. First, an extensive training program is required in order to prepare for practicing a profession, and this training is usually provided in an academic setting and results in an academic degree (most often an advanced academic degree). Second, the major focus of the training component is significantly intellectual. The development of intellectual skills differentiates a profession from a craft (e.g., bricklaying), where the major focus of training is on the development of physical skills. The intellectual skills include giving advice. Third, the trained skills provide an important service in society.

An extensive training program that results in the granting of an academic degree in biofeedback does not presently exist, although several academic settings offer course work and experience in biofeedback and neurofeedback. Nor is there presently any extensive intellectual skill training in biofeedback. Biofeedback is, however, providing a service in society and that service is likely to become more important over time as more professionals from various health care disciplines become aware of biofeedback and its usefulness as a "treatment of choice" for various conditions (DeLeon, 1998). So at present, biofeedback meets the requirements for one of the three features that characterize a profession as defined by Bayles (1988).

DeLeon (1998)—a long-time supporter of biofeedback and the AAPB, a member of Senator Daniel Inouye's staff, and a past president of the APA—has listed four features as necessary for determining whether an occupation can be deemed a profession. They are (1) whether or not the primary organization (in this case, the AAPB), considers its membership sufficiently trained to independently diagnose and treat patients; (2) whether or not the training programs offered are recognized within educational institutions; (3) whether or not an independent and reputable body of scientific knowledge exists upon which clinical practice is based; and (4) whether or not federal funds are allocated for the training of members of the occupation. It seems that the federal government will reimburse for the clinical services provided by those professionals whom it trains, but is reluctant to reimburse those for whom it will not fund training (DeLeon, 1998). DeLeon (1998) concluded that biofeedback does not meet these criteria for being deemed a profession, nor is it likely to do so in the future.

Developing Biofeedback as a Profession

Jack Wiggins, a past president of the APA, has said that being deemed "a profession" is primarily a political issue rather than a clinical one (cited in DeLeon, 1999). If that is the case, we must identify and deal with the political issues in a way that will not have a negative impact on the acceptability of biofeedback. A strong political barrier to biofeedback's becoming a profession may already exist. This barrier is related to the fact that, increasingly, licensing laws are changing to include "biofeedback" within the definition of the practice of specific professional disciplines—most notably psychology. This movement has been in part fueled by the tightening of health care dollars as managed care strives to reduce health care costs. Supposedly, it is easier to get reimbursed for services provided if one can show that the intervention is a legitimate activity for members of one's discipline. As such, many licensing laws have expanded the definition for what is included in the scope of practice for specific disciplines, to cover all the activities their members engage in that are ethically acceptable to the members of the discipline and that do not violate any existing law. To create a reputable and meaningful profession called "biofeedback" in such states will require mobilizing the support of existing health care professionals, or at least getting enough support so that these other professionals do not mobilize in opposition to the proposal of creating such a profession.

It may be extremely difficult to create a profession called "biofeedback" without putting in the time and effort to create the needed structure, especially without creating degree-granting programs in academic settings. At present, no academic setting offers a degree in biofeedback. The California School of Professional Psychology in San Diego, and the University of North Texas offer extensive training in biofeedback as part of other degree-granting programs (Glaros, 1998). Clearly, more such programs are needed, and at least one program is needed that will offer a degree in biofeedback per se. The more prestigious the academic program and faculty of that program are, the more likely it is that the degree will be considered reputable, and the more likely it is that other academic programs will create such degree programs. But is there a university that would be willing to offer a degree in biofeedback?

The AAPB's committee might well be encouraged to look at the issues related to what courses, course content, practica, and internship experiences might be needed for a degree-granting program in biofeedback. Looking at all of the characteristics suggested above as necessary for the creation of a profession could be overwhelming unless a long-term plan is created and the task is approached one step at a time.

If biofeedback is to become a reputable profession, much more than the knee-jerk reaction of creating a license will be needed. The support of many professionals from other professions that are already reputable will be required. Creating the right program and reputation for a new profession called "biofeedback" will take many years and resources. One cannot help wondering why licensed professionals would want to put resources into creating another profession that would compete with them for shrinking health care reimbursement dollars. It might be easier to ask, "Why do biofeedback providers who are not members of licensed professions not go back to school and get a degree in a reputable health care discipline that will allow them to become licensed and practice independently?" A number of individuals have gone back to school during the last several years to get degrees and later licenses. Doing so is a proactive behavior that is largely under the control of the individuals and thus doable. Creating a profession takes the coordinated effort of many individuals, and many factors may not be controllable.

In the meantime, biofeedback may best be described as an "emerging profession."

NOTES

1. This chapter is an amalgam of Chapters 8, 27, 28, 29, and 30, and parts of Chapter 38, from the second edition of this book (M. S. Schwartz & Associates, 1995). The primary reasons for needing to reduce these chapters and subsume them under one chapter were the needs to add new chapters to the book, update chapters, and reduce the length of the book. We extend much appreciation to R. Paul Olson, PhD, and Suzanne Kroon, BA, for their prior chapters (27 and 30, respectively). They will forever have our thanks. New information in the present chapter includes (1) the topics of coding, billing, and reimbursement; and (2) the topics of biofeedback as a separate profession and licensing.

2. The definition of "applied psychophysiology" was discussed extensively in 1999 in the journal *Applied Psychophysiology and Biofeedback, 24*(1), by Mark S. Schwartz, Sebastian Striefel, Barnard Engel, Edward Blanchard, Susan Middaugh, Kathie Wells, Peter Rosenfeld, Niels Birbaumer, Herta Flor, Steven Wolf, and David Hubbard.

3. See the second edition for examples/models of job descriptions. These have been omitted here for practical reasons.

4. Much of the material in this section is from R. Paul Olson's (1995b) work on the previous version of this chapter in the second edition. Appreciation is expressed to Paul for his work.

5. The service provided in this case should be described as relaxation therapy/psychotherapy, with psycho-physiological monitoring/measurement only or primarily for the therapist. Note that therapists often use the same biomedical instrumentation used with biofeedback to obtain psychophysiological information that enhances the therapist's provision of relaxation therapies. Consider the following guidelines:

1. Patients are not given direct or continuous biological feedback during sessions, except for very brief periods of about 3–5 minutes for introductory, illustrative, and educational purposes.
2. Most of each session (e.g., 45 minutes) involves activities customarily considered within the domain of psychotherapy (e.g., cognitive therapies, relaxation therapies). The written report identifies the session as being a psychotherapy session and specifically excludes biofeedback for the patient.
3. Descriptions of the physiological monitoring/measurements are given in the session reports, but in considerably less detail than for sessions that mostly involve direct biofeedback to and with the patient.

REFERENCES

The American Heritage dictionary for DOS (college ed.). (1992). Sausalito, CA: Writing Tools Group of Houghton Mifflin.

American Medical Association (AMA). (1998). *CPT coding manual.* Washington, DC: Author.

American Medical Association (AMA) (2002). *Current procedural terminology: CPT 2003.* Chicago: Author.

American Psychological Association (APA). (1987). *General guidelines for providers of psychological services.* Washington, DC: Author.

American Psychological Association (APA). (1993a). *Practice pointer: What to look for in your state utilization review law.* Washington, DC: Author.

American Psychological Association (APA). (1993b). *Practice pointer: The basics of Medicare audits.* Washington, DC: Author.

American Psychological Association (APA). (1993c). Record keeping guidelines. *American Psychologist, 48*(9), 984–986.

American Psychological Association (APA). (1995). *State Medicaid reimbursement standards for psychologists.* Washington, DC: Author.

American Psychological Association (APA). (2000, February). *Psychology: Promoting health and well being through high quality, cost-effective treatment.* Washington, DC: Author.

American Psychological Association. (2002). *Medicare handbook: A guide for psychologists.* [Online] Available: http//www.apa.org/practice/medtoc.html.

Bakal, D. (1999). *Minding the body: Clinical uses of somatic awareness.* New York: Guilford Press.

Bayles, M. D. (1988). The professions. In J. C. Callahan (Ed.), *Ethical issues in professional life.* New York: Oxford University Press.

Borgeat, F., Elie, R., & Castonguay, L. (1991). Muscular response to the therapist and symptomatic improvement during biofeedback for tension headache. *Biofeedback and Self-Regulation, 19*(2), 147–155.

Borgeat, F., Hade, B., Larouche, L. M., & Bedwani, C. N. (1980). Effects of therapist's active presence on EMG biofeedback training of headache patients. *Biofeedback and Self-Regulation, 5,* 275–282.

Borgeat, F., Hade, B., Larouche, L. M., & Gauthier, B. (1984). Psychophysiological effects of therapist's active presence during biofeedback as a single psychotherapeutic situation. *Psychiatric Journal of the University of Ottawa, 9*(3), 134–137.

Bregman, N. J., & McAllister, H. A. (1983). Voluntary control of skin temperature: Role of experimenter presence versus absence. *Biofeedback and Self-Regulation, 8,* 543–546.

The Charles Press handbook of current medical abbreviations (5th ed.). (1997). Bowie, MD: Charles Press.

Crider, A. B., & Glaros, A. G. (1999). A meta-analysis of EMG biofeedback treatment of temporomandibular disorders. *Journal of Orofacial Pain, 13*(1), 29–37.

DeLeon, P. H. (1998). Biofeedback—an independent profession? *Biofeedback, 26*(3), 4–5.

Dumouchel, B. D. (1985). *Patient's perceived control, therapist's presence/absence, and the optimization of biofeedback learning.* Unpublished doctoral dissertation. New York University.

Foxhall, K. (2000a, January). How would your practice records look to the FBI? *APA Monitor on Psychology,* pp. 1–6.

Foxhall, K. (2000b, October). New CPT codes will recognize psychologist's work with physical health problems. *APA Monitor on Psychology,* pp. 46–47.

Glaros, A. G. (1998). Is biofeedback a profession?: Some methods for answering the question. *Biofeedback, 26*(2), 4–6.

Kall, R. (1999). New Jersey biofeedback license initiative and biofeedback as a profession update. *Biofeedback, 27*(3), 5A.

Keatley, M. A. (1998). *Clinical outcome study in biofeedback.* Unpublished manuscript.

Miller, N. E. (1974). Introduction: Current issues and key problems. In N. E. Muller, T. X. Barber, L. V. Decara, J. Kamiya, D. Shapiro, & J. Stoyva (Eds.), *Biofeedback and self-control: 1973.* Chicago: Aldine.

Miller, N. E. (Chair). (1983, March). *Research model for evaluating clinical efficacy: A three system approach.* Symposium conducted at the Fourteenth Annual Meeting of the Biofeedback Society of America, Denver, CO.

Ochs, L. (1990). Rights and responsibilities of report writers: A preliminary personal statement of peer review criteria. *Biofeedback, 18*(4), 24–29.

Olson, R. P. (1995a). Definitions of biofeedback and applied psychophysiology. In M. S. Schwartz & Associates, *Biofeedback: A practitioner's guide* (2nd ed.). New York: Guilford Press.

Olson, R. P. (1995b). Models of practice: The delivery of biofeedback services. In M. S. Schwartz & Associates, *Biofeedback: A practitioner's guide* (2nd ed.). New York: Guilford Press.

O'Regan, B., & Hirsberg, C. (1993). *Spontaneous remission: An annotated bibliography.* Sausalito, CA: Institute of Noetic Sciences.

Osgood, C. E., Suci, G. J., & Tannenbaum, P. N. (1957). *The measurement of meaning.* Urbana: University of Illinois Press.

Perlin, M. J. (1982, March). *Legal regulation of biofeedback practice: The dawn of a new era.* Paper presented at the Thirteenth Annual Meeting of the Biofeedback Society of America, Chicago.

Perry, J. D. (2001). All biofeedback wins major victory in Medicare incontinence decision. *California Biofeedback, 17*(1), 7–8.

Schwartz, G. E. (1983). Research and feedback in clinical practice: A commentary on responsible biofeedback therapy. In J. V. Basmajian (Ed.), *Biofeedback: Principles and practice for clinicians* (3rd ed.). Baltimore: Williams & Wilkins.

Schwartz, M. S. (1981). Biofeedback Certification Institute of America: Blueprint Knowledge Statements. *Biofeedback and Self-Regulation, 6,* 253–262.

Schwartz, M. S. (1995). Professional communication. In M. S. Schwartz & Associates, *Biofeedback: A practitioner's guide* (2nd ed.). New York: Guilford Press.

Schwartz, M. S. (1999). What is applied psychophysiology?: Toward a definition. *Applied Psychophysiology and Biofeedback, 24*(1), 3–10.

Schwartz, M. S., & Associates. (1995). *Biofeedback: A practitioner's guide* (2nd ed.). New York: Guilford Press.

Schwartz, M. S., & Fehmi, L. (1982). *Application standards and guidelines for providers of biofeedback services.* Wheat Ridge, CO: Biofeedback Society of America.

Schwartz, M. S., & Gemberling, A. L. (1995). Therapist presence or absence. In M. S. Schwartz & Associates, *Biofeedback: A practitioner's guide* (2nd ed.). New York: Guilford Press.

Shellenberger, R., & Green, J. (1986). *From the ghost in the box to successful biofeedback training.* Greeley, CO: Health Psychology.

Stout, C. E. (1995). Mental health practices borrow ideas from business with positive results. In A. M. Christner & M. K. Arnold (Eds.), *Practice management for psychotherapists and counselors.* Providence, RI: Manisses Communication Group.

Striefel, S. (1995). Professional ethical behavior. In M. S. Schwartz & Associates, *Biofeedback: A practitioner's guide* (2nd ed.). New York: Guilford Press.

Striefel, S. (1999). Is the working definition of applied psychophysiology proposed by Schwartz too narrow/restrictive? *Applied Psychophysiology and Biofeedback, 24*(1), 11–20.

Striefel, S. (2000a). Telehealth uses in biofeedback and applied psychophysiology. *Biofeedback, 28*(2), 8–10.

Striefel, S. (2000b). Ethical and legal barriers in telehealth. *Biofeedback, 28*(2), 4–5, 10.

Striefel, S., Butler, F., Coxe, J. A., McKee, M. G., & Sherman, R. A. (1999). *Practice guidelines and standards of practice for providers of biofeedback and applied psychophysiological services.* Wheat Ridge, CO: Association for Applied Psychophysiology and Biofeedback.

Turk, D. C., & Melzack, R. (Eds.). *(1992). Handbook of pain assessment.* New York: Guilford Press.

Walters, D. (1999, June 30). *Board appoints committee to define steps necessary to establish biofeedback as a profession.* [Letter to membership]. Wheat Ridge, CO: Association for Applied Psychophysiology and Biofeedback.

Weiner, B. A., & Wettstein, R. M. (1993). *Legal issues in mental health care.* New York: Plenum Press.

Weiner, I. B. (1998). *Principles of psychotherapy* (2nd ed.). New York: Wiley.

Whitehouse, R. (1997). Suggested coding guidelines based on CPT code answers from the AMA. *Biofeedback, 25*(2), 8A–13A.

Whitehouse, R. (1998). CPT coding issues 1998 Update. *Biofeedback, 26*(2), 14A–17A.

Wickramasekera, I. (1999). The faith factor, the placebo, and AAPB. *Biofeedback, 27*(1), 1A–3A.

Zuckerman, E. L. (2003). *The paper office* (3rd ed.). New York: Guilford Press.

CHAPTER 38

Evaluating Research in Clinical Biofeedback

MARK S. SCHWARTZ
FRANK ANDRASIK

This chapter discusses select questions and issues for our readers to consider when they are evaluating biofeedback research. We hope that it will also serve to increase their awareness when conducting research and when reporting and interpreting clinical results.

THE GAP BETWEEN CLINICIANS AND RESEARCHERS: SOME SUGGESTIONS FOR CLOSING IT

Clinicians and researchers often appear as adversaries engaged in what seems to be the battle of the Hatfields and the McCoys. As Garmezy and Masten (1986) noted in a related paper, "the slings and arrows of these opposing camps have as yet to be put away as part of an arms reduction package" (p. 501).

Rosenfeld (1987) prepared an eloquent paper expressing his role as a mediator and champion of perspective. Reflecting upon the position of clinicians, he stated that they criticize findings obtained from "stripped-down experimental paradigms" that do not support the specific effects of biofeedback, partially due to the omission of "patient motivational factors." Practitioners sometimes claim that researchers ask either incorrect or unimportant questions. Some clinicians make accusations of inadequately conducted research and experimenter bias.

> Absence of evidence is not evidence of absence; one cannot in the end prove the null hypothesis. That is, a failed half-hearted attempt to find the needle in the haystack does *not* prove that it isn't there. One should really take a good look for it before giving up—if the needle has any value to one, that is. (p. 218; emphasis added)

On the other hand, exaggeration of clinical results is a claim often made by researchers. In all fairness, these problems are also present in other clinical, health, and educational settings (Garmezy & Masten, 1986; Hayes, Barlow, & Nelson-Gray, 1999).

Researchers and practitioners sometimes do not appreciate their dependency upon one another; nor do they see the benefits that would accrue from a productive alliance rather than an enduring antagonism between the camps. "To some extent, the disagreement is semantic [and due to] . . . much misrepresentation—probably due to mutual misunderstanding of the respective positions of the opponents" (Rosenfeld, 1987, p. 217). "Wisdom would dictate a recognition that there were contributions to be made by both talented clinicians *and* researchers" (Garmezy & Masten, 1986, p. 501).

Practitioners are hungry for knowledge about biofeedback, especially when it is relevant to clinical applications. They are hungry for good research and depend on it for answering a myriad of questions and increasing the credibility of clinical procedures. There is no substitute for good research. To quote again from Rosenfeld (1987),

> If biofeedback is to prosper, there must be acceptance by medical and scientific communities. This is ultimately necessary. . . . These . . . communities [ultimately] accept only one kind of evidence, scientific evidence. There [is] some disagreement as to what constitutes scientific evidence. (p. 217)

In turn, researchers need clinicians to help identify the questions requiring answers. Without widespread clinical applications, there would be far less need for research. Clinicians can often provide researchers with viewpoints and ideas on pertinent research questions and procedures. "Research resulting from such an alliance will foster the common goal of practitioner and [researcher] in improving the effectiveness of . . . therapeutic interventions" (Garmezy & Masten, 1986, p. 501).

Rosenfeld (1987) again provided optimism and encouragement: "I believe it is quite possible for clinicians and researchers together to provide scientific evidence" (p. 217). Later, he added that "researcher and clinician ought to begin talking *to* each other in advance of doing a study, rather than wasting time in a *posteriori* arguments" (p. 221; emphasis added).

Among the goals of this chapter are to help increase the sophistication and clinical usefulness of research, and to help consumers of that research. We favor anything that stimulates us all to work closely with one another toward improving the synergistic relationship of research, clinical applications, and reimbursement. Garmezy and Masten's (1986) directness is also helpful:

> The researcher who is uninformed of the observations depicted in clinical case accounts . . . is at risk for generating unsophisticated, inaccurate, and marginal studies. . . . The clinician equally uninformed about . . . developments in the areas of basic and applied science relevant to the clinical enterprise is at risk for rigidly adhering to a technique or model that can act as a conceptual straitjacket, containing the therapeutic effort. (p. 501)

Practitioners must be very knowledgeable about research methods and limitations, and researchers need to be well versed in clinical procedures and clinical practice. Neither can afford to have narrow or simplistic conceptualizations of biofeedback or other applied psychophysiological therapies. Journals and professional meetings need to extend their efforts to help consumers understand and evaluate research, and to place that research in conceptual and practical contexts. Typically, journal review articles and books that review the literature appear 1 or more years after the research has been published. Letters to the editor about research and issues appear infrequently. Some professionals might applaud seeing journal space devoted to editorial comments and critiques at the time an article is published.

The book by White and Tursky (1982) is a good example to follow, in that it provides a useful "round-table" discussion of each chapter. This is a valuable and refreshing book, and its format is one that journal editors and book publishers should consider more often.

We need to reduce the distrust of research that emerges among practitioners, and the responsibility for reducing this distrust resides in both camps. We encourage researchers to be mindful of the potential impact on clinical professionals of what they conclude, state, and imply. Everyone should willingly accept data from good research. This is valid regardless of whether the data conflict with clinicians' beliefs or practices. Practitioners also need to remember that it is very difficult to conduct excellent and clinically relevant research, and that even well-conducted research usually represents only a limited set of conditions.

So what are we all to do? Garmezy and Masten (1986) called for reason when they urged professionals to realize that both clinical relevance and mutual suspiciousness "can be overcome when clinician and scientist share a common regard for the other's area of activity, and a recognition that there are contributions to knowledge each can make to the common enterprise, namely to understand human behavior" (p. 502).

We hope that more researchers will become more aware of and responsive to the needs of their clinical peers. More instances of experienced clinicians and researchers working closely together would be very desirable.

CONSIDERATIONS IN EVALUATING AND USING RESEARCH RESULTS

The focus of this chapter now turns to questions and factors to consider when one is reading, evaluating, designing, conducting, writing about, or publishing research. These questions are subsumed under the rubrics of therapists, subjects,[1] therapy, individual-subject designs,[2] and data management. The list is not exhaustive. We encourage readers to review the emerging literature on the aptitude × treatment interaction model of therapy effectiveness (Holloway, Spivey, Zismer, & Withington, 1988; Dance & Neufeld, 1988; see also N. M. Schwartz & M. S. Schwartz, Chapter 3, this volume), as well as the critique of this model by Smith and Sechrest (1991/1992). Briefly, the model proposes interactions between the person and treatment that may account for outcomes. However, in terms of psychotherapy at least, Smith and Sechrest (1991/1992) criticized this type of research's potential for yielding dependable interactions. They presented stringent conditions for such research, and proposed that research adhering to their criteria would "uncover previously 'hidden' main effects more frequently than interactions" (p. 558). Many readers will also benefit from Maher's (1978/1992) guide to assessing research reports in clinical psychology.

Therapists

We begin by posing questions about therapists that merit consideration.

Competence

1. Who provided the therapy? Were the therapists and the investigator(s) graduate students or experienced clinicians?

2. What were the education, training, credentials, and experience of the therapists? Standardized information about the qualifications of therapists would be of considerable value if available to readers. Some researchers do have good clinical skills, characteristics, and experience. Some have even better skills and training than some clinical therapists. Nevertheless, failures to obtain or replicate therapeutic effects may not reflect a problem with the procedures. Differences may partly be related to different therapists. Therefore, do practitioner consumers know enough about the therapists to evaluate the relevance of the research results to themselves?

Investigator / Therapist Confidence and Bias

1. What do we know of each investigator's and therapist's beliefs about the therapy? Did the therapists have confidence in the therapy? Were the therapists required to conduct the research as research assistants or as a part of their clinical practice? Answers to these questions are often unclear, and resolving them is a complex and delicate matter. Investigators or therapists who are not confident in the therapy they are providing may communicate this indirectly or inadvertently to the subjects or patients. This can influence the style and content of the presentations to subjects and the way the therapists provide the therapy. We are not advocating that only "true believers" conduct therapy research. However, consumer professionals often want information about the beliefs of authors of the research and reviews. Acknowledging one's confidence and support or one's skepticism about a therapeutic strategy is desirable, appropriate, and honorable.

2. Does an investigator, reviewer, or clinician have a reputation for pushing one viewpoint? Wise consumers interpret research and reviews in the context of an author's other research and the way the author treats others' research and commentaries. Bias is sometimes very subtle. We quickly add that bias is inherently acceptable. An investigator or clinician without bias may be boring and unproductive. The issues are the degree of bias and the extent to which the bias interferes with impartiality.

3. Has an investigator, reviewer, or clinician ever reversed his or her position? This can enhance his or her credibility. If so, did the individual do this based on his or her own or others' research?

Consistency of Behavior and Adherence to Protocols

1. How do we know that the therapists followed the procedures for all patients in a given condition? A therapist may depart from a standard protocol when a patient/subject varies his or her behavior in certain ways. Are there provisions in the protocol for contingencies that arise during therapy? Did the therapists follow the therapy protocol outline as intended? Did the therapists report any departures from this outline to the research investigator(s)? Rather than implying distrust, these questions recognize a normal and understandable human condition. Therapists and research assistants do not always report to their supervisors all that occurs. They may not regard it as important, or they may expect disapproval from the supervisors.

Consistency may become a concern when the content of subjects' questions, comments, and informal talk differs during sessions. Therapists may respond differently to different subjects at different times. Certain of the following factors increase the chance of a therapeutically significant discrepancy among what an investigator planned, what occurred, and what a therapist reported: multiple therapists; the more the bias of the investigator is known to the therapist providing the therapy; the more the therapist is dependent upon the investigator for support and evaluation; the busier the supervisor is; the less supervision is provided; and the less specific protocol is, with fewer contingencies planned for. (See Yeaton & Sechrest, 1981, for a more in-depth discussion of treatment integrity.)

Specific Therapist Characteristics

1. Is there a description of therapist characteristics that could affect the attitudes and behaviors of the patients/subjects? These include age, sex, race, credibility, anxiety, friendliness, and appearance. This is another delicate issue; however, many professionals believe that therapist characteristics influence patient/subject attitudes, behaviors, and outcome. The point here is that many practitioners and researchers reading others' research want and need reports of such information.

Subjects

Subject Preparation for and Understanding of Therapy

1. How prepared for the therapy were the subjects? There is widespread agreement among professionals that patient education is important. It affects patients' attitudes about themselves and the therapy, and it affects compliance. Some published research either describes for readers the patient education content provided to the subjects, or lets readers know where this content is available. However, most studies report little or no such information. Readers want to know what the researchers communicated to the subjects, who told it to them, and what educational modalities were used. We ask that researchers at least summarize this information in the published paper and indicate where the details of the patient education can be found. The absence of it makes desirable comparisons among studies and therapy procedures more difficult.

2. What evidence was presented to support the assumption that the subjects understood, accepted, and learned the patient education content? Providing patient education does not assure adequate understanding, acceptance, learning, and mobilization for therapy. For example, did patients understand, accept, and learn the rationale for therapy and the procedures? Research that gives data about the knowledge understood, accepted, and learned will enjoy a better reception among readers.

Subject Motivation and Expectations

1. In many clinical and experimental situations, one independent variable may have no main therapeutic effect; however, when combined with another independent variable, the interaction leads to dependent variable changes. Rosenfeld (1987) pointed out that a feedback variable alone may not have an effect on physiological and symptom changes except when combined with another variable, such as motivation.

Thus practitioners want and need to know about motivational and expectancy variables. Indeed, many of the variables discussed in this chapter may be *necessary* for the "higher-order interactions" to occur. Consider therapist attitudes and confidence, patient education, the absence of other subject problems interfering with therapy, and specific therapy procedures. Consider also what information is available about the subjects' motivation for learning psychophysiological self-regulation and reducing their symptoms. Symptoms are often sufficient motivation, but in some instances the severity or frequency is not enough motivation. There are costs associated with receiving treatment, even in research studies that do not charge therapy fees. Such costs include travel, time away from work and other activities, and the like. One must balance the severity and frequency of the symptoms against all the costs that can affect motivation.

2. There is also the issue of "secondary gain." Did the investigator(s) assess the possibility of such variables among the subjects? Can we assume that the motivation of all subjects to reduce their symptoms was high? Was symptom reduction more motivating than competing factors? Randomization helps control for this variable, but with small samples and individual-subject designs, motivations competing with symptom reduction may compromise the results.

3. What were the expectations of subjects? Determining the subjects' expectations about the therapy should be part of most research, especially outcome studies.

Subjects' Attitudes toward Therapists

1. Did the subjects have confidence and trust in their therapists? What does the research paper tell us about the subjects' attitudes toward the therapists? Whether or not these attitudes affect outcome, to what degree, and under what conditions are empirical questions.

Other Medical and Psychological Problems of Subjects

1. What information is available about the subjects' other medical problems? Papers often include this information, but when a paper does not, the reader and journal reviewer/editor should request it.

2. What information do readers have about personality and psychopathology variables of potential importance (e.g., depression, absorption, locus of control, self-efficacy, anxiety, relaxation-induced anxiety, anger, and interpersonal comfort)?

3. What information do readers have about subjects' time use management?

Discrepancies between Self-Report Records and Verbal Reports

1. Self-report ratings are a valuable source of data, but they have limitations. Many people have difficulty following even simple instructions. Bias can influence their ratings, and their interpretations of ratings can also change over time. Changes in expectation during therapy stages may influence ratings. What did the investigators do to enhance the subjects' understanding of the instructions for symptom ratings?

2. Were there discrepancies between subjects' self-report symptom records and their verbal reports? Did the investigators assess and report discrepancies, and did they discuss and resolve them with the subjects?

Control of Relevant Variables

1. Were the experimental and control groups equated or otherwise controlled for potentially relevant variables? Many variables can differ among groups, including baseline and reactive physiological activity, initial responses to feedback, expectancies, understanding, attitudes toward therapy and therapists, frequency and severity of symptoms, number and intensity of stressors, and use of caffeine and nicotine. One cannot equate groups for all important variables. However, readers still want the information reported, as well as statistical analyses to assess their relative contribution.

Possible Prebaseline Improvement

1. Some patients show improvement after reassurance about the nonserious nature of their symptoms. Other patients improve in anticipation of receiving therapy soon. Therefore, were any of the subjects improving in their symptoms before baseline recording began or before starting therapy? Was the baseline period representative of subjects' symptom frequency and severity before the baseline?

2. Symptoms fluctuate over time for many conditions, and many patients seek assistance when symptoms are the most intense. Over time, the symptoms may lessen or "regress to the mean" in the absence of therapy. Could improvement be a function of expected fluctuation?

Therapy

Therapy Setting

1. The surroundings can influence the attitudes of subjects toward therapy. Where was the therapy conducted, and how did the subjects perceive it? If one intends to generalize the results to clinical settings, then the surroundings should approximate common clinical environments. Congested or otherwise unprofessional offices are ill suited for therapy. If a thera-

pist uses such an environment, then he or she should consider assessing the subjects' perceptions about the environment.

Specific Procedures

1. Subjects need opportunities to test their self-regulation abilities under conditions that at least approximate those of real life. Patients must apply their psychophysiological self-regulatory skills beyond a professional's office. What were the procedures for transfer of training and generalization of physiological self-regulation? How did the researcher(s) assess this transfer? Specific questions include whether each therapist conducted baseline and feedback phases with (a) each subject's eyes open and closed, (b) in varied body positions, (c) during and immediately after stressful activity without feedback, and (d) during and immediately after physical activity without feedback.

2. Were the subjects alone or with a therapist during the sessions?

3. How do readers know that the procedures described were the procedures performed? This is not easily answered. How involved were the investigator(s) in conducting the research protocol? How closely supervised were the therapists conducting the sessions? This question does not intend to imply intentional distortions of procedures and data. It is a reminder that distortions can and do occur for a variety of reasons, and that readers should at least be provided with some information about the supervision of the therapists.

4. A related question involves deviations from the protocol. What were the provisions in the protocol for various contingencies that might occur during therapy sessions? In clinical situations, one does not anticipate all events. Were there clear instructions for what a therapist was to do when such events occurred? Were departures from the protocol documented? Did the subjects avoid certain activities before therapy sessions? What do we know about what subjects were doing and thinking about during sessions?

Subject Application of Physiological Self-Regulation

1. How often and for how long did the subjects use the self-regulatory procedures in their daily lives? Were they using the procedures at the instructed times during their daily activities? It is not enough for authors to state that they instructed subjects to use the procedures in their daily lives. Documenting and reporting this information are desirable.

Symptom Records and Changes

1. How were the changes in symptoms assessed? Did the investigator(s) or therapists review the self-report symptom forms? What questions did the subjects answer during and after therapy and in later follow-up? Results can differ, depending on the answers to these questions.

2. Research reports should discuss the instructions. How careful were the instructions for the self-report records? Were the records complete? Did the report include information about whether there were data collection problems and, if so, how the investigators managed these problems?

3. There are multiple criteria for significant improvement, not all of which may be present for a specific subject. Were the self-report records analyzed sufficiently to determine whether different subjects improved with different symptom variables? Using one criterion for all subjects does not always reflect significant improvement for some subjects.

4. Were the reported symptomatic changes of clinical significance (Jacobson & Truax, 1992)? What was the operational definition of a clinically significant change? Was a combination of criteria used? How did the investigators' criteria match the subjects' perceptions?

Physiological Data and Changes

1. What were the criteria used to determine whether subjects developed physiological self-regulation? Note that researchers and clinicians sometimes use multiple criteria.

2. Were the physiological data reported in enough detail for the readers to know what occurred in different recording conditions? Summary data are often not enough to give readers useful information about the psychophysiological activity during different conditions.

Cognitive Factors in Subject Preparation and Therapy

1. How did the researchers cognitively prepare the subjects for biofeedback and other self-regulatory therapies? What were they told? Readers should look for details of the presentations. When presentations are lengthy, authors should indicate where they are available.

2. Recording and reporting the cognitive activity of subjects are useful endeavors. What did the subjects think about during the therapy sessions while using psychophysiological self-regulatory procedures? Did the study discuss the cognitive activity of the subjects?

Use of Cassette Relaxation Tapes

1. If the research used audiocassette relaxation tapes, then what were the details of the tapes? Patients, and presumably research subjects, have different perceptions of and reactions to different factors associated with tape-recorded relaxation procedures, such as content, voice, and tempo (see M. S. Schwartz, Chapter 13, this volume). Practitioners should look for information about these variables.

Controls and Assessment

1. Patients and subjects often initiate health improvement activities other than those specifically recommended and checked by practitioners. Were the effects of caffeine, nicotine, alcohol, and other dietary factors assessed before, during, and after therapy?

2. Were all pertinent medications checked and controlled for throughout the therapy and follow-up stages? Readers should look for sufficient details about medications.

3. Were life events and daily stress assessed before, during, and after therapy? Information about their presence, absence, and changes should be documented, because these factors can influence symptoms. Did the analyses control for their possible effects?

4. Aside from biofeedback and other methods of learning physiological self-regulation, what else occurred during the sessions?

5. What information is available about the occurrence and duration of periods of significant symptomatic improvement or remission in the past? For example, patients sometimes have periods of remission or reduction of symptoms during certain times of year (e.g., Raynaud's symptoms may lessen during warmer weather; symptoms may decrease during periods of lessened work responsibilities). Long follow-up periods help control for such factors.

Other Research Considerations

1. Readers should look for commonly reported information. This includes the number of sessions, age and sex of subjects, duration and severity of symptoms, randomized assignment to groups, sample sizes, proper statistics, and instrumentation and recording details. Also, readers should look for acceptable criteria for single-case designs.

2. Did the investigator(s) analyze differences between the subjects who were successful and those who were unsuccessful? This takes us to individual-subject experimental research.

Individual-Subject Experimental Research

Individual-subject research should be more commonly conducted and accepted by journals (see Andrasik, 2002). "One of the most difficult challenges for psychotherapy [biofeedback] research has been to demonstrate convincingly the link between what occurs in the treatment hour and patient change" (Jones, Ghannam, Nigg, & Dyer, 1993, p. 381). The relationship between process and outcome is typically unclear with group comparison designs or controlled clinical trials.

Hawkins (1989) has described the advantages of individual-subject experimental research. It permits comparison of the relative effects of different treatments for each individual (concerning direction, speed, pattern, and final level of effect). Practitioners receive quicker feedback on their efforts when individually graphed data are used. This feedback to therapists allows more information for therapists and chances to affect contingent changes in their behavior. For some therapists, "the more rapid feedback of data . . . leads to a greater enjoyment of and persistence at the tasks of research, at least for many of us" (Hawkins, 1989, p. 128).

Hawkins (1989) and others (Barlow, Hayes, Epstein, & Blanchard, 1977; Barlow & Hersen, 1984; Kratochwill, Mott, & Dodson, 1984; Jones, 1993) assert that individual-subject experimental designs potentially allow more generalization of results to natural settings than do most group research designs. Practitioners appreciate researchers' using group designs that also report individual data; however, typically these do not involve enough of the unique advantages of individual-subject experimental designs.

Data Management

Data management and mismanagement are serious topics. "Data mismanagement" refers to faulty quality control, documentation, or retention of data. Deficiencies in data management, even apparently minor ones, increase the risk that errors and omissions will occur and can make them difficult to detect. They can also interfere with data sharing and with secondary analyses of data sets, can render archived data sets inaccessible or uninterpretable, can make it difficult to confirm that data faithfully correspond to actual results of studies, and can prevent replication of statistical results (Freedland & Carney, 1992, p. 643). The problem is serious enough to prompt attention by major scientific organizations, universities, and congressional investigation. Federal regulations now exist, and further ones have been proposed (Office of Scientific Integrity Review, 1990). (See the Web sites in the "Resources" section for more information.)

Data mismanagement is not rare in biomedical research. However, there are no systematic studies of it in research fields other than in the realm of investigational drug trials. The full extent of the problem is not known, but there is anecdotal support for data mismanagement, at least in less standardized research and in research with less adequate funding (Freedland & Carney, 1992).

The focus here is on "honest error," up to and including what some consider "negligence." (This does not include the separate topic of willfully fabricating data and results—an occurrence uncommon in scientific research). Although "negligence is clearly unacceptable in scientific research" (Freedland & Carney, 1992, p. 640), the line is often unclear between unintentional errors, omissions, or inadequate data management on the one hand, and negligence or undue carelessness on the other. Freedland and Carney (1992) cite several references supporting the statement that researchers are accountable for careless practices and unintended deficiencies.

Even researchers who are well respected by peers can be unable "to reconstruct previously reported analyses of data from clinical databases . . . [and find it] . . . surprisingly difficult to determine which cases and . . . variables . . . [were] used, despite the fact that the original analyses . . . [were] performed with care" (Freedland & Carney, 1992, p. 641). However, these authors point out that except for U.S. Food and Drug Administration auditing of clinical trials since 1977, "audit worthiness" is a higher standard for data management than has been required of most research until recently.[3]

For the reasons described above, investigators, research assistants, and practitioners need to be conversant with this topic. Reading articles such as the one by Freedland and Carney (1992) is very enlightening. Planning, designing, and conducting research all call for understanding the problems and pitfalls of data management. This is especially true with the use of computer systems. There are many ways that unintentional negligence can occur with data management. Some readers may view this area as intimidating; however, an awareness of common deficiencies in data management helps prevent such negligence from occurring.

We include a brief summary of reasons for common mistakes in data management, and descriptions of some of these mistakes. The interested reader will refer directly to Freedland and Carney (1992) and to other references cited by them (e.g., Marshall, 1990; Office of Scientific Integrity Review, 1990; Racker, 1989). Interested readers can also consult experts, including those proficient with computers, interactive databases, and statistical analysis software.

Reasons for Common Deficiencies in Data Management

Reasons for data management deficiencies (Freedland & Carney, 1992) include the following:

1. There can be unintended side effects of technological progress in computers (e.g., statistical software that ends data management chores).

2. Computer users may have problems checking, documenting, and preserving their work carefully. These tasks can be tedious, time-consuming, and complicated. The tasks most likely to be problems are documentating and archiving the data for future access, interpretation, and analyses.

3. Some researchers are unable to diagnose subtle flaws in statistical results or adequate documentation, because of inadequate understanding of computer hardware and software. Achieving proficiency with computer programming and statistical packages usually requires considerable time and effort.

4. Also, data management is often very challenging and can be expensive, and smaller projects often have limited financial resources allocated for this.

Documentation of Data and Computer Programs

One needs accurate and permanent codebook-type information in the database, such as for variable names and subjects. Some software allows incorporation of this information with the data set. However, some software does not permit permanent documentation, or it stores the information in separate files from the data set. This can result in inadequate documentation of archived data sets. One can lose vital documentation from the original database. This can happen when one is exporting data to another software package or exporting data to another computer system. Regardless of how careful the original documentation may have been, translated versions may lack this necessary documentation.

Documentation of Analyses

Programming errors or "bugs" that do not violate software rules or other checks can escape detection by programmers and users of the program. Investigators do not always log essential information and cross-check statistical analyses. Thus statistical printouts may lack adequate documentation, and checking may involve undetected flaws that are difficult to trace. One needs a hard copy of the statistical analyses; otherwise, there is no hard evidence confirming the performance of these analyses. A hard copy permits others to review the analyses.

A similar problem directly related to biofeedback involves real-time data acquisition and processing of instrumentation-derived data. With computer-based biofeedback, there is often no hard copy of the data before the analyses. Often there are no notebook records or documentation of the details of sessions. Filtering, composite data, and analytic algorithms alter the original data and can produce untraceable statistical results.

Multiple Data Sets

Limitations of some computer resources dictate dividing data among multiple data sets often linked by advanced database technologies. One problem is updating and editing downstream data sets that do not automatically update upstream data sets.

Copies of Data Sets

The need for backup for data sets is vital and well known. However, there can be incomplete or unedited copies. Also, copies may not have adequate documentation; thus one might analyze the wrong copy or erase the corrected one accidentally. During the original active data-gathering and analysis phases, such problems are unlikely. However, months or years later, one could forget the intricate details of the backup and data set copies. This would make further use of the data a problem.

Computed Variables and Subsampling

Research sometimes classifies subjects on the basis of variables not within the data set. An example is basing classification on a composite of subjects' scores on multiple individual measures. Another example is classifying subjects according to individual items within the data set. One needs to save classified and computed scores permanently to prevent losing them. Also, one should update the master copy of the data set.

When reviewing research, some practitioner consumers may wonder about the data management. The only possible sources of this information are the investigators themselves and verification from journals—and the latter source does not yet exist. Journals could require verification and publish a statement to that effect as part of their policies. Such verification would be a major step forward.

FINAL COMMENTS AND FURTHER READING

This chapter has attempted to increase understanding of research, reviews, and clinical reports, and to help increase the sophistication and clinical usefulness of research. We have tried to remind readers of possible pitfalls, to point out the needs of practitioner consumers, and to stimulate productive discussions. We can well imagine some readers saying, "No research can possibly satisfy all these criteria." We partially agree. However, we encourage a concerted effort to address the questions and guidelines posed here. Practitioner consumers have a responsibility to ask these questions and the right to expect reasonable responses.

The research "facts" and "truths" of today often become the "myths" of tomorrow. Furthermore, even a well-controlled study probably contains some limitations, and other investigators may not replicate findings with different samples. As Rosenfeld (1987) pointed out, "We can and must do credible scientific research in the clinical setting" (p. 220). Practitioner consumers often want and need information that is missing from research reports. Individual-subject experimental designs are desirable and may be necessary. Quality assurance for data management is a major necessity for researchers and practitioner consumers.

High-quality and meaningful research, especially clinical research, is extremely difficult to design and conduct. The topics of research design, methodological considerations, pitfalls in human research, and related topics are covered well in other publications (we cite here only those not mentioned previously: Barber, 1976; Beck, Andrasik, & Arena, 1984; Andrasik & Attanasio, 1985; Green & Shellenberger, 1986a, 1986b; Kazdin, 1992; Kewman & Roberts, 1983; Ray, 1979; Ray, Raczynski, Rogers, & Kimball, 1979; Steiner & Dince, 1981, 1983; Taub, 1985). Also, the series of papers in a special 1987 issue of *Biofeedback and Self-Regulation* (Furedy, 1987; Shellenberger & Green, 1987; Furedy & Shulhan, 1987; Rosenfeld, 1987; Carlson, 1987) are very useful.

Lastly, evidence-based practice is now upon us. In 1993, David H. Barlow, then president of the Division of Clinical Psychology (Division 12) of the American Psychological Association, appointed a task force to identify "empirically validated treatments" (more recently, the terminology has changed to "empirically supported treatments") within clinical psychology. It was hoped that this effort would help educate therapists, third-party payers, and the public. In June 2001, a similar effort was launched within our field by Donald Moss, then president of the Association for Applied Psychophysiology and Biofeedback, and Jay Gunkelman, then president of the Society for Neuronal Regulation, who appointed a task force to develop standards on research methodology to use in determining the level of empirical support of treatments (Moss & Gunkelman, 2002). The task force extensively reviewed research articles on methodology and efficacy, guidelines developed by other agencies/societies, and documents addressing ethics in outcome research. Its efforts culminated in the development of a template designed to provide the field with a rigorous set of methodological standards to use in classifying applications at one of five levels of efficacy. The template and efficacy criteria may be found in La Vaque et al. (2002).

NOTES

1. The term "subjects" also refers to patients and clients who are part of clinical research.

2. "Single-case designs" and "single-subject designs" are the common terms (Barlow & Hersen, 1984). We agree with Hawkins's (1989) preference for the term "individual-subject designs" and adopt it for use here. His preference avoids the implications of application only to clinical cases or the use of only one subject in a study. He also steers away from the term "within-subject design," because "it does not discriminate the design from a group design in which subjects in all groups are measured across time" (p. 127).

3. Freedland and Carney (1992) note that during misconduct investigations, regulations of the U.S. Public Health Service (PHS) and the National Science Foundation (NSF) provide for data audits by the PHS Office of Scientific Integrity Review (1990) and the NSF Office of the Inspector General (NSF, 1988). (See the Web sites list in the Resources section.) In addition, there are proposals for routine or random audits by research institutions, funding agencies, and journals. These remain controversial and are not yet widely implemented (Culliton, 1988; Institute of Medicine, 1989; Rennie, 1989; Stewart & Feder, 1987).

RESOURCES

http://ethics.ucsd.edu/courses/ethics/resources/data.htm

Data acquisition, management, sharing and ownership; data management in biomedical research. Contact the Office of Research (ORI) at askORI@osophs.dhhs.gov for a copy of this conference report.

http://ori.dhhs.gov/html/publications/conference.asp

This Web site is for the Office of Research Integrity that contains handbooks and guidelines in MS Word and .pdf formats.

http://www.oig.nsf.gov/pub.htm

This Web site provides NSF Office of the Inspector General publications, including misconduct in science; 4201 Wilson Blvd, Suite 1135, Arlington, VA. Tel: 703-292-7100. Email: oig@nsf.gov. Hotline: 800-428-2189.

REFERENCES

Andrasik, F. (2002). The "Clinical Forum" in *Applied Psychophysiology and Biofeedback*, or something old, something new. *Biofeedback, 30*, 17–18.

Andrasik, F., & Attanasio, V. (1985). Biofeedback in pediatrics: Current status and appraisal. In M. L. Wolraich & D. K. Routh (Eds.), *Advances in developmental and behavioral pediatrics* (Vol. 6, pp. 241–286). Greenwich, CT: JAI.

Barber, T. (1976). *Pitfalls in human research: Ten pivotal points*. New York: Pergamon Press.

Barlow, D. H., Blanchard, E. B., Hayes, S. C., & Epstein, L. H. (1977). Single-case designs and clinical biofeedback experimentation. *Biofeedback and Self-Regulation, 2*, 221–239.

Barlow, D. H., & Hersen, M. (1984). *Single case experimental designs: Strategies for studying behavior change* (2nd ed.). New York: Pergamon Press.

Beck, J. G., Andrasik, F., & Arena, J. G. (1984). Group comparison designs. In A. S. Bellack & M. Hersen (Eds.), *Research methods in clinical psychology*. New York: Pergamon Press.

Carlson, J. G. (1987). Comments on the Furedy/Shellenberger–Green debate. *Biofeedback and Self-Regulation, 12*, 223–226.

Culliton, B. J. (1988). Random audit of papers proposed. *Science, 242*, 657–658.

Dance, K. A., & Neufeld, R. W. (1988). Aptitude–treatment interaction research in the clinical setting: A review of attempts to dispel the "patient uniformity" myth. *Psychological Bulletin, 104*, 192–213.

Freedland, K. E., & Carney, R. M. (1992). Data management and accountability in behavioral and biomedical research. *American Psychologist, 47*, 640–645.

Furedy, J. J. (1987). Specific versus placebo effects in biofeedback training: A critical lay perspective. *Biofeedback and Self-Regulation, 12*, 169–184.

Furedy, J. J., & Shulhan, D. (1987). Specific versus placebo effects in biofeedback: Some brief back-to-basic considerations. *Biofeedback and Self-Regulation, 12*, 211–215.

Garmezy, N., & Masten, A. S. (1986). Stress, competence, and resilience: Common frontiers for therapist and psychopathologist. *Behavior Therapy, 17*, 500–521.

Green, J., & Shellenberger, R. (1986a). Biofeedback research and the ghost in the box: A reply to Roberts. *American Psychologist, 41*, 1003–1005.

Green, J., & Shellenberger, R. (1986b). Clinical biofeedback training and the ghost in the box: A reply to Furedy. *Clinical Biofeedback and Health, 9*, 96–105.

Hawkins, R. P. (1989). Developing potent behavior-change technologies: An invitation to cognitive behavior therapists. *The Behavior Therapist, 12*, 126–131.

Hayes, S. C., Barlow, D. H., & Nelson-Gray, R. O. (1999). *The scientist practitioner: Research and accountability in the age of managed care* (2nd ed.). Needham Heights, MA: Allyn & Bacon.

Holloway, R. L., Spivey, R. N., Zismer, D. K., & Withington, A. M. (1988). Aptitude × treatment interactions: Implications for patient education research. *Health Education Quarterly, 15*, 241–257.

Institute of Medicine. (1989). *The responsible conduct of research in the health sciences* (Publication No. IOM-89-01). Washington, DC: National Academy Press.

Jacobson, N. S., & Truax, P. (1992). Clinical significance: A statistical approach to defining meaningful change in psychotherapy research. In A. E. Kazdin (Ed.), *Methodological issues and strategies in clinical research*. Washington, DC: American Psychological Association.

Jones, E. E. (Ed.). (1993). Single-case research in psychotherapy [Special section, seven articles]. *Journal of Consulting and Clinical Psychology, 61*, 371–430.

Jones, E. E., Ghannam, J., Nigg, J. T., & Dyer, J. F. P. (1993). A paradigm for single-case research: The time-series study of a long-term psychotherapy for depression. *Journal of Consulting and Clinical Psychology, 61*, 381–394.

Kazdin, A. E. (Ed.). (1992). *Methodological issues and strategies in clinical research*. Washington, DC: American Psychological Association.

Kewman, D. G., & Roberts, A. H. (1983). An alternative perspective on biofeedback efficacy studies: A reply to Steiner and Dince. *Biofeedback and Self-Regulation, 8*, 487–497.

Kratochwill, T. R., Mott, S. E., & Dodson, C. L. (1984). Case study and single-case research in clinical and applied psychology. In A. S. Bellack & M. Hersen (Eds.), *Research methods in clinical psychology*. New York: Pergamon Press.

La Vaque, T. J., Hammond, D. C., Trudeau, D., Monastra, V., Perry, J., & Lehrer, P. (2002). Template for developing guidelines for the evaluation of the clinical efficacy of psychophysiological interventions: Efficacy Template Taskforce. *Applied Psychophysiology and Biofeedback, 27*, 263–271.

Maher, B. A. (1992). A reader's, writer's, and reviewer's guide to assessing research reports in clinical psychology. In A. E. Kazdin (Ed.), *Methodological issues and strategies in clinical research*. Washington, DC: American Psychological Association. (Original work published 1978)

Marshall, E. (1990). A clash over standards for scientific records. *Science, 248*, 544–545.

Moss, D., & Gunkelman, J. (2002). Introduction to the task force report on methodology and empirically supported treatments. *Applied Psychophysiology and Biofeedback, 27*, 261–262.

Office of Scientific Integrity Review, U.S. Public Health Service (PHS). (1990). *Data management in biomedical research*. Washington, DC: Author.

Racker, E. (1989). A view of misconduct in science [Editorial]. *Nature, 339*, 91–93.

Ray, W. J. (Chair). (1979). *Evaluation of clinical biofeedback: Symposium conducted at the annual meeting of the Biofeedback Society of America* (Audiotape No. 224). New York: BMA Audio Cassettes.

Ray, W. J., Raczynski, J. M., Rogers, T., & Kimball, W. H. (1979). *Evaluation of clinical biofeedback*. New York: Plenum Press.

Rennie, D. (1989). Editors and auditors. *Journal of the American Medical Association, 261*, 2543–2545.

Rosenfeld, J. P. (1987). Can clinical biofeedback be scientifically validated?: A follow-up on the Green–Shellenberger–Furedy–Roberts debates. *Biofeedback and Self-Regulation, 12*, 217–222.

Shellenberger, R., & Green, J. (1987). Specific effects and biofeedback versus biofeedback-assisted self-regulation training. *Biofeedback and Self-Regulation, 12*, 185–209.

Smith, B., & Sechrest, L. (1992). Treatment of aptitude × treatment interactions. In A. E. Kazdin (Ed.), *Methodological issues and strategies in clinical research*. Washington, DC: American Psychological Association. (Original work published 1991)

Steiner, S. S., & Dince, W. M. (1981). Biofeedback efficacy studies: A critique of critiques. *Biofeedback and Self-Regulation, 6*, 275–288.

Steiner, S. S., & Dince, W. M. (1983). A reply on the nature of biofeedback efficacy studies. *Biofeedback and Self-Regulation, 8*, 499–503.

Stewart, W. W., & Feder, N. (1987). The integrity of the scientific literature. *Nature, 325*, 207–214.

Taub, E. (Chair). (1985). *Problems in clinical biofeedback research: Is misapplied scientific "rigor" misleading the public?: Symposium conducted at the annual meeting of the Biofeedback Society of America* (Audiotape No. BSA 85-22). Aurora, CO: Meyer Communications.

White, L., & Tursky, B. (Eds.). (1982). *Clinical biofeedback: Efficacy and mechanisms*. New York: Guilford Press.

Yeaton, W. H., & Sechrest, L. (1981). Critical dimensions in the choice and maintenance of successful treatments: Strength, integrity, and effectiveness. *Journal of Consulting and Clinical Psychology, 49*, 156–168.

PART XII

Frontier

The Frontier
and Further Forward

MARK S. SCHWARTZ
FRANK ANDRASIK

WRITER'S CRAMP: A TASK-SPECIFIC DYSTONIA

Etiologies, Features, Aggravating Factors, and Classification

The rare (one prevalence estimate is 69 per million; Nutt, Muenter, Aronson, Kurland, & Melton, 1988) and very disabling disorder writer's cramp is typically resistant to treatment. When a person with writer's cramp starts to write or attempts to continue writing after just a few words, there is excess gripping of the pen or pencil, with a subsequent inability to write at all.

> The hand may pronate, with ulnar deviation of the wrist and elevation of the elbow. Sometimes the thumb and index finger flex, so that they ride up the pen. Less commonly, the index finger or thumb, or both, extend to lift off the pen, which may fall from the grip. . . . Sudden jerks of the hand and arm may cause unintended strokes of the pen, or drive the nib through the paper. Tremor is common. (Marsden & Sheehy, 1990, p. 148)

Injury to the hand or arm immediately before symptom onset occurs in 5–10% of persons with writer's cramp. However, the onset is insidious in most patients. There are hints of inheritance in a small percentage of persons. Spontaneous remission for months or years reportedly occurs in about 5%, but relapse is also common. For about half of patients, writing difficulty is the only symptom. For many, there is progression to other manual acts. It is surprising that persons with writer's cramp can write shorthand without difficulty (Marsden & Sheehy, 1990).

Experts remain in disagreement about the etiology of writer's cramp. Some of this disagreement may result from the health care specialties of the investigators and the types of patients who seek their help. These divergent views result in different classifications of subtypes. Marsden and Sheehy (1990), for example, distinguish a "dystonic" from a "simple" type. In the dystonic type, there is involvement of other manual actions from the beginning. Persons with simple writer's cramp can complete other manual motor tasks without difficulty. These authors also distinguish a type they term "progressive" writer's cramp, which begins as simple writer's cramp. These persons develop difficulties with other hand actions, such as using eating utensils, shaving, threading a needle, and applying cosmetics. Although not clearly dystonic by Marsden and Sheehy's criteria, this type also often includes "subtle neurological signs." "A few [patients], particularly those with younger onset, . . . develop involuntary spontaneous dystonic muscle spasms" (p. 150) of the arm, neck, or other limbs. This is the basis for these authors' considering writer's cramp as a focal dystonia.

Different researchers may obtain different results in part because of treating patients with different features. Writer's cramp may not be a unitary disorder, and patient selection is probably very important. For diagnosing this disorder, Mishima, Kitagawa, Hara, and Nakagawa (1992) emphasize:

> The most basic and important point is that a patient has difficulty in hand movements only when writing. . . . If a patient has difficulty in a voluntary movement which is clearly different from handwriting, at the beginning . . . [the problem should] not be diagnosed as writer's cramp. When hand motions such as holding chopsticks and buttoning clothes, which include similar movements to writing, have gradually become disturbed . . . [the disturbance] can be diagnosed as writer's cramp. (p. 104)

These authors then distinguish types of writer's cramp on the basis of patients' scripts and surface electromyography (EMG). Some persons complain of a chronic disturbance but not one severe enough to prevent writing. They only want to preserve ideal writing. These individuals may not be good candidates for biofeedback (Mishima et al., 1992). Mishima et al. (1992) divide the patients with "objective" disturbance into three types. In the "spastic" type, muscle tension related to writing remains very high, thus preventing smooth movements. In the "tremor" type, there is tremulous movement when starting attempts to write. The third is the "dystonic" type, the most severe and most difficult to treat. There are "bizarre movements . . . such as flexion and/or a torsion of the wrist and an extension of the fingers, which never previously appeared during normal writing" (p. 105).

Some professionals link emotional factors (chiefly anxiety and anger) to the cause, persistence, and relapse of writer's cramp in some cases, although Marsden and Sheehy (1990) disagree. This link is not clear, and many professionals consider organic factors as primary. Some persons develop other more widespread neurological diseases (Marsden & Sheehy, 1990). However, practitioners often need to assess whether psychological factors are evident and treat them when relevant. For example, relapses reportedly occur during times of increased stress. Secondary gain from the symptom may be a factor complicating treatment in some persons.

Treatments

Reported treatments tried, all with mixed results, include altered grips on writing instruments, altered instruments, anticholinergic medications, beta-blockers, muscle relaxants, anxiolytics, botulinum toxin (Botox), aversion techniques with electrified pens, massed practice, relaxation therapies, systematic desensitization, operant shaping procedures, surface EMG (hereafter referred to simply as EMG) biofeedback, and various combinations. Writing aids (e.g., the Birdie and the Freedom Writer) can help but are not received well by some patients (Koller & Vetere-Overfield, 1989; O'Neill, Gwinn, & Adler, 1996). Botox is expensive, can lead to excessive weakness of muscles, and lasts only 4–6 months. Oral medications such as anticholinergics have negative side effects that typically outweigh their at best modest benefits.

An early review (Ince, Leon, & Christidis, 1986) of EMG biofeedback for writer's cramp concluded that despite results showing improvement in some patients, biofeedback reached "its near demise" as a treatment for writer's cramp. More recent reports of use of EMG biofeedback to treat writer's cramp show more promise, especially the studies of Murabayashi et al. (1992), Mishima et al. (1992), O'Neill et al. (1996), and Deepak and Behari (1999). Thus EMG biofeedback remains a logical and viable approach. (Candia et al., 1999, describe another behavioral approach—that of constraint-induced movement therapy—which has important implications for reorganizing cortical representation as well.) Marsden and Sheehy's (1990) recent review of etiology and treatment unfortunately ignored most of the literature on biofeedback available to that date. Reference was made only to one study with six subjects (Bindman & Tibbetts, 1977), and treatment effects were downplayed for three of the six patients. Other references of historical interest are Reavley (1975), Uchiyama, Lutterjohann, and Shah (1977), Rowan (1980), Cottraux, Juenet, and Collet (1983), Rubow (1983), and the aforementioned review by Ince et al. (1986).

Evaluation by Mishima et al. (1992) involved EMG from multiple sites, including the upper trapezius, forearm flexors and extensors, and hand muscles (e.g., the thenar eminence), while holding writing instruments during different types of writing. They reported 101 biofeedback sessions over 25 weeks for one 32-year-old male and 200 sessions for another 25-year-old male! However, these were very difficult cases, classed as dystonic, and both patients maintained improvement and work 1 year later.

Murabayashi et al. (1992) reported slightly better results for 8 cases of "tremor"-type writer's cramp than for 11 cases of "rigid"- or "stiffness"-type cramp. Of the 8 patients classed as having the tremor type, 2 showed marked improvement (25%), 2 showed moderate improvement (25%), and 2 showed mild improvement (25%). Of the 11 classed as having the rigid type, 1 improved markedly (9%), 3 showed moderate improvement (27%), and 3 were mildly improved (27%). There was no mention of response for their 1 patient classed as having the "dystonic" type. Of the 20 patients, 12 (60%) reported no difficulty writing, and 4 more (20%) reported only mild difficulty after treatment. Medications started before biofeedback did not have reported benefits; however, most patients continued one or more medications (17 took minor tranquilizers, 11 used beta-blockers mostly for tremor-type symptoms, and 3 used muscle relaxants). Autogenic relaxation procedures were used by 8 patients, mostly with tremor-type symptoms. Biofeedback involved 10 weekly sessions. Murabayashi et al. (1992) reported that the majority of those with tremor-type symptoms showed marked or moderate improvement with respect to muscle tension levels, but no information was provided about how this was determined. Of the 3 cases that showed further improvement among 13 patients followed for 1–46 months, 2 cases were classed as the stiffness type and 1 case classed as the tremor type. There is no information about categories of improvement. This important cumulative effect sometimes appears in other applications.

The dystonic type is the most severe and most difficult to treat. However, Mishima et al. (1992) reported successfully treating two cases they classified as dystonic. Treatment may also be effective for the spastic type (Mishima et al., 1992). Combining biofeedback with medication, such as a beta-blocker, may be effective for the tremor type.

The Deepak and Behari (1999) paper is also supportive and encouraging. They focused the EMG biofeedback on the large limb muscles (the brachioradialis, involved in forearm flexion, or the triceps). The 10 patients treated had dystonic postures and hypertrophy of the large muscles. They provided 4 or more biofeedback sessions (the average and range of sessions were not specified, but not many compared to those in the Japanese series) plus daily practice. Nine patients improved 37–93% in handwriting, discomfort reduction, and pain reduction. Seven of these showed more than 50% improvement.

Guidelines for Evaluation and Treatment

We recommend that biofeedback practitioners treating writer's cramp do the following:

- Obtain a medical/neurological evaluation, as well as a detailed history and description of the symptoms, all fine motor difficulties, and progression.
- Classify patients according to a system.
- Consider stepped care with brief intervention for recent-onset symptoms in a young patient.
- Prepare patients for the possibility of a lengthy treatment. Consider continuing treatment "as long as . . . symptoms appear to be . . . controllable" (Mishima et al., 1992, p. 111).
- Consider general relaxation, as well as deep relaxation (1–5+ minutes) of writing muscles between writing periods.
- Record and provide feedback from multiple EMG sites simultaneously (e.g., use at least two sites; five or more sites are ideal). Consider upper trapezius, deltoid, biceps, brachioradialis, forearm flexors and extensors, and abductor pollicis brevis or thenar eminence.
- Record during different types of writing (e.g., very slow vs. normal rate; simple figures and letters vs. sentences and paragraphs).
- Have patients use different writing instruments with different degrees of difficulty, such as ballpoint pen, pencils, and mechanical pencils, and different thicknesses of writing instruments.
- Start with nontargeted muscles—the secondary arm muscles and movements (e.g., triceps, brachioradialis)—and progress to muscles more involved with writing.
- Have patients start without holding a pen or pencil or holding it without intent to write.
- Have patients progress from writing of easier figures, symbols, and letters to more difficult attempts such as single words and sentences.
- Have patients progress from slow writing to faster writing.
- Include auditory and visual feedback.
- Ask patients to practice writing several times a day for 5–10 minutes each while relaxing all arm muscles.
- Include transfer-of-training procedures.
- Plan gradual relearning with successive approximations in small steps.
- Consider portable EMG biofeedback for augmenting home practice.
- Collect follow-up data to at least 1 year.

Appropriate treatment of selected persons with writer's cramp includes EMG biofeedback, which is often cost-efficient, acceptable to patients, and without side effects.

ESSENTIAL TREMOR

Essential tremor (ET) is very common (Metzer, 1994; Louis, Wendt, & Ford, 2000b). Louis et al. (2000b) report that at least mild and detectable tremor occurs in almost all older adults, and that in at least one activity it is of at least moderate amplitude in about one of three older adults. ET is the most prevalent idiopathic neurological movement disorder (Lundervold, Belwood, Craney, & Poppen, 1999); it is present in an estimated 14% of adults. The prevalence of ET increases significantly with age (Louis et al., 1995) and is slightly but consistently higher in men than in women (Salemi et al., 1994). The average age of onset is 45 years, but about 29% of patients show onset before age 30. Longer duration correlates with increased disability. A positive family history is reported in more than 60% of patients (Koller, Busenbark, & Miner, 1994). There is no known relationship with Parkinson's disease (Pahwa & Koller, 1993). Many patients with ET express social embarrassment about their condition (Pahwa et al., 1995). Metzer (1992) reported embarrassment, shame, and stress among 65–81% of patients. Persons with ET also have difficulties with activities of daily living (ADLs) and social situations.

Treatment for ET often involves pharmacological approaches. Drugs such as propranolol and primidone are reported to be helpful in about 40–65% of patients, as are benzodiazepines. However, this may be an overestimate of success (Bain et al., 1993), due to unreliable measures and problems with experimental methods (Lundervold et al., 1999). Alcohol ingestion is effective at reducing tremor in as many as 74% of patients (Koller et al., 1994). Thalamic stimulation and botulinum toxin (Botox) injections have also been used with varying success in treatment (Britton, 1995). Cognitive and behavioral therapies have been shown to be effective with patients who have a fear of showing bodily symptoms in public (Scholing & Emmelkamp, 1996).

Behavioral relaxation training for tremor management has been successfully used by Chung, Poppen, and Lundervold (1995) and Lundervold et al. (1999). Their treatment has led to statistically significant reductions in clinical and self-report tremor ratings, ADL disability, and social anxiety. In the 2000 study, Lundervold et al. reported on two patients aged 73 and 83, and provided good support for the efficacy of relaxation for ET in elderly persons. The methodological features of note in this work are the use of "extended baselines, a controlled, single-case experimental design, reliability of observations, systematic changes in multiple variables, and use of statistical tests . . . [and] use of a significant other to provide ratings" (p. 132). The authors also note that "relaxation . . . may serve as the first step in a multi-step biobehavioral rehabilitation model for ET" (p. 132).

About 50% of patients with ET have head tremor. This condition creates stress, embarrassment, decreased confidence, and anxiety. Horizontal movements are known as "no-no" tremor, and vertical movements are known as "yes-yes" tremor (Rapoport, Braun, Aviv, & Sarova, 1991). Most patients who experience ET of the head also have a tremulous pattern of activity known as "titubation" (Bradley, Daroff, Fenichel, & Marsden, 1996). Other muscles, such as those of speech and the lower extremities, are less often involved.

In a case study (Schwartz et al., 1997), a 60-year-old female who had had the "no-no" form of head ET for 11 years was treated using relaxation and physical therapy exercises within a single-case B-C-B-D design. Phase B was the combination of relaxation and physical therapy treatments. Phase C was physical therapy, which included axial extension of the neck, tensing and releasing upper back muscles, isometric neck strengthening, and stretching and range-of-motion exercises for the neck. Phase D was relaxation (guided instructions for passive relaxation, autogenic-type phrases, and diaphraghmatic breathing), augmented by four biofeedback sessions. The patient reported much embarrassment and social inhibition due to the tremor. She noted that stress (being with other people in social situations, as well as family stress) increased the tremor.

Symptom ratings on a 0–3 scale were kept over 45 days and involved 810 hours of symptom intensity assessment. Analysis of these ratings showed a statistically significant reduction of head-shaking symptoms in response to the combination of relaxation and physical therapy exercises versus either treatment alone ($p < .005$). The patient reported engaging in both types of procedures usually three times a day, every day. Her subjective global impression was a 60% overall improvement, and often 100% (i.e., she was able to go several hours a day, and sometimes a few days, without noticing any tremor).

Follow-up 5 months later involved 12 days of completing a symptom log. She reported continuing the relaxation and physical therapy for 2.5 months, but then stopping both because of her busy schedule and symptom progress. The average rating of symptom severity for the 12 days of logging was 0.32, with all ratings below 0.4. Home treatment, consisting of relaxation and physical therapy exercises, was instituted for 14 days, with considerable improvement reported. She was then asked to stop the relaxation procedures for 14 days to help isolate the source of effectiveness. After only 6 days the tremor had worsened, so relaxation was restarted and physical therapy exercises continued for 21 days. Physical therapy exercises were then stopped, but once again the tremors quickly worsened (after 4 days). Both treatments were then resumed.

Analysis of self-reported symptom ratings at posttreatment indicated not only significant reductions in tremor symptoms (as noted above), but also reduced anxiety and improved social functioning with a combination of daily relaxation and physical therapy exercises compared to either physical therapy alone ($p = .006$) or relaxation alone ($p = .005$). There was no significant difference in terms of treatment effect with regard to the first and third phases of treatment, when both relaxation and physical therapy occurred. The patient reported that her husband and other persons had commented favorably on her overall improvement. She was able to go to the beauty parlor with more confidence, less anxiety, and minimal tremor.

Select Considerations for Assessment and Treatment

We make the following suggestions for practitioners treating ET:

- Consider muscle relaxation therapies.
- Consider including EMG biofeedback-assisted procedures to help detect dysfunctional neuromuscular patterns and to correct sensorimotor functioning (Lundervold et al., 1999).
- Use a baseline of several days to a few weeks, if practical.
- Use multiple and reliable measures of tremor, if possible (e.g., the 10-point severity/disability scale developed by Bain et al., 1993). See also Montgomery and Reynolds (1991) for 10-point self-ratings, and Louis et al. (2000a) for other measures.)
- Use multiple raters, if practical.

IDIOPATHIC SCOLIOSIS

A creative biofeedback application involves an ambulatory device with computer chips and microprocessors to help the 2–4% of adolescents with idiopathic scoliosis—a lateral curvature of the spine that is severe enough to produce truncal deformity (Dworkin et al., 1985; Miller, 1985; Birbaumer, Flor, Cevey, Dworkin, & Miller, 1994). From 60% to 80% of people with the idiopathic type are female. The usual nonsurgical treatment is wearing a brace 23 hours a day for several years. Another technique is paraspinal electrical stimulation via surgical implantation or transcutaneous applications. However, this is not the treatment of choice for many adolescents. A third, more drastic option is spinal fusion surgery.

The biofeedback device and treatment work "by enhancing the patient's perceptions of incorrect posture and encouraging her to correct the position of her spine" (Dworkin et al., 1985, p. 2497). Biofeedback also provides "activation of specific groups of the patient's muscles to correct scoliotic curvature" and "develops learned muscle control through the patient's own nervous system rather than forcing contraction with extrinsic electric currents" (p. 2497).

For a description of the biofeedback device, the rationale, and its successful application for 12 adolescents with progressive idiopathic scoliosis, see the references above.

A major criterion for success is whether a patient passes through the adolescent growth period without significant progression of the curvature, thus avoiding treatments such as a rigid orthosis or surgery (Wong, Mak, Luk, Evans, & Brown, 2001). Birbaumer et al. (1994) successfully treated patients with both scoliosis and kyphosis, a forward curvature of the spine. A series of 13 patients in Hong Kong with progressive adolescent idiopathic scoliosis (Wong et al., 2001) indicated benefit for perhaps more than half of the patients. These authors reported that the scoliosis in most of the 13 patients remained under control after 18 months. Five completed their skeletal growth without curve progression. Four others were still wearing the device. Four of the other seven had curve deterioration and switched to a brace, and three others stopped the biofeedback early.

Patients typically prefer the postural training device to a rigid spinal orthosis, and most easily learn to use the feedback. For several advantages and disadvantages of the biofeedback device compared to the rigid orthosis, see Wong et al. (2001) and Dworkin et al. (1985). Advantages include the following: Adjustment is easy; the device is inconspicuous; no atrophy can occur, as with the rigid device; and it permits data recording for documentation. However, patients sometimes do not hear the audio feedback when ambient noise is high, or they are embarrassed by the tone with ambient quiet. Vibration feedback would have some advantages but certain limitations as well (e.g., increased energy consumption). Perhaps a combination of sequential vibration and a tone would be better if the battery energy problem could be solved. We look toward a more efficacious biofeedback application in the future.

DERMATOLOGICALLY RELATED CONDITIONS

There are several reports of applied psychophysiological interventions, including relaxation and biofeedback, for various dermatologically related conditions. Here we focus on hyperhidrosis, psoriasis, skin ulcers, and herpes, because these conditions have received the greatest research attention.[1] Preliminary work exists for eczema (McMenamy, Katz, & Gipson, 1998), and atopic dermatitis/neurodermatitis, and there is also a report on electric-burn-related pain (Bird & Colborne, 1980). The use of various applied psychophysiological therapies, including relaxation therapies and biofeedback, for dermatological disorders also receives support from the views that psychological or biobehavioral factors are thought to contribute to such disorders (Folks & Kinney, 1992; Sarti, 1998; Panconesi, Gallassi, Sarti, & Bellini, 1998; and Bilkis & Mark, 1998).

Hyperhidrosis

The hallmark of primary (idiopathic, essential) hyperhidrosis is excess perspiration of the palms, soles, and/or axillas, accentuated by mental stimuli more than by heat and exercise. It can be very distressing, is socially embarrassing, causes staining and rotting of clothing, can lead to social withdrawal, interferes with the grasping of objects, and affects writing on paper. It can even result in electric shock. Plantar hyperhidrosis (excessive sweating of the soles of the feet) can lead to unpleasant smells, friction blisters, infection, and rotting of socks and shoes.

White (1986) has reviewed the major medical treatments. One typically starts with a simple, safe, and inexpensive treatment such as aluminum chloride, which is often enough for axillary hyperhidrosis. White also noted that biofeedback and psychotherapy are worth considering for some patients. Reports of biofeedback treatment include those of Fotopoulos and Whitney (1978), Harris and Sieveking (1979), Duller and Gentry (1980), Farrar and Hartje (1987), Kawahara and Kikuchi (1992), and Alvarez, Cortes, and Rodriguez (1993).

Kawahara and Kikuchi (1992) treated five individuals (aged 16 to 25) with hyperhidrosis. The authors used a prototype device, a capsule air change method, providing visual feedback of sweating volume from dry nitrogen gas humidity data on the palm. They showed that three subjects could markedly inhibit sweating with feedback. In the first session, these three showed a paradoxical increase of sweat during feedback. One interpretation was that the feedback was initially stressful to the subjects. Inhibited sweat occurred during feedback in the next three to four sessions. The weekly sessions consisted of four 5-minute trials and 5-minute resting intervals. There were no controls, no self-reported symptom data, and no comparisons with conventional electrodermal biofeedback. However, the finding of inhibited sweat during feedback from a device measuring sweat is an important one.

Farrar and Hartje (1987) reported on five patients with hyperhidrosis. Treatment involved several methods of stress management, counseling, and a structured biofeedback program, involving multiple stressors and feedback stages. Feedback focused on skin conductance in addition to frontal EMG and hand temperature. They reported a 61% decrease of skin conductance and a 75% reduction of symptoms (ratings were collected four times a day). The report provided few other details about the data, and no controls were included. Combining several treatment components confounds interpretation of the role of biofeedback. However, the paper does support the idea that people with hyperhidrosis can reduce sweat during office procedures and during daily activities.

Alvarez et al. (1993) reported using skin conductance feedback and imagery with 25 recruited subjects who had had at least 10 years of palmar hyperhidrosis. Subjects made hourly ratings during a 2-week baseline and during treatment. The combined treatment was effective for the five subjects completing this approach, and the results once again show that it is possible to obtain significant improvements in sweating during office feedback procedures and in self-reported symptoms outside of therapy. However, the high dropout rate and methodological problems raise questions about the generality of effects. Furthermore, although the subjects were seen for a mean of nearly 18 sessions, treatment time varied considerably across individuals; thus the optimal number of sessions for benefit is not known.

We offer these suggestions for practitioners:

- Consider having patients use a self-report symptom log that provides time and situation samples and ratings of daily stressors.
- Monitor more than one body site in the office, and have patients do so in the log. For example, consider both hands, one hand and one foot, or axillary with one hand and/ or one foot.
- Careful placement of electrodes is important to ensure reliable data. For example, different degrees of pressure of Velcro-attached electrodes on the fingers can produce different data.

Psoriasis

Psoriasis is a condition where red lesions appear on the skin, and then multiply and scale over with silvery patches. Topical and oral medications and ultraviolet light are common treatments. Part of the rationale for applying biofeedback and other applied psychophysiological interventions for psoriasis involves the recognition that emotional factors and psychological stress can affect the onset and/or aggravation of symptoms (Keinan, Segal, Gal, & Brenner, 1995). After noting several studies that supported that association, Keinan et al. described their experience using a combination of relaxation and biofeedback (bifrontal EMG and skin temperature) modalities. Although there was no difference from before to after the 3 months of treatment, the authors pointed out that for psoriasis, "the best way to examine the net effect of any treatment is to compare the patient's condition to that of the same season in previous years" (p. 239). The group of 11 patients who received the combination treatment "reported considerably more improvement . . . relative to the same season of the previous year" (p. 239).

Practitioners should also note that the skin temperature focus in Keinan et al.'s study was on *cooling* the skin and especially the affected areas. Imagery in the suggestive relaxation procedures involved images of cooling from contact with ice, snow, or a cool breeze. (This is particularly interesting, because the study was conducted in Israel.) Twenty-four hours of biofeedback (two half-hour sessions per week) were provided, in addition to several weeks devoted to learning abbreviated progressive relaxation and suggestive cooling relaxation imagery.

Goodman (1994) reported a single case supporting the value of thermal biofeedback (13 sessions of 1 hour each) for psoriasis in a 56-year-old European American female for whom prior standard medical treatments had been unsuccessful over several years. All 11 psoriasis lesions disappeared. The size of these had been 2–6 centimeters. The patient reported no lesions and no use of medication at a 12-month follow-up. Treatment focused on *warming* of peripheral sites that varied over sessions; these included digit 2, then digit 5, and then web placements on the right and left hands. During the last two sessions, office stressors included intermittent cold breezes, conversation, and aversive distraction. Given that the opposite focis of thermal biofeedback were employed by Keinan et al. (1995) and by Goodman (1994), it is difficult to determine the role that temperature acquisition might be playing in mediating outcome.

Skin Ulcers

The application of biofeedback and related techniques to the treatment of skin ulcers has progressed considerably in recent years, due partly to the research on relaxation and biofeedback-assisted relaxation for foot ulcer healing among a group of patients with and without diabetes (Rice, Kalker, Schindler, & Dixon, 2001). In the second edition of this book, this application was only noted as another potential application as an adjunct to treating diabetic ulcers, based on the research of Shulimson, Lawrence, and Iacono (1986) and Guthrie, Moeller, and Guthrie (1983) who showed that this approach could result in increased skin temperatures among persons with diabetes. The work of Rice and Schindler (1992), who showed in patients with diabetes mellitus that biofeedback-assisted relaxation could help increase toe temperatures via vasodilation, was inadvertently overlooked.

The more recent investigation by Rice et al. (2001) was ambitious and had many excellent methodological features; the results were very supportive of the value of at least the combination of patient education, relaxation, and single-session thermal biofeedback. The treated group was compared to a control group that received the same standard medical wound care and biweekly office visits, plus "instructions to relax 15 to 20 minutes daily while off their feet and using a self-selected method" (p. 134) such as music, television, or daydreaming. As this constitutes the major and most recently published study, the findings are reported in detail:

- In the experimental (E) group, 14/16 (88%) showed healed ulcers, compared to 7/17 (41%) in the control (C) group.
- Of the 4 patients in the (C) group who later crossed over to the E group, all 4 showed complete healing.

- Healing rate was significantly faster for the E group.
- Ambulation ratings were significantly higher for the E group.
- Improved sensory nerve function in large myelinated fibers of the peroneal nerve was shown: The patients in the E group were able to perceive electric current at lower intensities at the end of treatment than at the start. This was assumed to be "due to better oxygenation of nerve endings through increased microvascular perfusion, brought about by decreased sympathetic muscle tone and peripheral vasodilation" (p. 139).
- Average warming within a session increased significantly for the E group from session 1 to session 2 at the end of the study, from 2°F to 5°F; thus more within-session warming occurred after treatment.

These dramatic results were documented with an ulcer-scoring measure, healing rates measured by changes in wound area, photographic documentation, ambulation measure, and ratings by podiatric physicians (who were unaware of group assignments) of clinically positive healing.

Useful information for practitioners that can be derived from this study includes the following:

- Patient commitment to comprehensive treatment is essential.
- Comprehensive treatment includes stopping smoking; avoiding trauma; complying with non-weight-bearing recommendations, topical medicine, and daily wound care; avoiding creating new wounds; and taking prescribed medications.
- Patient education includes fostering substantial responsibility for patients' own treatment, recommending lifestyle changes, teaching new skills, and providing encouragement.
- It is important to maintain close contact with physicians and allied health professionals who normally work with this condition.
- Rice et al. combined various relaxation procedures, such as progressive muscular relaxation, focused breathing, and phrases focused on feelings of warmth and heaviness. A 16-minute audiotape of instructions and phrases was provided.
- Portable devices were used to measure toe temperature on the volar side of great toe. Temperature logs were collected biweekly.
- Extra and altered patient education and instructions may be needed for some patients who have performance anxiety or who find relaxation procedures stressful for other reasons (e.g., consider deferring home measurements).

Rice et al. (2001) recognize the limitations of their small sample (especially the homogeneous ethnicity of the upper Midwest) but these do not detract from the value of the results. The authors provide logical reasons for including thermal biofeedback with relaxation (e.g., helping teach patients "the underlying concept of vascular physiology" (p. 134), and helping them "know that they were relaxing properly" (p. 139)). However, accomplishing this in one session—presumably (although this is not clearly stated) at the beginning of treatment and before relaxation procedures started—would be a lot to expect. The focus of the intervention was then on relaxing at least once a day 5 days each week during the 4–12 weeks needed for the ulcers to heal fully. Compliance with this was reported as very good. One can assume that these patients used the relaxation procedures more often then once a day, although this was not assessed.

Much more research is obviously needed, but this is a significant advance in an otherwise impoverished area for such a serious condition. Nonhealing or poorly healing foot ulcers occur with several medical problems that involve peripheral arterial disease. Perhaps some patients will at least be able to increase the success of medical/surgical procedures by utilizing similar approaches.

The report by Ward and Van Moore (1995) with finger ulcers and scleroderma is mentioned only because of the inclusion of biofeedback with medical, nonoperative treatment. One cannot separate the effects of the interventions that resulted in healed ulcers in 6 of 15 hands, and healing remaining at a 2-year follow-up.

In one study of solitary rectal ulcer syndrome, biofeedback was part of a behavioral approach that also included retraining of toileting, pelvic floor muscle coordination, posture, and the use of abdominal muscles during defecation (Vaizey, Roy, & Kamm, 1997). This British study reported on the role and usefulness of these therapies and procedures for a group of 13 consecutive patients with this syndrome, including 5 for whom prior surgical treatment had failed.

Herpes

The rationale for considering stress management interventions for recurrent herpes simplex is the presumed link between psychosocial stress and recurrences. Reports of applied psychophysiological treatments for reducing genital herpes outbreaks among people with frequent outbreaks are sparse (Longo, Clum, & Yeager, 1988; VanderPlate & Kerrick, 1985; Burnette, Koehn, Kenyon-Jump, Hutton, & Stark, 1991).

Burnette et al. (1991) used a multiple-baseline-across-subjects design with eight subjects to evaluate relaxation training. Five subjects were noted to improve; reductions in frequency of outbreaks ranged from 40%–93%. This study is impressive and encouraging. It involved self-report symptom baselines ranging from 13 to 30 weeks. All subjects reported very high baseline outbreak frequencies, averaging from approximately 2 to nearly 7 days per week. The number of office relaxation therapy sessions was only three for each subject, spaced over 3–6 weeks. The follow-up period was at least 3 months, during which time patients maintained their self-report symptom logs. The subjects reported using relaxation one or more times per day. The median was 5 days a week and ranged from almost 3 days a week to nearly daily.

The frequency and severity of herpes episodes decrease naturally over time. However, there are several reasons to attribute the observed changes to relaxation treatment. First, these subjects had long histories of herpes (2–14 years). Furthermore, the subjects recorded lengthy baseline symptom data, and the reductions occurred over a short time. One possible limitation concerns collateral medication use, which was not addressed. Presumably the subjects were not taking acyclovir (Zovirax).

We recommend that therapists consider providing relaxation therapy to patients for whom medication is either contraindicated or ineffective, or who continue to experience adverse effects or distress. We do not know the effects of relaxation on milder cases, or on patients for whom stress is less of a factor or is not a factor. For example, some recurrence of symptoms stems from physical irritation of the affected area; in such a case, a practitioner should consider more comprehensive applied psychophysiological interventions tailored to the patient. In conclusion, this application remains a frontier outpost for further development and consideration for selected patients.

MENOPAUSAL HOT FLUSHES

Another useful application for future development is treatment of menopausal hot flushes (HFs). Applied psychophysiological treatments may be of special value for those women for whom hormone therapy and/or pharmacotherapy are insufficient or contraindicated.

Estrogen remains the gold standard for treating HFs (Larson, 1996; Shuster, 2001). However, for women who do not take estrogen, treatments for HFs include the following (Shuster, 2001):

- Lifestyle modification, such as relaxation procedures, aerobic exercise, and avoiding smoking.
- Dietary restrictions, such as avoiding alcohol, caffeine, hot drinks, and spicy foods.
- Dietary additions, such as plant estrogens and soy.
- Dietary supplements, such as black cohosh, dong quai, chaste tree berry, red clover, wild yams, vitamin E, and DHEA.
- Nonhormonal prescription medications such as selective serotonin reuptake inhibitors, particularly venlaFaxine (Effexor).

Among women with HFs, perhaps more than half would choose a psychological therapy such as cognitive or relaxation therapy (Hunter & Liao, 1995). That study of 61 women reported that 60% of the 46 women asking for treatment chose a psychological option over hormone therapy. These women were more anxious, reported more stress management problems, and had lower self-esteem than those not seeking treatment. Those choosing psychological treatment were not much different from those choosing hormones, but some had concerns about medications (including past ineffectiveness), and several wanted skills to help control the HFs and life stressors. The study "highlights the need for the development of alternative treatment regimens for women seeking help for menopausal problems" (p. 101).

HFs occur in about 75% of women during menopause. Most have this symptom for at least 1 year, and 25–50% have it for more than 5 years (Berkow & Fletcher, 1992). The episodes usually last from a few seconds to at least several minutes. The term "menopause" literally means "last menstruation." In popular use, it refers to the years of gradual reduction of menstruation. The average age for the last menstruation is 50–51 in the United States, but these changes can start from about age 40 to about age 55. However, there are significant individual differences, and many women are asymptomatic. Estimates are that about 25% of women report no physiological changes except the gradual end of menstruation. About 25% of women report very bothersome changes. These include frequent night sweats, as well as embarrassment when the HFs and sweating occur during the day. The other 50% note only slight changes.

Many emotional and psychological symptoms accompany menopause; these include insomnia, fatigue, anxiety, and irritability. Other symptoms include dizziness, paresthesias, palpitations, tachycardia, urinary incontinence, nausea, constipation, diarrhea, myalgias, cold hands and feet, and headaches. One can attribute many of these to hormonal changes. However, psychological interventions are proper for many women with emotional problems and/or psychophysiological symptoms during the years of menopause. The potential role for applied psychophysiological interventions is logical.

The rationale for relaxation and biofeedback includes the dramatic changes in respiration that often precede the HFs (Woodward, Grevill, & Freedman, 1991), and that implicate the activation of the sympathetic nervous system in HF onset. Some women with HFs show a breathing pattern involving higher tidal volumes and fewer breaths per minute. These occur with feelings of breathlessness even during quiet rest. Breathing returns to lower tidal volume and more breaths per minute after the HFs. Other justifications include the emotional stress reactions of many women with HFs, and treatment for many of the specific symptoms associated with menopause. Often there is severe interference with sleep. Further justification stems from the effectiveness of relaxation and biofeedback for some of these symptoms associated with other conditions. Furthermore, some pharmacological interventions have limitations for some women.

Lee and Taylor (1987) reported an application of relaxation and biofeedback to HFs in one woman. The HFs had occurred many times each day for a year. Estrogen therapy was contraindicated because the patient had cancer, and anxiolytic medications were not helpful. Treatment involved four sessions of progressive relaxation and supportive counseling, and EMG biofeedback over 15 weekly sessions. HF frequency dropped from 24–30 per day in the first month (November in New York) to the range of 12–18 in the second month, 6–12 in the third month, and 0–6 per day for the next 3 months.

The clearest demonstration of success used slow and deep diaphragmatic breathing as the sole treatment (Freedman & Woodward, 1992b). This followed pilot work by Germaine and Freedman (1984) and careful methodological research to help justify this application and objectively document symptom changes (Freedman, 1989; Freedman & Woodward, 1992a; Freedman, Woodward, & Sabharwal, 1990; Woodward et al., 1991).

Freedman and Woodward (1992b) treated 11 postmenopausal women with 8 sessions of paced respiration. They compared this group with other groups of equal numbers receiving progressive muscle relaxation via live instruction or a placebo control procedure involving alpha electroencephalographic (EEG) feedback with eyes open. HF symptom changes were documented with 24-hour ambulatory recordings of sternal skin conductance level beyond 2 micromhos. These investigators showed in prior research that this criterion corresponded very well (86–95%) with patients' reports of HFs. Only the relaxed breathing group showed significant reductions of HF frequency, reduced respiration rate, and increased tidal volumes. The breathing measures supported the role of the breathing procedures. The HFs dropped from about 15 per day to about 10 per day. Respiration during office sessions dropped from about 14 to about 10 breaths per minute.

Finally, in six patients treated by Melin, Nedstrand, and Hammar (1997) with 12 relaxation therapy weekly groups, the number of HFs decreased an average of 73% (range = 59–100%) from the baseline period to a 6-month follow-up. Refinements and extensions of these treatments may result in even greater improvements.

ERYTHROMELALGIA

Erythromelalgia is a very rare disorder in its primary form.[2] Erythromelalgia involves sudden and intensive spastic dilation of blood vessels, or "paroxysmal vasodilation." The symptoms include burning pain, increased skin temperature, and redness. The feet, and less often the hands, are usually the sites of the symptoms. The terms for the name of this disorder come from Greek words meaning "red" (*erythros*), "extremities" (*melos*), and "pain" (*algos*). There are three different names for this condition. The original is "erythromelalgia," coined by Mitchell (1878), who described the first 16 cases. This term is in general use, although some writers argue for other terms such as "erythermalgia" and "erythmalgia." It can be idiopathic or secondary to other diseases. The idiopathic form is probably the more common and may have a better prognosis (Babb, Alarçon-Segovia, & Fairbairn, 1964). The origin of the primary form is unknown. The secondary form is associated with several diseases for which treatment can help the vasodilation. For further information, readers should consult Levine and Gustafon (1987), Michiels and van Joost (1988, 1990), Kurzrock and Cohen (1989), Davis, O'Fallon, Rogers, and Rooke (2000), or the sources listed in note 2.

Treatments and Natural History

Therapies include rest, elevation of the extremity, cold application, administration of vasoconstrictive medication or high doses of aspirin, and avoidance of exposure to ambient temperatures above about 85°F. Davis et al. (2000) conducted a long-term follow-up (average = nearly 9 years, range = 1–20 years) of 168 patients originally diagnosed at Mayo Clinic between 1970 and 1994. About 32% worsened, more than 26% reported no change, about 31% improved, and more than 10% reported complete resolution of symptoms. Of 163 of these patients, 97% reported intermittent patterns. Most cases involved the feet (88%), and over 25% involved the hands.

Biofeedback Cases

Only two cases reporting successful use of biofeedback could be located (Putt, 1978; Cahn & Garber, 1990). The Erythromelalgia Association's Web site (see note 2) refers to a few other patients who reportedly obtained some benefit from biofeedback, but these are not published reports.

Putt (1978) treated a woman with various relaxation procedures, administered in 13 sessions spaced over 11 weeks. The published account does not clearly describe or report direct temperature feedback to the patient, although there was implicit feedback from the therapist. The patient "expressed a fear of allowing her toes to warm because she became uncomfortable at about 32 degrees Centigrade [89.6°F]" (p. 628). She learned to warm her toe temperatures without symptoms. Her need for medication gradually decreased, and for 3 months she was symptom-free. The appearance of her toes and skin improved significantly. She tolerated foot temperatures of about 91–93°F. She then resumed smoking and had a partial relapse a few months later. However, her symptoms and medication use improved again after resuming office and home relaxation during 2 more months of treatment. Although we do not know enough of the treatment specifics, we have learned the following:

- Warming was the treatment.
- Treatment involved a variety of relaxation procedures.
- Thermal biofeedback played some role.
- There was probable improvement in symptoms and reduced medication.
- There was a probable relapse and improvement after repeated treatment.
- These patients fear warming, and care needs to be exercised with this approach.

In the other case report, Cahn and Garber (1990) "hypothesized that the painful symptoms may represent a rebound vasodilation" (p. 51). One therapy goal was avoiding large changes in temperature, rather than only avoiding warm temperatures. Another goal was to help the patient gradually warm her extremities without stimulating an attack. The multimodal treatment included thermal feedback, blood pulse volume feedback, respiration feedback, and multiple relaxation techniques. The authors believe that convincing the patient that "warm was good" was critical. After 1 year, she continued to have occasional attacks, but the severity decreased and there were significantly fewer episodes. Her foot temperatures consistently rose to over 90.0°F. Self-report records from June 1988 to July 1989 showed about 40–70 or more attacks per month in the first 3 months. This rate dropped to 5–10 attacks per month in the last 3 months—an improvement of more than 90%.

Implications

There is a chance that biofeedback might play a useful role in the treatment of some patients with this disorder. Selecting patients with the primary form is probably wiser. Collaboration with physicians who are knowledgeable about this disorder is obviously essential. Practitioners

should consider a minimum of two channels and preferably four or more temperature channels, because of the variability that occurs across digits and the need to check both feet and
both hands. Many sessions ovr many months should be expected. Practitioners might consider
providing at least some of this therapy pro bono or within a research project, because of the
embryonic stage of this treatment for this disorder and the length of time it involves.

NAUSEA AND VOMITING

Although there have been significant pharmaceutical advances in antiemetics, reports indicate that the anticipatory nausea/vomiting (N/V) reaction associated with chemotherapy still
remains a problem for a sizable minority of patients (Boakes, Tarrier, Barnes, & Tattersall,
1993; Chin, Kucuk, Peterson, & Ezdinli, 1992; Morrow et al., 1998). Dadds, Bovbjerg, Redd,
and Cutmore (1997) review imagery in human classical conditioning and state that "classical
conditioning offers the most comprehensive explanation of these phenomena" (p. 99). The
unconditioned stimulus is the chemotherapy; the unconditioned response is the initial N/V.
After repeated pairings, "previously neutral stimuli, such as medical and nursing staff and
hospital sights and smells, become CSs [conditioned stimuli] that are able to elicit a CR [con-
ditioned response]" (p. 99).

There is extensive and international research support for applied psychophysiological
treatments for anticipatory N/V associated with chemotherapy (Burish, Shartner, & Lyles,
1981; Shartner, Burish, & Carey, 1985; Carey & Burish, 1988; Greene, Seime, & Smith, 1991;
Burish & Jenkins, 1992; Vasterling, Jenkins, Tope, & Burish, 1993; Blasco, 1994; Marchioro
et al., 2000; Arakawa, 1995, 1997; Troesch, Rodehaver, Delaney, & Yanes, 1993). The treatments include primarily relaxation therapies, distraction methods, hypnosis, and guided imagery. Applied psychophysiological interventions—principally relaxation procedures and
hypnotic techniques—have also been useful for reducing N/V reactions to other causes and
medical conditions, such as general anesthesia and surgery (Enqvist, Bjorklund, Engman, &
Jakobsson, 1997). Whether or not practitioners use biofeedback to assist relaxation depends
on their preferences and on practical considerations. Research indicates that it is probably
not needed for most persons with these symptoms. However, relaxation and other methods
(e.g., distraction, hypnosis, immersive virtual reality) to reduce psychophysiological arousal
are applied psychophysiological approaches, and biofeedback has yet to be extensively studied with regard to potential benefits for selected patients.

STRESS-INDUCED VASOVAGAL SYNCOPE

"Syncope" is fainting or a sudden and brief loss of consciousness. Vasovagal syncope is
one type of fainting episode, which usually results from momentary insufficient blood supply to the brain. Common symptoms include nausea, weakness, visual blurring, sweating,
lightheadedness, and yawning. Vasovagal syncope is often attributed to "transient alterations in autonomic tone leading to sudden decreases in blood pressure and heart rate"
(McGrady, Bush, & Grubb, 1997, p. 63). In disposed persons, rapid changes in position/
posture and/or dehydration can precipitate syncope. Emotional stressors and a person's
reactions to these are also common major precipitants. Common examples of situations
and stimuli that prompt these behaviors and symptoms include the sight of blood; injections; pain; dental procedures; venipuncture; medical paraphernalia; and films or pictures
of medical diseases, illness, or accidents. One must establish the correct diagnosis and rule

out other causes for the syncope that require medical attention (various cardiovascular and noncardiovascular causes). Syncope also has many of the same features as phobic responses, and treatment will often include behavioral approaches. However, an important distinction is the syncope itself.

McGrady and Arqueta Bernal (1986) focused their intervention on relaxation procedures, frontal EMG, and hand temperature biofeedback. They combined these with cognitive-behavioral stress management and graduated exposure within a systematic desensitization model. A major part of the rationale for the presumed importance of the relaxation and bio-feedback was based on learning that before fainting, "the patient increased muscle tension for several minutes" (p. 24). His wife observed that he "went rigid" and tensed "his whole body." The sequence was stimulus → anxiety → increased muscle tension → sensations of weakness and limb heaviness → nausea and sweating → lightheadedness → syncope. Excess muscle tension was noted during resting baselines in the frontal and cervical neck regions, confirming the spouse's observations. The researchers also noted increased general tension and decreased hand temperature while the patient was talking about various stressors. They then reported substantial decreases in resting muscle tension, with levels reaching the relaxed range. Hand temperature increased up to 95°F.

The syncopal episodes occurred two or three times a year, and there was daily fear of fainting and anxiety episodes with presyncopal symptoms. At a 1-year follow-up, by contrast, there were no reported syncopal incidents. Before treatment, events would result in presyncopal symptoms or syncopal episodes. With relaxation procedures, these events resulted in asymptomatic reactions or successful management. For example, the patient could now receive a Novocain injection and dental treatment without problems.

Treatment by McGrady et al. (1997) included muscle relaxation with bifrontal EMG biofeedback, then finger temperature feedback with autogenic relaxation and diaphragmatic breathing. The rationale for the latter component included reducing autonomic arousal and reducing or preventing hyperventilation in stressful situations. The number of sessions ranged from 5 to 12 (average = 8.5). In each session, 20 of the 50 minutes involved patient education focused on identifying and recognizing presyncopal symptoms, identifying stressors that affected symptoms, and the functioning of the autonomic nervous system in regulating blood pressure and cerebral blood flow. Relaxation was implemented via printed scripts and cassette tapes that were used twice daily for 10–15 minutes and during presyncopal episodes. At the end of treatment, six of the seven patients with true syncope (those with loss of consciousness from seconds to minutes) reported no or rare syncope. Other autonomic symptoms were common for these patients; for three of these six patients, headache, lightheadedness, and dizziness, also decreased.

An interesting and detailed single-case study of the successful application of psychophysiological therapy was reported by Khurana, Lynch, and Craig (1997). They referred to it as "transactional psychophysiological therapy" and perceived it as "novel," which it was at the time it was done (about 14 years before publication—hence about 1983). The intervention was very successful. Frequency of episodes had increased from age 18, when the patient married, to age 31, just before treatment. The frequency was as great as 12 per day; episodes occurred primarily during standing (and sometimes when sitting), and were precipitated by a wide variety of activities, including emotional stress, ending physical activity, bowel movements, orgasm, strong smells, extreme heat, or alcohol. Hypotension was one of the symptoms. The authors observed that patients with syncope are not aware of their autonomic reactions during stress. To address this, they employed computer monitoring of cardiovascular responses during 28 weekly and then monthly sessions of psychodynamically oriented psychotherapy, which focused on avoiding excess arousal or reducing arousal. The patient "slowly began to learn what her body felt like when her blood pressure was going down . . . learned to recognize stress triggers that caused her pressure to fall . . . [and] learned methods of elevating pressure in the autonomic laboratory by doing simple mathematics, moving, talking, etc." (Khurana et al., 1997, p. 196). Today this therapy would be described as psychophysiological therapy with biofeedback and face-to-face psychotherapy. The term "biofeedback" was not mentioned once by Khurana et al. (1997)—but "a rose by any other name . . . "

The treatment components that are associated with improvements are unclear; support has been provided for all the types of relaxation used, multiple modalities of biofeedback, and psychophysiological therapy with psychotherapy. It is wise to tailor treatments for the specific patient. Caution is needed during the tensing portion of progressive muscle relaxation, because it can result in presyncopal sensations (McGrady & Arqueta Bernal, 1986). The results from these treatment packages are encouraging and support considering these alternative applied psychophysiological treatments for patients for whom pharmacotherapies are "ineffectual, poorly tolerated, or contraindicated" (McGrady et al., 1997, p. 64). Controlled, prospective studies are warranted. (See Kozak & Montgomery, 1981, Kozak & Miller, 1985, and Smith & Glass, 1989, for discussion of other case reports.)

SICKLE CELL CRISES

Sickle cell disease is a genetic anemic disease producing entrapment or sludging of red blood cells in small blood vessels. This restricts oxygenated blood from getting to parts of the body, and results in painful episodes or "crises." These crises include headaches or generalized pain in various parts of the body; other symptoms include shortness of breath and fever. More serious symptoms include kidney failure, strokes, and other permanent damage to organs. The frequency and timing of these crises vary among individuals. Some authorities consider emotional distress a possible factor increasing the risk of symptom crises in people with sickle cell disease. Emotional distress also may increase the risk of stress-related symptoms accompanying the crises. This is the rationale for considering applied psychophysiological interventions as adjuncts to treatment. Having the disease is a major source of stress, because of the increased vulnerability to infections and the potentially serious consequences of the disease.

Cozzi, Tryon, and Sedlacek (1987) reported a bold attempt to apply biofeedback and applied psychophysiological interventions as adjunctive therapy for this serious, chronic condition. Eight outpatients with sickle cell disease (ranging in age from 10 to 20 years) were provided six EMG and six thermal biofeedback sessions. A follow-up questionnaire at 6 months showed reduced headaches, less pain during crises, and less use of analgesics. Unfortunately, there were no improvements in hospitalizations or emergency room visits compared to the 6-month baseline before treatment.

Two prior investigations of applied psychophysiological interventions reported improvement in uncontrolled case studies of sickle cell disease (Thomas, Koshy, Patterson, Dorn, & Thomas, 1984; Zeltzer, Keller, Dash, & Holland, 1979). These reports involved a few sessions of thermal biofeedback and hypnosis or a treatment combination including hypnosis, relaxation, and cognitive strategies. See also Collins, Kaslow, Doepke, Eckman, and Johnson (1998) and Collins and Kaslow's Emery University Web site (http://www.emory.edu/PEDS/SICKLE/painmgt.htm) for a comprehensive, multidisciplinary approach to pain management for sickle cell syndrome pain. This approach involves biofeedback, self-hypnosis, relaxation therapy, and cognitive-behavioral interventions, in addition to analgesic medications, to manage vaso-occlusive pain episodes.

BENIGN ESSENTIAL BLEPHAROSPASM
AND OTHER OCULOMOTOR ABNORMALITIES

Applications for oculomotor abnormalities have a long history. The review by Rotberg and Surwit (1981) pointed toward the promise of these applications. Most of those publications were case studies. There are now experimental studies and replications of successful results for some applications. Nevertheless, these applications remain mostly on the frontier. Examples of applications with research support are the use of specialized biofeedback instruments and procedures for visual acuity (accommodation), strabismus, nystagmus, and amblyopia. Other applications include benign essential blepharospasm (BEB), intraocular pressure, and glaucoma. We admit being myopic about accommodation of biofeedback applications to visual acuity and most other applications for ophthalmic disorders. We have also avoided aligning our focus on strabismus and have oscillated about nystagmus. Collins et al. (1988), Trachtman (1987), Halperin and Yolton (1986), Hodes and Howland (1986), and Kaluza and Strempel (1995) are eye-opening references that will help readers improve their focus. We focus here on BEB.

BEB is one type of involuntary eyelid spasm. It typically involves bilateral, involuntary, forceful closure of the eyelids, with involvement of the orbicularis oculi muscles surrounding the eyes. Severity ranges widely with the worst cases resulting in functional blindness. Treatments include systemic medications for the underlying ocular surface disorder (such as dry eyes and blepharitis), botulinum toxin (Botox) injections, EMG biofeedback, and/or surgery.

Biofeedback as a treatment for BEB is described in reports by Peck (1977), Roxanas, Thomas, and Rapp (1978), Rowan and Sedlacek (1981), Brantley, Carnrike, Faulstich, and Barkemeyer (1985), Rotberg and Surwit (1981), and Murphy and Fuller (1984). Peck's (1977) case study reported marked decreases in spasm frequency and maintenance over a 4-month postfeedback period. Surwit and Rotberg (1984) reported that four of eight patients treated with EMG biofeedback achieved at least a 60% reduction in spasm frequency.

In current clinical practice, biofeedback is sometimes recommended in mild cases or in patients who are not responding to the best treatments. The primary current treatment is injections of minute quantities of Botox, which release the muscle spasms. When this therapy works, it lasts from a few weeks to several months and typically needs repeating (Anderson, Patel, Holds, & Jordan, 1998).

One case report (Craggs, Schwartz, & Kostick, 1999) supported the potential of extending the duration of the effect of Botox. A 70-year-old female with a 27-year history of BEB was needing Botox injections about every two to three months. She received 13 treatment sessions with passive relaxation, autogenic-type relaxation, diaphragmatic breathing, and EMG biofeedback involving bilateral orbicularis oculi, posterior neck, and bifrontal sites. When she felt increased stress, she tended to have increased bifrontal activity. When she attempted to open her eyes, she would raise her eyebrows in an attempt to lift her eyes open mechanically, causing activation of frontalis muscles. Feedback was provided to decrease this activity and to facilitate eye opening without significantly increasing frontalis activity. She also received cognitive-behavioral therapy involving reframing and assertiveness. The addition of this treatment component led her to go 32 weeks between injections, which was the longest period she had experienced in over 10 years of Botox treatment.

In summary, one still needs binoculars to view the location of biofeedback and related interventions on the frontier for oculomotor abnormalities, but they are still visible. Helpful Web sites include the following: http://www.blepharospasm.org/blepharp.html, http://www.steenhall.com/bspasm.html, and http://www2.truman.edu/shaffer/musculoskeletalinterventions.

COMPUTER-MEDIATED COMMUNICATIONS

A variety of computer-mediated communications (CMCs; Budman, 2000) will have an increasing impact on health care delivery in the next several years and far beyond.[3] Many examples are described in Barak (1999) and Budman (2000). Behavioral telehealth that includes biofeedback is a type of CMC and is emphasized here. One definition of "telehealth" is "the use of telecommunication and information technology to provide access to health assessment, intervention, consultation, supervision, education, and information across distance" (Nickelson, 1998, p. 527).

A good example of a practical system to provide real-time audio and video interactions that allow therapists to monitor and provide biofeedback services at remote sites, for persons who are located at substantial distances from properly qualified practitioners, is described by Folen, James, Earles, and Andrasik (2001). See the reference for details of this system. The cost for some such systems can be high, whereas this system is very economical and cost-effective for providing biofeedback. In this case, the central location for the system and practitioner was an Army base in Hawaii, and the remote stations were located at military bases in Korea, Japan, and Guam.

For an example of applied psychophysiology provided via the Internet with relaxation therapies and related stress management approaches, but without biofeedback, see Strom, Pettersson, and Anderson (2000). These authors provided Internet-based instructions to a group of recruited persons who reported various types of headaches. Their approach incorporated multiple treatments (mainly several types of relaxation procedures) assessments, e-mail interactions, and a log of symptoms and medications. Of the 20 who finished in the treatment group, half reported at least 50% improvement based on one end-of-the-day headache rating. This compared well to the 4% of the 25 in the waiting-list control (i.e., only 1 person in the control group met this criterion).

Selected features of the telehealth approach include the following:

- Technicians at remote sites need only limited training.
- Patients need selecting in part for their competence to interact with telehealth (e.g., those with significant vision or visuospatial limits are probably unsuited for this medium).
- Reliable hardware and software, with the capability to acquire, store, view, and manipulate physiological data signals in real time, are essential.
- Data transmission speeds from 19.2 K to 33.6 K are sufficient.
- Adequate Videophone systems, and built-in full-duplex speakerphones for hands-free communication, are important.
- Patient education materials need careful preparation and appropriate reading level.
- Compliance of remote patients needs special attention tailored to each individual.
- Extra attention to remote patients' diagnoses, other symptoms and problems, and special needs is necessary.
- Practitioners should adhere to the 10 interdisciplinary principles summarized below.

Additional issues that need resolving include licensure across state lines or "telehealth waiver" to practice in another state; consent by the remote patients for these services; and either courtesy staff credentialing at a hospital in another place, or a professional colleague at a remote hospital to assume responsibility for patients, legal liability coverage, and insurance coverage. Some insurance companies, including Medicare, are covering some telehealth services (e.g., psychotherapy) with several criteria, but most carriers have not addressed this.

Evaluation and management codes are required, and psychologists cannot use such codes for Medicare; thus they cannot bill Medicare for telehealth.

Anyone developing or providing telehealth-based services, including those within applied psychophysiology, should be aware of and comply with the "10 interdisciplinary principles for professional practice in telehealth" described in Reed, McLaughlin, and Milholland (2000, p. 172). These are briefly summarized here for reader convenience, but one should read the original for a better understanding.

1. Basic standards of professional conduct are not altered by the use of telehealth.
2. Confidentiality remains essential.
3. As in conventional treatment, clients must provide adequate informed consent.
4. Practitioners must adhere to basic assurances of high-quality care, in accordance with their discipline's clinical standards.
5. Each discipline must assure its members' competence in the delivery of services via telehealth.
6. Documentation requirements for telehealth services must include appropriate and adequate protections.
7. Clinical guidelines must be based on empirical evidence, when available.
8. The integrity and therapeutic value of the relationship between client and practitioner must be maintained and not diminished by telehealth.
9. Although professionals do not need additional licensing to provide services via telehealth technologies, they cannot provide services that otherwise are not legally or professionally authorized.
10. The safety of clients and practitioners must be ensured. Safe hardware and software, combined with user competence, are essential.

FUNCTIONAL VOICE DISORDERS

Functional voice disorders include hyperfunctional dysphonia. In these disorders, laryngeal-area EMG biofeedback, videoendoscopic feedback, relaxation, and related techniques are of value within a multicomponent treatment. Such treatment also includes voice therapy (Aronson, 1990).

Sime and Healey (1993) provide a report of therapy for a patient with a hyperfunctional voice disorder. The report reveals a creative use of EMG biofeedback as an adjunct in a successful combination of therapy techniques, including voice therapy with visual feedback and cognitive-behavioral therapy. A 45-year-old man needed to reduce the volume and duration of his verbal communication during presentations. Voice therapy with visual feedback from a computer-aided system (Goebel, 1986) helped significantly but was insufficient. The patient continued to strain the respiratory and vocal musculature by "trying to force the expression of too many words, too quickly, with too little expired air to maintain normal phonation" (p. 284).

The EMG electrodes were placed over the area of the infrahyoid muscles. Feedback showed the patient his excess muscle tension during rest and vocalization. It also showed the slow recovery of muscle tension after he had stopped talking. The EMG biofeedback helped identify the excess tension and reduce some of it. The EMG data also provided information for the patient and therapists about his progress.

Andrews, Warner, and Stewart (1986) showed successful use of laryngeal-area EMG biofeedback in five patients with hyperfunctional dysphonia. Feedback was provided from over the area of the pars recta site of the cricothyroid muscle. This muscle is the most superficial of the intrinsic laryngeal muscles. These treatments were in the context of a voice-training program. The study was unable to show a difference in outcome, compared to five matched patients receiving general relaxation.

Other references discussing the use of specialized voice feedback and at least laryngeal-area EMG biofeedback include Prosek, Montgomery, Walden, and Schwartz (1978), McFarlane and Lavorato (1984), Bastian and Nagorsky (1987), D'Antonio, Lotz, Chait, and Netsell (1987), Redenbaugh and Reich (1989), Allen, Bernstein, and Chait (1991), Stemple, Weiler, Whitehead, and Komray (1980), Watson, Allen, and Allen (1993), and Davids, Smith, and Montgomery (1996). Practitioners needing a textbook on voice disorders should consider the classic by Aronson (1990).

UNCONSCIOUS

Credible scientists have scrutinized the concept of the "unconscious," and have concluded that "the reality of the unconscious is no longer questionable" (Loftus & Klinger, 1992, p. 761). However, some academic psychologists go beyond skepticism and suggest that the concept "unconscious cognition" does not belong in psychology (Greenwald, 1992). The clinical, theoretical, and research implications of psychophysiological assessment and interventions for unconscious processes include many topics, with much overlap among them. Interested readers should consider the pertinent concepts and topics, discussion, and references listed in Schwartz (1995).

Readers interested in the unconscious and the relationships with biofeedback should read papers by Wickramasekera, many of which are listed among the references in his 1999 presidential address to the Association for Applied Psychophysiology and Biofeedback (AAPB). His theory is complex yet intriguing, and it has heuristic, clinical, and research value. In several prior papers summarized by Wickramasekera (1999), he has hypothesized and offered support for the position that

> the empirical efficacy of biofeedback in clinical symptom reduction is due to, at least, three mechanisms . . . [1] biofeedback temporarily increases trait hypnotic ability . . . and probably the patients' "openness" . . . to altered perceptions of the factors triggering and maintaining their clinical symptoms. Second, biomedical instruments used in biofeedback elicit a respondently conditioned mind–body therapeutic placebo response based on the memory of prior healing. . . . Third, biofeedback recruits one of the primary mechanisms of risk (high or low trait hypnotic ability) for stress disorders and reverses its direction of action. . . . (pp. 93–94)

PSYCHONEUROIMMUNOLOGY AND CANCER

Research supports the conclusion that biobehavioral factors and the brain influence the immune system (Gruber et al., 1993; Ader, Felten, & Cohn, 1991; Halley, 1991; O'Leary, 1990; Bovbjerg et al., 1990; Donaldson, 2000). Furthermore, there is support for the negative effects of stress on immunological activity (Ader et al., 1991; McDaniel, 1996). There is also support for the contention that biobehavioral strategies influence measurable immune system changes and are of potential therapeutic importance (for examples, see Gruber et al., 1993, and Halley, 1991). These strategies include relaxation and biofeedback. Examples of other behavioral interventions that are within the rubric of applied psychophysiology and could benefit the immune system include social support (Kiecolt-Glaser et al., 1985), guided imagery and relaxation (Gruber, Hall, Hersh, & Dubois, 1988; Gruber et al., 1993), immune system imagery (Rider et al., 1990), music-assisted cell-specific imagery (Rider & Achterberg,

1989), self-disclosure (Pennebaker, Kiecolt-Glaser, & Glaser, 1988), and visualization or mental imagery (Donaldson, 2000). Most of the studies reporting relaxation and biofeedback to be beneficial to the immune system involve various types of normal samples (Peavey, Lawlis, & Goven, 1985; McGrady et al., 1992). However, there are also reports with patient samples (Gruber et al., 1988, 1993).

Gruber et al. (1993) used an applied psychophysiological treatment package with 13 patients who had had modified radical mastectomies and were lymph-node-negative. This study combined relaxation procedures, guided imagery, and frontal EMG biofeedback in a controlled single-crossover design. Seven patients started treatment; the other six patients in a delayed-treatment group eventually participated in the treatment package. The intervention influenced immune function in immune assays in the desired direction, according to multiple pre–post comparisons. It produced "statistically significant effects primarily on T-cell populations including natural killer cells. Antibodies were minimally affected" (p. 14). Note that "several weeks to months were required for changes to reach statistical significance" (p. 14); this led to the speculation that "long-term effects of behavioral intentions . . . are cumulative" (p. 15). The investigators provided necessary and ethical cautions for interpreting their data. They also acknowledged the complex and unclear relationship between immune changes and reduced physiological activity; the relationship is not linear. They speculated on potential mechanisms and focused on altered plasma levels of cortisol.

Basic and essential questions and challenges to consider in this domain include the following:

- Do biobehavioral and central nervous system factors change the immune system in both undesired and desired directions? For example, Gregerson, Roberts, and Amiri (1996) reported that "high and low absorbers [as measured by the Absorption Scale] had diametrically opposite immune responses [mucosal immunoglobulin A in saliva] to relaxation with imagery" (p. 162) among a group of undergraduates.
- Can one help teach the immune system to make significant changes in desired directions with applied psychophysiological strategies such as relaxation and biofeedback?
- Can one elicit immunological changes among patients that reach statistical and clinical or "real-world" significance?
- Which immunological conditions and diseases respond to applied psychophysiological strategies?
- Do changes among patients last long enough to have long-term effects on preventing or reversing immunologically related diseases?
- Which applied psychophysiological strategies result in immunological changes that reach statistical and clinical significance?

The answer to at least the first two questions is clearly "Yes." The answers to the others remain more challenging and elusive.

One must continue to speculate about the mechanisms of change. For example, do these include the physiological relaxation; the cognitive changes associated with the relaxation and biofeedback procedures; changes in hormones, catecholamines, plasma levels of cortisol, or other chemicals; or some combination of these? This uncertainty is not different from that present with many interventions, including other applications of biofeedback and relaxation, many medications, and psychotherapies.

Major challenges remain in this field. Research must confirm results with more samples of patients and show the clinical significance of the immunological changes beyond statistical significance. Furthermore, research must clarify the active ingredients in the strategies. The frontier settlements for immunologically related disorders will remain for a long time.

The promise remains for a role for applied psychophysiology in effecting immunological changes of clinical significance; however, the complexities and challenges are monumental. The land is still untamed and replete with obstacles. Well-meaning inhabitants of the settlements still strive to find the formulas to bring this area into the heartland. Until that happens, prudent practitioners should be very cautious about applications and claims about results.

As a footnote to this topic, it is well worth noting that patients with advanced cancer can learn relaxation procedures taught by nurses or via audiotapes in an oncology ward, and that the benefits of these procedures include less cancer-related pain and increased comfort (Sloman, Brown, Aldana, & Chee, 1994). There is also a report supporting the use of relaxation therapies and imagery, or cognitive-behavioral therapy, for treatment-related pain among patients receiving bone marrow transplants (Syrjala, Donaldson, Davis, Kippes, & Carr, 1995).

INSOMNIAS AND OTHER SLEEP DISORDERS[4]

Insomnia, including psychophysiological insomnia, is extremely common, affecting between 9% and 12% of adults chronically (Morin et al., 1999). Insomnia contributes significantly to many other symptoms and disorders, and excess daytime sleepiness (often due to insomnia), interferes significantly with the efficient use of relaxation therapies, biofeedback, and other applied psychophysiological therapies for various symptoms and disorders. There are other sleep disorders for which relaxation therapies, relaxation assisted by EMG biofeedback, and other types of biofeedback have been used effectively.

Psychophysiological Insomnia

Various therapeutic relaxation procedures are used effectively to help people with psychophysiological insomnia improve sleep (Hauri & Esther, 1990). This conclusion has received much support from research dating back several decades (e.g., Freedman & Papsdorf, 1976). For reviews of behavioral/nonpharmacological interventions (including relaxation and many others), see Morin (1993), Rosen, Lewin, Goldberg, and Woolfolk (2000), and Morin et al. (1999).

Relaxation procedures are typically provided to alleviate sleep-onset insomnia, and sometimes to help people return to sleep after interruption. Part of the rationale is that many persons with psychophysiological insomnia are not aware of their tension or have difficulty letting go of tension and arousal. For many, relaxation procedures without biofeedback are sufficient, especially when provided appropriately and within the context of additional effective nonpharmacological/behavioral procedures including so-called sleep hygiene. For other persons, biofeedback (most commonly EMG biofeedback) provides useful additional information and help in learning to relax more efficiently and with more confidence (Hauri & Esther, 1990).

However, many persons with insomnia do not show excess physical tension or psychological anxiety: and they are sufficiently relaxed in bed, and can be uncomfortable trying to relax further (Hauri, Percy, Hellekson, Hartmann, & Russ, 1982; Hauri, 1991; Morin, 1993). Persons with insomnia, like those with other conditions, need to understand the rationale for the use of relaxation procedures, and to accept these techniques as appropriate for them. One implication is the importance of assessing a person's tension/arousal before recommending relaxation. Hauri (1991) reminds us that psychological, muscle, and sympathetic arousal correlate only modestly with each other; thus people often show elevated tension/arousal in some but not other areas.

In an ideal clinical practice, a practitioner could and would assess multiple types of tension in a person's own bed, at bedtime when the person is trying to start sleep (Hauri, 1991). Increased tension can and does exist under these conditions in some persons who are not excessively tense during the day. However advantageous this practice might be, it is not practical and, as Hauri (1991) states, is "cumbersome." He has described the procedures he uses in a book chapter (Hauri, 1991). He begins by monitoring one channel of frontal EMG and hand temperature while the patient reclines on a bed in his office. After observing the EMG and temperature for a period, he instructs the patient to "relax as deeply as possible, just as if you wanted to sleep," and continues his observations for another 5 minutes. The clinical questions he considers include the following (Hauri, 1991, p. 71):

- "Is the patient relaxed when no demands are made, but tenses considerably as soon as relaxation is demanded?"
- "Does the patient relax deeper and deeper over a course of 5 minutes, or does the patient become more and more tense as time progresses?"

Hauri (1991) reports starting with various relaxation procedures, sometimes with biofeedback assistance if there are signs of increased muscle tension or sympathetic arousal. He strongly recommends that patients initially avoid the use of relaxation procedures at bedtime in order to minimize failure experiences. When they develop the skills and confidence in their relaxation skills, he then shifts to using the relaxation at bedtime or later during the sleep period after sleep interruption.

The mechanisms by which relaxation therapies work are not clearly (or necessarily usually) due to muscle relaxation or other forms of cultivated low physiological arousal. The cognitive distraction or cognitive refocusing effects that result from focusing on somatic relaxation, as well as the effects of other cognitive-behavioral approaches are thought to have important roles in the mechanisms by which various relaxation procedures work (Borkovec & Fowles, 1973; Hauri, 1991; Morin et al., 1999; Edinger, Wohlgemuth, Radtke, Marsh, & Quillian, 2001). Focusing on relaxation procedures helps people focus away from such cognitive activities as worry, anxiety about not sleeping, review of the day's activities, and planning-related cognitions.

We inform patients that part of the rationale for the use of relaxation and cognitive refocusing procedures is as follows:

"Imagine yourself pinned down in an earthquake, or partially hidden behind enemy lines with enemy soldiers close by, and you need to remain awake for many hours beyond normal in order to survive. The natural biological method to remain awake is to use isometric muscle tension and cognitive activity to remain awake and sufficiently alert for lengthy periods. That's the 'good news.' The 'bad news' is that these 'hard-wired' features of our nervous systems also serve to keep us awake in the safety of our beds. Various relaxation and cognitive refocusing procedures allow the brain to allow sleep to start by sufficiently reducing the physical and psychological/cognitive tension and arousal."

There are, of course, many different treatment types and components for insomnia (Hauri & Linde, 1990; Morin, 1993; Ancoli-Israel, 1996). Multicomponent interventions are typical in clinical practice, but research has not always supported the superiority of multicomponent interventions compared to single components. For example, stimulus control procedures can be sufficient for some persons. One would typically not recommend relaxation procedures without other procedures, although for some persons relaxation alone or combined with a few biofeedback-assisted sessions might be sufficient.

Another type of biofeedback that has potential use for insomnia is EEG feedback (Hauri et al., 1982). They used theta and sensorimotor rhythm (SMR) feedback, each of which was helpful for different persons. Those with anxiety and tension benefited from theta but not

SMR, and only SMR was helpful for those who were already relaxed but still having sleep problems before treatment. We do not know how this approach compares with relaxation therapies, other forms of biofeedback, and other therapies.

Practice guidelines recommended by the American Academy of Sleep Medicine (Chesson et al., 1999) used the American Psychological Association's criteria for empirically validated treatments. The recommendations for treatment of chronic insomnia were as follows:

- Stimulus control is effective therapy with a high degree of clinical certainty.
- Muscle relaxation, paradoxical intention, and biofeedback are effective with a moderate degree of clinical certainty.
- Sleep restriction and multicomponent (cognitive) behavioral therapy are effective, but inconclusive or conflicting evidence or conflicting expert opinions exist.
- Sleep hygiene, imagery, and cognitive therapy each have insufficient evidence as a single therapy. However, sleep hygiene education is typically included with other interventions.

Recent research provides support for the value of relaxation treatment for older adults with primarily high daytime impairment or fatigue (Lichstein, Riedel, Wilson, Lester, & Aguillard, 2001), at least as measured by self-reported sleep. Sleep compression was more useful for older adults who were low in daytime fatigue. The average age of these adults was 68, and essentially all were aged from about 60 to 90.

Insomnia Secondary to Medical or Psychiatric Conditions

Cannici, Malcolm, and Peek (1983) used muscle relaxation alone in a successful treatment of long-term insomnia in a group of 15 patients with a variety of cancer diagnoses. This treatment led to better improvement than that for patients receiving routine care for cancer (which was not described). Sleep-onset latency was substantially reduced from about 2 hours to about 30 minutes and maintained at 3 months. Varni (1980) reported on the treatment of insomnia in a person with hemophilia.

Another useful recent study (Lichstein, Wilson, & Johnson, 2000) focused on patients with secondary insomnia, which is insomnia caused by a medical or psychiatric disorder. This includes a broad group of patients who have not previously been the focus of research with psychological interventions. With only 4 sessions combining relaxation and stimulus control procedures, this group of 54 older adults (aged 58 and above) showed substantial improvement in sleep and maintained it well at 3 months. For patients with chronic pain (primarily back or neck pain) and secondary insomnia, a multicomponent intervention including relaxation and cognitive therapy resulted in substantially improved sleep. The relaxation was an imagery-based method intended to distract the patients and refocus their cognitions.

Other Sleep Disorders: Further Out on the Frontier

The rationale for including the following symptoms and disorders includes the interesting findings for these conditions, the potential for successful use with other patients, and the potential heuristic value that (we hope) will result in further investigations and clinical experience. These two topics offer good examples of the rich possibilities of applied psychophysiological interventions for sleep problems. There is no intended implication that these treatments are equivalent or superior to other interventions (typically pharmacological) for these conditions. However, for some persons pharmacology is insufficient, carries risks or is contraindicated, is tolerated poorly because of side effects, or is resisted. For these persons, applied psychophysiology may be helpful.

Periodic Movements in Sleep

We know of only one case report (Ancoli-Israel, Seifert, & Lemon, 1986) on the use of biofeedback for periodic leg movements in sleep. The use of thermal biofeedback was associated with a reduction of leg kicks from a pretreatment average of 536 per night to 19.5 per night after therapy. The rationale for this approach was the observation that many patients with this problem report cold feet, and thus poor circulation may be contributing to the symptoms.

Night Terrors

In a single-case study of a 16-year-old male with a 9-year history of night terrors, Sadigh and Mierzwa (1995) used standard autogenic therapy in eight weekly 20-minute sessions to reduce the frequency of the night terrors from a 5-week baseline average of 4 episodes per week to zero in the last 3 weeks of the treatment and at follow-ups occurring at 24–26 weeks and at 50–52 weeks. No biofeedback was part of this treatment, but biofeedback-assisted autogenic therapy is appropriate for other conditions and could be appropriately considered in future cases and research.

OPTIMAL-FUNCTIONING BIOFEEDBACK AND APPLIED PSYCHOPHYSIOLOGY[5]

Biofeedback is sometimes viewed within much broader rubrics and philosophies even beyond applied psychophysiology (R. Kall, personal communication, March 2002). Optimal functioning is one aspect of these broader implications. For example, biofeedback is now being used with elite athletes (see Sime, Chapter 25, this volume) and musicians (see Zinn & Zinn, Chapter 24, this volume) to help them reach peak performance. Applications using virtual reality provide another example of frontier approaches.

Teaching physiological self-regulation as a basic life skill to children in schools is also still on the frontier (see Culbert & Banez, Chapter 31, this volume). The hope is that this could be helpful as a form of prevention. One of the hurdles and obstacles is lack of reimbursement for such interventions when recipients are healthy, or when the interventions are called "training" or "coaching." If the assumption or hypothesis is valid that learning and routinely applying psychophysiological self-regulation in childhood and early adulthood can result in improved functioning, then perhaps other sources of funding will be found to incorporate this into the schools. If various modalities of biofeedback significantly enhance the learning and maintenance of efficient psychophysiological skills for many children and other healthy young adults, then practical interventions and cost-efficient methods for their incorporation into childhood learning will emerge from the frontier. If these interventions reduce risks for some symptoms and illnesses later in life, then there could be more support for other sources of funding.

Advocates of using biofeedback for optimal functioning suggest that clinical practitioners can and should communicate to patients the "empowering nature of self-awareness and self-regulation" that can reverberate into other aspects of their lives beyond the symptoms for which they are seeking help (R. Kall, personal communication, April 2002). The additional potential benefits involve using self-regulation on a lifelong basis. Furthermore, another goal is for people to increase their self-efficacy or confidence that they have more control over themselves than they previously believed.

Fortunately, the advocates of broader conceptualizations and optimal-functioning applications remain aware that scientific methods are still needed, along with the art and philosophical aspects.

EEG FEEDBACK: A BRIEF COMMENT

Terms for EEG feedback include *"EEG biofeedback," "neurotherapy," "neurofeedback," "alpha–theta feedback,"* and others. (See Neumann, Strehl, & Birbaumer, Chapter 5, and the chapters in Part VI of this volume, for detailed discussions of instrumentation, applications, and research). Some of the bold attempts to treat various conditions and disorders with EEG feedback will remain on the frontier at least for a while. We expect that EEG feedback will be with us for a long time. In the second edition of this book, Mark S. Schwartz stated that he did not know whether many of the EEG feedback applications would emerge into the heartland or wither in the frontier, as did their ancestors. There are still controversies and complexities, but there is more supportive evidence that EEG applications are emerging from the frontier.

CONCLUSION

This chapter has noted various disorders and provides an expanded scope of applications. Inclusion here does not imply an expectation that further research will continue to support the efficacy of all these applications. The chapter does not purport to cover all possible applications.

In the years since the dawn of the term "biofeedback," participants at the annual meetings of the professional membership association (now the AAPB) have encountered many speculative ideas and claims about new applications. This field continues to attract advocates of bold and novel ideas. It allows the expression and cultivation of these ideas. It also allows criticism in the spirit of scientific debate. Biofeedback researchers and practitioners do not seek to dampen open inquiry and boldness. Had they done so, we would not have the many advances in knowledge and successful applications that are discussed here and elsewhere in this book. Although we all must remain open to new ideas, the burden of proof is on the advocates of those ideas. We close with Neal Miller's well-known admonition: "Be bold in what you attempt, but cautious in what you claim."

NOTES

1. Skin ulcers and herpes are included here because they involve the skin and often necessitate consultations by dermatologists. This does not imply the exclusion of other medical specialties or other classification systems for these conditions.

2. For more information, readers should consider contacting the Erythromelalgia Association, 4343 Roosevelt Way NE, Seattle, WA 98105, (206-632-0894; (http://www.erythromelalgia.org) or the National Organization for Rare Diseases (http://www.rarediseases.org). At Mayo Clinic Rochester, Thom W. Rooke, MD, Section of Vascular Medicine of the Department of Cardiovascular Diseases, as well as Mark D. P. Davis, MD, and Roy S. Rogers III, MD, of the Department of Dermatology, can provide information on this disorder.

3. CMCs include telehealth and behavioral telehealth, Web sites, CD-ROM and DVD programs, conferencing software, e-mail, bulletin boards, and others.

4. Prior editions of this book did not address insomnia directly as a set of conditions for at least some of which relaxation therapies and biofeedback can be useful in treatment. This was pointed out in a letter to Mark S. Schwartz from a South American health professional. Part of the rationale for omitting it was that although relaxation is very commonly used with some types of insomnia, biofeedback has not received much attention. Although relaxation therapies are often useful and sometimes crucial (and thus not part of the frontier), treatment of insomnia nearly always involves several other therapy recommendations, and quesitons about the use of biofeedback are the reason for including this topic in the present chapter. Schwartz was a little embarrassed about omitting insomnia in the second edition, because his friend and colleague Peter Hauri, PhD, one of the world's leading experts on insomnia, used relaxation therapies and biofeedback in his practice at the Mayo Clinic campus in Rochester, MN. We are pleased to include insomnia in this edition.

5. We "thank" Robert Kall, MA, for encouraging inclusion of a section on optimal functioning, and for generously sharing some insights that we refer to in this section as "personal communication."

REFERENCES

Writer's Cramp

Bindman, E., & Tibbetts, R. W. (1977). Writer's cramp—a rational approach to treatment. *British Journal of Psychiatry, 131,* 143–148.

Candia, V., Elbert, T., Altenmüller, E., Rau, H., Schäfer, T., & Taub, E. (1999). Constraint-induced movement therapy for focal hand dystonia in musicians [Letter]. *Lancet, ii*(353), 52.

Cottraux, J., Juenet, C., & Collet, L. (1983). The treatment of writer's cramp with multimodal behavior therapy and biofeedback: A study of 15 cases. *British Journal of Psychiatry, 142,* 180–183.

Deepak, K. K., & Behari, M. (1999). Specific muscle EMG biofeedback for hand dystonia. *Applied Psychophysiology and Biofeedback, 24,* 267–280.

Ince, L. P., Leon, M. S., & Christidis, D. (1986). EMG biofeedback for handwriting disabilities: A critical examination of the literature. *Journal of Behavior Therapy and Experimental Psychiatry, 17,* 95–100.

Koller, W. C., & Vetere-Overfield, B. (1989). Usefulness of a writing aid in writer's cramp. *Neurology, 39,* 149–150.

Marsden, C. D., & Sheehy, M. P. (1990). Writer's cramp. *Trends in Neurosciences, 13,* 148–153.

Mishima, N., Kitagawa, K., Hara, T., & Nakagawa, T. (1992). Treatment of writer's cramp with dystonic involuntary movements by biofeedback therapy. In K. Shirakura, I. Saito, & S. Tsutsui (Eds.), *Current biofeedback research in Japan.* Tokyo: Shinkoh Igadu Shuppan.

Murabayashi, N., Takekoshi, I., Takada, H., Igarashi, M., Nonaka, T., Tsuboi, K., Nakano, K., & Tsutshi, S. (1992). The effects of electromyogram biofeedback on writer's cramp. In K. Shirakura, I. Saito, & S. Tsutsui (Eds.), *Current biofeedback research in Japan.* Tokyo: Shinkoh Igadu Shuppan.

Nutt, J. G., Muenter, M. D., Aronson, A., Kurland, L. T., & Melton, L. J. (1988). Epidemiology of focal and generalized dystonia in Rochester, Minnesota. *Movement Disorders, 3,* 188–194.

O'Neill, M. E., Gwinn, K. A., & Adler, C. H. (1996). Biofeedback for writer's cramp. *American Journal of Occupational Therapy, 51,* 605–607.

Reavley, W. (1975). The use of biofeedback in the treatment of writer's cramp. *Journal of Behavior Therapy and Experimental Psychiatry, 6,* 335–338.

Rowan, D. C. (1980). *Behavioral approaches in the management of movement disorders.* Paper presented at the First World Congress on Behavior Therapy, Jerusalem, Israel.

Rubow, R. (1989, March). EMG biofeedback in the treatment of writer's cramp. In *Proceedings of the 20th Annual Meeting of the Association for Applied Psychophysiology and Biofeedback, San Diego.* Wheat Ridge, CO: Association for Applied Psychophysiology and Biofeedback.

Uchiyama, K., Lutterjohann, M., & Shah, M. D. (1977). Biofeedback-assisted desensitization treatment of writer's cramp. *Journal of Behavior Therapy and Experimental Psychiatry, 8,* 169–171.

Essential Tremor

Bain, P. G. Findley, L. J., Atchison, P., Behari, M., Vidaihet, M., Gresty, M., Rothwell, J. C., Thompson, P.D., & Marsden, C. D. (1993). Assessing tremor severity. *Journal of Neurology, Neurosurgery and Psychiatry, 56,* 868–873.

Bradley, W., Daroff, R., Fenichel, G., & Marsden, D. (1996). *Neurology in clinical practice* (Vol. 2). Boston: Butterworth-Heinemann.

Britton, T. (1995). Essential tremor and its variants. *Current Opinions in Neurology, 8,* 314–319.

Chung, W., Poppen, R., & Lundervold, D. (1995). Behavioral relaxation training for tremor disorders in older adults. *Biofeedback and Self-Regulation, 20*(2), 123–135.

Koller, W. C., Busenbark, K., & Miner, K. (1994). The relationship of essential tremor to other movement disorders: Report on 678 patients. Essential Tremor Study Group. *Annals of Neurology, 35,* 717–723.

Louis, E. D., Barnes, L. F., Wendt, K. J., Albert, S. M., Pullman, S. L., Yu, Q., & Schneier, F. R. (2000a). Validity and test–retest reliability of a disability questionnaire for essential tremor. *Movement Disorders, 15*(3), 516–523.

Louis, E. D., Marder, K., Cote, L., Pullman, S., Ford, B., Wilder, D., Tang, M., Lantigua, R., Gurland, B., & Mayeux, R. (1995). Differences in the prevalence of essential tremor among elderly African Americans, whites, and Hispanics in northern Manhattan, NY. *Archives of Neurology, 52*(12), 1201–1205.

Louis, E. D., Wendt, K. J., & Ford, B. (2000b). Senile tremor. What is the prevalence and severity of tremor in older adults? *Gerontology, 46*(1), 12–16.

Lundervold, D. A., Belwood, M. F., Craney, J. L., & Poppen, R. (1999). Reduction of tremor severity and disability following behavioral relaxation training. *Journal of Behavior Therapy and Experimental Psychiatry, 30,* 119–135.

Metzer, W. (1992). Severe essential tremor compared with Parkinson's disease in male veterans: Diagnostic characteristics, treatment, and psychosocial consequences. *Southern Medical Journal, 85,* 825–828.

Metzer, W. (1994). Essential tremor: An overview. *Journal of the Arkansas Medical Society, 90,* 587–590.

Montgomery, G. K., & Reynolds, N. C. (1991). Compliance, reliability, and validity of self-monitoring for physical disturbances of Parkinson's disease. *Journal of Nervous and Mental Disease, 178,* 636–641.

Pahwa, R., Busenbark, K., Swanson-Hyland, E. F., Dubinsky, R. M., Hubble, J. P., Gray, C., & Koller, W. C. (1995). Botulinum toxin treatment of essential head tremor. *Neurology, 45,* 822–824.

Pahwa, R., & Koller, W. (1993). Is there a relationship between Parkinson's disease and essential tremor? *Clinical Neuropharmacology, 16,* 30–35.

Rapoport, A., Braun, H., Aviv A., & Sarova, I. (1991). Combined resting–postural tremor of the head with a changing axis. *Movement Disorders, 6,* 261–262.

Salemi, G., Savettieri, G., Rocca, W., Meneghini, F., Saporito, V., Morgante, L., Reggio, A., Grigoletto, F., & Di Perri, R. (1994). Prevalence of essential tremor: A door-to-door survey in Terrasini, Sicily. Sicilian Neuro-Epidemiologic Study Group. *Neurology, 44,* 61–64.

Scholing, A., & Emmelkamp, P. (1996). Treatment of fear of blushing, sweating or trembling: Results at long-term follow-up. *Behavior Modification, 20,* 338–356.

Schwartz, M. S., Craggs, J. H., Brayshaw, G., Brazis, P. W., O'Brien, P., & Atkinson, E. (1997). The positive effect of relaxation therapy and physical therapy exercises on essential "no no" head tremor: A single case design. In *Proceedings of the 28th Annual Meeting of the Association for Applied Psychophysiology and Biofeedback, San Diego, CA.* Wheat Ridge, CO: Association for Applied Psychophysiology and Biofeedback.

Idiopathic Scoliosis

Birbaumer, N., Flor, H., Cevey, B., Dworkin, B., & Miller, N. E. (1994). Behavioral treatment of scoliosis and kyphosis. *Journal of Psychosomatic Research, 38,* 623–628.

Dworkin, B., Miller, N. E., Dworkin, S., Birbaumer, N., Brines, M. L., Jonas, S., Schwentker, E. P., & Graham, J. J. (1985). Behavioral method for the treatment of idiopathic scoliosis. *Proceedings of the National Academy of Sciences USA, 82,* 2493–2497.

Miller, N. E. (1985). Some professional and scientific problems and opportunities for biofeedback. *Biofeedback and Self-Regulation, 10,* 3–24.

Wong, M. S., Mak, A. F. T., Luk, K. D. K., Evans, J. H., & Brown, B. (2001). Effectiveness of audio-biofeedback in postural training for adolescent idiopathic scoliosis patients. *Prosthetics and Orthotics International, 25,* 60–70.

Dermatologically Related Conditions

General Review

Bilkis, M. R., & Mark, K. A. (1998). Mind–body medicine. Practical applications in dermatology. *Archives of Dermatology, 134,* 1437–1441.

Bird, E. L., & Colborne, G. R. (1980). Rehabilitation of an electrical burn patient through biofeedback. *Biofeedback and Self-Regulation, 5*(2), 283–287.

Folks, D. G., & Kinney, F. C. (1992). The role of psychological factors in dermatologic conditions. *Psychosomatics, 33,* 45–54.

McMenamy, C. J., Katz, R. C., & Gipson, M. (1988). Treatment of eczema by EMG biofeedback and relaxation training: A multiple baseline analysis. *Journal of Behavior Therapy and Experimental Psychiatry, 19*(3), 221–227.

Panconesi, E., Gallassi, F., Sarti, M. G., & Bellini, M. A. (1998). Biofeedback, cognitive-behavioral methods, hypnosis: "Alternative psychotherapy"? *Clinical Dermatology, 16,* 709–710.

Sarti, M. G. (1998). Biofeedback in dermatology. *Clinical Dermatology, 16*(6), 711–714.

Hyperhidrosis

Alvarez, L. M., Cortes, J. F., & Rodriguez, D. (1993, March). Cognitive-behavioral therapy for the treatment of palmar hyperhidrosis. In *Proceedings of the 24th Annual Meeting of the Association for Applied Psycho-*

physiology and Biofeedback, Los Angeles, CA. Wheat Ridge, CO: Association for Applied Psychophysiology and Biofeedback.

Duller, P., & Gentry, W. D. (1980). Use of biofeedback in treating chronic hyperhidrosis: A preliminary report. *British Journal of Dermatology*, *103*, 143–146.

Farrar, S., & Hartje, J. C. (1987, March). Hyperhidrosis: A successful methodology for treatment. In *Proceedings of the 18th Annual Meeting of the Biofeedback Society of America, Boston, MA*. Wheat Ridge, CO: Association for Applied Psychophysiology and Biofeedback.

Fotopoulos, S. S., & Whitney, P. S. (1978). Biofeedback in the treatment of psychophysiological disorders. *Biofeedback and Self-Regulation*, *3*(4), 331–361.

Harris, J., & Sieveking, N. (1979). Case study in hyperhidrosis. *American Journal of Clinical Biofeedback*, *2*(1), 31.

Kawahara, K., & Kikuchi, T. (1992). A study of palmar sweating biofeedback (A preliminary report). In K. Shirakura, I. Saito, & S. Tsutsui (Eds.), *Current biofeedback research in Japan*. Tokyo: Shinkoh Igaku Shuppan.

White, J. W., Jr. (1986). Treatment of primary hyperhidrosis. *Mayo Clinic Proceedings*, *61*, 951–956.

Psoriasis

Goodman, M. (1994). An hypothesis explaining the successful treatment of psoriasis and thermal biofeedback: A case report. *Biofeedback and Self-Regulation*, *19*(4), 347–352.

Keinan, G., Segal, A., Gal, U., & Brenner, S. (1995). Stress management for psoriasis patients: The effectiveness of biofeedback and relaxation techniques. *Stress Medicine*, *11*, 235–241.

Skin Ulcers

Guthrie, D., Moeller, T., & Guthrie, R. (1983). Biofeedback and its application to the stabilization of diabetes. *American Journal of Clinical Biofeedback*, *6*(2), 82–87.

Rice, B., Kalker, A. J., Schindler, J. V., & Dixon, R. M. (2001). Effect of biofeedback-assisted relaxation training on foot ulcer healing. *Journal of the American Podiatric Medical Association*, *91*(3), 132–141.

Rice, B. I., & Schindler, J. V. (1992). Effects of thermal biofeedback-assisted relaxation training on blood circulation in the lower extremities of a population with diabetes. *Diabetes Care*, *15*, 853–858.

Shulimson, A. D., Lawrence, P. F., & Iacono, C. U. (1986). Diabetic ulcers: The effect of thermal biofeedback-mediated relaxation training on healing. *Biofeedback and Self-Regulation*, *11*(4), 311–319.

Vaizey, C. J., Roy, A. J., Kamm, M. A. (1997). Prospective evaluation of the treatment of solitary rectal ulcer syndrome with biofeedback. *Gut*, *41*, 817–820.

Ward, W. A., & Van Moore, A. (1995). Management of finger ulcers in scleroderma. *Hand Surgery*, *20*(5), 868–872.

Herpes

Burnette, M. M., Koehn, K. A., Kenyon-Jump, R., Hutton, K., & Stark, C. (1991). Control of genital herpes recurrences using progressive muscle relaxation. *Behavior Therapy*, *22*, 237–247.

Longo, D. J., Clum, G. A., & Yaeger, N. J. (1998). Psychosocial treatment of recurrent genital herpes. *Journal of Consulting and Clinical Psychology*, *56*, 61–66.

VanderPlate, C. & Kerrick, G. (1985). Stress reduction of severe genital herpes virus. *Biofeedback and Self-Regulation*, *10*(2), 181–188.

Menopausal Hot Flushes

Berkow, R., & Fletcher, A. J. (1992). *The Merck manual of diagnosis and therapy* (16th ed.). Rahway, NJ: Merck.

Freedman, R. R. (1989). Laboratory and ambulatory monitoring of menopausal hot flashes. *Psychophysiology*, *26*, 573–579.

Freedman, R. R., & Woodward, S. (1992a). Elevated α_2-adrenergic responsiveness in menopausal hot flushes: Pharmacologic and biochemical studies. In P. Lomax & E. Schonbaum (Eds.), *Thermoregulation: The pathophysiological basis of clinical disorders*. Basel: Karger.

Freedman, R. R., & Woodward, S. (1992b). Behavioral treatment of menopausal hot flashes: Evaluation by ambulatory monitoring. *American Journal of Obstetrics and Gynecology*, *167*(2), 436–439.

Freedman, R. R., Woodward, W., & Sabharwal, S. (1990). Alpha$_2$-adrenergic mechanism in menopausal hot flushes. *Obstetrics and Gynecology, 76,* 573–578.

Germaine, L., & Freedman, R. R. (1984). Behavioral treatment of menopausal hot flushes: Evaluation by objective methods. *Journal of Consulting and Clinical Psychology, 52,* 1072–1079.

Hunter, M. S., & Liao, K. L.-M. (1995). Determinants of treatment choice for menopausal hot flushes: Hormonal versus psychological versus no treatment. *Journal of Psychosomatic Obstetrics and Gynecology, 16*(2), 101–108.

Larson, D. E. (Ed.). (1996). *Mayo Clinic family health book* (2nd ed.). New York: William Morrow.

Lee, C. T., & Taylor, D. N. (1987, March). Biofeedback, relaxation training and supportive counseling in the treatment of menopausal hot flush. In *Proceedings of the 18th Annual Meeting of the Association for Applied Psychophysiology and Biofeedback.* Wheat Ridge, CO: Association for Applied Psychophysiology and Biofeedback.

Melin, W. K., Nedstrand, E., & Hammar, M. (1997). Treatment of menopausal symptoms with applied relaxation: A pilot study. *Journal of Behavior Therapy and Experimental Psychiatry, 28*(4), 251–261.

Shuster, L. (2001). Office visit: Alternative treatments for hot flashes. *Supplement to Mayo Clinic Women's Healthsource* (MC2493–101).

Woodward, S., Grevill, H., & Freedman, R. R. (1991, March). Respiratory alterations during menopausal hot flashes. In *Proceedings of the 22nd Annual Meeting of the Association for Applied Psychophysiology and Biofeedback. Dallas.* Wheat Ridge, CO: Association for Applied Psychophysiology and Biofeedback.

Erythromelalgia

Babb, R. R., Alarçon-Segovia, D., & Fairbairn, J. P. (1964). Erythermalgia: Review of 51 cases. *Circulation, 2,* 136–141.

Cahn, T. S., & Garber, A. (1990, March). Biofeedback treatment of erythromelalgia: A case study. In *Proceedings of the 21st Annual Meeting of the Association for Applied Psychophysiology and Biofeedback, Washington, DC.* Wheat Ridge, CO: Association for Applied Psychophysiology and Biofeedback.

Davis, M. D. P., O'Fallon, W. M., Rogers, R. S., & Rooke, T. W. (2000). Natural history of erythromelalgia: Presentation and outcome in 168 patients. *Archives of Dermatology, 136,* 330–336.

Kurzrock, R., & Cohen, P. R. (1989). Erythromelalgia and myeloproliferative disorders. *Archives of International Medicine, 149,* 105–109.

Levine, A. M., & Gustafson, P. R. (1987). Erythromelalgia: Case report and literature review. *Archives of Physical Medicine and Rehabilitation, 68,* 119–121.

Michiels, J. J., & van Joost, T. (1988). Primary and secondary erythermalgia, a critical review [Editorial]. *Netherlands Journal of Medicine, 33,* 205–208.

Michiels, J. J., & van Joost, T. (1990). Erythromelalgia and thrombocythemia: A causal relation. *Journal of the American Academy of Dermatology, 22*(1), 107–111.

Mitchell, S. W. (1878). On a rare vaso-motor neurosis of the extremities, and on the maladies with which it may be confounded. *American Journal of Medical Science, 76,* 2–36.

Putt, A. M. (1978). Erythromelalgia—a case for biofeedback. *Nursing Clinics of North America, 13*(4), 625–630.

Nausea and Vomiting

Arakawa, S. (1995). Use of relaxation to reduce side effects of chemotherapy in Japanese patients. *Cancer Nursing, 18*(1), 60–66.

Arakawa, S. (1997). Relaxation to reduce nausea, vomiting, and anxiety induced by chemotherapy in Japanese patients. *Cancer Nursing, 20*(5), 342–349.

Blasco, T. (1994). Anticipatory nausea and vomiting: Are psychological factors adequately investigated? *British Journal of Clinical Psychology, 33,* 85–100.

Boakes, R. A., Tarrier, N., Barnes, B. W., & Tattersall, M. H. (1993). Prevalence of anticipatory nausea and other side-effects in cancer patients receiving chemotherapy. *European Journal of Cancer, 29A*(6), 866–870.

Burish, T. G., & Jenkins, R. A. (1992). Effectiveness of biofeedback and relaxation training in reducing the side effects of cancer chemotherapy. *Health Psychology, 11*(1), 17–23.

Burish, T. G., Shartner, C. D., & Lyles, J. N. (1981). Effectiveness of multiple muscle-site EMG biofeedback and relaxation training in reducing the aversiveness of cancer chemotherapy. *Biofeedback and Self-Regulation, 6*(4), 523–535.

Carey, M. P., & Burish, T. G. (1988). Etiology and treatment of the psychological side effects associated with cancer chemotherapy: A critical review and discussion. *Psychological Bulletin, 104*(3), 307–325.

Chin, S. B., Kucuk, O., Peterson, R., & Ezdinli, E. Z. (1992). Variables contributing to anticipatory nausea and vomiting in cancer chemotherapy. *American Journal of Clinical Oncology*, 15(3), 262–267.

Dadds, M. R., Bovbjerg, D. H., Redd, W. H., & Cutmore, T. R. H. (1997). Imagery in human classical conditioning. *Psychological Bulletin*, 122(1), 89–103.

Enqvist, B., Bjorklund, C., Engman, M., & Jakobsson, J. (1997). Preoperative hypnosis reduces postoperative vomiting after surgery of the breasts: A prospective, randomized and blinded study. *Acta Anaesthesiologica Scandinavica*, 41(8), 1028–1032.

Greene, P. G., Seime, R. J., & Smith, M. E. (1991). Distraction and relaxation training in the treatment of anticipatory vomiting: A single subject intervention. *Journal of Behavior Therapy and Experimental Psychiatry*, 22(4), 285–290.

Marchioro, G., Azzarello, G., Viviani, F., Barbato, F., Pavanetto, M., Rosetti, F., Pappagallo, G. L., & Vinante, O. (2000). Hypnosis in the treatment of anticipatory nausea and vomiting in patients receiving cancer chemotherapy. *Oncology*, 59(2), 100–104.

Morrow, G. R., Roscoe, J. A., Hynes, H. E., Flynn, P. J., Pierce, H. I., & Burish, T. (1998). Progress in reducing anticipatory nausea and vomiting: A study of community practice. *Supportive Care in Cancer*, 6(1), 46–50.

Shartner, C. D., Burish, T. G., & Carey, M. P. (1985). Effectiveness of biofeedback with progressive muscle relaxation training in reducing the aversiveness of cancer chemotherapy: A preliminary report. *Japanese Journal of Biofeedback Research*, 12, 33–40.

Troesch, L. M., Rodehaver, C. B., Delaney, E. A., & Yanes, B. (1993). The influence of guided imagery on chemotherapy-related nausea and vomiting. *Oncology Nursing Forum*, 20(8), 1179–1185.

Vasterling, J., Jenkins, R. A., Tope, D. M., & Burish, T. G. (1993). Cognitive distraction and relaxation training for the control of side effects due to cancer chemotherapy. *Journal of Behavioral Medicine*, 16(1), 65–80.

Stress-Induced Vasovagal Syncope

Khurana, R. K., Lynch, J. J., & Craig, F. W. (1997). A novel psychophysiological treatment for vasovagal syncope. *Clinical Autonomic Research*, 7, 191–197.

Kozak, M. J., & Miller, D. A. (1985). The psychophysiological process of therapy in a case of injury-scene-elicited fainting. *Journal of Behavior Therapy and Experimental Psychiatry*, 16, 139–145.

Kozak, M. J., & Montgomery, G. K. (1981). Multimodal behavioral treatment of recurrent injury-scene fainting (vasodepressor syncope). *Behavioral Psychotherapy*, 9, 316–321.

McGrady, A. V., & Argueta Bernal, G. A. (1986). Relaxation based treatment of stress-induced syncope. *Journal of Behavior Therapy and Experimental Psychiatry*, 17(1), 23–27.

McGrady, A. V., Bush, E. G., & Grubb, B. P. (1997). Outcome of biofeedback-assisted relaxation for neurocardiogenic syncope and headache: A clinical replication series. *Applied Psychophysiology and Biofeedback*, 22, 63–72.

Smith, M. S., & Glass, S. T. (1989). An adolescent girl with headache and syncope. *Journal of Adolescent Health*, 10, 54–56.

Sickle Cell Crises

Collins, M., Kaslow, N., Doepke, K., Eckman, J., & Johnson, M. (1998). Psychosocial interventions for children and adolescents with sickle cell disease (SCD). *Journal of Black Psychology*, 24, 418–432.

Cozzi, L., Tryon, W. W., & Sedlacek, K. (1987). The effectiveness of biofeedback-assisted relaxation in modifying sickle cell crisis. *Biofeedback and Self-Regulation*, 12(1), 51–61.

Thomas, J. E., Koshy, M., Patterson, L., Dorn, L., & Thomas, K. (1984). Management of pain in sickle cell disease using biofeedback therapy: A preliminary study. *Biofeedback and Self-Regulation*, 9, 413–420.

Zeltzer, L. K., Keller, J., Dash, J., & Holland, J. P. (1979). Hypnotically induced pain control in sickle cell anemia. *Pediatrics*, 69, 533–535.

Benign Essential Blepharospasm and Other Oculomotor Abnormalities

Anderson, R. L., Patel, B. C. K., Holds, J. B., & Jordan, D. R. (1998). Blepharospasm: Past, present and future. *Ophthalmic Plastic and Reconstructive Surgery*, 14(5), 305–316.

Brantley, P. J., Carnrike, C. L., Jr., Faulstich, M. E., & Barkemeyer, C. A. (1985). Blepharospasm: a case study comparison of trihexyphenidyl (Artane) versus EMG biofeedback. *Biofeedback and Self-Regulation*, 10(2), 173–180.

Collins, F. L., Pbert, L. A., Sharp, B., Smith, S., Gil, K. M., & Odom, J. V. (1988). Visual acuity improvement following fading and feedback training: I. Comparison of myopic and emmetropic volunteers. *Behaviour Research and Therapy, 26*(6), 461–466.

Craggs, J. H., Schwartz, M. S., & Kostick, D. A. (1999, April). Benign essential blepharospasm: Relaxation and biofeedback and frequency of Botox injections. A case report. In *Proceedings of the 30th Annual Meeting of the Association for Applied Psychophysiology and Biofeedback, Vancouver, BC.* Wheat Ridge, CO: Association for Applied Psychophysiology and Biofeedback.

Halperin, E., & Yolton, R. L. (1986). Ophthalmic applications of biofeedback. *American Journal of Optometry and Physiological Optics, 63*(12), 985–998.

Hodes, R. L., & Howland, E. W. (1986). Ocular and stabilization feedback: An evaluation of two EMG biofeedback control procedures. *Biofeedback and Self-Regulation, 6*(3), 375–388.

Kaluza, G., & Strempel, I. (1995). Effects of self-relaxation methods and visual imagery on IOP in patients with open-angle glaucoma. *Ophthalmologica, 209,* 122–128.

Murphy, J. K., & Fuller, A. K. (1984). Hypnosis and biofeedback as adjunctive therapy in blepharospasm: A case report. *American Journal of Clinical Hypnosis, 27*(1), 31–37.

Peck, D. F. (1977). The use of EMG feedback in the treatment of a severe case of blepharospasm. *Biofeedback and Self-Regulation, 2*(3), 273–277.

Rotberg, M. H., & Surwit, R. S. (1981). Biofeedback techniques in the treatment of visual and ophthalmologic disorders: a review of the literature. *Biofeedback and Self-Regulation, 6*(3), 375–388.

Rowan, G. E., & Sedlacek, K. (1981). Biofeedback in the treatment of blepharospasm: a case study. *American Journal of Psychiatry, 138*(11), 1487–1489.

Roxanas, M. R., Thomas, M. R., & Rapp, M. S. (1978). Biofeedback treatment of blepharospasm with spasmodic torticollis. *Canadian Medical Association Journal, 119*(1), 48–49.

Surwit, R. S., & Rotberg, M. (1984). Biofeedback therapy of essential blepharospasm. *American Journal of Ophthalmology, 98*(1), 28–31.

Trachtman, J. N. (1987). Biofeedback of accommodation to reduce myopia: A review. *American Journal of Optometry and Physiological Optics, 64*(8), 639–643.

Computer-Mediated Communication

Barak, A. (1999). Psychological applications on the Internet: A discipline on the threshold of a new millennium. *Applied and Preventive Psychology, 8,* 231–246.

Budman, S. H. (2000). Behavioral health care dot-com and beyond: Computer-mediated communications in mental health and substance abuse treatment. *American Psychologist, 55,* 1287–1300.

Folen, R. A., James, L. C., Earles, J. E., & Andrasik, F. (2001). Biofeedback via telehealth: A new frontier for applied psychophysiology. *Applied Psychophysiology and Biofeedback, 26,* 195–204.

Nickelson, D. W. (1998). Telehealth and the evolving health care system: Strategic opportunities for professional psychology. *Professional Psychology: Research and Practice, 29,* 527–535.

Reed, G. M., McLaughlin, C. J., & Milholland, K. (2000). Ten interdisciplinary principles for professional practice in telehealth: Implications for psychology. *Professional Psychology: Research and Practice, 31,* 170–178.

Strom, L., Pettersson, R., & Andersson, G. (2000). A controlled trial of self-help treatment of recurrent headache conducted via the Internet. *Journal of Consulting and Clinical Psychology, 68,* 722–727.

Functional Voice Disorders

Allen, K. D., Bernstein, B., & Chait, D. H. (1991). EMG biofeedback treatment of pediatric hyperfunctional dysphonia. *Journal of Behavior Therapy and Experimental Psychiatry, 22,* 97–101.

Andrews, S., Warner, J., & Stewart, R. (1986). EMG biofeedback and relaxation in the treatment of hyperfunctional dysphonia. *British Journal of Disorders of Communication, 21,* 353–369.

Aronson, A. E. (1990). *Clinical voice disorders* (3rd ed.) New York: Thieme.

Bastian, R. W., & Nagorsky, M. J. (1987). Laryugeal image biofeedback. *Laryngoscope, 97,* 1346–1349.

Davids, K., Smith, S., & Montgomery, D. D. (1996). Two case studies using EMG biofeedback treatment for laryngeal spasms and psychogenic hyperfunctional voice disorder. In *Proceedings of the 27th Annual Meeting of the Association for Applied Psychophysiology and Biofeedback, Albuquerque.* Wheat Ridge, CO: Association for Applied Psychophysiology and Biofeedback.

D'Antonio, L., Lotz, W., Chait, D., & Netsell, R. (1987). Perceptual-physiologic approach to evaluation and treatment of dysphonia. *Annals of Otology, Rhinology, and Laryngolgogy, 96,* 187–190.

Goebel, M. (1986). *A computer-aided fluency establishment trainer (CAFET).* Falls Church, VA: Annadale Fluency Clinic.

McFarlane, S. C., & Lavorato, A. S. (1984). The use of videoendoscopy in the evaluation and treatment of dysphonia. *Journal of Communication Disorders, 9*, 117–126.

Prosek, R. A., Montgomery, A. A., Walden, B. E., & Schwartz, D. M. (1978). EMG biofeedback in the treatment of hyperfunctional voice disorder. *Journal of Speech and Hearing Disorders, 43*, 282–294.

Redenbaugh, M. S., & Reich, A. R. (1989). Surface EMG and related measures in normal and vocally hyperfunctional speakers. *Journal of Speech and Hearing Disorders, 54*, 68–73.

Sime, W. E., & Healey, E. C. (1993). An interdisciplinary approach to the treatment of a hyperfunctional voice disorder. *Biofeedback and Self-Regulation, 18*, 281–287.

Stemple, J. C., Weiler, E., Whitehead, W., & Komray, R. (1980). Electromyographic feedback training with patients exhibiting a hyperfunctional voice disorders. *Laryngoscope, 90*, 471–476.

Watson, T. S., Allen, S. J., & Allen, K. D. (1993). Ventricular fold dysphonia: Application of biofeedback technology to a rare voice disorder. *Behavior Therapy, 24*, 439–446.

Unconscious

Greenwald, A. G. (1992). New look 3: Unconscious cognition reclaimed. *American Psychologist, 47*(6), 766–779.

Loftus, E. F., & Klinger, M. R. (1992). Is the unconscious smart or dumb? *American Psychologist, 47*(6), 761–765.

Schwartz, M. S., & Associates (1995). *Biofeedback* (2nd ed.). New York: Guilford Press.

Wickramasekera, I. (1999). How does biofeedback reduce clinical symptoms and do memories and beliefs have biological consequences?: Toward a model of mind–body healing. *Applied Psychophysiology and Biofeedback, 24*(2), 91–105.

Psychoneuroimmunology and Cancer

Ader, R., Felton, D. L., & Cohn, N. (Eds.), *Psychoneuroimmunology*. New York: Academic Press.

Bovbjerg, D. H., Redd, W. H., Maier, L. A., Holland, J. C., Lesko, L. M., Niedzwiechi, D., Rubin, S. C., & Hakes, T. B. (1990). Anticipatory immune suppression and nausea in women receiving cyclic chemotherapy for ovarian cancer. *Journal of Consulting and Clinical Psychology, 58*, 153–157.

Donaldson, V. W. (2000). A clinical study of visualization on depressed white blood count in medical patients. *Applied Psychophysiology and Biofeedback, 25*, 117–128.

Gregerson, M. B., Roberts, I. M., & Amiri, M. M. (1996). Absorption and imagery locate immune responses in the body. *Biofeedback and Self-Regulation, 21*, 149–165.

Gruber, B. L., Hall, N. R., Hersh, S. P., & Dubois, P. (1988). Immune system and psychological changes in metastatic cancer patients while using ritualized, relaxation and guided imagery. *Scandinavian Journal of Behavior Therapy, 17*, 25–46.

Gruber, B. L., Hersh, S. P., Hall, N. R. S., Waletzky, L. R., Kunz, J. F., Carpenter, J. K., Kverno, K. S., & Weiss, S. M. (1993). Immunological responses of breast cancer patients to behavioral interventions. *Biofeedback and Self-Regulation, 19*, 1–22.

Halley, F. M. (1991). Self-regulation of the immune system through biobehavioral strategies. *Biofeedback and Self-Regulation, 16*, 55–74.

Kiecolt-Glaser, J. K. Glaser, R., Williger, D., Stout, J., Messick, G., Sheppard, S., Richer, D., Romisher, S. C., Briner, W., Bonnell, G., & Donnerberg, R. (1985). Psychosocial enhancement of immunocompetence in a geriatric population. *Health Psychology, 4*, 25–78.

McDaniel, J. S. (1996). Stressful life events and psychoneuroimmunology. In T. W. Miller (Ed.), *Theory and assessment of stressful life events*. Madison, CT: International Universities Press.

McGrady, A., Conrad, P., Dickey, D., Garman, D., Farris, E., & Schumann-Brzezinski, C. (1992). The effects of biofeedback-assisted relaxation on cell-mediated immunity, cortisol, and white blood cell count in healthy adult subjects. *Journal of Behavioral Medicine, 15*(4), 343–354.

Peavey, B. S., Lawlis, F., & Goven, A. (1985). Biofeedback-assisted relaxation: Effects on phagocytic capacity. *Biofeedback and Self-Regulation, 10*(1), 33–47.

Pennebaker, J. W., Kiecolt-Glaser, J. K., & Glaser, R. (1988). Disclosure of traumas and immune function: Health implications for psychotherapy. *Journal of Consulting and Clinical Psychology, 56*, 239–245.

O'Leary, A. (1990). Stress, emotion, and human immune function. *Psychological Bulletin, 108*, 363–382.

Rider, M. S., & Achterberg, J. (1989). Effect of music-assisted imagery on neutrophils and lymphocytes. *Biofeedback and Self-Regulation, 14*, 247–257.

Rider, M. S., Achterberg, J., Lawlis, G. F., Goven, A., Toledo, R., & Butler, J. R. (1990). Effect of immune system imagery on secretory IgA. *Biofeedback and Self-Regulation, 15*, 317–333.

Sloman, R., Brown, P., Aldana, E., & Chee, E. (1994). The use of relaxation for the promotion of comfort and pain relief in persons with advanced cancer. *Contemporary Nurse, 3,* 6–12.

Syrjala, K. L., Donaldson, G. W., Davis, M. W., Kippes, M. E., & Carr, J. E. (1995). Relaxation and imagery and cognitive-behavioral training reduce pain during cancer treatment: A controlled clinical trial. *Pain, 63,* 189–198.

Insomnias and Other Sleep Disorders

Ancoli-Israel, S. (1996). *All I want is a good night's sleep.* St. Louis: Mosby.

Ancoli-Israel, S., Seifert, A. R., & Lemon, M. (1986). Thermal biofeedback and periodic movements in sleep: Patients' subjective reports and a case study. *Biofeedback and Self-Regulation, 11,* 177–188.

Borkovec, T., & Fowles, D. (1973). Controlled investigation of the effects of progressive and hypnotic relaxation on insomnia. *Journal of Abnormal Psychology, 82,* 153–158.

Cannici, J., Malcolm, R., & Peek, L. A. (1983). Treatment of insomnia in cancer patients using muscle relaxation training. *Journal of Behavior Therapy and Experimental Psychiatry, 14,* 251–256.

Chesson, A. L., Anderson, W. M., Littner, M., Davila, D., Hartse, K., Johnson, S., Wise, M., & Rafecas, J. (1999). Practice parameters for the nonpharmacologic treatment of chronic insomnia. *Sleep, 22,* 1128–1133.

Edinger, J. D., Wohlgemuth, W. K., Radtke, R. A., Marsh, G. R., & Quillian, R. E. (2001). Cognitive behavioral therapy for treatment of chronic primary insomnia: A randomized controlled trial. *Journal of the American Medical Association, 285,* 1856–1864.

Freedman, R., & Papsdorf, J. D. (1976). Biofeedback and progressive relaxation treatment of sleep-onset insomnia: A controlled, all-night investigation. *Biofeedback and Self-Regulation, 1,* 253–271.

Hauri, P. J. (1991). Sleep hygiene, relaxation therapy, and cognitive interventions. In P. J. Hauri (Ed.), *Case studies in insomnia.* New York: Plenum Press.

Hauri, P. J., & Esther, M. S. (1990). Insomnia. *Mayo Clinic Proceedings, 65,* 869–882.

Hauri, P. J., & Linde, S. (1990). *No more sleepless nights.* New York: Wiley.

Hauri, P. J., Percy, L., Hellekson, C., Hartmann, E., & Russ, D. (1982). The treatment of psychophysiological insomnia with biofeedback: A replication study. *Biofeedback and Self-Regulation, 7,* 223–235.

Lichstein, K. L., Riedel, B. W., Wilson, N. M., Lester, K. W., & Aguillard, R. N. (2001). Relaxation and sleep compression for late-life insomnia: A placebo-controlled trial. *Journal of Consulting and Clinical Psychology, 69,* 227–239.

Lichstein, K. L., Wilson, M. M., & Johnson, C. T. (2000). Psychological treatment of secondary insomnia. *Psychology and Aging, 15,* 232–240.

Morin, C. M. (1993). *Insomnia: Psychological assessment and management.* New York: Guilford Press.

Morin, C. M., Hauri, P. J., Espie, C. A., Spielman, A. J., Buysse, D. J., & Bootzin, R. R. (1999). Nonpharmacologic treatment of chronic insomnia. *Sleep, 22,* 1134–1156.

Rosen, R. C., Lewin, D. S., Goldberg, L., & Woolfolk, R. L. (2000). Psychophysiological insomnia: Combined effects of pharmacotherapy and relaxation-based treatments. *Sleep Medicine, 1,* 279–288.

Sadigh, M. R., & Mierzwa, J. A. (1995). The treatment of persistent night terrors with Autogenic training: A case study. *Biofeedback and Self-Regulation, 20,* 205–209.

Varni, J. W. (1980). Behavioral treatment of disease-related chronic insomnia in a hemophiliac. *Journal of Behavioral Therapy and Experimental Psychiatry, 11,* 143–145.

Index